Ultrasonography Examination

MW01079188

Notice

Medicine is an ever-changing science. As new research and clinical experience broaden our knowledge, changes in treatment and drug therapy are required. The authors and the publisher of this work have checked with sources believed to be reliable in their efforts to provide information that is complete and generally in accord with the standards accepted at the time of publication. However, in view of the possibility of human error or changes in medical sciences, neither the authors nor the publisher nor any other party who has been involved in the preparation or publication of this work warrants that the information contained herein is in every respect accurate or complete, and they disclaim all responsibility for any errors or omissions or for the results obtained from use of the information contained in this work. Readers are encouraged to confirm the information contained herein with other sources. For example and in particular, readers are advised to check the product information sheet included in the package of each drug they plan to administer to be certain that the information contained in this work is accurate and that changes have not been made in the recommended dose or in the contraindications for administration. This recommendation is of particular importance in connection with new or infrequently used drugs.

LANGE REVIEW

Ultrasonography Examination

Fourth Edition

Charles S. Odwin, BS, RT, PA-C, RDMS
Ultrasound Technical Consultant
Women's Health NCB Hospital
Physician Assistant in OB/GYN
Department of Obstetrics and Gynecology
North Central Bronx Hospital
Clinical Instructor, Emergency Medicine Residency Training Program
Jacobi Medical Center and Montefiore Medical Center
Bronx New York
Clinical Instructor, Diagnostic Medical Ultrasound
University of Medicine and Dentistry of New Jersey
School of Allied Health Professions
Newark, New Jersey

Arthur C. Fleischer, MD
Cornelius Vanderbilt Chair
Professor of Radiology and Radiological Sciences
Professor of Obstetrics and Gynecology
Chief, Diagnostic Sonography
Vanderbilt University Medical Center
Nashville, Tennessee

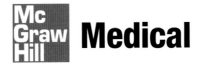

New York   Chicago   San Francisco   Lisbon   London   Madrid   Mexico City
New Delhi   San Juan   Seoul   Singapore   Sydney   Toronto

The McGraw·Hill Companies

LANGE REVIEW: Ultrasonography Examination, Fourth Edition

Copyright © 2012, 2004 by The McGraw-Hill Companies, Inc. All rights reserved. Printed in China. Except as permitted under the United States Copyright Act of 1976, no part of this publication may be reproduced or distributed in any form or by any means, or stored in a data base or retrieval system, without the prior written permission of the publisher.

Previous editions copyright © 1993, 1987 by Appleton & Lange.

4 5 6 7 8 9 10 DSS 20 19 18 17

Set ISBN 978-0-07-163424-3; Set MHID 0-07-163424-X
Book 978-0-07-149781-7; Book MHID 0-07-149781-1
CD ISBN 978-0-07-162954-6; CD MHID 0-07-162954-8

This book was set in Berkeley Old Style by Aptara, Inc.
The editors were Regina Y. Brown and Catherine A. Johnson.
The production supervisor was Catherine Saggese.
Project management was provided by Indu Jawwad, Aptara, Inc.
The designer was Mary McKeon.
RR Donnelley was printer and binder.

This book is printed on acid-free paper.

Library of Congress Cataloging-in-Publication Data

Lange review : ultrasonography examination / [edited by] Charles S. Odwin,
Arthur C. Fleischer. – 4th ed.
      p. ; cm.
   Ultrasonography examination
   Rev. ed. of: Appleton & Lange review for the ultrasonography
examination / [edited by] Carol A. Krebs, Charles S. Odwin, Arthur C.
Fleischer. c2004.
   Includes bibliographical references.
   ISBN-13: 978-0-07-149781-7 (pbk.)
   ISBN-10: 0-07-149781-1 (pbk.)
   I. Odwin, Charles S. II. Fleischer, Arthur C. III. Appleton & Lange
review for the ultrasonography examination. IV. Title: Ultrasonography
examination.
   [DNLM: 1. Ultrasonography–Examination Questions.   WN 18.2]

616.07'543076–dc23   2011035492

McGraw-Hill books are available at special quantity discounts to use as premiums and sales promotions, or for use in corporate training programs. To contact a representative, please e-mail us at bulksales@mcgraw-hill.com.

Dedication

*(Donna preparing for her lecture in the Mid 1990s
in Florida. The little square objects that she is
handling are slides. Photo courtesy of A.C. Fleischer.)*

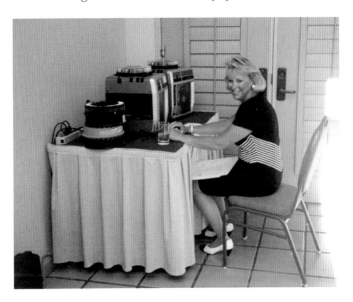

I would like to acknowledge the pride, professionalism, and enthusiasm of the late Donna Kepple, RT, RDMS, by dedicating this 4th edition of Lange Review: Ultrasonography Examination in her memory. Ms. Kepple was a prime example of how a caring and compassionate professional could combine technical expertise in sonography to enhance a patient's life and those that worked and interacted with her. Beginning in the early 1980s, Donna was one of the first students to graduate from our first Sonographer Training Program and then continue to excel at the local and national meetings. She touched not only her patients' lives, but those residents, medical students, and fellow sonographers nationwide that she came in contact with. She was a superb teacher, acting not only as Chief Sonographer for 18 years but was Program Director of our first "Era" of our sonography training program in 1982–1986. She was also involved in many sonographic societies, serving as an officer and in the American Registry of Diagnostic Medical Sonographers (ARDMS) and American Institute of Ultrasound in Medicine (AIUM), being recognized as "Sonographer of the Year" by AIUM 1996.

She exemplifies the impact of a dedicated, caring, and compassionate professional. On a lighter note she always insisted on being referred to as "sonographer" rather than "ultrasound technician." She leaves pleasant thoughts to those that knew her and an example of the impact that a committed medical professional can impart both to her patients and fellow professionals every day.

Contents

Contributors

Dunstan Abraham, MPH, PA-C, RDMS
Physician Assistant
Department of Surgery, Division of Urology
Lincoln Hospital and Medical Center
Bronx, New York
Clinical Instructor
Diagnostic Medical Sonography
School of Health Related Professions
University of Medicine and Dentistry of New Jersey
Newark, New Jersey

Endorectal Prostate Sonography

Ronald S. Adler, MD, PhD
Chief, Division of Ultrasound and Body Imaging
Department of Radiology and Imaging
Professor of Radiology
Weil Medical College of Cornell University
Hospital for Special Surgery
New York, New York

Musculoskeletal Ultrasound

Mark N. Allen, MBA, RDMS, RDSC, RVT
Senior Clinical Sales Specialist
Siemens Medical
Mountain View, California

Adult Echocardiography

Fernando Amador, RVT
Technical Director
Vascular Laboratory
Moses Division, Montefiore
New York, New York

Cerebrovascular Sonography
Peripheral Arterial Sonography

George L. Berdejo, BA, FSVS, RVT
Director, Vascular Ultrasound Services
Vascular Ultrasound Laboratory
Moses, North and Weiler Divisions of Montefiore
Bronx, New York

Cerebrovascular Sonography
Sonography of the Peripheral Veins
Peripheral Arterial Sonography

Teresa M. Bieker, MBA, RDCS, RDMS, RT, RVT
Lead Sonographer
Division of Ultrasound
University of Colorado Hospital
Denver, Colorado

Fetal Echocardiography

Joshua Cruz, RVT
Vascular Lab Manager
Heart and Vascular Center
Yale New Haven Hospital
New Haven, Connecticut

Cerebrovascular Sonography
Sonography of the Peripheral Veins
Peripheral Arterial Sonography

Arthur C. Fleischer, MD
Cornelius Vanderbilt Chair
Professor of Radiology and Radiological Sciences
Professor of Obstetrics and Gynecology
Chief, Diagnostic Sonography
Vanderbilt University Medical Center
Nashville, Tennessee

Sonography: Principles, Techniques, and Instrumentation
Abdominal Sonography
Sonography of the Thyroid and Scrotum
Obstetrical and Gynecologic Sonography and Transvaginal Sonography
3D Obstetric and Gynecologic Sonography: An Illustrative Overview

Carol A. Krebs, RT, RDMS, RVT
Ultrasound Consultant
Shreveport, Louisiana

Adult Echocardiography

Evan C. Lipsitz, MD
Associate Professor of Surgery
Albert Einstein College of Medicine
Chief, Division of Vascular and Endovascular Surgery
Department of Cardiovascular and Thoracic Surgery
Montefiore and the Albert Einstein College of Medicine
Medical Director, Vascular Diagnostic Laboratory
Moses Division, Montefiore
New York, New York

Cerebrovascular Sonography
Sonography of the Peripheral Veins
Peripheral Arterial Sonography

Lawrence E. Mason, MD
Director of Women's Imaging
Xray Associates of Louisville, LLC
Baptist Hospital East
Louisville, Kentucky

Breast Sonography

Marsha M. Neumyer, BS, FAIUM, FSDMS, FSVU, RVT
International Director
Vascular Diagnostic Educational Services
Vascular Resource Associates
Harrisburg, Pennsylvania

Abdominal Vascular Sonography

Charles S. Odwin, BS, RT, PA-C, RDMS
Ultrasound Technical Consultant, Women's Health
Physician Assistant, Department of Obstetrics and Gynecology
North Central Bronx Hospital
Clinical Instructor, Emergency Medicine Residency Training
    Program
Jacobi Medical Center and Montefiore Medical Center
Bronx, New York
Clinical Instructor, Diagnostic Medical Ultrasound
University of Medicine and Dentistry of New Jersey
School of Allied Health Professionals
Newark, New Jersey

Sonography: Principles, Techniques, and Instrumentation
Abdominal Sonography
Sonography: of the Thyroid and Scrotum
Obstetrical and Gynecologic Sonography and Transvaginal Sonography
Neurosonology

David A. Parra, MD
Assistant Professor of Pediatrics
Division of Pediatric Cardiology
Vanderbilt School of Medicine
Monroe Carell Jr. Children's Hospital
Nashville, Tennessee

Pediatric Echocardiography

Chandrowti Devi Persaud, RT, PA-C, RDCS, RDMS
Physician Assistant
Department of Obstetrics and Gynecology
Bronx-Lebanon Hospital Center
Bronx, New York

Neurosonology

Ronald R. Price, PhD
Director, Radiologic Sciences Division
Department of Radiology
Vanderbilt University, School of Medicine
Nashville, Tennessee

Sonography: Principles, Techniques, and Instrumentation

Cynthia A. Silkowski, MA, RVT, RDMS
Associate Professor and Chairperson, Department of Medical
    Imaging Sciences
Director, Diagnostic Medical Sonography
School of Health Related Professions, Newark, New Jersey
University of Medicine and Dentistry of New Jersey
Newark, New Jersey

Obstetrical and Gynecologic Sonography and Transvaginal Sonography

Amy E. Wilkinson, AMS, RDMS
Preceptor
Department of Radiology and Imaging
Academic Center for Musculoskeletal Ultrasound
The Hospital for Special Surgery
New York, New York

Musculoskeletal Ultrasound

Preface

Since publication of the 3rd edition of *Appleton and Lange's Review for the Ultrasonography Examination*, there have been many additional refinements in applications sonography. Foremost among these are 3D sonography, Doppler techniques, and musculoskeletal sonography. This new and updated 4th edition contains chapters including these topics.

The continuous expansion of sonographic techniques and clinical applications requires that sonographers continually update and expand their clinical skills. Sonographers now routinely perform 3D sonography, duplex and color Doppler studies, and detailed examination of the fetus and pelvic organs, and they provide vitally important guidance for interventional procedures using sonography. This rapid pace of innovation makes our field exciting and rewarding and, at the same time, demands that sonographers constantly improve their scanning skills.

It is the intention of this book to enable both students and experienced sonographers to enhance their knowledge base. Thus, it is much more than a study guide directed solely at passing a one-time test. It also provides a basis for the continuous study of diagnostic sonography.

I am confident that dedicated professional sonographers will continue to strive to improve the quality of life of their patients and loved ones by such a continuous and committed study. It is the editors' hope that this material can enhance and provide guidance for this process.

Arthur C. Fleischer, MD   Charles S. Odwin, RDMS
Nashville, TN   Riverdale, NY
June 2012   June 2012

Acknowledgments

The authors would like to express their gratitude to Catherine Johnson and Regina Brown of McGraw-Hill Publishers who guided the completion of this edition. Their commitment and guidance in this process is gratefully acknowledged. I would also like to express appreciation to Jill Trotter, RDMS, Director of the Sonographer Training Program at Vanderbilt, for her suggestions and guidance, and Aditi Desai (VSM IV) for her assistance with manuscript preparation. Vera Merriweather and Deborah Holland are thanked for their editorial assistance and John Bobbitt for his help with the images.

I would also like to thank Susan Gross, MD, Wendy Wilcox, MD, and Sharon Deans, MD from the North Central Bronx Hospital who were so kind to allow for a flexible work schedule, which provided the time needed to work on this edition.

The authors of each chapter are thanked for their expertise and assistance. Finally, we want to thank all of our sonographers and sonography students everywhere for providing the help and inspiration for this project.

Sonography: Principles, Techniques, and Instrumentation

Charles S. Odwin, Ronald R. Price, and Arthur C. Fleischer

Study Guide

WHAT IS ULTRASOUND?

Ultrasound is a longitudinal, mechanical wave that carries variations of quantities referred to as *acoustic variables*. Ultrasound is defined as an acoustic wave that has a frequency higher than the upper limit of human hearing. That limit is typically assumed to be above 20,000 cycles per second (or 20,000 Hz). The unit hertz (Hz) is the internationally accepted term for cycles per second.

Ultrasound waves are produced by oscillatory motion of particles in a medium, creating regions of compression and rarefaction. The continued movement of particles propagating through a medium is the result of collision between particles that make up the medium.

Ultrasound can be continuous or pulsed. In the *continuous* mode, the vibratory motions are produced by the source in an uninterrupted stream, whereas in the *pulsed* mode, the sound is delivered in a series of packets, or pulses. Almost all diagnostic ultrasound applications use *pulsed ultrasound*.

The following terms are commonly used in diagnostic medical sonography:

Longitudinal wave is a wave in which the particles of the medium are in a direction parallel to the wave propagation (as opposed to shear waves, also known as transverse waves, in which particles of the medium travel in a direction that is perpendicular to the wave propagation).

Mechanical wave is a wave that requires a medium in which to travel and, therefore, cannot propagate in a vacuum. *(not particles)*

Acoustic variable. Each of the following is considered an acoustic variable: *pressure, temperature, density, particle motion (distance)*. Note that all of these variables change as an acoustic wave passes through the medium.

Parameters of a wave (Fig. 1–1A). The following terms are common to all waves:

Cycle. A cycle is composed of one compression and one rarefaction, or a complete positive and negative change in an acoustic variable.

Frequency (*f*) is the number of cycles per second. Frequency describes how many times the acoustic variable (whether it be pressure, density, particle motion, or temperature) changes in one second. *Units:* hertz (Hz), megahertz (MHz).

$$\text{frequency } (f) = \frac{\text{propagation speed}}{\text{wavelength}}, \quad f = \frac{c}{\lambda}$$

1540m/sec / 50m (handwritten)

Period is the time it takes for 1 cycle to occur; the inverse of frequency. *Units:* seconds (s), microseconds (μs).

$$\text{period } (f) = \frac{1}{\text{frequency}}, \quad p = \frac{1}{f}$$

As the frequency increases, the period decreases. Conversely, as the frequency decreases, the period increases.

Wavelength (λ) is the distance the wave must travel in 1 cycle. Wavelength is determined by both the source of the wave and the medium in which it is propagating (Fig. 1–1B). *Units:* meters (m), millimeters (mm).

$$\text{wavelength } (f) = \frac{\text{propagation speed}}{\text{frequency}}, \quad \lambda = \frac{c}{f}$$

With a velocity or propagation speed (*c*) of 1,540 m/s, the wavelength of 1 MHz is 1.54 mm, of 2 MHz is 0.77 mm, and of 3 MHz is 0.51 mm.

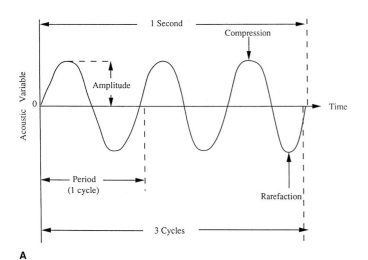

A

FIGURE 1–1A. The parameters of a wave. The frequency of this wave variable is 3 Hz (or cycles per second). A period is one complete cycle; therefore, this wave consists of three periods. *Note:* The vertical direction is compression and downward direction is rarefaction and both represent pressure and density. Otherwise, it represents a positive (upward) or negative (downward) change in the acoustic variable.

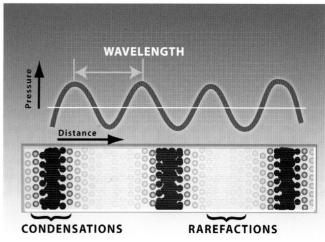

B

FIGURE 1–1B. A wavelength represents the distance between two adjacent wave peaks.

Propagation speed is the maximum speed with which an acoustic wave can move through a medium, determined by the density and stiffness of the medium. Propagation speed increases proportionally with the stiffness (i.e., the stiffer the medium, the faster the variable will travel). Density is the concentration of mass per unit volume, and propagation speed is inversely proportional to density. *Units:* meters/second (m/s), millimeters/microsecond (mm/μs).

$$\text{propagation speed } (f) = \sqrt{\frac{\text{elasticity (stiffness)}}{\text{density}}}, \quad c = \frac{e}{\rho}$$

It should be emphasized that *compressibility* is the opposite of stiffness. If compressibility increases, then the propagation speed decreases.

Propagation speed is greater in solids > liquids > gases. Propagation speed (c) is equal to frequency (f) times wavelength (λ) $\{c = f \times l\}$. Because the propagation speed is constant for a given medium, if the frequency increases, the wavelength will decrease. Conversely, if the frequency decreases, the wavelength will increase.

Example

If the frequency of an ultrasound wave traveling through soft tissue is increased from 5 to 10 MHz, what happens to the wavelength?

Steps to Solution:

$$\text{propagation speed} = 1{,}540 \text{ m/s or } 1.54 \text{ mm/μs}$$
$$\text{frequency} = 5 \text{ MHz}$$

$$\frac{\text{propagation speed}}{\text{frequency}} = \text{wavelength}$$

$$1.54 \text{ mm/μs} / 5 \text{ MHz} = 0.31 \text{ (mm)}$$
$$\text{frequency} = 10 \text{ MHz}$$
$$1.54 \text{ mm/μs} / 10 \text{ MHz} = 0.154 \text{ (mm)}$$

Doubling the frequency halves the wavelength in a given medium. Note how the wavelength gets smaller.

PARAMETERS USED TO DESCRIBE PULSED WAVES

Pulse repetition frequency (PRF) is the number of pulses per second. *Units:* hertz (Hz), kilohertz (kHz).

The PRF used depends on imaging depth. As the imaging depth increases, the PRF must decrease. This phenomenon is characteristic of the pulse-listening period-receiving cycle of the transducer. The longer it takes the returning signals (echoes) to come back to the transducer, the greater the interval between pulses. Therefore, the farther away a target, the longer the return trip, and the greater the interval between transmissions of the pulses wave.

Pulse repetition period (PRP) is the time from the beginning of one pulse to the beginning of the next (Fig. 1–2A). *Units:* seconds (s), milliseconds (ms).

$$\text{PRP} = \frac{1}{\text{PRF}}$$

The PRP increases as imaging depth increases. When depth decreases, the PRP decreases.

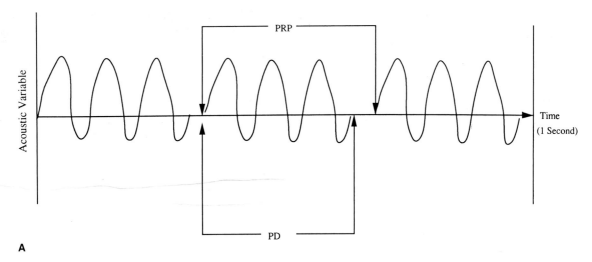

FIGURE 1–2A. Pulse repetition period (PRP).

Pulse duration (PD) is the time it takes for a pulse to occur: the period of the ultrasound in the pulse multiplied by the number of cycles in the pulse (see Fig. 1–2A). *Units:* seconds (s), milliseconds (ms), pulse duration = number of cycles (n) × period (p)

Duty factor is the fraction of time that the transducer is generating a pulse.

Maximum value: 1.0. In continuous wave, the transducer is always generating a pulse. A second transducer acts as the listening device.

Minimum value: 0.0. The transducer is *not* being excited (therefore, no pulse will be generated). In clinical imaging, using pulse-echo system the duty factor ranges from 0.001 to 0.01. *Units:* unitless.

$$\text{duty factor} = \frac{\text{PD (\mu s)}}{\text{PRP (ms)} \times 1{,}000}$$

Note: Because the duty factor is unitless, and PD is usually in microseconds, it is necessary to divide by 1,000 to cancel out the units in the formula. In using this formula, the units must match (PD and PRP both must be in seconds, milliseconds, or microseconds). If not, a correction factor, such as the 1,000 in the denominator, must be used.

The duty factor can also be computed by the following formula:

$$\text{duty factor} = \frac{\text{PD} \times (\text{PRF})}{1{,}000}$$

Spatial pulse length (SPL) is the distance over which a pulse occurs (Fig. 1–2B). *Unit:* millimeters (mm). Spatial pulse length (SPL) = wavelength (λ) × number of cycles in a pulse (n).

Amplitude is the maximum variation that occurs in an acoustic variable. It indicates the strength of the sound wave. To arrive at this variation, the undisturbed value is subtracted from the maximum value, and the unit for the acoustic variable is applied (Fig. 1–3). Peak-to-peak amplitude (P–P) is the maximum to minimum value.

Power is the rate of energy transferred. The power is proportional to the wave amplitude squared. *Unit:* watts (W).

$$\text{power} \sim \text{amplitude}^2$$

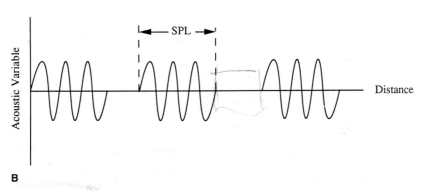

FIGURE 1–2B. Spatial pulse length (SPL).

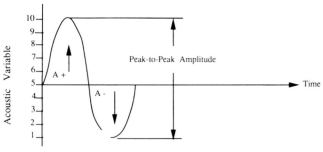

Max value = 10

Normal value = 5

Peak-to-Peak Amplitude = 9 (+ 5 + {-4}) = 5 + 4

FIGURE 1–3. A wave amplitude. Amplitude is equal to the maximum value minus the normal value. Peak-to-peak (P–P) amplitude is equal to the maximum plus absolute value of the minimum.

Intensity is the power in a wave divided by the area of the beam. *Unit:* watts per centimeter squared (W/cm²).

$$\text{intensity} = \frac{\text{power (W)}}{\text{area (cm}^2)}$$

Note: The intensity is proportional to the amplitude squared. If the amplitude doubles, then the intensity quadruples.

POWER AND INTENSITY

The ultrasound power and the intensity of the ultrasound beam are not identical, although the two terms are sometimes used interchangeably. The *ultrasound power* is the rate at which work is done; it is equal to the work done divided by the time required to do the work. The intensity is the power per unit area and represents the strength of the ultrasound beam. The intensities used in diagnostic medical ultrasound applications range from 1 to 50 mW/cm². Understanding of the ultrasound intensity is important when studying the biologic effects of ultrasound in tissue (discussed later in this chapter).

Intensities have both a peak value and an average value. The intensity of the sound beam as it travels through a medium varies across the beam (*spatial intensity*) and with time (*temporal intensity*).

Spatial peak (SP) is intensity at the center of the beam.

Spatial average (SA) is intensity averaged throughout the beam.

Temporal peak (TP) is maximum intensity in the pulse (measured when the pulse is on).

Temporal average (TA) is intensity averaged over one on-off beam cycle (takes into account the intensity from the beginning of one pulse to the beginning of next).

Pulse average (PA) is intensity averaged over the duration of the single pulse.

Six intensities result when spatial and temporal considerations are combined:

spatial peak–temporal peak	SPTP (highest)
spatial average–temporal peak	SATP
spatial peak–temporal average	SPTA (tissue heating)
spatial average–temporal average	SATA (lowest)
spatial average–pulse average	SAPA
spatial peak–pulse average	SPPA

In pulsed ultrasound, the TP is greater than the PA, which is greater than the TA. When using continuous-wave ultrasound, however, TP and TA intensities are the same.

Spatial peak intensity is related to SA by the beam uniformity ratio (BUR).

BUR is a unitless coefficient that describes the distribution of ultrasound beam intensity in space. The higher the SP, the more concentrated and the higher the SA, the less concentrated the intensity. *Units:* unitless.

$$\text{spatial average} = \frac{\text{spatial peak intensity (W/cm}^2)}{\text{beam uniformity ratio}}$$

$$\text{SA} = \frac{\text{SP}}{\text{BUR}}$$

$$\text{spatial peak} = \text{beam uniformity ratio} \times \text{spatial average}$$
$$= \text{BUR} \times \text{SA}$$

Temporal average intensity is related to TP by the duty factor (DF). *Units:* unitless.

$$\text{duty factor} = \frac{\text{temporal average}}{\text{temporal peak}}, \quad \text{DF} = \frac{\text{TA}}{\text{TP}}$$

Attenuation

Attenuation is the reduction of the sound beam's amplitude and intensity as it travels through a medium. This is why the echoes from deep structures are weaker than those from more superficial structures. The factors that contribute to attenuation are the following:

Absorption is the conversion of sound energy into heat. Absorption is the major source of attenuation in soft tissues.

Scattering. *Diffuse scattering* is the redirection of the sound beam after it strikes rough or small boundaries, when the wavelength is larger than the reflecting surface. Liver parenchyma and red blood cells represent diffuse scattering.

Reflection is the return of a portion of the ultrasound beam back toward the transducer (an echo). Of interest in diagnostic sonography is *specular reflection,* which occurs when the wavelength of the pulse is much smaller than the boundary it is striking, and the surface is smooth. The best examples of specular reflectors are the diaphragm, liver capsule, and gallbladder walls. Reflection of the ultrasound beam depends on the *acoustic impedance mismatch* at the boundary between two media (discussed in detail later in this chapter).

The unit in which attenuation is given is the decibel (dB). *The decibel is the unit of intensity ratio, or power; it is the quantity obtained by taking 10 times the log of the ratio of two intensities.*

$$\text{decibels (dB)} = 10 \log \frac{\text{final intensity}}{\text{initial intensity}}$$

Attenuation coefficient is the attenuation per unit length of sound wave travel. For soft tissue, it is approximately one-half of the operating frequency of the transducer; that is, for every centimeter per MHz, there is approximately 0.5 dB of attenuation. For example, if the operation frequency of a transducer is 5 MHz, then the attenuation coefficient is approximately 2.5 dB/cm.

$$\text{attenuation (dB)} = \text{attenuation coefficient (dB/cm)} \times \text{path length (cm)}$$

Note: Path length is the distance the sound beam travels in a medium. The actual calculation of decibel values is complex and need not be part of the sonographer's bank of common knowledge, but the sonographer should understand that because decibels are exponents, a small change in decibels can mean a large change in resulting values. The most useful way to handle these values is to memorize the commonly encountered ones (Table 1–1).

Example 1

The ultrasound beam produced by a 4 MHz transducer has an initial intensity of 20 mW/cm² after traveling through 3 cm of tissue. What is the intensity of the beam at the end of this path?

Given: Frequency is 4 MHz; original intensity is 20 mW/cm²; pathlength is 3 cm; attenuation coefficient is ½; frequency, i.e., ½; (4 MHz) = 2 dB/cm.

Then: If attenuation is attenuation coefficient × pathlength, then attenuation is 2 dB/cm × 3 cm = 6 dB. If attenuation is 0.25, then the decibel value is −6 dB.

(See Table 1–1.)

TABLE 1–1 • Decibel Values of Attenuation

Decibels (dB)	Value
−3	(1/2) 0.5
−6	(1/4) 0.25
−9	(1/8) 0.13
−10	(1/10) 0.10
−20	(1/100) 0.01
−30	(1/1,000) 0.001

To obtain the final intensity, multiply the intensity ratio by the original intensity:

$$20 \text{ mW/cm}^2 \times 0.25 = 5 \text{ mW/cm}^2$$

The intensity was, therefore, reduced to 25% of its original value. Another way to do this example is to note that a 3-dB reduction means halving a value. Because 6 dB = 3 dB + 3 dB, an attenuation of 6 dB reduces the power by one-half (20 W → 10 W), then by one-half again (10 W → 5 W).

Example 2

After passing through soft tissue media, an ultrasound beam has an initial intensity of 100 mW/cm². Calculate the amount of attenuation.

Given: Initial intensity is 100 mW/cm²; final intensity is 0.01 mW/cm².

Then: If decibels $= 10 \log \frac{0.01}{100} = 10 \log \frac{1}{10,000}$

$= 10 \, (-4) = 40 \text{ dB}$

Note: In strict mathematical terms, the 40 dB should be negative, but for our purpose, it can be simply stated as 40 dB of attenuation. The attenuation, therefore, was 40 dB (−40 dB).

The *half-intensity depth* is the distance at which the intensity will be one-half that of the original; the distance the sound beam will travel through a medium before its intensity is reduced by 50%. It is calculated by the formula:

$$\text{half-intensity depth} = \frac{3}{\text{attenuation coefficient (dB/cm)}}$$

The half-intensity depth can also be calculated from the frequency:

$$\text{half-intensity depth} = \frac{6}{\text{frequency (MHz)}}$$

The half-intensity depth is a good indicator of the frequency that should be selected to view different structures in the body. For example, if 50% of the intensity is gone before one reaches a certain depth, then it is obvious that deeper structures will receive less of the sound beam and, thus, generate weaker echoes. Therefore, to visualize deep structures it is necessary to use a lower frequency.

Time gain compensation (TGC) is an electronic compensation for tissue attenuation.

TGC near gain increases or decreases the echo brightness in the near field.

TGC far gain increases or decreases the echo brightness in the far field.

Overall gain increases or decreases the overall brightness in the image.

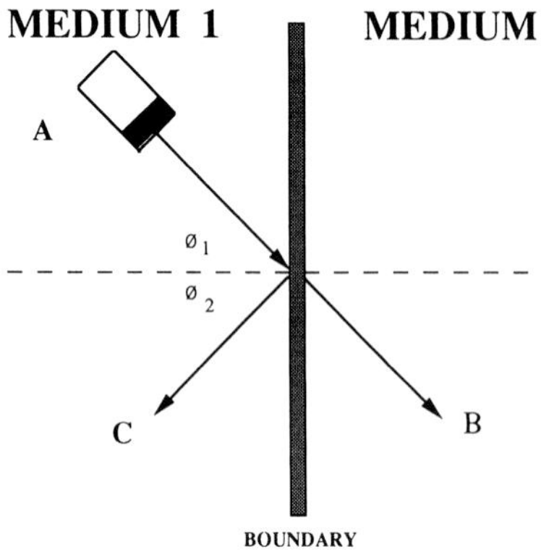

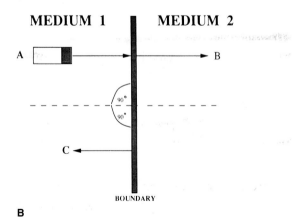

FIGURE 1–4A. (**A**) An oblique incidence striking a boundary; (**B**) refraction of the sound beam; (**C**) reflection of the sound beam. *Note:* An oblique incidence is *not* a normal incidence. A normal incidence is 90° (perpendicular). An incidence beam can be
1. Perpendicular (normal)
2. Oblique incidence (an incidence beam at an oblique angle) not perpendicular. The angle of incidence is the angle of any of the incidence beams.

Echoes

Echoes are the reflections of the sound beam as it travels through the media. An echo is generated each time the beam encounters an acoustic impedance mismatch, but its strength depends on a number of factors. One very important factor, the *angle of incidence,* is the angle at which the incident beam strikes a boundary. The angle of incidence is equal to the angle of reflection (Fig. 1–4A).

Perpendicular incidence is a beam traveling through a medium perpendicular to a boundary and encountering the boundary at a 90° angle (Fig. 1–4B). Perpendicular incidence is also known as *normal incidence.*[1] The portion of the beam

that is not reflected continues in a straight line; this is called *transmission.*

Perpendicular incidence will produce a reflection when the acoustic impedance changes at the boundary. *Acoustic impedance is the product of the density of a medium and the velocity of sound in that medium.*

Acoustic impedance (rayls) = density (kg/m)

$$\times \text{ propagation speed (m/s)}$$

$$Z = \rho \times c$$

At an acoustic impedance mismatch, the sound beam will proceed (transmission), be reflected, or both. The relationship between *perpendicular incidence* and the *intensity* of the echoes can be characterized by the following formulas:

$$\text{intensity reflection coefficient (IRC)} = \left(\frac{z_2 - z_1}{z_2 + z_1}\right)^2$$

$$\text{intensity reflection coefficient (IRC)} = \frac{\text{reflected intensity}}{\text{incident intensity}}$$

$$\text{intensity reflection transmission (ITC)} = \frac{\text{transmitted intensity}}{\text{incident intensity}}$$

The ITC can also be calculated by the formula:

$$\text{ITC} = 1 - \text{IRC}$$

$$\text{incident intensity} = \text{IRC} \times \text{incident intensity} + \text{ITC}$$
$$\times \text{incident intensity}$$

Example

Given two media, one with an acoustic impedance of 20 rayls and the other with an acoustic impedance of 40 rayls, calculate the intensity reflection coefficient (IRC), the intensity transmission coefficient (ITC), the reflected intensity, and the transmitted intensity. (Assume that the incident intensity is 10 mW/cm^2.)

$$Z_1 = 20 \text{ rayls}; Z_2 = 40 \text{ rayls}$$

$$\text{IRC} = \left(\frac{40 - 20}{40 + 20}\right)^2 = \left(\frac{20}{60}\right)^2 = \left(\frac{1}{3}\right)^2 = \frac{1}{9} = 0.11$$

Given: The IRC is 0.11

Then: ITC = 1 − IRC
ITC = 1 − 0.11 = 0.89

If the reflected intensity is equal to the IRC times the original intensity, then reflected intensity = 0.11 × 10 mW/cm^2 = 1.1 mW/cm^2.

If the transmitted intensity is equal to the ITC times the original intensity, then transmitted intensity = 0.89 × 10 mW/cm^2 = 8.9 mW/cm^2.

FIGURE 1–4B. The transmission of the perpendicular incidence sound beam, also called *normal incidence.* (**A**) Normal incidence striking a boundary perpendicularly; (**B**) the intensity transmitted; (**C**) reflection of energy at the boundary of medium 1 and medium 2. *Note:* Beam (**C**) actually travels back along the beam coming from (**A**), but it is depicted separately.

MEDIUM 1   (C= 4 m/s)   MEDIUM 2 (C= 2 m/s)

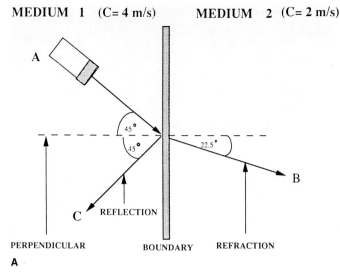

A

FIGURE 1–5A. In medium 1, the propagation speed is 4 m/s; in medium 2, the propagation speed is 2 m/s; therefore, the beam bends toward the normal plane. **(A)** Incidence striking a boundary; **(B)** refraction of the sound beam; **(C)** reflected beam.

MEDIUM 1   (C= 4 m/s)   MEDIUM 2   (C= 6 m/s)

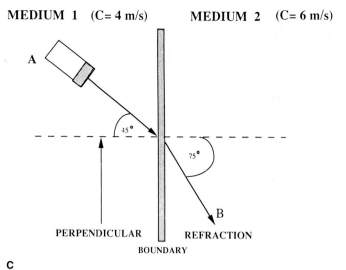

C

FIGURE 1–5C. In medium 1, the propagation speed is 4 m/s; in medium 2, the propagation speed is 6 m/s; therefore, the beam bends away from the normal angle. **(A)** Incidence striking a boundary; **(B)** refraction of the sound beam; **(C)** reflected beam.

Oblique incidence is an angle of incidence that is not 90° perpendicular to a boundary. The angle of transmission will be equal to the angle of incidence as long as the propagation speeds of the media on each side of the boundary are equal. If the propagation speeds are different, however, then the angle of incidence will not be equal to the angle of transmission. The change in direction, the difference in the angle of incidence and the angle of transmission (Fig. 1–5A, B, and C), is called *refraction* (Snell's law).

The angle of incidence is equal to the angle of reflection, but the angle of transmission is variable and can be calculated as follows:

angle of transmission = angle of incidence

$$\times \frac{\text{propagation speed (medium 2)}}{\text{propagation speed (medium 1)}}$$

$$\phi_1 = \text{angle of transmission}$$
$$\phi_1 = \text{angle of incidence}$$

$$\phi_2 = \phi_1 \times \frac{C_2}{C_1}$$

Note: The above equation is only an approximation; at larger angles, it is subject to larger error. To obtain true accuracy, use the full form of Snell's law:

$$\sin \phi_2 = \sin \phi_1 \times \frac{C_2}{C_1}$$

The *range equation* is the relationship between the round-trip travel time of the pulse and the distance to a reflector. This equation determines the position a reflector will have in depth on the display monitor.

distance to the reflector (mm) $= \frac{1}{2} \times$ propagation speed (mm/μs) $\times$ pulse round-trip time (μs)

If we assume the propagation speed to be constant at 1,540 m/s or 1.54 mm/μs, then one-half the propagation speed is equal to 0.77 mm/μs, and the formula can be simplified:

distance to the reflector $(d) = 0.77 \times$ pulse round-trip time (t)

MEDIUM 1   (C= 4 m/s)   MEDIUM 2   (C= 4 m/s)

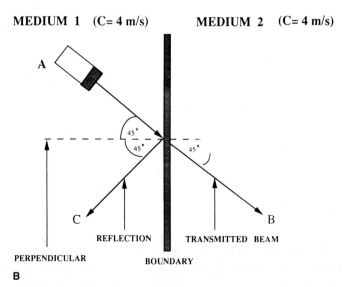

B

FIGURE 1–5B. In medium 1, the propagation speed is 4 m/s; in medium 2, the propagation speed is 4 m/s; therefore, the angle incidence will be equal to the angle of transmission with *no* refraction. **(A)** Incidence striking a boundary; **(B)** transmitted beam; **(C)** reflected beam.

If we assume that for every 13 μs the pulse travels 1 cm, then $d = t/13$. the value of (t) must be given in microseconds if the propagation speed is in millimeters per microseconds. The range equation defines the position a reflector will have in depth on the display monitor.

Contrast Agents and Tissue Harmonic Imaging

Contrast agents for ultrasound have included colloidal suspensions, emulsions, liquids, solid particles, and gas-filled microbubbles. At the present time, contrast agents based on gas-filled bubbles dominate those that are Food and Drug Administration-approved and in common clinical use. The first gas-filled microbubbles used air; however, agents that are more recent are microspheres containing trapped perfluorocarbon gas. The choice of a gas-filled structure to enhance reflectivity is obvious if we refer back to the intensity reflection coefficient (IRC). In the IRC, it is the difference between the acoustic impedance (Z) of the contrast agent and its surroundings that is important. By making the Z of the agent very small relative to the surrounding tissue (achieved by using a gas), the reflectivity of the agent becomes much greater than the surrounding tissue reflectivity.

Harmonic imaging is a result of the nonlinear propagation of the sound beam as it passes through tissue. Harmonic images were first recognized when imaging gas-filled contrast agents in which a portion of the energy being transmitted at a fundamental frequency (f) was being reflected (backscattered) at higher harmonic frequencies ($2f$, $3f$, etc.).

Later, it was recognized that harmonic frequencies were also being produced in tissues. The advantage of the harmonic beam is that it has less dispersion (narrower) than the fundamental frequency and also has smaller side lobes. The narrower beam results in increased lateral resolution, and the reduced side lobes reduce image clutter. Harmonic images are created by eliminating the fundamental frequency and selectively recording the higher-frequency echo components.

TRANSDUCERS

A *transducer* is a device that converts one form of energy to another. In diagnostic sonography, the transducer converts electrical energy to pressure energy (acoustic energy) and vice versa.

1. *Active element*
   A. *Piezoelectric principle* is the conversion of electrical energy to pressure energy and vice versa. Ultrasound (pressure energy) is generated by electric stimulation of the piezoelectric element causing expansions and contractions of the element, which, in turn, generate the ultrasound pulse. The resultant ultrasound pulse produces a similar distortion of the element and then converts back to an electric signal (Fig. 1–6).

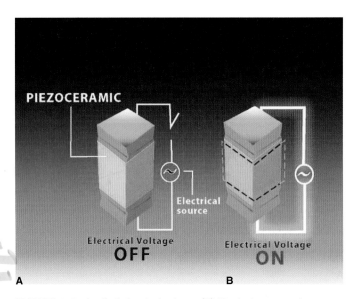

FIGURE 1–6. Applied electrical voltage. (**A**) Physical compression on the crystal will generate a potential difference across the faces of the crystal. The effect is called *piezoelectric effect*. (**B**) Voltage applied on the crystal will generate mechanical energy (ultrasound). The effect is called *reverse piezoelectric effect.*

B. *Material.* The active element can be *natural* (e.g., quartz, tourmaline, Rochelle salt) or *synthetic* (e.g., lead zirconate titanate [PZT], barium titanate, lithium sulfate). Synthetic elements are most commonly used in today's diagnostic equipment because of their availability and low cost. To turn one of these manufactured substances into a piezoelectric element, it is heated to its Curie point, or the temperature at which a ferroelectric material such as many piezoelectric materials, loses its magnetic properties. The dipoles within the material are then polarized with an electric current. When the element cools, the dipoles are fixed (Fig. 1–7). The material is cut and shaped, then housed in the transducer.

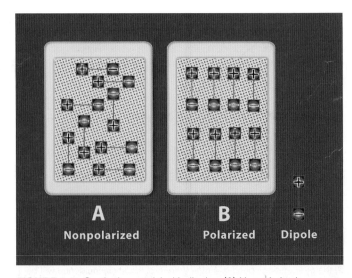

FIGURE 1–7. Synthetic material with dipoles. (**A**) Nonpolarized; (**B**) Polarized; (**C**) Dipole.

C. *Properties of elements (crystals).* The frequency of the acoustic wave produced by a standard pulsed-wave imaging system is determined by the *thickness* of the piezoelectric element and the *propagation speed* of the crystal. The propagation speed of the crystal is approximately three to five times greater than the speed of ultrasound in soft tissue, namely, 4 to 8 mm/μs. The thinner the crystal, the greater the frequency.

$$\text{frequency (MHz)} = \frac{\text{propagation speed of the crystal (mm/μs)}}{2 \times \text{thickness (mm)}}$$

The diameter of the crystal does not affect the pulse frequency; it does, however, determine the *lateral resolution.* Neither the impedance of the matching layer nor the thickness of the backing material is a primary determinant of ultrasound frequency.

In contrast to pulse wave, *the frequency of continuous-wave ultrasound is equal to the frequency of the electric voltage that drives the piezoelectric crystal.* In simpler terms, when the pulser of a continuous-wave system produces an electric signal with a frequency of 6 MHz, the frequency of the emitted acoustic signal will also be 6 MHz.

2. *Damping material (backing material)* is an epoxy resin attached to the back of the element that absorbs the vibrations and reduces the number of cycles in a pulse (Fig. 1–8). By reducing the number of cycles, the following are accomplished:

A. Pulse duration (PD) and spatial pulse length (SPL) are reduced. PD = number of cycles (n) × time (t), where t = period of ultrasound in pulse. SPL = number of cycles (n) × wavelength (λ).

By reducing these two factors, the axial resolution will be improved.

$$\text{axial resolution } (R_A) = \frac{\text{SPL}}{2}$$

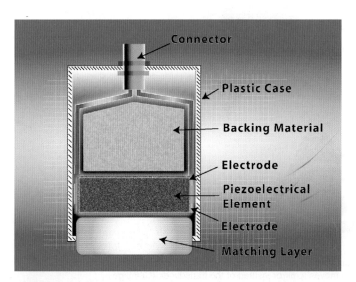

FIGURE 1–8. Components of a transducer.

B. *Bandwidth* (the width of the frequency spectrum) is increased by increasing the damping. When the bandwidth increases, the quality factor (Q factor) of the transducer decreases.

C. The duty factor is decreased.

3. *Matching layer* is a substance placed in front of the transducer element's face material to decrease the reflection at the transducer–tissue interface. The matching layer is necessary because the impedance difference between the transducer crystal and the soft tissue is so large that most of the energy will be reflected back at the skin surface. The matching layer provides an intermediate impedance, allowing transmission of the ultrasound beam into the body.

The thickness of the matching layer is usually equal to one-quarter of the wavelength.[1] Multiple layers are often used to avoid reflections caused by the variety of frequencies and wavelengths present in short pulses. In addition to the matching layer of the transducer, a *coupling gel* is used to form a transducer surface–skin contact that will eliminate air and prevent reflection at this boundary.

Bandwidth and Quality Factor

The transducer produces more than one frequency. For example, the operating frequency may be 3.5 MHz, but a spectrum of other frequencies are also generated, known as the *bandwidth.* The shorter the pulse, the more of these other frequencies are generated. Therefore, the bandwidth and the pulse length are inversely proportional; as the pulse length decreases, the bandwidth increases (Fig. 1–9). Continuous-wave ultrasound has a very narrow bandwidth.

If the bandwidth increases, the Q factor decreases. If, however, the operating frequency increases, the Q factor increases. A low Q factor indicates:

1. Broad bandwidth
2. Low operating frequency
3. Shortened pulse length
4. Uniform near field (Many frequencies in a pulse result in a more uniform intensity distribution.)

Types of Transducers

There are several ways to classify transducers; one is the way the sound beam is swept (or steered). This process can be either mechanical or electrical.

A *mechanical transducer* (Fig. 1–10) has a scan head that contains a single disk-shaped active element. One type of mechanical transducer is the *oscillatory* or *rotary type,* which has an element physically attached to a mechanical device to move it through a pathway (see Fig. 1–10A). A second type has an *oscillatory mirror* that mechanically moves while the element remains stationary (see Fig. 1–10B).

Focusing the beam produced by a mechanical transducer is achieved by curvature of the crystal, a curved lens on the

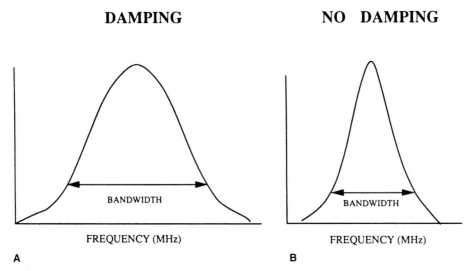

DAMPING   **NO   DAMPING**

BANDWIDTH

FREQUENCY (MHz)   FREQUENCY (MHz)

A   B

FIGURE 1-9. Bandwidth (**A**) with damping, (**B**) with no damping. *Note*: Damping increases bandwidth.

crystal, or the reflecting mirror. Focusing occurs at a *specific depth* on both the horizontal and vertical planes. To change the focal depth, the operator must select another transducer with the desired focal zone. The mechanical transducer produces a sector-shaped image (see Fig. 1–10C). *Mechanical transducers are mechanically steered (MS) and mechanically focused (MF).*

The *annular array* is a mechanical transducer. The transducer element consists of 5 to 11 rings of transducer elements mounted on a mechanically moved (steered) arm (Fig. 1–11).

The advantage of the annular array over the single element transducer is the presence of many elements, allowing for electronic focusing. By focusing transmission and reception of the ultrasound energy, greater depth resolution is achieved. The image produced by an annular array is also a sector. *Annular arrays are mechanically steered (MS) and electronically focused (EF).*

An *electronic transducer* is an assembly of multiple elements called an *array*. There are many types of arrays, each with a particular set of characteristics:

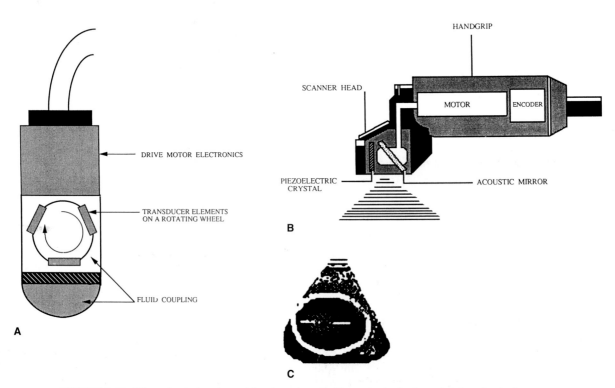

HANDGRIP

SCANNER HEAD

MOTOR   ENCODER

DRIVE MOTOR ELECTRONICS

PIEZOELECTRIC
CRYSTAL   ACOUSTIC MIRROR

TRANSDUCER ELEMENTS
ON A ROTATING WHEEL

B

FLUID COUPLING

A

C

FIGURE 1-10. (**A**) mechanical sector real-time transducer that is mechanically steered and mechanically focused. (**B**) A mechanical sector real-time transducer that moves a mirror instead of the transducer. (**C**) Image presentation from a mechanical sector.

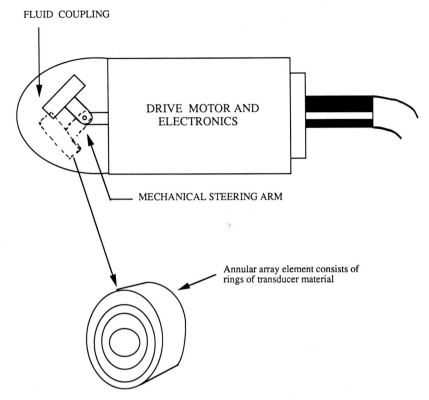

FLUID COUPLING

DRIVE MOTOR AND ELECTRONICS

MECHANICAL STEERING ARM

Annular array element consists of rings of transducer material

FIGURE 1–11. Annular array real-time transducer probe that contains four transducer rings (multielement) on a mechanically steered shaft.

Linear sequential array (linear array). Shown in Fig. 1–12. This type of transducer produces a rectangular image (Fig. 1–13B).

Curved array (radial array, convex array). The arrays of transducer elements are arranged with specific curvature (Fig. 1–14). Focusing the beam is achieved by internal and electronic focusing; there is no beam steering. The curved design of the transducer head creates a *sector* or *trapezoid image*.

Sector phased array (phased array). The voltage pulses are applied to the entire groups of elements with varying time delays. The beam can be electronically focused (EF) and steered (ES). The image format is sector (Fig. 1–15).

Focusing Techniques

Transducers can be either mechanically or electronically focused. *Mechanical focusing* is accomplished by using a curved crystal or an acoustic lens for each element. This type of focusing is usually applied to mechanical transducers and will improve lateral resolution by limiting the beam width.

There are two types of electronic focusing: transmit focusing and receive focusing.

Transmit focusing. Electronic focusing during transmission is accomplished by firing a group of elements with a small time delay (nanoseconds) between various elements in the group. The wavefront generated by each element in the

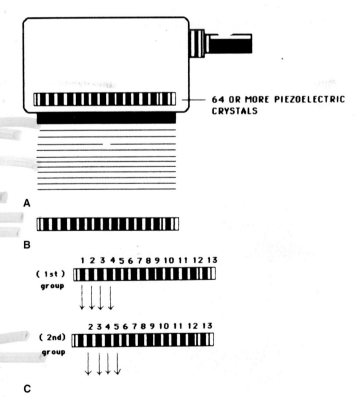

64 OR MORE PIEZOELECTRIC CRYSTALS

A

B

(1st) group   1 2 3 4 5 6 7 8 9 10 11 12 13

(2nd) group   2 3 4 5 6 7 8 9 10 11 12 13

C

FIGURE 1–12. Linear sequential array. (**A**) A real-time linear-array transducer. (**B**) Design of a linear segmental phased-array transducer. These transducers consist of a long strip of piezoelectric crystals divided into elements, that are arranged next to each other; (**C**) operation of a linear segmental phased-array transducer. The crystal elements are pulsed in groups of four in this example, with each group sending and receiving in succession.

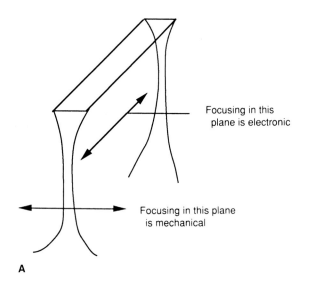
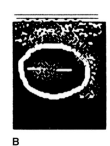

FIGURE 1–13. Linear sequential array. (**A**) Focusing in the plane of the long axis of the transducer is electronic; focusing in the plane perpendicular to the long axis is mechanical. (**B**) Image presentation from a linear phased array transducer. Note the rectangular image.

group will arrive at a specific point in space, resulting in a focused beam. Using transmit focus will improve lateral resolutions and create several possible focal zones. Multizone transmit focusing will result in a slower frame rate. If, for example, there are three focal zones, then the frame rate will be reduced as compared to a single focus zone. If the rate is very slow, then the image will flicker causing a "perceived" distortion of the image.

Received focusing. Electronic focusing of the received echoes, by electronically delaying the return of the signals to the processing system within the diagnostic unit, the optimum range of the focal zone can be extended. This process will enhance image clarity.

Sound Beam

A *sound beam* is the acoustic energy emitted by the transducer. The beam can be pulsed or continuous wave. *Ultrasound waves follow Huygens's principle, which states that the resultant beam is a combination of all sound arising from different sources (wavelets) on the transducer crystal face. Focusing is the superimposition (algebraic summation) of all sound waves in the beam.*[1–3] As the various wavelets within a beam collide, interference (constructive and destructive) results in the formation of a sound beam (Fig. 1–16).

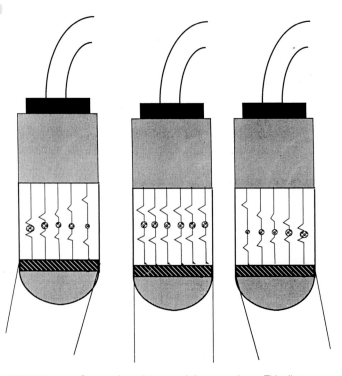

FIGURE 1–14. Curved linear array. The array of transducer elements are arranged with a specific curvature. There is no beam steering; focusing of the beam is achieved internally by mechanical and electronic means.

FIGURE 1–15. Sector phased array real-time transducer. This diagram illustrates how electronic pulses are used to steer the ultrasound beam.

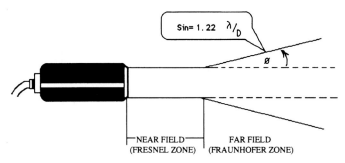

FIGURE 1–16. The ultrasound beam from an unfocused transducer.

Constructive interference. The waves are not in phase, producing a decrease in amplitude or even zero amplitude. Zero amplitude occurs if the out-of-phase waves completely cancel each other.

The beam is composed of a near zone, focal point, and a far zone.

1. *Near zone (near field or Fresnel zone)* is the portion of the sound beam in which the beam diameter narrows as the distance from the transducer increases until it reaches its narrowest diameter. This distance is the *near zone length* (NZL). At the far end of the NZL, the diameter of the beam is equal to one-half the diameter of the transducer. The NZL is also related to the frequency: increasing the frequency increases the NZL, and vice versa. Components of the beam of a focused transducer are shown in Fig. 1–17.

2. *Focal point* is the point at which the beam reaches its narrowest diameter. As the diameter narrows, the beam width resolution improves, becoming the best at the focal point. The *focal zone* is the distance between equal beam diameters that are some multiple of the diameter of the focal point (often two times the diameter of the focal point). The focal zone extends toward the transducer from the focal point, and toward the far zone. The *focal length* is the region of the beam from the transducer to the focal point.

3. *Far field (far zone or Fraunhofer zone)* is the portion of the sound beam (after the NZL) in which the diameter of the beam increases as the distance from the transducer increases. At a distance of two times the NZL, the beam diameter once again equals the diameter of the transducer. The divergence of the beam in the far field is inversely proportional to the crystal diameter and frequency. The larger the transducer element and the higher the frequency, the smaller the angle of divergence in the far field (Fig. 1–18A, B).

Resolution

There are two types of resolution: lateral and axial (Fig. 1–19A, B).

Lateral resolution (azimuthal, transverse, angular, or resolution) is equal to the beam diameter (see Fig. 1–19A). The distance between two interfaces has to be greater than the beam diameter (width) for the two interfaces to be resolved as separate entities. Lateral resolution applies to interfaces perpendicular to the direction of the sound beam. With an unfocused transducer, lateral resolution is best in the near field; with a focused transducer, the lateral resolution is best at the focal point. A transducer with a smaller diameter will improve lateral resolution as the beam diverges in the far zone. Transducers are sometimes designed with an acoustic lens in order to narrow the sound beam; this results in better lateral resolution.

Axial resolution (linear, range longitudinal, or depth resolution) is related to the SPL. Two interfaces at different depths will be distinguished from each other only if the distance between them is equal to or greater than one-half the SPL (see Fig. 1–19B).

$$\text{axial resolution} = \frac{\text{SPL}}{2}$$

To obtain maximum image quality, axial resolution (R_A) should be as small as possible. Axial resolution improves when wavelength or the number of cycles per second decreases (both of these factors are related to SPL). Frequency

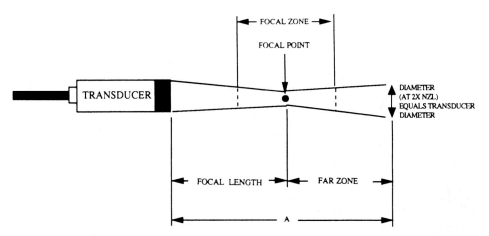

FIGURE 1–17. The components of the ultrasound beam in a focused transducer. Note that the diameter of the beam is equal to the diameter of the transducer face.

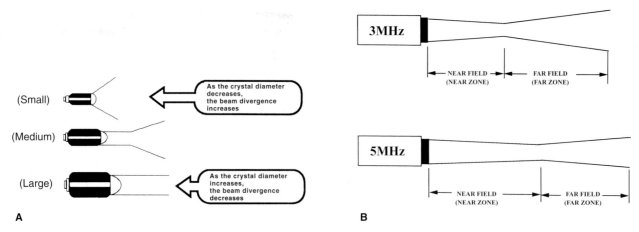

FIGURE 1–18. (**A**) Beam diversion with increasing crystal diameter. (**B**) Transducer crystal size shown in relationship to frequency. *Note:* The higher the frequency of the transducer, the smaller the beam diameter, and the longer the near-zone. The angle of beam divergences in the far field is smaller with a higher frequency transducer.

also affects the axial resolution. As the frequency increases, the wavelength decreases, thus the axial resolution improves. However, as the frequency increases, the depth of penetration decreases, creating a need to compromise resolution for adequate penetration into the tissues. This compromise is why the frequency range for diagnostic procedures is usually between 2 and 10 MHz.

Temporal Resolution

Temporal resolution is related to time and motion and is determined by frame rate. Video imaging with a frame rate greater than 30 images per second will give visual perception of full motion (real time). Less than 30 images per second will have a jerky image. Temporal resolution is improved by

- High frame rate
- Narrow sector

- Fewer pulses
- Low line density

IMAGING PROCESS

The components of a pulsed-echo diagnostic ultrasound system are the pulser, receiver, scan converter, and display (Fig. 1–20).

Pulser

The *pulser* produces an electric voltage that activates the piezoelectric element, causing it to contract and expand to produce the longitudinal compression wave (sound beam). A second function of the pulser is to signal the receiver and scan converter that the transducer has been activated. Each electric pulse generates an ultrasonic pulse. The number of ultrasonic pulses per second is defined as the *pulse repetition frequency*

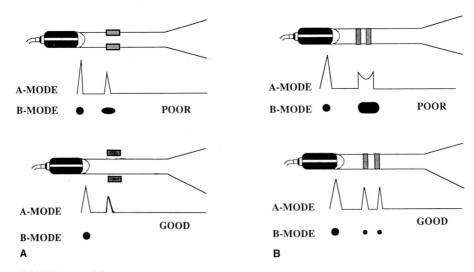

FIGURE 1–19. (**A**) *Lateral Resolution:* the ability of the ultrasound beam to separate two structures lying at a right angle (perpendicular) to the beam direction. Lateral resolution is also referred to as azimuthal, transverse, angular, or horizontal. (**B**) *Axial Resolution:* The ability of the ultrasound beam to separate two structures lying along the path of (parallel to) the beam direction. Axial resolution is also referred to as linear, longitudinal, depth, or range.

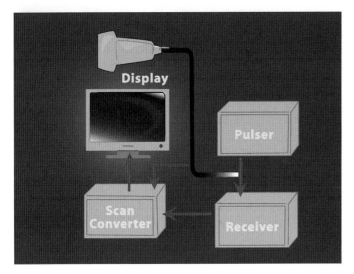

FIGURE 1–20. Components of a pulsed-echo ultrasound system.

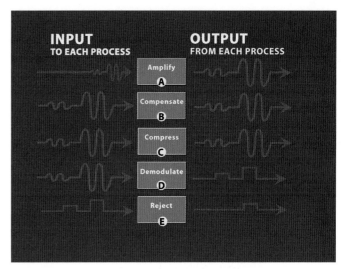

FIGURE 1–21. The five functions of the receiver. **(A)** Amplification of both pulses. **(B)** Compensation for the weaker pulses. **(C)** The difference between the pulse amplitudes is reduced. **(D)** The pulses are converted to another form. **(E)** The weaker pulse is rejected. *(Kremkaw FW. Diagnostic Ultrasound: Principles, Instruments, and Exercises. 3rd ed. Philadelphia: WB Saunders; 1989.)*

(PRF). With array transducers, the pulser is responsible for the delay and variations in pulse amplitude needed for electronic control of beam scanning, steering, and shaping. In improving the dynamic range of multielement transducers, the pulser suppresses grating lobes, a process termed *dynamic apodization.*[1]

Increasing the power output control of a system will raise the intensity by signaling the pulser to put out more voltage. To reduce the potential for harmful bioeffects, it is desirable to keep the power low. Therefore, to increase the number of echoes displayed, it is recommended that the operator increase the gain control, not the power.

Receiver

The receiver processes electric signals returned from the transducer (i.e., ultrasonic reflections converted into electric signals by the transducer). Processing involves amplification, compensation, compression, demodulation, and rejection (Fig. 1–21).

Amplification is the process that increases small electric voltages received from the transducer to a level suitable for further processing. This process is sometimes referred to as "over-all-gain" enhancement or increase. Gain is the ratio of output electric power to input electric power and is measured in decibels. *Dynamic range* is the range of values between the minimum and maximum echo amplitudes. It is the ratio of the largest power to the smallest power in the working range of the diagnostic unit. Dynamic range is also expressed in decibels.

Compensation is also referred to as gain compensation, swept gain, or time gain compensation. It is the mechanism that compensates for the loss of echo strength caused by the depth of the reflector. It allows reflectors with equal reflection coefficients to appear on the screen with equal brightness and to compensate, to a certain extent, for the effects of attenuation caused by greater depth. For the average soft

tissues, the attenuation coefficient is equal to one-half the frequency (expressed in decibels per centimeter).

Compression is the internal process in which larger echoes are equalized with smaller echoes. Compression decreases dynamic range.

Demodulation is the process of converting voltages delivered to the receiver to a more useful form. Demodulation is done by rectification (removal of negative components, replacement with positive values) and smoothing (averaging of the new wave form).

Rejection is also termed suppression or threshold. Rejection is the elimination of smaller amplitude voltage pulses produced by weaker reflections. This mechanism helps to reduce noise by removing low-level signals that do not contribute to meaningful information in the image.

Scan Converter (Memory)

The *scan converter*, or *memory*, transforms the incoming echo data into a suitable format for the display, storing all of the necessary information for the two-dimensional image. As the tissue is scanned, several images (frames) are acquired per second. Memory allows for a single scan consisting of one or more frames to be displayed. Most instruments have enough memory to store the last several frames scanned (cine loop). There are two types of scan converters (memories): analog and digital.

Analog scan converters are found in older machines, these consist of semiconductors arranged in square matrices. As the ultrasound pulse transverses the tissues, an electronic beam scans the square matrix. It is swept in the same direction as the beam in the body. The current within the electronic beam corresponds to the intensity of the returning echoes. If the echoes are weak, the current in the electronic beam is decreased and vice versa. The strengths of the electrical charges are precisely what are stored in the individual insulators of the matrix. These electronic charges have values that correspond to brightness levels. To read the stored images, the electronic beam is scanned across the stored matrix. The stored charge in each element affects the current in the electronic beam, and together these charges are used to vary the brightness of display.

Digital scan converters store image brightness values as numbers instead as of electrical charges. A digital scan converter consists of three components: an analog-to-digital (A–D) converter, which changes the voltages of received signals into numeric values; a digital memory, which stores these image echo values; and a circuit, which translates these stored numbers back into analog (voltage) values when needed (a digital-to-analog, or D–A, converter).

The digital memory component is the same as computer memory. Modern computers use circuits that have only two states: off and on. Within the computer these states may be represented; for example, by the absence or presence of electrical current, the open or closed condition of switches, or the direction of magnetization on a magnetic disk or tape. Each of these examples has two states, which the computer considers zero (0) or one (1). At first, it seems that this system, called the *binary number system*, or *binary*,[4] is not very useful for computing, but it can represent any number that the more common decimal system can. Instead of using increasing powers of 10, as the decimal system does, the binary system uses increasing powers of 2. In the decimal system, the right-most digit represents units, the next to the left tens, the next hundreds, etc. In the binary system, the rightmost binary digit or bit is ones, the next left twos, the next fours, the next eights, etc.[1] (Fig. 1–22).

Display

How is this system used to represent ultrasound images? Imagine that the image is divided into many small squares

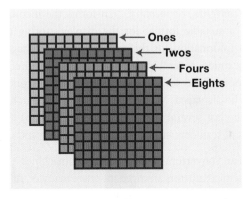

FIGURE 1–22. A 10 × 10 pixel, 4-bit-deep digital memory. *(Kremkaw FW. Diagnostic Ultrasound: Principles, Instruments, and Exercises. 3rd ed. Philadelphia: WB Saunders; 1989.)*

similar to a checkerboard. Each square is assigned a number that represents the ultrasound echo amplitude. For example, for white-on-black displays, the highest echo value is white, and the lowest is black (the reverse is true for black-on-white displays).[2] A square located in a part of the image that has the highest echo values (e.g., echoes in a gallstone) would be assigned a high number value, whereas, a square in the surrounding bile would receive a small number value. In color-flow imaging, each square would be assigned a number that represents the Doppler shift value. If the squares are made small enough, then the eye will not be able to see them as separate. Typically, ultrasound images are divided into 512 by 512 of these small squares.[1]

The squares are called picture elements, or *pixels*. The number 512 is a power of two (two to the ninth power) and also happens to fit well in a standard television frame. This number yields an image containing 262,144 pixels.

If each of these pixels could store only one binary value, then the results would be very much like an old bistable image, having only black and white values. Each pixel could be either black or white, with no gray values. To store gray scale images, each pixel must have more than one binary digit (or bit). For example, with three bits per pixel each pixel could represent eight different shades of gray. To calculate how many different shades of gray can be represented by a pixel containing a set number (n) of databits, the following formula can be applied:

$$\text{number of shades} = 2^n$$

The largest value that can be represented by a given number of bits is calculated by the formula:

$$\text{largest value of } n \text{ bits} = 2^n - 1$$

If, for example, we are considering three bits, we could represent eight different shades of gray with the largest gray value equal to seven.

Most ultrasound machines generate images with four to eight bits of gray scale (16 to 256 shades of gray). Color-flow Doppler machines need more bits to represent the various colors. Because the machine makes no distinction of color (to the machine, the image is merely an array of numbers), the color values are stored as a number value for each of three primary colors. Combinations of these three primaries (usually red, green, and blue) can yield almost any color.

Fig. 1–22 is an example of a 10 × 10 pixel matrix with 4 bits/pixel. To calculate how many bits an ultrasound image contains, the following formula can be applied:

$$\text{number of bits/image} = \text{number of image} \times \text{number of image columns} \times \text{number of bits/pixel}$$

or

$$\text{number of bits/image} = \text{total number of pixels} \times \text{number of bits/pixels}$$

In computer terminology, eight binary digits or eight bits equal 1 *byte*. To determine the number of bytes of memory an image requires, divide the number of bits per image by eight:

$$\text{number of bytes/image} = \frac{\text{number of bits per image}}{8}$$

Examples

If an image has 10 pixel columns and rows with 2 bits/pixels, then

$$\text{number of bits/image} = 10 \times 10 \times 2 = 200 \text{ bits}$$

$$\text{number of bytes/image} = \frac{200 \text{ bits/image}}{8} = 25 \text{ bytes}$$

If a 512 × 512 pixel image has 8 bits/pixel, then

$$\text{number of bits/image} = 512 \times 512 \times 8$$
$$= 2,097,152 \text{ bits}$$

$$\text{number of bytes/image} = \frac{2,097,152}{8} = 262,144 \text{ bytes}$$

Thus, a single image can contain over 2 million bits or more than 1/4 million bytes. To reduce the number of digits used to describe these values, multipliers are applied, such as kilo-, mega-, giga- (Table 1–2). These multipliers are not identical to their counterparts in the metric system, however. For example, 1 kilobit is not 1,000 bits, but 1,024 bits or 2 to the 10th power. For convenience, large numbers may be rounded (e.g., 262,144 bytes may be rounded to 260 kilobytes).

The image can be stored in the digital memory as numbers, but it cannot be viewed unless the numbers are converted back to an image. Otherwise, a large list of numbers is all that would be displayed. The third part of the digital scan converter does the following conversion. It takes the number values stored in the memory and changes them back into an analog voltage. The voltage varies the brightness of a spot on the cathode ray tube, generating an image that the human eye can interpret. The hardware that performs this function is the digital-to-analog (D–A) converter.

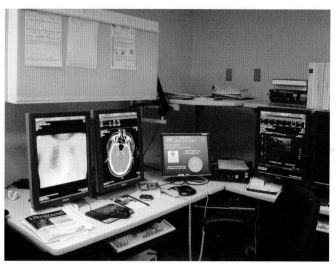

FIGURE 1–23. PACS web-based workstation for reading, archiving, and distribution of image via LCD flat screens.

DIGITAL IMAGING

Picture archiving and communications system, more commonly known as *PACS*, enables images such as x-ray, computed tomography (CT), and sonograms to be stored electronically and viewed on liquid crystal display (LCD) screens. The images can be manipulated to improve the ability to make diagnoses or to be transferred over a secure World Wide Web to be shared with other imaging experts. Fig. 1–23 shows PACS viewing and workstation.

Digital imaging and communicating in medicine, known as *DICOM*, is a standard protocol that makes digital information compatible with all manufacturing equipment.

CODED EXCITATION

Conventional ultrasound transducers are based on the principle that high-frequency ultrasound has difficulty penetrating deep into the body. A new digital technology called *coded excitation* provides good penetration and high resolution at the same time. When applied, this technique improves axial resolution, contrast resolution, signal-to-noise ratio, and penetration depth.

Pre-processing (write zoom) occurs during movement of the image called scanning and includes

- Before storage in the scan converter
- Time gain compensation (TGC)
- Write magnification
- Cannot be performed on a frozen image

Post-processing (read zoom) is the adjustment or changes to ultrasound images after storage in the scan converter, which include

- Any change after the freeze frame
- Measurements

TABLE 1–2 • Unit of Measurement in Computer Terminology			
Unit	**Prefix**	**Symbol**	**Quantity**
byte[a]	kilo-	K	1,000
byte	mega-	M	1,000,000
byte	giga-	G	1,000,000,000

[a]1 kilobyte equals 1,024 characters but can be rounded off to 1,000.

- Read magnification
- Contrast and brightness

Both pre-processing and post-processing are the manipulation of image data.

IMAGE QUALITY

A *frame* is a single image composed of multiple scan lines. To produce a dynamic or moving image, numerous frames are required. To freeze a frame, or stop the image to record or view it, the memory of the system is activated. The *frame rate* (FR) is the number of frames displayed or scanned per second. In most diagnostic medical sonography or echocardiography systems, the frame rate is usually 10–60 frames/s. If the display frame rate is below 20/s, then the real-time image appears to flicker, preventing the eye from integrating the images.

The pulse repetition frequency (PRF) is the number of pulses produced by the transducer in a given time period. It is related to the number of lines per frame and the frame rate by the formula:

$$\text{pulse repetition} = \text{lines per frame (LPF) frequency (PRF)} \times \text{frame rate (FR)}$$

The PRF, LPF, and FR are directly related to the propagation speed. The maximum effective velocity is 77,000 cm/s, or one-half the propagation speed of ultrasound in soft tissues (1,540 m/s or 154,000 cm/s). The one-half value results from the pulse having to make a round-trip to be received.

$$\text{depth} \times \text{LPF} \times \text{FR} = 77,000$$

Note: LPF × FR = PRF. Hence, the equation can also be stated

$$\text{depth} \times \text{PRF} = 77,000$$

Improving image quality by increasing the lines per frame will reduce the frame rate if the depth remains constant. Increasing the depth of penetration while maintaining a constant number of lines per frame also reduces the frame rate. The frame rate can be increased if the depth of penetration is decreased, assuming the LPF is constant.

The *display format* refers to how the image appears on the screen, as either a rectangular display or a sector display. A *rectangular display* image appears in the form of a rectangle. The width of the display is given in centimeters; the *line density* is expressed as the number of lines per centimeter. To determine the line density for a rectangular display the lines per frame are divided by the display width in centimeters.

$$\text{line density (lines/cm)} = \frac{\text{lines per frame (LPF)}}{\text{display width (cm)}}$$

A *sector display* yields a pie-shaped image. The scans form an angle so that the line density is expressed as lines per degree.

$$\text{line density (lines/degree)} = \frac{\text{lines per frame (LPF)}}{\text{sector angle (degrees)}}$$

The *scan converter*, electronic circuitry in the machine's display, transforms a rectangular or arc-shaped image into a rectangular video frame, and adds the text and graphics (such as depth markers).

Modes of Display

The *A-mode*, or amplitude mode, is a one-dimensional graphic display with vertical deflections of the baseline. The height of the deflection represents the amplitude, or strength, of the echo (y-axis); the distance in time is a function of where on the horizontal baseline the deflection occurs (x-axis).

The *B-mode*, or brightness mode, displays the echoes as variations in the brightness of a line of spots on the image. The position of the spot on the baseline is related to the depth of the reflecting structure; the brightness is proportional to the strength of the echo. Each row of spots represents information obtained from a single position of the transducer or scanning beam. When successive rows of these spots are integrated into an image, a B-scan is produced. In B-mode, the x-axis represents depth and the z-axis represents brightness. There is no y-axis in B-mode.

The *M-mode*, or motion mode, is a two-dimensional recording of the reflector's change in position, or motion, against time. The vertical axis represents depth and the horizontal represents time. Most M-modes display the brightness of the signal in proportion to the strength of the echo. This mode is most commonly used for the study of dynamic structures such as the heart.

ARTIFACTS

Unlike a Grecian urn, which is an *artifact* from a past culture, the term in diagnostic medical sonography has a very different implication. If refers to something seen on an image that does not, in reality, exist in the anatomy studied. An artifact can be beneficial to the interpretation of the image, or it can detract from this process. For example, certain artifacts are known to occur in cystic structures and are notably absent from a solid mass, and this information can therefore, be used in a beneficial way when determining the nature of a mass. Conversely, there are artifacts that can appear similar to the placenta, making delineation of the limits of the placenta more difficult. Artifacts can be subdivided by the physical principals that produce them; namely, resolution artifacts, propagation artifacts, attenuation artifacts, or miscellaneous artifacts.

Resolution Artifacts

Axial resolution is the failure to resolve two separate reflectors parallel to the beam.

Lateral resolution is the failure to resolve two separate reflectors perpendicular to the beam.

Speckle is scatter in tissues, causing interference effects referred to as *noise*.

Section thickness is the finite width of the beam producing extraneous echoes, or debris, in normal anechoic, or echo-free structures.

Propagation Artifacts

Reverberation is repetitive reflections between two highly reflective layers. The bouncing back and forth increases travel time, causing the signals to be displayed at different depths. The reverberations are seen on the image as equally spaced bands of diminishing amplitude.

Refraction is the change in direction of the sound beam as it passes from one medium to another. This phenomenon will cause a reflection to appear improperly positioned on the image.

Multipath. Because the returning signal does not necessarily follow the same path as the incident beam, the time required for some parts of the signal to return to the transducer will vary, causing reflections to appear at incorrect depths.

Mirror image is generated when objects present on one side of a strong reflector are also shown on the other side of the reflector. Such artifacts are commonly seen around the diaphragm. These types of artifacts produce a duplicated copy to appear incorrectly on the image.

Attenuation Artifacts

Shadowing is the reduction in echo strength of signals arising from behind a strong reflector or attenuating structure. Structures such as gallstones, renal calculi, and bone will produce shadowing.

Enhancement is an increase in the amplitude of echoes located behind a weakly attenuating structure. The increase pertains to the relative strength of the signals as compared with neighboring signals passing through more highly attenuating media. For example, stronger reflections may be seen behind a fluid-filled structure than behind a solid structure (e.g., the urine-filled bladder versus a solid tumor of the uterus).

Refraction or edge shadowing. The beam may bend at a curved surface and lose intensity, producing a shadow. If the beam is traveling from a higher velocity medium (less dense) to a low-velocity medium, a narrower shadow will be generated. Conversely, a sound beam traveling from a low-velocity medium to a higher one will project a wider shadow.

Miscellaneous Artifacts

Comet tail is produced by a strong reflector; similar in appearance to reverberation. The comet tail, however, is composed of thin lines of closely spaced discrete echoes. Comet tail artifacts frequently occur with the presence of gas bubbles, surgical clips, biopsy needle, or bullet fragments.

Ring down is thought to be caused by a resonance phenomenon and is associated with gas bubble. It also appears very similar to reverberation, producing numerous parallel echoes. Sometimes discrete echoes cannot be differentiated, giving the appearance of a continuous emission of sound.

Propagation speed error. Most diagnostic ultrasound equipment operates on the assumption that the speed of sound in the body is 1,540 m/s. This is not always true because different tissues have different propagation speeds. If the beam passes from a medium of one speed into a medium of a greater speed, then the calculated distance will be less than the actual distance, causing the echo to be erroneously displayed too close to the transducer. If the propagation speed decreases, then the echo will appear farther from the transducer than it actually is.

Side lobes are the result of the transducer element being finite in size. The difference in vibration at the center and edge results in acoustic energy emitted by the transducer flowing along the main axis of the sound beam. The energy that diverts from the main path is the cause of the side lobes, which will generate reflections at improper, off-axis locations in the image. Side lobes are created by a single crystal transducer. Apodization is a technical term for changing the shape of the ultrasound beam with different voltages. This is used to reduce both side lobes and grating lobes.

Grating lobes are seen with linear array transducers, which also produce off-axis acoustic waves as a result of the regular spacing of the active elements. All grating lobes will cause reflections to appear at improper, off-axis locations in the image. A grating lobe is created by multiple crystal transducers (arrays). Subdicing is a method of dividing the transducer elements into small elements. This is used to reduce grating lobes.

Range ambiguity. As noted earlier, the range equation relates the depth of a reflector to the propagation speed and the pulse round-trip time. The maximum depth (d_{max}) of a reflector that can be unambiguously recorded is:

$$d_{max} = \frac{1}{2} \times \text{propagation speed} \times \text{PRP}$$

Thus, the pulse repetition period (PRP) that controls the field-of-view (FOV) also determines the maximum depth of a reflector that can be unambiguously recorded. Echoes from a transmitted pulse that return after a time equal to the PRP will be erroneously recorded at a depth closer to the transducer.

QUALITY OF PERFORMANCE

To guarantee efficiency of performance, all ultrasound diagnostic equipment is tested under a quality assurance (QA) program. To ensure that the instrument is operating correctly and consistently, it is checked for the following:

1. Imaging performance
2. Equipment performance and safety

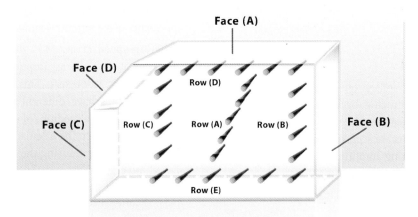

AIUM 100-mm test object

FIGURE 1–24. AIUM 100-mm test object.

3. Beam measurements
4. Acoustic output
5. Preventative maintenance (e.g., replacing worn parts before they actually fail)

AIUM TEST OBJECT

The American Institute of Ultrasound in Medicine (AIUM) has designed a test object specifically to measure imaging performance of an ultrasound system (Fig. 1–24). The AIUM test object is a "tank" consisting of a series of stainless steel rods, 0.75 mm in diameter, arranged in a specific pattern between two transparent plastic sides, with the other boundaries formed by thin, acrylic plastic sheets.[1,4] The tank is filled with a mixture of alcohol, an algae inhibitor, and water, which allows the propagation speed to approximate the speed of sound in soft tissues (1,540 m/s). The results obtained are not affected by normal fluctuations in room temperature; the speed varies less than 1% for a temperature variation of 5°Celsius (5°C).

The following factors are measured by the AIUM test object (Table 1–3):

TABLE 1–3 • Performance Measurements for the AIUM Test Object

Measurement	Row	Test Object Face	Parameter Tested
Dead zone	D	Face (A)	The distance measured between the transducer face and the first rod depicted
Lateral resolution	B	Face (B)	Linear measurement of the echoes produced by row D
Depth calibration	C or E	Face (A) or (B)	The distance measured between the first and the last line in Row E
Registration	E	Face (A), (B), (C), and (D)	Good Poor
Axial resolution	A	Face (A)	5-mm to 1-mm pins spaced at decreasing intervals of 1-mm in Row A
Digital calipers	E	Face (C)	A distance of 10 cm or 100 mm measured on the horizontal pins in Row E, indicating the digital calipers are functioning correctly
Liquid velocity	E	Face (C)	The cursors are positioned at the leading edge echo to the other end leading edge echo, on the horizontal pins in Row E. A 100-mm measurement indicates the liquid medium velocity is correct.

System sensitivity is measured by determining the weakest signal that the system will display.

Axial resolution is determined by placing the transducer on face A and scanning rod group (a). The six rods are separated by 4, 3, 2, and 1 mm, respectively. The system's axial resolution in millimeters is equal to the distance between the two closest yet distinguishable echoes.

Lateral resolution is measured by placing the transducer on face B and scanning rod group (b). The lateral resolution is equal to the distance between the two closest rods in this group.

Dead zone (ring-down) is the region of the sound beam in which imaging cannot be performed; the area closest to the transducer. To determine the extent of the dead zone, the transducer is placed on face A and rod group (d) is scanned. The distance from the transducer to the first rod imaged is equal to the length of the dead zone. The dead zone decreases with higher frequency and the region can be visualized with the application of an acoustic standoff gel. Position is between the transducer and the patient.

Range accuracy (depth accuracy) is measured by placing the transducer on face A and scanning rod group (e). For the system to be operating properly, the echoes should appear at their actual depths and spacings within 1 mm (the rods in this group are 2 cm apart). Checking the range accuracy ensures the accuracy of the internal calipers of the system.

In addition to the AIUM test object, other devices have been designed to measure different parameters of imaging performance. The *beam profiler* is designed to record three-dimensional reflection amplitude information. It consists of a pulser, receiver, transducer, and tank equipped with rods placed at different distances from the transducer.[1]

The transducer is pulsed and scanned across the rods. The fluctuation in amplitude of each reflection returning to the transducer is recorded in an A-mode pattern. The *hydrophone* is one of several devices that measure acoustic output; it consists of a small transducer element mounted on a narrow tube.[1] When used with an oscilloscope, the voltage produced in response to variations in pressure can be displaced and evaluated. The output produced by the hydrophone permits calculation of the period; pulse repetition period, and pulse duration. The hydrophone can also be used as a beam profiler.

Tissue/Cyst Phantom

This test device contains a medium that simulates soft tissue (Fig. 1–25A). Enclosed in the phantom are structures that mimic cysts and solid masses and a series of 0.375-mm targets, in two groups. Each group measures depth and angular resolution. The phantom is used to evaluate the ultrasound system and transducer performance. Sonographic equipment can be evaluated for scattering, attenuation, depth and axial resolution,

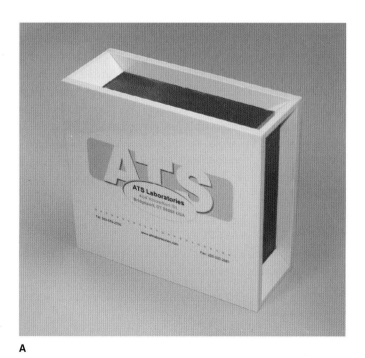

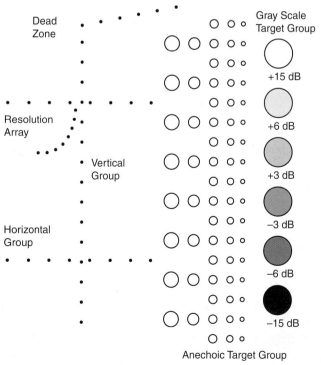

FIGURE 1–25 A. Multipurpose tissue/cyst phantom ATS Model 539 *(Courtesy of ATS Laboratories, Inc, St. Bridgeport, CT. Reprinted with permission.)* **B.** Drawing of anechoic target group ATS Model 539 *(Courtesy of ATS Laboratories Inc, St. Bridgeport, CT. Reprinted with permission.)*

vertical and horizontal distance calibration, and ring down.[5] Cyst-mimicking target structures are positioned vertically to permit a line-of-target group simultaneously (Fig. 1–25B).

Hydrophone

The first hydrophone was invented during World War I[6] and used for underwater echo detection. Hydrophones used in diagnostic ultrasound are used by engineers and physicists to measure or calculate

- Pressure amplitude
- Intensities
- Period and wavelength
- Pulse duration and pulse repetition period

Bioeffects

To date, there is no concrete evidence to support any truly detrimental bioeffects from the application of diagnostic ultrasound to human tissues.[1] The study of possible effects is ongoing, however, and the definitive answer has not been found. It is generally agreed that the potential value of the information obtained from the procedure far outweighs the possibility of deleterious effects. Greater study of the microscopic effects of sound on tissue will have to take place before additional conclusions can be reached. To clarify what is known to date, the potential bioeffects are categorized in two groups: thermal index and mechanical index. These indices are displayed on all new ultrasound monitors as two sets of acronyms, TI and MI (Fig. 1–26).

Thermal index (TI) is the ratio of total acoustic power that is required to cause a rise in temperature increase of 1°C. *TIs are produced primarily by the mechanisms of attenuation.* As a major component of attenuation, absorption by the tissue leads to a rise in tissue temperature. Increased temperatures can cause irreversible damage, depending on the extent of the

exposure. It is generally agreed that *exposure producing a maximum temperature of 1°C can be used without any effects. A rise in temperature of the tissues to 41°C or above is considered dangerous to a fetus. The longer that this temperature is maintained, the greater the potential risk for damage.*[1]

Temperature rise is dependent on tissue type, scanning time, and depth of tissue. Three types of thermal indices exist that correspond to different types of tissue:

TIS. Thermal index in soft tissue

TIB. Thermal index in bone

TIC. Thermal index in cranial bone

Mechanical index (MI) is an estimate of pressure amplitude that occurs in tissue. It is an indicator of potential cavitation.

Cavitation is the result of pressure changes in the medium causing gas bubbles to form; it can produce severe tissue damage. The two types of cavitation are stable cavitation and transient cavitation.

Stable cavitation involves microbubbles already present in tissue that respond by expanding and contracting when pressure is applied. These microbubbles can intercept and absorb a large amount of the acoustic energy. Stable cavitation can result in shear stresses and microstreaming in the surrounding tissues. In stable cavitation, these microbubbles tend to expand and contract without bursting.

Transient cavitation is dependent on the pressure of the ultrasound pulses. The tissue microbubbles expand and collapse violently. This type of cavitation can cause highly localized, violent effects involving enormous pressures, markedly elevated temperatures, shock waves, and mechanical stress. Cavitation may occur with short pulses and during the peak rarefactional pressure of the wave.[7] It has been shown that pulses with peak intensities of >3,300 W/cm^2 can induce cavitation in mammals.[1] Precise determination of when cavitation will occur is not currently within our capabilities. For specific conditions of homogeneous media, it is possible to estimate an index for the cavitation threshold. In transient cavitation, these microbubbles tend to expand and contract and burst. The collapse of the microbubbles causes a localized temperature elevation, which can reach a very high temperature.[7]

ALARA

ALARA (*as low as reasonably achievable*) is a principle recommended to minimize patient ultrasound exposure:

- Use a high receiver gain setting and a lower power output setting
- Avoid using high TI and MI values
- Minimize scanning time
- Use a higher frequency transducer when possible
- Use a focused transducer

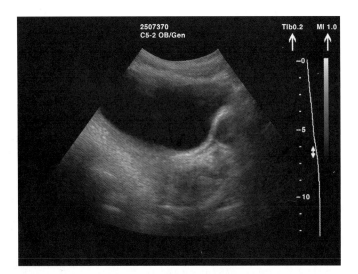

FIGURE 1–26. These indexes are displayed on all new ultrasound monitor as two sets of acronym TI and MI (white arrows).

- Avoid temperature elevation
- Avoid using spectral Doppler on early embryo when possible

The following guidelines are adapted from an official statement by the AIUM: *Bioeffects Considerations for the Safety of Diagnostic Ultrasound*. Bethesda, MD, American Institutes of Ultrasound Medicine, 1988. The reader is urged to read the full AIUM text.

Intensity. There are no independently confirmed significant biological effects in mammalian tissues exposed in vivo with unfocused transducers with intensities below 100 mW/cm^2 and below 1 W/cm^2 for focused transducers.

Exposure. Exposure times can be >1 s and <500 s for an unfocused transducer; and <50 s/pulse for a focused transducer. No significant bioeffects have been observed even at higher intensities than noted above (as long as the intensity × time product is <50 J/cm^2).

Thermal. A maximum temperature rise of 1°C is acceptable, but an increase in the *in situ* temperature to 41°C or greater is hazardous to fetuses.

Cavitation. Can result if pressure peaks are greater than 3,300 W/cm^2. However, it is not possible to specify a threshold at which cavitation will occur.

Randomized studies are the best method for assessing potential effects. *There are no independent confirmed biologic effects on patients or operators.*[1]

PATIENT CARE AND SAFETY

In order to identify and promote strategies to improve patient care and safety, hospital and health care schools are implementing training for health care workers in an effort to reduce the amount of medical errors. The national board in ultrasound now includes patient care and safety in the examination content outline.

Common causes for medical errors in ultrasound include the following:

- Wrong patient
- Wrong site
- Wrong procedure
- Missed diagnoses
- Missed pathology

In order to help in the reduction of scanning the wrong patient, the sonographer should first identify that the correct patient is present and then introduce him or herself to the patient with the employment ID visible to the patient.

Time Out: Immediately before Starting the Procedure with the Patient Present

- Check for the correct patient with name, date of birth and medical record number

- Check if clinical history corresponds to the requested examination
- Check if the examination requested is for the patient present
- Check for latex allergy

POST-PROCEDURE SAFETY CHECK

- Prior to the image being released to the physician or PACS, make sure it can be used for interpretation.
- Confirm that the side markers on the post-procedure images are correct.
- Check again to confirm that the images correspond to the correct patient.

INFORMED CONSENT

Informed consent is a written or verbal consent to undergo a medical or surgical treatment. The consent should include the following:

- What the procedure involves
- The benefits or risks of the procedure
- The right to refuse treatment
- Alternatives
- Witness to the consent
- Certified language line, for non-English patient

Patient can revoke consent at any time.[8]

UNIVERSAL PRECAUTIONS

Universal precautions are a set of precautions designed to prevent HIV, hepatitis B virus, and other blood-borne pathogens when providing health care. These precautions involve the utilization of protective barriers such as gloves, gowns, and masks. The following are applicable to universal precautions:

- Vaginal secretions
- Semen
- Amniotic fluid
- Cerebrospinal fluid
- Pleural fluid
- Peritoneal fluid

Feces, sweat, urine, and sputum do not apply to the universal precautions. The Centers for Disease Control and Prevention (CDC) recommends hand washing before and after procedures to reduce the spread of microorganisms. Hand washing should be done for at least 15–20 seconds with water and soap. This should be done even if gloves will be worn during a procedure.[8]

DISINFECTION OF THE TRANSVAGINAL TRANSDUCER

Transvaginal transducers are reusable instruments. Cross-contamination with reusable medical devices is possible if a precautionary method is not employed. The current methods used to prevent transmission of infection with transvaginal transducers include the use of

1. Cold chemical disinfectants
2. Disposable probe covers

Both methods are required to prevent cross-infection from the transducer because although the probe is covered, a microscopic tear in the cover could expose the transducer to bacteria or viruses from the vaginal mucosa. The piezoelectric crystal of the transducer is heat sensitive. Therefore, steam autoclaves should not be used because excessive heat could depolarize the transducer.[9]

DOPPLER COLOR-FLOW IMAGING INSTRUMENTATION

Color-flow imaging arrived on the medical scene in answer to a basic medical need: an ability to look at cardiovascular blood flow noninvasively. The technology emerged from the development of multigate Doppler systems, that first appeared in 1975.[10] Although these systems used color Doppler only inside an M-mode display, they established both the multigate approach and the use of color to encode motion. In 1983, the first real-time echocardiography color-flow system became commercially available.[11] The first commercial color-flow vascular imaging device followed in 1986. Since then, nearly all ultrasound manufacturers have added color-flow imaging capabilities to their product lines.

Because the ultrasound community had no terminology standards for displaying color-coded information, color-flow imaging (CFI) has acquired several alternate names including color Doppler imaging (CDI), color-flow Doppler, and angiodynography. In fact, CFI includes both Doppler and non-Doppler depictions of flow in color such as color velocity imaging (CVI).[12] Based on the number of instruments in use, however, Doppler-based CFI (DCFI) is the most common technology sonographers will see. In addition, CVI is not currently being produced or marketed. As a consequence, this chapter focuses only on DCFI instrumentation and how it fits into the major applications of imaging.

The current applications of DCFI are extensive and increasing vigorously. Basic and clinical research is extending the usefulness of this imaging modality. In addition, within the research departments of many ultrasound companies, new technologies are shaping the speed and capabilities of DCFI. As in other parts of ultrasound, understanding the instrumentation can go a long way toward understanding how to conduct clinical examinations and read the images.

The Essential Doppler Color-Flow Image

The primary feature of the color-flow image is its simultaneous depiction of stationary soft tissues in gray scale and moving soft tissues in color. For the most part, the moving soft tissue we are interested in is blood within the cardiovascular system. The technology, however, can be configured to provide a color depiction of myocardial motion as well as flowing blood.[13] Despite this special application, the gray scale and color relationship opens the use of DCFI for two major applications: echocardiography and vascular imaging. However, as you will discover, any moving echo source within and sometimes outside the scanning field can produce color in the image. Setting up the system correctly, however, can limit the color-flow information to moving blood.[11]

DCFI is the son of duplex imaging and Doppler multigate analysis. Duplex imaging is older than multigate analysis and has several different forms. It includes the combination of either a continuous-wave or a single-point (pulsed-Doppler) spectrum with an image.[14] The image can be an M-mode trace, a real-time B-mode image, or, almost paradoxically, a color-flow image. (The paradox is not real, however. DCFI and a single-point spectrum look at the same events, but they do so from different points of view. As a result, they can be profitably combined into a common presentation.)

Multigate analysis is a method of collecting Doppler data from several adjacent spatial locations. A multigate system analyzes each of several sampling sites for flow events using Doppler signal processing. The limitation on this form of signal processing is time. Multigate systems look at each of several sites serially; thus, as the number of sites increases, the time required to make a composite image also increases.[12] As a result, as the time needed to form a composite image frame *increases*, the corresponding image frame rate *decreases*.

Current machines use a number of modern signal-handling techniques to keep the image frame rates as high as possible. The essential color-flow presentation provides the following pieces of information directly from the image: (1) the existence of flow, (2) its location in the image, (3) its location in the anatomy, (4) its direction relative to the transducer, (5) its direction relative to the anatomy, and (6) its pattern over space and time.

Because the color image shows flow over space and time, we can use the image to locate specific characteristics within the flow pattern. For example, the higher-velocity flow segments (major streamlines and poststenotic jets) are visible within the heart and larger vessels. In addition, the image clearly shows the difference between a complex flow pattern resulting from anatomy and the poststenotic flow pattern (turbulence) associated with disease.[15]

The ability to clearly show the patterns of flow depends on advanced technologies focused on asking the right technological

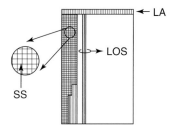

FIGURE 1–27. Sampling the scanning beams. LA is the linear array, SS is a sample site, and LOS represents the scanning lines sight. Each sampling site represents a position in the digital scan converter.

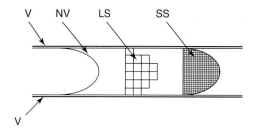

FIGURE 1–28. Flow image resolution and sampling intervals. V is the vessel wall, NV is the normal velocity profile, LS is the profile with large-interval sampling, and SS is the profile with small-interval sampling. The smaller the sampling, the better the depiction of flow.

questions. Everything comes together at the image, where we begin the discussion.

Doppler Color-Flow Imaging Technology
Producing an Image

DCFI begins by making a multigate image for both the gray-scale and the Doppler segments of the image. By design, the system divides each beam location in the scanning field into a series of small sampling sites, each of which translates into a specific location in the digital scan converter image.[16] Fig. 1–27 is an example of this division using a linear array. The digital scan converter design in the ultrasound machine determines the size and spacing of these sampling sites.[17]

The sampling intervals used to make the gray-scale and color segments of the DCFI depend on the image. For example, a gray-scale image requires sampling intervals no greater than one wavelength.[16] The gray-scale image rests on detection of the echo signal amplitudes, that the signal processing converts into gray-scale intensities. Sampling intervals that are greater than one wavelength simply do not display tissue texturing well enough to support good gray-scale imaging. To show the differences among tissues, a gray-scale image must show the differences among the various tissue textures.

Sampling for Doppler information has a different set of requirements. At the outset, Doppler signal processing requires more time than amplitude detection. For example, a single pulse–listen cycle can provide the information for a single gray-scale image line of sight (LOS). Doppler, however, requires anywhere from 4 to 100 pulse–listen cycles to build a single Doppler image LOS.[12] The increased time is needed to detect the phase shifts in the echo signals that encode the reflector motion. This extended sitting on a single LOS to detect motion is called *dwell time* or *ensemble time*. Practicalities will limit the dwell time on each LOS to a range of 4–32 cycles. As a result, the sampling intervals are usually larger and fewer than in conventional gray-scale imaging. The smallest Doppler sampling sites are at one-wavelength intervals. Often, to shorten the time to form one frame of the combined gray-scale and color real-time image, the Doppler sampling sites may be several wavelengths long. There is a limit here, too. Sampling sites larger than 1 mm provide a poor depiction of

vascular flow patterns. Fig. 1–28 shows how the sampling intervals can affect the depiction of flow patterns in a vessel.

The heart poses a different set of requirements. Because we do not need to see the same detailed flow patterns required in vascular imaging, color-flow echocardiography can use larger sampling intervals.[11] By reducing the time required to make the colored portion of an image, the combined frame rates can be accelerated enough to depict events in both adult and pediatric hearts. Even these techniques, however, may be inadequate. In these cases, the system can still obtain higher frame rates by limiting the flow interrogation to a smaller number of Doppler LOSs in the image. Limiting Doppler signal processing to a specific region of interest (ROI), or window, can help restore the frame rates to usable levels. Despite a limited ROI, the interrogation window can be moved to permit a look at flow over the entire FOV. At each Doppler sampling site, the DCFI system looks at the returning echo signals for changes in phase and the presence of Doppler shift frequencies.

Changes in phase. Changes in the phase or timing of an echo signal not only show that an echo source is moving but also reveal its direction of motion.[18] The ultimate reference for this motion is the transducer. As in duplex Doppler imaging, movement toward the transducer is called *forward* motion; movement away from the transducer is called *reverse* motion. The color-flow system encodes this directional information into color, typically red and blue. Fig. 1–29 shows this color

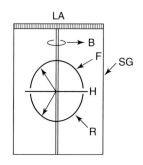

FIGURE 1–29. Color assignment to the direction of flow. LA is the linear array, B is the ultrasound beam, SG is the scanning field geometry, F is forward motion, R is a reverse motion, and H is a horizontal line. Flow vectors pointing on the F arc are all one color. Flow vectors pointing on the R arc are the opposite color. Anatomy further restricts blood flow to the geometry of the vessel.

assignment geometry for a linear array. These same rules apply to every ultrasound beam in either a sector or a linear scanning field. Because no universally accepted standard exists for assigning color to direction, most systems have a flow-reverse button that switches the color assignment. This often permits setting arterial flow in red and venous flow in blue. Obviously, in complex vascular patterns, this rule may not hold throughout the image. In this case, a pulsatile flow pattern usually identifies an artery from a vein with lower velocities and a respiratory dependence.

Doppler shift frequencies. Each Doppler image sampling site is a range gate that represents the position of the Doppler sample volume. If the sample volume is within a blood flow pattern, a spectrum of Doppler shift frequencies composes the resulting signal. The system, however, cannot display a frequency spectrum within each colored pixel that combines to form a color-flow image. Instead, most color-flow systems determine a representative frequency and encode this frequency into a color quality.[19]

All current color-flow systems use some form of average frequency to represent the Doppler shift frequency within a sample site. The average frequency is a good choice because it is less sensitive to noise than most alternatives. In some systems, the average frequency comes from an online spectral analysis.[19] In others, autocorrelation and signal-averaging techniques produce the average value. Regardless of the type of system, the signal processing encodes the average frequency into one of several color qualities.

Color has three inherent qualities we can use to encode information: hue, brightness, and saturation. The hue of a color represents its basic frequency or wavelength. For example, red and blue are different hues, and so are yellow and green. Some systems encode the Doppler shift frequency information into hue, presenting a variety of different colors, with each color representing a different average Doppler shift frequency.[11]

The brightness of a color represents its energy content. For example, increasing or decreasing the illumination on a color patch changes the brightness of the perceived color without changing its hue. Most DCFI designs use changes in hue rather than color brightness to encode the average frequency. At the same time, the brightness of the color may be modulated to smooth the color edges.

Saturation expresses the purity of a color. A color with 100% saturation is considered completely pure. For example, a pure or 100%-saturated red would appear on the display screen as a deep red. Changing the saturation means adding some white light to the color, thus, a less saturated red appears whiter. Many systems allow the user to choose color assignment rules including the use of color saturation to encode the average frequency information.[20] These color assignments make jets and major streamlines appear whiter than the surrounding color.

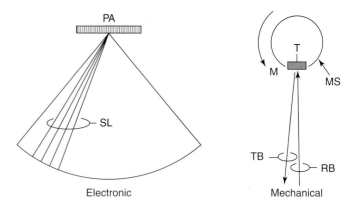

FIGURE 1–30. Electronic and mechanically steered beams. PA is a phased array, SL represents the scanning lines, MS is the mechanical scanning head, T is a transducer, M is the direction of motion, TB is the position of the transmit beam, and RB is the position of the receive beam. Electronic steering permits fixed positions for each scan line.

Beam Contributions to Sampling

Forming the ultrasound beam and the beam's subsequent motion has a strong role to play in making a color-flow image. Most DCFI systems use a phased-array, linear array, or curved linear array transducer. Only a few systems use a mechanical scan. This preference for electronic scanning is not merely a matter of chance.

The Doppler effect cannot distinguish between a moving ultrasound beam and a stationary echo source or a stable ultrasound beam with a moving echo source. Without special techniques to control the pattern of beam motion, a mechanical scanner has a steadily moving beam (see Fig. 1–30). This continuous motion means that the Doppler signal processing always sees some movement between the tissue echo sources and the ultrasound beam. This movement produces a set of low Doppler shift frequencies that can hide low blood flow velocities.

One clear advantage of the electronic systems is the formation of a stationary ultrasound beam (Fig. 1–30) in each LOS position. In this scanning pattern, a stationary beam appears at each LOS in the scanning plane.[21] Electronic beam forming and steering have a price as well, however. Every transducer, regardless of size, acts as if it were a hole or aperture in space. In this model (Fig. 1–31), the ultrasound comes from a point source behind the aperture. As the waves travel through the aperture, the waves and aperture interact to produce a diffraction pattern. Most of the energy comes through the aperture and forms a large central lobe of energy. The remaining energy diffracts into a set of *side lobes* that can broaden and smear the beam.

An array of transducer elements (whether linear or curved) produces a similar set of side lobes. Because these lobes come from the summation of side lobes from each transducer element as if from a diffraction grating, they are called *grating lobes*. When the electronic control positions the beam perpendicular to the array, the grating lobes can be relatively small. By using several different cancellation techniques, however, engineers can

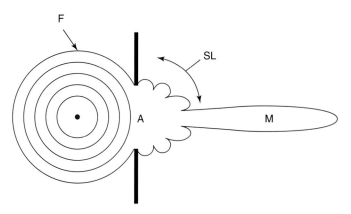

FIGURE 1-31. The transducer is a diffracting apertures. F is the virtual ultrasound field behind the aperture, A is the aperture, SL represents the diffraction side lobes, and M is the main beam. Each transducer including individual array elements acts as a diffracting hole in space.

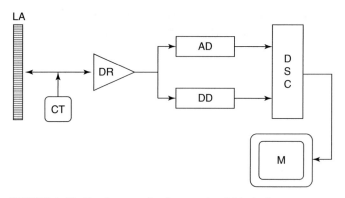

FIGURE 1-33. Synchronous signal processing. LA is the linear array, CT is a coherent transmitter, DR is a receiver, AD represents amplitude detection, DD represents Doppler detection, DSC is the digital scan converter, and M is the color monitor. Synchronous signal processing uses the same signal to make the gray-scale and Doppler images.

suppress the grating lobes as much as −60 dB (1/1,000th) or more below the main lobe of energy. When the steered beam points off to the side, however, the number and size of the grating lobes increase (Fig. 1–32).[11] Again, the result can be a smearing of the ultrasound beam and a loss of lateral resolution, a loss that can affect the accurate placement of color within an image.

Signal Processing

Once the echo signals are inside the machine, they face a diverse set of analyses. When and how these analyses occur will determine the character of the final color-flow image.

Within the Doppler-based machines, signal processing can take on two different forms. First, a system can use the same signal to make both the gray-scale and Doppler images. This is *synchronous* signal processing.[12] Alternatively, the system can use different signals to form the gray-scale and Doppler images. This is *asynchronous* signal processing.[12] Nearly all DCFI machines designed for vascular applications are now asynchronous, dividing the data collection between gray-scale imaging and color mapping to form each composite image frame.

Synchronous signal processing. Fig. 1–33 shows the basic organization of a synchronous signal-processing system. Replacing the linear array with a single transducer and replacing the B-mode image with an M-mode trace produced the earliest synchronous system: the M/Q system.[22,23] This system used the same signals to produce both an M-mode display and a point spectrum. All synchronous systems use the same transducer, coherent transmitter, and receiver because they extract different information from a common signal. After reception, the signals divide into two pathways: one for the gray-scale image, the other for the Doppler image. The system uses a priority function to place color properly within the gray-scale image.

To form image frames at speeds useful to echocardiography, most echocardiography color-flow systems use synchronous signal processing.[11] These systems use a phased array to form and steer the ultrasound beams (Fig. 1–34). Although beam steering spreads the beam because of grating lobes and side lobes, the effects of these beam distortions do not detract seriously from echocardiography images.

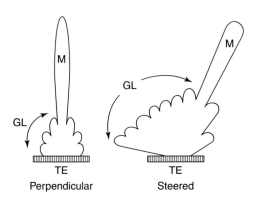

FIGURE 1-32. Grating lobe formation with beam steering. TE represents transducer elements, GL represents grating lobes, and M is the main lobe. Steering increases the formation of side lobes, smearing the ultrasound beam.

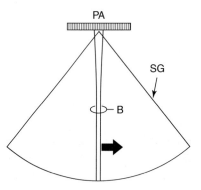

FIGURE 1-34. Formation of a phased array beam and steering. PA represents the phased array elements, B is the beam, SG is the scanning field geometry, and the arrow shows beam movement. The phased array has a limited aperture size that limits the focal point size and focal range. Thus, focusing is poorest at the edges of the sector.

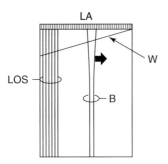

FIGURE 1–35. Scanning field organization in synchronous signal processing. LA is the linear array, LOS represents the scanning lines-of-sight, W is a wedge, B is the beam, and the arrow shows beam motion. The wedge provides a Doppler angle between the moving blood and the ultrasound beam.

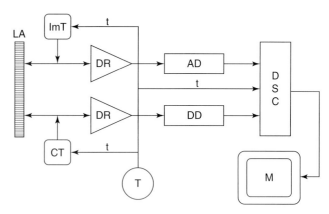

FIGURE 1–36. Asynchronous signal processing. LA is the linear array, ImT is the image transmitter, CT is the coherent transmitter, DR is a receiver, AD represents amplitude detection, DD represents Doppler detection, DSC is the digital scan converter, M is the color monitor, T is a common timer with control signals (t), and DR is the Doppler receiver. Asynchronous signal processing uses different signals for the gray-scale and color portions of the image.

In synchronous vascular imaging, the system shapes and focuses an ultrasound beam along an LOS perpendicular to the linear array. Fig. 1–35 shows the organization of such a system. The beam scans down the array to form a rectangular scanning field. Zone focusing on "transmit" and dynamic focusing on "receive" provide a narrow beam over the FOV.[24]

The system tests each sample site along each beam for flow. If flow exists, the corresponding image pixel becomes colored; if not, the pixel becomes gray scale. In this manner, the processing builds the image on a sample-site by sample-site basis.

Synchronous DCFI for the vascular system faces a Doppler angle requirement. Most of the vessels in the neck, arms, and legs are parallel, or nearly so, to the skin surface, which places an unsteered beam from a linear array 90° to the flow pattern. In this situation, the system can either beam-steer or use a wedge standoff to provide the necessary Doppler angle. A wedge standoff is a water-filled plastic device that slips on and off a linear array as needed. Despite the apparent simplicity of a wedge, most synchronous vascular imaging systems use electronic beam steering to provide the Doppler angle.

The physical simplicity of the wedge can be deceiving. For example, design engineers must consider not only beam formation, but also how the wedge may change the beam because of refraction, scattering from air bubbles, bacterial growth inside the wedge, and antiseptic treatments of the wedge that do not destroy the plastics that compose the wedge.

Asynchronous signal processing. Asynchronous signal-processing systems use different ultrasound beams and signals to create the composite gray-scale and Doppler images.

Asynchronous systems use separate transmitters for the gray-scale and Doppler portions of the image. Only the transducer array and a central coordinating timer are common to the separate signal pathways to the scan converter. Fig. 1–36 shows the organization of an asynchronous imaging system.

Most asynchronous systems use beam steering to obtain the Doppler image while keeping the gray-scale image beams perpendicular to the transducer. Fig. 1–37 shows how the two scanning fields overlay. Because the system uses two different transmitters, the Doppler carrier frequency can be different from the imaging frequency. For example, gray-scale imaging might be at 5.0 MHz and Doppler imaging at 3.0 MHz.

The operating cycle interweaves the Doppler and gray-scale beams to produce two separate images. This interweaving reduces the potential frame rates for the system. Because the sample sites for the two fields of view do not coincide, they cannot accumulate into a common memory in a simple manner. Instead, they pass to separate memories and finally overlay one over the other in the digital scan converter.

Because the two scanning fields have different orientations, the color and gray-scale imaging do not have a one-to-one correspondence over the composite image field (Fig. 1–37). Portions of the steered Doppler image are outside the gray-scale field, just as portions of the gray-scale scanning field are outside the Doppler scanning field. One way of keeping the overall image frame rate high is to confine the color signal processing to a small mobile window, or ROI. This technology arrangement is a common practice for all color-flow systems, both vascular and cardiac.

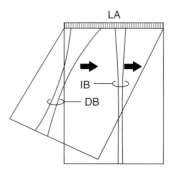

FIGURE 1–37. Scanning organization for asynchronous signal processing. LA is the linear array, DB is the Doppler beam, IB is the gray-scale beam, and the arrows show beam motion. Beam steering provides a Doppler angle for making the Doppler image. The operating Doppler and gray-scale frequencies can differ.

Amplitude signal processing (power Doppler imaging). Doppler signal processing is generally one of deriving the Doppler frequency components within a returning echo signal. Fast Fourier transform (FFT) analysis operates on the composite wave form and produces a range of discrete frequency components. Thus, an FFT provides two properties of these component signals for analysis and portrayal in color: (1) Doppler signal frequencies and (2) Doppler signal amplitudes. DCFI encodes the Doppler shift frequencies into color to show both the direction and the speed of blood flow. An alternative to frequency analysis is to determine the *power spectrum* of the Doppler signal amplitudes using the system directional (in-phase and quadrature) channels. Although this technique may have different trade names, the technology is most often called *amplitude* or *power Doppler* imaging.[15] Importantly, although the name of the technique includes the word *power*, it does not increase the *acoustic power* delivered to the patient. Rather, it is a different method of signal processing using normal signal amplitudes and output power values.

Signal processing for Doppler frequency information offers advantages and disadvantages. At the outset, frequency information shows both the direction and the relative velocity of the blood flow in the image. At the same time, it is very sensitive to noise, the Doppler angle, and is subject to high-frequency aliasing.

Power Doppler, on the other hand, is not as sensitive to system noise as frequency-based Doppler, but it is more sensitive to displaying flow boundaries. In addition, power Doppler is relatively angle independent and is nonaliasing. Because of these last three advantages, power Doppler can better show overall vascularity and better supports three-dimensional depictions of perfusion into organs and masses.[25]

Power Doppler, however, forfeits detailed flow information within the vessels. In addition, it is very sensitive to soft tissue motion and the so-called "flash artifact" produced by this motion. To date, much effort has gone into developing techniques that can suppress the flash artifact and improve power Doppler imaging.

Practical Issues
Cardiac Imaging Requirements
In general, viewing the heart with ultrasound requires intercostal and subcostal imaging with low-frequency ultrasound.[11] Parasternal DCFI naturally places the ultrasound beam approximately 90° to the flow pattern. As a result, apical and subcostal views of the heart are needed to place flow patterns parallel to the ultrasound beams. The phased-array and the short-radius curved linear arrays are the transducers of choice for viewing through these thoracic and abdominal windows. The sector angles range from 30° to 180°.

Because blood is a low attenuator (0.15 dB/cm per MHz), viewing the heart with ultrasound does not require the same sort of front-end design (delay lines and receivers) that vascular imaging requires. In addition, the high frame rates, combined with large fields of view, impose large sampling intervals on the cardiac image, and the scanning uses a sector format. All of these factors combine to make the cardiac color-flow device right for the heart and wrong for the vascular system.

Because the Doppler sampling intervals can be relatively large in echocardiography, detecting a regional turbulence is not always easy. To help locate flow disorganization (spectral broadening) for any sampling location, most cardiac systems determine not only the mean frequency at a sample site, but the signal variance as well.[11] In many cardiac devices, color-coding for an increasing variance introduces a green tint to the primary color.

Vascular Imaging Requirements
Vascular DCFI involves all available peripheral vessels, the large, upper thoracic vessels, and the deeper vessels in the abdomen. A linear array typically is used to view the peripheral vessels. This linear scanning field sets the stage for using changes in color to show changes in the direction of flow. In contrast, a sector scan of a linear vessel produces a continuously changing Doppler angle (Fig. 1–38) and, thus, continuously changing color. Instead, sector-scanning transducers, such as the phased-array and the curved linear array, are used to view abdominal vasculature. These transducers permit both subcostal and intercostal scanning to visualize the deeper abdominal vessels that may be within the rib cage.

The sector fields, however, make reading the images more difficult. Identifying arteries and veins requires knowing both the direction and the pulsatility of the flow. Large FOVs and longer processing times for the color-flow image often make the effective frame rates too low to permit an easy determination of pulsatility. Using a single-point spectrum and a color-flow image together as well as decreasing the ROI can yield information about vascular pulsatility.

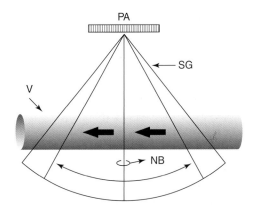

FIGURE 1–38. Vascular imaging with a sector scanning field. PA is a phased array, SG is the scanning field geometry, V is the vessel, and NB is the beam perpendicular to flow in the vessel (*arrows*). Because each beam position has a different Doppler angle, the colors in the image change rapidly.

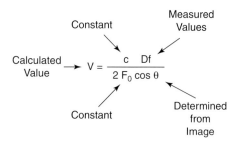

FIGURE 1–39. Calculation of velocity with the Doppler equation. V is the velocity, c is the ultrasound propagation velocity, Df is the Doppler shift frequency, F_o is the carrier frequency, and θ is the Doppler angle. Doppler machines measure frequency and calculate "true" velocity, V, based on an estimated Doppler angle entered by the sonographer.

Displays of Frequency and Velocity

All current color-flow images using Doppler are two-dimensional maps of the Doppler shift frequencies. After all, color flow uses Doppler, too.

Many systems show the color values in velocity (centimeters per second) rather than frequency (hertz). This sort of display suggests a direct measurement of velocity in color. As in all color-flow Doppler determinations of velocity, the values represent a solution to the Doppler equation (Fig. 1–39). In this display, however, the velocity is not the absolute velocity of the red cells. Instead, the image values represent the *closing velocity* along the ultrasound beam. Absolute velocities would require a continuous correction of all angles to the flow patterns throughout the image. Fig. 1–40 shows this closing velocity relationship.

Color-Flow Imaging Artifacts

Because DCFI incorporates both B-mode imaging and Doppler signal processing, it is subject to the same artifacts that affect ultrasound in general. Three primary sources of confusion in DCFI are (1) range ambiguity artifacts, (2) Doppler high-frequency aliasing, and (3) soft tissue vibrations.

Fig. 1–41 shows the organization of events required to obtain a range ambiguity artifact. The high power and faster frame rates typical of DCFI offer ample opportunities for this artifact.[26] In DCFI, the artifact appears as diffuse, nonpulsatile colors, suggesting flow that may not actually exist where it appears in the image.

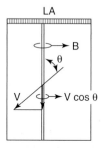

FIGURE 1–40. The closing velocity geometry. LA is the linear array, B is the ultrasound beam, V is the target velocity, and V cos θ is the closing velocity. Closing velocity is the component of motion along the ultrasound beam.

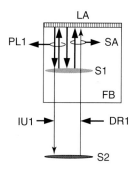

FIGURE 1–41. The range ambiguity artifact. LA is the linear array, PL1 is the initial pulse–listen cycle, IU1 is the incident ultrasound from PL1, S1 is a phantom echo source inside the field boundary (FB), S2 is a real echo source outside the scanning field, DR1 is the deeper returning echo, and SA represents the simultaneous arrival of the two echo signals. Range ambiguity occurs when echo sources outside the scanning field appear in the image.

In a pulsed Doppler system, the Doppler shift frequencies are being sampled at the pulse repetition frequency (PRF) of the system. High-frequency *aliasing* occurs when the Doppler shift frequency exceeds the system PRF sampling frequency. This aliasing limit is known as the *Nyquist limit*, which is PRF/2. When aliasing occurs in CFI, both the colors and the single-point Doppler spectra "wrap around" the display format (i.e., the high frequencies in one direction appear as lower frequencies in the opposite direction) and confuse the appearance of flow. To remove aliasing, a sonographer must either increase the PRF (shorten the FOV) or decrease the Doppler shift frequency associated with the highest velocity.[22] You can decrease the Doppler shift frequency by either decreasing the Doppler carrier frequency or moving the transducer to place the Doppler angle closer to 90°. Because of the increasingly pronounced error production with Doppler angles above 70°, however, it is better to choose a lower carrier frequency than to increase the Doppler angle above 70° (e.g., at 75°, the velocity calculation has an inherent error rate of 6.5%/degree; thus, an error of ±3° in estimating the true Doppler angle creates a velocity calculation error of ±19.5%).[6]

A not uncommon source of DCFI confusion is the mechanical vibration of soft tissues. For example, tissue vibrations can occur if a patient talks or if the blood flow happens to be producing a *bruit*, or noise.[27] These tissue vibrations can fill an image of an artery or vein with lots of color outside the vessel walls. The low-frequency pulse from the heart also can fill an abdominal image with a burst of color known as a *flash artifact*, which can cause problems for power Doppler as noted earlier.[25]

Applying the Technology to Real Images

Using these ideas of how the various color-flow systems work, we are now in a position to examine some examples of DCFI. They range from the depiction of flow within an M-mode recording to high-resolution imaging of the vascular system.

Fig. 1–42 shows the combination of an M-mode recording with DCFI. All motion in this image is referenced to the transducer as a closing velocity; that is, only as motion directly

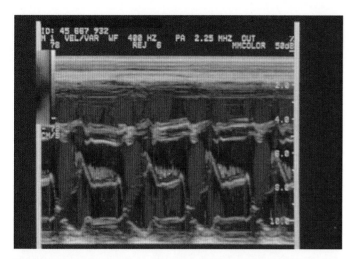

FIGURE 1–42. Color flow imaging of a mitral valve. The M-mode tracing views the mitral valve from the upper portion of the cardiac window, aimed down toward the mitral valve. Red is flow toward the transducer; blue is flow away. Closing velocity values (aliasing limits) appear on the color bar. The red flow between the interventricular septum and closed mitral valve is ejection through the left ventricular outflow tract. During ventricular filling, the blue–green flow along the anterior mitral valve leaflet is reversed, turbulent flow produced by an aortic regurgitation. Depth markers are at the right of the image, and an EKG trace provides timing at the bottom of the image. *(Reproduced with permission from Philips Healthcare.)*

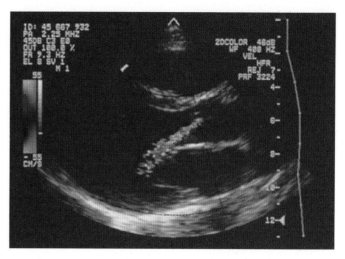

FIGURE 1–43. Cardiac color flow imaging. This parasternal long-axis view of the heart shows (from the top down) the right ventricle, the interventricular septum, and the left ventricle containing the mitral valve leaflets. Red is flow toward the transducer; blue is away. Closing velocity values (aliasing limits) appear on the color bar. The color-imaging window (blue boundary) shows a nonaxial blue–green turbulent jet (regurgitation) originating at the aortic root. Without color, the nonaxial quality of the jet could not be easily determined. *(Reproduced with permission from Philips Healthcare.)*

toward or away from the transducer. In this example, the Doppler frequencies have been calculated into closing velocities, which *do not* necessarily represent the true velocities of the cardiac blood flow. This system encodes the presence of spectral broadening by adding green to the primary directional colors. The green color flow in diastole demonstrates: (1) the presence of aortic regurgitation and (2) the ensuing turbulence as the left ventricle fills through an open mitral valve.

Determining the true flow pattern is easier with a two-dimensional image of the heart. Fig. 1–43 provides a clear view of the heart in long axis, with the color flow confined to the heart's chambers. Again, the Doppler frequency map is calculated into closing velocity values. This image shows a nonaxial regurgitating jet extending from the aortic root into the left ventricle. In this case, the color-flow images show not only the existence of the jet but also its nonaxial geometry.

Fig. 1–44 (normal carotid artery flow) depicts a normal carotid artery with an early synchronous DCFI system. The Doppler angle comes from a wedge standoff at the top of the image. The sampling rate in this image is at one-wavelength intervals (0.2 mm at 7.5 MHz) for both the gray-scale image and the color portion of the image. The internal flow pattern of the vessel shows a normal flow separation and reversal in the carotid bulb. The flow direction is from image right to left, away from the transducer, causing the vessel to appear red. The higher Doppler shift frequencies appear whiter, depicting the higher-velocity portions of the flow.

The beam steering that is typical of asynchronous signal processing changes the organization of a similar image of a normal carotid artery. This system depicts different average Doppler shift frequencies in different color hues. As in Fig. 1–45, however, the image clearly shows the flow separation and reversal (blue portion in the red vessel) that is typical of a normal carotid bulb. The beam steering in this image limits simultaneously showing flow and soft tissue anatomy throughout the image. Moving the color-flow processing window and changing the scanning position, however, permits a full interrogation of most vessels.

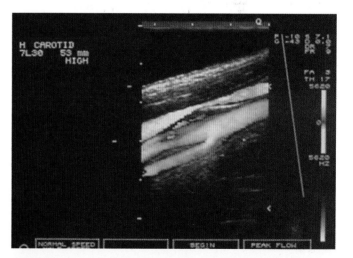

FIGURE 1–44. Color flow imaging of a carotid artery. The long-axis view of a normal carotid artery bifurcation shows the common carotid artery branching into internal (upper branch) and external (lower branch) carotid arteries. Flow is right to left, away from the transducer (red bar at the top of the image). The vessel above the carotid (blue) is the jugular vein. Within the carotid bulb is a normal flow separation and reversal (blue). Because higher Doppler shift frequencies are whiter, the major streamlines appear whiter in the image. The required Doppler angle comes from the wedge standoff (black triangular space at the top of the image). The peripheral dots are 1-cm markers, and the aliasing frequencies appear at the top and bottom of the color bar. *(Reproduced with permission from Siemens Healthcare, Malvern, PA.)*

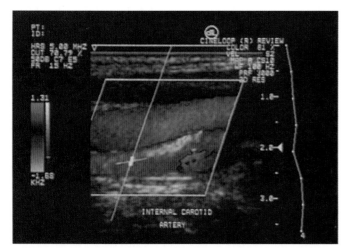

FIGURE 1–45. Color flow imaging of a carotid artery. The image shows the internal carotid artery and bulb. Flow in the artery (red) is from right to left, with a flow separation and reversal in blue. The major, nonaxial streamline (yellow) in the bulb is along the anterior wall. A small segment of aliasing (green) appears in the streamline. The more anterior blue vessel is the jugular vein. The Doppler angle in this image comes from beam steering. The white parallelogram shows the steering angle and the boundary for color signal processing in the image. The aliasing frequency limits appear on the color bar, with depth markers and a transmit focal point position on the right side of the image. *(Reproduced with permission from Philips Healthcare.)*

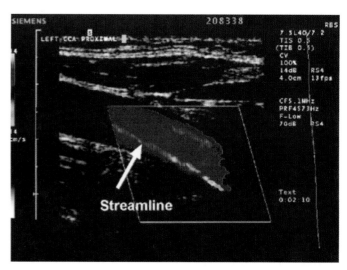

FIGURE 1–47. Color flow imaging of a common carotid artery. This artery has a curve that sends a major streamline (arrow) across the vessel lumen. Flow is from right to left toward the transducer. The upper red color bar represents motion toward the transducer. The flow deviation is about 15° steeper than the vessel wall. The vertical markers on the image left indicate 0.5-cm intervals. The aliasing closing velocities appear at the top and bottom of the color bar. *(Reproduced with permission from Siemens Healthcare, Malvern, PA.)*

Any highly vascular tissue or structure is a good candidate for DCFI when trying to separate out ambiguous anatomy. Flow within major fetal vessels appears in Fig. 1–46. This image is formed with a convex linear array, producing a sector image pattern. Because of the complexity of the vascular anatomy and the changing angle between the vessels and the beams, the immediate color encoding does not always indicate arteries and

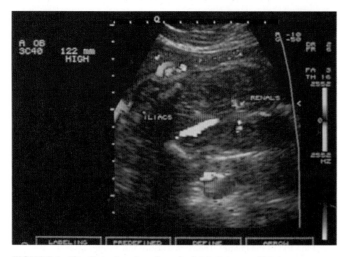

FIGURE 1–46. Color flow imaging of a fetal abdomen. This image shows the fetal aorta with renal and iliac branches. Flow away from the transducer is blue; flow toward the transducer is red. The peripheral dots are 1-cm markers, and the aliasing frequencies appear at the top and bottom of the color bar. A convex curved array forms a sector scanning field. *(Reproduced with permission from Siemens Healthcare, Malvern, PA.)*

veins. Instead, the vessel pulsatility and its position relative to internal anatomical landmarks tell the story. If the system frame rate is too slow, however, a single-point, pulsed Doppler spectrum will be the most reliable means of determining the pulsatile flow patterns of arteries and the steadier flow patterns of veins.

When wall disease in a vessel or simply vascular anatomy disturbs the flow pattern, a single-point spectrum cannot show the source or character of the disturbance. High-resolution DCFI, however, as shown in Fig. 1–47, clearly depicts not only curving vessel walls, but also a major streamline moving across the vessel in response to flow inertia.

In the presence of stenosis, the flow within the narrowing increases velocity. The narrowing also often appears in the image as a physical narrowing of the color distribution as the spatial signal processing maps a reduced lumen. Fig. 1–48 shows these two results, the narrowing of the color distribution and the acceleration (central green portion of the color in the lumen poststenosis) due to a carotid artery stenosis.

When frame rates are high enough and the Doppler sampling is fine enough, we begin to see some of the subtler flow physiology. For example, each pulse in the vascular system is a mechanical wave that travels down the vessels to be reflected at changes in hydraulic impedance. Fig. 1–49 shows the intersection of two traveling pulse waves: The red portion is the incident wave, and the blue portion is the reflected wave. The color-flow image and the Doppler spectrum show the connection between the triphasic flow pattern of this high-resistance vessel and the passing of forward and reversed pulse waves within the artery.

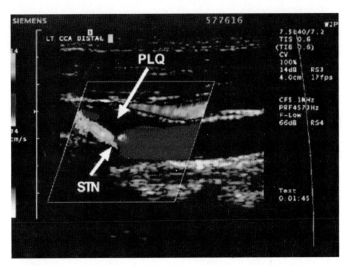

FIGURE 1–48. Color flow imaging of a carotid artery stenosis. This artery has a significant stenosis that is narrowing the flow channel (narrow color distribution), causing a poststenotic turbulence (mixed colors). Prestenotic flow is right to left, away from the transducer and colored red. The poststenotic flow is toward the transducer and colored blue. The markers on the image left are 0.5-cm intervals. The aliasing closing velocities appear at the top and bottom of the color bar. PLQ is a soft, anechoic plaque. STN is the narrowest region of the stenosis. *(Reproduced with permission from Siemens Healthcare, Malvern, PA.)*

Although power Doppler can fill an image with color as in Fig. 1–50, the processing loses the information about flow direction. As a consequence, the carotid arteries and the jugular vein have the same color. As the sampling approaches the vessel walls, the signals are coded for a decrease in signal brightness.

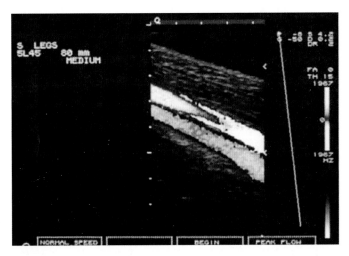

FIGURE 1–49. Color flow imaging of a superficial femoral artery and vein. These normal vessels show typical flow patterns during the cardiac and respiratory cycle. Arterial flow from left to right, and a distally reflected pulse wave (blue) arriving to cross the incident pulse wave (red). The superficial femoral vein (blue posterior vessel) is flowing right to left as flow and color fill the vein's residual lumen. This color flow image clearly shows the reversal of flow in a triphasic or biphasic flow pattern comes from a traveling pulse wave. The peripheral dots are 1-cm markers, and the aliasing frequencies appear at the top and bottom of the color bar. The black space at the top of the image is a wedge standoff. *(Reproduced with permission from Siemens Healthcare, Malvern, PA.)*

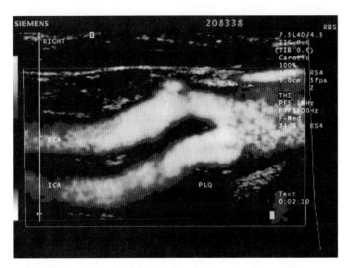

FIGURE 1–50. Power Doppler depiction of flow in a carotid artery. ECA is the external carotid; ICA is the internal carotid, PLQ is an anechoic plaque narrowing the carotid bulb. The depth marker on the image left shows 0.5-cm intervals. The upper right corner of the ROI includes a portion of the jugular vein flowing in opposite direction to the carotid arteries with the same color as the arteries. *(Reproduced with permission from Siemens Healthcare, Malvern, PA.)*

SUMMARY

DCFI is a combination of gray-scale anatomical information and a colored depiction of flow events. It is an integrated image of form and function, anatomy, and physiology. The color portion of the image is not an image of blood, however; it is an image of motion. Using power Doppler, the color can depict the presence of flow with great sensitivity, but without some flow details.

Within each Doppler color-flow system, the amplitudes of echo signals become gray-scale intensities, while the frequency content of the signals becomes color. The echo signals for both may be the same or different, even in carrier frequency. This imaging modality depends on the sophistication and speed of contemporary digital signal processing. It also is an imaging modality that is changing and will continue to change the fields of ultrasound and medicine.

References

1. Kremkau FW. *Diagnostic Ultrasound: Principles, Instruments.* 7th ed. St. Louis: Saunders Elsevier; 2006.

2. Edelman SK. *Understanding Ultrasound Physics.* 3rd ed. Woodlands, TX: EPS Inc.; 2005.

3. Pinkney N. *A Review of the Concepts of Ultrasound Physics and Instrumentation.* 4th ed. Philadelphia: Sonior; 1983.

4. Bushong SC, Archer RB. *Diagnostic Ultrasound: Physics, Biology, and Instrumentation.* St. Louis: Mosby-Year Book; 1991.

5. *Diagnostic Ultrasound: Test Equipment and Accessories.* New York: Nuclear Associates, Catalog U-2; 1991; 2-3.

6. Halpern GP. *A Naval History of World War 1. P343.* The United States Naval Institute; Annapolis, MD: Naval Institute Press; 1994.

7. Miele FR. *Essentials of Ultrasound Physics. The Board Review Book.* Forney, TX; Pegasus Lecturers and Inc. 2008.

8. Craig, M. *Essentials of Sonography and Patient Care*. 2nd ed. St. Louis: Saunders Elsevier; 2006.

9. Odwin C, Fleischer CA, Keepie D. Probe covers and disinfectant for transvaginal transducers. *J Diagnostic Med Sonogr* 1989; 6:130-135.

10. Fish PJ. Multichannel, direction resolving Doppler angiography. *Abstracts of 2nd European Congress of Ultrasonics in Medicine*. 72, 1975.

11. Omoto R, ed. *Color Atlas of Real-Time Two-Dimensional Doppler Echocardiography*. Tokyo: Shindan-ToChiryo; 1984.

12. Powis RL. Color flow imaging: understanding its science and technology. *J Diagnostic Med Sonogr* 1988; 4:236-245.

13. Gorcsan J. Tissue Doppler echocardiography. *Curr Opin Cardiol* 2000; Sept 15:323-329.

14. Burns PN. Instrumentation and clinical interpretation of the Doppler spectrum: carotid and deep Doppler. In: *Conventional & Color-Flow Duplex Ultrasound Course*. Proc AIUM Spring Education Meeting. 1989; 29-38.

15. Persson AV, Powis RL. Recent advances in imaging and evaluation of blood flow using ultrasound. *Med Clin North Am* 1986; 70:1241-1252.

16. Ophir J, Maklad NF. Digital scan converters in diagnostic ultrasound imaging. *Proc IEEE*. 1979; 67:654-664.

17. Atkinson P, Woodcock JP. *Doppler Ultrasound and Its Use in Clinical Measurement*. New York: Academic Press; 1982.

18. Goldstein A, Powis RL. Medical ultrasonic diagnostics in ultrasonic instruments and devices: reference for modern instrumentation, techniques and technology. In: Mason WP, Thurston RN, eds. *Physical Acoustics Series*. Vol. 23A. New York: Academic Press; 1999.

19. Powis RL. Color flow imaging technology. In: *Basic Science of Flow Measurement*. Proc Syllabus AIUM 1989 Spring Education Meeting. 1989; 27-33.

20. Merritt RBC. Doppler color flow imaging. *J Color Ultrasonogr* 1987; 15:591-597.

21. Havlice JF, Taenzer JC. Medical ultrasonic imaging: an overview of principles and instrumentation. *Proc IEEE* 1979; 67:620-641.

22. Powis RL, Powis WJ. *A Thinker's Guide to Ultrasonic Imaging*. Baltimore: Urban & Schwarzenberg; 1984.

23. Baker DW, Daigle RE. Noninvasive ultrasonic flow-metry. In: Hwang, NHC, Normann NA, eds. *Cardiovascular Flow Dynamics and Measurements*. Baltimore: University Park Press; 1977.

24. McDicken WN. *Diagnostic Ultrasonics: Principles and Use of Instruments*. 2nd ed. New York: John Wiley & Sons; 1981.

25. Murphy KJ, Rubin JM. Power Doppler: it's a good thing. *Semin Ultrasound CT MRI* 1997; Feb. 18:13-21.

26. Goldstein A. Range ambiguities in real-time. *Ultrasound* 1981; 9:83-90.

27. Middleton WD, Erickson S, Melson GL. Perivascular color artifact: pathologic significance and appearance on color Doppler US images. *Radiology* 1989; 171:647-652.

28. Shelly G, Cashman T. *Computer Fundamentals for an Information Age*. Brea, CA: Anaheim Publishing; 1984.

Questions

GENERAL INSTRUCTIONS: For each question, select the best answer. Select only one answer for each question unless otherwise specified.

1. Which of the following is the standard protocol for digital imaging that allows compatibility and communication between computers, workstations, and network hardware provided by various manufacturers of CT, MRI, and ultrasound equipment?

   (A) SDMS

   (B) PACS

   (C) AIUM

   (D) DICOM

   (E) ALARA

2. The spatial pulse length

   (A) determines the speed of ultrasound in tissue

   (B) usually increases with higher frequency

   (C) is improved with rectification

   (D) determines lateral resolution

   (E) usually decreases with higher frequency

3. Axial resolution is improved by

   (A) focusing

   (B) acoustic mirrors

   (C) acoustic lens

   (D) beam diameter

   (E) damping

4. Lateral resolution is improved by

   (A) ring-down

   (B) decreased beam diameter

   (C) spatial pulse length

   (D) imaging in the far zone

   (E) damping

5. The beam of an unfocused transducer diverges

   (A) because of inadequate damping

   (B) in the Fresnel zone

   (C) in the Fraunhofer zone

   (D) when the pulse length is long

   (E) at the dead zone

6. Reverberation artifacts are a result of

   (A) electronic noise

   (B) improper time gain compensation (TGC) settings

   (C) the presence of two or more strong reflecting surfaces

   (D) duplication of a true reflector

   (E) absence of echo information distal to a reflector

7. The recommendations for reducing the potential for bioeffects using the ALARA principle is to

   (A) increase receiver gain and decrease the power output

   (B) increase power output and decrease transducer frequency

   (C) decrease power output and increase scanning time

   (D) decrease scanning time when a patient has a maternal temperature and decrease overall gain and increase power output

   (E) use an unfocused transducer and increase the scan time

8. What technique can be employed to reduce grating side lobes?

   (A) depolarization

   (B) apodization

   (C) subsonic beam tapering

   (D) magnification

9. A technique that uses an ensemble of pulses to improve penetration and contrast resolution.

   (A) coded excitation

   (B) harmonic imaging

   (C) apodization

   (D) subdicing

   (E) magnification

10. A 75-year-old patient suffering from Alzheimer's disease arrived in the ultrasound department from the surgical ward for ultrasound of the right legs to rule out deep venous thrombosis. The patient has no name band. What is the most appropriate next step?

   (A) retrieve the name and medical record number from the chart that accompanied the patient.

   (B) return the patient to the ward for appropriate identification and tagging.

   (C) scan the patient now and retrieve identification later.

   (D) call the nurse on the floor by telephone to identify the patient.

   (E) put an ID wristband on the patient that matches the name sent to you.

Questions 11 through 15: Match the following group of wires with its function for the AIUM test object (Fig. 1–51).

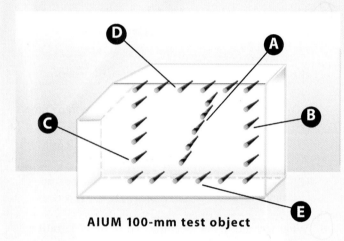

AIUM 100-mm test object

FIGURE 1–51.

B-mode a bright head (handwritten)

11. registration or B-mode alignment _____

12. axial resolution _____

13. lateral resolution _____

14. dead zone _____

15. depth calibration _____

16. **Decreasing the spatial pulse length**

   (A) reduces the field of view

   (B) reduces lateral resolution

   (C) improves axial resolution

   (D) improves lateral resolution

   (E) reduces axial resolution

17. How much will a 3.5 MHz pulse be attenuated after passing through 2 cm of soft tissue?

   (A) 7 dB

   (B) 3.5 dB

   (C) 17 dB

   (D) 1.75 dB

   (E) 5.3 dB

18. Propagation speed errors result in

   (A) reverberation

   (B) improper axial position

   (C) shadowing

   (D) a Doppler shift

   (E) all of the above

19. Enhancement is caused by

   (A) reduction in echo amplitude distally

   (B) propagation speed errors

   (C) Snell's law

   (D) weakly attenuating structures

   (E) duplication of echoes on the opposite side of a strong reflector

20. The Doppler shift frequency is

   (A) directly proportional to the velocity of the reflector

   (B) greater in pulsed Doppler systems

   (C) greater at high-intensity levels

   (D) dependent on the number of transducer elements being used

   (E) indirectly proportional to the velocity of the reflector

21. The number of frames per second necessary for a real-time image to be flicker free is

   (A) more than 15

   (B) less than 1

   (C) between 5 and 10

   (D) between 2 and 5

22. A non-English-speaking patient presented for an ultrasound-guided breast biopsy in which an informed consent is required. What is the most appropriate step to take?

    (A) get a family member who speaks the patient's language to be an interpreter.

    (B) use a sign-language interpreter licensed for the deaf and hearing impaired.

    (C) use any full-time employee who speaks that language as an interpreter.

    (D) get a physician who is scheduled to perform the ultrasound examination.

    (E) use a certified language line.

23. The intensity of the ultrasound beam is usually greater at the focal zone because of

    (A) decreased attenuation

    (B) smaller beam diameter

    (C) diffraction effects

    (D) a shorter duty factor

    (E) larger beam diameter

24. If the amplitude is doubled, the intensity is

    (A) doubled

    (B) cut in half

    (C) increased by four times

    (D) unchanged

    (E) decreased by four times

25. The attenuation for soft tissue is

    (A) increased with tissue thickness

    (B) determined by the slope of the TGC curve

    (C) increased with decreasing wavelength

    (D) unimportant when using digital scan converters

    (E) decreased with high frequency

26. The acoustic impedance of the matching layer

    (A) can be chosen to improve transmission into the body

    (B) must be much larger than the transducer material to reduce attenuation

    (C) is not necessary with real-time scanners

    (D) must be made with the same material as the damping material

    (E) must be smaller than the impedance of the tissue

27. Which of the following is necessary additional confirmation required to ensure that the patient you are about to scan is the correct patient?

    (A) which ward the patient is from

    (B) documented ultrasound request

    (C) what part to scan

    (D) date of birth

    (E) type of ultrasound study

28. If a patient's body fluids (blood or vaginal secretions) come into contact with the ultrasound machine, what would be the most appropriate action?

    (A) cancel the cases for the day and wait for the blood to dry before cleaning the machine.

    (B) document the date and time and call the biomedical department.

    (C) call the manufacturer of the ultrasound for advice.

    (D) use approved disinfectant solution to clean the machine.

    (E) the ultrasound machine should be regarded as contaminated waste and should be replaced with a new ultrasound machine.

29. The operating frequency

    (A) depends on the transducer's ring-down time

    (B) depends on the thickness of the crystal

    (C) is increased as the crystal diameter is decreased

    (D) depends on the strength of the pulser

    (E) all of the above

30. The period of an ultrasound wave is

    (A) the time at which it is no longer detectable

    (B) the number of times the wave is repeated per second

    (C) the time to complete one cycle

    (D) the speed of the wave

    (E) the peak pressure of the wave

31. The dynamic range of a system

    (A) is increased when specular reflectors are scanned

    (B) is decreased when shadowing is present

    (C) can be increased using coupling gel

    (D) is the ratio of smallest to largest power level that the system can handle

    (E) the difference between the smallest and largest signals measured

32. What term describes a digital imaging system that enables ultrasound, x-ray, MRI, and CT images to be stored electronically and viewed remotely on a workstation?

    (A) high-definition hormonic imaging
    (B) coded excitation digital imaging protocol
    (C) ALARA
    (D) DICOM
    (E) PACS

33. Increasing the pulse repetition period

    (A) improves resolution
    (B) increases the maximum depth that can be imaged
    (C) decreases the maximum depth that can be imaged
    (D) increases refraction
    (E) all of the above

34. Ultrasound bioeffects with an unfocused beam

    (A) do not occur
    (B) cannot occur with diagnostic instruments
    (C) are not confirmed below 100 mW/cm^2 spatial peak temporal average (SPTA)
    (D) are not confirmed above 1 W/cm^2 SPTA

35. When can an informed consent be revoked?

    (A) after 72 hours for an adult older than 21 years
    (B) at any time
    (C) only by a court order
    (D) cannot be revoked after signing, because it is a legally binding document
    (E) 24 hours after signing the document if the patient is currently hospitalized

36. What is the first thing you should do when a patient enters the ultrasound room?

    (A) introduce yourself with name and title
    (B) disinfect the transducer
    (C) turn on the ultrasound machine
    (D) check the ultrasound machine for electrical safety
    (E) find the protocol for the ultrasound procedure

37. How often should you disinfect the transvaginal transducer?

    (A) once a week
    (B) every day at the end of the work shift
    (C) only when the transducer probe cover is broken
    (D) if the patient has a vaginal infection or bleeding
    (E) after each use

38. Which of the following should be minimized in order to comply with the ALARA principle?

    (A) time gain compensation (TGC)
    (B) overall gain
    (C) frequency
    (D) transmit power
    (E) magnification

39. Which of the following best describes autocorrelation?

    (A) mathematical process in which a waveform is multiplied by a time-shifted version of itself.
    (B) the automatic correlation between the transmitted echo and the reflected echo.
    (C) the repositioning of the incident acoustic energy scattered back toward the source.
    (D) the continuously repeated display of a recorded image from memory.
    (E) a pulsed Doppler system that enables velocity measurements at several depths simultaneously.

40. What is the name of the mechanism of ultrasound bioeffects in which microbubbles oscillate without collapsing?

    (A) stable
    (B) ionization
    (C) thermal effect
    (D) fluid streaming
    (E) transient

41. Which of the following would not typically be related to ultrasound bioeffects?

    (A) power output
    (B) thermal index (TI)
    (C) examination time
    (D) high-frequency transducer
    (E) mechanical index (MI)

42. Harmonic frequencies are derived from

    (A) nonlinear wave propagation
    (B) perpendicular wave propagation
    (C) symmetrical wave propagation
    (D) proportional behavior
    (E) linear wave propagation

43. Which of the following has an effect on the propagation speed of the ultrasound?

    (A) high-frequency transducers

    (B) output power

    (C) angle of the ultrasound beam

    (D) tissue type

    (E) time gain compensation (TGC)

44. Which of the following is equivalent to the prefix giga?

    (A) 10^6

    (B) 10^{-6}

    (C) 10^9

    (D) 10^3

    (E) 10^{-9}

45. What percentage of intensity of an ultrasound pulse incident on an interface of 0.25 and 0.75 rayls is reflected?

    (A) 50%

    (B) 100%

    (C) 25%

    (D) 75%

    (E) 15%

46. Axial resolution can be improved by

    (A) higher frequency transducers

    (B) lower frequency transducers

    (C) larger transducers

    (D) poorly damped transducers

    (E) focusing the ultrasound beam in the near zone

47. When particle motion of a medium is parallel to the direction of a wave propagation, what is the wave being transmitted called?

    (A) longitudinal wave

    (B) shear wave

    (C) surface wave

    (D) electromagnetic wave

    (E) transverse wave

48. The wavelength in a material having a wave velocity of 1,500 m/s employing a transducer frequency of 5 MHz is

    (A) 0.3 mm

    (B) 0.3 cm

    (C) 0.6 mm

    (D) 0.6 cm

    (E) 3.0 cm

49. Which of the following determines the amount of reflection at the interface of two dissimilar materials?

    (A) the index of refraction

    (B) the frequency of the ultrasonic wave

    (C) Young's modulus

    (D) the difference in specific acoustic impedances

    (E) time gain compensation (TGC)

50. Which equation describes the relationship among wave propagation speed, wavelength, and frequency?

    (A) $V = f\lambda$

    (B) wavelength = 2(frequency × velocity)

    (C) $Z = pV$

    (D) wavelength = frequency + velocity

    (E) $\lambda = r \times f$

51. When a sound wave strikes a tissue interface at an oblique angle of incidence, what other condition must be present in order for refraction to occur?

    (A) a change in the angle of reflection

    (B) a difference in propagation speeds

    (C) a strong specular reflector

    (D) the presence of several small reflectors

    (E) normal incidence

52. The acoustic impedance of a material is

    (A) directly proportional to density and inversely proportional to velocity

    (B) directly proportional to velocity and inversely proportional to density

    (C) inversely proportional to density and velocity

    (D) equal to the product of density and velocity

    (E) unrelated to velocity and density

53. What is the average velocity of ultrasonic waves in soft tissue?

    (A) 1,540 m/s

    (B) 154,000 cm/s

    (C) 0.154 cm/μs

    (D) about one mile per second

    (E) all of the above

54. A soft tissue mass is measured to be 80 mm in diameter; what is the diameter in centimeters?

 (A) 80.00 cm

 (B) 8.0 cm

 (C) 4.0 cm

 (D) 0.8 cm

 (E) 0.08 cm

55. When a sound wave strikes a boundary between two tissues with a normal incidence, what other condition must be present in order for reflection to occur?

 (A) an oblique incidence

 (B) a difference in acoustical impedance

 (C) a weak non-specular reflector

 (D) a thick boundary

 (E) the two media must have identical impedances

56. Ultrasound transducers convert

 (A) mechanical to thermal energy and vice versa

 (B) thermal to cavitation energy and vice versa

 (C) electromagnetic to kinetic energy and vice versa

 (D) heat to electromagnetic energy and vice versa

 (E) mechanical to electrical energy and vice versa

57. The velocity of sound waves is primarily dependent on

 (A) angulation

 (B) reflection

 (C) the medium and the mode of vibration

 (D) frequency

 (E) acoustic power and the time gain compensation (TGC)

58. Increasing the frequency of an ultrasonic longitudinal wave will result in which of the following changes in the velocity of the wave?

 (A) an increase

 (B) a decrease

 (C) no change

 (D) a reversal

 (E) increase at first and then a decrease

59. Which of the following terms describes the change in direction of an ultrasonic beam when it passes from one medium to another in which elasticity and density differ from those of the first medium?

 (A) refraction

 (B) rarefaction

 (C) angulation

 (D) reflection

 (E) compression

60. A long near zone can be obtained by

 (A) using a higher-frequency transducer

 (B) adding a convex lens to the transducer

 (C) decreasing the diameter of the transducer

 (D) increasing the damping

 (E) using a low-frequency transducer

61. If a 2 MHz frequency is used in human soft tissue, what is the approximate wavelength?

 (A) 0.75 mm

 (B) 0.15 mm

 (C) 0.21 mm

 (D) 0.44 mm

 (E) 2.75 mm

62. What is the ratio of particle pressure to particle velocity at a given point within the ultrasonic field?

 (A) interference

 (B) impedance

 (C) incidence

 (D) interface

 (E) intensity

63. What is the following formula used to determine?

$$\frac{2 \times \text{velocity of reflector} \times \text{original frequency}}{\text{velocity of sound}}$$

 (A) shift in frequency caused by the Doppler effect

 (B) degree of attenuation

 (C) distance a wave front travels

 (D) amount of amplification necessary to produce diagnostic ultrasound

 (E) frequency related to wavelength

64. The principle that states that all points on a wavefront can be considered as point sources for the production of spherical secondary wavelets was postulated by

 (A) Doppler

 (B) Young

 (C) Huygens

 (D) Rayleigh

 (E) Snell

65. A 10-dB difference in signal intensity is equivalent to which of the following?

    (A) twofold
    (B) tenfold
    (C) 100-fold
    (D) 1000-fold
    (E) one-tenth

66. The level below which signals are *not* processed through an ultrasound receiver system is the

    (A) wall filter level
    (B) reject level
    (C) impedance level
    (D) dynamic range level
    (E) digitizing level

67. Term for signal dynamic range reduction.

    (A) rejection
    (B) compression
    (C) relaxation
    (D) elimination
    (E) sensitivity

68. An ultrasound system mode that displays an upward displacement from a baseline that is proportional to the strength of the echo.

    (A) A-mode
    (B) B-mode
    (C) B-scan
    (D) M-mode
    (E) C-mode

69. Which of the following is *not* a method for restricting the dynamic range of the ultrasound signal?

    (A) threshold
    (B) rejection
    (C) compression
    (D) relaxation

70. Which of the following types of scan converter is used in current ultrasound systems?

    (A) analog
    (B) digital
    (C) bistable
    (D) static
    (E) mechanical

71. Which of the following terms describes the fraction of time that pulsed ultrasound is actually on?

    (A) duty factor
    (B) frame rate
    (C) pulse repetition frequency
    (D) pulse repetition period
    (E) pulse stretching

72. Which of the following is a system performance parameter that is assessed using a multipurpose phantom to determine the minimum echo amplitude that can be detected?

    (A) compression
    (B) demodulation
    (C) gain
    (D) sensitivity
    (E) dead zone

73. Which of the following image shapes is produced by a linear sequenced array real-time transducer?

    (A) pie shape
    (B) rectangular
    (C) sector
    (D) triangular
    (E) trapezoidal shape

74. The major factor in determining the acoustic power output of the transducer is the

    (A) size of the transducer
    (B) magnitude of the pulser voltage spike
    (C) amount of amplification at the receiver
    (D) amount of gain
    (E) amount of magnification

75. Which two scan parameters may be used to indicate the potential for biological effects?

    (A) frame rate and field of view (FOV)
    (B) time gain compensation (TGC) and overall gain
    (C) pulse repetition frequency (PRF) and pulse repetition period (PRP)
    (D) thermal index and mechanical index
    (E) ensemble length and focal depth

76. Which of the following relates to bandwidth and operating frequency?

    (A) near zone
    (B) piezoelectric crystal
    (C) quality factor
    (D) far zone
    (E) matching layer

77. The extraneous beams of ultrasound not in the direction of the main axis specific to multielement transducer arrays are called

    (A) apodization zones
    (B) subdiced beams
    (C) Fraunhofer zones
    (D) harmonic lobes
    (E) grating lobes

78. The actual time from the start of the pulse to the end of the pulse is known as

    (A) pulse repetition frequency
    (B) pulse pressure
    (C) pulse repetition period
    (D) pulse duration
    (E) spatial pulse length

79. Arrange the given units in increasing order: nano, micro, milli, and centi.

    (A) $10^{-9}, 10^6, 10^2, 10^3$
    (B) $10^{-9}, 10^{-6}, 10^{-3}, 10^{-2}$
    (C) $10^{-9}, 10^6, 10^{-3}, 10^2$
    (D) $10^{-2}, 10^{-1}, 10^3, 10^{-3}$
    (E) $10^9, 10^6, 10^3, 10^2$

80. Specular reflection occurs when

    (A) the frequency is small compared with the wavelength
    (B) the object that causes the reflection is small relative to the wavelength
    (C) the reflector surface is large and smooth relative to the wavelength
    (D) the angle of incidence and the angle of reflection differ by at least 45°
    (E) irregular or rough interfaces resulting in sound waves traveling in many directions

81. The refractive index of water is slightly altered when a sound beam passes through it, thus causing compression and rarefaction of the water molecules.

The phenomenon is the basis for what technique used to make ultrasound beam measurements?

    (A) radiation force balance
    (B) Schlieren photography
    (C) impedance photography
    (D) autocorrelation
    (E) cross-correlation

82. Artifacts appearing as parallel, equally spaced lines are characteristic of

    (A) acoustic shadowing
    (B) off-normal incidence
    (C) specular reflection
    (D) reverberation
    (E) enhancement

83. An increase in reflection amplitude from reflectors that lie behind a weakly attenuating structure is called

    (A) the incidence angle
    (B) enhancement
    (C) the intensity reflection coefficient
    (D) the effective reflecting area
    (E) shadowing

84. The amount of dispersion in the far field of an ultrasound beam can be decreased by

    (A) using a transducer with a convex face
    (B) using a larger diameter transducer
    (C) decreasing the intensity of the beam in the near field
    (D) using a lower frequency transducer
    (E) using a smaller diameter transducer

85. Longitudinal or axial resolution is directly dependent on

    (A) depth of penetration
    (B) spatial pulse length
    (C) acoustic lens
    (D) the angle of incidence
    (E) ultrasound beam width

86. Which of the following ultrasound frequency spectrum is specifically equal to operating frequency divided by bandwidth?

    (A) frequency limit
    (B) Q-factor
    (C) resonant frequency
    (D) frequency duration
    (E) harmonic factor

87. The type of transducer that combines the technology of linear sequence and phased array to produce a trapezoidal-shaped image is called

(A) rectangular array

(B) multi-function array

(C) sector array

(D) linear curved array

(E) vector array

88. Which of the following is the *least* attenuating material to the transmission of ultrasound?

(A) muscle

(B) liver

(C) bone

(D) kidney

(E) urine

89. The ratio of the largest power to the smallest power that the ultrasound system can handle is the

(A) dynamic range

(B) overall gain

(C) rejection range

(D) amplification factor

(E) frequency factor

90. Ultrasound waves in tissues are called

(A) shear waves

(B) electromagnetic waves

(C) surface waves

(D) longitudinal waves

(E) transverse waves

Questions 91 through 99 refer to Fig. 1–52.

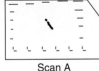 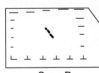 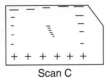

Scan A   Scan B   Scan C

FIGURE 1–52.

91. The row of wires in the middle are used to check

(A) lateral resolution

(B) axial resolution

(C) dead zone

(D) horizontal distance calibration

(E) all of the above

92. Which of the diagrams shows correct registration?

(A) scan A

(B) scan B

(C) scan C

(D) all of the above

(E) none of the above

93. The row of wires on top is used to check

(A) dead zone

(B) vertical distance calibration

(C) horizontal distance calibration

(D) axial resolution

(E) registration

94. The speed of ultrasound in the AIUM test object is equivalent to

(A) the speed of typical fatty tissue

(B) the speed of blood

(C) the speed of the thin, acrylic plastic

(D) the speed in soft tissue

(E) the speed of sound of the stainless steel rods within the test object

95. The row of wires on the bottom is used to check for

(A) axial resolution

(B) lateral resolution

(C) horizontal caliper check

(D) vertical distance calibration

(E) dead zone

96. Which of the following cannot be checked when the test object is scanned from the top only?

(A) axial resolution

(B) lateral resolution

(C) vertical distance calibration

(D) horizontal distance calibration

(E) dead zone

97. Which of the following parameters cannot be evaluated by the AIUM test object?

(A) gray scale

(B) dynamic range

(C) attenuation

(D) scattering characteristics

(E) all of the above

98. Scanning a test object from multiple sides could be used to check

    (A) gray scale
    (B) depth resolution
    (C) horizontal distance calibration
    (D) registration
    (E) all of the above

99. When using the AIUM test object, which of the following should be kept constant for comparisons?

    (A) output power
    (B) Time gain compensation (TGC)
    (C) reject
    (D) transducer, megahertz, and focus
    (E) all of the above

100. Which of the following types of cavitation can result in highly localized temperature elevation up to 10,000 degrees Kelvin?

    (A) transient
    (B) pressure
    (C) particle vibration
    (D) velocity
    (E) frequency

101. There are many types of natural and synthetic crystals that possess and exhibit piezoelectric properties. Which of the following are not natural?

    (A) tourmaline
    (B) quartz
    (C) Rochelle salt
    (D) lithium sulfate

102. Which one of the following materials would *not* be suitable as acoustic insulators for a pulse transducer backing?

    (A) cork
    (B) rubber
    (C) air
    (D) araldite loaded with tungsten powder
    (E) epoxy resin

103. When using a continuous-wave ultrasound, which of the following intensities are equal?

    (A) SPTP = SATP
    (B) SATP = SPTP
    (C) SATA = SATP
    (D) SPTP = SPPA

104. If the frequency of sound is below 20 Hz, what is it called?

    (A) infrasound
    (B) audible sound
    (C) ultrasound
    (D) x-rays
    (E) supersonic

105. If the frequency of sound is above 20 kHz, what is it called?

    (A) infrasound
    (B) ultrasound
    (C) audible sound
    (D) x-rays
    (E) subsonic

106. If the frequency of sound is between 20 Hz and 20 kHz, what is it called?

    (A) x-rays
    (B) audible sound
    (C) ultrasound
    (D) infrasound
    (E) supersonic

107. Which of the following is not among the spectrum of electromagnetic waves?

    (A) x-rays
    (B) ultrasound
    (C) ultraviolet
    (D) infrared
    (E) visible light

108. The term hertz denotes

    (A) strength of the ultrasound waves
    (B) the distance that ultrasound waves travel through a medium
    (C) the fraction of time that the transducer is transmitting a pulse
    (D) cycles per second
    (E) the pressure or height of a wave

109. Which one of the following Doppler interrogation of a vessel will possibly yield no Doppler shift?

    (A) 10°
    (B) 60°
    (C) 90°
    (D) 30°
    (E) 0°

110. Which of the following is an example of a transducer?

    (A) battery
    (B) loudspeaker
    (C) light bulb
    (D) human being
    (E) all of the above

111. When constant electrical voltage is applied across the thickness of a piezoelectric crystal, the crystal will

    (A) always increase in size
    (B) always decrease in size
    (C) vibrate
    (D) increase or decrease in size depending on the voltage polarity
    (E) cause a Curie temperature elevation and result in depolarization

112. The abbreviation 5 MHz denotes

    (A) five hundred thousand cycles per second
    (B) five hundred million cycles per second
    (C) 5,000 cycles per second
    (D) five million cycles per second
    (E) 5 Hz

113. The function of the damping material in the transducer housing is to

    (A) reduce pulse duration
    (B) improve axial resolution
    (C) reduce spatial pulse length
    (D) improve lateral resolution
    (E) A and B only
    (F) A and D only
    (G) A, B, and C only

114. What is the average speed of ultrasound in human soft tissue at 37°C?

    (A) 1,540 meters per second
    (B) 1,540 miles per second
    (C) 1,540 feet per second
    (D) 154,000 meters per minute
    (E) 1.54 centimeters per second

115. In physical science, the word *period* denotes

    (A) the pressure or height of a wave
    (B) the speed of a wave per cycle
    (C) the time it takes to complete a single cycle
    (D) the distance it takes for one cycle to occur
    (E) the number of times the wave is repeated per second

116. What direction is the motion of particles in a longitudinal wave

    (A) motion of particles is parallel to the axis of wave propagation
    (B) motion of particles is perpendicular to the axis of wave propagation
    (C) motion of particles travels counter-clockwise ellipse to the axis of wave propagation
    (D) motion of particles travels to the surface vibrating particles
    (E) motion of particles travels clockwise circle to the axis of wave propagation

117. What direction is the motion of particles in a transverse wave

    (A) motion of particles is parallel to the axis of wave propagation
    (B) motion of particles travels counter-clockwise ellipse to the axis of wave propagation
    (C) motion of particles is perpendicular to the axis of wave propagation
    (D) motion of particles travels to the surface vibrating particles
    (E) motion of particles travels clockwise circle to the axis of wave propagation

118. Ultrasound wave propagation causes displacement of particles in a medium. What are the regions of greatest particle concentration called?

    (A) reaction
    (B) compression
    (C) rarefaction
    (D) attenuation
    (E) reflection

119. Ultrasound wave propagation causes displacement of particles in a medium. What are the regions of lowest particle concentration called?

    (A) compression

    (B) condensation

    (C) compensation

    (D) attenuation

    (E) rarefactions

120. Which of the following disclosures cannot be made without an authorization signed by the patient?

    (A) reporting child abuse

    (B) response to court orders

    (C) request for medical records after drug treatment

    (D) reporting fraud or abuse of public funds

    (E) accidental gunshot wound

121. Which of the following is related to axial resolution

    (A) the ability to distinguish two objects separated in the direction of the ultrasound beam

    (B) the ability to distinguish two objects separated in the direction perpendicular to the ultrasound beam

    (C) the same as depth, longitudinal and range resolution

    (D) the same as azimuthal, angular, and transverse resolution

    (E) both A and D

    (F) both A and C

122. Which of the following is related to lateral resolution?

    (A) the same as depth, longitudinal and range resolution

    (B) the ability to distinguish two objects separated in the direction perpendicular to the ultrasound beam

    (C) the ability to distinguish two objects separated in the direction parallel to the ultrasound beam

    (D) the same as azimuthal, angular, and transverse resolution

    (E) both A and B

    (F) both B and D

Questions 123 through 128: Match the structures in Fig. 1–53 with the list of parts given.

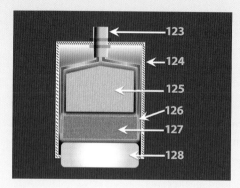

FIGURE 1–53.

123. _____ (A) matching layer

124. _____ (B) damping (backing) material

125. _____ (C) connector

126. _____ (D) piezoelectric element

127. _____ (E) plastic case

128. _____ (F) electrode

129. What does the arrow in Fig. 1–54 on the following page point to?

    (A) near gain

    (B) far gain

    (C) overall gain

    (D) power output

    (E) zoom-level controls

130. When making circumference measurements using electronic calipers in diagnostic ultrasound, the results are expressed in what type of unit?

    (A) millimeter or centimeter (cm)

    (B) centimeter squared (cm^2)

    (C) centimeter cubed (cm^3)

    (D) meter cubed (m^3)

    (E) millimeter cubed (mm^3)

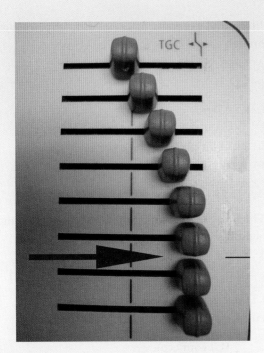

FIGURE 1–54.

131. **Implementation of apodization in diagnostic ultrasound systems requires**

(A) acoustic lens between each element

(B) different voltages to be applied to each element

(C) dividing the transducer elements into smaller elements

(D) depolarization of the transducer elements

(E) increasing the fundamental frequency

132. **This multipurpose phantom is used to evaluate what target group, arrow A (Fig. 1–55)?**

(A) ring down

(B) gray-scale and displayed dynamic range

(C) horizontal measurement calibration

(D) vertical measurement calibration

(E) axial resolution

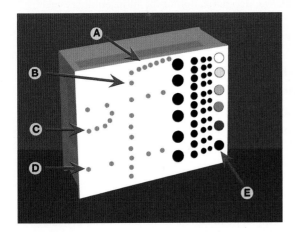

FIGURE 1–55.

133. **This multipurpose phantom is used to evaluate what target group, arrow B (Fig. 1–55)?**

(A) dead zone

(B) gray scale

(C) horizontal measurement calibration

(D) displayed dynamic range

(E) axial resolution

134. **This multipurpose phantom is used to evaluate what target group, arrow D (Fig. 1–55)?**

(A) dead zone

(B) gray scale

(C) lateral resolution

(D) displayed dynamic range

(E) axial resolution

135. **Which one of the following does _not_ improve temporal resolution?**

(A) low-line density

(B) higher frame rate

(C) narrowing the sector size

(D) fewer pulse per frame

(E) increasing depth

136. **Which of the following is true about the dynamic aperture when it is increased in size?**

(A) the beam will always focus at a greater depth.

(B) near-zone length increases.

(C) axial resolution increases.

(D) lateral resolution is unchanged.

(E) all of the above.

137. **Which of the following terms denotes the technique of dividing normal crystal elements into smaller elements?**

(A) coded excitation

(B) apodization

(C) aliasing

(D) subdicing

(E) autocorrelation

138. **Which of the following materials is used as a backing material in continuous-wave transducers?**

(A) epoxy resin

(B) tungsten

(C) ultrasound gel

(D) air

(E) barium sulfate

139. Which of the following converts Doppler shift information into visual analysis?

    (A) autocorrelation

    (B) hue

    (C) fast Fourier transform

    (D) reject control

    (E) saturation

140. The second harmonic frequency is

    (A) frequency of second reverberation echo

    (B) fundamental frequency plus the transmitted frequency

    (C) the same as the first transmitted frequency

    (D) twice the fundamental frequency

    (E) never recorded

141. If frequency is doubled, the wavelength will

    (A) double

    (B) increase by a factor of four

    (C) remain the same

    (D) become shorter by one-fourth

    (E) become shorter by one-half

142. If frequency is reduced by a factor of two, the wavelength will

    (A) double

    (B) increase by a factor of four

    (C) remain the same

    (D) become shorter by one-forth

    (E) become shorter by one-half

143. As frequency increases, the penetration will

    (A) decrease

    (B) increase

    (C) remain the same

144. In general, if frequency increases, the resolution will

    (A) decrease

    (B) increase

    (C) remain the same

145. For an unfocused transducer, if frequency increases, the beam width will

    (A) decrease

    (B) increase

    (C) remain the same

146. Ultrasound generally has most difficulty propagating through

    (A) lung

    (B) blood

    (C) bowel gas

    (D) IVP contrast

    (E) all of the above

    (F) A and C only

    (G) A and B only

147. Which of the following *can* be used as a coupling medium?

    (A) water

    (B) saline

    (C) water-soluble gel

    (D) aqueous gels

    (E) all of the above

148. Attenuation denotes

    (A) progressive weakening of the sound beam as it propagates through a medium

    (B) progressive decrease of speed of sound in the tissues

    (C) progressive redirection of the ultrasound beam following reflection

    (D) progressive bending of the ultrasound beam after crossing an interface

    (E) progressive decrease in frequency

149. The piezoelectric effect is the

    (A) depolarization of tissue following sonication

    (B) mechanical deformation of ultrasound crystal that results from a high voltage applied across the crystal thickness

    (C) the development of an electrical charge across the crystal thickness following deformation

    (D) the depolarization of the ultrasound crystal following heating

    (E) deformation of soft tissue following sonication

150. The reverse piezoelectric effect can be *best* described as

    (A) depolarization of tissue following sonication

    (B) mechanical deformation of ultrasound crystal that results from a high voltage applied across the crystal thickness

    (C) the development of an electrical charge across the crystal thickness following deformation

    (D) the depolarization of the ultrasound crystal following heating

    (E) deformation of soft tissue following sonication

151. **The parameter used to express attenuation coefficient is**

    (A) $\left(\dfrac{z_2 - z_1}{z_2 - z_1}\right)^2 \times 100$

    (B) 0.5 dB/cm/MHz

    (C) $z = pV$

    (D) $\dfrac{\sin i}{\sin r} = \dfrac{V_1}{V_2}$

152. **The ultrasound wave results in the transfer of which of the following through tissue?**

    (A) particles
    (B) matter
    (C) energy
    (D) mass
    (E) ionizing radiation

153. **The type of compressional wave in which the particles move back and forth parallel to the direction of wave propagation is known as**

    (A) longitudinal wave
    (B) heat waves
    (C) transverse wave
    (D) surface wave
    (E) electromagnetic wave

154. **Wavelength is a measure of**

    (A) time
    (B) voltage
    (C) distance
    (D) pulse duration
    (E) exposure

155. **Ultrasonic waves are**

    (A) compressional
    (B) x-ray
    (C) electromagnetic
    (D) solar
    (E) transverse

156. **Acoustic impedance is**

    (A) the amount of tissue × the speed of sound in tissue
    (B) the density of tissue × the speed of sound in tissue
    (C) the transducer frequency × the speed of sound in tissue
    (D) the distance from one interface to the next
    (E) mass per unit volume

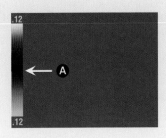

FIGURE 1–56.

157. **What does the arrow (A) point to in this color variance map (Fig. 1–56)?**

    (A) blood cells moving toward the transducer
    (B) blood cells moving away from the transducer
    (C) no Doppler shift
    (D) turbulent Doppler flow
    (E) laminar flow

158. **What is the typical frequency of medical ultrasound transducers?**

    (A) less than 20 Hz
    (B) less than 20 kHz
    (C) greater than 20 Hz but less than 20,000 Hz
    (D) greater than 20,000 Hz but less than 2,000,000 Hz
    (E) greater than 1 MHz

159. **Period is inversely proportional to**

    (A) velocity
    (B) power
    (C) wavelength
    (D) frequency
    (E) none of the above

160. **As the ultrasound beam becomes more perpendicular to an organ interface**

    (A) scattering becomes greater
    (B) there are more refracted echoes
    (C) there are fewer specular echoes
    (D) the received echoes will be larger
    (E) the received echoes will be smaller

161. **A decibel (dB) is proportional to the**

    (A) ratio of two sound intensities
    (B) sum of two sound intensities
    (C) amount of scattering
    (D) velocity of the sound wave
    (E) the difference between the transmitted and the received frequency

162. Axial resolution is also known as all of the following *except*

    (A) depth
    (B) range
    (C) azimuthal
    (D) longitudinal
    (E) radial

163. Which of the following has the highest sound velocity?

    (A) soft tissue
    (B) femur
    (C) air
    (D) water
    (E) blood

164. According to the AIUM, no significant biologic effects have been proved in mammals using a focused transducer with exposures of

    (A) SPTA intensities above 100 mW/cm^2
    (B) SPTA intensities below 100 mW/cm^2
    (C) SPTP intensities below 1 mW/cm
    (D) SATP intensities below 10 mW/cm^2
    (E) SPTA intensities below 1 W/cm^2

165. In addition to penetration, what does coded excitation improve?

    (A) frame rate
    (B) signal-to-noise ratio
    (C) lateral resolution
    (D) angular resolution
    (E) Doppler shift

166. Which of the following has the lowest intensity?

    (A) SPTP
    (B) SATP
    (C) SPTA
    (D) SATA
    (E) SPPA

167. What is the definition of the beam uniformity ratio?

    (A) the spatial average intensity divided by the spatial intensity
    (B) the spatial peak intensity divided by the spatial average intensity
    (C) the temporal average intensity divided by the spatial average intensity

    (D) the temporal peak intensity divided by the spatial peak intensity
    (E) none of the above

168. The duty factor of a pulsed echo system is normally less than

    (A) 5%
    (B) 100%
    (C) 1%
    (D) 25%
    (E) 99%

169. A shortened spatial pulse length results in

    (A) better lateral resolution
    (B) lower frequency
    (C) poorer axial resolution
    (D) better axial resolution
    (E) increased side lobes

170. The equation for measuring the relationship among propagation speed, frequency, and wavelength is

    (A) $\left(\dfrac{z_2 - z_1}{z_2 - z_1} \right)^2 \times 100$

    (B) $P = \dfrac{1}{f}$

    (C) $\lambda = \dfrac{c}{f}$

    (D) $\dfrac{\sin i}{\sin r} = \dfrac{V_1}{V_2}$

    (E) $Z = pc$

171. Attenuation of an ultrasound beam can occur by

    (A) divergence of the beam
    (B) scattering
    (C) reflection
    (D) all of the above

172. Which of the following units is used for an ultrasound attenuation coefficient?

    (A) dB/cm/MHz
    (B) dB/cm^2/Hz
    (C) cm/Hz/dB
    (D) m/dB/cm^3
    (E) dB/P/W/cm

173. If the transducer Q factor is low, which of the following is true about the bandwidth?

   (A) narrow
   (B) wide
   (C) Q and bandwidth are unrelated

174. Axial resolution can be improved by

   (A) reducing the spatial pulse length
   (B) increasing the spatial pulse length
   (C) lowering the transducer frequency
   (D) focusing

175. Which of the following primarily affects axial resolution?

   (A) beam width
   (B) spatial pulse length
   (C) aperture
   (D) acoustic lens
   (E) focusing

176. Which of the following may improve both axial and lateral resolution?

   (A) short pulse length
   (B) narrow beam width
   (C) increased beam diameter
   (D) increased transducer frequency

177. Which of the following is *not* another term for lateral resolution?

   (A) azimuthal
   (B) transverse
   (C) range
   (D) angular

178. What is the duty factor of continuous-wave Doppler?

   (A) less than 1%
   (B) 100%
   (C) greater than 100%
   (D) 50%
   (E) 10%

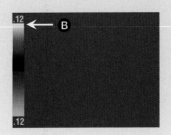

FIGURE 1–57.

179. What does the arrow (B) point to in this color variance map (Fig. 1–57)?

   (A) blood cells moving toward the transducer
   (B) blood cells moving away from the transducer
   (C) no Doppler shift
   (D) veins
   (E) arteries

180. Acoustic impedance may be expressed using which of the following units?

   (A) pascals
   (B) meters/dB
   (C) mW/cm^2
   (D) rayls
   (E) Hz

181. Which of the following is the *most* obvious application of C-mode?

   (A) cardiac imaging
   (B) 3D
   (C) pulsed-wave Doppler
   (D) 4D

182. The height of the vertical spike in an A-mode display corresponds to

   (A) the strength of the echo
   (B) the distance to the reflector
   (C) round-trip time of the echo
   (D) the pulse repetition frequency
   (E) Doppler shift

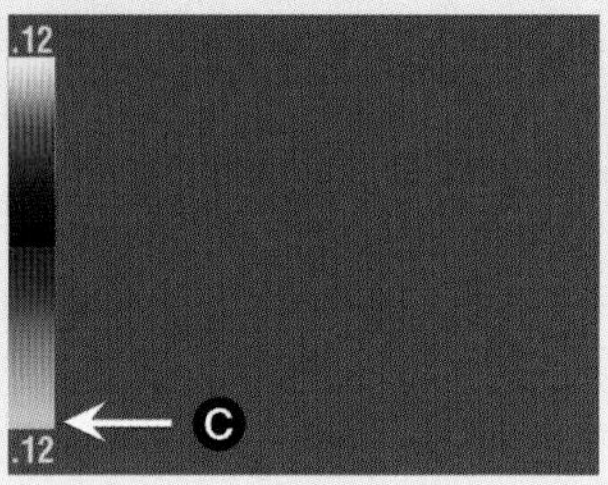

FIGURE 1–58.

183. What does the arrow (C) point to in this color variance map (Fig. 1–58)?

(A) blood cells moving toward the transducer

(B) blood cells moving away from the transducer

(C) no Doppler shift

(D) veins

(E) arteries

184. Which of the following equations is used for calculating the percentage of the reflected intensity at an interface?

(A) $R = \left(\dfrac{z_2 - z_1}{z_2 - z_1} \right)^2 \times 100$

(B) $R = \dfrac{Z_1 \times Z_2}{2}$

(C) $R = \sqrt{Z_1 + Z_2} \times \pi$

(D) $R = \dfrac{Z_1 \times Z_2}{Z_1 + Z_2}$

(E) $Z = pV$

185. The reflection coefficient between water and air is approximately:

(A) 1%

(B) 50%

(C) 75%

(D) 100%

(E) 0%

186. What happens to the ultrasound beam beyond the critical angle?

(A) 100% is transmitted

(B) 100% is reflected

(C) 75% is transmitted, 25% is reflected

(D) 75% is reflected, 25% is transmitted

(E) 100% refracted

187. Rayleigh scattering occurs if the particle dimensions are

(A) less than the wavelength

(B) greater than the wavelength

(C) equal to the wavelength

188. Which of the following will increase the dead-zone length?

(A) use of an acoustic standoff pad

(B) higher frequency transducer

(C) decreased spatial pulse length

(D) increased spatial pulse length

(E) increased output power

189. Power is defined as energy per unit

(A) mass

(B) distance

(C) time

(D) force

(E) work

190. The ability to resolve structures lying perpendicular to the axis of the ultrasound beam is called

(A) lateral resolution

(B) axial resolution

(C) depth resolution

(D) orthogonal resolution

191. In most soft tissues, the attenuation coefficient varies approximately

(A) inversely with frequency

(B) with the square of the frequency

(C) logarithmically with frequency

(D) directly with frequency

192. Ultrasound absorption in a medium results in

(A) conversion of ultrasound energy into heat

(B) dissipation of ultrasound energy into x-rays

(C) conversion of ultrasound energy into visible light

(D) dissipation of ultrasound energy into gamma rays

193. The typical value of one-way attenuation in soft tissue is

(A) 1 $dB/cm^2/Hz$

(B) 2 dB/cm/Hz

(C) 3 $dB/cm^2/MHz$

(D) 0.5 dB/cm/MHz

(E) 10 dB/mm/MHz

194. Which of the following produces false echoes that are occasionally seen in fluid-filled masses?

 (A) reflection
 (B) rarefaction
 (C) reverberation
 (D) diffraction
 (E) shadowing

195. Approximately what percentage of the ultrasound beam will be transmitted between fat and muscle?

 (A) 1%
 (B) 10%
 (C) 50%
 (D) 90%
 (E) 75%

196. Huygens' principle is used to describe

 (A) attenuation
 (B) refraction
 (C) the highest frequency in a waveform that can be represented by a sampled signal
 (D) wavefront
 (E) nonlinear propagation

197. Enhancement may occur posteriorly to structures that are

 (A) strong attenuators
 (B) weak attenuators
 (C) strong refractors
 (D) weak refractors

198. Sound attenuation in tissue may be expressed in terms of

 (A) half-value layer
 (B) millimeters per second
 (C) hertz
 (D) pascals
 (E) watts

199. Improper location of an echo may be attributable to

 (A) shadowing
 (B) Huygens's principle
 (C) spatial pulse length
 (D) propagation speed error
 (E) the dead zone

200. The range equation can be used to determine

 (A) the number of side lobes
 (B) the distance to a reflector
 (C) tissue attenuation
 (D) transducer pressure calibration
 (E) beam refraction

201. For a specular reflector

 (A) the angle of incidence is equal to the angle of reflection
 (B) the angle of incidence is greater than the angle of reflection
 (C) there is no dependence on beam angle
 (D) the angle of incidence is less than the angle of reflection
 (E) the surface is smaller than the wavelength

202. Which of the following is determined by the medium?

 (A) intensity
 (B) period
 (C) propagation speed
 (D) amplitude
 (E) frequency

203. Which of the following is *not* an acoustic variable?

 (A) density
 (B) pressure
 (C) temperature
 (D) force

204. Which of the following is an acoustic parameter?

 (A) wavelength
 (B) frequency
 (C) propagation speed
 (D) intensity
 (E) all of the above

205. What ultrasound method requires two active elements mounted side by side?

 (A) pulsed-wave Doppler
 (B) harmonic imaging
 (C) continuous-wave Doppler
 (D) spectral Doppler
 (E) power Doppler

206. The dimensionless index that indicates the likelihood of turbulence to occur is

    (A) rayls index
    (B) Bernoulli number
    (C) Poiseuille's index
    (D) Reynold's number
    (E) Rayleigh length

207. Which of the following arranges media in terms of propagation velocity, from lowest to highest?

    (A) air, fat, muscle, bone
    (B) bone, fat, air, muscle
    (C) bone, muscle, fat, air
    (D) muscle, air, fat, bone
    (E) air, muscle, bone, fat

208. As frequency increases, backscatter

    (A) decreases
    (B) does not change
    (C) increases
    (D) none of the above

209. What is the angle at which total reflection occurs called?

    (A) critical angle
    (B) refractive angle
    (C) reflectivity angle
    (D) diffraction angle
    (E) angle of incidence

210. The pulse repetition frequency

    (A) is the same as the pulse repetition period
    (B) is equal to the frame rate
    (C) increases when the depth of view increases
    (D) is equal to the number of scan lines per second

211. The units used for the duty factor are

    (A) rayls
    (B) hertz
    (C) dB/cm/MHz
    (D) unitless

212. The approximate value for the attenuation coefficient for 6 MHz ultrasound in soft tissue is

    (A) 3 dB/cm
    (B) 3 dB
    (C) 6 dB/cm
    (D) 6 dB

213. Normal incidence is the term used when the ultrasound beam strikes a boundary between two media at what angle?

    (A) parallel
    (B) orthogonal
    (C) any oblique angle
    (D) any obtuse angle

214. The amount of energy transmitted and/or reflected at the boundary between two media depends on

    (A) acoustic impedance mismatch
    (B) the frequency of the beam
    (C) the propagation speed of the first medium
    (D) the propagation speed of the second medium

215. Which of the following has a higher acoustic impedance coefficient?

    (A) solids
    (B) liquids
    (C) gas
    (D) clotted blood
    (E) fat

216. According to Snell's law, the transmission angle is greater than the incidence angle if the propagation speed

    (A) of medium 2 is greater than that of medium 1
    (B) of medium 1 is greater than that of medium 2
    (C) of the two media are equal
    (D) is calculated at 3 dB down

217. A reflected echo is received 39 μs after transmission; what is the depth of the interface?

    (A) 3 mm
    (B) 0.3 cm
    (C) 3 cm
    (D) 30 cm

218. The mirror image artifact is commonly seen around which of the following structures?

    (A) kidney
    (B) pancreas
    (C) spleen
    (D) diaphragm
    (E) blood cells

219. What type of artifact is seen with a bright tapering trail of echoes just distal to closely spaced strong reflectors?

(A) edge

(B) mirror image

(C) comet

(D) shadowing

(E) flash

220. Which of the following would be most likely to produce a comet tail artifact?

(A) liver–kidney interface

(B) spleen–kidney interface

(C) gas bubble–duodenum interface

(D) cystic mass–liver interface

221. The maximum Doppler shift frequency that can be sampled without aliasing is called

(A) second harmonic limit

(B) dispersion frequency limit

(C) Nyquist limit

(D) filter limit

222. The frequency bandwidth will typically be increased by

(A) increasing the quality factor

(B) increasing the pulse duration

(C) increasing the spatial pulse length

(D) increasing damping

(E) decreasing damping

223. The likelihood of aliasing in Doppler imaging can be reduced by

(A) increasing the pulse repetition frequency (PRF)

(B) increasing the Doppler angle

(C) shifting the baseline

(D) reducing the operating frequency

(E) all of the above

224. A reflected echo is received 52 μs after transmission; what is the depth of the interface?

(A) 2 cm

(B) 3 cm

(C) 4 cm

(D) 5 cm

225. Generally, ultrasound transducers have

(A) better axial resolution than lateral resolution

(B) better lateral resolution than axial resolution

(C) axial resolution and lateral resolution approximately equal

226. The pulse repetition frequency of an ultrasound unit is typically

(A) 1 Hz

(B) 10 Hz

(C) 100 Hz

(D) 1,000 Hz

(E) 10,000 Hz

227. What is the most common artifact in Doppler ultrasound?

(A) flash

(B) aliasing

(C) turbulent

(D) twinkle

(E) mirror

228. Approximately what percentage of the time is a typical pulsed ultrasound system capable of receiving echoes?

(A) 100%

(B) 99%

(C) 75%

(D) 50%

(E) less than 1%

229. If the frequency doubles, what happens to the wavelength?

(A) increases twofold

(B) increases fourfold

(C) decreases twofold

(D) decreases fourfold

(E) no change

230. Which of the following does not display a sector format?

(A) linear-sequenced array

(B) electronic-phased array

(C) annular phased array

(D) vector array

231. The equation for measuring acoustic impedance is

    (A) $\left(\dfrac{z_2 - z_1}{z_2 - z_1}\right)^2 \times 100$

    (B) $V = f\lambda$

    (C) Z (rayls) $= p$ (kg/m^3) $\times c$ (m/s)

    (D) $\dfrac{\sin i}{\sin r} = \dfrac{V_1}{V_2}$

232. Which of the following are most commonly used as an active element in ultrasound transducers?

    (A) lead zirconate titanate (PZT)

    (B) barium lead zirconate (BLZ)

    (C) lead metaniobate

    (D) quartz

    (E) polyvinylidene fluoride (PVDF)

233. An ultrasound pulse was transmitted from the transducer and strikes an interface and returns to the transducer. The transmitted and return time was 39 μs. What is the total distance traveled?

    (A) 2 cm

    (B) 3 cm

    (C) 4 cm

    (D) 5 cm

    (E) 6 cm

234. What is the total round-trip time in human tissue for reflected echo at a depth of 2 cm?

    (A) 6.5 μs

    (B) 13 μs

    (C) 26 μs

    (D) 39 μs

    (E) 52 μs

235. The pulse repetition frequency is

    (A) pulses emitted per second

    (B) time from the beginning of one pulse to the beginning of the next

    (C) time during which the pulse actually occurs

    (D) percentage of time the system is transmitting a pulse

236. Which of the following is the role of the pulser?

    (A) voltage generation to drive the transducer

    (B) gain adjustment for the receiver

    (C) beam focusing

    (D) beam steering

237. The type of artifact that produces a reduction in echoes distal to a highly reflective or highly attenuating structure is

    (A) enhancement

    (B) reverberation

    (C) shadowing

    (D) refraction

    (E) ring down

238. What is the Nyquist limit if the pulse repetition frequency is 18 kHz?

    (A) 2.5 kHz

    (B) 3.5 kHz

    (C) 5 kHz

    (D) 9 kHz

    (E) 18 kHz

239. Which of the following varies with distance from the transducer?

    (A) lateral resolution

    (B) frequency

    (C) axial resolution

    (D) spatial pulse length

240. In Figure 1–59, a period can be described by which number on the following diagram?

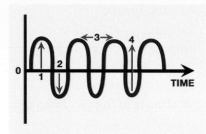

FIGURE 1–59.

    (A) #2

    (B) #1

    (C) #3

    (D) #4

241. Increasing axial resolution by increasing frequency also results in

    (A) decreased near-zone length

    (B) decreased penetration

    (C) decreased lateral resolution

    (D) decreased temporal resolution

242. **Reflection refers to**

    (A) the bending of the ultrasound beam as it crosses a boundary
    (B) narrowing the ultrasound beam
    (C) redirection of a portion of the ultrasound beam from a boundary
    (D) the scattering of the ultrasound beam in many directions

243. **If the transmitted frequency of the transducer is 3.5 MHz. What is the second harmonic frequency?**

    (A) 1.75 MHz
    (B) 3.5 MHz
    (C) 7 MHz
    (D) 2.5 MHz

244. **The term *bit* in computer science denotes**

    (A) binary digit
    (B) pixel
    (C) baud rate
    (D) matrix
    (E) picture element

245. **An 8-bit binary number is referred to as a**

    (A) byte
    (B) baud
    (C) pixel
    (D) voxel

246. **What is the purpose of employing an acoustic lens on transducers?**

    (A) decrease the spatial pulse length
    (B) increase the frequency bandwidth
    (C) steer the beam
    (D) narrowing of the ultrasound beam

247. **A needle or membrane hydrophone is used to measure**

    (A) pressure amplitude
    (B) mechanical index
    (C) thermal index
    (D) dead zone

248. **Viscosity is measured in units of**

    (A) megahertz
    (B) millimeters
    (C) poise
    (D) pascal
    (E) decibels

249. **Which one of the following will increase the speed of ultrasound?**

    (A) increased frequency
    (B) decreased frequency
    (C) increased tissue stiffness
    (D) decreased tissue stiffness

250. **The resistance to flow offered by a fluid in motion is called**

    (A) turbulence
    (B) eddies
    (C) variance
    (D) viscosity

251. **Autocorrelation is the mathematical process commonly used to detect**

    (A) aliasing
    (B) spectral dispersion
    (C) Doppler shifts
    (D) inertia

252. **A decrease in dynamic aperture results in**

    (A) increased temporal resolution
    (B) decreased lateral resolution
    (C) decreased the near-zone length
    (D) increased near-zone length

253. **Which one of the following would normally have the lowest viscosity?**

    (A) molasses
    (B) coupling gel
    (C) blood
    (D) water
    (E) mineral oil

254. **An 8-bit word microcomputer with 128K words of memory can store how many bits of data?**

    (A) 128
    (B) 1,000
    (C) 1,024
    (D) 128,000
    (E) 1,048,576

255. **Harmonics are created**

    (A) when the focal length is changed
    (B) when nonlinear oscillations occur in tissues
    (C) when acoustic lens are used
    (D) when the time gain compensation (TGC) is increased

256. Frequency compounding improves

(A) contrast resolution

(B) penetration depth

(C) temporal resolution

(D) lateral resolution

257. What is the unit for acoustic pressure?

(A) pascal

(B) poise

(C) torr

(D) erg

(E) watt

258. What does the horizontal axis (*x*-axis) on an M-mode display represent?

(A) amplitude

(B) brightness

(C) depth

(D) strength

(E) time

259. Which ultrasound frequency is commonly used in the clinical setting?

(A) 3.5 kHz

(B) 5 kHz

(C) 7 MHz

(D) 2.5 kHz

(E) 10 kHz

260. The ratio of the minimum to maximum signal amplitude that can be applied to a device without producing distortion is called

(A) Nyquist ratio

(B) dynamic range

(C) spectral range

(D) harmonic ratio

261. What does the vertical axis (*y*-axis) on an M-mode display represent?

(A) amplitude

(B) brightness

(C) depth

(D) strength

(E) time

262. Each binary digit can represent how many different digital memory states?

(A) 1

(B) 2

(C) 4

(D) 8

(E) 10

263. How many digits are utilized in a binary number?

(A) 1

(B) 2

(C) 4

(D) 10

264. What is the binary equivalent of the decimal number 30?

(A) 0110

(B) 1110

(C) 1001

(D) 1111

(E) none of the above

265. How many gray levels (echo amplitude levels) can a 4-bit deep digital scan converter store?

(A) 2

(B) 4

(C) 8

(D) 16

(E) 32

266. An ultrasound instrument that could represent 64 shades of gray would require how many bits memory?

(A) 8

(B) 6

(C) 4

(D) 16

(E) 24

267. What are the two categories of cavitation?

(A) turbulent and laminar

(B) stable and transient

(C) compression and rarefaction

(D) analog and digital

268. Which of the following functions are performed by the receiver in the ultrasound machine?

   (A) inspection, detection, correction, rejection, depression

   (B) randomization, amplification, modulation, rectification, limitation

   (C) amplification, compensation, compression, rejection

   (D) demodulation, contraction, band limitation, depolarization

269. A large amplitude voltage pulse from the pulser applied to the transducer results in

   (A) a long duration pulse from the transducer

   (B) a short duration pulse from the transducer

   (C) a small amplitude pressure pulse from the transducer

   (D) a large amplitude pressure pulse from the transducer

270. Voltage pulses from the pulser to the transducer are also used to

   (A) automatically adjust receiver gain

   (B) synchronize the receiver for the arrival time determination

   (C) adjust the gray-scale display dynamic range

   (D) determine field of view

271. The five major components of a pulse-echo ultrasound system are

   (A) flux capacitor, image memory, transducer, scan arm, amplifier

   (B) synchronizer, pulser, receiver, display, power supply

   (C) image memory, display, scan arm, time gain compensation (TGC) control, foot switch

   (D) transducer, receiver, image memory, pulser, display

   (E) amplification, compression, freeze, demodulation, reject

272. Transducers may be focused by internal focusing and external focusing. These are accomplished by

   (A) crystal thickness and/or by adding water path offset

   (B) concave transducer elements and/or by using an acoustic lens

   (C) "doping" the crystal with metal ions and/or by added damping

   (D) adjustment of frequency and/or crystal diameter

273. Which unit is used to specify the Q factor (quality factor)?

   (A) pascal

   (B) poise

   (C) Nyquist

   (D) Fresnel

   (E) none of the above

Questions 274 through 282: Match each term in Column A with the correct definition in Column B.

COLUMN A

274. acoustic shadow _____

275. acoustic enhancement _____

276. anechoic _____

277. artifact _____

278. echogenic _____

279. hyperechoic _____

280. hypoechoic _____

281. interface _____

282. sonolucent _____

COLUMN B

(A) without echoes

(B) echoes of lower amplitude than surrounding tissues

(C) the boundary between two media having different acoustic impedances

(D) an echo that does not correspond to a real structure

(E) reduction in echo amplitudes within a region distal to a strongly attenuating structure

(F) the property of a medium allowing easy passage of sound: low attenuation (echo-free)

(G) an increase in echo amplitudes within a region distal to a weakly attenuating structure

(H) echoes of higher amplitude than the normal surrounding tissues

(I) a structure that produces echoes

283. Which of the following is a commonly used backing material for continuous-wave Doppler transducers?

   (A) epoxy resin

   (B) cork

   (C) metal powder

   (D) tungsten powder

   (E) no backing material

284. Which one of the following is *not* associated with continuous-wave Doppler?

   (A) no backing material

   (B) no Nyquist limit

   (C) aliasing

   (D) no TGC

   (E) two transducers

285. The strength of the echo in B-mode ultrasound is displayed as

    (A) *y*-axis deflection
    (B) *x*-axis position
    (C) pixel brightness
    (D) decibels

286. Ultrasound cannot travel in which one of the following?

    (A) intravenous pyelogram (IVP) contrast
    (B) solid tissue
    (C) vacuum
    (D) blood
    (E) bone

287. Lambda (λ) represents

    (A) period
    (B) wavelength
    (C) frequency
    (D) velocity
    (E) intensity

288. The time it takes to complete a single cycle is called

    (A) period
    (B) wavelength
    (C) frequency
    (D) velocity
    (E) amplitude

289. A wave vibration at 20 cycles per second has a frequency of

    (A) 20 MHz
    (B) 20 Hz
    (C) 20 kHz
    (D) 120 kHz
    (E) 20,000 MHz

290. A wave vibrating at 1 million cycles per second has a frequency of

    (A) 1 GHz
    (B) 1 kHz
    (C) 1 MHz
    (D) 100 MHz
    (E) 1,000 MHz

291. A damaged active element in a mechanical transducer may result in

    (A) a horizontal band of signal dropout at a particular depth
    (B) the loss of an entire image
    (C) a reduced frame rate
    (D) a vertical line of dropout extending from the top to the bottom of the image

Questions 292 through 294: Match the question in Column A with the correct answer in Column B.

COLUMN A

292. Which statement best describes A-mode? _____

293. Which statement best describes B-mode? _____

294. Which statement best describes M-mode? _____

COLUMN B

(A) a graphic presentation with vertical spikes arising from a horizontal baseline; the height of the vertical spikes represents the amplitude of the deflected echo

(B) a two-dimensional image of internal body structures displayed as dots; the brightness of the dots is proportional to the amplitude of the echo; the image is applicable to both real-time and static scanners

(C) one-dimensional presentation of moving structures displayed in a pie-shaped or rectangular image; the image is applicable only to real-time scanners

(D) a graphic presentation of moving structures in a waveform; the display is presented as a group of lines representing the motion of moving interfaces versus time

295. A long dead zone may indicate

    (A) a fluid-filled mass
    (B) a short spatial pulse length
    (C) high tissue temperature
    (D) detached backing material
    (E) a high-frequency transducer was used

296. The frame rate in ultrasound is strongly affected by

    (A) transducer frequency
    (B) focal method
    (C) cavitation
    (D) spatial pulse length
    (E) imaging depth

297. Doppler signals and velocities cannot be measured at what Doppler angle?

   (A) 90°
   (B) 30°
   (C) 40°
   (D) 50°
   (E) 60°

298. A device used to visualize the dead zone.

   (A) radiation force balance
   (B) analog-digital converter
   (C) acoustic standoff
   (D) Schlieren camera

299. The intensity of the ultrasound beam from a pulsed-echo system

   (A) is measured in watts
   (B) is constant at all depths
   (C) will depend upon the beam diameter
   (D) is constant in time

300. Whose principle states that all points on an ultrasound waveform can be considered as point sources for the production of secondary spherical wavelets?

   (A) Doppler
   (B) Curie
   (C) Huygens
   (D) Nyquist
   (E) Snell

301. The fraction of time that a pulsed ultrasound system is actually producing ultrasound is called the

   (A) duty factor
   (B) Curie factor
   (C) frame rate
   (D) transmission factor
   (E) power

302. Real-time ultrasound transducers can be classified as

   (A) annular, sector, linear, and static scanners
   (B) sector scanners, vector, and annular
   (C) phased, linear, annular, and vector
   (D) linear sequenced array and vector

303. The speed at which ultrasound propagates within a medium depends primarily on

   (A) its frequency
   (B) the compressibility of the medium
   (C) its intensity
   (D) the thickness of the medium
   (E) aperture of the transducer

304. An artifact that results from a pulse that has traveled two or more round-trip distances between the transducer and the interface is called

   (A) a multipath
   (B) a side lobe
   (C) reverberation
   (D) scattering
   (E) mirror image

305. The ratio of output of electric power to input electric power is termed

   (A) power
   (B) intensity
   (C) gain
   (D) voltage
   (E) frequency

306. Multipath artifacts result from

   (A) echoes that return directly to the transducer
   (B) shotgun pellets
   (C) echoes that take an indirect path back to the transducer
   (D) sound wave propagates through a medium at a speed other than soft tissue
   (E) small amplitude echoes resulting from electrical interference

307. What type of noise is associated with Doppler shift?

   (A) clutter
   (B) speckle
   (C) flash
   (D) harmonics
   (E) aliasing

308. To achieve the best possible digital representation of an analog system, the echo signals should undergo

    (A) postprocessing
    (B) preprocessing
    (C) rectification
    (D) amplification
    (E) mechanical impedance

309. Near-zone length may be increased by increasing

    (A) wavelength
    (B) wavelength and bandwidth
    (C) small transducer aperture
    (D) high frequency and large diameter transducer
    (E) low frequency and small diameter transducer

Questions 310 through 319: Match each term in Column A with the correct definition in Column B.

COLUMN A

310. density _____
311. propagation _____
312. frequency _____
313. power _____
314. duty factor _____
315. bandwidth _____
316. acoustic impedance _____
317. absorption _____
318. quality factor _____
319. intensity _____

COLUMN B

    (A) rate at which work is done
    (B) mass divided by volume
    (C) conversion of sound to heat
    (D) number of cycles per unit time
    (E) density multiplied by sound propagation speed
    (F) range of frequencies contained in the ultrasound pulse
    (G) the fraction of time that the ultrasound pulse is on
    (H) progression or travel
    (I) operating frequency divided by bandwidth
    (J) power divided by area

320. Which of the following is a true definition for a highly damped transducer?

    (A) increased efficiency, sensitivity, and spatial pulse length
    (B) decreased efficiency, sensitivity, and spatial pulse length
    (C) increased efficiency and sensitivity, but decreased spatial pulse length
    (D) decreased efficiency, but increased sensitivity and spatial pulse length
    (E) no change in efficiency or sensitivity only in spatial pulse length

321. Gain compensation is necessary due to

    (A) reflector motion
    (B) gray scale
    (C) attenuation
    (D) resolution
    (E) none of the above

322. The frequency bandwidth may be determined by which of the following?

    (A) spectral analysis
    (B) Schlieren system
    (C) hydrophone analysis
    (D) cathode analysis
    (E) refraction

323. Which of the following is *not* true of power output?

    (A) bioeffects concerns
    (B) does not affect signal-to-noise ratio
    (C) can be used to change the brightness of the entire image
    (D) alters patient exposure
    (E) should be decreased first if the image is too bright

324. What is the gray-scale resolution for a 5-bit digital instrument that has a dynamic range of 42 dB?

    (A) 1.9 dB
    (B) 3 dB
    (C) 1.3 dB
    (D) 0.07 dB
    (E) 13.0 dB

325. If it takes 0.01 seconds for a pulse emitted by the transducer to reach an echo source of soft tissue, what distance must the pulse travel to be recorded?

    (A) 1,540 cm
    (B) 30.8 m
    (C) 15.4 m
    (D) 1.54 m
    (E) 20.8 m

326. An artifact that is produced from interaction of the incident beam with a curved surface and that results in an acoustic shadow is referred to as

    (A) a ghost artifact
    (B) an edge artifact
    (C) a comet tail artifact
    (D) a ring down artifact
    (E) enhancement artifact

327. An artifact that results from refraction of the ultrasound beam at a muscle–fat interface and that gives rise to double images is called

(A) a split image artifact

(B) an edge artifact

(C) a comet tail artifact

(D) a ring down artifact

(E) speckle artifact

328. An artifact that would *least* likely produce a pseudo-mass is

(A) a comet tail artifact

(B) a multipath artifact

(C) a mirror image artifact

(D) a slide lobe artifact

(E) ghost artifact

329. Split image artifact is more noticeable in

(A) athletic patients and mesomorphic habitus patients

(B) patients with underdeveloped rectus muscle

(C) mesomorphic habitus patients and patients with underdeveloped rectus muscle

(D) all of the above

330. Select the *least* likely cause or causes for a split image artifact.

(A) abdominal scar

(B) lateral margins of the rectus muscles

(C) gas bubble

(D) refraction of the sound beam at a muscle–fat interface

(E) superficial abdominal skin keloids

331. What is the *most* likely cause for a beam thickness artifact?

(A) metallic surgical clips

(B) gas bubble

(C) partial volume effect

(D) shotgun pellets

(E) abdominal scar

332. Beam thickness artifact is primarily dependent on

(A) position of the patient

(B) gas bubble

(C) beam angulation

(D) gravity

(E) body fat

333. Which of the following is *not* true for side-lobe artifact?

(A) caused by multiple side lobes of the transducer

(B) direction is different from the main beam

(C) may be diffuse or specular in appearance

(D) the side-lobe beam is stronger than the primary beam

(E) apodization is used to reduce side lobe artifact

334. Which of the following is *least* likely to produce an acoustic shadow?

(A) bone interface

(B) metallic surgical clips

(C) gallstones

(D) gas interface

(E) calcifications

335. The most common type of artifact encountered in patients with shotgun wounds is

(A) comet tail artifact

(B) multipath artifact

(C) mirror image artifact

(D) side lobe artifact

(E) wound-skin artifact

336. The type of reverberation echo that usually results from a small gas bubble and appears as a high-amplitude echo occurring at regular intervals is called a

(A) multipath artifact

(B) mirror image artifact

(C) side lobe artifact

(D) ring-down artifact

(E) flash artifact

337. The amount of splitting that occurs in a split image artifact for a given structure

(A) can be calculated using Snell's law

(B) cannot be calculated because it is an artifact

(C) can be calculated using the equation $Z = pV$

(D) can be calculated using a 5 MHz transducer with the equation: split (m/s) = $D\pi/T$

(E) can be calculated using Luez's law

338. The first vertical deflection on the A-mode that corresponds to the transducer face is called

    (A) bistable
    (B) side lobe
    (C) main bang
    (D) gain
    (E) x-axis

339. The type of real-time system that employs a combination of electronic and mechanical means is called

    (A) wobbler sector real-time
    (B) rotating wheel real-time
    (C) annular-array real-time
    (D) linear-sequenced array
    (E) vector array

340. If the amount of acoustic coupling medium is insufficient, what changes could result?

    (A) A decrease in amplitude of the returning echo.
    (B) A increase in amplitude of the returning echo.
    (C) The transducer will slide on the skin easier.
    (D) No effect on the image.
    (E) An increased penetration into the tissue.

341. A technique in which scan lines are directed in multiple directions and then combined together to create one image is called?

    (A) spatial compounding
    (B) elastography
    (C) coded excitation
    (D) combined operating mode
    (E) clutter

Questions 342 through 344: Each diagram represents modes of operation used in diagnostic ultrasound.

342. Identify the type of mode displayed in the following diagram (Fig. 1–60).

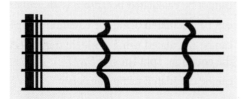

FIGURE 1–60.

    (A) B-mode
    (B) A-mode

    (C) M-mode
    (D) C-mode
    (E) QB-mode

343. Identify the type of mode displayed in the following diagram (Fig. 1–61).

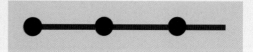

FIGURE 1–61.

    (A) B-mode
    (B) A-mode
    (C) M-mode
    (D) C-mode
    (E) QB-mode

344. Identify the type of mode displayed in the following diagram (Fig. 1–62).

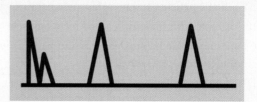

FIGURE 1–62.

    (A) B-mode
    (B) A-mode
    (C) M-mode
    (D) C-mode
    (E) QB-mode

345. The undesired effects of diagnostic ultrasound on human soft tissue as a result of interaction with the ultrasound beam are called

    (A) sensitivity effects
    (B) biologic effects
    (C) neurologic effects
    (D) radiation poisoning
    (E) electromagnetic effect

346. What is the average propagation speed of ultrasound in soft tissue?

    (A) 1,540 m/s
    (B) 1.54 mm/μs
    (C) 0.154 cm/μs
    (D) one mile per second
    (E) all of the above

Questions 347 through 350: Identify the regions on the diagram (Fig. 1–63) below by filling in the blanks.

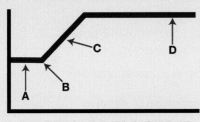

DIAGRAM OF TGC CURVE

FIGURE 1–63.

347. slope _____

348. delay _____

349. far gain _____

350. near gain _____

Questions 351 through 360: Match each term in Column A with the correct definition in Column B.

COLUMN A

351. attenuation _____

352. elastography _____

353. bit _____

354. cavitation _____

355. coupling medium _____

356. damping _____

357. gray scale _____

358. matching layer _____

359. pixel _____

360. static imaging _____

COLUMN B

(A) picture element
(B) the production and behavior of microbubbles within a medium
(C) progressive weakening of the sound beam as it travels through a medium
(D) a liquid placed between the transducer and the skin
(E) the number of intensity levels between black and white
(F) imaging technique to assess tissue stiffness
(G) binary digit
(H) a method of reducing pulse duration by electrical or mechanical means
(I) single-frame imaging
(J) plastic material placed in front of the transducer face to reduce the reflection at the transducer surface

361. The intensity of ultrasound is measured in

(A) kg/m^3
(B) N/m^2
(C) Hz

(D) W/cm^2
(E) MHz

362. The imaging technique that allows previous hidden structures beneath highly attenuating objects to become visible is called

(A) spatial compounding
(B) elastography
(C) coded excitation
(D) combined operating mode
(E) clutter

363. The acronym SPTA denotes

(A) static probe transmission amplitude
(B) static probe transmission absorption
(C) spatial peak temporal average
(D) sound propagation temperature artifact

Questions 364 through 370: Match the quantity in Column A with the correct unit in Column B.

COLUMN A

364. density _____

365. speed _____

366. frequency _____

367. work _____

368. intensity _____

369. wavelength _____

370. attenuation _____

COLUMN B

(A) W/cm^2
(B) kg/m^3
(C) mm
(D) m/s
(E) Joule (J)
(F) Hz
(G) dB

371. The general range of intensities in diagnostic ultrasound is

(A) $0.5 \ W/cm^2$–$2.0 \ W/cm^2$ SPTA
(B) $0.002 \ W/cm^2$–$0.5 \ W/cm^2$ SPTA
(C) $50 \ W/cm^2$–$100 \ W/cm^2$ SPTA
(D) $100 \ W/cm^2$ SPTA to $1,000 \ W/cm^2$ SPTA
(E) the general range of intensities in diagnostic ultrasound is unknown

372. The general range of intensities in therapeutic ultrasound is

(A) $0.5 \ W/cm^2$–$2.0 \ W/cm^2$ SPTA
(B) $0.002 \ W/cm^2$–$0.5 \ W/cm^2$ SPTA
(C) $50 \ W/cm^2$–$100 \ W/cm^2$ SPTA
(D) $20.5 \ W/cm^2$–$30.0 \ W/cm^2$ SPTA
(E) the general range of intensities in therapeutic ultrasound is unknown

373. Which of the following characteristics does *not* apply to diagnostic ultrasound at normal diagnostic intensity levels?

   (A) noninvasive
   (B) atraumatic
   (C) ionizing
   (D) nontoxic
   (E) absorption

374. What is the most common result of high-intensity ultrasound?

   (A) cavitation
   (B) brain damage
   (C) fetal developmental anomalies
   (D) heat
   (E) mitosis of cells

375. In the study of bioeffects, what does cavitation denote?

   (A) production and behavior of gas bubbles
   (B) necrosis
   (C) cell membrane rupture
   (D) chromosome breakage
   (E) mitosis of cells

376. What are the two types of cavitation?

   (A) silent and noisy
   (B) micro and macro
   (C) membrane and nonmembrane
   (D) stable and transient
   (E) heat and absorption

377. An instrument used to detect frequency shift is called

   (A) Doppler
   (B) real-time
   (C) A-mode
   (D) static scanner
   (E) hydrophone

378. Specular reflections

   (A) occur when the interface is larger than the wavelength
   (B) occur when the interface is smaller than the wavelength
   (C) arise from interfaces smaller than 3 mm
   (D) are not dependent on the angle of incidence
   (E) occur at irregular surface interfaces

379. Nonspecular reflections

   (A) occur when the interface is larger than the wavelength
   (B) occur when the interface is smaller than the wavelength
   (C) arise from mirror-like surfaces
   (D) are beam-angle dependent
   (E) occur at a smooth boundary

380. The acronym SATA denotes

   (A) static amplitude transmission average
   (B) spatial average temporal average
   (C) spatial average tissue absorption
   (D) sound attenuation transmission average
   (E) safety accuracy in tissue acoustic

381. The acronym SPPA denotes

   (A) static probe power average
   (B) static probe transmission absorption
   (C) spatial peak pulse average
   (D) sound propagation performance average
   (E) safety parameters and protocols for acoustics

382. Which mode is *not* applicable to a Doppler instrument?

   (A) A-mode
   (B) pulsed
   (C) continuous
   (D) audible
   (E) duplex

383. Which of the following transducers would be *most* useful for imaging superficial structures?

   (A) 5 MHz, short-focus
   (B) 3 MHz, long-focus
   (C) 5 MHz, long-focus
   (D) 2.5 MHz, short-focus
   (E) 3.5 MHz, short-focus

384. Which of the following transducers would be *most* useful for good penetration on an obese patient?

   (A) 5 MHz, short-focus
   (B) 3 MHz, long-focus
   (C) 5 MHz, long-focus
   (D) 2.5 MHz, short-focus
   (E) 10 MHz, long-focus

385. The digital memory represents a picture element called a

(A) pixel

(B) electrons

(C) real-time

(D) matrix

(E) phosphors

386. How many shades of gray can the human eye distinguish?

(A) about 16 shades

(B) between 150 and 250 shades

(C) more than 512 shades

(D) more than 1,000 shades

(E) 256 shades

387. The most recent digital storage employs what size memory?

(A) $512 \times 512 \times 8$-bit deep and 256 shades

(B) $64 \times 64 \times 2$-bit deep

(C) $128 \times 128 \times 4$-bit deep

(D) $16 \times 16 \times 2$-bit deep

(E) $30 \times 30 \times 6$-bit deep and 16 shades

388. Which of the following is a disadvantage of pulsed-wave (PW) Doppler relative to continuous-wave (CW) Doppler?

(A) It is unidirectional.

(B) The Doppler shift depends on frequency.

(C) It is subject to "aliasing".

(D) It does not provide in-depth information.

389. Which of the following does not utilize gain?

(A) duplex imaging

(B) real-time system

(C) continuous-wave Doppler

(D) color Doppler

(E) all of the above

390. What is the effect of ultrasound absorption on tissues at normal intensity levels?

(A) dissipation of heat by conduction

(B) significant temperature elevations

(C) proliferation of tissues

(D) necrosis

(E) cavitation

391. Which of the following is *not* an advantage of continuous-wave Doppler?

(A) ability to measure very high velocities

(B) the absence of aliasing

(C) small probe size

(D) ability to use high frequency

(E) range ambiguity

392. Turbulent flow is most likely to occur in which one of the following situations?

(A) high velocities and acute anemia

(B) small diameter and high viscosity

(C) small diameter and high hematocrit

(D) large diameter, low velocity, and polycythemia

(E) large diameter, low velocity, and low viscosity

393. Which one of the following can be used to decrease the likelihood of aliasing on aspectral analysis?

(A) using higher transducer frequency

(B) decreasing the pulse repetition frequency (PRF)

(C) decreasing the Doppler shift

(D) lowering the baseline

394. Temporal resolution is decreased with all of the following *except*

(A) wide sector

(B) shallow imaging

(C) high line density

(D) increased 2D depth

(E) lower frame rate

395. Which one of the following *most* likely is a contributor to aliasing?

(A) high frequency

(B) continuous Doppler

(C) high pulse repetition frequency (PRF)

(D) slow blood velocity

(E) lower frequency

396. Digital memory can be visualized as

(A) squares on a checkerboard

(B) a transducer

(C) an electron beam

(D) a hydrophone

(E) a beam of light

397. A region that is anechoic is displayed as

    (A) echo-free
    (B) echogenic
    (C) hyperechoic
    (D) hypoechoic
    (E) isoechoic

398. A region that is hyperechoic is

    (A) anechoic
    (B) echogenic
    (C) echo-free
    (D) transonic
    (E) isoechoic

399. Which of the following cannot be measured by a hydrophone?

    (A) acoustic pressure
    (B) spatial pulse length
    (C) impedance
    (D) intensity
    (E) period

400. The hydrophone is made up of

    (A) algae inhibitor and alcohol to mimic soft tissue speed
    (B) small transducer elements
    (C) acrylic plastic sheets
    (D) gelatin and vinyl chloride
    (E) stainless steel pins

401. Bioeffects at medium intensity levels on laboratory animals have resulted in

    (A) cancer
    (B) death
    (C) growth retardation
    (D) no effects
    (E) tissue necrosis

402. Which of the following is the *least* likely cause for attenuation?

    (A) absorption
    (B) reflection
    (C) refraction
    (D) scattering
    (E) bone

403. Absorption refers to

    (A) bending of the sound beam crossing a boundary
    (B) conversion of sound to heat
    (C) redirection of a portion of the sound from a boundary beam
    (D) redirection of the sound beam in several directions
    (E) conversion of heat to sound

404. Diffraction refers to

    (A) spreading-out of the ultrasound beam
    (B) conversion of sound to heat
    (C) redirection of a portion of the sound from a boundary beam
    (D) bending of the sound beam crossing a boundary
    (E) the narrowing of the sound beam

405. Scattering refers to

    (A) bending the sound beam crossing a boundary
    (B) conversion of sound to heat
    (C) redirection of a portion of the sound from a boundary beam
    (D) redirection of the sound beam in several directions
    (E) all of the above

406. The method for sterilizing transducers is

    (A) heat sterilization
    (B) steam
    (C) recommended by the transducer manufacturer
    (D) autoclave
    (E) ethylene oxide

407. An example of an acoustic window is

    (A) liver interface
    (B) rib interface
    (C) tissue/air interface
    (D) tissue/bone interface
    (E) none of the above

408. The binary number 1010 equals the decimal number

    (A) 10
    (B) 11
    (C) 110
    (D) 200
    (E) 101

409. **What are the lowest intensity measurements that are used in diagnostic ultrasound?**

    (A) SPPA

    (B) SATP

    (C) SPTP

    (D) SAPA

    (E) SATA

410. **What is the intensity that is used in diagnostic ultrasound to measure the potential biological effects in mammalian tissue?**

    (A) SATA

    (B) SPTA

    (C) SPTP

    (D) SAPA

    (E) SATP

411. **Which is the recommended orientation for a transverse scan?**

    (A) all transverse scans should be viewed from the patient's feet.

    (B) all transverse scans should be viewed from the patient's head.

    (C) all transverse scans should be viewed lateral from the patient's right side.

    (D) all transverse scans should be viewed lateral from the patient's left side.

    (E) there is no standard image orientation for transverse scans.

412. **What is the recommended orientation for longitudinal scans?**

    (A) the patient's head to the right of the image and feet to the left of the image

    (B) the patient's head to the left of the image and feet to the right of the image

    (C) the patient's head to the top (anterior) of the image and feet to the bottom (posterior) of the image

    (D) scans should be viewed from the patient's feet

    (E) there is no standard image orientation for longitudinal scans

413. **Demodulation is a function performed by which of the following?**

    (A) pulser

    (B) amplifier

    (C) receiver

    (D) transmitter

    (E) transducer

414. **Which of the following statements about ultrasound waves is *not* true?**

    (A) ultrasound waves are mechanical vibrating energy.

    (B) ultrasound waves can be polarized.

    (C) ultrasound waves are not part of the electromagnetic spectrum.

    (D) ultrasound waves cannot travel in a vacuum.

    (E) ultrasound waves are longitudinal waves.

415. **The transducer crystal *most* likely to be employed in high-frequency work, above 18 MHz, is**

    (A) lithium sulfate

    (B) lead zirconate titanate

    (C) Rochelle salt

    (D) quartz

    (E) barium titanate

416. **Lead zirconate titanate has which of the following advantages over other ceramic materials?**

    (A) easy to shape

    (B) effective at low voltage

    (C) inexpensive

    (D) greater temperature stability

    (E) all of the above

417. **All of the following statements about a linear-phased transducer is true *except*?**

    (A) produces a sector image

    (B) the sound beam is focused electronically

    (C) has multiple-focusing capability

    (D) elements are fired in successive groups

    (E) all scan lines are perpendicular to the transducer face

418. **How many shades of gray can be displayed using a scan converter with 8 bits per memory element?**

    (A) 16

    (B) 30

    (C) 128

    (D) 256

    (E) 525

419. **The highest intensity measurements used in diagnostic ultrasound denoted by which of the following?**

    (A) SATA

    (B) SATP

    (C) SPTA

    (D) SPTP

    (E) SPPA

420. **What is the difference between real-time ultrasound and x-ray fluoroscopy?**

    (A) ultrasound does not always require contrast media.

    (B) fluoroscopy has potential biologic effects; whereas, ultrasound has no known biologic effects at normal intensity level.

    (C) ultrasound is nonionizing.

    (D) ultrasound cannot travel in a vacuum and x-rays can travel in a vacuum.

    (E) all of the above.

421. **Which of the following contrast media used in x-rays can obscure the propagation of ultrasound?**

    (A) barium sulfate ($BaSO_4$) for upper GI examination

    (B) hypaque for IVP examination

    (C) LOCA intravenous injection dyes

    (D) Telepaque for oral cholecystogram

    (E) all of the above

Questions 422 through 430: Match each term in Column A with the correct definition in Column B.

COLUMN A

422. acoustic lens _____

423. pixel _____

424. sector _____

425. acousto-optical converter _____

426. side lobe _____

427. wavefront _____

428. rayl _____

429. Snell's law _____

430. Doppler effect _____

COLUMN B

    (A) unit of impedance

    (B) the portion of the sound beam outside of the main beam

    (C) picture element

    (D) pie shaped

    (E) a change in frequency as a result of reflector motion between the transducer and the reflector

    (F) a device that changes sound waves into visible light patterns

    (G) the ratio between the angle of incidence and the refraction

    (H) imaginary surface passing through particles of the same vibration as an ultrasound wave

    (I) a device used to focus sound beams

431. **Lateral resolution is equal to**

    (A) the wavelength

    (B) the beam diameter

    (C) the near-zone length

    (D) the wave number

    (E) damping material

432. **Which of the following materials is *not* used to make acoustic lenses?**

    (A) aluminum

    (B) Perspex (acrylic plastic)

    (C) polystyrene

    (D) ethylene oxide

    (E) all of the above

433. **Ultrasound beams can be focused and defocused with the use of**

    (A) a concave or convex mirror

    (B) acoustic lenses

    (C) both A and B

    (D) ultrasound beam cannot be focused; only light can be focused

    (E) all of the above

434. **What is the normal range of wavelength in medical application?**

    (A) 0.77–0.15 mm

    (B) 1.5–5.4 mm

    (C) 2–5 mm

    (D) 5.5–15 mm

    (E) 0.1–1.0 mm

435. **Which of the following cannot be distinguished on diagnostic ultrasound?**

    (A) tissue

    (B) solid mass

    (C) individual cells

    (D) male and female genitalia

    (E) nerve

436. **Density is defined as**

    (A) unit of impedance

    (B) force divided by area

    (C) force multiplied by displacement

    (D) mass per unit volume

    (E) unit of pressure

437. **Ultrasound absorption is directly proportional to**

    (A) viscosity

    (B) frequency

    (C) distance

    (D) increased collagen content

    (E) all of the above

438. The confirmed bioeffect(s) on pregnant women with the use of real-time diagnostic instruments is (are)

(A) brain damage
(B) fetal developmental anomalies
(C) growth retardation
(D) no known effect
(E) lung hemorrhage

439. The confirmed bioeffects on pregnant mice exposed to continuous-wave ultrasound in a laboratory setting have resulted in

(A) cancer
(B) death
(C) hemorrhage
(D) necrotic tissue
(E) no known effect

440. Which of the following combinations of frequency and intensity would *most* likely result in cavitation?

(A) high frequency and low intensity
(B) low frequency and high intensity
(C) high frequency and high intensity
(D) low frequency and low intensity
(E) intensity has no effect on cavitation

Questions 441 through 448: Match each term in Column A with the correct definition in Column B.

COLUMN A	COLUMN B
441. in vivo _____	(A) an in vivo phenomenon characterized by erythrocytes within small vessels stopping the flow and collecting in the low pressure regions of the standing wave field
442. in vitro _____	
443. spectral analysis _____	
444. viscoelasticity _____	(B) elimination of small amplitude echo
445. rejection _____	(C) a process of acoustic energy absorption
446. relaxation _____	(D) energy transported per unit time
447. real cell stasis _____	(E) tissue cultures in a test tube
448. acoustic power _____	(F) a method of analyzing a waveform
	(G) the property of a medium characterized by energy distortion in the medium and irreversibly converted to heat
	(H) living human tissue

449. Which of the following statements about bioeffects is (are) unconfirmed?

(A) ultrasound exposure in humans is accumulative.
(B) most harmful bioeffects that occurred in experimental conditions have been confirmed in humans in a clinical setting.
(C) intensity, frequency, and exposure time used on experimental animals were compatible to those used in a clinical setting.
(D) continuous wave used in experimental studies gives the same tissue exposure as pulsed ultrasound used in a clinical setting.
(E) the exposure of pregnant women to high intensity levels resulted in growth retardation of their offspring.
(F) all of the above are false or unconfirmed.

450. The number of known human injuries resulting from diagnostic medical ultrasound exposure is

(A) 2,500 in England
(B) 115 in the United States
(C) 1,500 in Japan
(D) 5 cases in last 10 years
(E) no exposure injuries in humans have been reported

451. What is the distinction between real-time scans and B-scans?

(A) no distinction; real-time scans are B-scans.
(B) Real-time scans display gray-scale images, whereas B-scans display bistable images.
(C) Real-time scans exhibit motion images, whereas B-scans exhibit static images.
(D) B-scans are specific for static scanners; real-time scans are not.

452. Transonic regions are always

(A) echo-free
(B) anechoic
(C) echogenic
(D) uninhibited to propagation
(E) isoechoic

453. Which of the following is *not* related to real-time?

(A) A-mode
(B) static imaging
(C) dynamic imaging
(D) M-mode
(E) color Doppler

454. Which of the following is *not* a component of the time gain compensation (TGC) curve?

    (A) gray scale
    (B) far gain
    (C) knee
    (D) delay
    (E) slope

455. The range of pulse repetition frequencies used in diagnostic ultrasound is

    (A) 4–15 kHz
    (B) 2.5–10 MHz
    (C) 2.5–3.5 kHz
    (D) 10–15 MHz
    (E) 0.5–4 MHz

456. The spatial pulse length is defined as the product of the _____ multiplied by the number of _____ in a pulse.

    (A) cycles; frequency
    (B) frequency; velocity
    (C) wavelength; cycles
    (D) frequency; wavelength
    (E) amplitude; distance

457. Which of the following is (are) one-dimensional?

    (A) B-mode and A-mode
    (B) A-mode and M-mode
    (C) B-mode
    (D) static imaging
    (E) color Doppler

458. When multiple images are created over time and organized to create one image, this is known as which of the following?

    (A) harmonic imaging
    (B) spatial compounding
    (C) autocorrelation
    (D) frequency compounding
    (E) fast Fourier transform (FFT)

459. Which imaging modality is audible?

    (A) x-ray
    (B) ultrasound
    (C) Doppler
    (D) computed tomography (CT)
    (E) harmonic imaging

460. Which mode requires two crystals: one for transmitting and one for receiving?

    (A) A-mode
    (B) M-mode
    (C) continuous-wave mode
    (D) pulse-echo mode
    (E) power Doppler

Question 461 through 464: Fill in the blanks by correlating with the letters in Fig. 1-64

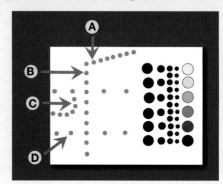

FIGURE 1–64.

461. (A) _____

462. (B) _____

463. (C) _____

464. (D) _____

465. The normal range of intensities used in Doppler instruments is

    (A) 0.2–400 W/cm^2
    (B) 0.2–400 mW/cm^2
    (C) 400–800 mW/cm^2
    (D) 800–900 mW/cm^2
    (E) 2.0–100 W/cm^2

466. If the media boundary is moving toward the source, the reflected sound wave will have

    (A) a higher frequency than the incident frequency
    (B) a lower frequency than the incident frequency
    (C) no change in frequency
    (D) be delayed
    (E) aliasing

467. If the media boundary is moving away from the source, this will result in

    (A) a higher frequency than the incident frequency
    (B) a lower frequency than the incident frequency
    (C) no change in frequency
    (D) aliasing
    (E) delayed sound

468. A Doppler instrument that can distinguish between positive and negative shifts is called

(A) bistable

(B) a modulator–demodulator

(C) bidirectional

(D) a polarized shifter

(E) Nyquist limit

469. Which statement about Doppler application is *not* true?

(A) Doppler color has slower velocities that are represented by lighter hues

(B) Doppler is within the audible range

(C) Doppler instruments use both pulsed and continuous wave

(D) Doppler can display an image

(E) Doppler cosine of 90° is zero

Questions 470 through 474: Match the time gain compensation (TGC) controls in Column A with the control functions in Column B.

COLUMN A

470. near gain _____

471. far gain _____

472. slope _____

473. delay _____

474. knee _____

COLUMN B

(A) control used to suppress or increase echoes in the far field

(B) control used to suppress or increase echoes in the near field

(C) control used to delay the start of the slope

(D) control the upward incline of the TGC, used to display an even texture

(E) controls the point where the slope ends

475. The range of frequencies contained in an ultrasound pulse is called

(A) intensity

(B) bandwidth

(C) power

(D) spatial pulse length

(E) duty factor

476. Which quantity is unitless?

(A) Q-factor

(B) volume

(C) intensity

(D) force

(E) period

477. Which of the following would be *most* likely to cause acoustic enhancement?

(A) a solid mass

(B) a urine-filled bladder

(C) a calcified mass

(D) a gallstone

(E) echogenic fluid

478. Which of the following would be *most* likely to cause acoustic shadowing?

(A) gallbladder

(B) a fluid-filled mass

(C) surgical clips

(D) urinary bladder

(E) echogenic fluid

479. Which of the following is not related to the sonographic description of blood flow?

(A) laminar

(B) pooling

(C) parabolic

(D) plug

(E) disturbed

480. The greatest Doppler angle is achieved

(A) when the beam strikes a vessel at a sharp right angle

(B) when the beam strikes a vessel perpendicular

(C) when the beam strikes a vessel at a 30° angle

(D) when the beam strikes a vessel at a 70° angle

(E) when the beam strikes a vessel at an orthogonal angle

481. If the power output of an amplifier is 100 times the power at the input, what is the gain?

(A) 10 dB

(B) 20 dB

(C) 30 dB

(D) 40 dB

(E) 60 dB

482. Which control is used to minimize the effects of attenuation?

(A) reject

(B) field-of-view

(C) frame rate

(D) time gain compensation

(E) depth

483. When an ultrasound beam passes obliquely across the boundary between two materials, what will occur if there is a difference in acoustic impedance in the two materials?

    (A) reflection, impedance

    (B) reflection, density

    (C) refraction, impedance

    (D) refraction, propagation speed

    (E) no change

484. A decreased pulse duration leads to which of the following?

    (A) better axial resolution

    (B) decreased spatial resolution

    (C) decreased longitudinal resolution

    (D) better lateral resolution

    (E) none of the above

485. What is the reflected intensity from a boundary between two materials if the incident intensity is 1 mW/cm^2 and the impedances are 25 and 75?

    (A) 0.25 mW/cm^2

    (B) 0.33 mW/cm^2

    (C) 0.50 mW/cm^2

    (D) 1.00 mW/cm^2

    (E) 100 mW/cm^2

486. The near-zone length of an unfocused transducer depends on

    (A) frequency and thickness

    (B) frequency and diameter

    (C) resolution and field of view

    (D) diameter and field of view

    (E) Time gain compensation

487. The frequency of a transducer depends primarily on which of the following?

    (A) overall gain

    (B) the speed of ultrasound

    (C) the element diameter

    (D) the element thickness

    (E) near and far gain

488. An ultrasound beam with a normal incident will experience no

    (A) attenuation

    (B) refraction

    (C) reflection

    (D) absorption

    (E) demodulation

489. What is the average speed of propagation of ultrasound in soft tissue?

    (A) 1,540 ft/s

    (B) 1.54 dB/cm

    (C) 1.54 mm/μs

    (D) 1,540 mW/cm^2

    (E) one mile per minute

490. The duty factor for a system with a pulse duration (PD) of 5 μs and a pulse repetition period (PRP) of 500 μs is

    (A) 0.1%

    (B) 0.5%

    (C) 1.0%

    (D) 10.0%

    (E) 100%

491. What increases the acoustic energy that a patient receives?

    (A) high frequency

    (B) wavelength

    (C) gain

    (D) examination time

492. Frequency is a significant factor in

    (A) propagation speed

    (B) tissue compressibility

    (C) tissue attenuation

    (D) transducer diameter

    (E) all of the above

493. In a pulse-echo system, a 3.5 MHz beam of 2 cm of tissue will be attenuated by

    (A) 3.5 dB/cm

    (B) 7.0 dB/cm

    (C) 3.5 dB

    (D) 7.0 dB

    (E) 30.0 dB

494. The characteristic acoustic impedance of a material is equal to the product of the material density and

    (A) path length

    (B) wavelength

    (C) frequency

    (D) propagation speed

    (E) power

495. In what area of a stenotic blood vessel does the maximum velocity of blood occur?

(A) within the stenosis
(B) before the stenosis
(C) after the stenosis
(D) before and after the stenosis
(E) one cm after the stenosis

496. For normal incidence, if the intensity reflection coefficient is 30%, the intensity transmission coefficient will be

(A) 15%
(B) 30%
(C) 60%
(D) 70%
(E) 100%

497. Turbulent flow is possible when blood flow exceeds what Reynolds number?

(A) 100
(B) 200
(C) 1,500
(D) 2,000
(E) 10

498. The range equation relates

(A) frequency, velocity, and wavelength
(B) frequency, velocity, and time
(C) distance, velocity, and time
(D) distance, frequency, and time
(E) incidence, reflection, and refraction

499. Which of the following predicts the onset of turbulent flow?

(A) dosimetry
(B) acoustic pressure
(C) Reynolds number
(D) wall thump
(E) flow detector

500. The Doppler shift frequency is zero when the angle between the receiving transducer and the flow direction is

(A) 0°
(B) 45°
(C) 90°
(D) 180°
(E) 190°

501. Turbulence flow occurs at what area of a stenotic blood vessel?

(A) within the stenosis
(B) before the stenosis
(C) after the stenosis
(D) before and after the stenosis
(E) all of the above

502. The dynamic range of a pulse-echo ultrasound system is defined as

(A) the ratio of the maximum to the minimum intensity that can be processed
(B) the range of propagation speeds
(C) the range of gain settings allowed
(D) the difference between the transmitted and the received ultrasound frequency
(E) none of the above

503. The thermal paper printer is not working, what is the first step?

(A) call the manufacturer for service
(B) check for a paper jam
(C) call biomedical services
(D) call the ultrasound supervisor
(E) call environmental services

504. The time gain or depth gain compensation control

(A) compensates for attenuation effects
(B) compensates for increased patient scan time
(C) compensates for machine malfunctions
(D) compensates for video-image drifts
(E) all of the above

505. A digital scan converter is essentially a

(A) radio receiver
(B) video monitor
(C) television set
(D) computer memory
(E) optical media

506. An increase in peak rarefactional pressure could result in which of the following?

(A) increased thermal index
(B) hypothermia of biological tissue
(C) necrotic tissue
(D) inertial cavitation
(E) cancer

507. Acoustic enhancement can be observed when scanning

    (A) highly attenuating structures
    (B) weakly attenuating structures
    (C) highly reflective structures
    (D) structures with large speed differences
    (E) surgical clips

508. Ultrasound depth penetration is inversely related to

    (A) period
    (B) propagation speed
    (C) magnification
    (D) frequency
    (E) aperture

509. Lateral resolution

    (A) is affected by the beam diameter
    (B) is affected by aperture size and acoustic lens
    (C) is improved at the focal zone
    (D) is improved with increased frequency
    (E) all of the above

510. If the lines per degree in a mechanical sector scanner remain constant, a decreased sector angle can result in

    (A) decreased resolution
    (B) increased frame rate
    (C) decreased frame rate
    (D) increased resolution
    (E) no change

511. What letter represents a group of nylon lines used to evaluate horizontal distance accuracy in this tissue-equivalent phantom (Fig. 1–65)?

    (A) line A
    (B) line B
    (C) line C
    (D) line D
    (E) line E

512. What letter represents a group of nylon lines used to evaluate range accuracy in this tissue-equivalent phantom (Fig. 1–65)?

    (A) line A
    (B) line B
    (C) line C
    (D) line D
    (E) line E

513. The advantages of continuous wave (CW) include all of the following *except*

    (A) ability to measure very high velocities
    (B) ability to use high frequencies
    (C) no aliasing
    (D) range ambiguity
    (E) no Nyquist limit

514. If the gain of an amplifier is 18 dB, what will the new gain setting be if the gain setting is reduced by one-half?

    (A) 9 dB
    (B) 36 dB
    (C) 15 dB
    (D) 0.5 dB
    (E) 18 dB

515. Decreasing the pulse repetition period

    (A) decreases spatial resolution
    (B) decreases axial resolution
    (C) decreases the maximum depth imaged
    (D) increases the maximum depth imaged
    (E) none of the above

516. The AIUM 100-mm test object is used to evaluate all of the following *except*

    (A) registration
    (B) dead zone
    (C) range accuracy
    (D) azimuthal resolution
    (E) attenuation

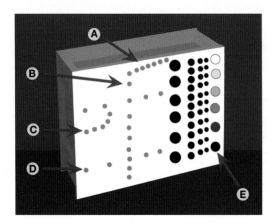

FIGURE 1–65.

517. A 3.5 MHz transducer is used on a patient with the ultrasound wave propagating the various tissues listed below. Which one will have the longest wavelength?

(A) muscle

(B) blood

(C) water

(D) fat

(E) lungs

518. What type of resolution is degraded in the presence of grating lobes and side lobes?

(A) lateral

(B) axial

(C) temporal

(D) range

(E) contrast

519. Spatial compounding improves the quality of the image in several ways *except*

(A) reducing the amount of reverberation and shadowing in the image

(B) reduced clutter artifacts

(C) structures previously hidden beneath distal acoustic shadow can be visualized

(D) creating multiple images in a single angle

520. A 7.5 MHz transducer is used on a patient with the ultrasound wave propagating various tissues listed below. Which one will have the shortest wavelength?

(A) muscle

(B) blood

(C) water

(D) fat

(E) lungs

521. The ability of a system to detect low-amplitude echoes accurately is referred to as

(A) resolution

(B) sensitivity

(C) accuracy

(D) dynamic accuracy

(E) registration accuracy

522. The primary mechanisms whereby ultrasound can produce biologic effects are

(A) thermal and cavitation

(B) absorption and reflection

(C) reflection and transmission

(D) photon energies and ultraviolet

(E) gamma rays and molecular electron

523. The near-zone length of a transducer depends on

(A) propagation speed and frequency

(B) frequency and transducer diameter

(C) field of view and transducer diameter

(D) magnification

(E) time gain compensation

524. The AIUM Committee on Biological Effects in 1991 stated what biologic effects with the use of ultrasound intensities below SPTA 100 mW/cm^2?

(A) has small amount reported cases of cancer of the fetal kidneys

(B) has no confirmed effects in mammalian

(C) result in maternal leukemia in mothers who had multiple sonograms during pregnancy

(D) mammalian effects was minimal

(E) minimal amount of neurological defects in sonographers after 20 years

525. The intensity of a focused beam is generally

(A) constant

(B) highest at the transducer surface

(C) highest at the focal zone

(D) lowest at the transducer surface

(E) lowest at the focal zone

526. The wavelength of a 5 MHz wave passing through soft tissue is approximately

(A) 0.1 mm

(B) 0.3 mm

(C) 0.5 mm

(D) 1.0 mm

(E) 3.0 mm

527. An echo that has undergone an attenuation of 3 dB will have an intensity that is _____ than its initial intensity.

(A) three times smaller

(B) three times larger

(C) two times smaller

(D) two times larger

(E) one time larger

528. Linear array transducers are commonly called

    (A) vector

    (B) phased

    (C) convex

    (D) annular

    (E) sequential

529. A 5 MHz transducer used in a pulse-echo system will generally produce

    (A) a wide band of frequencies centered at 5 MHz

    (B) frequencies only at 5 MHz

    (C) frequencies only at 5 MHz or multiples of 5 MHz

    (D) a wide band of frequencies above 5 MHz

    (E) a narrow band of frequencies centered at 5 MHz

530. The transducer _____ determines its _____.

    (A) diameter; intensity

    (B) damping; lateral resolution

    (C) thickness; sensitivity

    (D) thickness; resonance frequency

    (E) width; power

531. The axial resolution of a transducer can be improved with _____ but at the expense of _____.

    (A) increased damping; sensitivity

    (B) frequency; lateral resolution

    (C) focusing; sensitivity

    (D) focusing; lateral resolution

    (E) beam width; lateral resolution

532. A material that changes its dimensions when an electric field is applied is called which of the following?

    (A) piezoelectric

    (B) acoustic-optics

    (C) RAID

    (D) acoustic insulator

    (E) damping element

533. The process of making the impedance values on either side of a boundary as close as possible to reduce reflections is known as which of the following?

    (A) damping

    (B) refracting

    (C) matching

    (D) compensating

    (E) acoustic insulator

534. Which of the following data medium has the largest storage capacity used in diagnostic ultrasound?

    (A) flash drive

    (B) CD

    (C) magneto-optical

    (D) DVD

    (E) RAID

535. Shadowing occurs with

    (A) highly attenuating structures

    (B) large changes in propagation speed

    (C) low frequencies more often than with high frequencies

    (D) weak reflectors

    (E) highly propagated structures

536. Reverberation artifacts

    (A) occur most often at high frequencies

    (B) occur with multiple strong reflecting structures

    (C) occur only with real-time arrays

    (D) cannot occur in color Doppler systems

    (E) are more frequently seen in solid masses

537. A transducer with a large bandwidth is likely to have

    (A) good axial resolution

    (B) a large ring-down time

    (C) poor resolution

    (D) a high Q factor

    (E) poor axial resolution

538. The region of the ultrasound beam from the focus to beam diversion is called which of the following?

    (A) Fraunhofer zone

    (B) Fresnel zone

    (C) focal zone

    (D) divergence zone

    (E) acoustic focus

539. Refraction will not occur at an interface

    (A) when high frequencies are used

    (B) if the acoustic impedances are equal

    (C) if the propagation speeds are significantly different

    (D) with normal incidence of the ultrasound beam

    (E) when the propagation speed of the two media is the same

540. Acoustic power output is determined primarily by

(A) the diameter of the transducer

(B) the thickness of the transducer

(C) the pulser voltage spike

(D) focusing

(E) time gain compensation

541. Specular reflections occur when

(A) the reflecting object is small with respect to the wavelength

(B) the reflecting surface is large and smooth with respect to the wavelength

(C) the reflecting objects are moving

(D) the angle of incidence and angle of reflection are unequal

(E) diffuse reflection creates backscatter

542. The angle at which an ultrasound beam is bent as it passes through a boundary between two different materials is described mathematically by which of the following?

(A) Huygen's principle

(B) Curie's principle

(C) Snell's law

(D) Nyquist limit

(E) Rayleigh principle

543. What type of transducer is composed of multiple ring-shaped elements?

(A) annular

(B) linear sequential arrays

(C) trapezoidal

(D) phased array

(E) vector

544. The percentage of an ultrasound beam reflected at an interface between gas and soft tissue is approximately

(A) 90–100%

(B) 70–80%

(C) 45–55%

(D) 10–25%

(E) >1%

545. The percentage of an ultrasound beam reflected at an interface between fat and muscle is approximately

(A) 90–100%

(B) 70–80%

(C) 45–55%

(D) 15–25%

(E) 1–10%

546. Which of the following is a reason to use an acoustic standoff?

(A) to reduce tissue attenuation

(B) to move the focal zone closer to the skin surface

(C) to allow a lower frequency transducer to be used

(D) to move the focal zone deeper in the body structure

(E) to visualize deep image structures

547. Ultrasound waves in tissue are referred to as

(A) shear waves

(B) transverse waves

(C) vibrational waves

(D) longitudinal compression waves

(E) ultraviolet waves

548. High-frequency transducers have

(A) shorter wavelengths and less penetration

(B) longer wavelengths and greater penetration

(C) shorter wavelengths and greater penetration

(D) longer wavelengths and less penetration

549. When the piezoelectric crystal continues to vibrate after the initial voltage pulse, this is referred to as

(A) ring-down time

(B) pulse delay

(C) pulse retardation

(D) overdamping

(E) depolarization

550. Annular phased arrays, unlike linear phased arrays,

(A) can be dynamically focused

(B) electronically focus in two dimensions rather than one

(C) can be used in Doppler systems

(D) can achieve high frame rates

(E) electronically focus in one dimension

551. Which group is arranged in the correct order of increasing propagation speed?

(A) gas, bone, muscle

(B) bone, muscle, gas

(C) gas, muscle, bone

(D) muscle, bone, gas

(E) bone, tendon, muscle, blood, lungs

552. The lower useful range of diagnostic ultrasound is determined primarily by _____, whereas, the upper useful range is determined by _____.

    (A) resolution; penetration
    (B) scattering; propagation speed
    (C) cost; resolution
    (D) scattering; resolution

553. Convert the number 125,000,000,000 to engineering notation.

    (A) 125×10^{-11}
    (B) 1.25×10^{11}
    (C) 1.25×10^{-11}
    (D) 125×10^9
    (E) 125×10^6

554. Which of the following is true?

    (A) SPTA is always equal to or greater than SPTP
    (B) SPTP is always equal to or greater than SPTA
    (C) SATA is always equal to or greater than SATP
    (D) SPTA is always equal to or greater than SATP

555. A beam-intensity profile is often mapped with

    (A) dosimetry
    (B) acousto-optics
    (C) a hydrophone
    (D) AIUM test object
    (E) calorimeter

556. If the direction of flow is perpendicular to the sound beam, what is the velocity and cosine?

    (A) velocity is 1 and the cosine is 1
    (B) velocity is 0.87 and the cosine is 0.87
    (C) velocity is 0.5 and the cosine is 0.5
    (D) velocity is −1.0 and the cosine is −1.0
    (E) velocity is zero and the cosine is zero

557. The technique of passing an ultrasound beam through water so that compression and rarefaction of the water molecules allow the beam pattern to be measured is referred to as the

    (A) Doppler method
    (B) Schlieren method
    (C) hydrostatic method
    (D) water-density method
    (E) acousto-optics

558. Pulse duration is the _____ for a pulse to occur.

    (A) space
    (B) range
    (C) intensity
    (D) time
    (D) distance

559. A 10 MHz Doppler transducer is used with a PRF of 2,000 Hz with an image depth of 12 cm. What is the Nyquist frequency?

    (A) 20 Hz
    (B) 24 dB
    (C) 1 kHz
    (D) 1 dB
    (E) 2,000 Hz

560. What is the unit of measure of SPTA?

    (A) dB
    (B) W/cm^2
    (C) W
    (D) Hz
    (E) MHz

561. The piezoelectric properties of a transducer will be lost if the crystal is heated above the

    (A) crystal point
    (B) dynamic range
    (C) Curie point
    (D) dead zone
    (E) Nyquist limit

562. If the amplitude of a wave is increased threefold, the intensity will

    (A) decrease threefold
    (B) increase threefold
    (C) increase ninefold
    (D) increase sixfold
    (E) intensity does not change with the increase in amplitude

563. Which of the following is used to improve the signal-to-noise ratio?

    (A) output power
    (B) near gain
    (C) far gain
    (D) receiver gain

564. If the frequency is increased, the _____ will be _____.

    (A) velocity; increased

    (B) attenuation; decreased

    (C) velocity; decreased

    (D) velocity; unchanged

565. Beam steering is achieved in a linear phased array by

    (A) mechanical motion

    (B) electronic time-delay pulsing

    (C) an acoustic lens

    (D) dynamic focusing

566. Dynamic focusing

    (A) is made possible by array-based systems

    (B) is made possible by acoustic lens

    (C) is not possible in a linear-switched array

    (D) is often used in single-element systems

567. Adjusting the overall gain will increase or decrease the brightness of the image due to which of the following?

    (A) amplification of the receiver voltage

    (B) magnification

    (C) amplification of the transmitted pulse

    (D) temperature of the tissue

    (E) kinetic energy

568. Sound will travel _____ in 1 μs in soft tissue.

    (A) 1,540 m

    (B) 1.54 cm

    (C) 1.54 mm

    (D) 0.75 mm

    (E) one mile per minute

569. The arrow in Fig. 1–66 points to which of the following?

    (A) ring-down artifact

    (B) mirror image artifact

    (C) side lobe artifact

    (D) ghost artifact

    (E) distal acoustic shadow

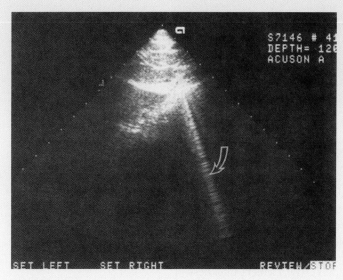

FIGURE 1–66.

570. In the image in Fig. 1–67, that represents a tissue-equivalent phantom, what do the small open arrowheads point to?

    (A) rods for measuring dead zone

    (B) parallel rods used for horizontal calibration

    (C) rods used for axial resolution

    (D) rods used for measuring registration

    (E) simulated cystic mass

571. In the image in Fig. 1–67, that represents a tissue-equivalent phantom, what does the curved open arrow point to?

    (A) a dead zone

    (B) a simulated solid lesion

    (C) a ghost artifact

    (D) a side lobe artifact

    (E) a simulated cystic mass

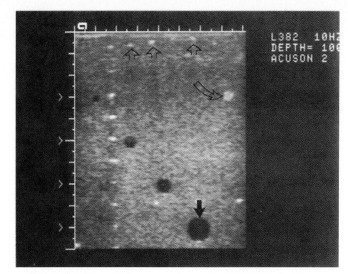

FIGURE 1–67.

572. In the image in Fig. 1–67, that represents a tissue-equivalent phantom, what does the solid black arrow point to?

    (A) a ghost artifact
    (B) a dead zone
    (C) a simulated cyst
    (D) a side lobe artifact
    (E) a simulated solid mass

573. What determines the frequency of the transducer?

    (A) beam shape
    (B) aperture
    (C) matching layer
    (D) element thickness
    (E) time gain compensation

574. At the present time, most ultrasound contrast agents are based upon

    (A) radiopaque media
    (B) higher viscosity liquids
    (C) iodine contrast media
    (D) gas-filled microbubbles
    (E) barium sulfate

575. Microspheres filled with which of the following materials are currently used as an ultrasound contrast agent?

    (A) xenon
    (B) perfluorocarbon
    (C) iodine
    (D) gadolinium
    (E) barium sulfate

576. As the pulse repetition frequency is increased, what is the potential effect?

    (A) depth of view increases
    (B) depth of view decreases
    (C) repetition period increases
    (D) poor spatial resolution
    (E) decreased frame rate

577. Acoustic clutter and ghosting artifact can be eliminated with

    (A) magnification
    (B) time gain compensation
    (C) acoustic power
    (D) autocorrelation
    (E) wall filter

578. What type of noise arises from small amplitude sound waves that interfere with each other?

    (A) clutter
    (B) speckle
    (C) electrical
    (D) signal processing
    (E) spurious reflections

579. Duplex imaging combines gray scale with Doppler and can appear as

    (A) M-mode and spectrum
    (B) B-mode and spectrum
    (C) color-flow imaging and spectrum
    (D) all of the above

580. Doppler color-flow imaging produces an image composed of

    (A) tissue echoes in gray scale and blood echoes in color
    (B) moving soft tissue echoes in gray scale and blood motion in color
    (C) stationary tissues in gray scale and moving tissues in color
    (D) stationary tissues in gray scale and stationary blood in color

581. Color Doppler imaging is a term used to describe

    (A) a form of color-flow imaging
    (B) a form of magnetic resonance imaging
    (C) a new form of imaging relying on high-speed propagation velocities in soft tissues
    (D) a form of detecting flow with lasers

582. The Doppler effect occurs

    (A) only to waves traveling more than 1,000 m/s
    (B) only to ultrasound waves with intensities greater than 500 mW/cm^2, SPTA
    (C) to all waves coming from a moving wave source
    (D) in ultrasound, but only when the targets are moving faster than 1.0 m/s

583. Doppler effect depends on

    (A) the carrier frequency, the angle between echo source velocity and beam axis, and the reflectivity of blood
    (B) the closing velocity between transducer and tissue, carrier frequency, and ultrasound propagation velocity
    (C) the lowest Doppler-shift frequency detectable and the highest frequency without aliasing
    (D) the largest change in acoustical impedance within the moving blood

584. **To calculate blood velocity using color-flow imaging, a sonographer must**

    (A) place a sample volume in the major streamline or jet within the vessel and set an angle correction parallel to the vessel wall

    (B) assume that all flow is parallel to the vessel wall

    (C) locate the major streamline and place the sampling angle at 60° to the vessel wall

    (D) place a sample volume in the major streamline or jet and set the angle correction parallel to the streamline

585. **To preserve gray-scale texture, digital sampling for gray-scale images must be at intervals of**

    (A) 0.6 mm

    (B) one wavelength or less

    (C) 1.0 mm

    (D) 3 dB

586. **To preserve flow detail, digital Doppler sampling intervals for a vascular color-flow image must be at intervals of**

    (A) 1–2 mm

    (B) 1–2 cm

    (C) one wavelength or more but less than 1 mm

    (D) −6 dB

587. **Gray-scale tissue texture in a color-flow imaging system depends on**

    (A) transmit focusing only

    (B) receive focusing only

    (C) the product of transmit and receive focusing

    (D) the speed at which the ultrasound beam is moved by the scanhead

588. **The shape of the sample volume in pulsed Doppler has a major effect on the content of the Doppler signal.**

    (A) true

    (B) false

589. **To form the color patterns in a Doppler color-flow image, a color-flow system samples down each Doppler image line of sight for**

    (A) the amplitude of the Doppler signal

    (B) the velocities of red blood cells

    (C) the average Doppler shift frequency

    (D) the velocity spread within the sample site

590. **The Doppler portion of a color-flow image is a map of red-cell velocities.**

    (A) true

    (B) false

591. **Separating moving soft tissue from moving blood in a color-flow image tests for**

    (A) Doppler signal amplitudes only

    (B) tissue signal amplitudes only

    (C) Doppler signal frequencies only

    (D) the relationship between the amplitudes and frequencies of the Doppler signals

592. **A curving vessel within a color-flow image shows color in the vessel when the beam and vessel are parallel but shows no color, as the vessel turns perpendicular to the beam. The loss of color means that**

    (A) the vessel is occluded

    (B) the vessel is open, but the blood velocity is too low to complete the image

    (C) the dark region is diseased

    (D) the Doppler effect works only when the vessel is parallel to the ultrasound beam.

593. **The smallest vessels that appear in a color-flow image are about 1 mm in diameter. The smaller vessels are absent because**

    (A) arterial blood velocities are too low in vessels that are less than 1 mm in diameter

    (B) the smaller vessels are shadowed by the surrounding soft tissue

    (C) soft tissue does not have many vessels that are less than 1 mm in diameter

    (D) the smaller vessels do not reflect ultrasound as well as the larger vessels do

594. **The color-flow image provides information on (1) the existence of flow, (2) the location of flow in the image, (3) flow direction relative to transducer, (4) the maximum flow velocity.**

    (A) all of the above

    (B) 1, 3, and 4

    (C) 3 and 4

    (D) 1, 2, and 3

595. Detecting flow in a color-flow imaging system depends on the detection of

    (A) changes in Doppler signal amplitude

    (B) changes in Doppler signal frequency content

    (C) changes in echo signal phase and frequency content

    (D) changes in echo signal phase

596. One begins reading a color-flow image by

    (A) determining the maximum systolic frequency

    (B) knowing the position of the scan plane on the patient's body

    (C) knowing the direction of flow relative to the transducer

    (D) determining the Doppler carrier frequency

597. Changes in the Doppler shift frequencies within a color-flow image sample site appear in the image as

    (A) nothing; the image only shows changes in phase

    (B) different colors (hues)

    (C) different levels of color saturation (purity)

    (D) different colors (hues) or different levels of saturation (purity)

598. A Doppler color-flow image can show changes in the frequency content at a Doppler sample site by

    (A) changes in gray scale

    (B) changes in saturation

    (C) changes in color hue

    (D) the introduction of green markers

599. Cardiac color-flow imaging shows changes in the frequency content of the Doppler sample site by

    (A) changes in color

    (B) changes in saturation

    (C) changes in color texture

    (D) the introduction of red markers

600. Color-flow imaging systems determine the maximum Doppler shift frequency at each sample site.

    (A) true

    (B) false

601. A measurement of the peak systolic frequency in a carotid artery with a single-point spectrum will be lower than a measurement of the color-encoded frequency at the same point.

    (A) true

    (B) false

602. The synchronous signal processing uses a Doppler carrier frequency that is the same as the imaging center operating frequency.

    (A) true

    (B) false

603. Asynchronous signal processing in color-flow imaging requires the same frequency for both Doppler and gray-scale imaging.

    (A) true

    (B) false

604. Beam steering in asynchronous color-flow imaging is used to provide

    (A) a Doppler angle significantly less than 90° to typical blood flow

    (B) a way of looking at the same soft tissue targets at an angle different from the perpendicular beams

    (C) an enlarged Doppler beam to improve Doppler sensitivity

    (D) improved Doppler sensitivity to smaller vessels

605. The mechanical wedge in synchronous color-flow imaging is used to provide

    (A) improved penetration through impedance matching

    (B) improved beam focusing for the gray-scale image

    (C) an attenuation system to remove side lobes

    (D) a Doppler angle between the typical flow patterns in vessels

606. The ability to see flow in deep vessels is limited by the fact that

    (A) blood has scattering units that are about the same size as soft tissue

    (B) blood is moving faster than the surrounding tissues

    (C) blood has an extremely low attenuation rate

    (D) blood reflectivity is about 40–60 dB below that of soft tissue

607. Levels of output power and intensity for color-flow imaging are generally higher than those for conventional gray-scale imaging.

    (A) true

    (B) false

608. Because Doppler signal processing requires more energy, synchronous signal processing always produces Doppler power levels that are higher than those for gray-scale imaging.

    (A) true
    (B) false

609. In general, tissue ultrasonic intensity levels are higher for single-point spectra than for color-flow imaging with the same system.

    (A) true
    (B) false

610. Moving from gray-scale only to full-screen color-flow imaging in a system means that the image frame rate will probably do which of the following?

    (A) decrease
    (B) increase
    (C) stay the same
    (D) color signal processing has no effect on frame rate

611. Color-flow imaging in the heart uses larger Doppler sampling intervals to increase the image frame rate than vascular imaging.

    (A) true
    (B) false

612. Cardiac color-flow imaging also works well in the vascular system because the design can handle the high attenuation rates in cardiac imaging.

    (A) true
    (B) false

613. Sampling intervals for cardiac color-flow imaging and vascular color-flow imaging are similar.

    (A) true
    (B) false

614. Cardiac color-flow imaging is limited with a mechanical sector scanner because

    (A) the cardiac attenuation rate is too high
    (B) the ultrasound beams are always moving
    (C) the beam has a fixed focal point
    (D) the beam has too many side lobes

615. The phased-array sector scanner and the linear array share common beam forming properties of
    (1) a stationary beam at each line of sight,
    (2) increased grating lobes with beam steering,
    (3) three-dimensional dynamic focusing on receive,
    (4) the same aperture sizes for dynamic focusing.

    (A) 1 and 2
    (B) 1, 2, and 4
    (C) 2, 3, and 4
    (D) all of the above

616. Color-flow imaging in the peripheral vascular system typically uses

    (A) the phased sector scan
    (B) the linear array scan
    (C) the curved linear scan
    (D) a combination of A and B

617. Color-flow imaging in the heart typically uses

    (A) the phased sector scan
    (B) the linear array scan
    (C) the curved linear scan
    (D) a combination of A and C

618. You are imaging a small vessel using 7.5 MHz DCFI with the lowest displayable velocity of 6.0 cm/s. Changing only the carrier frequency to 5.0 MHz will change the *lowest* displayable velocity to

    (A) 1.5 cm/s
    (B) 9 cm/s
    (C) 6.0 cm/s; the vessel does not change
    (D) 15 cm/s

619. Doppler color-flow imaging is unique because it does not have a major problem with high-frequency aliasing.

    (A) true
    (B) false

620. Both the color and a point spectrum in a stenosis show high-frequency aliasing. One strategy for removing the aliasing involves

    (A) doing nothing; aliasing cannot be removed from the system
    (B) decreasing the system PRF
    (C) decreasing the carrier frequency
    (D) decreasing the Doppler angle toward zero

621. Increasing the output power levels and PRF to increase penetration and frame rates opens the system to which of the following artifacts?

    (A) high-frequency aliasing
    (B) loss of low velocities
    (C) tissue mirroring
    (D) range ambiguity

622. The color-coding of red arteries and blue veins and the slow high-resolution frame rates makes the identity of arteries and veins in the abdomen direct and easy.

    (A) true
    (B) false

623. Turbulence in a vascular color-flow image appears as

    (A) a mottled pattern of colors
    (B) a mottled pattern of red and blue with changing saturations
    (C) a mottled green region
    (D) A or B

624. Turbulence in a cardiac color-flow image appears as

    (A) a mottled pattern of colors
    (B) a mottled pattern of red and blue with changing saturations

    (C) a bright red region
    (D) a mottled green region

625. Power Doppler imaging is so named because

    (A) it increases output power for image improvement
    (B) it encodes the power spectrum of the Doppler signal into color
    (C) it uses the phase of the amplitude to detect flow
    (D) none of the above

626. Power Doppler imaging is limited because

    (A) it has a serious aliasing problem
    (B) it does not work with low carrier frequencies
    (C) it does not show the directionality of vessel flow
    (D) A and B

627. Power Doppler imaging is a good choice when you

    (A) want to show tissue perfusion
    (B) want to show tissue velocity
    (C) want to easily separate blood flow from simple tissue motion
    (D) A and B

Answers and Explanations

At the end of each explained answer, there is a number combination in parentheses. The first number identifies the reference source; the second number or set of numbers indicates the page or pages on which the relevant information can be found.

1. **(D)** The acronym DICOM stands for digital imaging and communication in medicine, which are the standards for distributing and viewing all kinds of medical images and files. This is the universal standard protocol that allows digital information to be compatible with all medical manufacturing equipment. *(2:148)*

2. **(E)** An ultrasound pulse takes up physical space in length and therefore is referred to as spatial pulse length. Spatial pulse length is defined as the product of the number of cycles in the pulse and its wavelength. This is generally shorter for higher frequencies since the wavelength is shorter. *(2:25)*

3. **(E)** Axial resolution, also called longitudinal, range, or depth resolution, is determined by the wavelength, damping, and frequency. Axial resolution improves with increased frequency. Damping (backing) material causes the number of cycles per pulse to decrease, thus improving axial resolution. *(2:76–81; 24:41)*

4. **(B)** Lateral resolution is defined as having the ability to distinguish between two structures that are in a plane that is perpendicular to sound path and is improved by reducing the beam diameter by focusing with acoustic lens or acoustic mirrors or using higher frequency transducer. *(2:79; 24:45)*

5. **(C)** The beam of an unfocused transducer diverges in the Fraunhofer zone. *(1:351)*

6. **(C)** Reverberation artifacts are present when two or more strong reflectors are located within the beam with decreasing intensity. Reverberation artifacts occur between the face of the transducer and a specular reflector. *(2:263; 20:598)*

7. **(A)** The acronym ALARA denotes "as low as reasonably achievable." This principle was implemented to reduce the risk while obtaining diagnostic images. Minimize scanning time when possible, increase the gain and decrease the power output, use the highest frequency transducer when possible, and use a focus transducer. *(2:322; 18:231)*

8. **(B)** The grating side lobes are reduced by apodization, subdicing, and harmonic imaging. *(2:105; 18:190)*

9. **(A)** Coded excitation uses digitally coded pulses to provide good penetration and high resolution at the same time. It also improves signal-to-noise ratio, axial resolution, and contrast resolution. *(2:92)*

10. **(B)** Patient identification errors have a significant negative impact on patient safety. Return the patient to the ward for appropriate identification and tagging. *(19:97)*

11. **(A, B, C, D, E)** All rods must be used to check registration accuracy. *(18:21; 21:282–283)*

12. **(A)** See Fig. 1–24 and Table 1–3, Study Guide. *(18:21; 21:282–283)*

13. **(B)** See Fig. 1–24 and Table 1–3, Study Guide. *(18:21; 21:282–283)*

14. **(D)** See Fig. 1–24 and Table 1–3, Study Guide. *(18:21; 21:282–283)*

15. **(C or E)** See Fig. 1–24 and Table 1–3, Study Guide. *(18:21; 21:282–283)*

16. **(C)** Decreasing the spatial pulse length improves axial resolution. Axial resolution is equal to one-half of the spatial pulse length. *(2:25)*

17. **(B)** A rule of thumb approximating the attenuation coefficient of a reflected echo in soft tissue is 0.5 dB/cm/MHz. Thus, the attenuation coefficient will be one-half the operating frequency.

    attenuation (dB) = attenuation coefficient (dB/cm)
    × path length (cm)
    dB = 1.75 dB/cm × 2 cm = 3.5 dB
    (2:30–32)

18. **(B)** Improper axial (along-the-beam) position *(2:43–44)*

19. **(D)** Weakly attenuating structures *(2:277)*

20. **(A)** Directly proportional to the velocity of the reflector *(2:170–171)*

21. **(A)** The frame rate is between 15 and 30 frames per second (fps). Color Doppler has a slower frame rate, about 15 fps. *Note:* The scan converter in most modern systems turns the scanning frame rate (which is the subject of this question) into a display frame rate (or video frame rate), which is usually faster (30 video fps). This is done by displaying the same scan frame more than once if the scan frame is less than video rate. CRT television monitors have an image rate of 30 fps using 525 horizontal lines. Most ultrasound departments today use LCD flat-panel display using 60 fps and a resolution of 720 pixels to 1,080 pixels. *(1:363; 2:143)*

22. **(E)** Use a certified language line *(19:41)*

23. **(B)** Smaller beam diameter. Intensity is defined as power per unit beam area; as the beam area decreases, the intensity increases. *(18:135)*

24. **(C)** Increased by four times. Intensity equals the square of the amplitude. *(2:28)*

25. **(A)** Increased with tissue thickness. Attenuation is the product of the attenuation coefficient and path length. Attenuation is associated with frequency, tissue characteristic, and depth. High frequency has high attenuation and poor penetration. Tissues such as bone and air have high attenuation when compared to water. (2:22)

26. **(A)** The matching layer is located between the active element and the skin. Both the matching layer and the acoustic gel reduce the reflection of ultrasound at the surface. The matching layer is chosen to be at a value approximately equal to the mean of impedances of the material on either side of it. (2:59; 18:190)

27. **(D)** After confirming that the patient name and medical record number are correct, an additional confirmation is the date of birth. (19:96–97)

28. **(D)** Use approved disinfectant (16:130–135)

29. **(B)** Depends on crystal thickness. Thickness equals one-half the wavelength. (2:55–56)

30. **(C)** The time taken to complete one cycle (one wavelength) (2:20; 18:20)

31. **(D)** Ratio of smallest to largest power level (18:257–262)

32. **(E)** Picture archiving and communications systems (PACS) provides the ability of digital images to be transmitted over the internet or viewed on workstations. This is not be confused with Digital Imaging and Communication in Medicine (DICOM), which is a standard to permit communication of information between manufacturers. (2:145–148)

33. **(B)** Increases the maximum depth that can be imaged (20:209; 18:51)

34. **(C)** Are not confirmed below 100 mW/cm² SPTA for unfocused beam and are not confirmed below 1 W/cm² (1,000 mW/cm²) SPTA for focused beam (2:325)

35. **(B)** The patient has the right to consent to or refuse any treatment by the hospital. A patient can revoke an uninformed consent at any time. (19:181)

36. **(A)** The first step is to introduce yourself to the patient with your employment ID and title visible. The second step is to be sure you have the right patient. The third step is to explain the ultrasound procedure to the patient. (8:70)

37. **(E)** The transvaginal transducer should be disinfected and covered with a probe cover after each patient. (16:130–135)

38. **(D)** Reduce the transmit power. The ALARA principle also suggests minimizing scanning time when possible, increasing the gain, and using the highest frequency transducer when possible. (2:322; 18:231)

39. **(A)** A mathematical process in which a waveform is multiplied by time-shift versions of itself. (2:188; 10:15)

40. **(A)** Stable cavitation occurs when the oscillation of the microbubbles does not collapse. (2:328; 20:622)

41. **(D)** The least likely possible potential ultrasound bioeffect is high-frequency transducers. Low-frequency transducers have a higher potential for bioeffects. (2:394)

42. **(A)** Harmonic frequency sound waves are derived from nonlinear or asymmetrical wave propagation. (2:105–108; 20:664–665)

43. **(D)** Propagation speed is determined by the tissue medium. Different tissue media have different propagation speeds. The speed is highest in solids and lowest in gases. The average propagation speed in soft tissue is 1,540 m/s. (2:20; 20:96–97)

44. **(C)** The prefix "giga" denotes 1,000,000,000 or 10^9, which is a unit of measurement in the metric system. (18:6)

45. **(C)** Twenty-five percent. The reflection coefficient (R) is equal to

$$R = \left(\frac{z_2 - z_1}{z_2 - z_1}\right)^2 = \left(\frac{0.75 - 0.25}{0.75 - 0.25}\right)^2 = 0.25,$$

where z_1 and z_2 are the acoustic impedances of each material. (1:366)

46. **(A)** Higher frequency transducers usually produce shorter spatial pulse lengths and thus improve axial resolution. (2:76–81)

47. **(A)** Longitudinal wave. In this type of wave, the motion in which the particle displaces in the medium is parallel to the direction of wave propagation. Transverse waves is the particle displacement perpendicular to the direction of wave propagation. (2:18; 10:153; 20:82–83)

48. **(A)** 0.3 mm (18:33)

$$\text{wavelength (mm)} = \frac{\text{velocity (mm/µs)}}{\text{frequency (M}} \quad = \frac{\overline{1.5}}{} = 0.3 \text{ mm}$$

49. **(D)** The difference in specific acoustic impedances. The fraction of sound reflected at an interface (r) is given by

$$R = \left(\frac{z_2 - z_1}{z_2 - z_1}\right)^2,$$

where z_1 and z_2 are the acoustic impedances of the boundary material. (2:37–38; 8:16)

50. **(A)** V or C = propagation velocity (cm/s)

f = frequency (cycles/s)

λ = wavelength (cm)

$V = f\lambda$ (2:20; 18:21–23)

51. **(B)** There are two conditions in which refraction occurs. First is an oblique incidence and the second is when the propagation speeds of the two media are different. Refraction is described by Snell's law, which relates the incident angle (θ_i) to the transmitted angle (θ_t) to the relative velocities of the two media making up the interface. (2:39; 18:89–99)

$$\frac{\sin \theta_i}{\sin \theta_t} = \frac{C_1}{C_2} \quad (1:367)$$

52. **(D)** Equal to the product of density and velocity for longitudinal waves (2:36–37; 20:153)

53. **(E)** The speeds of ultrasound in soft tissue are 1,540 m/s, 154,000 cm/s, 1.54 mm/μs, 0.154 cm/μs, or one mile per second. (2:20; 18:35)

54. **(B)** 8.0 cm. To change millimeters (mm) into centimeters (cm), move the decimal point one space to the left, and to change centimeters to millimeters, move the decimal point one space to the right. Recall that 10 mm = 1 cm. (18:5; 20:40)

55. **(B)** There are two conditions in which reflection occurs. First is a normal incidence and the second is a difference in acoustic impedances. (18:93)

56. **(E)** Ultrasound transducers convert mechanical energy to electrical energy and electrical energy to mechanical energy. (10:154)

57. **(C)** The medium (tissue) through which the sound is being transmitted and the mode of vibration determines the propagation speed. The speed is not affected by frequency. Ultrasound travels faster in solids and slower in gases. (18:34; 20:96)

58. **(C)** No change. The velocity of sound propagation depends on the material through which it is being transmitted and is independent of frequency. (18:34; 20:96)

59. **(A)** Refraction (2:38–39)

60. **(A)** Using a higher-frequency transducer. The near-zone length (x) is given by

$$x = \frac{r^2}{\lambda},$$

where r is the radius of the transducer, and λ is the wavelength. Thus, a longer near-zone length is achieved by increasing the transducer diameter or increasing the frequency. (2:140)

61. **(A)** 0.75 mm. The wavelength can be determined by using the following equation:

$$\lambda = \frac{u}{f}$$

v = propagation velocity (m/s)

f = frequency (Hz)

λ = wavelength (m)

For example, $\lambda = \dfrac{1,500 \text{ meters per second}}{2 \text{ MHz}}$

$$\lambda = \frac{1.5 \times 10^3 \text{ meters per second}}{2 \times 10^6 \text{ cycles per second}}$$

$$\lambda = 0.75 \times 10^{-3} \text{ meters}$$

$$\lambda = 0.75 \text{ mm}$$

(2:8; 12:2)

62. **(B)** Impedance

$$Z \text{ (impedance) for longitudinal waves} = \frac{\text{particle pressure}}{\text{particle velocity}}$$

(5:13)

63. **(A)** Doppler-shift formula (2:270–273)

64. **(C)** Huygens (10:71)

65. **(B)** Tenfold difference in intensity or power (2:30–33)

66. **(B)** Threshold, negative, or reject level (1:376)

67. **(B)** Compression (2:108)

68. **(A)** A-mode is amplitude modulation that is a graphical presentation of an upward displacement along a baseline. The upward displacement is the vertical axis (y-axis) representing the amplitude of the echo, and the horizontal axis (x-axis) represents depth. A-mode is a one-dimensional scan, which is obsolete on modern ultrasound imaging. (10:11; 18:157)

69. **(D)** Relaxation processes are modes by which ultrasound may be attenuated in passing through a material. Suppression or threshold is another name for rejection. (2:79–85; 18:229)

70. **(B)** Digital scan converter (3:31)

71. **(A)** The fraction of time that pulsed ultrasound is actually on is the duty factor. (2:25; 18:58)

72. **(D)** Sensitivity (18:360)

73. **(B)** Linear array transducers produce a rectangular image. (Sector scanners produce a pie-shaped image.) (2:55)

74. **(B)** Magnitude of the voltage spike applied to the transducer by the pulser (18:214)

75. **(D)** Thermal index (TI) and mechanical index (MI) (2:326–327; 18:372–375)

76. **(C)** Quality factor, or Q factor, is equal to the operating frequency divided by the bandwidth. (1:36)

77. **(E)** Grating lobes result from multielement structures of transducer arrays. Side lobes are similar to grating lobes

but are created by mechanical or single element transducers. (1:189; 20:69)

78. **(D)** Pulse duration (18:47)

79. **(B)** 10^{29}, 10^{-6}, 10^{-3}, 10^{-2} (18:6)

80. **(C)** Specular reflection occurs when the ultrasound strikes a large, smooth mirror-like surface, which is angle dependent and relative to the wavelength of the wave. (20:148)

81. **(B)** Schlieren technique of measurement (1:362)

82. **(D)** Reverberation (2:263)

83. **(B)** Enhancement (2:277)

84. **(B)** Using a larger diameter transducer. The dispersion angle in the far field (θ) is given as: sin θ = 1.22 λ/d, where λ is the wavelength, and d is the diameter of the transducer. The angle can be reduced by using either a larger transducer or a higher frequency (smaller wavelength). (1:364)

85. **(B)** Spatial pulse length (2:64)

$$\text{axial resolution (mm)} = \frac{\text{spatial pulse length (mm)}}{2}$$

86. **(B)** Quality factor (Q factor)

$$Q = \frac{f_0}{f_2 - f_1},$$

where f_0 is the central resonance frequency and $(f_2 - f_1)$ is the frequency bandwidth. (1:360; 2:53)

87. **(E)** Vector array is the name applied to the type of transducer technology that converts the image format from a linear array (rectangular) to trapezoidal-shaped image. (2:73; 20:272–279)

88. **(E)** Ultrasound resistant to propagate and the speed in which it travels depends on the density, elasticity, and temperature of the medium (tissue type). Ultrasound travels with least resistance in fluid with low viscosity. Urine has lower viscosity than blood. (2:20–22, 160)

89. **(A)** Dynamic range (10:48)

90. **(D)** Ultrasound waves are longitudinal waves, compressional, and mechanical waves. (2:18)

91. **(B)** Axial resolution (18:355)

92. **(C)** Scan C (18:356)

93. **(A)** Dead zone (18:355)

94. **(D)** The AIUM test object is filled with a mixture of alcohol, an algae inhibitor, and water, which allows the propagation speed to approximate the speed of sound in soft tissue (1,540 m/s). (18:355)

95. **(C)** Horizontal caliper check (18:355–356)

96. **(B)** Lateral resolution (18:356)

97. **(E)** Attenuation, echogenicity, solid and cystic mass, gray scale, and scattering characteristics cannot be evaluated by the AIUM test object. These characteristics can best be evaluated by the tissue equivalent phantom. (18:356–357)

98. **(D)** Registration (18:356)

99. **(E)** When using the AIUM test object, the output power, time gain compensation (TGC), reject, transducer frequency, and focus should be kept constant for comparisons. (2:306–307)

100. **(A)** There are two types of cavitation: stable and transient. Transient cavitation results in a violent collapse of microbubbles, which can cause localized temperature elevations as high as 10,000 degrees Kelvin. (20:90, 646–647)

101. **(D)** Lead zirconate titanate, barium titanate, lithium sulfate, lead metaniobate, and ammonium dihydrogen phosphate are not natural. (2:55; 18:117)

102. **(C)** Air. Cork, rubber, epoxy resin, and tungsten powder in araldite are good acoustic insulators. Water and air are not suitable acoustic insulators for pulse ultrasound transducers. Most transducers used in therapeutic or continuous-wave Doppler ultrasound do not use backing material. (18:121; 20:81–85)

103. **(C)** The intensities for continuous wave are equal (SATA = SATP and SPTA = SPTP). (24:125)

104. **(A)** Infrasound (subsonic) is below the limit of human hearing with a frequency less than 20 Hz. (20:111)

105. **(B)** Ultrasound has a frequency above 20,000 Hz. (20:111)

106. **(B)** Audible sound range from 20 Hz to 20,000 Hz (20:111)

107. **(B)** The electromagnetic spectrum is a large family of electromagnetic waves. Light, x-rays, and infrared, and ultraviolet rays are among its spectrum; ultrasound is not. (1:1–3)

108. **(D)** Hertz (Hz) is the internationally accepted term for cycles per second (cps). (2:18; 20:93)

109. **(C)** A 90° interrogation with a vessel will possible yield no Doppler shift because the cosine for 90° is zero. (24:74)

110. **(E)** All of the answers given are correct. (2:55; 20:234)

111. **(D)** Increase or decrease depending on the polarity applied (20:234–237)

112. **(D)** 1 mega = 1 million. Therefore, 5 MHz = 5 million cycles per second or 5 million Hz. (18:21–22)

113. **(G)** The damping material reduces pulse duration and spatial pulse length and, as a result, improves axial resolution. (2:57–58)

114. **(A)** Velocity of ultrasound transmitted through a medium depends on the properties of the medium: (1) temperature, (2) elasticity, and (3) density. The speed of ultrasound varies with temperature. However, temperature/velocity in human soft tissue can usually be ignored because body temperature is usually constant within a narrow range, for example, 94°F (low) to 106°F (high). The velocity of ultrasound in soft tissue at 37°C or 98.6°F (core body temperature) is 1,540 m/s. (3:3; 20:114–121)

115. **(C)** Period is the time it takes to complete a single cycle. The distance it takes for one cycle to occur is a wavelength. (3:3; 20:201)

116. **(A)** Particle motion is parallel to (or in the same direction of) the axis of wave propagation (20:83–88)

117. **(C)** Particle motion is perpendicular to the axis of wave propagation (20:83–88)

118. **(B)** Compression (2:17)

119. **(E)** Rarefactions (2:17)

120. **(C)** All gunshot or stab injuries, child abuse, or fraud are reportable without consent from the patient. The request for patient medical records warrants an authorization signed by the patient. (19:64)

121. **(F)** both A and C (18:112)

122. **(F)** both B and D (18:149)

123–128. See Fig. 1–8 in the Study Guide. (1:367; 2:98)

129. **(B)** Far gain (2:99–100)

130. **(A)** The unit for circumference is millimeter (mm) or centimeter (cm). The unit for area is square centimeter (cm^2), and the unit for volume is cubic centimeter (cm^3). (18:5)

131. **(B)** Apodization is used with array transducers to decrease the grating lobes. The grating lobes are reduced by different high voltages that excited the elements. (20:1004)

132. **(A)** The ring down or dead zone is evaluated by scanning the group of targets located at the top of the phantom close to the transducer. (18:355)

133. **(E)** Axial resolution is evaluated by scanning the group of targets located parallel to the ultrasound beam main axis. (18:355)

134. **(C)** Lateral resolution is evaluated by scanning the group of targets located perpendicular to the ultrasound beam main axis. (18:355)

135. **(E)** Deeper imaging decreases frame rate and results in a decrease in temporal resolution. (2:139–140; 18:196)

136. **(B)** An increase in aperture or frequency will increase the near-zone length. If the aperture size is increased, the resolution will decrease. Aperture refers to the size of the transducer surface. (2:74; 20:253)

137. **(D)** Subdicing is a technique of dividing the transducer elements into smaller elements, and as a result, the grating lobe artifact is reduced. (18:341)

138. **(D)** Continuous-wave (CW) Doppler transducers emit sound waves constantly and therefore do not need a backing material. However, when a backing material is required, air is used to allow much more energy into a forward direction toward the patient. This is due to the acoustical impedance mismatch between air and the piezoelectric crystal. (24:40)

139. **(C)** Fast Fourier transform (FFT) uses a mathematical technique to make the conversion from Doppler shift information into visual spectral analysis. (24:77)

140. **(D)** Harmonic frequency is twice the fundamental frequency. Harmonic frequency produces harmonic imaging, which is a new advancement in diagnostic ultrasound. There are currently two types of harmonic imaging: tissue harmonics and contrast harmonics. Tissue harmonics are created by reflections from tissue that are twice the transmitted frequency (fundamental frequency). Harmonic imaging improves the image quality and eliminates the grating lobe artifacts. Contrast agents are taken orally or by injection. The microbubbles acts as harmonic oscillator and contrast enhanced echo signals giving higher harmonics. (2:105; 18:263–264)

141. **(E)** If frequency increases, the wavelength decreases. (2:20)

142. **(A)** If frequency decreases, the wavelength increases. (2:20)

143. **(A)** As frequency increases, the penetration decreases. (2:25–26)

144. **(B)** As frequency increases, the resolution increases. (2:20–27)

145. **(A)** Higher frequency transmits shorter pulse and narrower beam width. (2:79)

146. **(F)** Air and barium sulfate ($BaSO_4$). The contrast material used for intravenous pyelogram (IVP) and blood does not prevent the propagation of ultrasound. (18:35; 20:121)

147. **(E)** A coupling medium is a liquid medium placed between the transducer and the skin to eliminate air gap. Air has a reflection coefficient approaching 100%, which results in almost zero transmission. Water or saline can also be used, but they dry out faster than gel. (2:60)

148. **(A)** The progressive weakening of the sound beam as it travels. Attenuation occurs because of (1) absorption, (2) reflection, and (3) scatter. Barium sulfate and air impair ultrasound transmissions. (2:32–33)

149. **(C)** When crystals are subjected to pressure resulting in an electrical charge on their surfaces, it is called a piezoelectric effect. (18:117)

150. **(B)** When crystals are subjected to electrical impulse and generate ultrasound as a result, it is called a reverse piezoelectric effect. *(18:117)*

151. **(B)** Attenuation is the amount of energy lost per unit of depth into the tissue. The parameter used to express the energy loss is the decibel (dB). Attenuation coefficient is directly related to frequency. The parameter used to express attenuation coefficient is 0.5 dB/cm/MHz. *(24:29)*

152. **(C)** Waves carry energy from one place to another through a medium. *(19:13–14)*

153. **(A)** A mechanical (longitudinal) wave causes particles to oscillate in the direction of the wave propagation. *(20:83–84)*

154. **(C)** Wavelength is the distance between two identical points on the waveform. *(2:19)*

155. **(A)** Ultrasonic waves are mechanical, longitudinal, and compressional waves that require a medium for propagation. *(20:83–84)*

156. **(B)** Acoustic impedance is defined as the density of tissue × the speed of sound in tissue ($Z = pc$). *(2:35)*

157. **(C)** The black region in the middle of the color map is the base line and wall filter and represent no Doppler flow. *(18:312)*

158. **(E)** Ultrasound is above 20,000 cycles per second (Hz) and is above the audible range of sound. However, in the clinical settings, ultrasound transducers are in the megahertz range. (1–20 MHz). *(20:111)*

159. **(D)** The equation for period is

$$\text{period} = \frac{1}{\text{frequency}}$$

(14:2; 18:22)

160. **(D)** The direction of the returning echo is related to the beam angle. The more perpendicular the beam gets to an organ interface, the greater the portion of the reflected echo that will be received by the transducer. *(2:35–36)*

161. **(A)** A decibel is the ratio of two sound intensities, highest to lowest (or vice versa). *(10:39)*

162. **(C)** Azimuthal is another name for *lateral* resolution. *(18:112)*

163. **(B)** The femur is a bone that has the highest sound velocity because of its stiffness. *(2:35)*

164. **(E)** No significant biologic effects have been proved in mammals exposed using a focused transducer below 1 W/cm² or 100 mW/cm² spatial peak temporal average (SPTA) for unfocused transducers. *(2:334; 20:658)*

165. **(B)** Coded excitation provides good penetration and high resolution while at the same time also improves axial resolution, contrast resolution, and signal-to-noise ratio. *(2:92; 10:28)*

166. **(D)** SATA has the lowest intensity because the intensity is averaged over the whole beam profile (SA), and over the whole duration of exposure (TA). *(2:30)*

167. **(B)** The beam uniformity ratio is defined as the spatial peak intensity (measured at the beam center) divided by the spatial average intensity (the average intensity across the beam). *(2:29–30)*

168. **(C)** The duty factor is the fraction of time the transducer is emitting sound. In a pulsed echo system, it is normally less than 1%. *(2:25)*

169. **(D)** Axial resolution is defined as one-half the spatial pulse length. Therefore, the shorter the spatial pulse length, the better the axial resolution. *(18:111)*

170. **(C)** Propagation speed (mm/μs); f = frequency (cycle/s) and λ wavelength (mm) *(24:8)*

171. **(D)** Attenuation of an ultrasound beam can occur by divergence of a beam, scattering, and reflection. It can also occur by absorption. *(18:296)*

172. **(A)** Attenuation coefficient of sound is determined by knowing dB/cm/MHz and then multiplying that quantity by the frequency expressed in MHz. *(2:32–33)*

173. **(B)** Transducer Q factor (quality factor) is equal to the operating frequency divided by the bandwidth. Therefore, if the transducer Q factor is low, the bandwidth is wide. *(18:123)*

174. **(A)** Axial resolution can be improved by shortening pulse length, increasing damping, and a higher-frequency transducer. *(18:111–116)*

175. **(B)** Axial resolution is primarily affected by spatial pulse length. Because the spatial pulse length is the product of wavelength, reducing the wavelength or increasing the frequency will affect axial resolution. *(2:76–81; 18:111–116)*

176. **(D)** Increasing transducer frequency will improve both lateral and axial resolution but decrease depth of penetration. *(2:76–81; 18:111–116)*

177. **(C)** Range resolution is another name for *axial* resolution. *(18:148)*

178. **(B)** The duty factor is the fraction of time that sound is being emitted from the transducer. In continuous wave, the sound is being emitted 100% of the time. *(2:25)*

179. **(A)** The arrow (B) points to blood cells moving toward the transducer. *(18:312)*

180. **(D)** Acoustic impedance is calculated as $Z = p \times c$ and measured with units of rayls. The average soft tissue impedance is 1,630,000 rayls. *(18:86; 20:170)*

181. **(C)** Constant depth mode (C-mode). Its application is pulsed-wave Doppler. *(20:369–370)*

182. **(A)** The height of the vertical spike corresponds to the strength of the echo received by the transducer (y-axes). *(18:157)*

183. **(B)** The arrow (C) points to blood cells moving away from the transducer. *(18:312)*

184. **(A)** The correct equation for calculating reflection percentage is

$$R = \left(\frac{Z_2 - Z_1}{Z_2 + Z_1} \right)^2 \times 100$$

(31:14–15)

185. **(D)** The reflection coefficient between water and air interface is 100%. Air prevents the sound from entering the body. It is for this reason that a coupling gel is necessary. *(20:144–152)*

186. **(B)** Beyond the critical angle, 100% of the sound beam is reflected and 0% is transmitted. *(20:153)*

187. **(A)** Rayleigh scattering occurs when the particle size is smaller than a wavelength (for ultrasound typically in the 1-mm range). *(20:149)*

188. **(D)** The least likely way to decrease the dead zone (main bang) is to increase pulse length. The dead zone is decreased with high frequency, short pulse length, and increasing the output power and acoustic standoff pad. *(18:355)*

189. **(C)** Power is defined as the rate at which work is done or energy is transferred (energy per unit time). *(2:269)*

190. **(A)** Lateral resolution is the minimum separation between two reflectors perpendicular to the sound path. *(2:76–81)*

191. **(D)** In most soft tissues, the attenuation coefficient increases directly with frequency. As frequency is increased, the attenuation coefficient increases, thereby limiting depth of perception. *(2:32–33)*

192. **(A)** Absorption is the conversion of ultrasound energy into heat. Absorption, scattering, and reflection are all factors of attenuation. *(2:32–33)*

193. **(D)** The rule of thumb for attenuation in soft tissue is 0.5 dB/cm/MHz. Therefore, an ultrasound beam of 1 MHz frequency will lose 0.5 dB of amplitude for every centimeter traveled. *(2:32–33)*

194. **(C)** Reverberation produces false echoes. *(2:263)*

195. **(D)** The acoustic impedance mismatch between fat and muscle is small; therefore, approximately 90% of the sound beam is transmitted. *(20:174)*

196. **(D)** Huygens's principle states that all points on a wavefront can be considered as a source for secondary spherical wavelets. *(20:269)*

197. **(B)** Enhancement is the "burst of sound" visualized posterior to weak attenuations. *(2:277)*

198. **(A)** Half-value layer (HVL—sometimes called half-intensity depth) is defined as the thickness of tissue that reduces the beam intensity by one-half. *(10:70)*

199. **(D)** Propagation speed error. The ultrasound machine assumes a speed of 1,540 m/s. If the sound passes through a medium of a different velocity, the result is an error in the range equation. *(2:267)*

200. **(B)** The range equation explains the distance to the reflector, which is equal to one-half of the propagation speed × the pulse round-trip time. *(2:338)*

201. **(A)** For a specular reflector, the angle of incidence is equal to the angle of reflection. This type of reflection occurs from a surface, which is larger than the wavelength. *(20:148)*

202. **(C)** Propagation speed is determined by the medium. The transducer determines amplitude, period, intensity, and frequency. *(20:120–121)*

203. **(D)** Acoustic variables include density, pressure, temperature, particle motion, and distance. *(18:12)*

204. **(E)** Acoustic parameters include frequency, power, intensity, period, amplitude, wavelength, and propagation speed. *(18:12)*

205. **(C)** Continuous-wave Doppler requires two active elements mounted side by side. One element transmits and the other receives the echoes. *(18:303)*

206. **(D)** Reynold's number is a dimensionless index that indicates the likelihood of turbulence to occur. *(20:767)*

207. **(A)** A is correct, with the propagation velocity in this order respectively: 331 m/s, 1,450 m/s, 1,585 m/s, and 4,080 m/s. *(18:35)*

208. **(C)** Backscatter is increased by increasing frequency and increasing heterogeneous media. *(2:39)*

209. **(A)** Critical angle is the angle at which sound is totally reflected and none is transmitted. *(10:37)*

210. **(D)** The pulse repetition frequency (PRF) is the number of pulses occurring per second. The PRF is inversely proportional to the pulse repetition period. The PRF and depth of view are inversely related and the PRF is equal to the number of scan lines per second. *(18:55; 24:9)*

211. **(D)** The duty factor is the fraction of time that the transducer is emitting a pulse. It is unitless. *(18:58)*

212. **(A)** The attenuation coefficient is the attenuation per unit length of sound travel. Its typical value is 3 dB/cm, for 6 MHz sound in soft tissue (0.5 dB/cm/MHz × 6 MHz = 3 dB/cm). *(2:32–33)*

213. **(B)** Normal incidence is also known as orthogonal, perpendicular, right angle, or 90°. At normal incidence, sound may be reflected or transmitted in various degrees. *(2:36; 18:89)*

214. **(A)** The difference (mismatch) of acoustic impedance between two media is what determines how much energy will be transmitted or reflected. *(20:170)*

215. **(A)** Acoustic impedance is equal to the product of the density of a substance and the velocity of sound. The propagation speed in solids is higher than that in liquids, and the propagation speed in gas is low. The increase in propagation speed is caused by increasing stiffness of the media, not by the density. *(2:36)*

216. **(A)** According to Snell's law,

$$\frac{\sin i}{\sin r} = \frac{V_1}{V_2},$$

the transmission angle is proportional to the incidence angle times the medium 2 propagation speed divided by the medium 1 propagation speed. *(2:39)*

217. **(C)** The depth of the interface is 3 cm. Ultrasound equipment is programmed at 1.54 mm/μs, and because the average speed in soft tissue is known, the depth and time can be calculated using the following equation:

$$\text{depth (mm)} = \frac{1.54 \text{ mm/μs} \times \text{transmitted and reflected time (μs)}}{2}$$

This equation is called range equation.

Another method is using the 13-μs rule. This rule states that for every 13 μs of transmitted time, the reflected interface is 1 cm depth; therefore, 26 μs is 2 cm depth and 39 μs is 3 cm depth. *(18:106)*

218. **(D)** The mirror image artifact duplicates a structure on the other side of a strong curved reflector,e.g., the diaphragm and pleura. *(2:265)*

219. **(C)** The comet tail is a bright tapering trail of echoes just distal to a strongly reflecting structure. The greater the acoustic impedance mismatch, the greater the possibility of this artifact to occur. *(5:7)*

220. **(C)** The acoustic impedance mismatch between tissue and gas is very great; therefore, it may produce the comet tail artifact. *(5:7)*

221. **(C)** Aliasing occurs when the Doppler shift frequency exceeds one-half of the pulse repetition frequency (PRF). This is known as Nyquist limit. *(2:340)*

222. **(D)** By increasing damping, one also increases the bandwidth. Bandwidth is the range of frequency involved in a pulse. *(2:57–58)*

223. **(E)** All of the above *(2:340)*

224. **(C)** Using the range equation 13-μs rule, $4 \times 13 = 52$ μs. Therefore, the depth is 4 cm for 52 μs *(18:106)*

225. **(A)** An ultrasound transducer generally can resolve reflectors along the sound path better than it can resolve those perpendicular to it. *(2:76–81)*

226. **(D)** The number of electrical pulses produced per second is typically 1,000 Hz. *(2:22–23)*

227. **(B)** The most common artifact in Doppler ultrasound is aliasing. *(2:340)*

228. **(B)** With a typical PRF of 1,000 Hz, each pulse–receive interval is 1 ms (1,000 μs) long. Because an average pulse is 1 μs long, this leaves 999 μs for receiving. 999/1,000 is 99.9%. *(9:190)*

229. **(C)** Frequency equals velocity divided by wavelength. Because velocity is standard at 1,540 m/s, doubling the frequency will result in decreasing the wavelength by one-half. *(2:45)*

230. **(A)** Real-time transducers display two formats: sector and rectangular. The linear-sequenced array transducer displays a rectangular format. *(2:66–73)*

231. **(C)** Z is the acoustic impedance; p is the material density; and c is the propagation speed. Z (rayls) = p (kg/m^3) × c (m/s). *(25:28)*

232. **(A)** Lead zirconate titanate (PZT) is a ceramic material with piezoelectric properties. It is most commonly used in transducers because of its greater efficiency and sensitivity. *(20:236)*

233. **(E)** The pulse travels to the interface and back to the transducer, the total time for the distance travel is 39 μs. Using the 13 μs rule, $3 \times 13 = 39$ μs; therefore, the depth of the reflector is 3 cm. The total distance traveled is $2 \times 3 = 6$ cm. *(18:106)*

234. **(C)** The total round-trip time in human tissue for reflected echo at a depth of 2 cm is 26 μs. *(18:106)*

235. **(A)** Pulse repetition frequency (PRF) is the number of pulses emitted per second. *(2:22–23)*

236. **(D)** The pulser produces the electric voltage pulses; this, in turn, drives the transducer to emit ultrasound pulses. It also tells both the memory and the receiver when the ultrasound pulses were produced. *(2:22–23)*

237. **(C)** Shadowing is a useful artifact that helps with diagnosis. The ultrasound beam striking a highly reflective or highly attenuating structure causes this artifact. *(2:267)*

238. **(D)** PRF 18 kHz = 9 Nyquist limit *(2:281)*

239. **(A)** Lateral resolution is dependent on beam diameter, which varies with distance from the transducer. *(2:76–81)*

240. **(C)** A period is the time it takes for one full cycle to occur. *(20:93)*

241. **(B)** Half-intensity depth decreases with increasing frequency. As frequency increases, the wavelength decreases both axial and lateral resolution. *(2:76–81)*

242. **(C)** Redirection of a portion of the sound beam from a boundary *(3:5)*

243. **(C)** 7 MHz. The transmitted frequency is called the fundamental frequency. The second harmonic frequency is twice the fundamental frequency. *(18:263)*

244. **(A)** Bit is an acronym for binary digit and represents the basic digital unit for storing data in the main computer memory. *(7:8.1)*

245. **(A)** Eight bits equal 1 byte. A bit is a unit of data in binary notation and assumes one of two states: "on" representing the number 1, or "off" representing the number 0. *(7:136)*

246. **(D)** The purpose of using an acoustic lens on transducers is to narrow the ultrasound beam, which improves lateral resolution. *(18:151)*

247. **(A)** The needle or membrane hydrophone is used to measure pressure amplitude, wavelength, intensity, and pulse repetition frequency *(2:319)*

248. **(C)** Viscosity is measured in units of *poise* or *kilograms per meter-second* (kg/m-s). *(2:160)*

249. **(C)** The speed of ultrasound is dependent on bone, muscle, soft tissue, and fat, which make up the medium. The speed is not dependent on the range of frequency or output power. If stiffness increases, speed increases, and if density increases, speed decreases. *(18:35–37)*

250. **(D)** The resistance to flow offered by a fluid in motion is called viscosity. *(2:160–161)*

251. **(C)** Autocorrelation is the mathematical process commonly used to detect Doppler shifts in color Doppler instruments. *(2:188)*

252. **(C)** A decrease in frequency or transducer aperture size will decrease the near-zone length (Fresnel zone). *(18:140)*

253. **(D)** Water has the lowest viscosity. *(2:160; 18:280)*

254. **(C)** While the symbol k represents kilo or 1,000 in metric, in computer terminology K = 1,024. Then, the amount that can be stored in memory is 128 × 1,024 × 8 bits = 1,048,576 bits, referred to as 1 megabit. *(7:8.1–8.17)*

255. **(B)** Harmonics frequencies are created when structures undergo nonlinear oscillations. These nonlinear vibrations can occur both in tissue as well as with microbubbles used as contrast agents. Harmonics frequencies are multiples of the fundamental frequency, e.g., twice that of the fundamental frequency. *(2:41, 105–108; 18:263, 266)*

256. **(A)** Frequency compounding reduces speckle and as a result, improves image contrast. *(20:366)*

257. **(A)** The unit for acoustic pressure is pascal (Pa). *(18:12)*

258. **(E)** The horizontal (or *x*-axis) on the M-mode display represents time. *(18:161)*

259. **(C)** 7 MHz. Diagnostic ultrasound transducers used in the clinical setting range from 2.5 MHz to 10 MHz. Ultrasound frequencies in the kilohertz range are not useful in diagnostic range. *(18:21)*

260. **(B)** The ratio of the minimum to maximum signal amplitude that can be applied to a device without producing distortion is called dynamic range. *(10:48)*

261. **(C)** The vertical (*y*-axis) on the M-mode display represents depth of the reflector. *(18:161)*

262. **(B)** Two: off or on. "Off" represented by the number 0. "On" represented by the number 1. *(20:62)*

263. **(B)** Two (0 or 1) *(20:62)*

264. **(E)** The number 30 is represented by 011110. To convert from decimal to binary, repeatedly divide by two and note the remainder.

30 ÷ 2 = 15 remainder 0	3 ÷ 2 = 1 remainder 1
15 ÷ 2 = 7 remainder 1	1 ÷ 2 = 0 remainder 1
7 ÷ 2 = 3 remainder 1	0 ÷ 2 = 0 remainder 0

(2:121–123)

265. **(D)** The binary system, which is used in digital scan converter memory, is based on the powers of two. For four bits, 2^4 ($2 \times 2 \times 2 \times 2$) or 16 different gray levels can be represented. Another way of looking at this is to list all possible states:

0000	0100	1000	1100
0001	0101	1001	1101
0010	0110	1010	1110
0011	0111	1011	1111

There are 16 possible unique states. *(2:121–123)*

266. **(B)** Digital memory, where the electronic components are either on (1) or off (0), is based on the binary number system. We can say that the number of discrete levels possible, N, is equal to 2 raised to the power of that number of bits. $N = 2^n$. Therefore, to make 64 shades of gray would require 2^6 bit memory.

$$(2 \times 2 \quad 4 \times 2 \quad 8 \times 2 \quad 16 \times 2 \quad 32 \times 2 = 64)$$

. 2   3   4   5   6   *(19:32)*

267. **(B)** The acoustic output with potential for producing cavitational effects in tissue is characterized by the mechanical index (MI). Cavitation is classified as either stable or transient. *(2:328; 18:374–375)*

268. **(C)** The receiver processes echoes detected by the transducer. These echoes may be amplified (gain), compensated for depth (TGC), compressed (to fit into the dynamic range of the system), and rejected (eliminating low-level signals). *(18:291)*

269. **(D)** The greater the pulse amplitude (electronic voltage applied to the transducer), the greater the amplitude of the ultrasound pulse provided by the transducer. *(2:57; 20:234–235)*

270. **(B)** The pulser produces electric voltage pulses that drive the transducer and serve to synchronize the receiver so that the arrival time of returning echoes can be accurately determined. *(20:234–235)*

271. **(D)** Components of a pulse-echo system include the *pulser* that produces the electrical pulse, which drives the *transducer*. For each reflection received from the tissue by the transducer, an electrical voltage is produced that goes to the *receiver*, where it is processed for display. Information on transducer position and orientation is delivered to the *image memory*. Electric information from the memory drives the *display*. *(18:221–213)*

272. **(B)** Transducers may be focused by using a curved piezoelectric transducer element (internal focusing) or by using an acoustic lens. *(18:151–152)*

273. **(E)** Quality factor (Q factor) is equal to the operating frequency divided by the bandwidth and is unitless. *(2:26–27)*

274. **(E)** Reduction in echoes from a region distal to an attenuating structure *(2:267)*

275. **(G)** An increase in echoes from a region distal to a weakly attenuating structure or tissue *(2:277)*

276. **(A)** A structure that is echo-free; not necessarily cystic unless there is good through transmission. A solid mass can be anechoic but will not have good through transmission. *(19:922)*

277. **(D)** An echo that does not correspond to the real target *(20:593)*

278. **(I)** A structure that possesses echoes *(10:50)*

279. **(H)** Echoes of higher amplitude than the normal surrounding tissues *(10:72)*

280. **(B)** Echoes of lower amplitude than the normal surrounding tissues *(10:72)*

281. **(C)** The surface forming the boundary between two media having different acoustic impedances *(19:4)*

282. **(A and F)** A structure without echoes and with low absorption; not necessarily cystic unless there is good through transmission. *Sonolucent* is a misnomer for *anechoic*. *(10:132)*

283. **(E)** Air. There are numerable backing materials used for damping. Pulse-echo transducer backing materials are: (1) epoxy resin, (2) tungsten, (3) cork, and (4) rubber. Continuous-wave Doppler transducers have little or no backing materials. *(2:57; 18:304)*

284. **(C)** Aliasing *(18:319–310)*

285. **(C)** Brightness of pixel *(18:161)*

286. **(C)** For ultrasound to propagate a medium, it must be composed of particles of matter. A vacuum is a space empty of matter; therefore, ultrasound cannot travel in a vacuum. *(8:13)*

287. **(B)** Wavelength *(6:5)*

288. **(A)** Period *(18:20)*

289. **(B)** Hertz (Hz) represents cycles per second (cps). Therefore, 20 cps = 20 Hz. *(6:5)*

290. **(C)** 1 MHz *(6:5)*

291. **(B)** Mechanical transducers have only one crystal, so this will result in total image loss. *(18:12)*

292. **(A)** A-mode is a shortened form of amplitude mode. This mode is presented graphically with vertical spikes arising from a horizontal baseline. The height of the vertical spikes represents the amplitude of the deflected echo. *(18:157–161)*

293. **(B)** B-mode is a shortened form of brightness modulation. This mode presents a two-dimensional image of internal body structures displayed as dots. The brightness of the dots is proportional to the amplitude of the echo. B-mode display is employed in all two-dimensional images, static or real-time. *(18:157–161)*

294. **(D)** M-mode is short for time-motion modulation. This mode is a graphic display of movement of reflecting structures related to time. M-mode is used almost exclusively in echocardiography. *(18:157–161)*

295. **(D)** A long dead zone may indicate a detached backing material. The use of a high-frequency transducer or a short pulse duration will typically decrease the dead zone. *(18:361)*

296. **(E)** The frame rate in ultrasound is determined by image depth and the speed of sound in the medium. *(18:194)*

297. **(A)** Doppler signals and velocities cannot be measured with perpendicular incidence (90°). *(18:300)*

298. **(C)** The technique used to visualize the dead zone is acoustic standoff. *(18:361)*

299. **(C)** The intensity of the ultrasound beam depends on the beam diameter. Intensity is defined as the beam power divided by the beam cross-sectional area. *(2:27–28)*

300. **(C)** Huygens principle *(20:369)*

301. **(A)** The fraction of time that a pulsed ultrasound is actually producing ultrasound is called the duty factor.

$$\text{duty factor (DF)} = \frac{\text{pulse duration (PD)}}{\text{pulse repetition period (PRP)}}$$

(2:25)

302. **(C)** Real-time ultrasound instrumentation is classified as phased, linear, annular, and vector. *(2:66–74; 20:278–279; 25:55)*

303. **(B)** The speed at which ultrasound propagates within a medium depends primarily on the compressibility of the medium. *(2:20–22)*

304. **(C)** The reverberation artifact occurs when two or more reflections are present along the path of the beam. This gives rise to multiple reflections, which will appear behind one another at intervals equal to the separation of the real reflectors. *(3:40; 2:263)*

305. **(C)** Gain is the ratio of electric power. Gain governs the electric compensation for tissue attenuation and is expressed in decibels (dB). *(2:94; 9:89)*

306. **(C)** Multipath reverberation artifacts result from sound reflected from a highly curved specular surface when the echo takes an indirect path back to the transducer. *(18:345)*

307. **(A)** Doppler shift artifacts are called clutter. Clutter is eliminated by wall filters. *(18:320)*

308. **(B)** Echo signals that are in analog format as they emerge from the receiver are transferred to a digital format by an analog-to-digital (A–D) converter. Preprocessing then produces the best possible digital representation of the analog signal. *(2:101)*

309. **(D)** By increasing frequency (MHz) (*f*) and/or transducer diameter (mm), the near-zone length (mm) is increased, as shown in the equation:

$$\text{near zone length} = \frac{(\text{transducer diameter})^2 \, f}{6}$$

(2:63–65)

310. **(B)** Mass divided by volume *(2:17)*

311. **(H)** Progression or travel *(2:20)*

312. **(D)** Number of cycles per unit time *(2:18–19)*

313. **(A)** Rate at which work is done *(10:105)*

314. **(G)** The percentage of time the system is transmitting a pulse *(2:25)*

315. **(F)** Range of frequencies contained in the ultrasound pulse *(2:26–27)*

316. **(E)** Density multiplied by sound propagation speed *(2:35–36)*

317. **(C)** Conversion of sound to heat *(2:38–39)*

318. **(I)** Operating frequency divided by bandwidth *(2:27)*

319. **(J)** Power divided by area *(2:27–28)*

320. **(B)** The damping material reduces spatial pulse length, efficiency, and sensitivity. *(2:57–58)*

321. **(C)** Gain is electric compensation for tissue attenuation. *(20:326)*

322. **(A)** Spectral analysis allows the determination of the frequency spectrum of a signal. *(6:16)*

323. **(B)** The output power is a knob on the ultrasound equipment that is used to increase or decrease the brightness of the entire image; increasing the power output improves the signal-to-noise ratio, and increasing this output also increases patient exposure with potential bioeffect concerns. *(18:232)*

324. **(C)** Gray-scale resolution is the ability of a gray-scale display to distinguish between echoes of slightly different amplitudes or intensities. The first step in this problem is to figure out how many shades of gray are contained in a 5-bit digital system. The total number of shades of gray is 32 ($2^5 = 32$). The next step is to divide the dynamic range (42 dB) by the number of levels. This will give the number of decibels per level. 42 dB ÷ 32 gray levels = 1.3 dB/gray level. *(2:109–121)*

325. **(B)**

$$\text{Distance} = \text{velocity} \times \text{time}$$
$$= 1{,}540 \text{ m/s} \times 0.01 \text{ s}$$
$$= 15.4 \text{ m}$$

However, 0.1 seconds is only the time to reach the echo source. The time of the round-trip must be calculated by multiplying by 2. Round-trip distance = 15.4 m × 2 = 30.8 m. *(4:2)*

326. **(B)** An edge artifact. Edge shadowing results from refraction and reflection of the ultrasound beam on a rounded surface, for example, the fetal skull. *(13:42)*

327. **(A)** A split image artifact (ghost artifact) may produce duplication or triplication of an image, resulting in ultrasound beam refraction at a muscle–fat interface. *(11:29–34; 12:49–52)*

328. **(A)** Multipath, mirror image, and side lobe artifacts are most likely to produce a pseudomass. A comet tail artifact is least likely. *(13:27–43)*

329. **(A)** Split image artifact is more noticeable in athletic and mesomorphic habitus patients. *(12:49–52)*

330. **(C)** Split image artifact (ghost artifact) is *not* caused by a gas bubble. The most likely cause is refraction of the sound beam at a muscle–fat interface. The artifact is more evident at an interface between subcutaneous fat and abdominal muscle or between rectus muscles and fat in the pelvis. The artifact can also be produced by an abdominal scar or superficial abdominal skin keloids. *(11:29–34; 12:49–52)*

331. **(C)** The most likely cause of beam thickness artifact is partial volume effect. This type of artifact occurs most often when the ultrasound beam interacts with a cyst or other fluid-filled structures. *(13:27–45)*

332. **(C)** Beam thickness artifacts depend on beam angulation, not gravity. Therefore, if an image of the gallbladder has what appears to be sludge, a change in the patient's position relative to the beam could differentiate pseudosludge caused by artifact from layering of biliary sludge. *(13:27–45)*

333. **(D)** Side lobe artifacts are weaker than the primary beam. *(13:27–45; 25:180)*

334. **(B)** Shotgun pellets and metallic surgical clips produce a trail of dense continuous echoes. Bone, gas, calcifications, and gallstones produce a distal acoustic shadow. *(13:27–45)*

335. **(A)** The most common type of artifact observed in patients with shotgun pellets or metallic surgical clips are comet tail artifacts. This type of reverberation artifact is characterized by a trail of dense continuous echoes distal to a strongly reflecting structure. *(10:30; 14:225–230)*

336. **(D)** A ring-down artifact is characterized sonographically as high-amplitude parallel lines occurring at regular intervals distal to a reflecting interface. This type of artifact is commonly associated with bowel gas. *(15:21–28)*

337. **(A)** It is possible to calculate the displacement in split images by using Snell's law. *(11:29–34)*

338. **(C)** The first large vertical reflection at the start of the A-mode is called "main bang," or transducer artifact. *(3:26–27)*

339. **(C)** Annular-array real-time uses a combination of mechanical and electronic devices. The annular array is used for dynamic focusing; the mechanical part for beam steering. *(2:66–74; 20:261–272)*

340. **(A)** A decrease in the amplitude of the returning echo and also a decrease in the amount of transmitted sound: these result in a fade-away picture. The combination of the coupling medium and matching layers enables passage and return of echoes from the body to the transducer. *(3:52; 2:60)*

341. **(A)** Spatial compounding *(24:94)*.

342. **(C)** M-mode stands for time-motion modulation. This mode displays a graphic representation of motion of reflecting surfaces. It is used primarily in echocardiography. *(3:44)*

343. **(A)** B-mode stands for brightness modulation. This mode displays a two-dimensional view of internal body structures in cross section or sagittal section. The images, displayed as dots on the monitor, result from interaction between ultrasound and tissues. The brightness of the dots is proportional to the amplitude of the echo. Real-time equipment uses B-mode. *(3:44; 18:159)*

344. **(B)** A-mode stands for amplitude modulation. This mode displays a graphic representation of vertically reflected echoes arising from a horizontal baseline. The height of the vertical reflection is proportional to the amplitude of the echo, and the distance from one vertical reflection to the next represents the distance from one interface to another. A-mode is one-dimensional. The horizontal baseline is the x-axis and the vertical reflection represents the y-axis. *(3:26, 44; 18:157)*

345. **(B)** The effects of ultrasound on human soft tissue are called bioeffects, or biologic effects. *(2:319; 20:622)*

346. **(E)** The speed of ultrasound in soft tissue is 1,540 meters per second (1,540 m/s), 1.54 millimeters per microsecond (1.54 mm/µs), 0.154 cm/µs, or one mile per second. *(2:20; 18:35)*

347. **(C)** Slope

348. **(B)** Delay

349. **(D)** Far gain

350. **(A)** Near gain *(6:299–318; 18:224)*

351. **(C)** Progressive weakening of the sound beam as it travels through a medium *(2:30)*

352. **(F)** A new imaging technique used to assess tissue stiffness. This is based on a well-established principle that malignant tissue is stiffer than benign tissue *(25:92)*

353. **(G)** Binary digit *(2:121–123)*

354. **(B)** The production and behavior of microbubbles within a medium *(2:328–330)*

355. **(D)** A liquid placed between the transducer and the skin *(2:41)*

356. **(H)** A method of reducing pulse duration by mechanical or electrical means *(2:57–58)*

357. **(E)** The number of intensity levels between black and white *(2:118)*

358. **(J)** Plastic material used in front of the transducer face to reduce the reflection at the transducer surface *(2:59–60)*

359. **(A)** Picture element *(2:112–113)*

360. **(I)** Single-frame imaging *(2:218–220)*

361. **(D)** W/cm^2 *(6:242)*

362. **(A)** Spatial compounding *(24:94)*

363. **(C)** Spatial peak temporal average *(2:29–32)*

364. **(B)** kg/m^3 *(2:20–23)*

365. **(D)** m/s *(2:20)*

366. **(F)** Hz *(2:18)*

367. **(E)** Joule (J) *(2:261; 20:1009)*

368. **(A)** W/cm^2 *(2:29–32)*

369. **(C)** Wavelength can be expressed in millimeter (mm) or meter (m). One millimeter is one thousandth of a meter (0.001 m). *(2:20; 18:32)*

370. **(G)** dB *(2:30–31)*

371. **(B)** 0.002 W/cm^2–0.5 W/cm^2 SPTA *(6:250)*

372. **(A)** 0.5 W/cm^2–2.0 W/cm^2 SPTA *(6:250)*

373. **(C)** Under normal intensity ranges, diagnostic ultrasound is atraumatic, nontoxic, noninvasive, and nonionizing. It is nonionizing because the intensity in diagnostic ultrasound range is not sufficient to eject an electron from an atom. *(10:26)*

374. **(D)** Heat. However, at the diagnostic intensity range, the heat produced has no known effect. *(10:26)*

375. **(A)** The production and behavior of gas bubbles (microbubbles) is called cavitation. Cavitation occurs when dissolved gases grow into microbubbles during the negative pressure phase of ultrasound wave propagation. There are two types of cavitation, stable and transient. Stable cavitation is a phenomenon in which microbubbles are formed and persist in a diameter with the passing pressure variations of the ultrasound wave. In transient cavitation, the microbubbles continue to grow in size until they collapse, producing shock waves. *(2:320–330)*

376. **(D)** There are two types of cavitation, stable and transient. Stable cavitation is a phenomenon in which microbubbles are formed and persist. In transient cavitation, the microbubbles continue to grow in size until they collapse. *(2:320–330)*

377. **(A)** Doppler *(2:6)*

378. **(A)** When an interface is smooth, or "mirror-like," or larger than the wavelength, it is called a specular reflector. When the ultrasound beam strikes a specular reflector, the angle of reflection can be a critical factor when performing sonograms. The maximum amount of reflected echo occurs when the transducer is perpendicular to the interface. *(3:6, 12)*

379. **(B)** When an interface is smaller than the wavelength, usually less than 3 mm, it is called a nonspecular reflector. Nonspecular reflectors are not beam-angle dependent. *(3:6, 12)*

380. **(B)** Spatial average temporal average *(6:242; 18:71)*

381. **(C)** Spatial peak pulse average *(6:242; 18:71)*

382. **(A)** Because Doppler instruments are used for moving structures, A-mode imaging does not apply. The Doppler instrument employs pulsed or continuous waves. The frequency ranges from 20 cps to 20,000 cps, which is amplified by a loudspeaker; thus, the resulting sound is audible. *(18:294)*

383. **(A)** 5 MHz, short-focus. The choice of focal zone depends on what structure is to be imaged. The choice of transducer frequency depends on the amount of penetration and/or resolution needed. High-frequency transducers display good axial resolution but reduced tissue penetration. For superficial structures, a high-frequency transducer is most useful; for deep structures, low frequency is most useful. *(2:82)*

384. **(B)** 3 MHz, long-focus. See explanation for Question 383. *(2:82)*

385. **(A)** Pixel is short for picture element. *(3:32)*

386. **(A)** Under normal circumstances, and depending on the lighting conditions, the human eye can distinguish as many as 16 shades of gray. The human eye can differentiate more color shades than gray shade. Current ultrasound systems can produce 256 shades of color, which is beyond the levels of the human lens under normal conditions. *(2:129; 3:32)*

387. **(A)** 512 × 512 × 8-bit deep with 256 shades *(2:112)*

388. **(C)** "Aliasing" results when the velocity exceeds the pulse repetition frequency (PRF). Aliasing is an artifact seen in pulse Doppler ultrasound. Aliasing *never emerges with continuous-wave Doppler*. *(18:309)*

389. **(C)** Continuous-wave Doppler does not have time-gain compensation. *(18:303)*

390. **(A)** As ultrasound propagates through body tissue, it undergoes attenuation, which is the progressive weakening of the sound wave as it travels. The causes of attenuation are:
    1. absorption
    2. reflection
    3. scattering

    When the sound wave is absorbed, it is then converted to heat. The heat generated from absorption is mostly removed by conduction. Cavitation does not occur at normal intensity levels. *(3:5, 28; 8:74)*

391. **(E)** One of the major disadvantages of continuous-wave Doppler is range ambiguity. *(24:75)*

392. **(A)** Turbulence is most likely to occur with a larger diameter, higher velocity, and lower viscosity. Anemia is a decrease in the amount of red blood cells causing the blood to have a decrease in viscosity. Therefore, a low

hematocrit or acute anemia is related to lower viscosity. Polycythemia is an increase in the number of red blood cells causing the blood to have an increase in viscosity. *(24:66–68)*

393. **(C)** Decreasing the Doppler shift, increasing the pulse repetition frequency (PRF), adjusting the spectral baseline, or using a lower frequency can be used to decrease the likelihood of aliasing. *(24:76)*

394. **(B)** Temporal resolution is increased by shallow imaging, high frame rate, narrow sector, and low-line density. *(18:205; 20:218)*

395. **(A)** Aliasing is most likely to occur with high-frequency transducers, low pulse repetition frequency (PRF), and faster blood velocity. Aliasing does not occur in continuous-wave Doppler. *(18:307)*

396. **(A)** Digital memory can be visualized as squares on a checkerboard in which echoes are stored in a square corresponding to the location of the scanning plane. *(2:109–113)*

397. **(A)** Echo-free *(18:330)*

398. **(B)** Echogenic *(18:330)*

399. **(C)** Impedance cannot be measured by a hydrophone. *(2:319)*

400. **(B)** The hydrophone is made up of piezoelectric transducer elements and a membrane made of polyvinylidene fluoride (PVDF). *(2:315–319)*

401. **(C)** When ultrasound was applied for 2–3 minutes on laboratory animals, the results were growth retardation and hemorrhage. These effects were observed in laboratory animals, not humans, and with continuous-wave ultrasound. *(6:251)*

402. **(C)** Refraction is least likely associated with attenuation. Refraction is the bending of the sound beam as it crosses an acoustic impedance mismatch. *(2:30; 3:5)*

403. **(B)** Conversion of sound to heat *(3:5)*

404. **(A)** The spreading out of an ultrasound beam is referred to as diffraction. *(3:5; 9:48)*

405. **(D)** Redirection of the sound beam in several directions *(2:215; 3:5; 9:60)*

406. **(C)** The transducer's piezoelectric ceramic is heat sensitive and should not be subjected to excessive heat sterilization because the crystal in the transducer housing could become depolarized and loses it piezoelectric properties. Transducers are made up of a variety of materials, including plastic, crystals, bounding seals, steel, or metal casing, but they are not all constructed alike. A disinfectant that is safe for some transducers may be destructive to others. The recommended method for sterilizing transducers is available from the manufacturer's user manual or from the manufacturer's technical support department.

Any product used on transducers against the manufacturer instructions or precautionary measures could result in damage to the transducer and loss of the transducer warranty. *(16:130–131)*

407. **(A)** An acoustic window is a pathway through which the sound beam travels without interference. Examples are the liver and urinary bladder. *(22:77)*

408. **(A)** The decimal number 10 may also be represented by the binary number 1010. *(2:96)*

409. **(E)** The lowest intensity measurements used in diagnostic ultrasound is SATA. *(18:71)*

410. **(B)** The intensity used in diagnostic ultrasound to measure the potential biological effects in mammalian tissue is SPTA. *(18:71)*

411. **(A)** All images of transverse scans should be viewed from the patient's feet, in supine or prone positions. *(22:86)*

412. **(B)** In longitudinal (sagittal) scans, the images are presented with the patient's head to the left of the image and feet to the right of the image in both supine and prone positions. *(22:86)*

413. **(C)** Within the receiver, a number of signal-processing functions take place: amplification, compensation, demodulation, compression, and rejection. *(2:84)*

414. **(B)** Because the particles in ultrasound waves oscillate in the same direction of wave propagation, no plane is defined. Therefore, ultrasound waves cannot be polarized. *(2:17–18; 20:81–86)*

415. **(D)** Quartz is the transducer crystal most likely to be employed. *(2:55; 20:234–236)*

416. **(E)** All of the above *(2:55; 20:234–236)*

417. **(E)** The sound beam from a linear phased-array transducer is electronically transmitted in outward direction to produce a sector shape image. *(18:167–168; 24:47; 25:51)*

418. **(D)** Two hundred fifty-six (256), or the number 2 raised to the power of 8 (the number of bits per memory element): $256 = 2^8$. *(2:116–123)*

419. **(D)** The highest intensity measurements used in diagnostic ultrasound are SPTP. *(18:71)*

420. **(E)** Both ultrasound and fluoroscopy evaluate moving structures in movie-like appearance. However, ultrasound is nonionizing because its intensity is insufficient to eject an electron from the atom. Fluoroscopy is ionizing and results in potential biologic effects. X-ray fluoroscopy is produced in vacuum tubes, which is a space without matter. Ultrasound needs matter in order to propagate. *(8:13; 20:83)*

421. **(A)** The contrast media used for roentgenographic oral cholecystogram (x-ray of the gall bladder) and nous

pyelogram (x-rays of the kidneys) do not obscure the propagation of ultrasound. Barium sulfate ($BaSO_4$) for upper gastrointestinal examination obscures the propagation of ultrasound. *(8:13)*

422. **(I)** A device used to focus sound beams *(2:65)*

423. **(C)** Picture element *(2:112, 116)*

424. **(D)** Pie shaped *(2:68)*

425. **(F)** A device that changes sound waves into visible light patterns acoustic-optics (Schlieren). *(18:367)*

426. **(B)** The portion of the sound beam outside of the main beam *(18:189)*

427. **(H)** Imaginary surface passing through particles of the same vibration as an ultrasound wave *(2:209–217)*

428. **(A)** Unit of impedance *(2:35–36)*

429. **(G)** The ratio between the angle of incidence and the refraction *(2:39)*

430. **(E)** A change in frequency as a result of reflector motion between the transducer and the reflector *(2:6)*

431. **(B)** The lateral resolution is defined as being equal to the beam diameter. *(2:76–79)*

432. **(D)** Perspex, aluminum, and polystyrene can be used to make acoustic lenses. Ethylene oxide is a gas, not a material used for lenses. *(20:249–250)*

433. **(C)** Both ultrasound and light can be focused and defocused by mirrors and lenses. *(18:151–153)*

434. **(A)** 0.77–0.15 mm (2–10 MHz transducer) *(2:19)*

435. **(C)** Individual cells cannot be identified because they are smaller than the wavelength used in the medium. Advancement in ultrasound allows depiction of nerve. This new methodology uses ultrasound to aid in nerve blocks. *(2:322)*

436. **(D)** Mass per unit volume *(18:13)*

437. **(E)** The longer the distance traveled, the greater the absorption. Absorption increases with increased frequency, and the amount of frictional force encountered by the propagating sound wave (viscosity) determines the amount of absorption. Absorption in the body also tends to increase in collagen content. *(18:82; 20:642)*

438. **(D)** There are no confirmed biologic effects on human tissue exposed to intensities used in the diagnostic range below 100 m/Wcm^2. However, laboratory experiments on pregnant mice with intensities far greater than that used in the diagnostic range resulted in growth retardation in the offspring of the mice. *(2:333; 6:251)*

439. **(C)** Pregnant mice exposed to continuous-wave ultrasound, for 2–3 minutes, experienced hemorrhage, neurocranial damage, and growth retardation. *(2:325)*

440. **(B)** A combination of low frequency and high intensity is most likely to cause cavitation resulting in tissue damage. *(6:250)*

441. **(H)** Living human tissue *(18:369)*

442. **(E)** Tissue cultures in a test tube *(18:369)*

443. **(F)** A method of analyzing a waveform *(2:229)*

444. **(G)** The property of a medium characterized by energy distortion in the medium and irreversibly converted to heat *(10:157)*

445. **(B)** Elimination of small amplitude echo *(10:120)*

446. **(C)** A process of acoustic energy absorption *(10:120)*

447. **(A)** An in vivo phenomenon characterized by erythrocytes within small vessels stopping the flow and collecting in the low-pressure regions of the standing wave field *(2:3–12)*

448. **(D)** Energy transported per unit time *(10:10)*

449. **(F)** All of the statements are false or unconfirmed at the present time. Experimental studies were conducted on pregnant mice, not pregnant women. The intensity, frequency, and exposure time were far greater than those used in a diagnostic setting. Continuous ultrasound was used in many of the experiments. *(2:319–329)*

450. **(E)** At present, there are no known exposure injuries in humans in the clinical setting. Injuries have been reported only in laboratory animals. *(2:319–329)*

451. **(A)** No distinction. All real-time scans are B-scans, and both static and real-time instruments employ B-mode. *(13:44–45)*

452. **(D)** The word transonic implies a region uninhibited to the propagation of ultrasound. An echo-free (anechoic) region does not guarantee the region to be transonic. For example, a homogenous solid mass can be echo-free but not transonic. Conversely, a region can exhibit echoes and be transonic. *(10:152)*

453. **(B)** Real-time is also referred to as dynamic imaging. A-mode and M-mode are also real-time modes. A static imaging cannot be changed or moved. *(10:171)*

454. **(A)** The TGC is composed of near gain, delay, slope, knee, and far gain. *(22:58–61)*

455. **(A)** The range of pulse repetition frequencies used in diagnostic ultrasound is 4–15 kHz. *(2:89)*

456. **(C)** Wavelength, cycles. The spatial pulse length (SPL) is defined as the product of the wavelength multiplied by the number of cycles in a pulse. *(17:61)*

457. **(B)** A-mode and M-mode *(2:143; 18:157–161)*

458. **(B)** Spatial compounding is a sequential averaging of frames that view anatomy from different angles. This creates multiple images over time and organizes them to

create one image. Frequency compounding is a combination of echo data from the same location but different frequencies. *(2:114; 10:65, 135)*

459. **(C)** Ultrasound and x-rays are inaudible. Doppler instruments employ an audio mode (20–20,000 Hz). *(18:22, 294)*

460. **(C)** Continuous-wave mode. Continuous-wave mode requires two crystals, one for transmitting and the other for receiving. *(18:303)*

461. **(A)** Ring-down (dead zone) *(20:708–709)*

462. **(B)** Vertical measurement calibration *(20:708–709)*

463. **(C)** Axial-lateral resolution *(20:708–709)*

464. **(D)** Horizontal measurement calibration *(20:708–709)*

465. **(B)** 0.2–400 mW/cm^2 *(2:172–173)*

466. **(A)** Higher frequency than the incident frequency *(2:172)*

467. **(B)** Lower frequency than the incident frequency *(2:172)*

468. **(C)** Bidirectional *(2:128)*

469. **(A)** Doppler color has faster velocities that are represented by lighter color or hue *(2:186)*

470. **(B)** Control used to suppress or increase echoes in the near field *(18:224)*

471. **(A)** Control used to suppress or increase echoes in the far field *(18:224)*

472. **(D)** Control the upward incline of the TGC. Used to display an even texture throughout an organ *(18:224)*

473. **(C)** Control used to delay the start of the slope *(18:224)*

474. **(E)** Controls the point where the slope ends *(18:224)*

475. **(B)** Bandwidth is the range of frequencies contained in an ultrasound pulse. *(2:26)*

476. **(A)** The Q factor is unitless. *(2:27)*

477. **(B)** The urine-filled bladder is characterized by sharp posterior walls and distal acoustic enhancement. The enhancement is associated with low attenuation. Solid and calcified masses demonstrate a different phenomenon, distal attenuation, the degree of which is determined by the attenuating properties of the mass. *(8:11–12)*

478. **(C)** Surgical clips, calcified masses, gallstones, or any high reflective or attenuating structure can produce an acoustic shadow. This results from failure of the sound beam to pass through the object. The urinary bladder, gallbladder, and any fluid-filled structure will demonstrate acoustic enhancement. In some circumstances, both acoustic enhancement and acoustic shadowing can be seen, for example, a gallbladder with stones. *(8:11–12)*

479. **(B)** Pooling not related to the sonographic descriptions of blood flow. Blood is classified into five different flow characteristics (1) plug flow, (2) parabolic flow, (3) laminar flow, (4) disturbed flow, and (5) turbulence flow. *(2:162–163)*

480. **(C)** When the beam strikes a vessel at a 30° angle. Doppler angle is the angle between the direction of propagation of the ultrasound beam and the direction of flow. Unlike real-time imaging of the abdominal organs in which the best images are obtained when the ultrasound beam has a perpendicular incidence, Doppler has minimum shift at 90° (perpendicular) incidence, and a maximum shift when the transducer is oriented parallel to the direction of flow, even though parallel transducer orientation is not possible in most cases. Doppler application employs a Doppler angle of 30°–60° with respect to the vessel. *(18:299–300)*

481. **(B)** 20 dB *(18:75–76)*

$$dB = 10 \log\left(\frac{\text{power out}}{\text{power in}}\right)$$
$$= 10 \log(100) = 20 \text{ dB}$$

(34:3)

482. **(D)** Time-gain compensation (TGC) *(18:224)*

483. **(D)** Refraction, propagation speed. Refraction occurs in oblique incident and if the propagation speed is different between the two media. *(18:99)*

484. **(A)** Better axial resolution. Axial resolution is related to the length of the pulse. The shorter the pulse, the better the axial resolution. *(2:76–81)*

485. **(A)** 0.25 mW/cm^2. The reflection fraction R: *(1:366)*

$$R = \left(\frac{Z_2 - Z_1}{Z_2 + Z_1}\right)^2 = \left(\frac{75 - 25}{75 + 25}\right)^2 = 0.25$$

486. **(B)** Frequency and diameter. Near-zone length (NZL) is the same as the Fresnel zone:

$$NZL = \frac{D^2}{4\lambda},$$

where D is diameter transducer (cm), and λ is wavelength (cm). *(2:63–65)*

487. **(D)** The element thickness. The operating frequency is determined by the element thickness, the thinner the element the higher the frequency.

$$\text{thickness} = \frac{1}{2} \text{ wavelength} \quad (2:56)$$

488. **(B)** Refraction does not occur with normal incidence or when the propagation speed of the two media is the same. Refraction is described by Snell's law, which relates

the incident angle (ϕ_i) and the transmitted angle (ϕ_t) to the relative velocities of the two media.

$$\frac{\sin \phi_t}{\sin \phi_t} = \frac{V_1}{V_2}$$

When there is normal incidence, $\phi_i = 0$, and the sound will only change velocity and will not be bent. *(18:99)*

489. **(C)** 1.54 mm/µs or 1,540 m/s *(18:35)*

490. **(C)** 1.0%

$$DF = \frac{PD}{PRP} = \frac{5}{500} = \frac{1}{100} = 1\%$$

(2:25)

491. **(D)** The amount of acoustic exposure is determined by the intensity of the ultrasound beam and the amount of examination time. *(24:126)*

492. **(C)** Tissue attenuation. Tissue attenuation increases and penetration decreases with increased frequency. *(2:32–33)*

493. **(C)** 3.5 dB
total attenuation = attenuation coefficient × path length

$$dB = 1.75 \text{ dB/cm} \times 2 \text{ cm}$$
$$= 3.5 \text{ dB}$$

The attenuation coefficient in dB/cm is by a rule of thumb equal to one-half the frequency in MHz; i.e., at 3.5 MHz, the attenuation coefficient is 1.75 dB/cm. *(2:32–33)*

494. **(D)** Propagation speed *(2:20–22)*

495. **(A)** Maximum velocity occur within the stenosis. *(18:282)*

496. **(D)** 70%

100% = percentage reflected + percentage transmitted *(2:36)*

497. **(D)** Turbulent flow is possible when blood flow exceeds of Reynolds number of 2,000. *(2:163)*

498. **(C)** Distance, velocity, and time

$$\text{distance} = \text{velocity} \times \text{time}$$

(2:338)

499. **(C)** Reynolds number *(2:163)*

500. **(C)** 90°

$$\text{Doppler shift frequency} = \frac{2fV}{C}\cos\theta,$$

where V = velocity of blood flow; f, transducer frequency; C, velocity of sound. Because cos 90° is 0, the Doppler shift frequency is 0. *(2:172)*

501. **(C)** Turbulence is a non-laminar flow, with flow in randomized and in multiple directions. Turbulence flow occurs beyond (distal) the obstruction in a stenotic blood vessel. *(2:163)*

502. **(A)** The ratio of the maximum to the minimum intensity that can be processed. *(18:257)*

503. **(B)** If the thermal paper printer is not working, the first step is to check for a jam in the printer. *(18:251)*

504. **(A)** Compensates for attenuation effects *(2:100–101)*

505. **(D)** Computer memory *(2:101–103)*

506. **(D)** An increase in the peak rarefactional pressure could result in inertial cavitation. Mechanical index (MI) indicates the likelihood of cavitation. *(2:329, 357; 20:1012)*

507. **(B)** Weakly attenuating structures *(2:30)*

508. **(D)** Ultrasound depth penetration is inversely related to frequency. As frequency increases, penetration decreases. *(2:25–26)*

509. **(E)** Lateral resolution is affected by beam diameter, aperture, acoustic lens, focal zone, and frequency. Higher frequencies improve both axial and lateral resolution. *(18:148–153)*

510. **(B)** Increased frame rate. If the line density is kept constant, then the number of lines per image will decrease, making the time required per image smaller. *(18:194–195)*

511. **(D)** Line D. The transducer is placed on top of the tissue-equivalent phantom. The ultrasound beam is perpendicular to the group of nylon lines horizontal to the axis of the sound beam. This group is used to evaluate horizontal distance accuracy. *(20:708–709)*

512. **(B)** The transducer is placed on top of the tissue-equivalent phantom. The ultrasound beam is parallel to the group of nylon lines vertical to the axis of the sound beam. This group is used to evaluate range accuracy or vertical depth calibration. *(18:362)*

513. **(D)** The advantages of continuous-wave include the ability to measure very high velocities, higher frequency, no aliasing, and no Nyquist limit. The disadvantage is range ambiguity. *(18:303–309)*

514. **(C)** 15 dB. For every change of 3 dB, the intensity will change by a factor of 2. *(2:30–32)*

515. **(C)** Decreases the maximum depth imaged. The pulse repetition period (PRP) is the length of time allowed to collect echoes for each image line; a short PRP means less image depth. *(18:52)*

516. **(E)** The AIUM 100-mm test object is not used to evaluate attenuation, scattering, echo-texture, gray scale, and cystic and solid mass. *(18:355–356)*

517. **(A)** All ultrasound regardless of frequency travels at the same propagation speed if traveling in the same medium. It is the medium that determines the speed of ultrasound.

Ultrasound travels faster in solids and slower in gases. Fast medium has long wavelength and slow medium has short wavelength. (*18:34–35*)

518. **(A)** Lateral resolution (*18:189*)

519. **(D)** Spatial compound imaging is a technique that improves the image quality with scan lines directed in multiple directions created over time and then averaged together to create one image. The benefits of compound imaging are the reduction of reverberation and shadowing and to visualized structures hidden beneath high attenuation. (*20:366; 25:92*)

520. **(E)** All ultrasound regardless of frequency travels at the same propagation speed if traveling in the same medium. It is the medium that determines the speed of ultrasound. Ultrasound travels faster in solids and slower in gases. Fast medium has long wavelength and slow medium has short wavelength. Gas and air in the lungs are slow medium and therefore have a short wavelength. (*18:34–35*)

521. **(B)** Sensitivity (*18:360*)

522. **(A)** Thermal and cavitation. Thermal or heating effects are normally unmeasurable with diagnostic instruments. Further cavitation is also unlikely at current diagnostic levels. Cavitation refers to the growth and behavior of gas bubbles produced in tissue by ultrasound. (*2:327–328*)

523. **(B)** Frequency and transducer diameter. High frequencies and/or large diameter transducers produce long near-zone (Fresnel zone) lengths. (*2:62–63*)

524. **(B)** No evidence of independently confirmed biological effects in mammalian below SPTA 100 mW/cm^2 (*20:643*)

525. **(C)** Highest at the focal zone. This is true because the intensity is equal to the power/beam area, and the beam area is smallest at the focal zone. (*2:62–63*)

526. **(B)** 0.3 mm (*2:19*)

$$\lambda = \frac{V}{f} = \frac{1.54 \text{ mm/μs}}{5 \text{ MHz}}$$

$$\lambda = 0.3 \text{ mm}$$

(*2:8*)

527. **(C)** Two times smaller. A 3-dB attenuation change would correspond to a factor-of-2 reduction; that is, one-half. For each decrease in intensity of 3 dB, the intensity is decreased by one-half. Thus, for 6-dB attenuation, the intensity is decreased by one-fourth. (*1:356*)

528. **(B)** Linear-phased array is commonly called phased array. Linear-phased array has a sector-shaped image and linear sequential array is a rectangular image. (*2:68; 18:185*)

529. **(A)** A wide band of frequencies centered at 5 MHz (*1:360*)

530. **(D)** Thickness, resonance frequency. Specifically, thickness equals one-half wavelength, where wavelength is velocity divided by frequency. (*1:358*)

531. **(A)** Increased damping, sensitivity. Increased damping does improve axial resolution by making the spatial pulse length shorter; however, the result is to make the transducer less sensitive to small echoes. (*1:360*)

532. **(A)** Piezoelectric (*2:55–57*)

533. **(C)** Matching. Usually a matching layer is added to the front surface of the transducer acoustic impedance intermediate between the impedance of the transducer and that of soft tissue. (*1:370*)

534. **(E)** RAID is an acronym for redundant array of independent disks. RAID is an alternative to a large storage system that requires speedy data transfer rate and security. The main archive device for PACS server is RAID. (*23:97*)

535. **(A)** Highly attenuating structures (*2:30*)

536. **(B)** Occur with multiple strong reflectors. Reverberation artifacts are present when two or more strong reflectors are located in the beam. One of these may be the transducer itself. The sound, in essence, gets trapped between these reflectors. Reverberation artifacts are displayed as equally spaced echoes often seen in fluid-filled mass. (*2:263*)

537. **(A)** Good axial resolution. A large bandwidth is equivalent to a short spatial pulse length. (*1:360*)

538. **(A)** Fraunhofer zone. The far zone is also known as the Fraunhofer zone; this is the region from the focus and extending to beam diversion. (*18:135*)

539. **(D)** With normal incidence of the ultrasound beam. At oblique incidence, a sound beam will be bent if there is a change in propagation speed across the boundary. With normal incidence, however, the beam will either slow down or speed up, but will not bend. (*18:99*)

540. **(C)** The pulser voltage spike. The larger the applied voltage, the greater the deformation of the crystal and, consequently, the amplitude of the pressure wave produced. However, a larger crystal (same thickness) experiencing the same voltage will produce more acoustic energy. (*18:212–213*)

541. **(B)** The reflecting surface is large and smooth with respect to the wavelength. Reflectors whose boundaries are smooth relative to the wavelength behave as mirrors and reflect all frequencies equally. Small reflectors (diffuse or nonspecular) scatter the sound in all directions and show a frequency dependence. (*18:79*)

542. **(C)** Snell's law (*2:39*)

543. **(A)** Annular phased array has multiple ring-shaped elements. (*18:176*)

544. **(A)** 90–100%. Because the acoustic impedance of gas is so much smaller than that of soft tissue, there is almost 100% of the energy reflected. (*1:366*)

545. **(E)** 1–10%

$$Z_{fat} = 1.38$$
$$Z_{muscule} = 1.70$$
$$R = \left(\frac{1.70 - 1.38}{1.70 + 1.38}\right)^2 = 0.011 \ (1.1\%)$$

where *R* is the percentage of beam reflected. (*1:366*)

546. **(B)** Focal zone can be moved to the skin surface. The acoustic standoff (waterpath) is normally positioned between the transducer and the patient skin to allow visualization of superficial structures. Superficial structures are sometimes difficult to image due to the dead zone. High-frequency transducer and acoustic standoff are used to image structures in the dead zone. (*18:361*)

547. **(D)** Longitudinal compression waves. Longitudinal implies that the variation in the pressure occurs in the direction of propagation. This is opposed to a transverse wave, where variations occur perpendicular to the propagation. Transverse waves can occur in bone. (*2:18; 20:83*)

548. **(A)** Shorter wavelength and less penetration. The wavelength is inversely related to the frequency, and the attenuation is directly related to frequency.

$$\text{half-intensity depth (cm)} = \frac{3 \ dB}{f},$$

where *f* is the frequency in MHz. (*2:18–21*)

549. **(A)** Ring-down time. A long ring-down time is undesirable. It increases the spatial pulse length and, thus, decreases axial resolution. (*1:360*)

550. **(B)** Electronically focus in two dimensions rather than one. An annular phased array can be focused dynamically in two dimensions. A linear array can be focused dynamically only in the plane of the array. In the slice-thickness direction, perpendicular to the array plane, focusing is achieved by shaping the transducer elements or by acoustic lens. This is often referred to as double focusing. (*18:176–180*)

551. **(C)** Gas, muscle, bone. This ordering proceeds along increasing stiffness or lack of compressibility. Therefore, gas is slow, with an increasing order to the fastest, which is bone. (*18:35*)

552. **(A)** Resolution, penetration. At low frequencies, the axial resolution becomes unacceptable (<1 MHz), whereas at high frequencies, the depth of penetration in the body becomes prohibitively small (10 MHz). (*18:21–22*)

553. **(B)**. Engineering notation, also known as scientific notation, is a shorthand way of writing very large or very small numbers. The first step is to put a decimal after

the first digit and drop the zeroes. For the given number 125,000,000,000, the coefficient is 1.25. To find the exponent, count the number of places from the decimal to the end of the number. This should be 11 places. The number 125,000,000,000 is written 1.25×10^{11}. (*18:6*)

554. **(B)** SPTP is always equal to or greater than SPTA. SPTP refers to spatial peak–temporal peak, and SPTA refers to spatial peak–temporal average. In all cases, peak values will be at least as great as the average values by definition. For continuous-wave ultrasound, there is no variation of the intensity in time, and peak values will be equal. (*2:28–30*)

555. **(C)** A hydrophone. A hydrophone is a small piezoelectric crystal that is moved in front of a transducer in a manner so that the beam pattern is mapped. A radiation force balance is used to quantify the total beam power. Other phantoms can be used to give qualitative estimates of beam profiles. (*2:315, 319*)

556. **(E)** When the direction of flow is perpendicular, 90°, to the sound beam, the velocity and cosine are zero. (*18:300*)

557. **(B)** Schlieren method. Schlieren photography gives a two-dimensional photograph of the beam pressure profile. (*1:362*)

558. **(D)** Time. Pulse duration is equal to the period of a wave times the number of waves in a pulse, usually microseconds in length. (*18:47–48*)

559. **(C)** Nyquist frequency is one-half of the pulse repetition frequency (PRF). The PRF given was 2,000 Hz; therefore, the Nyquist frequency is 1 kHz (1,000 Hz). (*18:306–309*)

560. **(B)** W/cm^2. SPTA refers to intensity, which is power (watts) per unit beam area (cm^2). (*2:29*)

561. **(C)** Curie point. Crystals heated above the Curie point lose their piezoelectric property. The Curie point for quartz is 573°C and for PZT is 328°C. (*1:358*)

562. **(C)** Increase ninefold. $I = A^2 = (3)^2 = 9$, where *I* is intensity, and *A* is amplitude. (*1:388*)

563. **(A)** Increasing the output power improves the signal-to-noise ratio. Increasing the receiver gain amplification does not change the signal-to-noise ratio. (*18:231*)

564. **(D)** Velocity, unchanged. The velocity is essentially independent of frequency and is rather dependent upon the physical properties of the medium. (*18:34*)

565. **(B)** Electronic time-delay pulsing. The delay pulsing of the array elements can be used to form a wavefront directed at different angles. Pulsing can also be used to focus the beam at different depths. (*18:167*)

566. **(A)** Is made possible by array-based systems. Dynamic focusing is possible only with array-based systems because it is necessary to monitor individually echoes received from each location. (*2:66–67*)

567. **(A)** Amplification of the receiver voltage *(18:231)*

568. **(C)** 1.54 mm. The velocity of ultrasound in soft tissues is 1.54 mm/μs. *(2:35)*

569. **(A)** Ring-down artifact. The arrow points to a ring-down artifact produced most probably by gas bubbles resulting in a tail of reverberation echoes. *(15:21–28)*

570. **(A)** Rods for measuring dead zone (ring-down). The small open arrowheads point to a rod group used in measurement of the transducer dead zone. *(6:261–276)*

571. **(B)** A simulated solid lesion *(6:261–276)*

572. **(C)** A simulated cyst *(6:261–276)*

573. **(D)**.The thickness of active element. The frequency of the transducer is determined by the thickness of the active element and the speed of sound in the active element. *(18:126–127)*

574. **(D)** Most contrast agents contain gas-filled microbubbles that are stabilized by protein or lipid shell. The earliest agents used air-filled bubbles. More recently, perfluorocarbon gas is used. *(2:41)*

575. **(B)** Perfluorocarbon *(2:41)*

576. **(B)** As the pulse repetition frequency (PRF) increases the depth of view decreases. *(18:55)*

577. **(E)** Acoustic clutter and ghosting artifact can be eliminated with wall filter. Clutter results from tissue, heart wall, or vessel wall motion. *(2:297; 18:320; 20:545–547)*

578. **(B)** Speckle is a form of acoustic noise that appears in close proximity to the transducer as random variation signal giving the impression of tissue texture but not corresponding to true anatomic tissue. *(18:347; 20:168)*

579. **(D)** All of the above. Color-flow images can be used to position a single-point, pulsed-Doppler, sample volume, as is the case with more conventional duplex imaging. *(30:1241)*

580. **(C)** Stationary tissue in gray-scale and moving tissues in color. All moving tissues in a color-flow imaging can produce color. Thus, stationary tissues are in gray scale, whereas moving tissues, including blood, are in color. *(28:236)*

581. **(A)** A form of color-flow imaging. Color-flow imaging includes both Doppler and non-Doppler forms of imaging. *(28:236; 30:1241; 34:27)*

582. **(C)** To all waves coming from a moving wave source. The Doppler effect happens to all waves coming from a moving source, regardless of propagating velocity or power levels. *(37:172)*

583. **(B)** The closing velocity between transducer and tissue, carrier frequency, and ultrasound propagation velocity. The Doppler equation looks like the following:

$$Df = 2(f_0/c) \, V \cos \theta,$$

where f_0 is the carrier frequency, c is the propagation velocity, and θ is the Doppler angle. $V \cos \theta$ is the closing velocity between the transducer and moving tissue. *(37:173)*

584. **(D)** Place a sample volume in the major streamline or jet and set the angle correction parallel to the streamline. Because the color pattern shows the location of the major streamline or jet, calculating velocity requires correction relative to the flow geometry, not the vessel. *(37:195)*

585. **(B)** One wavelength or less. This is necessary for textural information to reach the display in a digital scan converter. *(32:654)*

586. **(C)** One wavelength or more but less than 1 mm. Digital sampling for vascular flow information requires such an interval because larger intervals cannot show the flow patterns within the vessel. *(28:236)*

587. **(C)** The product of transmit and receive focusing. The effective beam width results from the mathematical product of both functions. *(36:620; 38:155)*

588. **(A)** True. The sample volume and flow interact in a manner that depends on the geometry of the sample volume. *(33:9)*

589. **(C)** The average Doppler shift frequency. At each sample site, the color-flow system determines the average Doppler shift frequency. *(28:236)*

590. **(B)** False. At each sample site, the system determines the average Doppler shift frequency. The display is then either these average frequencies or, in some cases, the calculated closing velocity. This velocity is the rate at which the flow is approaching or moving away from the transducer along the line of sight. *(28:236)*

591. **(D)** The relationship between the amplitudes and frequencies of the Doppler signals. The system will then avoid coloring strong slow-moving echo sources (tissue) but still color moderately fast weak echo sources (blood). *(39:647)*

592. **(B)** The vessel is open, but the blood velocity is too low to complete the image. As the vessel curves away from the beam, the Doppler frequencies become too low to be portrayed. The completeness of a color-flow image depends on the velocity of the blood flow and the Doppler angle. *(27:19, 44)*

593. **(D)** The smaller vessels do not reflect ultrasound as well as the larger vessels do. Every living cell in the body is no more than two cell layers away from a red blood cell. The

smaller vessels, however, are not sufficiently echogenic and vanish from the color display first because of their small echo signals. (*34:7*)

594. **(D)** 1, 2, and 3. Color provides information about the existence of flow, its location in the image, its location in the anatomy, the direction of the flow relative to the transducer, the direction of flow within the vessel, the flow pattern within the vessel, and the pulsatility of the flow. It does not indicate the velocity of the flow. (*30:1245*)

595. **(D)** Changes in echo signal phase. As with all directional Doppler systems, color-flow systems detect the existence of motion with a change in echo signal phase. By measuring the direction of the phase change, the system shows whether the direction of motion is toward or away from the transducer. (*33:34*)

596. **(B)** Knowing the position of the scan plane on the patient's body. The expected flow pattern in any vessel comes from knowing how the scan plane is positioned on the patient. For example, the patient's head is always placed on the image left in long axis scans, and the patient's right side is on the image left in cross-sectional scans. (*37:407*)

597. **(D)** Different colors (hues) or different levels of saturation (purity). The average frequency within each Doppler sample site is portrayed as a change in either color saturation (purity or whiteness) or hue (color). The object is to use the color to show flow patterns within the vessel lumen or heart chambers. (*27:44*)

598. **(C)** Changes in color hue. The variance in Doppler frequencies can be shown with a change in hue, such as green tones with increasing variance. (*9:27; 28:236*)

599. **(A)** Changes in color. Cardiac systems change color hues (frequencies) along red and blue lines to show changes in Doppler shift frequencies. Broadening frequencies in a sample site become shades of green. (*27:44*)

600. **(B)** False. Because only one frequency can come to the screen for each Doppler image pixel, all current systems use some estimate of the mean frequency. (*28:236*)

601. **(B)** False. Because color uses the average frequency at each location, the maximum systolic frequency will always be greater than the mean value. (*28:236; 34:27; 35:591*)

602. **(A)** True. Because synchronous signal processing uses the same echo signal for both Doppler and gray-scale signal processing, the frequency must be the same. (*28:236*)

603. **(B)** False. Asynchronous signal processing can, and often does, use different frequencies for the gray-scale image and the Doppler image. For example, it could image at 5.0 MHz and have a Doppler carrier of 3.0 MHz. (*28:236*)

604. **(A)** A Doppler angle significantly less than 90° to typical blood flow. All Doppler imaging requires a Doppler angle. In asynchronous systems that do not use a wedge, the angle comes from beam steering. (*37:173*)

605. **(D)** A Doppler angle between the typical flow patterns in vessels. Synchronous systems that keep the beams perpendicular to the transducer array (angiodynography) use a mechanical wedge to obtain the Doppler angle to the flow pattern of the vessel. (*28:236; 34:27*)

606. **(D)** Blood reflectivity is about 40–60 dB below that of soft tissue. The fact that blood reflectivity is about 1/100th to 1/1,000th that of soft tissues translates into reflectivities that are much lower than those of soft tissues. (*33:18*)

607. **(A)** True. Because the reflectivity of blood is low, many color-flow systems improve color penetration by greatly increasing the power of the transmitted Doppler output. (*28:236*)

608. **(B)** False. Synchronous signal-processing systems are limited by the power levels of the common transmitter used for both gray-scale imaging and Doppler imaging. As a result, imaging with and without Doppler produces similar power levels. (*9:27; 28:236*)

609. **(A)** True. The single-point spectrum requires the ultrasound beam to linger over its position longer than is the case in either real-time gray-scale imaging or color-flow imaging. (*9:27; 28:236*)

610. **(A)** Decrease. Color-flow imaging requires dwelling on each line of sight for as few as four pulse–listen cycles to as many as 32 pulse–listen cycles. Various systems have different dwell times. The typical end result is a reduction in image frame rate for color-flow imaging. (*28:236*)

611. **(A)** True. Real-time color-flow imaging of the heart requires relatively high frame rates. In general, Doppler requires dwelling on each line of sight for some period of time. In addition, each Doppler sample site requires processing time to extract the average Doppler shift frequency. Restoring suitable cardiac frame rates requires decreasing the number of color-flow lines of sight and the number of samples along each line. (*9:27; 37:17*)

612. **(B)** False. Cardiac color-flow imaging does not work well for vascular imaging because the Doppler sampling intervals are too large. Imaging the heart also involves a problem with reflectivities, not with tissue attenuation. (*27:236*)

613. **(B)** False. Doppler sampling for vascular imaging may be well below intervals of 1 mm. In contrast, sampling for echocardiography may be at intervals of several millimeters or more. (*27:17*)

614. **(B)** The ultrasound beams are always moving. This is the case because mechanical systems lack a special motor that could move the beam in small steps. Because Doppler signal processing is keyed to relative movement and the beam is always moving, color does not work well in mechanical systems. (*27:17*)

615. **(A)** 1 and 2. The linear phased array and the phased linear array have stationary ultrasound beams at each line of sight in the scanning plane. Both arrays also have increased grating lobes with beam steering. They do not have three-dimensional dynamic focusing or apertures necessarily of the same size. *(2:21; 34:27)*

616. **(B)** The linear array scan. The linear array with a rectangular scanning field is the geometry used for vascular imaging. The sector-scanning geometry makes reading color ambiguous in the straighter segments of a vessel. *(27:44)*

617. **(D)** A combination of A and C. Color-flow imaging of the heart uses the phased-array sector scan and the curved-linear array sector scan. These scanheads permit cardiac imaging from intercostal and subcostal windows. *(27:41)*

618. **(B)** 9 cm/s. Lowering the Doppler carrier frequency means that the same Doppler shift frequency requires a higher velocity to be just visible. *(38:280)*

619. **(B)** False. Like all pulsed Doppler systems, color systems will alias when the Doppler frequencies exceed the PRF sampling limit. *(33:37)*

620. **(C)** Decreasing the carrier frequency. This moves all Doppler frequencies downward and may bring the high aliasing frequencies below the aliasing limit. *(37:192)*

621. **(D)** Range ambiguity. High frame rates (high PRF) and high output power permit structures from outside the field of view to enter the image as a range ambiguity artifact. *(39:83)*

622. **(B)** False. The large fields of view for abdominal imaging slow the frame rate. In addition, vessel anatomy goes in all directions. Sorting out arteries and veins requires the spectrum to determine pulsatility. *(35:591)*

623. **(D)** A or B. In vascular color-flow imaging, turbulence appears as broken streamlines. The image then takes on a mottled appearance either in color or in color saturation. *(36:591)*

624. **(D)** A mottled green region. In color-flow echocardiography, the sampling intervals are too large to show turbulence. As a result, the system determines the spectral variance at each sampling site and expresses increased turbulence (increased variance) with increasing tones of green. *(27:12)*

625. **(B)** It encodes the power spectrum of the Doppler signal into color. Power Doppler looks at only the amplitudes of the Doppler signals in the I and Q channels. *(40:13)*

626. **(C)** It does not show the directionality of vessel flow. Power Doppler uses only the amplitudes of the signals in the I and Q channels. Without phase information, power Doppler cannot show the direction of flow. *(41:14)*

627. **(A)** Want to show tissue perfusion. Power Doppler will show wherever the system detects Doppler signal amplitudes. Thus, the color will distribute according to this signal map for both arteries and veins. *(41:16)*

References

1. Curry T, Dowdey J, Murry R Jr. *Christensen's Physics of Diagnostic Radiology*. 4rd ed. Philadelphia: Lippincott Williams & Wilkins; 1990.

2. Kremkau FW. *Diagnostic Ultrasound: Principles, Instruments*. 7th ed. St. Louis, MO: Saunders Elsevier; 2006.

3. Bartrum R, Crow H. *Real-time Ultrasound: A Manual for Physicians and Technical Personnel*. Philadelphia: WB Sanders; 1983.

4. Pinkney N. *A Review of the Concept of Ultrasound Physics and Instrumentation*. Philadelphia: Sonior; 1983.

5. Ziskin MC, Thickman DI, Goldberg NJ. The comet tail artifact. *J Ultrasound Med*. 1982; 1:1

6. Powis R, Powis W. *A Thinker's Guide to Ultrasonic Imaging*. Baltimore: Urban & Schwarzenberg; 1984.

7. Shelly G, Cashman T. *Computer Fundamentals for an Information Age*. Brea, CA: Anaheim Publishing; 1984.

8. Hagen-Ansert S. *Textbook of Diagnostic Ultrasonography*. 6th ed. Vol 1. St. Louis, MO: Mosby Elsevier; 2006.

9. Skelly A: Beyond 100 mW/cm^2. In: *A Bioeffects Primer: Part 1— Fundamentals*. Vol 1. No 5. Philadelphia: JB Lippincott; 1985.

10. Ziskin MC. *American Institute of Ultrasound in Medicine: Recommended Ultrasound Terminology*. 3rd ed. Laurel, MD: AIUM; 2008.

11. Sauerbrei E. The split image artifact in pelvic ultrasonography: The anatomy and physics. *J Ultrasound Med*. 1985; 29-34.

12. Buttery B, Davison G. The ghost artifact. *J Ultrasound Med*. 1984; 49-52.

13. Laing F. Commonly encountered artifacts in clinical ultrasound. In: Raymond H, Zwiebel W, eds. *Seminars in Ultrasound: Physics 4(1)*. New York: Grune & Stratton; 1983.

14. Thickman D, Ziskin M, Goldenberg J, et al. Clinical manifestations of the comet tail artifact. *J Ultrasound Med*. 1983; 225-230.

15. Avruch L, Cooperberg P. The ring-down artifact. *J Ultrasound Med*. 1985; 21-28.

16. Odwin C, Fleischer AC, Kepple DM, et al. Probe covers and disinfectants for transducers. *J Diag Med Sonogr*. 1990; 6:130-135.

17. Bushong SC, Archer BR. *Diagnostic Ultrasound: Physics, Biology, and Instrumentation*. St. Louis: Mosby-Year Book; 1991.

18. Edelman SK. Understanding Ultrasound Physics. 3rd ed. Woodlands, TX: EPS, Inc; 2005.

19. Craig, M. *Essentials of Sonography and Patient Care*. 2nd ed. St. Louis: Saunders Elsevier; 2006.

20. Miele FR. *Ultrasound Physics and Instrumentation*. 4th ed. Forney, TX: Pegasus Lectures Inc; 2006.

21. Hedrick WR, Hykes DL, Starchman DE. *Ultrasound Physics and Instrumentation*. 3rd ed. St. Louis, MO: Mosby; 1994.

22. Wicks J. Howe K. *Fundamentals of Ultrasonographic Technique*. Chicago: Yearbook; 1983.

23. Oakley, J. *Digital Imaging: A Primer for Radiographers, Radiologists and Health Care Professionals*. New York: Cambridge; 2003.

24. Hugehes S, Goss S. *National Certification Exam Review: Sonography Principles and Instrumentation*. Texas: SDMS; 2009.

25. Kremkau FW. *Diagnostic Ultrasound: Principles, Instruments*. 8th ed. St. Louis, MO: Saunders Elsevier; 2011

26. Fish PJ. Multichannel, direction resolving Doppler angiography. *Abstracts of 2nd European Congress of Ultrasonics in Medicine*. 1975; 72.

27. Omoto R, ed. *Color Atlas of Real-Time Two-Dimensional Doppler Echocardiography*. Tokyo: Shindan-ToChiryo; 1984.28.

28. Powis RL. Color flow imaging: understanding its science and technology. *JDMS*. 1988; 4:236-245.

29. Gorcsan J. Tissue Doppler echocardiography. *Curr Opin Cardiol*. 2000; Sept 15:323-329.

30. Burns PN. Instrumentation and clinical interpretation of the Doppler spectrum: carotid and deep Doppler. In: *Conventional & Color-Flow Duplex Ultrasound Course*. Proc AIUM Spring Education Meeting. 1989; 29-38.

31. Persson AV, Powis RL. Recent advances in imaging and evaluation of blood flow using ultrasound. *Med Clin North Am*. 1986; 70:1241-1252.

32. Ophir J, Maklad NF. Digital scan converters in diagnostic ultrasound imaging. *Proc IEEE*. 1979; 67:654-664.

33. Atkinson P, Woodcock JP. *Doppler Ultrasound and Its Use in Clinical Measurement*. New York: Academic Press; 1982.

34. Goldstein A, Powis RL. Medical ultrasonic diagnostics in ultrasonic instruments and devices: reference for modern instrumentation, techniques and technology. In: Mason WP, Thurston RN, eds. *Physical Acoustics Series*. Vol. 23A. New York: Academic Press; 1999.

35. Powis RL. Color flow imaging technology. In: *Basic Science of Flow Measurement*. Proc Syllabus AIUM 1989 Spring Education Meeting. 1989; 27-33.

36. Merritt RBC. Doppler color flow imaging. *J Color Ultrasonog*. 1987; 15:591-597.

37. Havlice JF, Taenzer JC. Medical ultrasonic imaging: an overview of principles and instrumentation. *Proc IEEE*. 1979; 67:620-641.

38. Baker DW, Daigle RE. Noninvasive ultrasonic flowmetry. In: Hwang, NHC, Normann NA, eds. *Cardiovascular Flow Dynamics and Measurements*. Baltimore: University Park Press; 1977.

39. McDicken WN. *Diagnostic Ultrasonics: Principles and Use of Instruments*. 2nd ed. New York: John Wiley & Sons; 1981.

40. Murphy KJ, Rubin JM. Power Doppler: It's a good thing. *Semin Ultrasound CT MRI*. 1997; Feb. 18:13-21.

41. Goldstein A. Range ambiguities in real-time. *Ultrasound*. 1981; 9:83-90.

42. Middleton WD, Erickson S, Melson GL. Perivascular color artifact: pathologic significance and appearance on color Doppler US images. *Radiology*. 1989; 171:647-652.

2

Adult Echocardiography

Mark N. Allen and Carol A. Krebs*

Study Guide

INTRODUCTION

Echocardiography has evolved into a highly specialized field of ultrasound. It originally began with M-mode techniques and developed into two-, three-, and even four-dimensional imaging combined with Doppler and color-flow capabilities. Innovative technical advances, such as transesophageal examinations and contrast agents, added yet further diagnostic capabilities. Echocardiology serves as an ideal noninvasive method to examine cardiac anatomy in the normal as well as abnormal states. The combination of anatomical and functional information provided by echocardiography makes it the diagnostic method of choice in a variety of clinical situations.[1]

The heart is an extremely complex organ, and echocardiography provides a variety of techniques that can be applied to obtain comprehensive information about a very dynamic organ. When performing an echocardiographic examination, it is important to consider not only the two-dimensional imaging information but also the Doppler and color-flow findings.[1] These techniques are performed as an integral part of an echocardiographic examination and should be used to complement one another.

TECHNIQUES AND INSTRUMENTATION

Transthoracic Exam

Real-time imaging combined with M-mode and Doppler are the foundation of the basic echocardiographic examination. Electrocardiography (ECG) provides timing for electrical events, which are used in making measurements and calculations. There are specific protocols established by each laboratory that govern the performance and interpretation of the examination. These protocols usually include the guidelines recommended

by the American Society of Echocardiography (ASE). The positions are specifically designed for viewing specific heart structures. The structures viewed from the various positions and windows are listed in the following sections.

Left Parasternal Long-Axis View

- Anterior right ventricular free wall
- Right ventricular cavity
- Interventricular septum, including membranous portion
- Left ventricle
- Left ventricular posterior wall
- Mitral valve and apparatus
- Left ventricular outflow tract
- Aortic valve—left and noncoronary cusps
- Aortic root
- Left atrium
- Descending thoracic aorta
- Coronary sinus
- Pericardium

Right Ventricular Inflow View

- Obtained by starting in a left parasternal long-axis view and angling anteriorly
- Right atrium
- Right ventricle
- Tricuspid valve and apparatus (chordae tendineae and papillary muscles)

Parasternal Short-Axis View

- Left ventricle—all wall segments
- Aortic valve—all three cusps

*This chapter is reprinted from the third edition of Appleton & Lange Review for the Ultrasonography Examination.

- Pulmonic valve
- Tricuspid valve
- Right atrium
- Right ventricle
- Main pulmonary artery (left and right branches)
- Interatrial septum
- Pericardium
- Left atrium

Apical Four-Chamber View

- Left ventricle (septal wall, apex, lateral wall)
- Right ventricle
- Left atrium
- Right atrium
- Mitral valve—anterior and posterior leaflets
- Tricuspid valve
- Interatrial and interventricular septae
- Pulmonary veins

Apical Two-Chamber View

- Left ventricle (anterior wall, inferior wall, apex)
- Left atrium and left atrial appendage
- Coronary sinus
- Mitral valve

Apical Long-Axis View

- Left ventricle (septum, posterior wall, apex)
- Left atrium
- Aortic valve
- Ascending aorta
- Mitral valve (both leaflets) and apparatus
- Right ventricle (small portion)

Apical Four-Chamber View with Aorta

- Left ventricle (septal wall, apex, lateral wall)
- Right ventricle
- Left atrium
- Right atrium
- Atrioventricular valves
- Aortic valve
- Ascending aorta/left ventricular (LV) outflow tract

Subcostal Four-Chamber View

- Left ventricle (septal wall, lateral wall)
- Right ventricle
- Left atrium
- Right atrium
- Atrioventricular valves

- Interatrial septum
- Interventricular septum

Subcostal Short-Axis View

- Left ventricle—short axis
- Right ventricle
- Tricuspid valve
- Pulmonic valve
- Right ventricular outflow tract
- Main pulmonary artery

Subcostal Inferior Vena Cava View

- Inferior vena cava
- Hepatic veins
- Right atrium

Suprasternal View

- Ascending aorta
- Aortic arch
- Descending aorta
- Left common carotid artery
- Left subclavian artery
- Innominate artery
- Right pulmonary artery

Stress and Pharmacologic Examination

Stress echocardiography can be performed using a treadmill, supine or upright bike, and pacing techniques or using such pharmacologic agents as dobutamine, adenosine, or dipyridamole. The combination of echocardiography, ECG, and stress has been used since the 1980s. The use of exercise ECG only is unreliable in such subgroups of patients as women or patients who have a history of myocardial infarction or coronary bypass surgery, as well as in patients on certain medications such as antiarrhythmic agents, diuretics, and antidepressive agents. In addition, exercise ECG is unreliable in patients with certain arrhythmias, such as left bundle branch block or other repolarization abnormalities, and valvular heart disease.

The ischemic cascade is a series of events that take place with an ischemic episode (see Table 2–1).

The fact that systolic changes occur before ECG changes and patient symptoms, the addition of imaging techniques to the exercise ECG improves the diagnostic accuracy of the test.

Myocardial ischemia occurs when the regional oxygen supply is insufficient to meet the body's demand. When the myocardial blood flow reserve becomes inadequate, such as during exercise or inotropic stimulation, it results in ischemia and impaired myocardial function. Coronary artery stenoses may have little or no effect in the resting state but become manifested during stress or exercise. Therefore, evaluation of patients with exercise has become a standard part of the echocardiographic examination.

TABLE 2–1 • Ischemic Cascade

Imbalance in supply and demand	Myocardial perfusion is decreased by obstructed coronary vessel
Decreases in LV compliance	Changes in diastolic function occur such as slowed relaxation, increased L stiffness and increased end-diastolic pressure (LVEDP)
Decreased or changes in systolic function	Segmental or regional wall motion abnormalities develop
ECG changes develop	Significant changes in ST segment (elevation or depression)
Patient symptoms	Chest pain

Exercise echocardiography has evolved as a test ideally suited for the evaluation of patients with coronary artery disease (CAD) or valvular heart disease. It is a cost-effective, reliable tool for detecting the presence, extent, and distribution of coronary stenosis. Echocardiography rapidly detects regional wall motion at rest and after exercise, which allows highly accurate predictions of the extent and distribution of CAD.[1] Other capabilities of stress echocardiography include the following:

- Assessment of LV size and ejection fraction
- Identification of thrombus or aneurysm that may have resulted from previous myocardial infarction (MI)
- Identification of other causes of chest pain unrelated to vascular obstruction, such as hypertrophic cardiomyopathy, aortic dissection, or pericardial disease
- The evaluation of valvular heart lesions, especially if used in conjunction with Doppler echocardiography

Indications for stress echocardiography include: (1) screening of new patients for CAD, (2) assessing states before and after intervention, (3) determining prognosis after myocardial infarction, and (4) evaluating hemodynamic significance of valvular heart disease.[1]

Contraindications include: (1) recent myocardial infarction, (2) unstable angina, (3) potentially life threatening dysrhythmias, (4) acute pericarditis, (5) severe hypertension, (6) acute pulmonary embolism, and (7) critical aortic valve stenosis. Interpretation of the test includes the evaluation of the patient's blood pressure, ECG, symptoms, and the echocardiographic response to exercise. The LV myocardial segments are divided into three perfusion zones, each dictated by coronary artery anatomy. The left anterior descending artery, or LAD, supplies the anterior, septal, and apex. The left circumflex coronary artery supplies the posterolateral segments but may also sup-

ply the inferior segments depending on dominance. The right coronary artery, or posterior descending artery (PDA), supplies the inferior segments.

An exercise echocardiogram is considered positive if any of these three findings are present: (1) there is an exercise-induced wall motion abnormality, (2) there is an increase in LV volume, or (3) there is a decrease in global LV ejection fraction. The greater the wall motion abnormality, the more severe the disease. There are many factors that affect wall motion abnormalities. Perhaps the most important of these include the duration of exercise; the less exercise the patient does, the less likely the patient will achieve an adequate heart rate. A list of false positives and false negatives follows below in Table 2–2.

Contrast Echocardiography

The use of contrast agents has gained widespread use in the field of echocardiography. Their uses range from the evaluation of left and right heart structures and function, enhancements of regurgitant and stenotic lesions, enhanced assessment of pulmonary artery pressures, presence of various shunts such as patent foramen, ASD and VSDs and other shunts, and patency coronary artery perfusion.[1]

Contrast agents come in many forms from the simplest, such as agitated saline solution, to complex agents composed of perfluorocarbon shells (or other substances) filled with gases. These later forms of contrast agents hold special promise not only in aiding in the identification of cardiac structures and function, but more recently in the evaluation of myocardial perfusion imaging. Currently (at the time of this writing), contrast agents are only approved by the Food and Drug Administration (FDA) in the evaluation of LV opacification and not for the evaluation of myocardial perfusion imaging. Still, research continues in the use of microbubbles to help identify coronary distribution.

TABLE 2–2 • False Positives and Negatives

False-Negative Exams	False-Positive Exams
Mild coronary artery disease	Cardiomyopathies
Inability to reach maximal heart rate	Inadequate exercise
Presence of extensive collateral vessels (improves flow to diseased area)	Preexisting myocardial dysfunction Left ventricular hypertrophy Left ventricular fibrosis Aging of the heart High blood pressure (220/110 mm Hg) Severe hypertension

Internal contrast or spontaneous echo contrast (SEC) is the discrete reflections in the blood within the cardiac chambers or vessels without the injection of contrast media. SEC is observed when blood becomes echogenic in a region of decreased flow. It is not seen with shear rates greater than 40 seconds. SEC may be seen in normal states as well as abnormal conditions. SEC has the potential to induce embolic events caused by thrombus formation.[1] As technology and equipment improve, visualization of SEC may become more prevalent, even in totally healthy patients.

Contrast agents in the form of microbubbles range in size from 0.1 to 8.0 μm. These tiny spheres are strong reflectors of ultrasound but are small enough to pass through the capillary bed. The microbubbles must be small to avoid harmful effects, must remain tiny after injection, and must stay in the circulation long enough to be detected by ultrasound. The reflective property of the microbubbles comes from the material within the bubbles or spheres, which is usually gas or air bodies. Because of the acoustic impedance of the air or gas versus blood, there is a strong signal. Other factors that affect reflective properties are:

- Transmitted frequency
- Microbubble diameter
- Microbubble concentration
- Microbubble survival rate

The microbubble eventually disappears through natural processes of the body. Table 2–3 lists the currently available agents in the United States and their potential uses.

Transesophageal Examination

Transesophageal echocardiography (TEE) is another echocardiographic technique routinely used to evaluate cardiac structure and function. It is performed by a physician with specialized training in TEE performance and interpretation.[1] TEE examinations provide complete evaluation of all regions of the heart, including the great vessels. Although it is considered more invasive than a transthoracic or surface echocardiogram, it is a relatively simple procedure tolerated by most patients.

Atrial paced TEE is performed by attaching a flexible silicone-coated pacing catheter to the TEE probe. Pacing is increased incrementally to 85% of patient age predicted maximum heart

scale. LV function is monitored by TEE examination at baseline, as well as during and immediately after maximal pacing. This technique has a high sensitivity and specificity for detection of CAD and a high success rate of 90–100% of patients.[1]

TEE plus pharmacologic agents is used to assess CAD and has proved to be feasible and accurate. At each stage of dobutamine infusion, it is important to use longitudinal and transverse planes to optimize visualization of all wall segments.

There are several advantages of using TEE, that include the following:

- TEE provides higher resolution than the transthoracic echocardiographic (TTE) exam because of the use of the transesophageal window, that allows the use of higher frequencies. The transducer is mounted on a flexible gastroscope that is sufficient in length to be advanced down the esophagus. It is positioned behind the posterior wall of the left ventricle.
- TEE provides additional viewing of structures that are often not seen well on the TTE exam in technically difficult studies. These structures include the posterior cardiac structures such as the aorta, atria, left atrial appendage, and cardiac valves.
- TEE provides "off-axis planes" in addition to the standard planes, which often provides a clearer view of the anatomy or anomalies.

There are contraindications to performing the TEE examination. These include: esophageal tumors or tumors of the mouth, esophageal stenosis or strictures, diverticulum, esophageal varices, perforated viscus, gastric volvulus or perforation, active gastrointestinal tract bleeding, and patient refusal or unwillingness to cooperate.[1] Occasionally, the TEE probe cannot be easily passed and should never be forced.

Table 2–4 lists the indications for TEE.

CARDIAC ANATOMY

To become proficient in the techniques of echocardiography, a thorough understanding of cardiac anatomy is essential. One must know the normal structures and be able to recognize normal variants from pathologic states. One must also understand the anatomic orientation of the heart within the chest cavity.

The heart is a cone-shaped, hollow, fibromuscular organ located in the middle mediastinum between the lungs and the pleurae. It has a base, apex, and multiple surfaces and borders. It is enclosed within the pericardium. The pericardium is made of fibrous and serosal components. The fibrous pericardium is the tough outer sac that completely surrounds the heart but does not adhere to it. The serosal component is the inner layer, which has two components. The visceral, or epicardial, layer adheres to the surface of the heart and makes up the epicardium and the serosal pericardium, which is the outer or parietal layer.

TABLE 2–3 • Microbubble Agents		
Available Agents	**Manufacturer**	**Uses (FDA approved)**
Optison	Amersham	• LV opacification
Definity	Bristol-Myers Squibb	• LV opacifcation

TABLE 2–4 • Indications for TEE

Left ventricular function	• Regional wall motion abnormalities • Global LV function
Endocarditis	• Valvular vegetations • Valvular strands
Valvular disorders/pathology	• Mitral valve prolapse • Mitral, aortic, pulmonic, tricuspid stenosis • Mitral, aortic, pulmonic, tricuspid regurgitation • Flail leaflets • Torn chordal structures
Pericardial disease	• Pericarditis • Pericardial fluid • Tamponade
Aortic abnormalities	• Presence and extent of arteriosclerotic disease • Traumatic aortic rupture • Aortic dissection • Nondissecting aneurysms
Shunts (atrial, ventricular, other)	• Atrial septal defects • Ventricular septal defects • Patent foramen ovale • Atrial septal aneurysms
Source of embolus	• Can help identify patients at risk for stroke • Used to screen patients for cardioversion • Allows interrogation of left atrial appendage
Right heart function	• Monitoring during and after open heart surgery

The serosal pericardium lines the inside surface of the fibrous pericardium. Within the serosal layers is a thin film of pericardial fluid. The purpose of the pericardium is to (1) reduce friction with cardiac movement; (2) allow the heart to move freely with each beat, facilitating ejection and volume changes; (3) contain the heart within the mediastinum, especially during trauma; and (4) serve as a barrier to infection.[1]

The average adult heart measures approximately 12 cm from the apex to the base, 8–9 cm transversely in the broadest diameter, and 6 cm anterior–posterior. The weight varies in males ranging from 280–340 g and in females from 230–280 g. Cardiac weight is approximately 0.45% of total body weight in men and 0.40% of total body weight in women.[1,2]

The heart is divided into four chambers: two atria and two ventricles. The external surface contains numerous grooves and sulci. The coronary or atrioventricular groove separates the atria from the ventricles and contains the main trunk of the coronary arteries and coronary sinus. The interventricular groove separates the right and left ventricles. The anterior interventricular groove runs on the anterior surface and contains the descending branch of the left coronary artery. The posterior interventricular groove lies on the diaphragmatic surface of the heart and contains the posterior interventricular descending coronary artery and the middle cardiac vein. The interatrial grooves separate the atria. The interatrial grooves are shallow and less prominent than the other grooves. The interatrial, atrioventricular, and posterior interventricular grooves meet and form the crux of the heart. The terminal groove or sulcus terminalis demarcates the true atrium and the venous component of the right atrium. These external grooves are filled with fatty tissue that varies with overall body fat and increases with age.[1]

There are basically two important types of heart valves: the semilunar and the atrioventricular. Semilunar valves are the aortic and the pulmonary. Atrioventricular valves are the tricuspid and the mitral.

Numerous pathologies can affect the heart in the adult. These disease states can cause a variety of primary as well as secondary anatomical changes in the heart. Knowing what these changes are greatly enhances the echocardiographic examination. Once the student has an understanding of the heart anatomy, the echocardiographic images are better understood. The basic two-dimensional echocardiographic views are illustrated in Figs. 2–1 to 2–8. These figures are from the American Society of Echocardiography and are the accepted nomenclature for two-dimensional imaging.

Left Ventricle

Anatomy. The left ventricle is the largest cardiac chamber, accounting for 75% of the heart mass. It consists of two papillary muscles, has trabeculations in the apex, and a smooth-walled basal area. Its end-diastolic diameter is 3.6–5.6 cm, and its end-systolic diameter is 2.3–4.0 cm. Normal fractional shortening (difference between diastolic and systolic diameters is:

$$FS = \frac{LV\,Dd\text{-}LVLVIDS}{LVIDd}$$

Normal LV wall thickness in diastole ranges from 0.6–1.1 cm.

Hemodynamics. The ventricle receives oxygenated blood from the left atrium and pumps it through the aortic valve to the body by way of arteries, arterioles, and capillaries. Its systolic pressure is 100–120 mm Hg.

Echocardiographic Views. Almost all the standard views allow visualization of at least part of the left ventricle. The apical views allow examination of the apex, which can be difficult to see in other views. The maximum internal dimensions are seen at end systole and should be taken at the peak posterior motion of the interventricular septum (see Table 2–5).

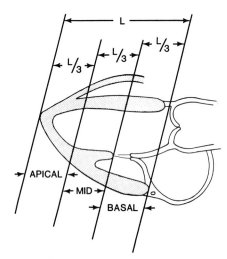

FIGURE 2–1. Parasternal long-axis view of the heart demonstrating the method of subdividing the myocardial walls along the long axis (L) into three regions of equal length using the left ventricular papillary muscles as landmarks. *(Reproduced with permission from Henry WL, DeMaria A, Feigenbaum H, et al: Report of the American Society of Echocardiography Committee on Nomenclature and Standards: Identification of myocardial wall segments. November, 1982: 1–15.)*

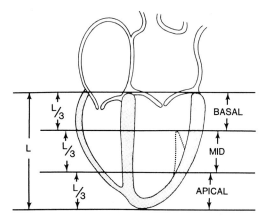

FIGURE 2–2. Apical four-chamber view of the heart demonstrating the method of subdividing the myocardial walls into three regions using the left ventricular papillary muscles as landmarks. *(Reproduced with permission from Henry WL, DeMaria A, Feigenbaum H, et al: Report of the American Society of Echocardiography Committee on Nomenclature and Standards: Identification of myocardial wall segments. November, 1982: 1–15.)*

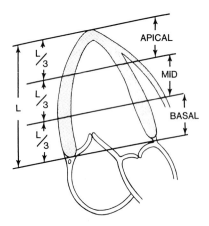

FIGURE 2–3. Apical long-axis view of the heart demonstrating the method of subdividing the myocardial walls into three regions of equal length. *(Reproduced with permission from Henry WL, DeMaria A, Feigenbaum H, et al: Report of the American Society of Echocardiography Committee on Nomenclature and Standards: Identification of myocardial wall segments. November, 1982: 1–15.)*

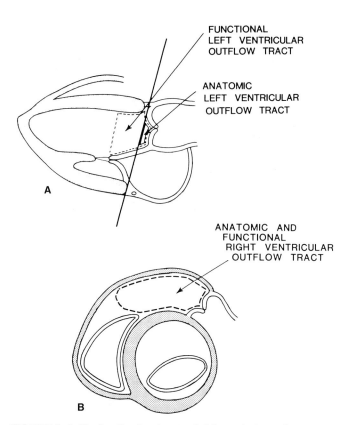

FIGURE 2–4. The functional and anatomic left ventricular outflow tracts of the heart are diagrammed in the upper panel (**A**), whereas the functional and anatomic right ventricular outflow tract is illustrated in the bottom panel (**B**). *(Reproduced with permission from Henry WL, DeMaria A, Feigenbaum H, et al: Report of the American Society of Echocardiography Committee on Nomenclature and Standards: Identification of myocardial wall segments. November, 1982: 1–15.)*

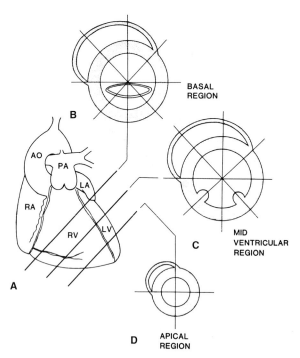

FIGURE 2–5. Diagram of the heart (**A**) and the short-axis views of the basal region (**B**), midventricular region (**C**), and apical region (**D**). *(Reproduced with permission from Henry WL, DeMaria A, Feigenbaum H, et al: Report of the American Society of Echocardiography Committee on Nomenclature and Standards: Identification of myocardial wall segments. November, 1982: 1–15.)*

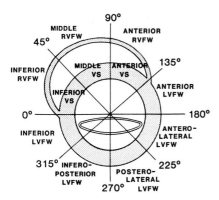

FIGURE 2–6. Short-axis view of the basal region of the heart demonstrating the method of subdividing the myocardial walls into segments using a coordinate system consisting of eight lines that are 45° apart. With this system, the left ventricular free wall (LVFW) is divided into five segments, whereas the ventricular septum (VS) and right ventricular free walls (RVFW) are subdivided into three segments each. *(Reproduced with permission from Henry WL, DeMaria A, Feigenbaum H, et al: Report of the American Society of Echocardiography Committee on Nomenclature and Standards: Identification of myocardial wall segments. November, 1982: 1–15.)*

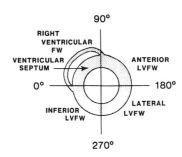

FIGURE 2–8. Short-axis view of the apical region of the heart demonstrating the method of subdividing the myocardial walls into segments using a coordinate system consisting of four lines that are 90° apart. With this system, the left ventricular free wall (LVFW) is subdivided into three segments, whereas the ventricular septum and right ventricular free wall (FW) are subdivided into one segment each. *(Reproduced with permission from Henry WL, DeMaria A, Feigenbaum H, et al: Report of the American Society of Echocardiography Committee on Nomenclature and Standards: Identification of myocardial wall segments. November, 1982: 1–15.)*

Left Atrium

Anatomy. The left atrium is a smooth-walled sac, the walls of which are thicker than those of the right atrium. The chamber receives four pulmonary veins: two (sometimes three) on the right and two (sometimes one) on the left. The interatrial septum divides the left and right atria. It is thinnest in its central portion, the fossa, and varies in thickness elsewhere due to fat deposits. These normally increase with age. The left auricle, or left atrial appendage, arises from the upper anterior part of the left atrium and contains small pectinate muscles. The average dimension of the chamber in the adult is 29–38 mm.

Hemodynamics. The mean pressure in the left atrium ranges from 1 to 10 mm Hg. Oxygenated blood flows from the lungs

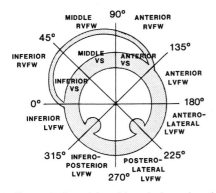

FIGURE 2–7. Short-axis view of the midventricular region of the heart demonstrating the method of subdividing the myocardial walls into segments using a coordinate system consisting of eight lines that are 45° apart. With this system, the left ventricular free wall (LVFW) is divided into five segments, whereas the ventricular septum (VS) and right ventricular free walls (RVFW) are subdivided into three segments each. *(Reproduced with permission from Henry WL, DeMaria A, Feigenbaum H, et al: Report of the American Society of Echocardiography Committee on Nomenclature and Standards: Identification of myocardial wall segments. November, 1982: 1–15.)*

TABLE 2–5 • TEE Left Ventricle Examination

Views	Structures/Walls
Long-axis (LAX)	• Septum • Posterior wall • Papillary muscles • Trabeculations
Short-axis (SAX)	• Septum (inferior, mid, anterior) • Lateral wall • Posterior wall • Inferior wall
Apical four chamber	• Apex • Lateral wall • Septum • Papillary muscles
Apical two chamber	• Apex • Posterior wall • Anterior wall
Apical long-axis	• Apex • Septum • Posterior wall
Subcostal four chamber	• Apex • Septum • Lateral wall
Subcostal short-axis	• Septum • Lateral wall • Posterior wall • Inferior wall

and enters the atrium through the pulmonary veins. As left atrial pressure increases over that of the left ventricle, the mitral valve opens, and blood then passes through the mitral valve and enters the left ventricle.

Echocardiographic Views. Maximal dimensions should be measured at end-systole. Measurements may be made from the leading edge of the posterior wall of the aorta to the leading edge of the posterior wall of the left atrium. This chamber is best seen from the parasternal long- and short-axis views; however, it also can be seen from the apical and subcostal views. In the left parasternal long-axis view, the descending aorta can be seen from running posteriorly to the left atrium. Care must be given when measuring the diameter of the left atrium so that the descending aorta is not included in the measurement because this will give an erroneous left atrial diameter. The left atrial appendage can be seen from the transthoracic two-chamber and parasternal short-axis views.

TEE can also be used to evaluate this area and is typically carefully evaluated in patients where the source of embolus is a consideration or when patients may be scheduled for cardio-version.

Right Atrium

Anatomy. The right atrium has two parts: an anterior portion and a posterior portion. The two portions are separated by a ridge of muscle called the crista terminalis. This area is typically not well seen from the transthoracic approach.

The smooth-walled posterior portion of the atrium is derived from the embryonic sinus venosus and receives the inferior and superior vena cavae. Guarding the opening (ostium) of the inferior vena cava is a thin fold of tissue called the eustachian valve, which is sometimes large and complex and forms a network of tissues known as the network of Chiari. The coronary sinus also enters the right atrium anteriorly to the inferior vena cava. The coronary sinus also can be guarded by a thin fold of tissue called the Thebesian valve.

The anterior portion, that represents the embryonic right atrium, is extremely thin and is trabeculated. The right atrial appendage, or right auricle, arises from the superior portion of the right atrium and contains pectinate muscle. The dimensions of the right atrium in adults range from 26 to 34 mm.

Hemodynamics. Deoxygenated blood from the body, head, and heart flows into the right atrium through the inferior vena cava, the superior vena cava, and the coronary sinus, respectively. When pressures in the right atrium increase above the pressures in the right ventricle, the tricuspid valve opens, allowing the blood to flow forward into the right ventricle. Mean pressures in this chamber range from 0 to 8 mm Hg.

Echocardiographic Views. Apical views are best for assessing the right atrium. Others include the subcostal and, to a lesser extent, the parasternal short-axis views.

Right Ventricle

Anatomy. The right ventricle is divided into a posterior inferior inflow portion and an anterior superior outflow portion. The inflow portion contains the tricuspid valve and is heavily trabeculated. The outflow portion, also called the infundibulum, gives rise to the pulmonary trunk. The subpulmonic area is smooth walled.

The right ventricle contains numerous papillary muscles that anchor the tricuspid valve. The ventricle contains numerous bands of muscle. One band, the moderator band, is readily seen in the apex of the ventricle by two-dimensional imaging. Internal diameters range from 7 to 26 mm.

Hemodynamics. Systolic pressures range from 15 to 30 mm Hg, and diastolic pressures range from 0 to 8 mm Hg.

Echocardiographic Views. The right ventricle is seen best from the apical and subcostal views. It also can be seen from the left parasternal long- and short-axis views and right ventricular inflow view.

Aorta

Anatomy. The aorta arises from the base of the heart and enters the superior mediastinum, where it almost reaches the sternum, then courses obliquely backward and to the left over the left bronchus. It then becomes the descending aorta and courses downward anterior to and slightly left of the vertebral column. The aorta is highly elastic and has three layers: (1) a thin inner layer called the tunica intima, (2) a thick middle layer called the tunica media, and (3) a thin outer layer called the tunica adventitia. The diameter of the aortic root measures 2.5–3.3 cm.

Hemodynamics. Maximal velocities of blood flow in adults are 1.0–0.7 m/s.

Echocardiographic Views. The aortic root is seen from the parasternal views. A good portion of the ascending aortic arch can be seen by beginning with the transducer in a standard left parasternal long-axis view and sliding the probe up an intercostal space. The ascending aorta, aortic arch, and descending aorta can be seen from the suprasternal view. As was mentioned earlier, part of the descending aorta also can be seen behind the left atrium in the long-axis view. The subcostal views allow visualization of the aortic root and valve.

Main Pulmonary Artery

Anatomy. The main pulmonary artery is located superior to and originates from the right ventricle. Immediately after leaving the pericardium, it bifurcates into a right pulmonary artery and a left pulmonary artery that enter the right and left lung, respectively.

Hemodynamics. This artery delivers deoxygenated blood from the right ventricle to the lungs. Flow velocities range from 0.6 to 0.9 m/s.

Echocardiographic Views. The artery is best seen from the parasternal short-axis view.

Mitral Valve

Anatomy. The mitral valve is an atrioventricular valve. It is located between the left atrium and the left ventricle and it is a thick yellow-white membrane that originates at the annulus fibrosus, a fibrous ring that surrounds the orifice of the valve. The valve has an anterior leaflet and a posterior leaflet, both of which have sawtooth-like edges. Both leaflets are attached to papillary muscles by chordae tendineae. The surface on the atrial side of the valve is smooth, whereas the surface on the ventricular side is irregular the normal mitral valve area is 4–6 cm^2.

Hemodynamics. Flow velocities across the valve range from 9.6 to 1.3 m/s. The valve's function is to prevent backflow of blood from the left ventricle into the left atrium.

Echocardiographic Views. The mitral valve is best seen from the long- and short-axis parasternal views and the apical view. Doppler measurements are best obtained from the apical four- and two-chamber views.

Aortic Valve

Anatomy. The aortic valve consists of three pocket-shaped, thin, smooth cusps named according to their location in relation to the coronary arteries. The cusp near the left coronary artery is the left coronary cusp, the cusp near the right coronary artery is the right coronary cusp, and the cusp that is not near a coronary artery is the noncoronary cusp. Because of its lunar, or half-moon shape, the aortic valve is referred to as semilunar. The normal aortic valve area is 3–4 cm^2.

Hemodynamics. The function of the aortic valve is to prevent backflow of blood from the aorta into the left ventricle. The velocity of flow ranges from 1.0 to 1.7 m/s.

Echocardiographic Views. The valve is best seen from the parasternal views. It also can be seen from the apical four-chamber view with anterior angulation. The best Doppler measurements are obtained from the apical four-chamber view with anterior angulation, from the right parasternal window, and from the suprasternal view.

Tricuspid Valve

Anatomy. The tricuspid valve is an atrioventricular valve. It is located between the right atrium and ventricle. The atrial side is smooth, whereas the ventricular side is irregular. As in the mitral valve, it is a thick yellow-white membrane that originates at the annulus fibrosus, a fibrous ring that surrounds the orifice of the valve. The valve has three leaflets—anterior, posterior, and medial—all of which are sawtooth-like in appearance. Each leaflet is attached to papillary muscles by chordae tendineae.

Hemodynamics. The function of this valve is to prevent backflow of blood from the right ventricle to the right atrium. The velocity of flow ranges from 0.3 to 0.7 m/s.

Echocardiographic Views. The valve is best seen from the parasternal short-axis, parasternal four-chamber, apical four-chamber, and subcostal views. Measurements are best obtained in the parasternal four-chamber view. The best Doppler measurements are taken from the parasternal short-axis and apical four-chamber views.

Pulmonic Valve

Anatomy. The pulmonic valve consists of three thin, smooth pocket S-shaped cusps. Because of its shape, this valve, like the aortic valve, is called semilunar.

Hemodynamics. The function of this valve is to prevent backflow of blood from the main pulmonary artery to the right ventricle. The velocity of flow ranges from 9.6–0.9 m/s.

Echocardiographic Views. The pulmonic valve is best seen from the parasternal short-axis view. The best Doppler recordings are taken from the left parasternal short axis.

PHYSIOLOGY

The heart functions as a pump to distribute blood to the body. In order for blood to be adequately distributed, the blood pressure must be maintained. Pressure and flow are controlled by a complex control mechanism that responds to the metabolic requirements of the body.

There are two fluid pumps within the heart, one on the right and one on the left, lying side by side. The right side supplies the pulmonary circulation. From the lungs, blood returns to the left side and ultimately supplies the body via the systemic circulation. The volume pumped by both sides is equal to

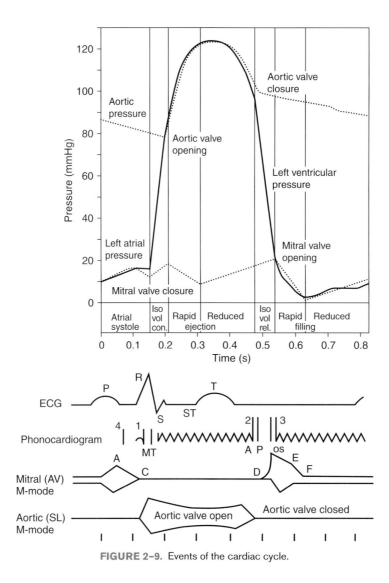

FIGURE 2–9. Events of the cardiac cycle.

ensure normal circulation of flow. The blood is pumped from the ventricles during systole and received during diastole, the relaxation phase. The cardiac cycle includes all of the electrical and mechanical events that occur during the cycle of one heartbeat (see Fig. 2–9). Each side of the heart has specific characteristics and functions, which are listed below.

RIGHT HEART CHARACTERISTICS AND FUNCTIONS

- Blood returns to the right atrium from the superior and inferior vena cava.
- Right heart supplies the pulmonary circulation.
- Normal pressure in the right ventricle is approximately 22 mm Hg.
- Blood returning to the right heart has a lower oxygen saturation (75%).
- Contains the tricuspid valve which closes during right ventricular systole and contained blood in right ventricle

is propelled out of right ventricle outflow tract through the open semilunar pulmonic valve to the pulmonic circulation.

LEFT HEART CHARACTERISTICS AND FUNCTIONS

- Left ventricular pressure is approximately 120 mm Hg.
- Blood pumped from the left ventricle has a high oxygen saturation (95–100%).
- Left atrium receives blood from the lungs through the pulmonary veins in the back of the left atrium.
- During left atrial systole, the mitral valve opens and allows blood in the left atrium to be propelled into the left ventricle. When ventricular systole occurs, the mitral valve closes and blood is propelled out of the left ventricle through the outflow tract.

The blood supply to the heart is derived from the right and left coronary arteries and their respective tributaries (see Fig. 2–10).

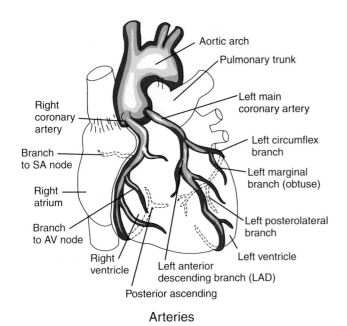

FIGURE 2–10. Anatomic drawing of the heart and vessels.

CONDUCTION SYSTEM OF THE HEART/INTRINSIC INNERVATION OF THE HEART

The conduction system of the heart is responsible for the initiation, propagation, and coordination of the heartbeat. Fig. 2–11 demonstrates this system.

The sinoatrial node (SA) is also called the pacemaker of the heart. It provides the bursts of electrical impulses that are conducted throughout the walls of the heart. The activation

conduction is from the sinoatrial node to the atrioventricular (AV) node, where it is slows and delays. The impulse is conducted to the ventricles by way of the atrioventricular bundle and the right and left bundle branches. It becomes continuous with the fibers of the Purkinje network. The ventricles contract and blood is ejected to the pulmonic and systemic circulation. The heart contains its own intrinsic conduction system; however, its rate is modified by the autonomic nervous system. Fibers from both the sympathetic and the parasympathetic nervous systems are received by the heart. Sympathetic nervous system fibers are received by the atria via the right and left vagus nerves, which contribute to the control of the sinoatrial and atrioventricular nodes. The parasympathetic nerves are derived from the vagus and come off in the neck as vagal cardiac nerves. They connect to the sinoatrial node. Stimulation of the parasympathetic nervous system fibers to the heart causes the following:

- Decrease in the heart rate
- Retardation of transmission between the atria and ventricles
- Decrease in the force of contraction
- Decrease in conduction rate of the nodes and atria

The sympathetic and parasympathetic nervous systems have opposite effects on the heart. The reflex center for both is in the medulla oblongata.

DISEASES AFFECTING THE VALVES

Anomalies or diseases of the valves can be divided into two main categories. Valve anomalies that occur in fetal development are

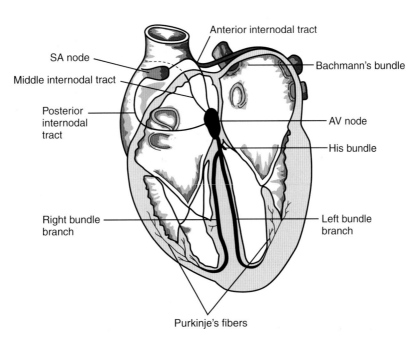

FIGURE 2–11. Intrinsic conduction system of the heart.

known as congenital anomalies. Valve anomalies that develop after fetal development or in the adult stages are referred to as acquired valve disease. This latter category can be further divided into rheumatic and nonrheumatic heart disease.

Mitral Valve Disease

Stenosis. Mitral valve stenosis results primarily from rheumatic disease. The valves may not become involved for many decades following rheumatic fever. Congenital mitral stenosis can occur but is extremely rare.

M-mode findings include (1) a flattened E–D slope (reduced diastolic filling), (2) anterior motion of the posterior leaflet, (3) thickened leaflets, and (4) an absent A wave in the absence of atrial fibrillation. Two-dimensional imaging also indicates thickening and shows doming of the leaflets in diastole.

Doppler measurements reveal a reduced rate of decrease in diastolic flow (reduced diastolic slope), a higher than normal peak velocity of flow, and spectral broadening on Doppler display. Secondary findings and complications include left atrial dilatation, pulmonary hypertension, a left atrial clot, and an exaggerated diastolic dip of the interventricular septum.[3] Color Doppler shows turbulent LV inflow.

Stenosis–Severity of Mitral Stenosis (Valve Area)

Normal	$4-6 \text{ cm}^2$
Mild	$1.6-2.0 \text{ cm}^2$
Moderate	$1.1-1.5 \text{ cm}^2$
Severe	1.0 cm^2 or less

Regurgitation. Mitral regurgitation (shunting back and forth of blood) can occur as a result of mitral annular calcification, rheumatic mitral disease, flail mitral valve leaflet, conditions that may stretch the mitral annulus, such as cardiomyopathies, myocardial infarction, mitral valve vegetations or other masses on the mitral valve or within the left atrium, papillary dysfunction, and mitral valve prolapse. The hallmark sign of regurgitation is a systolic murmur, most often maximal over the LV apex.

M-mode findings include (1) increased size of the left atrium, (2) exaggerated motion of the interventricular septum, (3) pulsations of the left atrial wall, and (4) preclosure of the aortic valve during systole. The first three findings are the result of volume overload.

Two-dimensional imaging reveals an increase in the size of the left atrium and exaggerated motion of the interventricular septum—all of which are the result of volume overload. In addition, pulsations of the left atrial wall and preclosure of the aortic valve during systole are observed.

Doppler may be used to evaluate the regurgitant fraction. Color Doppler displays the turbulent jet in the left atrium and is useful for estimating the severity of regurgitation.

Prolapse. (Protrusion or buckling of the mitral leaflets into the left atrium in systole.) The classic clinical findings in mitral valve prolapse are a systolic click (a sound that corresponds with the posterior displacement of the mitral valve leaflet into the left atrium) and a late systolic murmur (a sound that corresponds with the resulting mitral regurgitation that often occurs because of the prolapsing leaflets).

M-mode findings include late systolic posterior displacement of the anterior and posterior leaflets and anterior motion of the mitral valve in early systole. To achieve the best views for making the diagnosis, the ultrasound beam should be perpendicular to the valve from the parasternal windows. The two-dimensional findings reveal that the valve is bowing into the left atrium and, in many cases, thickened.

Flail Leaflet. The most common cause of flail leaflet is rupture of the chordae tendineae, which often occurs secondarily to myocardial infarction. Rupture of papillary muscle is a less common etiology.

M-mode findings indicate coarse diastolic fluttering and systolic fluttering of the leaflet and visualization of part of the leaflet in the left atrium. Two-dimensional imaging indicates protrusion of the flail leaflet into the left atrium, non-coaptation of the two leaflets, and a systolic and coarse diastolic motion of the flail leaflet. Doppler measurements indicate harsh, turbulent mitral regurgitation.

Annular Calcification. Mitral annular calcification results from the deposition of calcium in the annulus of the mitral valve. This is normally associated with aging. This condition can be caused by mitral regurgitation, conduction abnormalities, aging, or obstruction of the LV outflow (LVOF) tract.

M-mode findings reveal high-density echoes between the valve and the posterior wall of the left ventricle. Two-dimensional imaging reveals high-density bright echoes between the valve and the posterior wall of the left ventricle.

Aortic Valve Disease

Stenosis (versus Sclerosis). The cause of stenosis of the aortic valve can be congenital, the result of rheumatic heart disease, or degeneration. Degenerative disease is the most common cause of aortic valve stenosis. Clinical symptoms include chest pain, shortness of breath, and syncope. These symptoms do not present until the aortic valve stenosis becomes moderate to severe. Patients with aortic valve stenosis often present with a harsh systolic murmur heard at the right sternal border, which often radiates to the carotids.

The normal aortic valve has three leaflets. In congenital or rheumatic stenosis, the body of the cusps may appear to be thin and pliable, but the cusp tips are tethered, resulting in a systolic doming effect that is best seen in the early systole from a left parasternal or apical long-axis view. In degenerative stenosis, the cusps frequently appear to be bright reflectors with little or no discernable cusp separation. Because of the increased pressure from the valve stenosis, the walls of the left ventricle become thickened or hypertrophied.

M-mode findings indicate thickened cusps and restricted excursion of the cusps to <1.5 cm. Continuous-wave Doppler is used in the apical long-axis or apical "five"-chamber views to evaluate the velocity across the valve. The peak instantaneous and mean aortic gradients are recorded. The continuity equation is commonly used to evaluate the severity of the aortic valve stenosis by calculating the valve area. This equation is based on the principle of "conservation of mass." All blood flow going across the LVOT must be equal to the blood flow across the aortic valve. By determining the flow in the LVOT, the flow in the aortic valve can also be determined. This is measured by calculating the velocity integral of flow in the LVOT and at the aortic valve leaflet tips. The diameter of the LVOT is also measured to obtain a cross-sectional area. The continuity equation is as follows: Flow 1 = Flow 2, where Flow 1 = LVOT VTI × LVOT CSA and Flow 2 = AV VTI × AV CSA. The aortic valve area, or AVA, is calculated by dividing LVOT VTI × LVOT CSA by AV VTI. It is important to note that the LVOT VTI is obtained using pulsed-wave Doppler, whereas the AV VTI is obtained using continuous wave Doppler. The LVOT diameter is a two-dimensional measurement. Current equipment normally performs this calculation for the user, but an understanding of these principles is important. The normal aortic valve area is 2.5–4.5 cm^2. The normal diameter of the LVOT ranges from 1.8 to 2.4 cm with an LVOT VTI of 18–22 cm (see Table 2–6). Color Doppler can also be used to help identify aortic valve stenosis by demonstrating turbulent flow in the ascending aorta.

Parasternal Long- and Short-Axis Views.

These views can be used to help evaluate the aortic valve cusps, making measurements of the LV walls in M-mode or two-dimensional planes. The diameter of the LVOT is usually taken from a left parasternal long-axis view, although the apical long-axis view may also be used.

Apical Views.

The apical views are used to obtain Doppler measurements across the valve because the blood flow is parallel to the sound beam and, therefore, well suited to obtain maximal and accurate blood velocities.

Regurgitation.

The effects of regurgitation on atria, ventricles, and cardiac vessels result in dilatation of the left ventricle. The condition can be caused by any one of the following: congenital (bicuspid cusp), rheumatic heart disease (the most common cause in adults), or degeneration of the leaflet caused by infection or aortic dilatation (Marfan syndrome).

M-mode findings reveal fluttering of the interventricular septum and diastolic fluttering of the mitral valve. Two-dimensional imaging indicates fine diastolic fluttering of the aortic valve, diastolic fluttering of the mitral valve, and fluttering of the interventricular septum. Spectral Doppler studies reveal diastolic flow, which appears above the baseline when in an apical position.

Tricuspid Valve Diseases

Stenosis.

Stenosis of the tricuspid valve is most often caused by rheumatic heart disease. It can be caused by other conditions, which include systemic lupus erythematosus (SLE), carcinoid heart disease, Löffler's endocarditis, metastatic melanoma, and congenital heart disease.[1] In stenotic disease of the tricuspid valve, the effects on atria, ventricles, and vessels cause dilatation of the right atrium.

M-mode findings indicate a reduced diastolic slope and thickening and decreased separation of the leaflets. Two-dimensional imaging reveals the most specific finding, systolic doming, as well as thickening of the leaflets. In Doppler measurements, the sample is placed in the right ventricle, and the results indicate turbulent diastolic flow and slowed reduction in the velocity of flow during diastole.

Doppler is used to qualify and quantitate the severity of stenosis.

Regurgitation.

Regurgitation is a common abnormality associated with the tricuspid valve in adults.[1] The primary cause of regurgitation is secondary to pulmonary hypertension. In rare cases, the condition can be caused by rheumatic heart disease, prolapse of the valve, or carcinoid heart disease. A secondary effect is dilatation of the right atrium and ventricle. Continuous-wave Doppler is used to measure the velocity of the regurgitant jet. Pulmonary artery pressure may be calculated by adding the pressure gradient across the tricuspid

TABLE 2–6 • Criteria Range for Aortic Valve Stenosis

	Mild Aortic Stenosis	Moderate Aortic Stenosis	Severe/Critical Aortic Stenosis
Peak gradient	16–36 mm Hg	37–79 mm Hg	>80 mm Hg
Mean gradient	<20 mm Hg	21–49 mm Hg	>50 mm Hg
Valve area	1.1–1.9 cm^2	0.75–1.0 cm^2	<0.74 cm^2

valve to right atrial pressure (normally 5–10 mm Hg). Generally, a TR (tricuspid valve regurgitation) velocity at 3 m/s or greater indicates pulmonary hypertension.

M-mode findings indicate a dilated right ventricle and anterior motion of the interventricular septum during isovolumetric contraction. Two-dimensional imaging reveals incomplete closure and diastolic fluttering of the leaflets, ruptured chordae, dilatation of the right ventricle, and flattening of the interventricular septum. With Doppler measurements, turbulent flow can be detected in the right atrium during systole.

Pulmonic Valve Disease

Stenosis. The causes of pulmonic valve disease are atherosclerosis, infections, endocarditis, and papillary fibroma. This disease is extremely rare in adults. Continuous-wave Doppler reveals velocities greater than 2 m/s in the main pulmonary artery. Color Doppler reveals turbulent flow distal to the pulmonic valve.

Regurgitation. M-mode findings reveal fluttering of the tricuspid leaflets, and Doppler measurements reveal early diastolic high-velocity, turbulent flow. The cause can be pulmonary hypertension or bacterial endocarditis or secondary to pulmonary valvotomy.

Endocarditis

Endocarditis is an inflammation of the endocardium characterized by vegetations on the surface and in the endocardium.[1]

Types. Endocarditis can be caused by either bacteria or vegetation (fungus-like growth) and, depending on the infecting organism, is classified as acute or subacute. Although the disease can occur in the endocardium of the heart, the infection usually affects the endocardium in specific valves and is more likely to affect the left heart than the right. Infection of the tricuspid and pulmonic valves is usually the result of intravenous (IV) drug abuse.

Bacterial Endocarditis. Predisposing factors for bacterial endocarditis include dental procedures, tonsilloadenoidectomy, cirrhosis, drug addiction, surgery, and burns. Infectious endocarditis is mainly caused by two groups of bacteria: staphylococci and streptococci.[1]

Nonbacterial Endocarditis. Among the nonbacterial forms of the disease are SLE and fungal (mycotic), nonbacterial thrombotic, Löffler's, marantic, and Libman–Sacks endocarditis. The most common manifestation of SLE is vegetation. Although this nonbacterial form of endocarditis primarily involves the mitral valve, it also can affect the mural endocardium. The mycotic form of the disease is usually subacute and can be caused by a variety of fungi—most commonly *Candida*, *Aspergillus*, and *Histoplasma*. In the thrombotic form of nonbacterial endocarditis, the vegetation consists of fibrin and other blood elements.

Löffler's endocarditis is characterized by a marked increase of eosinophils. It primarily affects men in their forties who live in temperate climates. The disease affects both ventricles equally. Thickening of the inflow portions of the ventricles and the apices can be observed, as can formation of mural thrombi. Hemodynamically, diastolic filling is impaired because of increased stiffness of the heart. Atrioventricular valve regurgitation is a typical finding.

In the marantic form of the disease, the vegetation is nondestructive and sterile. It occurs in patients with malignant tumors and primarily affects the valves on the left side of the heart. Embolus is the most serious complication.

Libman–Sacks endocarditis is characterized by vegetation or verrucae on the echocardium.

Hemodynamic Mechanisms. One common cause of subacute infectious endocarditis occurs when a high velocity jet consistently hits a surface. Damage results when blood from a high-pressure area flows to a low-pressure area; this is called the Venturi effect. The site where vegetation has formed will usually be in the low-pressure area. When the mitral valve is involved and mitral regurgitation is present, the atrial side of the leaflets is the susceptible area. In this case, the high-pressure area is the ventricle, and because the mitral leaflets fail to coapt, the low-pressure area is the atrial side of the leaflets. The atrial wall that bears the brunt of the regurgitation also may become infected.

When the aortic valve is involved and aortic insufficiency is present, the aorta is the high-pressure area, and the ventricle is the low-pressure area. Vegetations tend to form on the ventricular side of the aortic cusps because the cusps do not close completely in aortic regurgitation. The section of the ventricular wall hit by the regurgitant jet also may be damaged.

In ventricular septal defects (VSDs), the high-pressure area is the left ventricle in left-to-right shunting and the low-pressure area is the right ventricular side of the defect. The right ventricular wall directly across from the defect also can suffer damage and become prone to vegetation.

The presence of a mass on any valve leads to a diagnosis of infection caused by vegetation. However, echocardiography cannot differentiate between a new and an old infection. M-mode patterns indicate shaggy echoes on the infected valve and detect 52% of vegetations. TEE is the imaging modality of choice.

Aortic Valve. Vegetation is seen best in diastole and is attached to the ventricular side of the cusps. This condition can cause reduced cardiac output and acute aortic regurgitation. The best views for two-dimensional imaging are the left parasternal long and short axes.

Mitral Valve. Predisposing factors to vegetational infection of the mitral valve include mitral valve prolapse, rheumatic valvulitis, and dysfunction of the papillary muscles with secondary mitral regurgitation and mitral annular calcification. Infection occurs most commonly on the atrial side of the leaflet.

The best views include the left parasternal short and long axes; the apical two- and four-chamber views also can be used. Vegetations as small as 2 mm in diameter are detectable or can be as large as 40 mm in diameter. Whereas M-mode imaging detects 14–65% of the vegetation, two-dimensional imaging detects 43–100%. Differential diagnoses include myomas, lipomas, and fibromas.

Tricuspid or Pulmonic Valve. Infections of the tricuspid or pulmonic valves are usually caused by intravenous (IV) drug abuse. Such infections are less common than left-sided infections; however, when they occur on the tricuspid valve, the infections can become larger than is typical of left-sided infections. They rarely occur on the pulmonic valve.

Prosthetic Valves

Types. Two types of prosthetic valves are available: mechanical and bioprosthetic. The mechanical types are ball-in-cage, disc-in-cage, and tilting-disc valves. The Starr–Edwards valve is the most common ball-in-cage type. The best view for observing excursion of the ball is the apical view when in the mitral and aortic positions. The disc-in-cage valve has less excursion than the ball-in-cage type. The most common type of tilting-disc valve is the Bjork–Shiley, which consists of one disc that tilts. The less common St. Jude valve contains two tilting discs.

All bioprosthetic valves are made from biological tissue, which include heterografts or xenografts (porcine tissue or bovine pericardial tissue), homografts (human cryopreserved from autopsy), and allografts (patient's own tissue).[1] The most common bioprosthetic valve is the xenograft. A porcine heterograft is the most commonly used tissue; porcine pericardial tissue also can be used. Human homografts and fascia lata tissue are sometimes used as valves.

Malfunctions. The following factors cause both types of prosthetic valves to malfunction: thrombi, regurgitation, stenosis, dehiscence, and vegetation.

Thrombi. Blood clots, the most common cause of valve malfunction, reduce the effective orifice and impair motion of the ball, disc, or leaflet tissue. Their major complication is the potential for an embolus. Two-dimensional imaging is the echocardiographic technique of choice for detecting the presence of a clot. The limitation of the technique is the masking effect produced by the highly reflective nature of the prosthetic valves. In the Bjork–Shiley mitral prosthesis, there is a rounding to the E point on M-mode.

Regurgitation. Regurgitation can occur through the valve or around the sewing ring. Doppler echocardiography is the procedure of choice for detecting the problem. When masking is a problem from apical views, color Doppler is especially useful. Color-flow Doppler not only allows spatial orientation but also demonstrates the direction of blood jets. Secondary echocardiographic findings for aortic prosthetic regurgitation include: (1) fluttering of the mitral valve, (2) fluttering of the interventricular septum, and (3) evidence of volume overload in the left ventricle. Doppler echocardiography also is a procedure of choice for detecting paravalvular leaks with a high degree of sensitivity and specificity. In the Bjork–Shiley mitral valve, an early diastolic bump is noted by M-mode and two-dimensional imaging.

Stenosis. All prosthetic valves have some degree of obstruction. Doppler echocardiography can detect a valve with moderate to severe stenosis.

Dehiscence. In dehiscence, the valve becomes detached from its sewing bed. Disruption of suture lines securing the prosthesis to the sewing ring is usually the cause. The result is severe regurgitation, heart failure, or both, which can be detected by a Doppler examination. Two-dimensional imaging demonstrates an unusual rocking motion away from its normal excursion. Cinefluoroscopy can be helpful in assessing abnormal rocking motion.

Vegetation. As was mentioned earlier, vegetation is difficult to assess with echocardiographic techniques because it is often masked by the highly reflective properties of the prosthesis. These infections are usually found on bioprosthetic valves, are extremely mobile, and are more common in the aortic than in the mitral position.

Degeneration. Degeneration is most common in the bioprosthetic valves and usually occurs as a result of calcification of the area where the valve is joined to the surrounding tissue.

DISEASES AFFECTING THE PERICARDIUM

The pericardium is composed of two layers. The inner layer is a serous membrane called the visceral pericardium, which is attached to the surface of the heart. This layer folds back upon itself to form an outer fibrous layer called the parietal pericardium. Between the two layers is the pericardial space, which is filled with a thin layer of fluid throughout. The functions of the pericardium are to (1) fix the heart anatomically,[1] (2) prevent excessive motion during changes in body position, (3) reduce friction between the heart and other organs, (4) provide a barrier against infection, and (5) help maintain hydrostatic forces on the heart. Pericardial disease can be caused by any one of the following: malignant disease that spreads to the pericardium, pericarditis, acute infarction, cardiac perforation during diagnostic procedures, radiation therapy, SLE, or postcardiac surgery.

Effusion

In the normal pericardium, the pressure within the pericardial space is similar to that in the intrapleural pressure and lower than the right and LV diastolic pressures. Increased intrapericardial pressure depends on three factors: the volume of the effusion, the rate at which fluid accumulates, and the characteristics of the pericardium. The normal intrapericardial space contains 15–50 mL of fluid, and it can tolerate the slow addition of as much as 1–2 L of fluid without increasing the intrapericardial pressure. However, if the fluid is added rapidly, the intrapericardial pressure increases dramatically.

Pericardial effusion can be diagnosed using M-mode and two-dimensional techniques. Three diagnostic criteria can be used: (1) posterior echo-free space, (2) obliteration of echo-free space at the left atrioventricular groove, and (3) decreased motion of the posterior pericardial motion.

Cardiac tamponade results when intrapericardial pressures increase. This problem is characterized by increased intracardiac pressures, impaired diastolic filling of the ventricles, and reduced stroke volume. The following echocardiographic findings are associated with cardiac tamponade:

- Increased dimensions of the right ventricle during inspiration
- Decreased mitral diastolic slope (E–F)
- Decreased end-diastolic dimension of the right atrium or ventricle
- Posterior motion of the anterior wall of the right ventricle
- Collapse of the right ventricular free wall
- Diastolic collapse of the right atrial wall
- Increased flow velocities across the tricuspid pulmonic valve during inspiration

Several findings can create a false-positive diagnosis of pericardial effusion:

- Epicardial fat located on the anterior wall
- Misinterpretation of normal cardiac structures such as the descending aorta or coronary sinus
- Other abnormal cardiac or noncardiac structures
- Confusion of pleural effusions with pericardial effusions

Pericardial effusion can be differentiated from pleural effusion in several ways. First, in pericardial effusion, a large amount of fluid can collect posterior to the heart without any anterior collection. Second, pericardial effusion tapers as it approaches the left atrium; a pleural effusion does not. Third, if both types of effusion occur simultaneously, a thin echogenic line should be noted between the two collections of fluid. And fourth, the descending aorta lies posterior to a pericardial effusion, whereas it lies anterior to a pleural effusion.

Pericarditis

Pericarditis comes in two forms: acute and constrictive. In acute pericarditis, the pericardium is inflamed. This form of the disease has a variety of etiologies: idiopathic causes, viruses, uremia, bacterial infections, acute myocardial infarction, tuberculosis, malignancies, and trauma. Echocardiography reveals thickening of the pericardium, with or without pericardial effusion.

In constrictive disease, the pericardium thickens and restricts diastolic filling of the heart chambers. As in the acute form, it has a variety of causes: tuberculosis, hemodialysis used to treat chronic renal failure, connective tissue disorders (e.g., SLE, rheumatoid arthritis), metastatic infiltration, radiation therapy to the mediastinum, fungal or parasitic infections, and complications of surgery. Echocardiographic findings may include:

- Thickened pericardium
- Flattening of the LV wall in mid and late systole
- A rapid mitral valve E–F slope
- Exaggerated anterior motion of the interventricular septum
- Mid-diastolic premature opening of the pulmonic valve
- Inspiratory dilatation of hepatic veins and the inferior vena cava
- Inspiratory leftward motion of the interatrial and interventricular septa

DISEASES AFFECTING THE MYOCARDIUM

The term cardiomyopathy is used to describe a variety of cardiac diseases that affect the myocardium. Cardiomyopathies have been classified into three categories: (1) hypertrophic, which may or may not obstruct the LV outflow tract, (2) dilated, and (3) restrictive. The classification depends on the anatomical characteristics of the LV cavity as well as systolic ejection and diastolic-filling properties of the left ventricle.

Hypertrophic Cardiomyopathy

Hypertrophic cardiomyopathy is characterized by concentric or asymmetric LV hypertrophy, which results in an increase in LV mass, with normal or reduced dimensions of the LV cavity. Normal systolic function usually is preserved. Although asymmetric hypertrophy can occur anywhere within the left ventricle, the most common site is the proximal portion of the ventricular septum near the outflow tract. Asymmetric septal hypertrophy can be diagnosed when the ratio of septal thickness to posterior wall thickness is 1.3:1.0. When asymmetric hypertrophy is present, obstruction most frequently occurs. Concentric hypertrophy may or may not lead to obstruction. A number of names are used to describe the obstructive forms of cardiomyopathy, including idiopathic hypertrophic subaortic stenosis, muscular subaortic stenosis, asymmetric septal hypertrophy, and hypertrophic obstructive cardiomyopathy.

Several echocardiographic findings, when found in conjunction, are highly specific for the diagnosis of obstructive cardiomyopathy. M-mode and two-dimensional findings include systolic anterior motion of the mitral valve, asymmetric septal hypertrophy, premature midsystolic closure of the aortic valve, septal hypokinesis, and anterior displacement (and its size) of the mitral valve. The left ventricle may be small to normal in size.

Doppler examination reveals a decreased E wave to mitral flow with an exaggerated A wave. These findings suggest a decrease in diastolic compliance and an increase in LV end-diastolic pressures. In aortic flow, there is a midsystolic reduction of velocity. Fifty percent of patients demonstrate regurgitation in the mitral valve. Pulsed-wave Doppler is used to determine the obstructed area. At rest, systolic anterior motion of the mitral valve may not be demonstrated. Because this motion is a diagnostic indication for this disease, provocative maneuvers are used to bring it out. Such techniques include the Valsalva maneuver and amyl nitrate and IV isoproterenol administration.

Dilated Cardiomyopathy

Dilated cardiomyopathy is characterized by globally reduced systolic function, with an ejection fraction of less than 40%, increased end-systolic and end-diastolic volumes, and, eventually, congestive heart failure. M-mode findings include increased end-diastolic and end-systolic dimensions of the left ventricle, reduced septal and posterior wall excursion, increased E point-to-septal separation, decreased aortic root movement, and a structurally normal aortic valve that opens slowly and drifts closed during systole because of reduced cardiac output. The principal two-dimensional echocardiographic findings include LV dilatation and dysfunction, abnormal closure of the mitral valve, and dilatation of the left atrium. The abnormal closure of the aortic valve also is noted. Mitral regurgitation is a frequent Doppler finding in dilated cardiomyopathy. Hemodynamically, the left ventricle demonstrates signs of increased diastolic pressure in the left ventricle and decreased compliance. The walls of the left ventricle are normal in size. The right heart also may become enlarged as a result of the increased diastolic pressures in the left heart. The most common complication of dilated cardiomyopathy is the formation of thrombi and a potential cardiac source of emboli.

Dilated cardiomyopathies can be the result of a familiar or X-linked cardiomyopathy, pregnancy, systemic hypertension, ingestion of toxic agents such as alcohol or other drugs, and a variety of viral infections. They also can be of an unknown cause, or idiopathic. This form of cardiomyopathy also can be found in severe CAD.

Restrictive Cardiomyopathy

Restrictive cardiomyopathy falls into two categories: endomyocardial fibrosis and infiltrative myocardial disease, which includes amyloidosis, sarcoidosis, hematochromatosis, Pompe's disease, and Fabry's disease. The characteristic feature of restrictive cardiomyopathy is increased resistance to LV filling. The associated cardiac findings include elevated diastolic pressure in the left ventricle, hypertension and enlargement of the left atrium, and secondary pulmonary hypertension. The echocardiographic features include an increase in the thickness and mass of the LV wall, a small-to-normal-sized LV cavity, normal systolic function, and pericardial effusion. Restrictive cardiomyopathies

are most common in East Africa; they account for only 5% of noncoronary cardiomyopathies in the Western world.

Endomyocardial fibrosis involves formation of fibrotic sheets of tissue in the subendocardium. These sheets vary in thickness and result in increased stiffness of the ventricles. The bright reflective characteristic of this tissue is easily seen with two-dimensional echocardiography. Other characteristic echocardiographic findings include a normal-sized left ventricle, increased thickness of the LV wall, thrombus, and left atrial enlargement, which usually occurs because of elevated diastolic pressure of the left ventricle. The right heart is normal in size, with mildly reduced systolic function and increased wall dimensions. Tricuspid regurgitation is present because of the pulmonary hypertension that occurs as a result of elevated pressures in the left heart.

There are two basic varieties of endomyocardial fibrosis. One form, found primarily in temperate regions, results from hypereosinophilia and is, therefore, termed hypereosinophilic syndrome. This syndrome, also referred to as Löffler's endocarditis parietalis fibroplastic or Löffler's endocarditis, mainly affects men in their 40s and is characterized by increased eosinophils of more than 1,500/mm.[4] The second form, obliterative endomyocardial fibrosis,[4] occurs primarily in subtropical climates and is especially common in Uganda and Nigeria. It accounts for 10–20% of all cardiac deaths in those countries. Large pericardial effusions are typical in this cardiomyopathy.

Diastolic Dysfunction

The importance of diastolic function has become apparent over recent years. Many patients with symptoms of congestive heart failure (shortness of breath, edema) have normal systolic function. The inability of the left ventricle to relax properly can result in diastolic heart failure. This is often seen in patients with hypertrophic cardiomyopathies and similar conditions. Doppler echocardiography is the diagnostic tool of choice for evaluating diastolic function.

CARDIAC MASSES

Benign Tumors

Myxomas. Myxomas are neoplasms that arise from the endocardial tissue and typically arise from the left atrium.[1] They are the most common type of benign tumor, accounting for 30–50% of all benign tumors. Three times as many females as males are affected, and 90% of the tumors are found in the atria: 75–86% are found in the left atrium; 9–20% in the right atrium; and 5–11% in the right atrium or left ventricle but rarely in both atria. Ninety percent of myxomas are pedunculated; the most common site of attachment is the interatrial septum near the fossa ovalis. This tumor may be hereditary (autosomal dominant).

M-mode findings reveal echoes behind the anterior leaflet of the mitral valve. Two-dimensional imaging reveals an echogenic mass in the affected chamber. The echo may be brightly echogenic to sonolucent because of hemorrhage or necrosis.

The clinical findings include the following: symptoms similar to those of mitral valve disease, embolic phenomena, no symptoms, symptoms similar to those of tricuspid valve disease, sudden death, pericarditis, myocardial infarction, symptoms similar to pulmonic valve disease, and a fever of unknown origin.

Rhabdomyomas. Rhabdomyoma is a benign tumor derived from striated muscle most commonly associated with tuberous sclerosis. It is also called myocardial hamartoma, and the most common cardiac tumor found in infants and children. In 90% of the cases, multiple rhabdomyomas are involved. The tumor is yellow gray in appearance, ranges from 1 mm to several centimeters in diameter, and most commonly involves the ventricles. Large tumors may lead to intracavitary obstruction resulting in death.

Lipomas. Lipomas are benign tumors usually containing mature fat cells. They are the second most common benign tumors of the heart. They affect people of all ages and are found equally often in males and females. Most of these tumors are sessile. Fifty percent are located in the subendocardium, and 25% are intramuscular. The most common sites are the left ventricle, right atrium, and interatrial septum.

Fibromas. Fibromas occur in the connective tissue and contain fibrous connective tissue. They are usually well circumscribed and the second most common benign tumors found predominantly in children (most of whom are younger than 10 years of age). Almost all of these tumors occur in the ventricular myocardium. On the echocardiogram, they typically present as large masses within the interventricular system.

Angiomas. Angiomas are extremely rare. They may occur in any part of the heart.[5]

Teratomas. Teratomas are extremely rare and occur more often in children. They contain all three germ cell layers. They are found most frequently in the right heart but also can occur in the interatrial or interventricular septum.[5]

Malignant Tumors

Primary Cardiac Tumors. Angiosarcomas usually occur in adults and are twice as common in men than in women. They are the fourth most common primary tumors but the most common malignant cardiac tumors. They are soft tissue tumors of the blood vessels and are usually found in the right atrium; the most common site is the interatrial septum. Other primary cardiac tumors are rhabdomyosarcomas, fibrosarcomas, lymphosarcomas, and sarcomas of the pulmonary artery.

Secondary Metastatic Tumors. Metastatic and secondary tumors usually invade the right heart and are far more common than primary tumors. Usually they are clinically silent. However, they can cause superior vena cava syndrome because of obstruction, supraventricular arrhythmias, myocardial infarction, cardiomegaly, congestive heart failure, or nonbacterial endocarditis, bronchogenic carcinomas, breast carcinomas, malignant melanomas, and leukemias. Spread of these tumors varies. Bronchogenic carcinomas spread via the lymphatic channels, and metastases of malignant melanomas spread through the blood. Usually metastases involve the pericardium or the myocardium.[5]

Cardiac Thrombi

Left Ventricular Thrombi. Thrombi of the left ventricle occur in myocardial infarctions, LV aneurysms, and cardiomyopathies. They usually form in the apex of the ventricle. Two-dimensional imaging can diagnose clots with 90% sensitivity and specificity. Echocardiography reveals that the clot has distinct margins, is usually located near an akinetic or dyskinetic area, and may protrude within the ventricle or move with the adjacent wall. Protruding thrombi tend to be more echo dense than mural thrombi, whereas mural thrombi have a layered appearance and are often echolucent along the endocardial border.

Thrombi form within the first 4 days after an infarction and occur in 30% of all anterior wall infarctions; they rarely occur in inferior wall infarctions. If they do not dissolve spontaneously, they may disappear with the use of anticoagulants.

Left Atrial Thrombi. Thrombi usually form in the left atrium in the presence of mitral valve disease (stenosis), an enlarged left atrium, and atrial fibrillation—conditions that predispose to blood stasis. The most common site is the atrial appendage. The echocardiographic appearance of these thrombi varies. In many cases, they are attached to the atrial wall and can be round or ovoid in shape. Their borders are often well defined, they demonstrate mobility, and their texture is uniform. Occasionally, a thrombus appears as a flat immobile mass or as a free-floating ball.

Thrombi of the Right Heart. Most thrombi form in the right heart in the presence of right ventricular infarction, cardiomyopathies, or cor pulmonale. They usually are immobile, heterogeneous sessile masses. In addition, secondary thrombi may occur. Their source is embolization from deep-vein thrombosis. Echocardiography typically reveals a long, serpentine, apparently free-floating mass with no obvious site of attachment. Patients are at a much higher risk for an embolus when the thrombus in any area of the heart is protruding or free floating.

Other Cardiac Masses. Because a number of foreign objects can mimic a thrombus, one must be aware of their presence and location. For example, right-heart catheters are often seen in both the right atrium and the right ventricle. These appear as highly reflective linear echoes.

Normal cardiac structures also can mimic intracardiac masses. The moderator band seen in the apex of the right ventricle appears as a thick muscular band extending from the free wall of the right ventricle to the interventricular septum. Occasionally, a prominent eustachian valve can be seen in the right atrium at the junction of the inferior vena cava. It appears as a thin, long, mobile structure in the right atrium, which also may contain thin filamentous structures known as the Chiari network that is a remnant of embryonic structures. The left ventricle also may contain long thin fibers known as false tendons or ectopic chordae tendineae. These filamentous structures traverse the left ventricle and typically are brightly reflective structures of no clinical significance.

DISEASES OF THE AORTA

Aortic Dilatation

The aorta is considered dilated when its diameter is >37 mm. The average diameter of the adult aorta is 33–37 mm. M-mode measurements of the aorta should be taken at the level of the aortic annulus and the sinus of Valsalva. Aortic dilatation is seen most frequently in patients with annuloaortic ectasia or Marfan syndrome. In these patients, the medial layer of the aorta weakens, and the aorta dilates. The dilatation occurs not only in the wall of the aorta, but in the aortic annulus as well. This often leads to aortic insufficiency because the cusps of the aorta are unable to coapt during closure. Two-dimensional echocardiography can easily detect a dilated aorta.

Aortic Aneurysm

An aortic aneurysm can occur anywhere along the thoracic aorta. The most common sites are the arch and descending aorta, with most occurring just beyond the left subclavian artery. Aneurysms of the thoracic aorta often extend into the abdominal aorta. There are several types of aneurysms, that include; saccular (sack-like dilatation), fusiform (spindle-shaped aneurysm), and dissecting (separation of the arterial wall creating a false and true lumen).

A dissecting aortic aneurysm results from intimal tears of the aortic wall. The driving force of the blood destroys the media further and strips the intimal layer from the adventitial layer. Aortic dissections are classified according to the area and extent of the intimal tear. Type I tears extend from the ascending aorta and continue beyond the arch. Type II tears also begin a few centimeters from the aortic valve but are confined to the ascending aorta. Type III tears begin in the descending aorta, usually just distal to the origin of the left subclavian artery. More than 90% of patients with dissecting aneurysms experience severe pain. Dissections occur twice as often in men as in women and usually in the sixth and seventh decade of life. M-mode findings reveal extra linear echoes within the aorta. Two-dimensional imaging is the echocardiographic tool of choice. Two-dimensional imaging allows visualization of the intimal flap, which divides the true lumen of the aorta from the false lumen. Color-flow Doppler can be invaluable in localizing the site of intraluminal communication. Other echocardiographic evidence for dissection includes aortic regurgitation—the most commonly noted complication. Doppler is useful for detecting disturbed flow patterns in the LV outflow tract. The left ventricle may become enlarged because of volume overload from the aortic regurgitation; pericardial effusion can be noted, and left pleural effusion also may be noted. The diagnosis of dissection should be made when an intima flap is seen in more than one view.

Aneurysms that occur in the sinus of Valsalva are best seen using two-dimensional imaging. They are observed most easily in the short-axis view during diastole. Rupture usually occurs in the right side of the heart, but it also can occur in the left heart and interventricular septum. Sinus of Valsalva aneurysms can be acquired or congenital in nature.

CONGENITAL HEART DISEASE

Aortic Stenosis

Abnormalities of the LV outflow tract are the most common congenital heart disease found in the adult population. Obstruction can occur at the subvalvular, supravalvular, or valvular level. Congenital abnormalities of the aortic valve occur in 1% of the population, with a higher prevalence among males. The most common malformation of the aortic valve is a bicuspid valve. Aortic coarctation, VSD, and isolated pulmonic stenosis are associated with the condition. As the valve ages, it becomes fibrotic and may calcify. By the fourth decade, 50% of all bicuspid aortic valves become stenotic.

Subvalvular stenosis also can occur. There are two types of subvalvular stenosis: discrete and subaortic. In discrete stenosis, a thin membrane obstructs the outflow tract or a more fibromuscular ridge obstructs the flow of blood. Subaortic stenosis, too, is more common in males. Aortic regurgitation is a frequent finding in subaortic stenosis. Discrete subvalvular stenosis is primarily an acquired rather than a congenital problem when it is present in adults.

Supravalvular stenosis also can be classified into two categories. The most frequent supravalvular narrowing is found in the ascending aorta just above the valve. Less frequently, the obstruction involves the ascending aorta, the aortic arch, and the descending aorta. Supravalvular obstruction can be a familial finding, but it also can be sporadic or as a result of rubella infection. When found in association with mental retardation, a diagnosis of Williams syndrome can be made.

Patients with congenital outflow obstruction usually present with LV systolic hypertension and develop concentric LV hypertrophy. The physical examination reveals a harsh systolic ejection murmur over the right parasternal border. Echocardiography has become the diagnostic tool of choice in making this diagnosis. M-mode echocardiography reveals a thickened valve with an eccentric closure line. Normally, the closure line of the aortic valve is centrally located. In a bicuspid aortic valve, however, the closure line is displaced toward either the anterior or the posterior wall of the aorta. Two-dimensional echocardiography reveals systolic doming of the cusps, which is seen in the left parasternal long-axis view. The left parasternal short-axis view reveals the presence of only two cusps. Pulsed-wave Doppler echocardiography can localize the area of obstruction and determine what type of obstruction is present. Continuous-wave Doppler examination allows quantification of peak and mean pressure gradients across the obstruction. Color-flow Doppler examination allows assessment of blood flow direction.

Atrial Septal Defects

Atrial septal defects (ASDs) are the second most common congenital abnormality found in adults. There are three classifications of ASDs, depending on their location: ostium secundum defects, ostium primum defects, and sinus venosus defects. Ostium secundum defects make up 70% of all ASDs found in adults. These are located near the fossa ovalis. Women are three times more likely than men to have this defect. Twenty percent of patients with this type of ASD have mitral valve prolapse. Other associated findings include mitral or pulmonic stenosis and atrial septal aneurysm. When an ASD and mitral stenosis exist simultaneously, the condition is called Lutembacher's syndrome. In isolated mitral stenosis, the left atrium is dilated because the valve area is reduced. With ASD, the blood can escape across the atrial defect, thereby preserving the size of the left atrium.

Fifteen percent of all ASDs are of the ostium primum type. These defects occur in the region of the ostium primum or the lower portion of the atrial septum. A commonly associated finding is a clefted anterior mitral valve leaflet.

Sinus venosus ASDs account for the other 15%. The defects occur in the upper portion of the atrial septum near the orifice of the inferior vena cava. The most common finding associated with this defect is partial anomalous pulmonary venous drainage.

Two-dimensional and M-mode echocardiography reveal a volume overload in the right heart. Findings indicative of right-sided volume overload include a dilated right ventricle and a flattening of the septum in diastole. Two-dimensional imaging of the atrial septum allows direct visualization and localization of the defect. The views most commonly used to assess the atrial septum include the parasternal short-axis, the apical four-chamber, and the subcostal views. The latter view is the best one for visualizing the atrial septum. In addition to the secondary findings already described, two-dimensional imaging allows direct visu-alization of the defect. In septal defects, a dropout of echoes is noted in the area of the defect. On echocardiography, the dropout of echoes is characterized by a bright echo perpendicular to the atrial septum. This finding has been described as the T sign.

Doppler echocardiography also can help detect ASDs. In the absence of elevated pressures in the right heart, blood flows from the higher-pressure left ventricle to the lower-pressure right heart. In the subcostal view, a pulsed Doppler sample gate can be placed in the right heart near the atrial septum. The spectral display will reveal turbulent flow toward the transducer in late systole and throughout diastole. Color-flow Doppler allows visualization of the interatrial shunt by superimposing a color coding on a two-dimensional image.

Contrast echocardiography can be used when imaging and Doppler are unable to identify the atrial defect clearly. When used in conjunction with two-dimensional imaging, 92–100% of ASDs can be detected. Contrast agents injected into a vein enter the right heart, which is often highly opacified. In the presence of an ASD, small amounts of contrast material can be seen crossing the atrial septum into the left atrium and to the left ventricle. When the shunt is left to right, which is normally the case, a negative contrast effect can be noted. Contrast enhancement can be increased by having the patient perform the Valsalva maneuver, or cough.

Patent Foramen Ovale

Patent (open) foramen ovale can be found in 27% of older patients. Left-to-right shunting does not normally occur when pressures are normal. A potential complication of the condition is paradoxical embolus.

Ventricular Septal Defects

VSDs are the most common defects found in infants and children. In the adult, ASDs are much more common. VSDs fall into two major classifications: muscular septal defects and membranous defects. Like ASDs, VSDs are classified according to the region involved.

Muscular Septal Defects. Muscular septal defects are entirely surrounded by muscle. Outlet defects occur in the most superior portion of the septum and make up part of the outflow region of the left ventricle. They are also referred to as outflow defects, subpulmonic or infundibular defects, or bulbar defects. These defects are bordered by the trabecular septomarginalis (right ventricular septal band) and the pulmonary valve annulus. Thus, they are the most difficult VSDs to image and are best seen from the subcostal and high parasternal positions.

A special form of outlet defect occurs above the crista supraventricularis. This defect is known as supracristal ventricular defect; it is also referred to as the doubly committed subarterial defect because of its proximity to both semilunar valves. This defect also is best seen from the subcostal and high parasternal positions. Associated findings in this defect include: (1) aortic valve prolapse because of lack of support, usually involving the right coronary cusp, (2) dilatation of the right coronary sinus of Valsalva, and (3) aortic insufficiency. The defect is usually small.

Inlet ventricular defects are bordered superiorly by the tricuspid valve annulus, apically by the tips of the papillary muscles, and anteriorly by the trabecula septomarginalis. They are also referred to as endocardial cushion defects, retrocristal defects, sinus defects, and inflow defects, which can be seen in several planes, including the parasternal, apical, and subcostal views. Because these defects are usually large, they can be confused with a double-inlet ventricle.

Trabecular defects are bordered by the chordal attachments of the papillary muscle to the apex. They extend from the smooth outlet septum to the inlet septum, are heavily trabeculated, and are usually large. They also can be multiple. These defects typically lead to hypertension of the right ventricle and may produce a right-to-left shunt if the pressures in the right heart exceed those in the left. A special type of muscular septal defect that occurs in the muscular septum is characterized by numerous small defects resembling Swiss cheese. This "Swiss cheese" defect occurs primarily in the apex.

Membranous Defects. Membranous septal defects occur in the region bordered by the inlet and outlet septums and the junctions between the right and noncoronary cusps of the aortic valve. This part of the septum is located at the base of the heart. Defects in this area are often referred to as perimembranous because they usually involve part of a surrounding muscular septum. Almost all planes can be used to image these defects, which occur more frequently than the muscular varieties.

Using two-dimensional imaging allows visualization of the septum. When the defect is large, a dropout of echoes is appreciated. In addition, a T artifact is observed. When imaging does not allow localization of the defect, color-flow Doppler can be used. High-velocity turbulent flow usually can be seen as a mosaic color pattern in the area of the jet. Contrast echocardiography also can be used to localize the defect. Agitated solution can be injected into the right heart through a peripheral vein. Even a few bubbles seen entering the left ventricle are indicative of a right-to-left shunt when right-sided pressures are slightly elevated.

Tetralogy of Fallot

In adults, tetralogy of Fallot is the primary congenital disease producing cyanosis. In this condition, four specific findings are noted. The aorta overrides the perimembranous VSD. Infundibular or valvular pulmonic stenosis is present, resulting in right ventricular hypertrophy. M-mode criteria for diagnosing tetralogy of Fallot include a break in the continuity of the anterior wall of the aorta from that of the interventricular septum as well as a narrowing of the right ventricular outflow tract. Two-dimensional imaging, however, allows direct visualization of the cardiac anatomy and is, therefore, the echocardiographic

procedure of choice. Imaging often allows visualization of the VSD and gives valuable information about the amount of aortic override. Doppler echocardiography allows quantification of gradients across the obstruction of right ventricular outflow.

Pulmonic Stenosis

Eighty percent of all congenital obstructions of right ventricular outflow occur at the level of the pulmonic valve. The valve is often thickened with fusion of the cusps and can be seen doming in systole. Right ventricular hypertrophy occurs as a result of the increased resistance to flow. Two-dimensional imaging allows visualization of the valve, which usually appears thickened and with reduced excursion.

Persistent Ductus Arteriosus

Persistent ductus arteriosus (PDA) occurs when the ductus fails to close after birth. In utero, communication exists between the pulmonary circulation and the systemic circulation, the purpose of which in fetal circulation is to direct the flow of desaturated blood away from the coronary and cerebral circulation and toward the placenta. The ductus is located near the isthmus of the aorta near the origin of the left subclavian artery; it extends to the left pulmonary artery just beyond the bifurcation. In the absence of elevated pulmonary pressures, blood flows from the aorta to the pulmonary artery. In adults, the most common symptom of a PDA is dyspnea on exertion. In persistent ductus, the increased blood flow to the lungs results in dilatation of the pulmonary arteries, the left atrium and ventricle, and the aorta. If pulmonary pressure increases, the blood flow may reverse and travel from the pulmonary circulation toward the aorta. This condition is known as Eisenmenger's complex and is characterized by right-to-left shunting.

Coarctation of the Aorta

Coarctation is a stricture or contraction of the aorta. Twice as many men as women are likely to have coarctation of the aorta. Most patients with this condition are asymptomatic. The coarctation is manifested as LV hypertension. On physical examination, a systolic murmur can be heard. The most common site of narrowing occurs in the thoracic aorta just distal to the left subclavian artery. This condition is often found in association with other congenital abnormalities such as VSD, PDA, a bicuspid aortic valve, and mitral valve abnormalities. It is the most common cardiac malformation found in Turner's syndrome.

The suprasternal notch offers the best view of the ascending aorta, the arch, and the descending aorta. Direct visualization of the coarctation is possible using two-dimensional imaging. Doppler echocardiography typically reveals increased velocities across the site of coarctation.

Ebstein's Anomaly

Ebstein's anomaly is characterized by downward displacement of the anterior or septal leaflet of the tricuspid valve into the right ventricle. As a result, the ventricle becomes "atrialized" and loses some of its pumping capacity. Associated findings include secundum-type ASDs, pulmonic stenosis or atresia, VSD, and mitral valve prolapse. Symptoms may not be evident until the patient is between 30 and 40 years of age. The most common complication of this abnormality is failure of the right ventricle.

The M-mode criterion for this anomaly includes visualization of a large tricuspid valve leaflet, simultaneously seen with the anterior leaflet of the mitral leaflet. A delay time in closure of the tricuspid valve of 80 m/s or more to that of closure of the mitral valve is the second M-mode finding. Two-dimensional imaging allows direct visualization of the anatomy. Specific findings in imaging include an apically located tricuspid leaflet and a functionally small right ventricle. Ebstein's anomaly can be diagnosed if the leaflet is displaced 20 mm or more.

HYPERTENSIVE DISEASE

Systemic Hypertension

There are two basic types of systemic hypertension: essential or idiopathic and secondary hypertension. Both affect the diastolic and systolic pressure. The classification of blood pressure is shown in Table 2–7.

The cause of essential hypertension is unknown. Although several mechanisms may come into play, no specific cause has been well described. Secondary hypertension results in high blood pressure associated with any of the following: renal disease, endocrine disease, coarctation of the aorta, pregnancy, neurological disorders, acute stress, increased intravascular volume, alcohol and other drug abuse, increased cardiac output, and rigidity of the aorta.

TABLE 2–7 • Classification of Blood Pressure

Range (mm Hg)	Category
Diastolic	
<85	Normal blood pressure
85–89	High normal blood pressure
90–104	Mild hypertension
105–114	Moderate hypertension
≥115	Severe hypertension
Systolic, when diastolic blood pressure is <90 mm Hg	
<140	Normal blood pressure
140–159	Borderline isolated systolic hypertension
≥160	Isolated systolic hypertension

Reprinted with permission from The 1984 Report of the Joint National Committee on Detection, Evaluation, and Treatment of High Blood Pressure. Arch Intern Med. 144, May, 1984.

The hemodynamic properties of systemic hypertension, whatever the cause, are similar. Initially cardio output increases, as does fluid volume. This increased fluid volume is transferred to the various organs and tissues. Once tissues receive more blood than they need, the blood vessels that deliver the blood constrict. This is known as vasoconstriction, which is an intrinsic property of such systemic vessels as arterioles, and the bicep increases in size when one does curls, so do the arteries. If this state continues, the vessels continue to exert resistance on the incoming blood (peripheral resistance). As a result, the heartbeats gain greater resistance and the vessel themselves become thicker.

As is the case with any muscle, hypertrophy occurs when stress is exerted. Similar to the bicep increasing in size when one does curls, the heart also increases in size as it is forced to pump blood against increased peripheral resistance. Therefore, the main echocardiographic findings are increased muscle mass of the heart, especially the left ventricle. By M-mode criteria, the walls of the left ventricle are thick. The principal Doppler findings include (1) decreased transmitral E wave, (2) increased A wave, and (3) increased A-to-E-wave ratios.

Pulmonary Hypertension

In normal physiology, the pulmonary blood flow allows passage of blood to the lungs for three basic functions: oxygenation, filtration, and pH balance by excreting carbon dioxide. Blood coming in from the various tissues and organs of the body is directed to the right heart through the superior and inferior vena cavae. Once this deoxygenated blood enters the right atrium, it passes through the tricuspid valve into the right ventricle across the pulmonic valve and into the main pulmonary artery, which bifurcates into a left and right branch and directs blood to the left and right lobes of the lungs. Normally the pulmonary circulation offers little resistance to blood flow. The normal peak systolic pressure ranges from 18 to 25 mm Hg, and the normal diastolic pressure ranges from 6 to 10 mm Hg. Pulmonary artery pressure in excess of 30 mm Hg systolic pressure and 20 mm Hg diastolic pressure represents elevated pulmonary pressures, or pulmonary hypertension.

As with systemic hypertension, pulmonary hypertension has two basic forms: primary and secondary. Primary pulmonary hypertension—also known as idiopathic, essential, or unexplained pulmonary hypertension—has no known discernible cause. Secondary pulmonary hypertension can be the result of any one of the following factors:

- Increased resistance to pulmonary venous drainage
- Elevated LV diastolic pressure
- Left atrial hypertension (mitral stenosis)
- Pulmonary parenchyma disease
- Pulmonary venous obstruction (cor triatriatum or pulmonary veno-occlusive disease

Cor triatriatum is a congenital abnormality in which the common embryonic pulmonary vein is not incorporated into the left atrium. Instead, the pulmonary veins empty into an accessory chamber and communicate with the left atrium through a small opening. The result is obstruction of pulmonary venous flow that simulates mitral stenosis. In pulmonary veno-occlusive disease, the veins and venules of the lung become fibrotic. M-mode findings reveal an absent or decreased A wave in the absence of right ventricular failure: a lack of respiratory variation in the A wave; an extended pre-ejection period; midsystolic closure of the pulmonic valve, also known as midsystolic notch; and reduced ejection time of the right ventricle. Two-dimensional imaging indicates a dilated pulmonary artery and abnormalities in interventricular septal motion.

Doppler measurements reveal the following: a decreased acceleration time, a longer pre-ejection period, a shorter ejection time, and tricuspid regurgitation. The acceleration time is the time interval between the onset of flow and the peak systolic flow. In pulmonary hypertension, the velocity of blood flow increases rapidly and peaks early in systole. This measurement is made by identifying the beginning of the Doppler signal and the peak velocity of the same signal. The time between the two is the acceleration time.

The pre-ejection period is the time interval between the onset of the QRS complex to onset of flow in the pulmonary artery. In pulmonary hypertension, this time period increases.

Ejection time is the time from the onset of flow to the cessation of flow. In pulmonary hypertension, this time period becomes shorter. This measurement is made by taking the time between the beginning and the end of the Doppler signal.

Tricuspid regurgitation occurs in the majority of patients with elevated pressures in the pulmonary artery. Continuous-wave Doppler can be used to localize the regurgitant jet and obtain the peak transtricuspid gradient using the modified Bernoulli equation. The peak gradient is the difference in systolic pressure between the right atrium and right ventricle. Estimation of the pulmonary pressures is accomplished by adding the right atrial pressures, which are determined by visual inspection of the jugular venous pulse. A more common way is to add the constant "10" to the peak systolic transtricuspid gradient. When stenosis of the pulmonic valve is present, however, one cannot determine pulmonary artery pressures using the peak transtricuspid regurgitant gradient.

CORONARY ARTERY DISEASE

The normal right and left coronary arteries supply the heart muscle with oxygenated blood (see Table 2–8). The left coronary artery originates from the left coronary sinus of Valsalva, which bifurcates into two branches: the anterior interventricular or descending branch, also known as the left anterior descending branch, and the circumflex branch. The right coronary artery originates from the right coronary sinus of Valsalva.

The coronary anatomy can vary considerably in humans. In 67% of cases, the right coronary artery is the dominant artery. In these cases, this artery supplies the parts of the left ventricle and septum. In 15% of cases, the left coronary artery is the dominant one and supplies blood to all of the left ventricle and septum. In 18% of cases, the two arteries are equal; this situation is called the balanced coronary arterial pattern.

Abnormal Wall Motion

When the blood supply to the heart muscle is interrupted, the muscle is damaged and immediate changes in motion can be observed. The affected area can be identified using the various echocardiographic views. The wall segment should be identified using the American Society of Echocardiography's recommendation (see the section on Normal Anatomy).[6]

TABLE 2–8 • Normal Branches of the Coronary Arteries

Coronary Artery	Major Branches	Area Supplied
Left coronary	Left anterior descending	Anterior left ventricular wall Anterior two-thirds of apical septum Anteroapical portions of left ventricle Anterior-lateral papillary muscle Midseptum Bundle of His Anterior right ventricular papillary muscle
	Circumflex*	Lateral left ventricular wall Left atrium
Right coronary	Numerous branches	Anterior right ventricular wall Posterior third (or more) of the interventricular septum Diaphragmatic wall of right ventricle Atrioventricular node

*If the circumflex terminates at the crux of the heart, it supplies the entire left ventricle and interventricular septum.

Complications of Ischemic Heart Disease

Ventricular Aneurysm. One complication of ischemic heart disease is ventricular aneurysm. Although aneurysm can form in any part of the left ventricle, more than 80% form in the apex and are the result of an anterior infarction. Of the 5–10% that form in the posterior wall, nearly half are false aneurysms.

The echocardiographic appearance of aneurysms includes thin walls that do not thicken in systole, a bulging wall, and dyskinetic motion to the affected area.

There are three types of ventricular aneurysms: anatomically true, functionally true, and anatomically false aneurysms. An anatomically true aneurysm is composed of fibrous tissue, may or may not contain a clot, and protrudes during both diastole and systole. Its mouth is wider or as wide as its maximum diameter, and its wall is the former LV wall. An anatomically true aneurysm almost never ruptures once healed. A functionally true aneurysm also consists of fibrous tissue but protrudes only during ventricular systole.

An anatomically false aneurysm always contains a clot. Its mouth is considerably smaller than its maximum diameter, and it protrudes during both systole and diastole and may even expand. Its wall is composed of parietal pericardium. Because a false aneurysm often ruptures, immediate surgery is usually required.

Ventricular Septal Defect. A VSD occurs when a rupture occurs in the septum. Several echocardiographic techniques can be used to make the diagnosis. Two-dimensional imaging allows direct visualization of the defect. With contrast echocardiography with imaging, contrasting material can be seen filling the right ventricle and entering the left ventricle as blood moves back and forth through the defect. Negative contrast effect also can be noted. Doppler measurements can detect turbulent high-velocity signals on the right side of the ventricular septum. The best views include the left parasternal long- and short-axis views and the apical four-chamber view. Color Doppler can demonstrate communication between the left and right ventricles. The color jet appears as a mosaic pattern of high-velocity flow.

Thrombus. Thrombus, the most common complication of infarction, usually occurs in the apex in areas of dyskinesia. It can be laminar, lay close to the wall of the ventricle, or protrude into the cavity and be highly mobile. The diagnosis should be made when the thrombus is seen in several views.

Valve Dysfunction. An infarction is most likely to affect the mitral valve. Mitral regurgitation results if the papillary muscle is ruptured, if it becomes fibrosed, or if the mitral annulus is affected, resulting in incomplete closure of the leaflets.

Right Ventricular Involvement. Involvement of the right ventricle occurs primarily when the infarction is in the inferior wall or when the proximal right coronary artery is obstructed. Echocardiography reveals that the ventricle is dilated and its free wall moves abnormally.

References

1. Allen MN, *Echocardiography*. 2nd ed. New York: Lippincott; 1999.

2. *Gray's Anatomy*. Williams PL, Warwick R, Dyson M, eds. 37th ed. New York: Churchill Livingstone; 1989.

3. Driscoll DJ, Fuster V, McGoon DC. Congenital heart disease in adolescents and adults: atrioventricular canal defect. In: Brandenburg RO, Fuster V, Giulani ER, et al., eds. *Cardiology: Fundamentals and Practice*. Chicago: Year Book Medical Publishers; 1987.

4. *Report of the American Society of Echocardiography Committee on Nomenclature and Standards Identification of Myocardial Wall Segments*. 1982.

5. Braunwald E. *Heart Disease: A Textbook of Cardiac Medicine*. 3rd ed. Philadelphia: WB Saunders; 1988.

6. Feigenbaum H. *Endocardiopathy*. 4th ed. Philadelphia: Lea & Febiger; 1986.

Questions

GENERAL INSTRUCTIONS: For each question, select the best answer. Select only one answer for each question unless otherwise specified.

1. **Which heart groove or sulci separates the atria from the ventricles?**

   (A) interventricular

   (B) interatrial

   (C) anterior interventricular

   (D) coronary or atrioventricular

   Identify the coronary arteries in Fig. 2–12.

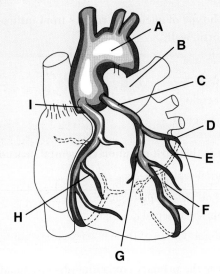

FIGURE 2–12. Anatomic drawing of the heart and vessels.

2. _____ left posterolateral branch

3. _____ left circumflex branch

4. _____ pulmonary trunk

5. _____ left marginal branch

6. _____ atrioventricular node branch

7. _____ left main coronary artery

8. _____ right coronary artery

9. _____ aortic arch

10. _____ left anterior descending branch

11. **Which of the following is *not* an indication for stress echocardiography?**

    (A) screening of new patients for coronary artery disease

    (B) assessing states before and after intervention

    (C) determining prognosis after myocardial infarction

    (D) unstable angina

12. **Which of the following cardiology examination requires a physician to perform?**

    (A) echocardiography

    (B) stress echocardiography

    (C) transesophageal echocardiography

    (D) color-flow Doppler

13. **What is the purpose of the pericardium?**

    (A) allow the heart to move freely with each beat

    (B) facilitating ejection and volume changes

    (C) contain the heart within the mediastinum

    (D) serve as a barrier to infection

    (E) all of the above

14. **What is the largest cardiac chamber?**

    (A) right atrium

    (B) right ventricle

    (C) left atrium

    (D) left ventricle

15. **The left atrium receives how many pulmonary veins?**

    (A) one

    (B) two

    (C) three

    (D) four

16. **What is crista terminalis?**

    (A) anterior portion of the right atrium

    (B) posterior portion of the right atrium

    (C) a ridge of muscle separating the right atrium

    (D) a heart groove or sulci

17. Which valve is located between the left atrium and the left ventricle?

    (A) tricuspid

    (B) mitral

    (C) aortic

    (D) foramen ovale

18. Which of the following is *not* a right heart characteristic and/or function?

    (A) supplies blood to the pulmonary circulation

    (B) normal pressure in the ventricle is approximately 140 mm Hg

    (C) blood returning to the right heart has a lower oxygen saturation

    (D) contains the tricuspid valve

19. Mitral valve stenosis results primarily from which of the following?

    (A) atherosclerosis

    (B) endocarditis

    (C) hypertension

    (D) rheumatic disease

20. Vegetations are more commonly associated with which of the following?

    (A) pulmonary hypertension

    (B) aneurysms

    (C) endocarditis

    (D) mitral valve disease

21. Which of the following is not a type of bioprosthetic heart valve?

    (A) xenograft

    (B) heterograft

    (C) homograft

    (D) Bjork–Shiley valve

22. Which of the following would indicate pericardial effusion?

    (A) 5–10 mL of fluid

    (B) 10–15 mL of fluid

    (C) 15–50 mL of fluid

    (D) 75–100 mL of fluid

23. The term cardiomyopathy is used to describe which of the following?

    (A) pericardial effusion

    (B) variety of cardiac diseases that affect the pericardium

    (C) variety of cardiac diseases that affect the myocardium

    (D) variety of cardiac diseases that affect the endocardium

24. What is the most common type of benign tumor of the heart?

    (A) myxoma

    (B) rhabdomyoma

    (C) lipoma

    (D) fibroma

25. What is the most common malignant cardiac tumor?

    (A) teratoma

    (B) rhabdomyoma

    (C) carcinoma

    (D) angiosarcoma

26. Which type of aneurysm results from intimal tears of the aortic wall?

    (A) saccular

    (B) fusiform

    (C) pseudo

    (D) dissecting

27. What is the most common congenital heart disease?

    (A) atrial septal defects

    (B) ventricular septal defects

    (C) muscular septal defects

    (D) abnormalities of the left ventricular outflow tract

28. What is the primary congenital disease in adults that produces cyanosis?

    (A) pulmonic stenosis

    (B) coarctation of the aorta

    (C) persistent ductus arteriosus

    (D) tetralogy of Fallot

29. Which of the following is *not* a characteristic of cardiomyopathy?

    (A) dilatation

    (B) pericarditis

    (C) restrictive

    (D) hypertrophic

30–36. **Identify the structures in Fig. 2–13.**

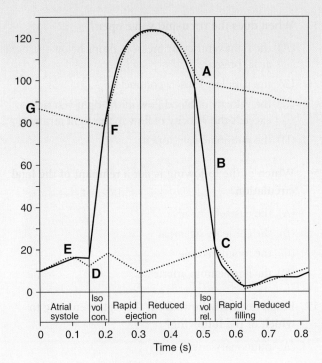

FIGURE 2–13. Events of the cardiac cycle.

30. _____ aortic valve closure

31. _____ aortic valve opening

32. _____ aortic pressure

33. _____ left ventricular pressure

34. _____ mitral valve closure

35. _____ left atrial pressure

36. _____ mitral valve opening

37. **In stenotic diseases of the tricuspid, which of the following is dilated?**

(A) left atrium

(B) left ventricle

(C) right atrium

(D) right ventricle

38. **In tricuspid valve disease, what is the primary cause of regurgitation?**

(A) carcinoid heart disease

(B) prolapse of the valve

(C) rheumatic heart disease

(D) secondary to pulmonary hypertension

39. **Which of the following is not a type of endocarditis?**

(A) Ebstein's anomaly

(B) bacterial

(C) mycotic

(D) Löffler's

40. **Which of the following is *not* a clinical symptom associated with aortic valve stenosis?**

(A) chest pain

(B) dyspnea on exertion

(C) shortness of breath

(D) syncope

41. **Which of the following is the bicuspid valve with two major leaflets?**

(A) tricuspid valve

(B) aortic valve

(C) pulmonic valve

(D) mitral valve

42. **What is a classic finding in mitral valve prolapse?**

(A) systolic doming

(B) fluttering of the mitral valve

(C) pulmonary edema

(D) a systolic click

43. **What is the most common cause of a flail leaflet?**

(A) rupture of the chordal tendineae

(B) rupture of the papillary muscle

(C) annular calcification

(D) congenital defect

44. **Which cardiac examination provides the highest resolution?**

(A) transthoracic echocardiography

(B) contrast transthoracic echocardiography

(C) stress echocardiography

(D) transesophageal echocardiography

45. **In which cardiac sinus is a thin fold of tissue guard called the thebesian valve?**

(A) sinus of Morgagni

(B) aortic sinus

(C) coronary sinus

(D) sinus of Valsalva

46. **What is the average length of an adult heart?**

    (A) 12 cm

    (B) 8–9 cm

    (C) 6 cm

    (D) 16 cm

47. **The atrioventricular node is located in which trinagular region of the right atrium?**

    (A) posterior region

    (B) anterior region

    (C) triangular region

    (D) triangle of Koch

48. **Which vessel drains the head and parts of the upper extremities?**

    (A) aorta

    (B) superior vena cava

    (C) inferior vena cava

    (D) portal venous system

49. **Which of the following views would *best* demonstrate all four cardiac chambers simultaneously?**

    (A) left parasternal

    (B) right parasternal

    (C) subcostal

    (D) suprasternal

50. **Which of the following is used to denote the three orthogonal planes for two-dimensional echocardiographic imaging?**

    (A) long axis, short axis, and four chamber

    (B) apical, subcostal, and parasternal

    (C) suprasternal, right sternal border, and left sternal border

    (D) anterior, posterior, and coronal

51. **Which of the following abnormalities are usually *best* demonstrated with the subcostal four-chamber view?**

    (A) atrial septal defects and ventricular septal defects

    (B) mitral regurgitation and tricuspid regurgitation

    (C) mitral stenosis and tricuspid stenosis

    (D) aortic insufficiency and pulmonic insufficiency

52. **Which of the following terms is used to describe the control that suppresses near-field echoes and enhances the intensity of the far-field echoes?**

    (A) attenuation

    (B) time-gain compensation

    (C) reject

    (D) compression

53. **When does the tricuspid valve open?**

    (A) the right ventricular pressure drops below the right atrial pressure

    (B) the papillary muscle contracts

    (C) the velocity of blood flow in the right ventricle exceeds the velocity of flow in the right atrium

    (D) the pulmonic valve opens

54. **Which of the following is *not* a remnant of the fetal circulation?**

    (A) the eustachian valve

    (B) the coronary ligament

    (C) the foramen ovale

    (D) the ligamentum arteriosus

55. **Blood normally flows from the right ventricle to which of the following?**

    (A) pulmonary artery

    (B) aorta

    (C) right atrium

    (D) pulmonary vein

56. **A pulmonary vein is normally attached to which of the following?**

    (A) right ventricle

    (B) left ventricle

    (C) left atrium

    (D) right atrium

57. **Which of the following statements regarding cardiac anatomy is false?**

    (A) The heart tends to assume a more vertical position in tall thin people and a more horizontal position in short, heavy people.

    (B) The ligamentum arteriosum runs from the left pulmonary artery to the descending aorta.

    (C) The coronary arteries arise from the sinuses within the pockets of the left and right coronary cusps of the aortic valve.

    (D) The left ventricle constitutes most of the ventral surface of the heart.

58. Left ventricular ejection time can be assessed from an M-mode echocardiogram by measuring the distance between which of the following?

(A) aortic valve opening and closing points

(B) mitral D and C points

(C) R wave and T wave

(D) mitral valve closure and aortic valve opening

59. Often, what is the best two-dimensional view for examining patients with chronic obstructive pulmonary disease?

(A) parasternal

(B) apical

(C) suprasternal

(D) subcostal

60. What are the two best transducer positions for Doppler investigation of systolic blood flow across the aortic valve?

(A) parasternal and suprasternal

(B) apical and right sternal border

(C) suprasternal and subcostal

(D) subcostal and apical

61. When should the size of the left atrium be measured on the M-mode?

(A) at end-systole

(B) at the peak of the R wave

(C) with the onset of aortic valve opening

(D) at the beginning of the P wave

62. Doming of any cardiac valve on two-dimensional echocardiography is consistent with which of the following?

(A) regurgitation

(B) decreased cardiac output

(C) stenosis

(D) congenital malformation

63. Two-dimensional images are best obtained when the ultrasound beam is directed _____ to the structure of interest. Doppler signals are best obtained when the ultrasound beam is directed _____ to the flow of blood.

(A) oblique; perpendicular

(B) parallel; perpendicular

(C) perpendicular; parallel

(D) perpendicular; oblique

64. Right ventricular systolic pressure overload can be caused by which of the following?

(A) pulmonary insufficiency

(B) an atrial septal defect

(C) aortic stenosis

(D) pulmonary hypertension

65. Left ventricular measurements should be obtained from the parasternal long-axis view at the level of which of the following?

(A) mitral valve annulus

(B) tips of the mitral leaflets

(C) chordae tendineae

(D) papillary muscle

66. Which of the following cannot cause paradoxical interventricular septal motion?

(A) left bundle branch block

(B) postpericardiotomy

(C) left ventricular volume overload

(D) severe tricuspid regurgitation

67. In a patient with volume overload of the right ventricle, the onset of ventricular systole is likely to show the interventricular septum moving

(A) toward the right ventricular free wall

(B) toward the left ventricular wall

(C) laterally

(D) not at all

68. A murmur that is associated with a thrill is likely to be which of the following?

(A) organic in origin

(B) insignificant

(C) functional

(D) the result of an atrial septal defect

69. The Valsalva maneuver and the inhalation of amyl nitrite are techniques that are sometimes used during an echocardiographic examination when checking for which of the following?

(A) mitral valve prolapse or systolic anterior motion of the mitral valve

(B) aortic stenosis or mitral stenosis

(C) aortic stenosis or aortic regurgitation

(D) a ventricular septal defect or pulmonic stenosis

70. Clubbing of the fingers and nail beds is a sign of which of the following?

    (A) cyanotic heart disease
    (B) Marfan syndrome
    (C) Barlow syndrome
    (D) increased cardiac output

71. Even though two-dimensional echocardiography has largely replaced M-mode echocardiography for cardiac diagnosis, M-mode still has the advantage of which of the following?

    (A) defining spatial relationships of cardiac structures
    (B) providing enhanced temporal resolution
    (C) providing dynamic assessment of the velocity of blood flow
    (D) providing superior lateral resolution

72. When attempting a parasternal short-axis view, if the left ventricle appears oval rather than circular, where should the echocardiographer move the transducer?

    (A) medially
    (B) laterally
    (C) to a higher intercostal space
    (D) to a lower intercostal space

73. A Doppler tracing of the mitral valve in which the A point is higher than the E point indicates which of the following?

    (A) high cardiac output
    (B) low cardiac output
    (C) decreased left ventricular compliance
    (D) high left ventricular end-diastolic pressures

74. Which of the following is usually not a secondary finding in patients with mitral stenosis?

    (A) a dilated left atrium
    (B) a dilated right atrium
    (C) a left ventricular thrombus
    (D) a left atrial thrombus

75. Which of the following is most likely to *not* be demonstrated on the Doppler signal obtained from the apex in a patient with mitral stenosis?

    (A) an increased diastolic peak velocity
    (B) spectral broadening
    (C) a decreased E–F slope
    (D) a peak gradient occurring in late diastole

76. Torn chordae tendineae will cause which of the following?

    (A) aortic insufficiency
    (B) myocardial infarction
    (C) mitral insufficiency
    (D) mitral stenosis

77. Which of the following cannot produce false-positive signs of mitral valve prolapse on an M-mode?

    (A) pericardial effusion
    (B) premature ventricular contractions
    (C) improper placement of the transducer
    (D) hypertrophic obstructive cardiomyopathy

78. Which of the following is a secondary echocardiographic finding in mitral regurgitation?

    (A) a dilated left atrium
    (B) left ventricular hypertrophy
    (C) a hypokinetic left ventricle
    (D) a dilated aortic root

79. The degree of mitral regurgitation is best estimated by measuring which of the following?

    (A) width and length of the systolic jet by color Doppler
    (B) peak velocity of the continuous-wave Doppler systolic mitral signal
    (C) pressure half-time of the continuous-wave Doppler diastolic signal
    (D) integral of the continuous-wave systolic curve

80. Which of the following is least likely to occur as a sequela of rheumatic fever?

    (A) mitral stenosis
    (B) mitral insufficiency
    (C) aortic stenosis
    (D) pulmonic stenosis

81. The two-dimensional echocardiogram of a patient with combined mitral and aortic stenosis is most likely to demonstrate which of the following?

    (A) a dilated left atrium and left ventricular hypertrophy
    (B) a dilated left atrium and a dilated left ventricle
    (C) a small left atrium and a small left ventricle
    (D) systolic anterior motion of the mitral valve and left ventricular hypertrophy

82. **Why is the M-mode of the mitral valve in mitral stenosis often missing an A wave?**

    (A) high initial diastolic pressures in the left ventricle

    (B) concurrent atrial fibrillation

    (C) decreased compliance of the left ventricle

    (D) a dilated left atrium

83. **A Doppler tracing that demonstrates a late diastolic mitral inflow velocity (A point) that is higher than the initial diastolic velocity (E point) can be seen with which of the following pathologies?**

    (A) aortic insufficiency

    (B) hypertrophic cardiomyopathy

    (C) mitral regurgitation

    (D) a ventricular septal defect

84. **If the two-dimensional examination demonstrates a markedly dilated and hyperkinetic left ventricle and a left atrium of normal size, one should suspect the presence of which of the following?**

    (A) mitral regurgitation

    (B) aortic regurgitation

    (C) a ventricular septal defect

    (D) aortic stenosis

85. **Which group of echocardiographic findings would give a definitive diagnosis of mitral stenosis?**

    (A) a decreased E–F slope, a dilated left atrium, and a small left ventricle

    (B) a thickened mitral valve, a dilated left atrium, and a small left ventricle

    (C) a decreased E–F slope, a thickened mitral valve, and diastolic doming of the mitral valve

    (D) a thickened mitral valve and a mitral diastolic velocity >1.5 m/s

86. **A patient with mitral stenosis will usually not have which of the following?**

    (A) a diastolic rumble on auscultation

    (B) an increased E–F slope on M-mode

    (C) a history of rheumatic fever

    (D) a dilated left atrium

87. **To obtain the true circumference of the mitral valve, one should obtain a short-axis view at the level of which of the following?**

    (A) papillary muscle

    (B) chordae tendineae

    (C) tips of the mitral leaflets

    (D) mitral annulus

88. **Which of the following is not a secondary echocardiographic finding of mitral stenosis?**

    (A) a dilated left atrium

    (B) a dilated right atrium

    (C) a dilated left ventricle

    (D) a left atrial thrombus

89. **Which of the following is a successful mitral valve commissurotomy *least* likely to demonstrate?**

    (A) doming of the mitral valve

    (B) mitral valve thickening

    (C) an increase in pressure half-time

    (D) a dilated left atrium

90. **Which of the following can be suggested by left ventricular dilatation in a patient with mitral stenosis?**

    (A) severe mitral stenosis

    (B) concomitant mitral regurgitation

    (C) aortic stenosis

    (D) hypertrophic cardiomyopathy

91. **Early diastolic closure of the mitral valve is usually a sign of which of the following?**

    (A) severe acute aortic regurgitation

    (B) a left bundle branch block

    (C) poor function of the left ventricle

    (D) first-degree A–V block

92. **Which one of the following conditions cannot accelerate degenerative calcification of the mitral annulus?**

    (A) systemic hypertension

    (B) aortic stenosis

    (C) hypertrophic obstructive cardiomyopathy

    (D) a ventricular septal defect

93. **A mitral valve pressure half-time of 220 ms is consistent with which of the following mitral valve areas?**

    (A) 0.6 cm^2

    (B) 1 cm^2

    (C) 2.2 cm^2

    (D) 5 cm^2

94. Echocardiographic findings of significant aortic stenosis do *not* include which of the following?

    (A) reduced separation of the aortic valve cusp

    (B) diastolic fluttering of the anterior mitral leaflet

    (C) Doppler systolic velocities greater than 4 m/s

    (D) thickened left ventricular walls

95. Which of the following causes the left ventricular walls to appear thick on an echocardiogram?

    (A) mitral stenosis

    (B) aortic insufficiency

    (C) mitral regurgitation

    (D) systemic hypertension

96. The presence of a systolic ejection murmur should alert one to look for which of the following?

    (A) a ventricular septal defect

    (B) mitral regurgitation

    (C) aortic stenosis

    (D) patent ductus arteriosus

97. Which of the following statements regarding a bicuspid aortic valve is false?

    (A) The problem is a congenital one.

    (B) It may be associated with aortic stenosis.

    (C) It is often seen in conjunction with mitral stenosis.

    (D) It may be associated with coarctation of the aorta.

98. The continuity equation is used to calculate the _____. It is most helpful in patients with _____.

    (A) mitral valve area; mitral stenosis

    (B) aortic valve area; poor left ventricular function

    (C) aortic valve velocity; systemic hypertension

    (D) degree of shunting; a ventricular septal defect

99. In patients with combined aortic stenosis and aortic insufficiency, which of the following parameters is *best* for assessing the severity of aortic stenosis?

    (A) the maximum pressure gradient

    (B) the mean pressure gradient

    (C) the high pulse-repetition frequency

    (D) the analog waveform

100. Which of the following two-dimensional views will best illustrate a color Doppler jet of aortic insufficiency?

    (A) the apical long-axis view

    (B) the suprasternal view

    (C) the subcostal fine-chamber view

    (D) the short-axis view of the base

101. Which of the following is a secondary echocardiographic sign of aortic stenosis?

    (A) a thickened aortic valve

    (B) left ventricular hypertrophy

    (C) a hyperdynamic left ventricle

    (D) a dilated left ventricle

102. Which of the following is consistent with an M-mode finding of fine diastolic fluttering of the anterior mitral leaflet?

    (A) aortic insufficiency

    (B) mitral stenosis

    (C) atrial fibrillation

    (D) a prolonged heart rate

103. Diastolic velocity signals were detected in a patient's left ventricular outflow tract using pulsed Doppler. They could be detected between the tip of the anterior mitral leaflet and the aortic valve from the parasternal position. Which of the following can be said about this finding?

    (A) normal

    (B) consistent with severe mitral regurgitation

    (C) consistent with severe aortic regurgitation

    (D) consistent with moderate aortic regurgitation

    (E) consistent with moderate mitral regurgitation

104. The referring physician hears an Austin–Flint murmur. What is the M-mode echocardiogram of this patient most likely to demonstrate?

    (A) a thickened mitral valve with a decreased E–F slope

    (B) fine diastolic fluttering and possible flattening of the anterior mitral leaflet

    (C) a thickened aortic valve with a decreased opening

    (D) systolic posterior motion of the tricuspid valve

105. Which of the following is the best approach for obtaining the maximum aortic velocity in patients with aortic stenosis?

    (A) left sternal border

    (B) left supraclavicular region

    (C) subcostal region

    (D) right sternal border view

106. The best way to rule out an aortic dissection is with which of the following?

    (A) M-mode echocardiography

    (B) transthoracic two-dimensional imaging

    (C) color Doppler

    (D) transesophageal echocardiography

107. Which echocardiographic finding is *not* associated with tricuspid insufficiency?

    (A) a dilated right atrium

    (B) tricuspid prolapse

    (C) a dilated right ventricle

    (D) a thickened anterior right ventricle wall

108. A tricuspid regurgitant velocity of 4 m/s indicates the presence of which of the following?

    (A) tricuspid stenosis

    (B) severe tricuspid regurgitation

    (C) a flail tricuspid leaflet

    (D) pulmonary hypertension

109. Which of the following regarding tricuspid stenosis is *not* true?

    (A) It occurs as a sequela to rheumatic fever.

    (B) Doppler echocardiography demonstrates a decreased pressure half-time.

    (C) Two-dimensional echocardiography shows diastolic doming, and M-mode reveals a decreased E–F slope.

    (D) It is usually seen as part of the aging process.

110. A peripheral contrast injection into the arm of a patient with severe tricuspid regurgitation is likely to demonstrate which of the following?

    (A) contrast in the pulmonary veins during diastole

    (B) right-to-left shunting

    (C) contrast in the inferior vena cava during ventricular systole

    (D) left-to-right shunting

111. If the physician suspects carcinoid heart disease, the echocardiographer should pay special attention to which of the following?

    (A) mitral valve

    (B) tricuspid valve

    (C) inferior vena cava

    (D) interatrial septum

112. Which of the following can be calculated using the velocity of a tricuspid regurgitant jet?

    (A) the severity of tricuspid regurgitation

    (B) right ventricular systolic pressure

    (C) the severity of pulmonic regurgitation

    (D) left atrial pressure

113. Coarse systolic fluttering of the pulmonic valve with an extremely high systolic velocity in the right ventricular outflow tract is most likely to be found in a patient with which of the following?

    (A) pulmonic regurgitation

    (B) paradoxical interventricular septal motion

    (C) infundibular pulmonic stenosis

    (D) pulmonary hypertension

114. Which of the following is the most common window used to record peak pulmonic systolic velocity?

    (A) suprasternal

    (B) apical

    (C) right parasternal

    (D) left parasternal

115. The pulmonic valve is located where in relation to the aortic valve?

    (A) cranial and lateral

    (B) caudal and lateral

    (C) cranial and medial

    (D) caudal and medial

116. Which one of the following echocardiographic findings is *not* associated with pulmonic stenosis?

    (A) right ventricular hypertrophy

    (B) M-mode demonstration of a steep pulmonic A wave

    (C) midsystolic notching noted on M-mode

    (D) systolic pulmonic Doppler velocities >3 m/s

117. Valvular vegetations are best detected with which of the following?

    (A) M-mode echocardiography

    (B) two-dimensional echocardiography

    (C) Doppler echocardiography

    (D) contrast injection

118. A 30-year-old intravenous drug abuser presents with an embolus to the right leg. The presence of which of the following is the most likely cause of the embolic event?

    (A) a left atrial myxoma

    (B) mitral valve vegetation

    (C) a right ventricular thrombus

    (D) a myocardial abscess

119. Color Doppler assessment of prosthetic heart valves is especially helpful when checking for which of the following?

    (A) presence of valve stenosis

    (B) presence of paravalvular regurgitation

    (C) presence of a clot

    (D) valve area

120. Which of the following describes a normally functioning Starr–Edwards valve?

    (A) may exhibit high Doppler velocities

    (B) will echocardiographically resemble a bioprosthetic valve

    (C) has a major and a minor orifice

    (D) may exhibit mild to moderate regurgitation

121. Which of the following describes a Bjork–Shiley?

    (A) an example of a mechanical heart valve

    (B) an example of a bioprosthetic heart valve

    (C) not noticeable on the two-dimensional image

    (D) a surgical procedure used to correct for transposition of the great vessels

122. Which of the following echocardiographic examinations is best used for evaluating the function of a prosthetic valve?

    (A) M-mode echocardiography

    (B) high-pulse repetition-frequency Doppler echocardiography

    (C) transesophageal echocardiography

    (D) contrast echocardiography

123. Which one of the following is *not* an example of a mechanical prosthetic valve?

    (A) St. Jude

    (B) Bjork–Shiley

    (C) Starr–Edwards

    (D) Hancock

124. To check for prosthetic valve dehiscence, what should the echocardiographer look for?

    (A) decreased valve excursion

    (B) an abnormal mass of echoes on the valve

    (C) abnormal rocking motion of the valve

    (D) Doppler evidence of stenosis

125. A 26-year-old woman with significant mitral insufficiency is about to receive a mitral valve replacement. Why are the surgeons most likely to use a porcine valve?

    (A) It tends to last longer.

    (B) It preserves myocardium better.

    (C) It often makes anticoagulation unnecessary.

    (D) It obstructs flow less.

126. Why are prophylactic antibiotics often recommended for individuals with mitral valve prolapse who are undergoing dental or surgical procedures?

    (A) These patients are at a higher risk for endocarditis.

    (B) To prevent possible mitral regurgitation.

    (C) To prevent pneumonia.

    (D) Incisions on patients with mitral valve prolapse usually take longer to heal.

127. One can be reasonably certain that a large amount of pericardial effusion is present by noting which of the following?

    (A) echocardiographic signs of cardiac tamponade

    (B) a crescent-shaped pattern on the short-axis view

    (C) a "swinging heart" on the two-dimensional examination

    (D) a posterior echo-free space

128. Which of the following is true concerning constrictive pericarditis?

    (A) It impairs diastolic filling.

    (B) It is sometimes referred to as "Dressler's syndrome."

    (C) It is detected by noting increased echogenicity of the pericardium.

    (D) It is usually associated with a large pericardial effusion.

129. When is cardiac tamponade most likely to occur?

    (A) Pressure in the pericardial cavity rises to equal or exceed the diastolic pressure in the heart.

    (B) There is a small pericardial effusion.

    (C) There is a large chronic pericardial effusion.

    (D) The pericardium becomes a sheath of fibrous tissue that interferes with diastolic filling.

130. Which one of the following statements about pericardial effusion is false?

    (A) Pericardial effusion may be confused with epicardial fat.

    (B) An effusion may accumulate anteriorly without accumulating posteriorly.

    (C) A pericardial effusion can consist of blood or clear fluid.

    (D) In Dressler's syndrome, a pericardial effusion develops as a result of renal disease.

131. A 38-year-old woman with a history of breast cancer is referred for an echocardiogram because she is experiencing shortness of breath. Which of the following is the echocardiogram most likely to reveal?

    (A) metastasis to the left atrium

    (B) metastasis to the right atrium

    (C) a left atrial myxoma

    (D) a pericardial effusion

132. Which one of the following cannot lead to a false-positive diagnosis of pericardial effusion on M-mode?

    (A) the descending aorta

    (B) a calcified mitral annulus

    (C) ascites

    (D) mitral valve prolapse

133. A false-negative sign of tamponade may occur in patients with which of the following?

    (A) pulmonic stenosis

    (B) a pleural effusion

    (C) mitral regurgitation

    (D) loculated effusions

134. Why does the pericardium appear as an extremely bright linear structure on the echocardiogram?

    (A) It is a thick structure.

    (B) It is a fibrous band.

    (C) There is a large acoustic mismatch between lung tissue and pericardial tissue.

    (D) It contains calcium.

135. Which two echocardiographic techniques are useful when evaluating for the presence of pericardial effusion?

    (A) increasing reject and decreasing frame-rate

    (B) decreasing time-gain control and increasing overall gain

    (C) decreasing overall gain and increasing depth setting

    (D) increasing reject and decreasing depth setting

136. Which structure often aids in differentiating a pericardial effusion from a pleural effusion on two-dimensional examination?

    (A) liver

    (B) inferior vena cava

    (C) pleural sac

    (D) descending aorta

137. Flat mid-diastolic motion of the posterior wall on an M-mode echocardiogram suggests which of the following?

    (A) constrictive pericarditis

    (B) left ventricular volume overload

    (C) myocardial infarction

    (D) dilated cardiomyopathy

138. What is the most striking echocardiographic feature of patients with an absent pericardium?

    (A) excessive cardiac motion

    (B) absence of bright linear pericardial echoes

    (C) hypokinesis of the heart

    (D) dyskinetic motion of the heart

139. What is the effect of systemic hypertension on the heart?

    (A) thickening of the right ventricular free wall

    (B) decreased systolic function of the left ventricle

    (C) reduced compliance of the left ventricle

    (D) right ventricular dilatation

140. Which of the following is not an echocardiographic sign of outflow tract obstruction in hypertrophic cardiomyopathy?

    (A) midsystolic notching of the aortic valve

    (B) left ventricular hypertrophy

    (C) systolic anterior motion of the mitral valve

    (D) high systolic velocity in the left ventricular outflow tract

141. A definitive diagnosis of amyloid heart disease is best made with which of the following?

    (A) M-mode echocardiography

    (B) transthoracic echocardiography

    (C) transesophageal echocardiography

    (D) endomyocardial biopsy

142. Which of the following cannot cause dilated (congestive) cardiomyopathy?

    (A) coronary artery disease

    (B) sarcoidosis

    (C) viral myocarditis

    (D) long-term alcohol abuse

143. Which of the following is *not* an echocardiographic finding seen in dilated cardiomyopathy?

    (A) increased systolic velocity in the left ventricular outflow tract

    (B) dilated chambers

    (C) global hypokinesis

    (D) an increased E point-to-septal separation

144. Which of the following is true concerning cardiac contusion?

    (A) It is more likely to affect the right ventricle than the left ventricle.

    (B) It is the same as a myocardial infarction.

    (C) It occurs when there is underlying coronary artery disease.

    (D) It leads to hypercontractility of the left ventricle.

145. A 64-year-old man presents with an acute myocardial infarction of the anterior wall and an embolus to the right leg. Before beginning the examination, the echocardiographer should suspect the possibility of which one of the following (choose the most likely diagnosis)?

    (A) an apical aneurysm with a mural thrombus

    (B) mitral stenosis and a left atrial clot

    (C) a right ventricular infarct with a clot

    (D) vegetation on the mitral or aortic valve

146. Which one of the following echocardiographic findings is not consistent with diastolic dysfunction of the left ventricle?

    (A) M-mode demonstration of a mitral valve B notch

    (B) M-mode demonstration of a high mitral A wave

    (C) two-dimensional demonstration of an ejection fraction lower than 50%

    (D) Doppler demonstration of a mitral valve E-to-A ratio >1.0

147. Akinesis of the anterior left ventricular wall is most likely to indicate obstruction of which of the following arteries?

    (A) right coronary artery

    (B) left circumflex artery

    (C) left anterior descending artery

    (D) posterior descending artery

148. Which of the following is true concerning pseudoaneurysms?

    (A) They are usually hyperkinetic.

    (B) They have a low risk of rupture.

    (C) They have walls comprised of endocardium, myocardium, epicardium, and pericardium.

    (D) They have a narrow neck.

149. An increased E point-to-septal separation is usually a good indicator of which of the following?

    (A) high end-diastolic pressures in the left ventricle

    (B) a reduced ejection fraction

    (C) high initial diastolic pressures

    (D) poor compliance of the left ventricle

150. Which of the following best describes a segment of the left ventricle that lacks systolic wall thickening and motion?

    (A) hypokinetic

    (B) akinetic

    (C) dyskinetic

    (D) aneurysmal

151. Aneurysms in the inferior wall of the left ventricle may be associated with all of the following *except*

    (A) an increased E point-to-septal separation

    (B) thrombus formation

    (C) mitral regurgitation

    (D) occlusion of the left anterior descending coronary artery

152. The echocardiogram of a patient with a ruptured papillary muscle will exhibit which of the following?

    (A) mitral valve prolapse

    (B) severe mitral regurgitation

    (C) some degree of aortic insufficiency

    (D) dyskinesis of the posterior left ventricular wall

153. Which of the following describes stress echocardiography?

    (A) It is used instead of standard stress testing.

    (B) It is used in the study of acoustic properties of the myocardium.

    (C) It allows for visualization of myocardial perfusion.

    (D) It is used in diagnosing ischemic heart disease.

154. Which of the following statements regarding left atrial myxomas is *not* true?

(A) They usually attach to the interatrial septum.

(B) They may be pedunculated.

(C) They do not recur once they are surgically removed.

(D) Clinically, they can mimic mitral stenosis.

155. The QP/QS ratio is used to evaluate the severity of which of the following?

(A) pulmonic stenosis

(B) ventricular septal defects

(C) aortic stenosis

(D) systemic hypertension

156. Which of the following would best describe the pulsed Doppler pattern of a patent ductus arteriosus if the sample volume were placed in the pulmonary artery from a short-axis view of the base of the heart?

(A) systolic flow below baseline

(B) continuous flow (systolic and diastolic) above baseline

(C) diastolic flow above baseline

(D) a biphasic systolic flow pattern below baseline

157. Which of the following is the best way to detect a small atrial septal defect?

(A) two-dimensional echocardiography

(B) contrast injection echocardiography

(C) M-mode echocardiography

(D) pulsed-wave Doppler echocardiography

158. What is the most common type of atrial septal defect?

(A) primum

(B) secundum

(C) fenestrated

(D) sinus venosus

159. Which of the following is consistent with a ventricular septal defect with right-to-left shunting?

(A) Ebstein's anomaly

(B) tetralogy of Fallot

(C) Eisenmenger's syndrome

(D) a double-outlet right ventricle

160. Which of the following is not associated with Ebstein's anomaly?

(A) an abnormally large tricuspid valve

(B) infundibular pulmonic stenosis

(C) "atrialization" of the right ventricle

(D) an atrial septal defect

161. The echocardiogram of a patient with an endocardial cushion defect might exhibit which of the following?

(A) a muscular ventricular septal defect and tricuspid valve vegetation

(B) a hypokinetic left ventricle and mitral valve vegetation

(C) overriding of the aorta and subpulmonic stenosis

(D) ostium primum atrial septal defect and an inlet ventricular septal defect

162. An echocardiographic diagnosis of coarctation of the aorta can be made by detecting a high-velocity Doppler jet in which of the following?

(A) left branch of the pulmonary artery

(B) aortic arch, proximal to the subclavian artery

(C) descending thoracic aorta

(D) abdominal aorta

163. Which of the following is *not* one of the four principal components of tetralogy of Fallot?

(A) a ventricular septal defect

(B) an override of the aorta

(C) an obstruction of pulmonary blood flow

(D) an atrial septal defect

164. Which of the following describes cor triatriatum?

(A) It is a fairly common congenital abnormality.

(B) It is a congenital malformation in which a fibrous membrane divides the left atrium into an upper and lower chamber.

(C) It results in mitral stenosis.

(D) It is a condition in which the pulmonary veins drain into the right atrium.

165. Which of the following echocardiographic findings is most commonly associated with left bundle branch block?

(A) left ventricular hypertrophy

(B) a hypercontractile interventricular septum

(C) paradoxical septal motion

(D) a dilated left ventricle

166. The echocardiographic pattern of the mitral valve in Fig. 2–14 is consistent with which of the following?

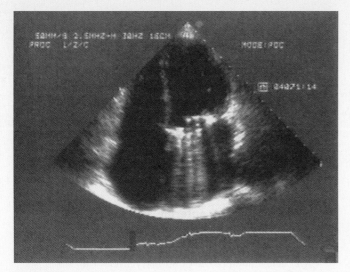

FIGURE 2–14. Apical four-chamber view.

(A) mitral stenosis

(B) mitral valve vegetation

(C) a mechanical prosthetic valve

(D) a calcified mitral valve annulus

167. The M-mode pattern in Fig. 2–15 suggests which of the following about the ejection fraction of the left ventricle?

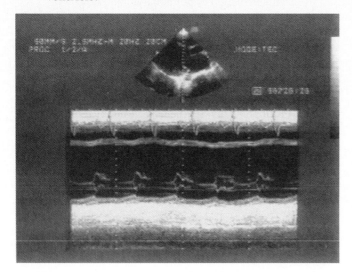

FIGURE 2–15. M-mode echocardiogram at the level of the mitral valve.

(A) normal

(B) mildly increased

(C) significantly increased

(D) significantly decreased

168. What other hemodynamic information could be derived from the M-mode (Fig. 2–15)?

(A) cardiac output is increased

(B) left ventricular end-diastolic pressure is increased

(C) the systolic ejection period is prolonged

(D) atrial flutter is present

169. The Doppler tracing in Fig. 2–16 demonstrates which of the following?

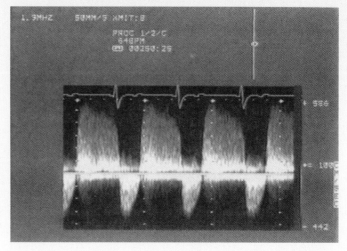

FIGURE 2–16. Continuous-wave Doppler tracing obtained from the apical position.

(A) aortic stenosis and aortic insufficiency

(B) mitral stenosis and mitral regurgitation

(C) tricuspid stenosis and tricuspid regurgitation

(D) mitral stenosis and aortic stenosis

170. The echocardiographic findings in Fig. 2–17 indicate that the patient probably has a history of which of the following?

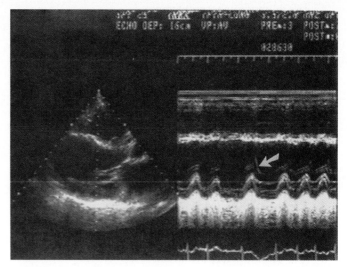

FIGURE 2–17. Split-screen display of a two-dimensional long-axis (left) and a correlating M-mode pattern (right). Note M-mode scan plane indicated by cursor (arrow).

(A) hypertension

(B) diabetes mellitus

(C) rheumatic fever

(D) coronary artery disease

171. **What is the arrow in Fig. 2–17 pointing to?**

   (A) a side-lobe artifact
   (B) papillary muscle
   (C) chordae tendineae
   (D) the anterior mitral leaflet

172. **Fig. 2–18 demonstrates echoes within the left ventricular cavity. These echoes are which of the following?**

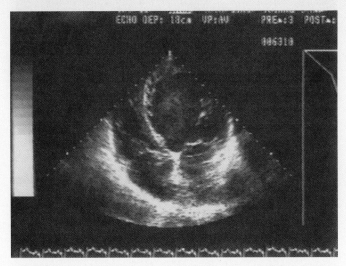

FIGURE 2–18. Apical four-chamber view showing a dilated left ventricle.

   (A) artifactual
   (B) caused by a mural thrombus
   (C) caused by stagnant blood
   (D) caused by a high near-gain setting

Questions 173 through 179: Match the numbered structures in Fig. 2–19 with the correct term given in Column B.

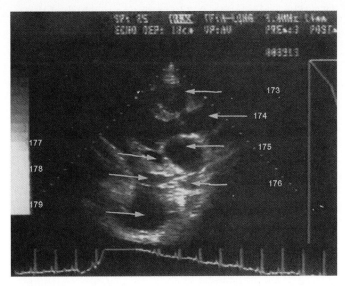

FIGURE 2–19. Parasternal long-axis view with an increased depth setting.

COLUMN A	COLUMN B
173. _____	left ventricle
174. _____	coronary sinus
175. _____	left atrium
176. _____	right ventricle
177. _____	pericardial effusion
178. _____	descending aorta
179. _____	pleural effusion
	aortic root
	right atrium

180. **What is demonstrated in Fig. 2–20?**

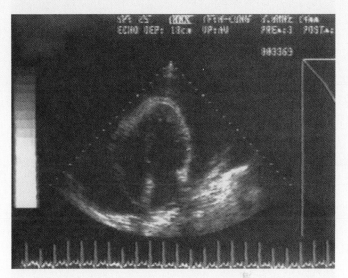

FIGURE 2–20. Apical four-chamber view.

   (A) a large pleural effusion
   (B) pneumomediastinum
   (C) ascites
   (D) a large pericardial effusion

181. **The echocardiographic examination of this patient should include analysis of the motion of which of the following?**

   (A) interventricular septum
   (B) right ventricular wall
   (C) left ventricular wall
   (D) tricuspid valve

182. Color Doppler interrogation of the aortic valve shown in Fig. 2–21 is most likely to demonstrate which of the following?

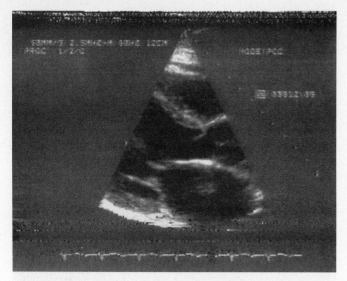

FIGURE 2–21. Narrow sector parasternal long-axis view.

(A) a narrow diastolic jet directed at the anterior mitral leaflet

(B) a diastolic jet filling the left ventricular outflow tract and extending deep into the left ventricle

(C) a normal pattern of blood flow

(D) a narrow systolic jet directed at the anterior mitral leaflet

183. The arrow in Fig. 2–22 is pointing to which of the following?

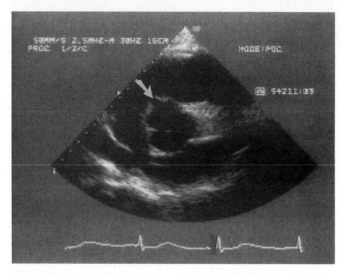

FIGURE 2–22. Short-axis view of the base of the heart.

(A) a fistula between the aorta and right ventricle

(B) the coronary sinus

(C) the left main coronary artery

(D) the origin of the right coronary artery

184. The right ventricular outflow tract is located medial to the arrow in Fig. 2–22.

(A) true

(B) false

185. The contrast study in Fig. 2–23 shows which of the following?

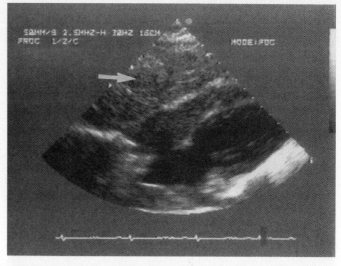

FIGURE 2–23. Subcostal four-chamber view with contrast injection.

(A) left-to-right shunting at the atrial level

(B) no shunting of blood

(C) right-to-left shunting at the atrial level

(D) right-to-left shunting at the ventricular level

186. A secondary finding noted on Fig. 2–23 is a moderate-sized pericardial effusion.

(A) true

(B) false

187. The arrow in Fig. 2–23 is pointing to which of the following?

(A) lung tissue

(B) liver parenchyma

(C) a mediastinal tumor

(D) the spleen

188. The absence of an A wave and midsystolic notching of the pulmonic valve on the M-mode in Fig. 2–24 is consistent with which of the following?

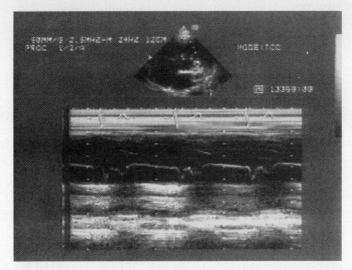

FIGURE 2–24. M-mode of the pulmonic valve.

(A) pulmonic stenosis

(B) tricuspid stenosis

(C) mitral stenosis

(D) pulmonary hypertension

189. What other abnormality should be ruled out in the presence of the abnormality noted on the M-mode of the tricuspid valve in Fig. 2–25?

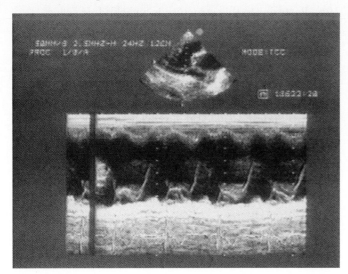

FIGURE 2–25. M-mode of the tricuspid valve.

(A) tricuspid stenosis

(B) pulmonary hypertension

(C) mitral valve prolapse

(D) atrial septal defect

190. An 85-year-old woman with a long history of chest pain is sent for an echocardiogram. The M-mode of the mitral valve is shown in Fig. 2–26. The M-mode of the aortic valve would be likely to demonstrate which of the following?

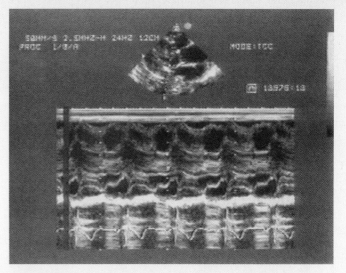

FIGURE 2–26. M-mode echocardiogram at the level of the mitral valve.

(A) diastolic fluttering

(B) delayed opening

(C) midsystolic notching

(D) systolic fluttering

191. An extremely tall, slender young man was referred for an echocardiogram because he has a murmur. Echocardiographic findings in Fig. 2–27 include which of the following?

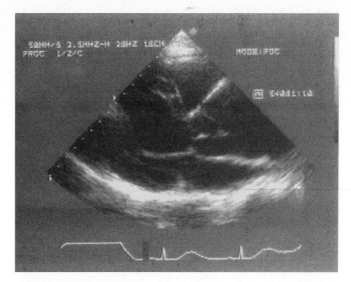

FIGURE 2–27. Parasternal long-axis view.

(A) a bicuspid aortic valve

(B) a cleft mitral valve

(C) a dilated aortic root

(D) left ventricular hypertrophy

192. **Which echocardiographic view would be best for further evaluation of this abnormality?**

    (A) the long-axis suprasternal view

    (B) the short-axis view of the base of the heart

    (C) the apical four-chamber view

    (D) the subcostal four-chamber view

193. **The left ventricle in Fig. 2–28 demonstrates which of the following?**

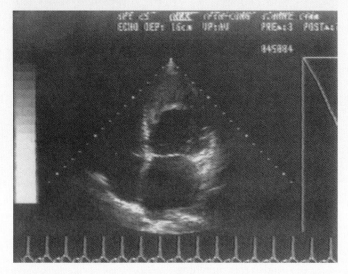

FIGURE 2–28. Apical four-chamber view.

    (A) hypertrophic cardiomyopathy

    (B) an infiltrative tumor

    (C) a large apical thrombus

    (D) a myxoma

194. **Which of the following is true about the mitral valve shown in Fig. 2–29?**

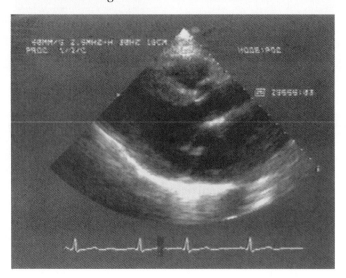

FIGURE 2–29. Parasternal long-axis view.

    (A) it is normal

    (B) it is flail

    (C) it is stenotic

    (D) it is prolapsing

195. **What is the arrow in Fig. 2–30 pointing to?**

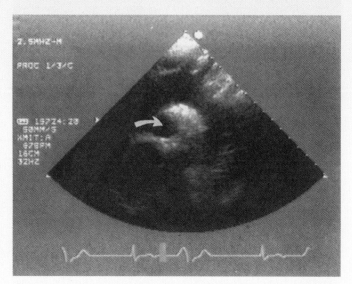

FIGURE 2–30. Suprasternal notch long-axis view of the aorta and transverse arch.

    (A) left subclavian artery

    (B) right pulmonary artery

    (C) superior vena cava

    (D) left pulmonary vein

196. **Posterior to this structure is an echo-free space, which represents which of the following?**

    (A) the left atrium

    (B) a pleural effusion

    (C) pericardial effusion

    (D) the superior vena cava

197. The curved arrow in Fig. 2–31 is directed at which of the following?

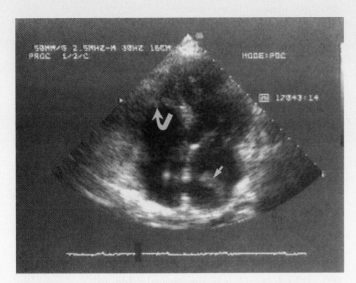

FIGURE 2–31. Apical four-chamber view.

(A) a pacemaker wire

(B) the Chiari network

(C) false chordae tendineae

(D) the moderator band

198. The straight arrow in Fig. 2–31 is pointing to a structure that most likely represents which of the following?

(A) a right atrial myxoma

(B) a left atrial thrombus

(C) the left pulmonary vein

(D) the eustachian valve

199. The echocardiographic findings in the long-axis view presented in Fig. 2–32 include which of the following?

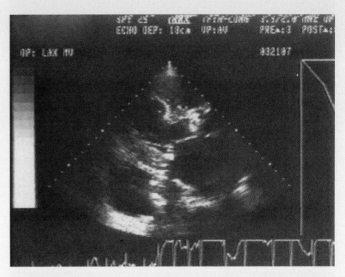

FIGURE 2–32. Parasternal long-axis view with slightly increased depth setting.

(A) a dilated left atrium, mitral stenosis, and a pericardial effusion

(B) aortic stenosis, a calcified mitral annulus, and basal septal hypertrophy

(C) a dilated coronary sinus, left ventricular hypertrophy, and mitral valve vegetation

(D) a dilated aortic root, a dilated left ventricle, and a thickened mitral valve

200. What are these findings most consistent with?

(A) rheumatic heart disease

(B) congenital heart disease

(C) subacute bacterial endocarditis

(D) an aged heart

201. The mitral valve diastolic waveforms in Fig. 2–33C are not uniform. Which of the following causes this?

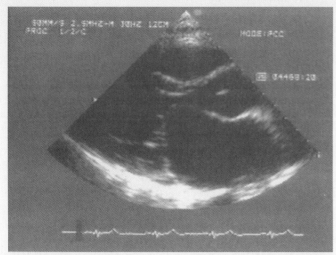

A

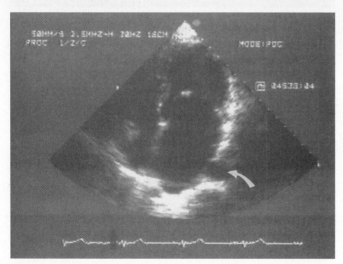

B

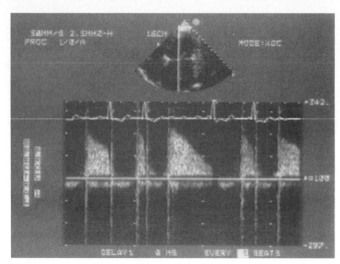

C

FIGURE 2–33. (**A**) Parasternal long-axis view; (**B**) apical four-chamber view; (**C**) continuous-wave Doppler tracing of mitral inflow from the apical position.

(A) high end-diastolic pressure of the left ventricle

(B) faulty technique

(C) inspiration

(D) atrial fibrillation

The following study is of a 58-year-old woman who vaguely remembers a childhood illness that included pain in her joints. She presented with a transischemic attack and atrial fibrillation. For questions 202 through 204, refer to Fig. 2–33A, B, and C.

202. What does the mitral valve demonstrate?

(A) systolic prolapse

(B) diastolic doming

(C) myxomatous degeneration

(D) hyperkinesis

203. Which chamber is significantly dilated?

(A) the left atrium

(B) the left ventricle

(C) the right atrium

(D) the right ventricle

204. What is most likely to be revealed by auscultation of this patient?

(A) a midsystolic click

(B) a systolic ejection murmur

(C) a systolic rumble

(D) an opening snap

205. What is the arrow in Fig. 2–33B pointing to?

(A) coronary sinus

(B) inferior vena cava

(C) descending aorta

(D) left pulmonary vein

206. The pressure half-time derived from the Doppler tracing of the mitral valve in Fig. 2–33C can be used to estimate which of the following?

(A) the mitral valve area

(B) the mitral valve gradient

(C) the severity of aortic insufficiency

(D) the ejection fraction

A 52-year-old woman presents with chronic dyspnea. Chest x-ray reveals cardiomegaly. For questions 207 through 210, refer to Fig. 2–34A and B.

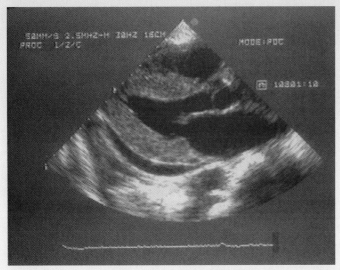

A

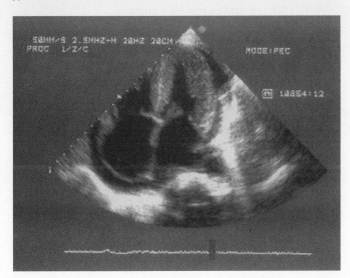

B

FIGURE 2–34. (**A**) Parasternal long-axis view; (**B**) apical four-chamber view.

207. **What is the most striking feature of this echocardiogram?**

   (A) left atrial compression

   (B) mitral valve doming

   (C) left ventricular hypertrophy

   (D) right ventricular dilatation

208. **Which of the following are additional findings on this echocardiogram?**

   (A) a dilated aortic root, mitral valve prolapse, and a dilated coronary sinus

   (B) a thickened mitral valve, a prominent inter-atrial septum, a small left ventricle, and pericardial effusion

   (C) a calcified mitral annulus, an extracardiac mass, and pleural effusion

   (D) left atrial dilatation, systolic anterior motion of the mitral valve, and a thickened aortic valve

209. **Given all the above information, what is the most likely diagnosis?**

   (A) hypertrophic obstructive cardiomyopathy

   (B) Marfan syndrome

   (C) endomyocardial fibrosis

   (D) amyloid cardiomyopathy

210. **The best way to substantiate this diagnosis is by obtaining which of the following?**

   (A) a computed tomographic scan

   (B) an endomyocardial biopsy

   (C) a cardiac catheterization

   (D) an electrocardiogram

A 64-year-old man sustained a myocardial infarction 1 week before this echocardiogram. He developed congestive heart failure and became hypotensive. A new murmur was detected on auscultation. For questions 211 through 215, refer to Fig. 2–35A and B.

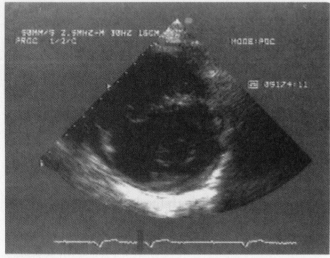

A

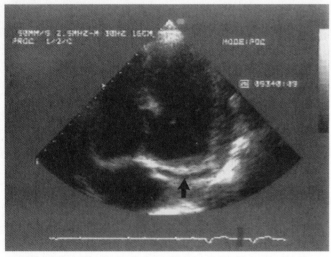

B

FIGURE 2–35. (**A**) Parasternal short-axis view at the level of the papillary muscles; (**B**) modified apical four-chamber view: The transducer is angled posteriorly and the depth setting is decreased.

211. **What does the echocardiogram reveal?**

    (A) dilated cardiomyopathy

    (B) ventricular septal defect

    (C) cleft mitral valve

    (D) pseudoaneurysm

212. **Which of the following would be most helpful in confirming the diagnosis?**

    (A) color-flow Doppler imaging

    (B) M-mode echocardiography

    (C) continuous-wave Doppler imaging

    (D) pulsed-wave Doppler imaging

213. **The arrow in Fig. 2–35B is pointing to a linear structure called which of the following?**

    (A) coronary sinus

    (B) left anterior descending coronary artery

    (C) left pulmonary vein

    (D) left circumflex coronary artery

214. **What does this linear structure contain?**

    (A) serous fluid

    (B) deoxygenated blood

    (C) oxygenated blood

    (D) air

215. **In Fig. 2–35B, in what direction would the transducer need to be directed to visualize the left ventricular outflow tract?**

    (A) anteriorly

    (B) medially

    (C) laterally

    (D) inferiorly

A 34-year-old woman is extremely nervous at the time of the examination. She states that she often experiences chest pain and palpitations. Auscultation reveals a systolic murmur. For questions 216 through 219, refer to Fig. 2–36A and B.

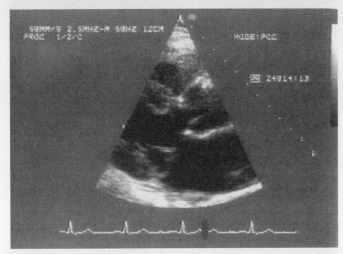

A

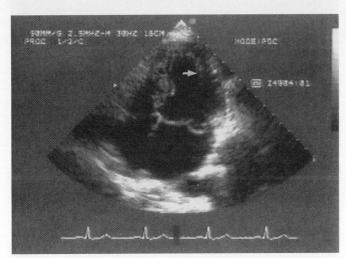

B

FIGURE 2–36. (**A**) Narrow sector parasternal long-axis view; (**B**) apical four-chamber view.

216. What does the mitral valve demonstrate?

(A) diastolic doming

(B) prolapse of the anterior leaflet

(C) prolapse of the posterior leaflet

(D) systolic anterior motion

217. Continuous-wave Doppler evaluation of the mitral valve from the apical position would most likely demonstrate which of the following?

(A) a systolic curve below baseline >3 m/s

(B) a diastolic signal above baseline with a decreased pressure half-time

(C) a systolic curve above baseline <3 m/s

(D) a diastolic curve below baseline >3 m/s

218. The arrow in Fig. 2–36B is pointing to the posterior wall of the left ventricle.

(A) true

(B) false

219. The dropout of echoes in the interatrial septum in Fig. 2–36B is most likely which of the following?

(A) a primum atrial septal defect

(B) a secundum atrial septal defect

(C) artifactual

(D) the result of interatrial septal prolapse

A 23-year-old man was referred for an echocardiogram because a systolic ejection murmur was heard on auscultation. For questions 220 through 223, refer to Fig. 2–37A and B.

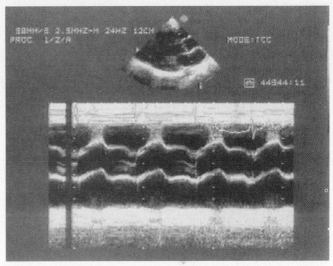

A

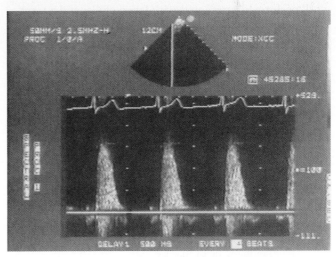

B

FIGURE 2–37. (**A**) M-mode tracing at the aortic valve level; (**B**) Continuous-wave Doppler tracing of aortic flow from the right sternal border (calibration marks are 1 m/s).

220. **What does the M-mode of the aortic valve in Fig. 2–37A demonstrate?**

   (A) slight thickening of the valve with a normal opening

   (B) the absence of aortic valve echoes

   (C) systolic fluttering of the aortic valve

   (D) a thickened aortic valve with a markedly decreased opening

221. **According to the Doppler tracing in Fig. 2–37B, what is the approximate peak aortic gradient using the simplified Bernoulli formula?**

   (A) 4 mm Hg

   (B) 16 mm Hg

   (C) 36 mm Hg

   (D) 100 mm Hg

222. **Which of the following is the most likely diagnosis for this patient?**

   (A) aortic valve vegetation

   (B) congenital aortic stenosis

   (C) moderate aortic insufficiency

   (D) rheumatic heart disease

223. **Two-dimensional examination of the aortic valve is most likely to demonstrate which of the following?**

   (A) systolic doming

   (B) a mass of echoes in the left ventricular outflow tract

   (C) diastolic doming

   (D) four aortic cusps

A 38-year-old woman, who recently had extensive dental work performed, presented with fever, chills, and a trans-ischemic attack. Auscultation revealed a grade 2/6 systolic murmur. For questions 224 through 229, refer to Fig. 2–38A, B, and C.

224. **Which of the following best describes the mitral valve?**

   (A) normal

   (B) doming

   (C) exhibiting shaggy irregular echoes

   (D) flail

225. **What is the most likely diagnosis for this patient?**

   (A) rheumatic heart disease

   (B) subacute bacterial endocarditis

   (C) ruptured papillary muscle

   (D) mitral valve prolapse

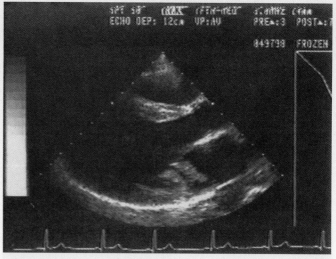

A

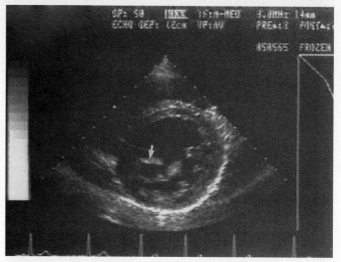

B

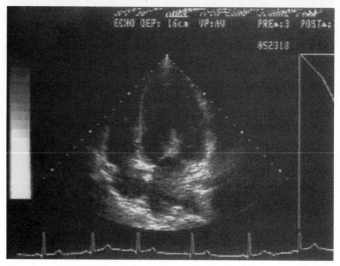

C

FIGURE 2–38. (**A**) Parasternal long-axis view; (**B**) parasternal short-axis view at the papillary muscle level; (**C**) apical four-chamber view.

226. Which of the following best describes the mitral valve excursion?

    (A) reduced
    (B) increased
    (C) normal
    (D) absent

227. Which of the following is most likely to be demonstrated on apical continuous-wave Doppler examination of the mitral valve?

    (A) systolic waveform below baseline
    (B) diastolic waveform below baseline
    (C) diastolic waveform above baseline >3 m/s
    (D) systolic waveform above baseline

228. By referring to all three echocardiographic views presented in this case, one could suggest which of the following about the mass of echoes on the mitral valve?

    (A) it is stationary
    (B) it prolapses into the left atrium
    (C) it prolapses into the left ventricle
    (D) it prolapses into the left atrium and left ventricle

229. What does the arrow in Fig. 2–38B point to?

    (A) a mural thrombus
    (B) the posteromedial papillary muscle
    (C) vegetation
    (D) a cleft mitral valve

Answers and Explanations

At the end of each explained answer, there is a number combination in parentheses. The first number identifies the reference source; the second number or set of numbers indicates the page or pages on which the relevant information can be found.

1. **(D)** The coronary or atrioventricular groove separates the atria from the ventricles. Within this groove lies the main trunk of the coronary arteries and the coronary sinus. *(31:13)*

2. **(F)** *(31:378)*

3. **(D)** *(31:378)*

4. **(B)** *(31:378)*

5. **(E)** *(31:378)*

6. **(H)** *(31:378)*

7. **(C)** *(31:378)*

8. **(I)** *(31:378)*

9. **(A)** *(31:378)*

10. **(G)** *(31:378)*

11. **(D)** Indications for stress echocardiography do not include unstable angina. In fact, this is a contraindication for stress echocardiography. *(31:138)*

12. **(C)** Transesophageal echocardiography (TEE) is performed by a physician with specialized training in TEE performance and interpretation. TEE is routinely used to evaluate cardiac structure and function, although it is considered more invasive than a transthoracic or surface echocardiogram. *(31:209)*

13. **(E)** The purpose of the pericardium is to (1) reduce friction with the cardiac movement, (2) allow the heart to move freely with each beat, facilitating ejection and volume changes, (3) contain the heart within the mediastinum, especially during trauma, and (4) serve as a barrier to infection, whereas the grooves or sulci separate the heart chambers and contain the vessels. *(31:12, 13)*

14. **(D)** Left ventricle. In the adult, the left ventricle is larger and has an outer wall that is 8–12 mm thick. *(31:16)*

15. **(D)** There are four pulmonary veins, two from each lung. They carry oxygenated blood from the lungs to the left atrium of the heart. *(31:14)*

16. **(C)** The right atrium has two parts: an anterior portion and a posterior portion. These two portions are separated by a ridge of muscle called the crista terminalis. *(Study Guide: 106)*

17. **(B)** The mitral valve is an atrioventricular valve that is located between the left atrium and the left ventricle. *(31:14, 15)*

18. **(B)** The normal pressure in the right ventricle is approximately 15–30 mm Hg. *(Study Guide: 106)*

19. **(D)** Mitral valve stenosis results primarily from rheumatic disease. The valves may not become involved for many decades following rheumatic fever. Other rare causes include congenital mitral stenosis, calcification of the mitral annulus that involves the mitral leaflets, thrombus, vegetations, atrial myxomas, and parachute mitral valve deformity. *(31:241)*

20. **(C)** Endocarditis. Endocarditis is caused by bacterial, yeast, or fungal infections that seed and grow on the valves of the heart, papillary muscles, and in some cases, the endocardial surface of the ventricles. Vegetations, commonly associated, form as a result of complex interactions between the immune system, the coagulation system, hemodynamic forces, and the invading microorganisms. *(31:477)*

21. **(D)** Bjork–Shiley is a tilting disc valve that is a mechanical prosthetic valve. The xenograft, heterograft, homograft, and allograft are all bioprosthetic heart valves. *(31:310, 311)*

22. **(D)** The normal intrapericardial space contains 15–50 mL of fluid. In cases of pericardial effusion as the fluid is added rapidly, the intrapericardial pressure increases dramatically. Initially, pericardial effusion is recognized in the posterior basal region, and as it increases, it occurs medially and laterally and involves the apex. *(31:489)*

23. **(C)** The term cardiomyopathy is used to describe a variety of cardiac diseases that affect the myocardium. Cardiomyopathies affect an otherwise structurally normal heart and are classified into three categories: hypertrophic, dilated, and restrictive. *(31:586)*

24. **(A)** Myxoma is the most common benign tumor of the heart. Almost 75% of all primary tumors are benign, with myxomas accounting for almost half of this group. They can occur in all age groups. *(31:463)*

25. **(D)** Angiosarcomas are the most common malignant cardiac tumors of the heart. They usually occur in adults and are more frequent in men. They are soft tissue tumors of the blood vessels and lymphatic endothelium. *(31:467)*

26. **(D)** A dissecting aneurysm results from intimal tears of the aortic wall. The driving force of the blood destroys the media and strips the intimal layer from the adventitial layer. They are classified as a Type I, II, or III, according to the area and extent of the intimal tear. *(31:606, 607)*

27. **(D)** Abnormalities of the left ventricular outflow tact are the most common congenital heart disease in the adult population, with obstruction occurring at the subvalvular, supravalvular, or valvular level. *(Study Guide)*

28. **(D)** In adults tetralogy of Fallot is the primary congenital disease producing cyanosis. It comprises four defects: aorta overriding intraventricular septum IVS, ventricular septal defect (VSD), infundibular stenosis, and right ventricular hypertrophy. *(31:549)*

29. **(B)** Pericarditis is not a characteristic of cardiomyopathy. Cardiomyopathy is a term describing a variety of cardiac diseases affecting the myocardium. They are classified into three categories according to the characteristics. The categories are hypertrophic, dilated, and restrictive. *(31:586–588)*

30. **(A)** *(31:28)*

31. **(F)** *(31:28)*

32. **(G)** *(31:28)*

33. **(B)** *(31:28)*

34. **(D)** *(31:28)*

35. **(E)** *(31:28)*

36. **(C)** *(31:28)*

37. **(C)** Right atrium. In stenotic disease of the tricuspid valve, the effects on atria, ventricles, and vessels cause dilatation of the right atrium. Tricuspid stenosis is most often caused by rheumatic heart disease but can also be caused by such other conditions as: systemic lupus erythematosus, carcinoid heart disease, Löffler's endocarditis, metastatic melanoma, and congenital heart disease. *(31:295, 296)*

38. **(D)** In tricuspid valve disease, the primary cause of regurgitation is secondary to pulmonary hypertension. In rare cases, regurgitation can be caused by rheumatic heart disease. *(31:297)*

39. **(A)** Ebstein's anomaly of the tricuspid valve is a condition where the tricuspid valve leaflets are displaced toward the apex of the right ventricle. *(31:571)*

40. **(B)** Dyspnea on exertion. Clinical symptoms of aortic valve stenosis include chest pain, shortness of breath, and syncope. Most patients do not develop these classic symptoms until the degree of aortic stenosis is moderate to severe. *(31:277)*

41. **(D)** The mitral valve has two major leaflets and is the only cardiac valve with this characteristic; therefore, it is occasionally called the bicuspid valve. *(31:15)*

42. **(D)** The classic clinical finding in mitral valve prolapse is a systolic click, which corresponds with the posterior displacement of the mitral valve leaflet into the left atrium,

and a late systolic murmur, which corresponds with the resulting mitral regurgitation that often occurs because of the prolapsing leaflets. *(31:263)*

43. **(A)** The most common cause of flail leaflet is rupture of the chordae tendineae, which often occurs secondary to myocardial infarction. Rupture of the papillary muscle is a less common etiology. The chordae tendineae support the leaflets and prevent them from prolapsing during systole. *(31:19)*

44. **(D)** Transesophageal echocardiography provides complete evaluation of all regions of the heart, including the great vessels. It provides higher resolution because of the transesophageal window, allowing the use of higher-frequency transducers. *(31:92)*

45. **(C)** The coronary sinus is guarded by the thebesian valve. This valve is often continuous with the eustachian valve. *(31:18)*

46. **(A)** The average length of an adult heart is 12 cm, width 8–9 cm in the broadest diameter, and 6 cm at its narrowest portion. The weight is roughly 280–340 g in men and 230–280 g in women. Cardiac weight is approximately 0.45% of total body weight in men and 0.40% of total body weight in women. *(31:12, 13)*

47. **(D)** The atrioventricular node and its atrial branches are located in a triangular zone lying between the attachment of the septal leaflet of the tricuspid valve, the anteromedial orifice of the coronary sinus, and the tendon of Todaro. It is referred to as the triangle of Koch. *(31:17)*

48. **(B)** Superior vena cava. The blood circulates through the body and returns to the heart to be transported to the lungs for reoxygenation. The inferior vena cava drains the trunk and lower extremities and the superior vena cava drains the head and parts of the upper extremities. *(31:17)*

49. **(C)** Subcostal. Standard parasternal and suprasternal views do not demonstrate all four cardiac chambers. Only the apical and subcostal windows allow visualization of all cardiac chambers. *(1:80)*

50. **(A)** Long axis, short axis, and four chamber. The American Society of Echocardiography has standardized two-dimensional views of the heart into three basic orthogonal planes for which all views can basically be categorized. *(2:212)*

51. **(A)** Atrial septal defects and ventricular septal defect. If the ultrasound beam is not oriented perpendicular to the interatrial and interventricular septum, there may be false dropout of echoes. The subcostal approach allows the ultrasound beam to be perpendicular to the cardiac chambers, thereby allowing a better demonstration of atrial or ventricular septal defects. In addition, any gap noted in the interatrial or interventricular septum when the subcostal four-chamber view is used should be considered real. *(1:92)*

52. **(B)** Time-gain compensation. The time-gain compensation control allows the echocardiographer to selectively increase or decrease the gain at different depths of tissue. The objective is to achieve a uniform echocardiographic image without artifactually adding or eliminating information. *(3:52)*

53. **(A)** The right ventricular pressure drops below the right atrial pressure. The atrioventricular valves open when ventricular pressure drops below atrial pressure. *(3:38)*

54. **(B)** The coronary ligament. This ligament defines the bare area of the liver and is the only choice that does not represent a remnant of fetal circulation. *(4:30)*

55. **(A)** Pulmonary artery. The right side of the heart pumps deoxygenated blood through the pulmonary artery to the lungs for reoxygenation. (The pulmonary artery is the only artery in the body that carries deoxygenated blood.) *(3:9)*

56. **(C)** Left atrium. Four pulmonary veins transport oxygenated blood from the lungs to the left atrium. (The pulmonary veins are the only veins in the body that carry oxygenated blood.) *(3:9)*

57. **(D)** The left ventricle constitutes most of the ventral surface of the heart. The right ventricle, though less muscular than the left ventricle, dominates the ventral surface of the heart. *(3:25)*

58. **(A)** Aortic valve opening and closing points. Left ventricular ejection time—the time it takes for blood to be ejected from the left ventricle—can be obtained from an M-mode tracing of the aortic valve by measuring the time interval between opening and closing of the valve. *(3:156)*

59. **(D)** Subcostal. Lung expansion in patients with chronic obstructive pulmonary disease often obliterates the apical and parasternal position. This lung expansion also tends to shift the heart inferiorly, making the subcostal view the best approach for scanning the heart. *(5:79)*

60. **(B)** Apical and right sternal border. The most common windows used to record systolic blood flow across the aortic valve are the apical, right parasternal, and suprasternal. *(6:128)*

61. **(A)** At end-systole. M-mode measurements of the left atrium, left ventricle, and right ventricle are done at a point when the chambers are at their largest. The left atrium is largest at end-systole. *(3:82)*

62. **(C)** Stenosis. Doming is a main two-dimensional feature of any stenotic valve. The valve domes when it opens because the commissures are fused, causing the body of the valve to separate more widely than the tips. *(1:251)*

63. **(C)** Perpendicular, parallel. Because of the differences in transducer orientation for optimum two-dimensional and Doppler studies, one rarely obtains excellent quality images and waveforms simultaneously and may have to relinquish quality in one to obtain excellent-quality images in the others. *(1:104)*

64. **(D)** Pulmonary hypertension. The constant pressure overload of pulmonary hypertension causes right ventricular hypertrophy until the ventricle fails, at which point the right ventricle wall dilates. *(3:217)*

65. **(C)** Chordae tendineae. Left ventricular dimensions have been standardized to be obtained at the level of the chordae tendineae. *(7:1072)*

66. **(C)** Left ventricular volume overload. Right ventricular volume overload may cause paradoxical interventricular septal motion (anterior motion of the interventricular septum at the onset of systole). *(1:164)*

67. **(A)** Toward the right ventricular free wall. Right ventricular volume overload causes paradoxical septal motion, whereby the septum moves toward the right side of the heart in systole rather than toward the left side of the heart. *(1:164)*

68. **(A)** Organic in origin. A thrill is a murmur that produces a vibratory sensation when palpated. It is almost always organic in origin. *(8:51)*

69. **(A)** Mitral valve prolapse or systolic anterior motion of the mitral valve. The Valsalva maneuver and the inhalation of amyl nitrite decrease left ventricular volume and reduce the diameter of the left ventricular outflow tract, thereby stimulating mitral valve prolapse or systolic anterior motion of the mitral valve. *(3:222)*

70. **(A)** Cyanotic heart disease. Clubbing occurs when there is widening and cyanosis of the distal ends of the fingers and toes. *(9:18)*

71. **(B)** Providing enhanced temporal resolution. M-mode is still used in many laboratories to take measurements and to evaluate events that occur too rapidly for the eye to perceive such as diastolic fluttering of the anterior mitral leaflet. This is the case because M-mode provides far better temporal (time) resolution than does two-dimensional echocardiography and allows for better analysis of intracardiac events. *(3:78)*

72. **(C)** To a higher intercostal space. If the transducer is placed too low relative to the position of the heart, the sector plane passes obliquely through the left ventricle, producing an ovoid image. *(3:110)*

73. **(C)** Decreased left ventricular compliance. This situation, referred to as reversed E-to-A ratio, indicates decreased left ventricular diastolic compliance. Conditions that cause this include left systemic hypertension, hypertrophic cardiomyopathy, and coronary artery disease. *(3:240)*

74. **(C)** A left ventricular thrombus. Left ventricular function is not impaired in mitral stenosis. Because thrombi tend to form in areas of poor blood flow, the likelihood of finding a left ventricular thrombus is low. *(1:489)*

75. **(D)** A peak gradient occurring in late diastole. The peak gradient in mitral stenosis usually occurs in early diastole. *(10:132)*

76. **(C)** Mitral insufficiency. Ruptured chordae tendineae always result in mitral regurgitation, the onset of which is often abrupt and acute. *(3:189)*

77. **(D)** Hypertrophic obstructive cardiomyopathy. This causes anterior motion of the mitral valve. It is not a source of confusion for mitral valve prolapse, in which the mitral valve moves posteriorly in systole. *(11:211)*

78. **(A)** A dilated left atrium. This is a secondary sign of mitral regurgitation. The left ventricle usually dilates as well and becomes hyperkinetic in response to the volume overload. *(1:266)*

79. **(A)** Width and length of the systolic jet by color Doppler. Color Doppler provides a spatial display of regurgitant flow. Quantification of the severity of mitral regurgitation is based roughly on the size and configuration of the regurgitant jet. *(12:87)*

80. **(D)** Pulmonic stenosis. The pulmonic valve is the valve that is least likely to be deformed by rheumatic fever. When pulmonic stenosis is noted on an echocardiogram, it is usually a congenital abnormality rather than a sequela of rheumatic fever. *(9:1711)*

81. **(A)** A dilated left atrium and left ventricular hypertrophy. Mitral stenosis causes the left atrium to dilate, and aortic stenosis leads to left ventricular hypertrophy. *(3:186, 206)*

82. **(B)** Concurrent atrial fibrillation. Mitral stenosis often leads to atrial fibrillation. The A wave of the mitral valve corresponds to the P wave on the electrocardiogram. Because the P wave is absent in atrial fibrillation, the A wave will be absent as well. *(11:333)*

83. **(B)** Hypertrophic cardiomyopathy. Under normal circumstances, the mitral E point, which represents rapid ventricular filling, is higher than the mitral A point, which corresponds to atrial contraction. This relationship between the two points is altered when there is decreased left ventricular compliance (as is the case with hypertrophic cardiomyopathy). *(6:155)*

84. **(B)** Aortic regurgitation. Aortic regurgitation causes a left ventricular volume overload pattern on the echocardiogram (a dilated and hypercontractile left ventricle). Mitral regurgitation usually causes dilatation of both the left atrium and the left ventricle. *(5:231)*

85. **(C)** A decreased E–F slope, a thickened mitral valve, and a mitral distal velocity >1.5 m/s. Both thickening of the mitral valve and a reduced E–F slope must be noted to be sure the pathology is mitral stenosis. Diastolic doming of the mitral valve also is a specific sign of mitral stenosis. *(1:251)*

86. **(B)** An increased E–F slope on M-mode. One M-mode criterion for mitral stenosis is a decreased E–F slope. *(1:249)*

87. **(C)** Tips of the mitral leaflets. The mitral valve is funnel shaped, with the true orifice at the narrow end. Measurement of the size of the orifice should therefore be done at the tips of the leaflets at the point where the chordae tendineae merge with the body of the valve. *(3:161)*

88. **(C)** A dilated left ventricle. Unless there is concomitant mitral regurgitation, the size of the left ventricle will be normal or smaller than normal. *(13:64)*

89. **(C)** An increase in pressure half-time. A successful mitral valve commissurotomy should lead to a decrease in the pressure half-time. The other findings will usually remain, although the left atrium may decrease slightly in size. *(13:65)*

90. **(B)** Concomitant mitral regurgitation. Pure mitral stenosis leads to a dilated left atrium and a normal or smaller-than-normal left ventricle. Aortic stenosis and hypertrophic cardiomyopathy cause the left ventricular walls to appear thickened. Only concomitant mitral regurgitation will cause left ventricular dilatation as well. *(1:139)*

91. **(A)** Severe acute aortic regurgitation. Severe acute aortic insufficiency can cause an elevated left ventricular diastolic pressure, which, in turn, causes the mitral valve to close early. *(1:295)*

92. **(D)** A ventricular septal defect. Such conditions as systemic hypertension that stress the area of the mitral annulus can lead to premature calcification of the mitral annulus. *(9:1035)*

93. **(B)** 1 cm^2. Studies by Hatle and coworkers found that a mitral valve with an area of 1 cm^2 exhibits a Doppler pressure half-time of 220 m/s. *(14:1096)*

94. **(B)** Diastolic fluttering of the anterior mitral leaflet. This is a finding of aortic insufficiency. *(3:210)*

95. **(D)** Systemic hypertension. This produces pressure overload of the left ventricle that, in turn, leads to left ventricular hypertrophy. Choices B and C cause a left ventricular volume overload pattern on the echocardiogram (dilated and hyperkinetic left ventricle). *(15:104)*

96. **(C)** Aortic stenosis. A systolic ejection murmur can be heard with this disorder. *(3:204)*

97. **(C)** It is often seen in conjunction with mitral stenosis. A bicuspid aortic valve is a congenital abnormality in which one of the aortic commissures is fused, leading to the formation of two aortic cusps instead of the usual three. Bicuspid valves tend to become stenotic in adulthood. Although they are sometimes seen in conjunction with coarctation of the aorta, a bicuspid valve and mitral stenosis have no direct association. (3:202)

98. **(B)** Aortic valve area, poor left ventricular function. When aortic stenosis is found in conjunction with a poorly moving left ventricle, standard estimations of the degree of aortic stenosis will be inaccurate. The continuity equation compensates for ventricular hypocontractility, allowing for a more accurate estimate of the aortic valve area. (3:207; 16:105)

99. **(B)** The mean pressure gradient. Aortic insufficiency may cause a high initial instantaneous gradient. When there is combined aortic stenosis and insufficiency, the mean pressure gradient is more specific for estimating the severity of aortic stenosis. (6:137)

100. **(A)** The apical long-axis view. All Doppler procedures are best performed with the ultrasound beam directed parallel to the flow of blood. Of the choices presented, the apical long-axis view provides the optimum angle to image acquisition. (1:104)

101. **(B)** Left ventricular hypertrophy. Aortic stenosis causes pressure overload of the left ventricle. This overload leads to left ventricular hypertrophy. (11:203)

102. **(A)** Aortic insufficiency. The anterior mitral leaflet flutters rapidly when hit by an aortic insufficiency jet. These oscillations are best detected by M-mode. Atrial fibrillation causes coarse diastolic fluttering of the anterior mitral leaflet. (1:294)

103. **(D)** Consistent with moderate aortic regurgitation. The grading of aortic insufficiency with Doppler echocardiography is similar to the grading method used in cardiac catheterization laboratories. An aortic insufficiency jet that extends from the aortic valve to the tips of the anterior mitral leaflet is consistent with moderate aortic regurgitation. (17:339)

104. **(B)** Fine diastolic fluttering and possible flattening of the anterior mitral leaflet. An Austin–Flint murmur represents functional mitral stenosis caused by inhibition of anterior leaflet motion resulting from compression by a strong aortic insufficiency jet. This would appear on M-mode as fine diastolic fluttering of the anterior mitral leaflet with inhibition of opening. (9:77)

105. **(D)** Right sternal border view. When obtainable, the right sternal border approach is usually best for acquiring maximum aortic valve velocities. The patient is turned onto his or her right side, and the Doppler probe is directed into the aortic root. (18:89)

106. **(D)** Transesophageal echocardiography. Because of the high-resolution images it provides of the thoracic aorta, transesophageal echocardiography has been highly successful in evaluating patients with suspected aortic dissection. (19:216)

107. **(D)** A thickened anterior right ventricle wall. Thickening of the right ventricular walls is usually caused by right ventricular pressure overload. Tricuspid insufficiency causes right ventricular volume overload. (1:162)

108. **(D)** Pulmonary hypertension. The right ventricular systolic pressure in this ventricle is approximately 74 mm Hg (using the formula $4V^2 + 10$). Because right ventricular pressures are basically equal to pulmonary artery pressures, the pulmonary artery pressure in this instance is roughly 74 mm Hg, thus indicating the presence of pulmonary hypertension. (3:161)

109. **(D)** It is usually seen as part of the aging process. Tricuspid stenosis is a rare condition that usually occurs as a sequela to rheumatic fever. Its echocardiographic findings are similar to those of mitral stenosis. (3:198)

110. **(C)** Contrast in the inferior vena cava during ventricular systole. With severe tricuspid regurgitation, the regurgitant volume extends all the way back into the right atrium and sometimes into the inferior vena cava as well. By injecting contrast, this regurgitant volume can be "seen" with M-mode or two-dimensional echocardiography. (1:305)

111. **(B)** Tricuspid valve. The echocardiographer should pay special attention to this valve because carcinoid heart disease presents as thickening and rigidity of the tricuspid valve leaflets. Severe tricuspid regurgitation is usually detected with Doppler. (1:305)

112. **(B)** Right ventricular systolic pressure. By using the modified Bernoulli equation and an estimate of jugular venous pressure, systolic pressure in the right ventricle can be determined. (3:112)

113. **(C)** Infundibular pulmonic stenosis. This is caused by hypertrophied muscle bands in the right ventricular outflow tract. Echocardiographically, it can be distinguished from valvular pulmonic stenosis by noting a step-up in Doppler velocities proximal to the pulmonic valve. In addition, the muscular ridge produces turbulence of blood, which hits the pulmonic valve and causes it to flutter. (1:393)

114. **(D)** Left parasternal. Pulmonary artery flow velocities are usually obtained from the left parasternal short-axis view at the level of the aortic root. (10:80)

115. **(A)** Cranial and lateral. This relationship is best appreciated from the short-axis view of the base of the heart. (3:27)

116. **(C)** Midsystolic notching noted on M-mode. Midsystolic notching is a sign of pulmonary hypertension. (3:388)

117. **(B)** Two-dimensional echocardiography. The spatial orientation of two-dimensional echocardiography provides for a better assessment of the size, location, and motion of valvular vegetations. (3:277)

118. **(B)** Mitral valve vegetation. Intravenous drug abusers have an increased incidence of endocarditis because of microorganisms that enter the bloodstream via unsterile needles. Vegetations usually form on the valves of the right side of the heart, but they may settle on left-sided valves as well. One complication of valvular vegetation is an embolic event. (3:276)

119. **(B)** Presence of paravalvular regurgitation. The spatial orientation of color Doppler allows for a quick assessment of blood flow in the region surrounding the prosthetic valve. (12:141)

120. **(A)** May exhibit high Doppler velocities. The normal Doppler velocities across any prosthetic valve will be slightly higher than those of a native valve. A Starr–Edwards, or ball-in-cage, valve tends to exhibit the highest velocities. (3:349)

121. **(A)** An example of a mechanical heart valve. The Bjork–Shiley is a tilting-disc mechanical heart valve. (3:314)

122. **(C)** Transesophageal echocardiography. This is a major application in the evaluation of prosthetic heart valves, particularly in the mitral position. (3:358)

123. **(D)** Hancock. This valve is an example of a heterograft (bioprosthetic) valve. (3:334)

124. **(C)** Abnormal rocking motion of the valve. Valve dehiscence refers to a condition in which the prosthetic valve loosens or separates from the sewing ring and causes an abnormal rocking motion and a paravalvular leak. (3:346)

125. **(C)** It often makes anticoagulation unnecessary. Mechanical valves require constant anticoagulation. Women during childbearing years would, therefore, be more likely to receive a bioprosthetic valve, which would not require anticoagulation. (20:1392)

126. **(A)** These patients are at a higher risk for endocarditis. Because bacteremias occur during dental or surgical procedures, prophylactic antibiotics are often administered to susceptible patients (such as mitral valve prolapse patients) in an attempt to prevent bacterial endocarditis. (20:1151)

127. **(C)** A "swinging heart" on the two-dimensional examination. Excessive motion of the heart can sometimes be noted with massive pericardial effusion. (1:558)

128. **(A)** It impairs diastolic filling. The rigid and fibrotic pericardial sac impairs diastolic filling of the cardiac chambers. (3:268)

129. **(A)** Pressure in the pericardial cavity rises to equal or exceed the diastolic pressure in the heart. Tamponade occurs when intrapericardial pressures rise and impair cardiac filling. Although cardiac tamponade is usually seen in association with a large pericardial effusion, a small effusion may cause tamponade if the rate of accumulation of pericardial fluid exceeds the ability of the pericardium to accommodate the increased volume. (15:213)

130. **(D)** In Dressler's syndrome, a pericardial effusion develops as a result of renal disease. Dressler's syndrome, also known as postmyocardial infarction syndrome, is the development of pericardial effusion 2–10 weeks after infarction. (9:1287)

131. **(D)** A pericardial effusion. Neoplasms from the thoracic region often lead to pericardial effusion. (20:1254)

132. **(D)** Mitral valve prolapse. The descending aorta, a calcified mitral annulus, and ascites can cause echo-free spaces that may be misleading on an echocardiogram. Although a large effusion in which the heart exhibits excessive motion may lead to false mitral valve prolapse, which will not lead to a false-positive diagnosis of pericardial effusion. (1:552)

133. **(A)** Pulmonic stenosis. Diastolic collapse of the right ventricular walls is a good indicator of tamponade. Pulmonic stenosis, or any other form of right ventricular pressure overload, leads to thickening of the right ventricular walls. A thickened wall is unlikely to collapse in diastole. (1:565)

134. **(C)** There is a large acoustic mismatch between lung tissue and pericardial tissue. A greater mismatch between two structures results in brighter reflected echoes from the interface between them. Because there is an extremely large acoustic mismatch between lung (air) and pericardium (tissue), the interface created by the two will cause a bright echo to appear on the echocardiogram. (1:2)

135. **(C)** Decreasing overall gain and increasing depth setting. Decreasing the gain allows for differentiation between the pericardium and epicardium, and increasing the depth setting helps define the borders of the effusion. (11:249)

136. **(D)** Descending aorta. Because the descending aorta lies posterior to the pericardial effusion and anterior to the pleural effusion, it often aids in differentiating between the two. (1:554)

137. **(A)** Constrictive pericarditis. The pericardium limits cardiac motion. When the pericardium is surgically removed (e.g., in constrictive pericarditis), the heart expands and exhibits excessive motion. (1:575)

138. **(A)** Excessive cardiac motion. Again, because the pericardium limits cardiac motion, the heart exhibits excessive motion when the pericardium is surgically removed. (1:575)

139. **(C)** Reduced compliance of the left ventricle. Systemic hypertension causes pressure overload of the left ventricle. As in all pressure-overload situations (e.g., aortic stenosis), the left ventricle hypertrophies and may become noncompliant, leading to diastolic dysfunction. (11:273)

140. **(B)** Left ventricular hypertrophy. This condition can be present in the absence of an obstruction. (1:522)

141. **(D)** Endomyocardial biopsy. Several echocardiographic signs are suggestive of amyloid heart disease, but a definitive diagnosis can be made only with an endomyocardial biopsy performed in the catheterization laboratory. (20:1215)

142. **(B)** Sarcoidosis. This is an infiltrative process that can lead to restrictive cardiomyopathy. (11:317)

143. **(A)** Increased systolic velocity in the left ventricular outflow tract. Velocities are low because of decreased cardiac output. (3:230)

144. **(A)** It is more likely to affect the right ventricle than the left ventricle. Cardiac contusion may be seen following a blunt trauma to the chest (such as a steering-wheel injury). Because the right ventricle is the most anterior structure of the heart, it is the one most susceptible to injury. (3:301)

145. **(A)** An apical aneurysm with a mural thrombus. Apical aneurysms sometimes develop following an anterior wall myocardial infarction. Because aneurysms are a likely site for thrombus, choice A is the most likely answer. (1:489)

146. **(C)** Two-dimensional demonstration of an ejection fraction lower than 50%. The ejection fraction is a measure of systolic left ventricular function. (20:51)

147. **(C)** Left anterior descending artery. This artery supplies the anterior wall of the left ventricle and the anterior portion of the interventricular septum. (3:237)

148. **(D)** They have a narrow neck. The best way to differentiate a true aneurysm from a pseudoaneurysm is to look at the width of its neck. Pseudoaneurysms tend to have a narrow neck because they result from a tear in the myocardium. (1:486)

149. **(B)** A reduced ejection fraction. An E point-to-septal separation of more than 10 mm correlates with a reduced ejection fraction. (11:205)

150. **(B)** Akinetic. Lack of systolic thickening and motion is referred to as akinesis. (11:287)

151. **(D)** Occlusion of the left anterior descending coronary artery. Blood to the inferior wall of the left ventricle is usually supplied by the right coronary artery. (1:467; 21:93)

152. **(B)** Severe mitral regurgitation. Doppler interrogation of a patient with ruptured papillary muscle will usually demonstrate this condition. (3:249)

153. **(D)** It is used in diagnosing ischemic heart disease. Stress echocardiography is used as an adjunct to standard stress testing in diagnosing patients with suspected coronary artery disease. Resting wall motion is compared to wall motion during and after stress. (3:250)

154. **(C)** They do not recur once they are surgically removed. Although characterized as a benign tumor, a myxoma may recur if some cells remain after excision of the tumor. (20:1285)

155. **(B)** Ventricular septal defects. The QP/QS ratio refers to the ratio of pulmonary-to-systemic blood flow. It can be calculated echocardiographically to determine the magnitude of left-to-right shunting of blood. (6:161)

156. **(B)** Continuous flow (systolic and diastolic) above baseline. Shunting of blood from the aorta to the pulmonary artery occurs in both systole and diastole. (18:220)

157. **(B)** Contrast injection echocardiography. Even a small atrial septal defect can be detected by noting the presence or absence of microbubbles. (1:406)

158. **(B)** Secundum. Atrial septal defects occur most commonly in the area of the foramen ovale, where they are termed ostium secundum defects. (3:381)

159. **(C)** Eisenmenger's syndrome. In this syndrome, the pulmonary vascular resistance is equal to or greater than the systemic vascular resistance, leading to right-to-left shunting. (20:589)

160. **(B)** Infundibular pulmonic stenosis. In Ebstein's anomaly, the tricuspid valve is large and partially adherent to the walls of the right ventricle so that the valve orifice is displaced apically. Therefore, most of the right ventricle functions as part of the right atrium. It is frequently associated with an atrial septal defect. Infundibular pulmonic stenosis is not part of the spectrum of this disorder. (3:406)

161. **(D)** Ostium primum atrial septal defect and an inlet ventricular septal defect. Endocardial cushion defects occur when the atrial and ventricular components of the cardiac septum fail to develop properly. (3:381)

162. **(C)** Descending thoracic aorta. Coarctation of the aorta is a constrictive malformation of the aortic arch, usually located just distal to the origin of the left subclavian artery. The obstruction increases the velocity of blood flow beyond the point of constriction. (3:396)

163. **(D)** An atrial septal defect. The fourth component is right ventricular hypertrophy. (3:421)

164. (B) It is a congenital malformation in which a fibrous membrane divides the left atrium into an upper and lower chamber. Cor triatriatum is a rare abnormality in which an embryonic membrane in the left atrium fails to regress. It can be detected echocardiographically by noting a linear echo traversing the left atrium. Doppler echocardiography will detect high-velocity flow across a hole in the membrane. *(3:402; 22:53)*

165. (C) Paradoxical septal motion. Left bundle branch block often causes this motion. *(1:231)*

166. (C) A mechanical prosthetic valve. This high echogenicity of the mitral valve is characteristic of a mechanical prosthetic valve. *(3:347)*

167. (D) It is significantly decreased. The M-mode demonstrates a dilated and hypokinetic left ventricle. The markedly increased E point-to-septal separation is consistent with a decreased left ventricular ejection fraction. *(23:140)*

168. (B) Left ventricular end-diastolic pressure is increased. There is a mitral valve B notch, which is consistent with high end-diastolic pressure in the left ventricle. *(24:69)*

169. (A) Aortic stenosis and aortic insufficiency. The systolic waveform below baseline is consistent with moderate aortic stenosis. A mitral regurgitation waveform would be wider and is usually of higher velocity. The diastolic waveform above baseline is too high a velocity to be caused by mitral or tricuspid stenosis and is consistent with aortic insufficiency. *(6:78)*

170. (D) Coronary artery disease. The interventricular septum is hypokinetic and more echogenic than the posterior left ventricular wall. These findings are consistent with an old myocardial infarction. *(1:478)*

171. (C) Chordae tendineae. The M-mode cursor in this long-axis view is directed beyond the tips of the mitral leaflets at the level of the chordae tendineae—the level at which left ventricular measurements are obtained. *(11:12)*

172. (C) Caused by stagnant blood. The cloud of fuzzy smoke-like echoes in the left ventricle is the result of blood stasis. It is usually seen when there is a severe decrease in left ventricular contractibility. *(1:492)*

173–179. If you are having a difficult time orienting yourself to an echocardiographic image, find a structure that is easy for you to recognize and work your way from there. For example, if you can identify the aortic root, you can then follow the anterior wall of the root as it continues into the interventricular septum. The posterior wall of the root will follow into the anterior mitral leaflet, and so on. **173.** Right ventricle. **174.** Aortic root. **175.** Left atrium. **176.** Descending aorta. **177.** Left ventricle. **178.** Pericardial effusion. **179.** Pleural effusion. *(1:558)*

180. (D) A large pericardial effusion. A massive circumferential pericardial effusion is demonstrated in this four-chamber view. *(11:253)*

181. (B) Right ventricular wall. The presence of tamponade should be ruled out in patients with pericardial effusion, especially a massive one. A fairly specific echocardiographic sign of tamponade is diastolic collapse of the right ventricle, the right atrium, or both. *(25:561)*

182. (B) A diastolic jet filling the left ventricular outflow tract and extending deep into the left ventricle. This long-axis view demonstrates a flail right coronary cusp of the aortic valve. The cusp is seen extending into the left ventricular outflow tract in diastole. Color Doppler would be likely to demonstrate severe aortic insufficiency, which choice B describes. *(12:100)*

183. (D) The origin of the right coronary artery. With slight superior angulation from a standard short-axis view of the aortic valve, the ostia and proximal segments of the right coronary artery can be visualized. *(11:23)*

184. (B) False. The right ventricular outflow tract is located lateral to the origin of the right coronary artery. *(1:102)*

185. (A) Left-to-right shunting at the atrial level. There is a washout effect in the right atrium as blood from the left side of the heart enters the contrast-filled right atrium. *(11:355)*

186. (B) False. A pericardial effusion would appear on a subcostal four-chamber view as an echo-free space anterior to the right ventricle. *(11:251)*

187. (B) Liver parenchyma. To obtain a subcostal four-chamber view, the transducer is placed on the abdomen and angled in a cephalic direction. Therefore, liver parenchyma will occupy the near field of the image. *(3:129)*

188. (D) Pulmonary hypertension. An absent A wave and midsystolic notching (flying W sign) are consistent with this condition. *(3:388)*

189. (C) Mitral valve prolapse. The M-mode in Fig. 2–25 demonstrates late-systolic tricuspid valve prolapse. Tricuspid valve prolapse almost always occurs in patients with concomitant mitral valve prolapse. *(1:305)*

190. (C) Midsystolic notching. Fig. 2–26 is an example of systolic anterior motion of the mitral valve. This is one classic echocardiographic sign of hypertrophic obstructive cardiomyopathy. The midsystolic obstruction of the left ventricular outflow tract will often be demonstrated on the M-mode of the aortic valve as well as by midsystolic notching. *(26:6)*

191. **(C)** A dilated aortic root. This patient exhibits characteristic findings of Marfan syndrome, a connective tissue disorder. There is a linear echo near the aortic valve suggesting aortic root dissection, another complication of Marfan syndrome. This syndrome often causes ascending aortic dilatation as well as myxomatous degeneration of the aortic and mitral valves. (11:242)

192. **(A)** The long-axis suprasternal view. Because the aortic root is dilated, echocardiographic evaluation should follow the length of the aorta to determine the extent of the aneurysm. The suprasternal long-axis view allows for visualization of the aortic arch and the proximal portion of the descending aorta. Further investigation should include a modified apical two-chamber view for evaluating the thoracic aorta and a subcostal approach for interrogating the abdominal aorta. (3:121, 137)

193. **(C)** A large apical thrombus. This thrombus is seen filling the apex, with a piece of the medial segment protruding into the left ventricle. Most thrombi are associated with anterior infarctions and are located in the apex in the majority of cases. (1:489)

194. **(B)** It is flail. The tip of the posterior leaflet can be seen protruding into the left atrium, which is consistent with a flail mitral valve. (27:1383)

195. **(B)** Right pulmonary artery. The artery is seen in its short axis. (11:36)

196. **(A)** The left atrium. This atrium can sometimes be visualized posterior to the right pulmonary artery on the suprasternal long-axis view. (11:36)

197. **(D)** The moderator band. This is a muscular strip located in the apical third of the right ventricle. It is sometimes misdiagnosed as a right ventricular apical thrombus. (3:117, 294)

198. **(B)** A left atrial thrombus. This is seen protruding into the left atrium. (The bright linear echo in the right atrium originates from a pacemaker wire.) (1:592)

199. **(B)** Aortic stenosis, a calcified mitral annulus, and basal septal hypertrophy. The aortic valve is markedly calcified; there is a bright echo posterior to the mitral valve, representing a calcified mitral annulus; and the base of the interventricular septum is hypertrophied. The posterior echo-free space represents pleural effusion, as opposed to a pericardial effusion, because it does not taper at the descending aorta. (1:345, 283)

200. **(D)** An aged heart. When seen together, these findings usually indicate signs of aging. (9:1658)

201. **(D)** Atrial fibrillation. The electrocardiogram at the top of the Doppler tracing indicates this fibrillation. The variations from beat to beat reflect the altering lengths in diastolic filling periods that occur with atrial fibrillation. (11:333)

202. **(B)** Diastolic doming. The mitral valve is bulging into the left ventricle in diastole because the valve is stenotic and cannot accommodate all the blood available for delivery into the left ventricle. (1:251)

203. **(A)** The left atrium. Even without using the centimeter markers as a gauge, one can determine that the left atrium is dilated. In the long-axis view, the aortic root and left aorta should be approximately the same size. The apical four-chamber view is extremely useful for assessing relative chamber size. The right and left atria should be roughly the same size (although the left atrium is usually slightly larger), and they should be smaller than the ventricles. (11:368)

204. **(D)** An opening snap. The opening snap often affords the first clue to the diagnosis of mitral stenosis. (20:185)

205. **(C)** Descending aorta. A portion of the aorta can be seen lying behind the left atrium on the apical four-chamber view. (1:98)

206. **(A)** The mitral valve area. The pressure half-time, or the time it takes for the initial pressure drop of the mitral valve to be halved, can be used to measure the mitral valve area. A pressure half-time of 220 ms has been shown to correlate with a valve area of 1 cm^2. (18:117)

207. **(C)** Left ventricular hypertrophy. The left ventricular walls are thickened and exhibit increased echogenicity. (28:188)

208. **(B)** A thickened mitral valve, a prominent interatrial septum, a small left ventricle, and pericardial effusion. The mitral valve and interatrial septum are slightly thickened, there is a small-to-moderate-sized pericardial effusion, and the left ventricle is small. (1:535)

209. **(D)** Amyloid cardiomyopathy. This patient exhibits classic features of this disease. The infiltrative process of the disease causes thickening of the ventricles, interatrial septum and valves. Pericardial effusion is another finding sometimes associated with this disease. (3:232)

210. **(B)** An endomyocardial biopsy. This has been shown to be helpful in identifying amyloid cardiomyopathy. (3:232)

211. **(B)** Ventricular septal defect. The short-axis and modified four-chamber views demonstrate a gap in the posterior aspect of the midsection of the interventricular septum. Given the patient's history and the irregular borders on the echocardiogram, one can assume that this defect is acquired rather than congenital. (29:506)

212. **(A)** Color-flow Doppler imaging. This is particularly useful for quickly determining the location and quantifying the extent of abnormal blood flow in patients with ventricular septal defects. (3:243)

213. **(A)** Coronary sinus. When imaged from the apical two-chamber view, the coronary sinus appears as a circular structure in the atrioventricular groove. By rotating to a four-chamber view and angling posteriorly, one can follow the coronary sinus as it courses along the length of the posterior atrioventricular groove. (20:29)

214. **(B)** Deoxygenated blood. The coronary sinus carries venous blood to the right atrium. (30:211)

215. **(A)** Anteriorly. By tilting the scan plane anteriorly from this posteriorly directed apical four-chamber view, the aorta and left ventricular outflow tract can be imaged. (3:131)

216. **(C)** Prolapse of the posterior leaflet. The posterior mitral leaflet bulges beyond the plane of the mitral annulus, which is consistent with prolapse. (3:189)

217. **(A)** A systolic curve below baseline >3 m/s. Mitral valve prolapse, especially to the degree shown in this study, is most likely to be accompanied by some degree of mitral regurgitation, which is detected from the apical window with Doppler echocardiography by noting a systolic curve below baseline usually >3 m/s. (6:74)

218. **(B)** False. The arrow is pointing to the lateral wall of the left ventricle. (11:25)

219. **(C)** Artifactual. A dropout of echoes in the interatrial septum is not an uncommon finding when visualized from the apical four-chamber view. If this were a true atrial septal defect, a T sign would likely be noted. (1:404)

220. **(A)** Slight thickening of the valve with a normal opening. This thickening is noted best in diastole. The leaflets appear to open widely in systole. (They open in close proximity to the walls of the aortic root.) (1:279)

221. **(C)** 36 mm Hg. Using the simplified Bernoulli equation, the peak aortic gradient can be obtained by squaring the peak velocity (in this case 3 m/s) and then multiplying by 4. (18:23)

222. **(B)** Congenital aortic stenosis. In this disorder, the valve may be thin or minimally thickened, and M-mode may demonstrate a normal opening if the cursor was directed at the body of the leaflets rather than at the restricted tips. The best way to determine if congenital aortic stenosis is present is by noting Doppler evidence of increased velocities across the valve. (1:384)

223. **(A)** Systolic doming. This occurs in congenital aortic stenosis because the body of the leaflets expands to accommodate systolic flow while the tips of the leaflets restrict blood flow. (Normally, the tips of the aortic valve open wide and lie parallel to the aortic root in systole.) (1:383)

224. **(C)** It is exhibiting shaggy irregular echoes. The mitral valve has a mass of shaggy echoes with irregular borders attached to it. (3:277)

225. **(B)** Subacute bacterial endocarditis. Because of the patient's history and the echocardiographic demonstration of an irregular mass attached to the mitral valve, this is the most likely diagnosis. (20:1141)

226. **(B)** Increased. Unlike calcium, which tends to inhibit valve opening, vegetations are likely to increase valve excursion. Because calcium and vegetations can look similar, echocardiographically this difference can aid in the diagnosis. (3:277)

227. **(A)** Systolic waveform below baseline. A mitral valve vegetation will usually cause the mitral valve to be regurgitant. Mitral regurgitation can be detected by continuous-wave Doppler from the apical four-chamber view by noting systolic flow below baseline. (6:74)

228. **(D)** It prolapses into the left atrium and left ventricle. In Fig. 2–38A, the mass is in the left atrium. In Fig. 2–38B and C, the mass appears in the left ventricle. Therefore, one could deduce that the mass is prolapsing into the left atrium in systole and into the left ventricle in diastole. (1:312)

229. **(B)** The posteromedial papillary muscle. On the opposite wall of the left ventricle, one can see the anterolateral papillary muscle. Between the two papillary muscles, the tip of the mitral valve vegetation can be seen protruding into the left ventricle. (3:113)

References

1. Feigenbaum H. *Echocardiography*. 4th ed. Philadelphia: Lea & Febiger; 1986.

2. Henry WL, DeMaria A, Gramik R. *Nomenclature and Standardization in Two-Dimensional Echocardiography*. Raleigh, NC: American Society of Echocardiography; 1980.

3. Craig M. *Diagnostic Medical Sonography: A Guide to Clinical Practice. Vol. 2. Echocardiography*. Philadelphia: JB Lippincott; 1991.

4. Cosgrove DO, McCready VR. *Ultrasound Imaging: Liver, Spleen, Pancreas*. New York: John Wiley & Sons; 1982.

5. Weyman AE. *Cross-Sectional Echocardiography*. Philadelphia: Lea & Febiger; 1982.

6. Kisslo J, Adams D, Mark DB. *Basic Doppler Echocardiography*. New York: Churchill Livingstone; 1986.

7. Sahn DJ, DeMaria A, Kisso J, Weyman A. Recommendations regarding quantitation in M-mode echocardiography: results of a survey of echocardiographic measurements. *Circulation*. 1978; 58:1072-1083.

8. Sokolow M, McIlroy MB, Cheitlin MD. *Clinical Cardiology*. 5th ed. Norwalk, CT: Appleton & Lange; 1990.

9. Braunwald E. *Heart Disease: A Textbook of Cardiovascular Medicine*. 3rd ed. Philadelphia: WB Saunders; 1988.

10. Goldberg SJ, Allen HD, Marx GR, Flinn CJ. *Doppler Echocardiography*. Philadelphia: Lea & Febiger; 1985.

11. Harrigan P, Lee R. *Principles of Interpretation in Echocardiography*. New York: John Wiley & Sons; 1985.

12. Kisso J, Adams DB, Belkin RN. *Doppler Color-Flow Imaging*. New York: Churchill Livingstone; 1988.

13. Salcedo E. *Atlas of Echocardiography*. 2nd ed. Philadelphia: WB Saunders; 1985.

14. Hatle L, Angelsen B, Tromsdal A. Noninvasive assessment of atrioventricular pressure half-time by Doppler ultrasound. *Circulation*. 1979; 60:1096-1104.

15. Gravanis MB. *Cardiovascular Pathophysiology*. New York: McGraw-Hill; 1987.

16. Popp RL. Echocardiography. *N Engl J Med*. 1990; 323:101-109.

17. Aobanu J, et al. Pulsed Doppler echocardiography in the diagnosis and estimation of severity of aortic insufficiency. *Am J Cardiol*. 1982; 49:339-343.

18. Hatle L, Angelsen B. *Doppler Ultrasound in Cardiology: Physical Principles and Clinical Applications*. Philadelphia: Lea & Febiger; 1985.

19. Currie PJ. Transesophageal echocardiography: new window to the heart. *Circulation*. 1989; 80:215-218.

20. Hurst JW. *The Heart,* 6th ed. New York: McGraw-Hill; 1986.

21. Wasser HJ, Greengart A, et al. Echocardiographic assessment of posterior left ventricular aneurysms. *J Diagn Med Sonography*. 1986; 2:93-95.

22. Driscoll DJ, Fuster V, McGoon DC. Congenital heart disease in adolescents and adults: atrioventricular canal defect. In: Brandenburg RO, Fuster V, Giulani ER, et al., eds. *Cardiology: Fundamentals and Practice*. Chicago: Year Book Medical Publishers; 1987.

23. D'Cruz IA, Lalmalani GG, et al. The superiority of mitral E point-ventricular septum separation to other echocardiographic indicators of left ventricular performance. *Clin Cardiol*. 1979; 2:140.

24. D'Cruz IA, Kleinman D, Aboulatta H, et al. A reappraisal of the mitral B-bump (B-inflection): its relationship to left ventricular dysfunction. *Echocardiography*. 1990; 7:69-75.

25. Williams GJ, Partidge JB, Right ventricular diastolic collapse: an echocardiographic sign of tamponade. *Br Heart J*. 1983; 49:292.

26. Doi YL, McKenna WJ, et al. M-mode echocardiography in hypertrophic cardiomyopathy: diagnostic criteria and prediction of obstruction. *Am J Cardiol*. 1980; 45:6-14.

27. Child JS, Skorton DJ, Taylor RD, et al. M-mode and cross-sectional echocardiographic features of flail posterior mitral leaflets. *Am J Cardiol*. 1979; 44:1383-1390.

28. Sigueira-Filho AG, Cunha CL, Tajik AJ, et al. M-mode and two-dimensional echocardiographic features in cardiac amyloidosis. *Circulation*. 1981; 63:188-196.

29. Chandraratna PAN, Balachandran PK, Shah PM, Hodges M. Echocardiographic observations on ventricular septal rupture complicating myocardial infarction. *Circulation*. 1975; 51:506-510.

30. Berne RM, Levy MN. *Cardiovascular Physiology*. 4th ed. St. Louis: CV Mosby; 1981.

31. Allen MN. *Diagnostic Medical Sonography: A Guide to Clinical Practice Echocardiography*. 2nd ed. Philadelphia: Lippincott; 1999.

3

Pediatric Echocardiography

David A. Parra*

Study Guide

INTRODUCTION

Effective echocardiographic evaluation of congenital heart disease requires an appreciation of malformation severity and cardiovascular hemodynamics. In the current clinical practice, two-dimensional (2-D) echocardiography is the primary tool for imaging and involves the use of every modality available. Anatomy should be carefully delineated because malformations frequently occur in combination rather than as isolated lesions. Doppler techniques provide information about shunt patterns, flow volumes, gradients through obstructions, and severity of regurgitation. Color-flow Doppler facilitates rapid detection of flow abnormalities and qualitative assessment of such flow characteristics as direction, timing, and degree of turbulence. Pulsed-wave (PW) Doppler provides range (spatial) resolution of flow patterns. Quantification of high-velocity flows requires the use of continuous-wave (CW) Doppler. M-mode is used primarily to evaluate subtle movements and to measure chamber, vessel, and wall size. Contrast echocardiography is useful in the demonstration of intracardiac and extracardiac shunts, particularly in cases in which 2-D and color-flow imaging are suboptimal.

The study outline is intended as a guide for the entry-level pediatric echocardiographer and, as such, includes malformations that occur with relative frequency as well as those that occur rarely but are relatively straightforward. The outline includes a definition of the anatomic malformation, a list of variants, the hemodynamic effect of the lesion, characteristic clinical findings, key echocardiographic concepts, the natural history of the disease, commonly associated cardiac malformations, interventional catheterization techniques, and palliative as well as corrective surgical procedures. Complex malformations such as single ventricle, double-inlet ventricle, and double-outlet ventricle are beyond the scope of this chapter. For information regarding these malformations, the reader is referred to more extensive texts.

Sample examination questions are provided following the text to give the reader an appreciation of the scope of knowledge required to perform routine diagnostic pediatric echocardiograms. The questions are *not* intended to be a comprehensive review but to assist the reader in determining what needs to be studied in greater detail.

For discussions of normal anatomy, general scanning technique, echocardiographic physics and instrumentation, and acquired heart disease that are not specific to the pediatric population, the reader is referred to other chapters within this book. Acquired pathologies that occur in the pediatric as well as adult population include mitral valve prolapse, rheumatic heart disease, cardiac masses, cardiomyopathies, pericardial effusions, and bacterial endocarditis. Evaluation of ventricular function in the pediatric population is identical to that of the adult population and, therefore, will not be repeated within this chapter.

SEGMENTAL ANATOMY

When evaluating congenital heart disease, the echocardiographer begins by determining whether the heart within the thorax is located mostly in the left chest (levocardia), right chest (dextrocardia), or directly posterior to the sternum (mesocardia). The direction in which the apex is pointing is also noted. The echocardiographer should demonstrate segmental anatomy by delineating situs, ventricular looping, and great vessel relationship. This will allow an accurate description of cardiac anomalies and can be used to compare with other imaging modalities.

*Michael W. Yates wrote the previous edition version of this chapter.

171

This may be done by documenting anatomic landmarks for each chamber and vessel, as follows:

1. Atrial situs[1,2]

   A. Determined by

   (1) Positions of the atria as proven by anatomic landmarks

   a. Right atrium

   - Presence of Eustachian valve

   - Right atrial appendage (broad connection to atrium)—parasternal or subcostal sagittal views

   - Entrance of superior vena cava and inferior vena cava (the superior vena cava is not a reliable marker of the right atrium, as it may drain into the left atrium; inferior vena cava may also be interrupted), and coronary sinus

   b. Left atrium

   - Left atrial appendage (tubular, with narrow connection)—parasternal long- or short-axis, subcostal, apical four-chamber views

   - Entrance of pulmonary veins—posterior subcostal coronal plane (pulmonary veins are not reliable marker of the left atrium due to potential anomalous drainage)

   B. Types

   (1) Solitus—normal

   - Right atrium is right sided; receives the inferior vena cava, superior vena cava, and coronary sinus

   - Left atrium is left sided and receives the pulmonary veins

   - Descending aorta to the left; inferior vena cava to the right

   (2) Inversus—mirror image visceral placement

   - Very rare

   (3) Left atrial isomerism—double left-sidedness

   - Both atria have left atrial morphology

   - Seventy percent have interrupted inferior vena cava with dilated azygos vein located posterior to the aorta on the same side of the spine or direct hepatic vein drainage into atria bilaterally (2-D transverse subcostal views; confirm venous versus arterial structures by Doppler from sagittal views)

   - Usually have polysplenia

   - Frequently have complex cardiac anomalies

   (4) Right atrial isomerism—double right-sidedness

   - Inferior vena cava located anterior to the aorta on the same side of the spine

   - Usually have asplenia

   - Frequently have other cardiac lesions

2. Ventricular connection (looping)[3–5]

   A. Determined by positions of the ventricles as proven by anatomic landmarks

   (1) Right ventricle

   - Trabeculated endocardial surface

   - Tricuspid valve (three leaflets)

     — annulus inserts more apically than the mitral valve

     — chordal insertion into ventricular septum or free wall

   - Moderator band

   (2) Left ventricle

   - Smooth endocardial surface

   - Mitral valve (two leaflets)

   - Two prominent papillary muscles

   B. Types

   (1) Dextro—right ventricle to the right

   (2) Levo—right ventricle to the left

3. Great vessel relationship[1]

   A. Types

   (1) Dextro—aortic valve to the right and posterior of the pulmonic valve

   (2) Levo—aortic valve to the left of the pulmonic valve

   B. Determined by positions of the great arteries as proven by anatomical landmarks

   (1) Pulmonary artery

   - Bifurcates soon after exiting the heart

   - Posterior course from base of the heart

   (2) Aorta

   - Superior course from base of the heart, to form aortic arch

   - Coronary arteries

NORMAL HEMODYNAMICS[6]

Chamber/vessel	Mean	Diastolic	Systolic
Right atrium		<9 mm Hg	<9 mm Hg
Right ventricle		<7 mm Hg	<30 mm Hg
Pulmonary artery	<20 mm Hg		<30 mm Hg
Left atrium	<12 mm Hg		<17 mm Hg
Left ventricle		<12 mm Hg	<140 mm Hg (within 5 mm Hg of arm pressure)
Aorta	Determined by blood pressure cuff on arm		

IMPORTANT DOPPLER CALCULATIONS

1. Conversion of frequency shift into velocity by use of the Doppler equation[7]
2. Estimation of pressure gradient by application of the modified Bernoulli equation[7]
3. Determination of flow volume[8]
4. Determination of pulmonary to systemic flow ratio, referred to as Q_p; Q_s[9–11]
5. Estimation of valve area by use of the continuity equation[12]

ESTIMATION OF PULMONARY ARTERY PRESSURE

The development and progression of elevated pulmonary artery pressure is of concern in any patient with congenital heart disease. Pulmonary artery pressures rise in response to increased flow volume or pressure as pulmonary vascular resistance becomes elevated. Increased flow volume or high pressure causes the intimal and medial layers of the pulmonary arterioles to hypertrophy, thereby increasing pulmonary vascular resistance. With prolonged exposure to high-flow volume or pressure, the patient develops pulmonary hypertension and eventually pulmonary vascular obstructive disease, which is irreversible. When pulmonary artery pressures exceed systemic pressures, blood flow through intracardiac and extracardiac shunts reverses, so that they become pulmonary-to-systemic or right-to-left shunts. Mixing of deoxygenated blood with oxygenated blood leads to cyanosis. The right ventricle eventually fails because of the increased resistance against which it must work to eject blood. Pulmonary vascular disease that results from prolonged increased volume and pressure to the pulmonary vascular bed from a systemic to pulmonary (left to right) shunt is referred to as Eisenmenger's syndrome.[13]

Echocardiographic Signs of Elevated Pulmonary Artery Pressure (Pulmonary Hypertension)

- Dilated right atrium[14] and ventricle with thickened right ventricular free wall
- Disappearance of the "a" wave on the pulmonic valve M-mode[15,16]
- Midsystolic closure of the pulmonic valve on M-mode, also known as the "flying W"[17]
- Tricuspid and/or pulmonic regurgitation in the absence of structural abnormalities of the valves[18]

Estimation of Systolic Pulmonary Artery Pressure

- Peak tricuspid regurgitation gradient plus 7 mm Hg (assumed central venous pressure)[18,19]

- Enhancement of tricuspid regurgitation Doppler tracing by use of echocardiographic contrast[20]

Estimation of Diastolic Pulmonary Artery Pressure

- End-diastolic pulmonary regurgitation gradient plus 7 mm Hg (assumed central venous pressure)[21]
- Pulmonary artery diastolic pressure = 0.49 × PA systolic pressure (from peak TR gradient)[22]

Estimation of Mean Pulmonary Artery Pressure

- Acceleration time (AcT) divided by ejection time (ET) flow through the right ventricular outflow tract as recorded by PW Doppler[23]

SIMPLE SHUNT LESIONS

Persistent Patent Ductus Arteriosus

Anatomy. The ductus arteriosus is a vessel connecting the left pulmonary artery to the descending aorta (immediately distal to the level of the left subclavian artery) that allows blood to bypass the pulmonary circulation during fetal life. Shortly after birth, this vessel should close so blood can enter the pulmonary circulation to be oxygenated. When the vessel remains patent, it is referred to as a persistent patent ductus arteriosus.

Hemodynamics. During fetal life, pulmonary vascular resistance is higher than systemic vascular resistance; therefore, pulmonary pressure is higher than systemic pressure, so blood flows from the pulmonary artery to the descending aorta. After birth, pulmonary vascular resistance decreases and becomes much lower than systemic vascular resistance. The reversal in pressure differences between the pulmonary and systemic circulations causes a reversal of flow through a persistently patent ductus arteriosus, so that the blood from the descending aorta enters the pulmonary circulation. The resulting increase in pulmonary flow continues into the left atrium as a volume overload, causing the left atrium and ventricle to dilate. The magnitude of the systemic to pulmonary shunt is determined by the difference between the pulmonary and systemic vascular resistances, the difference in pulmonary artery and descending aortic pressures, and by the luminal diameter and length of the ductus arteriosus.[6]

Clinical Presentation.[6,24] Patients are usually asymptomatic if ductus is small; in cardiac failure if the shunt is large.

- Physical exam: bounding pulses (moderate to large patent ductus arteriosus)
- Auscultation: systolic murmur in infants, continuous murmur at older age
- ECG (electrocardiogram): variable

- Chest x-ray: enlarged pulmonary artery and aorta, increased vascular markings, ductus "bump" off the descending aorta (large ductus)

Key Echocardiographic Concepts

- Demonstrate position, size, and course of patent ductus arteriosus in 2-D and color
- 2-D visualization of the ductus entering the pulmonary artery (parasternal short-axis or high parasternal view)[25,26]
- 2-D visualization of the ductus entering the descending aorta (suprasternal notch or high parasternal view)[27,28]
- Continuous flow in the pulmonary artery by PW or color-flow Doppler[29,30]
- Diastolic flow reversal in the descending aorta distal to the left subclavian artery by PW or color-flow Doppler[12,31]
- Demonstration of shunt by contrast echocardiography[25,32]
- Left atrial to aortic root ratio (LA/Ao ratio) greater than 1.2 in the absence of left ventricular failure[32]
- Estimation of pulmonary artery pressure by determining the pressure gradient through the duct by CW Doppler and subtracting this value from the systolic blood pressure[12]
- Demonstrate arch sidedness, assess for possible coarctation or LPA stenosis

Populations at Increased Risk[6]

- Preterm infant
- Infant born at altitudes >4,500 m above sea level
- Rubella syndrome
- Family history
- Complex congenital heart disease[13]

Natural History.[6] A large shunt may cause congestive heart failure, failure to thrive, and recurrent respiratory infections. Pulmonary vascular obstructive disease will develop if left untreated.

Treatment[6]

- Indomethacin: to close ductus medically
- Device (Amplatzer, Helix) closure by interventional catheterization[33]
- Surgical ligation
- Prostaglandin E$_1$: to keep ductus patent in the presence of a "duct-dependent" lesion, in which the ductus is necessary to provide pulmonary or systemic circulation

Postoperative Echocardiographic Evaluation. Left atrial and ventricular size should regress to normal. Color-flow or PW Doppler should be used to check for residual shunting.

Assessment of the aortic arch and branch pulmonary arteries is essential to determine residual obstruction or inadvertent impingement of the LPA or descending aorta

Other Systemic to Pulmonary Shunts
Echocardiographic Concepts

- PW Doppler documentation of diastolic descending aortic flow reversal to evaluate patency of the shunt
- Localization of shunt by PW Doppler (determines the level at which the diastolic reversal begins)
- Visualization of shunt on 2-D and color-flow Doppler

Types

A. Aortopulmonary window: a defect in the walls of the ascending aorta and main pulmonary artery resulting in blood shunting between these structures; Doppler findings are similar to those of persistent patent ductus arteriosus, except reversal of flow may be detected in the ascending as well as descending aorta.[12]

B. Surgically Created Systemic to Pulmonary Shunts[6,34]

1. Blalock–Taussig: subclavian artery to pulmonary artery (classic BT shunt), currently the shunt of choice is the modified BT shunt (Gore-Tex tube from the innominate artery to pulmonary artery) on side opposite the aortic arch; modified versions may be placed on either side.
2. Central: anastomosis or conduit between the pulmonary artery and aorta
3. Potts: descending aorta to pulmonary artery; difficult to control size; older technique
4. Waterston: ascending aorta to right pulmonary artery; difficult to control size; older technique
5. Glenn (cavopulmonary shunt): superior vena cava to right main pulmonary artery; occlusion may lead to various complications; including superior vena cava syndrome

Atrial Septal Defects

Anatomy. Atrial septal defect is incomplete septation of the atrial septum that results in a "hole" or communication through which blood can flow directly from one atrium to the other. Types of atrial septal defects, as determined by physical location, are listed below.[26,35]

- Secundum: area of the foramen ovale; most common
- Primum: posterior, near the atrioventricular valves; associated with cleft mitral valve and mitral regurgitation
- Sinus venosus: posterior and superior, near the entrance of the superior vena cava; associated with anomalous right pulmonary venous return into the right atrium
- Coronary sinus: area of the entrance of the coronary sinus; rare; associated with persistent left superior vena cava, absent coronary sinus, and complex congenital heart disease.[36]

Hemodynamics. Blood is "shunted" from the higher pressure left atrium to the lower pressure right atrium causing a volume overload and, therefore, dilation of the right atrium, right ventricle, and pulmonary arteries. Doppler interrogation reveals blood flow through the interatrial septum and increased flow velocities through the tricuspid and pulmonic valves.

Clinical Presentation.[6,24] Patients are usually asymptomatic.

- Physical exam: systolic impulse may be felt at the lower left sternal border
- Auscultation: fixed splitting of the second heart sound, systolic crescendo–decrescendo (ejection) murmur that is heard best at upper left sternal border (relative pulmonary stenosis)
- ECG: right ventricular hypertrophy
- Chest x-ray: enlarged heart and increased pulmonary vascular markings

Key Echocardiographic Concepts

- Visualization of defect on 2-D and with color-flow Doppler (subcostal long and short, parasternal short axis, and apical four-chamber views)[26,30]
- Determine defect location and size and relationship with surrounding structures (atrioventricular valves, pulmonary and systemic veins) for possible device closure
- PW Doppler tracing characteristic of left to right shunt through an atrial septal defect[37]
- Degree of right atrial and ventricular dilatation to estimate severity of shunt
- PW Doppler technique to calculate $Q_p:Q_s$ (i.e., magnitude of the shunt)
- Use of echocardiographic contrast to confirm the presence of a shunt[38,39]

Associated Disease[24,32]

- Mitral valve prolapse
- Left ventricular inflow obstruction (Lutembacher's syndrome—rare and associated with rheumatic heart disease)
- Subaortic stenosis
- Atrial septal aneurysm
- Partial anomalous pulmonary venous return

Natural History[6,24]

- May close spontaneously
- Symptoms occur in the second decade of life
- Pulmonary vascular obstructive disease may develop, usually in adulthood

Treatment

- Device closure by interventional catheterization (in secundum defects with adequate rims)
- Elective surgical patch closure with pericardial or Teflon patch
- Elective surgical suture closure

Postoperative/Device Closure Echocardiographic Evaluation

- Right atrial and ventricular size should regress to normal.
- Color flow, PW Doppler, or contrast echo[40] should be used to check for residual shunting around the patch
- Visualization of device and possible migration, obstruction of neighboring structures, perforation or rupture of cardiac structures[41–43]

Ventricular Septal Defects

Anatomy. A communication exists between the ventricles as a result of incomplete septation. Type is determined by location, as listed below.[26,44]

- Perimembranous: including the membranous septum and frequently portions of the muscular septum directly under the aortic valve
- Malalignment: the aorta or pulmonary artery overrides the interventricular septum
- Inflow (atrioventricular canal, endocardial cushion): posterior, at the level of the atrioventricular valves
- Doubly committed subarterial (subpulmonic, supracristal): immediately proximal to the pulmonic valve, in the right ventricular outflow tract
- Muscular: in the body of the ventricular septum; may be localized at the apex or in the anterior, mid, or posterior portion of the muscular septum
- Left ventricular to right atrial shunt: rare; mimics tricuspid regurgitation[45]

Hemodynamics. Blood from the higher-pressure left ventricle courses through the communication into the lower-pressure right ventricle. The greatest volume of blood is shunted during systole, when the pressure difference between the ventricles is most pronounced. Because the pulmonic valve is open during systole, the high-velocity jet from the left ventricle proceeds through the right ventricle directly into the pulmonary artery. The pulmonary vasculature, therefore, is affected more by the increased volume and pressure than the right ventricle. The increased blood volume proceeds into the left atrium and ventricle causing dilatation of these chambers.

The degree of shunting depends on the pulmonary vascular resistance.

Clinical Presentation.[24] Patients usually are asymptomatic if the defect is small, but may present in cardiac failure if the shunt is moderate to large.

Small ventricular septal defect

- Physical exam: palpable thrill over the chest
- Auscultation: harsh holosystolic murmur; variably split second heart sound

Moderate to large ventricular septal defect

- Physical exam: failure to thrive, prominent precordium; left ventricular heave; tachypnea, tachycardia, hepatomegaly
- Auscultation: low-pitched holosystolic murmur; gallop
- ECG: left ventricular hypertrophy with or without right ventricular hypertrophy
- Chest x-ray: dilated pulmonary artery, pulmonary vessels, left atrium, left ventricle

Key Echocardiographic Concepts

- Visualization of defect on 2-D (size and location) and of the shunt (jet) by color-flow Doppler[26,30,46]
- Relationship of ventricular septal defect with neighboring structures (tricuspid, aortic, and pulmonary valves)
- Systolic flow into the right ventricle through the interventricular septum by PW or CW Doppler[10,47]
- Evidence of shunt by contrast echocardiography[44]
- Estimation of right ventricular pressure by determining the pressure gradient through the ventricular septal defect by CW Doppler and subtracting this value from the systolic blood pressure[48]
- Restrictive versus nonrestrictive ventricular septal defect[13]
- Estimation of the magnitude of the shunt by calculation of the $Q_p:Q_s$ by Doppler technique, and mostly by determination of size of left cardiac chambers

Associated Disease

- Multiple ventricular septal defects may occur
- Aortic insufficiency (particularly with doubly committed subarterial and perimembranous types)[26,49]
- Membranous subaortic stenosis[45]

Natural History[6,13]

- Small defects may close spontaneously
- Risk of developing endocarditis
- Aneurysms of tricuspid valve tissue may partially or completely occlude perimembranous ventricular septal defects[44]
- Doubly committed subarterial ventricular septal defects may develop coronary cusp herniation (prolapse) and subsequent aortic insufficiency of increasing severity[49]
- Development of pulmonary vascular obstructive disease if a significant defect remains open
- Increased risk of progression of pulmonary vascular obstructive disease if closure is delayed beyond 2 years of life.

Treatment

- Elective surgical stitch or patch closure
- Repair of aortic valve herniation

Postoperative Echocardiographic Evaluation

- Left atrial and ventricular size should regress to normal[32]
- Assess for peripatch residual shunts by PW Doppler, color flow, or contrast echo[40,13,29]
- Assess for patch dehiscence[32]

Atrioventricular Septal Defects

Anatomy. A spectrum of malformations that occur at the crux of the heart where the atrioventricular valves, interatrial septum, and interventricular septum intersect. These malformations may also be referred to as endocardial cushion defects or atrioventricular canals. Any combination of the following malformations may exist. When there is atrial, ventricular, and atrioventricular valve involvement, the patient is said to have a complete atrioventricular septal defect[50]:

- Primum atrial septal defect
- Inlet ventricular septal defect
- Atrioventricular valve malformation: including cleft mitral valve, single atrioventricular valve, overriding atrioventricular valve, straddling atrioventricular valve
- Common atrium: interatrial septum is completely absent (associated with atrial isomerism)

Hemodynamics. The defects are generally large; therefore, equalization of pressures may occur between chambers, resulting in bidirectional shunting through septal defects. The right heart is dilated because of increased volume or pressure. Atrioventricular valve regurgitation may cause atrial dilatation.

Clinical Presentation.[6,24] Patients are usually symptomatic during infancy.

- Physical exam: failure to thrive, fatigue, dyspnea, heart failure, recurrent respiratory infections
- Auscultation: variety of murmurs
- ECG: left-axis deviation, biventricular hypertrophy
- Chest x-ray: gross cardiomegaly with increased vascular markings

Key Echocardiographic Concepts

- 2-D evaluation of size, location, and additional ventricular and atrial septal defects
- Relative right ventricular and left ventricular size by 2-D[50]
- Atrioventricular valve competency by PW or color-flow Doppler[10]
- Structure of the atrioventricular valves, particularly chordal attachments[44]
- Assessment of spacing of the left ventricle papillary muscles
- Assessment of atrial and/or ventricular unbalance
  - Visualize atrioventricular valve annulus and inflow into the ventricle by color (four-chamber view) and

- Distribution of atrioventricular valve over the ventricles (subcostal view)[51]
- Assessment of pulmonary artery pressure by Doppler methods

Associated Disease[6,32,50]

- Left heart and aortic obstructive lesions
- Secundum atrial septum defects
- Muscular ventricular septal defects
- Atrial isomerisms

Natural History

- Pulmonary vascular obstructive disease develops at an early age[24]

Treatment.[6] Surgery is usually done during the first year of life

- Elective surgical repair of atrioventricular valves and patch closure of septal defects
- Pulmonary artery band: surgical palliation in which supravalvular pulmonary stenosis is created to limit blood flow to the pulmonary vascular bed to retard progression of pulmonary vascular disease

Postoperative Echocardiographic Evaluation

- After definitive repair, evaluate ventricular function, check for residual shunts and assess competency of atrioventricular valves.
- After pulmonary artery banding, determine the anatomic position of the band and the pressure gradient across it by CW Doppler.

OBSTRUCTIVE LESIONS

Left Ventricular Outflow Obstructions

Anatomy. Various types ·of obstruction are listed below.[6,13,26,32]

- Bicuspid aortic valve: one of the commissures remains fused; the most common type of congenital heart disease; frequently hemodynamically insignificant until adulthood
- Unicuspid aortic valve: in place of a valve, there is a membrane with an orifice
- Discrete subaortic stenosis: membrane or ridge in the left ventricular outflow tract; may also affect the anterior leaflet of the mitral valve
- Dynamic subaortic stenosis (idiopathic hypertrophic subaortic stenosis, hypertrophic obstructive cardiomyopathy): thickened interventricular septum; genetically transmitted
- Tunnel aortic stenosis: diffuse narrowing of the left ventricular outflow tract; rare

- Supravalvular aortic stenosis: localized or diffuse narrowing of the ascending aorta, generally just distal to the sinuses of Valsalva; usually associated with Williams syndrome

Hemodynamics. Obstruction increases resistance to flow out of the left ventricle. The left ventricle must, therefore, generate higher systolic pressures to force the blood past the obstruction. This pressure overload results in thickening of the left ventricular walls.

Clinical Presentation.[6,24] Patients are usually asymptomatic unless obstruction is severe.

- Physical exam: anacrotic notch and prolonged upstroke in peripheral arterial pulse; left ventricular lift and precordial systolic thrill may be palpable
- Auscultation: ejection click and systolic ejection murmur, narrowed splitting of the second heart sound; reversed splitting of the second heart sound if obstruction is severe
- ECG: left ventricular hypertrophy
- Chest x-ray : dilated ascending aorta

Key Echocardiographic Concepts

General Concepts

- High-velocity turbulent jet distal to obstruction by PW or color-flow Doppler[8,7,29]
- Increased thickness of left ventricular walls[32]
- Prolonged time to peak velocity (acceleration time to left ventricular ejection time ratio >0.30 suggests pressure >50 mm Hg, >0.55 requires surgery)[7]
- Estimation of pressure gradient through the obstruction by CW Doppler-peak systolic pressure gradient >75 mm Hg and a mean gradient >50 mm Hg with a normal cardiac output is critical aortic stenosis and a surgical emergency[2,6,7]
- Estimation of valve area by continuity equation—area less than 0.5 cm^2 is critical aortic stenosis and a surgical emergency[6]

Valve area:

- Mild stenosis: effective orifice area >1.4 cm^2
- Moderate stenosis: effective orifice area 1.0–1.4 cm^2
- Severe stenosis: effective orifice <1.0 square cm[52]
- Calculation of left ventricular wall stress[32]
- Estimation of left ventricular pressure as posterior left ventricular wall thickness at end systole divided by end-systolic diameter multiplied by 225[53]

Bicuspid Aortic Valve

- Delineation of configuration of cusps and commissural fusion by 2-D

- Doming of cusps on 2-D
- Aortic eccentricity index greater than 1.5 determined by M-mode[32]

Discrete Subaortic Stenosis[26,32]

- 2-D visualization of the membrane from the parasternal long-axis or apical five-chamber and subcostal coronal view
- Premature closure or midsystolic notch on the aortic valve M-mode or PW Doppler tracing
- Coarse systolic fluttering of the aortic cusps on M-mode
- Increased velocity of flow proximal to the aortic valve by PW and color-flow Doppler and development of aortic insufficiency

Dynamic Subaortic Stenosis[54]

- 2-D demonstration of distribution of myocardial thickening
- Late systolic peak on CW Doppler tracing

Tunnel Aortic Stenosis

- 2-D visualization of diffusely narrow left ventricular outflow tract, hypoplastic aortic valve with thick cusps, and hypoplastic ascending aorta[26]

Associated Disease[6]

- Bicuspid aortic valve: aortic insufficiency, coarctation of the aorta and ventricular septal defect
- Unicuspid aortic valve: aortic insufficiency
- Discrete subaortic stenosis: aortic insufficiency

Natural History[6]

- Obstruction usually progresses
- Development of aortic regurgitation

Treatment.[6,13] Patients are generally prophylaxed and may be restricted from participating in competitive sports depending on the degree of stenosis.

- Valvular aortic stenosis: intervention when peak systolic pressure gradient exceeds 75 mm Hg or mean gradient exceeds 50 mm Hg or orifice size decreases to 1 cm^2 of body surface area
  - Percutaneous balloon valvuloplasty[55]
  - Commissurotomy
  - Aortic valve replacement
- Discrete subaortic stenosis: surgical resection of the membrane
- Supravalvular aortic stenosis: surgical resection of obstruction when pressure gradient exceeds 50 mm Hg
- Tunnel aortic stenosis: left ventricular to descending aorta valved conduit,[56] Konno procedure (widening of aortic root and left ventricular outflow tract)

Postoperative Echocardiography Evaluation. Evaluate for residual or restenosis and aortic insufficiency.

Coarctation of the Aorta

Anatomy. There is a discrete or diffuse narrowing of the aorta, most commonly located immediately distal to the left subclavian artery in the area of the ductus arteriosus. Infrequently, the coarctation will occur proximal to the ductus arteriosus or a portion of the aortic arch may be hypoplastic. In either of these cases, patency of the ductus arteriosus may be necessary to perfuse the descending aorta and maintain life.[6]

Hemodynamics. Obstruction to flow at the level of the coarctation results in a build-up of pressure proximal to the obstruction and decreased flow distal to it.[13] Left ventricular walls thicken in response to increased resistance. A high-velocity jet through the obstruction may weaken the aortic wall immediately distal to the obstruction causing post-stenotic dilatation.

Clinical Presentation.[6,24] Presentation varies according to age. In the neonate, the patient may present with heart failure and shock after the ductus arteriosus has closed. Older patients are usually asymptomatic and are treated for hypertension.

- Physical exam: systemic hypertension, with systolic blood pressure much higher in the upper extremities than in the lower extremities[13]; weak femoral pulses; upper body may be more well developed than the lower body
- Auscultation: systolic murmur along the left sternal border transmitting to back and neck; bruits from collateral vessels in older children
- ECG: right ventricular hypertrophy in symptomatic infants; left ventricular hypertrophy in older children
- Chest x-ray: inverted "3" sign at level of coarctation; prominent descending aorta; rib notching in children older than 8 years

Key Echocardiography Concepts

- 2-D evaluation of arch anatomy, including branching and size of branches, measurement of proximal and distal arch diameters, isthmus diameter and proximal descending aortic diameter[57]
- Evaluation of flow in the patent ductus arteriosus
- Evaluation of left ventricular morphology (inflow and outflow) and ventricular size and function
- 2-D visualization of obstruction within the aortic lumen[58,59]
- Determination of gradient by CW Doppler tracing through the coarctation[60]
  - Velocity of flow proximal to the obstruction should be taken into consideration[10]
- Decreased pulsatility on the PW Doppler tracing of the descending aorta (blunted acceleration and slow

deceleration of flow that does not return to baseline during diastole)[10]

Associated Disease[6,59]

- Bicuspid aortic valve (found in as many as 50% of patients with coarctation of the aorta)
- Additional levels of left heart obstruction
- Ventricular septal defects
- Transposition of the great arteries
- Double-outlet right ventricle

Natural History. If unrelieved, as many as 80% of patients die before reaching the age of 50 years.[6]

Neonatal coarctation (ductal dependent systemic blood flow lesion) will present in shock after closure of the ductus

Treatment.[6,13] Early repair seems to decrease probability of residual systemic hypertension.

- Surgical resection of constricted area and primary anastomosis (end to end) or subclavian artery flap to widen aortic lumen. Surgery is the dominant treatment for native coarctation in the neonate.
- Balloon angioplasty and stent placement are commonly used for treatment of native coarctation in older children and adults, and to treat recurrent coarctation.[61,62]

Postoperative Echocardiographic Evaluation

- Assessment of the lumen size and pressure gradient in the area of the re-anastomosis
- PW Doppler spectral tracing of the descending aortic flow may continue to appear somewhat blunted

Hypoplastic Left Heart Syndrome

A spectrum of left-sided hypoplasia in which the left atrium, mitral valve, left ventricle, aortic valve, and aorta may be hypoplastic, stenotic, or atretic. Frequently associated with an atrial septal defect through which pulmonary venous return flows into the right atrium and a patent ductus arteriosus, which in turn supplies the descending aorta.[26]

This is a ductal dependent systemic blood flow lesion.

Treatment[63]

- Prostaglandins started in the immediate neonatal period to ensure patency of the ductus arteriosus and maintain systemic blood flow
- Norwood procedure
- Cardiac transplantation

Pulmonary Stenosis

Anatomy. Obstruction may occur at various levels along the right ventricular outflow tract and the pulmonary arterial system. Types are listed below.[6,24]

- Valvular stenosis: fusion or dysplasia of cusps
- Infundibular stenosis: hypertrophy of muscle bands in the right ventricular outflow tract; usually associated with a ventricular septal defect or valvular pulmonary stenosis[26]
- Double-chamber right ventricle: hypertrophied anomalous muscle bundles in the right ventricle, effectively dividing the right ventricle into two chambers with a communication between them; associated with valvular pulmonary stenosis, perimembranous ventricular septal defects, and subaortic stenosis[44,64]
- Peripheral pulmonary stenosis: may occur as a distinct shelf in the pulmonary artery, discrete narrowing of the pulmonary artery branches, or as diffuse tapered narrowing of the pulmonary artery branches[65]

Hemodynamics. Increased resistance to right ventricular outflow results in a pressure overload to this chamber. The right ventricular walls thicken. Blood flow into the pulmonary arterial system is at high velocity and turbulent. Eddy currents produced distal to the obstruction may cause poststenotic dilatation of the pulmonary artery.[26]

Clinical Presentation.[6] Patients are usually asymptomatic.

- Auscultation: systolic ejection murmur
- ECG: right ventricular hypertrophy
- Chest x-ray: prominent pulmonary artery trunk; large right atrium

Key Echocardiographic Concepts

- 2-D visualization and measurement of pulmonary valve annulus in candidate for balloon angioplasty of valvular stenosis[66]
- 2-D visualization of anomalous muscle bundle and orifice from parasternal and subcostal views[66]
- Measure the diameter of main and branch pulmonary arteries
- Doppler estimation of pressure gradient from all available positions[67]
- Assess right ventricular function, free wall hypertrophy, systolic pressure (based on TR jet estimation)
- Assess tricuspid valve morphology and annulus size
- Determine the presence of a ductus arteriosus
- Accentuation of the "a wave" on M-mode[6]

Natural History[6]

- Increased risk of endocarditis
- Mild valvular and peripheral stenosis (right ventricular pressure <50 mm Hg and a pressure gradient of <40 mm Hg) is considered benign and may or may not progress.

- Severe stenosis (right ventricular pressure >100 mm Hg and a pressure gradient >60 mm Hg) requires relief.[68]
- Infundibular stenosis and anomalous muscle bundles tend to become progressively more obstructive.

Treatment. When the patient becomes symptomatic or pressure gradient exceeds 60 mm Hg[13]

- Balloon valvuloplasty: to relieve valvular and peripheral stenosis[55]
- Surgical valvotomy[6]
- Surgical resection of infundibular muscle or anomalous muscle bundles

Postoperative Echocardiographic Evaluation

- Assess patency of area of former obstruction
- Assess presence and severity of pulmonary insufficiency

Pulmonary Atresia with Intact Ventricular Septum

Anatomy. There is an imperforate membrane or thick fibrous band in place of a pulmonary valve or complete absence of the main pulmonary artery in the absence of a ventricular septal defect.[65,69]

Hemodynamics. Life is dependent on a persistent patent ductus arteriosus. Main and branch pulmonary arteries are usually normal in size.

Clinical Presentation.[6] Severe cyanosis and hypoxemia are seen in the neonate.

- Auscultation: possibly the murmur of a persistent ductus arteriosus
- ECG: right ventricular hypertrophy; right-axis deviation
- Chest x-ray: decreased pulmonary vascular markings

Key Echocardiographic Concepts[6,66]

- 2-D delineation of anatomy
  - Right ventricular outflow tract, location, and size of main pulmonary artery and branches (subcostal coronal and parasternal short axis)
  - Assessment of tricuspid valve anatomy and annulus diameter (annulus predicts outcome—z score of <3 associated with lower likelihood of tolerating right ventricular decompression)[70,71]
  - Associated malformations
- Contrast echocardiography to delineate anatomy
- Doppler and color-flow delineation of flow patterns

Associated Disease[66]

- Persistent ductus arteriosus
- Atrial septal defect or patent foramen ovale

- Malformations of the tricuspid valve
- Coronary arterial sinusoids (interrogate myocardium by color and Doppler at low Nyquist limit)

Natural History

- Death when the persistent ductus arteriosus closes or becomes insufficient to sustain minimal blood oxygenation requirements[6]

Treatment[6,13]

- Prostaglandin: to keep the ductus arteriosus patent
- Palliation with a surgically created systemic to pulmonary shunt
- Surgical reconstruction and/or placement of prosthetic valve
- May need to follow single ventricle palliative route (Glenn–Fontan)

Postoperative Echocardiographic Evaluation

- Evaluate patency of systemic to pulmonary shunt
- Evaluate patency of reconstructed area

Left Ventricular Inflow Obstruction

Anatomy. Left ventricular inflow is obstructed by a membrane in the left atrium or a decrease in the mitral orifice size. Various forms exist, as listed below.[26,44]

- Cor triatriatum: rare; left atrial membrane immediately superior to the fossa ovalis and left atrial appendage
- Supravalvular ring: more common than cor triatriatum; left atrial membrane immediately superior to the mitral valve annulus; usually associated with other mitral valve anomalies[36,72]
- Valvular mitral stenosis: rare; dysplastic valve leaflets, chordae and papillary muscles
- Parachute mitral valve: all chordae insert onto a single papillary muscle
- Arcade mitral valve: chordae insert onto multiple papillary muscles; may be regurgitant
- Double orifice mitral valve: rare; tissue bridge divides mitral valve into two halves and chordae from each half inserting onto a particular papillary muscle; may be regurgitant; associated with atrioventricular malformation[73]
- Mitral valve hypoplasia: small mitral valve annulus and leaflets
- Mitral Atresia: imperforate mitral valve may be associated with a large ventricular septal defect, straddling tricuspid valve, or double-outlet right ventricle

Hemodynamics. Obstruction to left ventricular inflow results in a buildup of pressure in the left atrium causing it to dilate. Pulmonary veins become congested because they cannot empty easily into the left atrium.

Clinical Presentation[6]

- Physical exam: history of recurrent respiratory infections
- Auscultation: diastolic murmur heard best at the apex
- ECG: left atrial enlargement
- Chest x-ray: left atrial enlargement; increased pulmonary vascular markings; right heart enlargement

Key Echocardiographic Concepts

- Delineation of anatomy by 2-D:
  Supravalvar area (cor triatriatum/supravalvar mitral ring)
  Annulus size
  Anatomy of papillary muscles
- Doppler estimation of pressure gradient
- Estimation of orifice size by application of the continuity equation

Associated Disease[6]

- Other levels of left heart obstruction
- Secundum and primum atrial septal defects
- Transposition of the great arteries
- Double-outlet right ventricle

Natural History. The degree of obstruction depends on the valve area, the cardiac output, and the heart rate.[74] Left ventricle inflow obstruction eventually develops into pulmonary vascular obstructive disease.[7]

Treatment[6,74]

- Valvular: balloon valvuloplasty (in attempt to delay surgery); commissurotomy or valve replacement
- Cor triatriatum and supramitral ring: surgical excision of membrane[66]

Postoperative Echocardiographic Evaluation

- Evaluate residual stenosis and regurgitation

Tricuspid Atresia

Anatomy. A dense band of tissue replaces the tricuspid valve preventing direct communication between the right atrium and ventricle. A large atrial septal defect or patent foramen ovale must coexist to provide an outlet to the right atrium (obligatory shunt).[44] The right ventricle is usually small.[13]

Type I: Normally related great arteries; ventricular septal defect or patent ductus arteriosus is path of pulmonary blood flow.

Type II: Transposed great arteries; ventricular septal defect is the path for systemic blood; any restriction causes subaortic stenosis.[75]

Hemodynamics. Deoxygenated systemic venous blood returns to the right atrium and is shunted into the left atrium, where it mixes with oxygenated pulmonary venous return. This mixing of deoxygenated blood with the pulmonary venous return results in a desaturation of the oxygenated blood and, therefore, cyanosis. The right atrium and left heart are generally dilated because of increased flow volume. Because the right ventricle receives blood only indirectly through a ventricular septal defect, it is generally small.[24]

Clinical Presentation.[6,24] Patients are cyanotic with a history of hypoxic spells.

- Physical exam: clubbing of the fingers; delayed growth; hyperactive cardiac impulse at the apex
- Auscultation: single first heart sound; no murmur
- ECG: left ventricular hypertrophy; left axis deviation
- Chest x-ray: decreased vascular markings

Key Echocardiographic Concepts

- 2-D visualization of dense fibrous band across tricuspid annulus and absence of tricuspid valve leaflets
- Dilated right atrium[44]
- Atrial septal defect (determine size and effective shunting) or single atrium
- Small right ventricle or right ventricular outflow tract
- Relationship of great arteries (normally related versus dextro-transposition of the great arteries)

Associated Disease[6,24]

- Atrial septal defect or patent foramen ovale
- Ventricular septal defect and pulmonary stenosis
- Pulmonary atresia
- Transposition of the great vessels (coarctation is common in this group—30%)[75]

Natural History

- Early death without intervention[6]

Treatment[1]

- Pulmonary artery band (surgical palliation to restrict flow to the pulmonary bed)
- Systemic to pulmonary shunt (surgical palliation to increase flow to the pulmonary bed)
- Balloon atrial septostomy (interventional catheterization to increase interatrial shunting)
- Park blade septostomy (interventional catheterization to increase interatrial shunting)
- Fontan procedure: definitive physiologic correction; the right atrium is connected to the pulmonary artery by placement of a patch or conduit in the hope of increasing pulmonary flow[35]

Postoperative Echocardiographic Evaluation

- Assess for right atrial contractility and adequacy of flow through the pulmonary artery

Tricuspid Hypoplasia/Stenosis

Anatomy. There is a small tricuspid valve annulus, usually associated with critical pulmonary stenosis, pulmonary atresia with intact interventricular septum, or Ebstein's anomaly.[44]

Imperforate Tricuspid Valve

Anatomy. Membrane exists in place of a tricuspid valve, which may be surgically opened.[44]

MALFORMATION OF THE TRICUSPID VALVE

Ebstein's Anomaly of the Tricuspid Valve

Anatomy. The septal leaflet is tethered to the interventricular septum and attaches at least 8 mm distal to the tricuspid valve annulus.[32] Other tricuspid leaflets may also adhere to the ventricular wall and be dysplastic.[76] This malformation results in a large "functional" right atrium and small "functional" right ventricle. In Ebstein's anomaly, the tricuspid valve is "off-set" relative to the anterior leaflet of the mitral valve >0.8 mm/m^2.[77] The dysplastic nature of the leaflets and chordae prevents effective coaptation resulting in varying degrees of tricuspid insufficiency and stenosis.[44] Contractility of the right ventricle is affected by its size.

Hemodynamics. The right atrium is dilated because of the volume overload that results from the tricuspid regurgitation. The size of the right ventricle varies with the severity of tricuspid valve leaflet displacement.

Clinical Presentation.[6,24,76] Cyanosis, dyspnea, or exertion, and profound weakness or fatigue may be present.

- Physical exam: prominent left chest
- Auscultation: systolic and diastolic murmurs; loud, widely split first heart sound—"sail sound"; triple or quadruple rhythm
- ECG: right atrial hypertrophy; right bundle branch block; Wolff–Parkinson–White syndrome; paroxysmal supraventricular tachycardia
- Chest x-ray: enlarged heart; decreased pulmonary vascular markings; right atrial enlargement

Key Echocardiographic Concepts

- 2-D delineation of the anatomy of the tricuspid valve and degree of displacement and tethering of each leaflet from parasternal short axis, apical four-chamber and subcostal long- and short-axis views[78]
- Determination of the size of the functional right ventricle— if less than 35% of the size of the anatomic right ventricle, prognosis is poor[32]
- Severity of tricuspid regurgitation

- Tricuspid valve closure delayed greater than 90 m/s after mitral valve closure on M-mode[32]

Associated Disease[6,76,78]

- Persistent patent ductus arteriosus
- Atrial septal defect or patent foramen ovale with right to left shunting
- Mitral valve prolapse
- Pulmonary stenosis
- Pulmonary atresia with intact ventricular septum
- Congenitally corrected transposition of the great vessels
- Ventricular septal defect

Natural History[6,76,78]

- Increased risk of endocarditis
- Prognosis is better with a larger functional right ventricle
- Prognosis is good if the child survives infancy but generally is poor if there are associated lesions

Treatment[6,76,78]

- Annuloplasty: repair of the valve annulus to make it smaller
- Valve replacement
- Valve repair
- Plication of some of the atrialized portion of the right ventricle

Postoperative Echocardiographic Evaluation

- Assess right ventricular function and residual tricuspid insufficiency and/or stenosis

COMPLEX CONGENITAL HEART DISEASE

Tetralogy of Fallot

Anatomy. In this malformation, a large anterior malaligned ventricular septal defect is associated with malalignment of the aorta, so that the aortic root overrides the septal defect. The malalignment of the aortic root contributes to the infundibular pulmonary stenosis that occurs as part of this malformation.[66]

Hemodynamics. The large size of the ventricular septal defect allows equalization of left and right ventricular pressures, so that the shunting through the defect is bidirectional. The overriding aorta receives blood from both ventricles, thereby mixing deoxygenated with oxygenated blood.

Clinical Presentation.[6,24] Cyanosis and a history of "tet spells" (transient cerebral ischemia resulting in limpness, paleness, and unconsciousness); history of squatting may present.

- Physical exam: prominent left chest, "clubbing" of fingers in older patients, right ventricular heave

- Auscultation: single second heart sound; systolic ejection murmur
- ECG: right ventricular hypertrophy; right axis deviation
- Chest x-ray: boot-shaped heart with decreased vascular markings

Key Echocardiographic Concepts[66]

- Assessment of cardiac position
- Assessment of atrial level communication and pulmonary venous return
- 2-D visualization of large perimembranous ventricular septal defect and assessment of degree of aortic override
- 2-D assessment of degree and levels of right ventricular outflow obstruction
- Size of pulmonary valve annulus and morphology
- Size of pulmonary artery and branches from high parasternal short axis and suprasternal notch views (aneurysmally dilated in cases of absent pulmonic valve)[79]
- Thickened RV free wall
- 2-D delineation of coronary artery (rule out anomalous origin of LAD from the right coronary artery or other prominent branches crossing the right ventricular outflow tract) and aortic arch anatomy to determine surgical approach[80]

Associated Disease[6,32,66,79]

- Valvular pulmonary stenosis or pulmonary atresia
- Congenitally absent pulmonic valve
- Right-sided aortic arch
- Atrioventricular malformation (Ebstein's malformation, mitral stenosis, common atrioventricular valve)
- Coronary artery anomalies
- Persistent left superior vena cava

Natural History.[6] Severe infundibular stenosis may result in a fatal "tet spell," in which the infundibulum becomes totally occluded. Recognition and surgical treatment have had a tremendous impact on the natural history of this disease, leaving now a population of adults with repaired tetralogy of Fallot that needs adequate imaging for follow-up.

Treatment[6]

- Palliation by surgical creation of a systemic to pulmonary shunt
- Patch closure of ventricular septal defect and possible myomectomy of the right ventricular outflow tract, pulmonary valvotomy (valve sparing technique) or transannular patch repair

Postoperative Echocardiographic Evaluation

- Evaluation of patency of surgically created systemic to pulmonary shunt

- Evaluation of residual right ventricular outflow obstruction and residual shunting around ventricular septal defect patch
- Evaluation of ventricular function
- Evaluation of degree of pulmonary regurgitation

Transposition of the Great Arteries

Anatomy. The aorta arises from the embryologic right ventricle, and the pulmonary artery arises from the embryologic left ventricle. Terminology is listed below.

- D-transposition of the great arteries (D-TGA, frequently referred to simply as transposition of the great arteries or complete transposition): the ventricles are concordant with the atria; however, the aorta originates from the right ventricle and the pulmonary artery originates from the embryologic left ventricle.
- Congenitally corrected transposition of the great arteries (L-transposition): ventricular inversion with the great vessels originating from the incorrect ventricle; blood flow sequence is normal; however, there is a high incidence of associated congenital heart disease.

Hemodynamics

- D-TGA: Blood flows in two parallel circuits. It flows from the systemic veins into the right atrium, through the tricuspid valve, into the right ventricle and out the aorta, to return again through the systemic veins. Pulmonary venous return flows into the left atrium, through the mitral valve into the left ventricle, and out the pulmonary artery, to return again through the pulmonary veins. In short, deoxygenated blood flows in a continuous loop, and oxygenated blood flows in a separate continuous loop. Unless a communication exists between the systemic and pulmonary circulations (i.e., an obligatory shunt), this situation is incompatible with life. In the newborn period, a left-to-right shunt occurs at the level of the foramen ovale and through a persistent ductus arteriosus, allowing mixing of oxygenated with deoxygenated blood.
- Congenitally corrected TGA: Blood flows in the normal sequence—from the systemic veins into the right atrium, through the mitral valve into the left ventricle, and out the pulmonary artery, returns to the left atrium via the pulmonary veins, courses through the tricuspid valve, into the right ventricle and out the aorta.

Clinical Presentation for D-TGA.[6,24] Newborns become cyanotic, as the ductus arteriosus closes.

- Physical exam: normal weight, healthy-looking infant
- Auscultation: no murmurs; single second heart sound
- ECG: right ventricular hypertrophy
- Chest x-ray: cardiomegaly; narrow mediastinum (egg on a string); increased vascular markings

Key Echocardiographic Concepts[81]

- Identify situs by delineating anatomic atrial landmarks on 2-D
- Identify ventricular morphology (embryologic origins) by delineating anatomic landmarks on 2-D
- Identify great vessel morphology and relationship (will course in parallel fashion)
- Identify and evaluate magnitude of shunt through the obligatory shunt defect(s)
- Delineate coronary artery anatomy for consideration of surgical approach[80]
- Identify and evaluate associated congenital heart disease

Associated Disease for D-TGA[32,81]

- Patent ductus arteriosus: obligatory shunt; most commonly associated with heart disease
- Aortic arch anomalies: coarctation, hypoplastic segment, interrupted aortic arch
- Atrial septal defect or patent foramen ovale: obligatory shunt
- Ventricular septal defect: obligatory shunt; with or without juxtaposed atrial appendages
- Outflow tract obstruction: fixed or dynamic; morphology of aortic and pulmonary valves; degree of aortic or pulmonary regurgitation
- Straddling atrioventricular valve: chordae from one atrioventricular valve attach into both ventricles
- Atrioventricular malformation: rare
- Pulmonary origin of coronary artery

Natural History. Patients with D-TGA must be palliated or repaired on an emergent basis because occlusion of the obligatory shunt would result in immediate death. The mortality rate in the absence of intervention is 95% at the end of 2 years of life.[16]

Patients with congenitally corrected transposition may never know they have congenital heart disease unless there is associated congenital heart disease, in which case, the natural history is determined by the associated disease.

Treatment[6,32,34]

Prostaglandin E₁ Treatment. Palliation; to keep ductus arteriosus patent until arterial switch can be performed.

Balloon Atrial Septostomy (Rashkind Procedure). Palliative interventional catheterization technique in which a distended balloon catheter is torn across a patent foramen ovale or small atrial septal defect creating a large atrial septal defect. Atrial level shunt is the most important site for adequate mixing.

Surgical Atrial Septectomy (Blalock–Hanlon Operation). Palliation

Arterial Switch (Jatene Procedure). Surgical procedure in which the great arteries are taken off their trunks and moved so that each is re-anastomosed to the trunk that will restore a normal blood flow sequence; coronary arteries also are removed and re-implanted into the neoaorta.

Rastelli Procedure (Intraventricular Repair and Extracardiac Conduit). Surgical procedure in which a tunnel is constructed through a large ventricular septal defect so that the left ventricular outflow is directed to the aortic valve and a valved conduit is placed between the right ventricle and pulmonary artery.

Mustard Procedure (Atrial Switch). The atrial switch (Mustard and Senning, see below) is no longer performed as a first line of choice for surgical repair; however, many adult patients with this type of repair survive. Surgical excision of the interatrial septum and placement of a baffle made of pericardium or synthetic material to redirect right atrial flow through the mitral valve into the left ventricle and allow pulmonary venous return to flow around the baffle into the tricuspid valve.

Senning Procedure (Atrial Switch). Surgical reconstruction of the atrial wall and interatrial septum to create an intra-atrial baffle redirecting venous flow through the atria.

Postoperative Echocardiographic Evaluation. Evaluation of left ventricular function.

- Balloon atrial septostomy: 2-D visualization of definitive tear in the interatrial septum and calculation of atrial septal defect size to interatrial septal length ratio[16]
- Arterial switch operation: evaluate anastomotic sites of great arteries for possible constriction, assess intracardiac shunting and regional wall motion and coronary artery flow[6]
- Mustard and Senning procedures: rule out superior vena cava or pulmonary venous obstruction and baffle leaks[6,12] by PW Doppler, color-flow Doppler, or contrast echocardiography[40]

Truncus Arteriosus

Anatomy.[6,24] A rare malformation in which a single large great artery (common trunk) arises from the heart through a single semilunar valve and receives outflow from both ventricles. In most cases, the common trunk overrides the large ventricular septal defect, which must be present. The valve of the common trunk frequently has more than three cusps. Pulmonary circulation occurs in one of the following ways:

- Type I: main pulmonary trunk arises from the common trunk (usually from the posterior aspect) and bifurcates into right and left branches
- Type II: right and left pulmonary arteries arise separately from the left posterolateral aspect of the common trunk
- Type III: right and left pulmonary arteries arise separately from lateral aspects of the common trunk
- Type IV: no pulmonary arteries exist; pulmonary circulation is through bronchiole arteries arising from the descending aorta

Hemodynamics.[6] The large ventricular septal defect causes equalization of pressures between the ventricles. Flow into the pulmonary circulation is at systemic pressures because the pulmonary arteries arise from the aorta, and there is no pulmonary valve. There may be decreased flow to the pulmonary circulation if there is stenosis of the pulmonary branches or in Type IV.

Clinical Presentation.[6,24] Patients are cyanotic.

- Physical exam: early congestive heart failure or hypoxic spells
- Auscultation: single second heart sound; systolic ejection click and murmur
- ECG: biventricular hypertrophy
- Chest x-ray: cardiomegaly; biventricular enlargement; wide mediastinum

Key Echocardiographic Concepts

- 2-D delineation of anatomy:
  - Presence of atrial communication
  - Location and size of ventricular septal defect
  - Atrioventricular valve anatomy
  - Morphology of truncal valve
  - Evaluation of size of pulmonary arteries
  - Additional sources of pulmonary blood flow
  - Aortic arch anatomy and branching
  - Coronary artery anatomy (relation to pulmonary artery and truncal valve leaflets)
  - Associated lesions
- Color-flow and PW Doppler:
  - Truncal valve (rule out stenosis or insufficiency)
  - Pulmonary arteries (suprasternal notch views may be most helpful)
- Assessment of function and size of ventricles

Associated Disease.[6] Usually, truncus arteriosus is an isolated lesion.

- Right aortic arch
- Truncal valve stenosis and/or insufficiency
- Aortic arch anomalies
- Persistent patent ductus arteriosus
- Coronary ostial anomalies
- Absence of a branch pulmonary artery on the side of the arch
- Persistent LSVC
- Anomalous pulmonary venous connections

Natural History.[6] If left untreated, death in infancy from heart failure or later from pulmonary vascular obstructive disease will result. Without intervention, survival beyond 1 year is unusual.

Treatment[6]

- Complete surgical repair involves closure of the ventricular septal defect and removal of the pulmonary arteries from the aorta and placement of a valved conduit between the right ventricle and pulmonary arteries. If coarctation or interrupted aortic arch is present, these are corrected at the same time.

Postoperative Echocardiographic Evaluation

- Evaluate truncal valve (now aortic valve) function
- Evaluate competency of the conduit valve and evaluate pulmonary artery branches for stenosis
- Look for residual lesions (ventricular septal defects)
- Ventricular size and function
- Evaluate aortic arch

ANOMALIES OF THE CORONARY ARTERIES

Kawasaki Syndrome (Mucocutaneous Lymph Node Syndrome)

Definition. Kawasaki disease is an acute systemic vasculitis of unknown cause. It is a common form of acquired heart disease in the pediatric population. The acute phase of the illness features microvascular angiitis, endarteritis, and perivascular inflammation of coronary arteries. The subacute phase may have persistent panvasculitis of the coronary arteries. The convalescent phase shows resolution of the microvascular angiitis replaced by intimal thickening of the coronary arteries. In addition, the inflammatory process may involve pericarditis, myocarditis, and endocarditis.[82]

The proximal branches seem to be most frequently involved. Distal aneurysms may occur in addition, although rarely without proximal involvement.[83]

Clinical Presentation.[84] There is no diagnostic test for Kawasaki disease, so the diagnosis is made clinically. It begins as a febrile illness of more than 5 days in children between 1 and 5 years. In addition to the fever, at least four of the following five findings are noted:

- Physical exam: (1) nonexudative bilateral conjunctivitis; (2) dry, fissured lips, strawberry tongue; (3) polymorphous truncal rash; erythema of palms and soles; (4) desquamation of fingertips and toes; (5) anterior cervical lymphadenopathy of 1.5 cm or greater.

Diagnosis can be made with fewer than four of five criteria in the presence of echocardiographic evidence of coronary involvement.

TABLE 3–1 • Echocardiographic Views Used to Evaluate Coronary Artery Anatomy

Coronary Artery	Echocardiographic View
Proximal right, left main, proximal left anterior descending, proximal left circumflex	Parasternal short axis High parasternal short axis (caudal angle) Subcostal four coronal
Distal right coronary	Subcostal coronal (acute margin of heart) Subcostal short axis (sagittal) Posterior apical four chamber (posterior atrioventricular groove)
Posterior descending	Parasternal short axis Subcostal coronal Apical four chamber
Left circumflex	Parasternal short Parasternal long Subcostal sagittal
Distal left anterior descending	Parasternal long Parasternal short Subcostal coronal

(Data from references 5 and 46.)

- Lab tests: elevated white count, platelet count, erythrocyte sedimentation rate, α_2-globulin, immunoglobulin E, transaminase, and lactic acid dehydrogenase
- ECG: infrequent, minimal changes

Key Echocardiographic Concepts

Acute Phase[80,85]
- Left ventricular dysfunction
- Valvular regurgitation
- Pericardial effusion

Convalescent Phase
- 2-D demonstration of saccular or fusiform coronary aneurysms (Table 3–1)
- Segmental wall motion abnormalities

Natural History. The majority of aneurysms resolve; however, those with diameters larger than 8 mm are at increased risk for thrombosis, which may result in myocardial infarction.[85] Other factors related to aneurysm regression are age younger than 1 year at diagnosis, saccular aneurysm, and distal aneurysm location. Giant aneurysms are more frequently associated with late sudden death from infarction.

Follow Up. Serial echocardiographic exams are performed at 2 weeks and again at 6–8 weeks after diagnosis. This is the time at which transient changes in coronary ectasia or dilatation will resolve or that aneurysms obtain their maximal size.

Imaging of coronary arteries should be performed with the highest transducer frequency possible.

Treatment. Patients are treated with intravenous immunoglobulin and high-dose aspirin per day until defervescence, and then the aspirin is changed to a low dose for 6–8 weeks to decrease risk of thrombosis.

With persistent aneurysms, coronary angiography is indicated at intervals to determine whether coronary artery bypass surgery is indicated.[6]

Anomalous Origin of the Left Coronary Artery

Anatomy. A rare malformation in which the left coronary artery originates from the main pulmonary artery rather than from the aortic root.[80]

Hemodynamics. In the newborn period, the myocardium of the left ventricle is inadequately perfused with oxygen because the blood flowing into the left coronary artery is deoxygenated blood from the pulmonary artery when pulmonary vascular resistance is high; however, this does not cause ischemia. During the transitional period, when pulmonary vascular resistance and pressure decrease, flow in the left coronary becomes retrograde (from right coronary to left coronary via collaterals) and left coronary artery perfusion pressure decreases. This is the usual stage at presentation. Some may pass this stage and present as adults once myocardial ischemia is produced from "steal" phenomenon (left coronary artery drains right coronary blood into the pulmonary artery).

Clinical Presentation.[80] It is symptomatic in infancy.
- Physical exam: irritable, dyspneic, tachypneic
- Auscultation: mitral insufficiency murmur
- ECG: left ventricular hypertrophy with anterolateral myocardial infarction and deep Q wave in lead I and aVL
- Chest x-ray: enlarged heart

Key Echocardiographic Concepts[80]
- 2-D visualization of left coronary artery originating from the pulmonary artery
- 2-D visualization of a dilated right coronary artery originating from the right sinus of Valsalva
- PW Doppler or color-flow demonstration of diastolic flow entering the main pulmonary artery just distal to the pulmonary valve
- Decreased left ventricular contractility
- Mitral insufficiency

Natural History. In the absence of intervention, permanent myocardial damage occurs.

Treatment. Surgery to reimplant the left coronary artery into the aortic root is recommended.[80]

Coronary Arteriovenous Fistula

Anatomy. A variably tortuous coronary artery courses along the surface of the heart or within the myocardium to empty into a cardiac chamber or great vessel. Generally, it is the right coronary artery (60%) that is involved, and the site of drainage is usually a right heart structure.[80]

Hemodynamics. Rather than perfusing the myocardium, blood from the coronary artery flows into the cardiac chamber or vessel into which it empties. The amount of blood that is "stolen" from the myocardium is small, evidenced by the rare presentation of myocardial ischemia. The physiology is more of a shunt and if fistula is large may cause symptoms of volume overload even in infancy.

Clinical Presentation. Generally, patients remain asymptomatic and are diagnosed after investigation of a murmur or incidentally during echocardiographic exam.[84,86]

- Auscultation: atypical continuous murmur

Key Echocardiographic Concepts[87]

- 2-D demonstration of a dilated coronary artery
- 2-D demonstration of origin, course, and site of drainage of the fistula
- Color-flow Doppler visualization and PW Doppler confirmation of a continuous, turbulent jet entering a cardiac chamber or great vessel in a location in which shunt lesions do not enter
- PW Doppler demonstration of turbulent late systolic, early diastolic flow in a dilated coronary artery supplying the fistula

Natural History[87]

- Spontaneous closure may occur
- Bacterial endocarditis
- Congestive heart failure due to volume overload and myocardial ischemia

Treatment. Elective surgical ligation of the fistula.[87]

Postoperative Echocardiographic Evaluation. Check for residual flow through the fistula.

VENUOUS MALFORMATIONS

Persistent Left Superior Vena Cava

Anatomy. In this relatively common malformation (0.5% of the general population and 3–5% of patients with congenital heart disease), a superior vena cava persists in the left chest and travels in front of the left pulmonary artery and between the left atrial appendage and left pulmonary veins. The left superior vena cava may empty into coronary sinus (62%), pulmonary venous atrium (21%), common atrium (17%), or rarely into a left-sided pulmonary vein. In most cases, there is also a right superior vena cava, and in 45–60% of cases, a communication exists between the two superior venae cavae.[88]

Hemodynamics. Systemic venous blood returns to the cardiac chamber to which the left superior vena cava connects. Deoxygenated blood mixes with oxygenated blood (right to left shunt) if the left superior vena cava drains into a left heart structure.

Key Echocardiographic Concepts[35]

- 2-D and color-flow visualization of the left superior vena cava (from a high left parasagittal view)
- Dilated coronary sinus
- Contrast echocardiography to assess for unroofed coronary sinus or drainage into the left atrium[89]
- Absent or small innominate vein

Associated Disease[88]

- Atrial septal defect
- Complex congenital heart disease

Total Anomalous Pulmonary Venous Return

Anatomy. All of the pulmonary veins drain into systemic venous channels. The types of anomalous drainage are listed below.[35,90]

- Supracardiac: pulmonary veins drain in a confluence behind the left atrium and through a vertical vein empty into the innominate vein, superior vena cava, or occasionally the azygous vein. The vertical vein travels usually in front of the pulmonary artery.
- Cardiac: pulmonary veins drain into the right atrium or coronary sinus
- Infracardiac: pulmonary veins form a collection behind the heart and by a common vein descend below the diaphragm and empties into the portal vein, ductus venosus or hepatic vein, reentering the heart through the inferior vena cava. On echocardiogram there is the appearance of an inverted Christmas tree.
- Mixed: a combination of any of the above

Hemodynamics. There is increased flow into a systemic vein, right atrium, or coronary sinus,[90] and ultimately, the right heart. There is an obligatory right-to-left shunt at the atrial level with complete mixing (all chambers will have the same saturation)[24,91]

Clinical Presentation Without Obstruction.[24]   There is mild cyanosis; usually asymptomatic.

- Physical exam: poor growth; prominent left chest; right ventricular heave and hepatomegaly
- Auscultation: fixed, widely split second sound
- ECG: right ventricular hypertrophy
- Chest x-ray: enlarged right heart; increased pulmonary vascular markings; snowman- or figure 8-shaped mediastinum

Clinical Presentation in the Presence of Obstruction.[24]   Patients are acutely ill; there is cyanosis; symptomatic with respiratory distress during the newborn period.

- Physical exam: tachypnea; dyspnea; right ventricular failure
- Auscultation: no murmurs
- ECG: right ventricular hypertrophy
- Chest x-ray: normal size heart; increased pulmonary vascular markings

Key Echocardiographic Concepts[36,90]

- Determine the number of pulmonary veins, their connections, and drainage by 2-D and color Doppler
- Visualization of all systemic venous return to the heart including left innominate vein, superior vena cava, inferior vena cava, and coronary sinus
- Assessment of position and patency of the atrial septum
- Color-flow Doppler interrogation of anomalous venous structures to rule out obstruction, direction of flow direction, as well as restriction of the atrial septum by color-flow and spectral Doppler
- Assessment of right ventricular dysfunction and right ventricular or pulmonary hypertension

Associated Disease

- Atrial septal defect

Natural History.[24]   Obstruction of the common vein or entry into a systemic venous structure will result in pulmonary edema and right heart failure, complete obstruction will cause death. Eventually, pulmonary vascular obstructive disease will develop.

Treatment.   Surgical anastomosis of the common vein with the left atrium and closure of the atrial communication are the indicated treatment.

Postoperative Echocardiographic Evaluation

- Assessment of right ventricular size and function
- Evaluate area of anastomosis and individual pulmonary veins to rule out obstruction. Usually apical views are the best for assessment of the pulmonary venous confluence; individual veins are best seen in subcostal, high parasternal, and suprasternal views.
- Evaluation of right heart and pulmonary artery pressure

TRANSESOPHAGEAL ECHOCARDIOGRAPHY

Transesophageal echocardiography (TEE) is a more invasive echo technique that requires sedation of the patient. A biplane or multiplane echo probe, similar to an endoscope, allows visualization of the heart from the esophagus and stomach. Most of the ultrasound's limiting factors are removed in this technique like lung and bone, allowing for much better imaging and resolution.

Indications: TEE is becoming a standard of care in the operating room during pediatric cardiovascular procedures. It enables the surgeon to delineate anatomy before surgery and evaluate repair effectiveness after surgery and is known to demonstrate anatomic details missed by transthoracic imaging and alter the surgical plan.[92] TEE allows the probe to be left in the patient for the entire procedure with continuous monitoring, although images and hemodynamics are better assessed once reduced or the patient is off cardiopulmonary bypass. Comparison of the preoperative and postoperative left ventricular systolic function has proved helpful in perioperative medical management. Intraoperative TEE is most commonly performed by the echocardiographer or an anesthesiologist.

Routine TEE is performed in cases where acceptable images are not obtained by transthoracic echocardiography (TTE) due to poor acoustic windows (large patients, open chest after surgery, etc.). TEE is superior to TTE in most of these cases, allowing better visualization of valve apparatus, interatrial septum, and most other cardiac structures. Anterior structures such as the right ventricular outflow tract, pulmonary valve, or anterior muscular ventricular septal defects or structures close to an adjacent airway (like the left pulmonary artery and transverse aortic arch) can be difficult to visualize.

TEE is invaluable in situations where assessment of intracardiac vegetations or thrombus is required in patients with poor echocardiographic windows, as well as in the guidance of catheterization procedures such as device closure of atrial and ventricular septal defects or stenting and ballooning complex venous baffles or outflow tract obstruction.[93]

The review of the guidelines for TEE in children is beyond the scope of this chapter but may be accessed by the interested reader from the American Society of Echocardiography.[94]

HYPERTENSION

Long recognized as a contributor to heart disease in adults, hypertension is being diagnosed much more frequently in pediatric patients than in the recent past. Echocardiography is required to assess the effect on the heart.

Clinical Presentation

- Normally asymptomatic and usually noted during routine examinations

Hemodynamics

- In adults, systolic and diastolic pressures may be elevated.

Key Echocardiographic Findings

- Long-standing hypertension can result in left ventricular hypertrophy and increased left ventricular mass, resulting in impaired left ventricular filling.
- Careful evaluation of the patency of the aortic arch is required to exclude clinically unrecognized coarctation of the aorta

Natural History

- Untreated hypertension will result in myriad cardiac abnormalities, including left ventricular outflow obstruction, coronary artery disease, stroke, and kidney failure.

CHEST PAIN AND FATIGUE

Chest pain and fatigue are fairly common complaints among older children and adolescents. The cause is seldom cardiac and usually not serious. However, if cardiac causes are present, they are generally serious.

Causes of Cardiac Chest Pain in Children

1. Congenital coronary abnormalities (rare, associated with exercise, explained by ischemia)
   a. Anomalous coronary origin (left main coronary artery from right coronary artery—left main coronary artery is compressed between great vessels)
   b. Coronary fistula (rare—may cause ischemia from steal phenomenon)
2. Acquired coronary disease
   a. Kawasaki's disease (residual critical narrowing of coronary arteries)
   b. Emboli
3. Aortic stenosis
4. Cardiomyopathy
   a. Hypertrophic cardiomyopathy
   b. Dilated cardiomyopathy
5. Pericarditis
6. Rhythm abnormalities

As previously stated, these are rare, but their seriousness requires that the echo exam for chest pain in children must be accurate and comprehensive. Particular attention should be paid to the coronary arteries.

Fatigue in children is also rarely cardiac related, but some cardiac findings may include the following:

- Dilated cardiomyopathy
- Hypertrophic cardiomyopathy
- Shunts
- Aortic stenosis
- Pulmonic stenosis

As in cases of chest pain, a complete echo exam is required to rule out any cardiac source.

References

1. Anderson R, Ho SY. Echocardiographic diagnosis and description of congenital heart disease: anatomic principles and philosophy. In: St. John Sutton M, Oldershaw PJ, eds. *Textbook of Adult and Pediatric Echocardiography and Doppler.* Boston: Blackwell Scientific; 1989:573-606.

2. Silverman NS, Araujo LML. An echocardiographic method for the diagnosis of cardiac situs and malpositions. *Echocardiography.* 1987; 4:35-57.

3. Foale R, Stefanini L, Rickards A, et al. Left and right ventricular morphology in complex congenital heart disease defined by two-dimensional echocardiography. *Am J Cardiol.* 1982; 49:93.

4. Sutherland GR, Smallhorn JF, Anderson RH, et al. Atrioventricular discordance: cross-sectional echocardiographic morphological correlative study. *Br Heart J.* 1983; 50:8.

5. Tani L, Ludomirsky A, Murphy DJ, et al. Ventricular morphology: echocardiographic evaluation of isolated ventricular inversion. *Echocardiography.* 1988; 5:39-42.

6. Adams FH, Emmanouilides GC, Riemenschneider TA, eds. *Moss' Heart Disease in Infants, Children, & Adolescents.* 4th ed. Baltimore: Williams & Wilkins; 1989.

7. Hatle L, Angelsen B. *Doppler Ultrasound in Cardiology: Physical Principles and Clinical Applications.* 2nd ed. Philadelphia: Lea & Febiger; 1985.

8. Sahn DJ, Valdes-Cruz LM. Ultrasound Doppler methods for calculating cardiac volume flows, cardiac output and cardiac shunts. In: Kotler MN, Steiner RM, eds. *Cardiac Imaging: New Technologies and Clinical Applications.* Philadelphia: FA Davis; 1986:19-31.

9. Cloez JL, Schmidt KG, Birk E, Silverman NS. Determination of pulmonary to systemic blood flow ratio in children by a simplified Doppler echocardiographic method. *J Am Coll Cardiol.* 1987; 11:825-830.

10. Stevenson JG. Doppler evaluation of atrial septal defect, ventricular septal defect, and complex malformations. *Acta Paediatr Scand.* 1986; 329 (suppl):21-43.

11. Stevenson JG. The use of Doppler echocardiography for detection and estimation of severity of patent ductus arteriosus, ventricular septal defect and atrial septal defect. *Echocardiography.* 1987; 4:321-346.

12. Silverman NH, Schmidt KG. The current role of Doppler echocardiography in the diagnosis of heart disease in children. *Cardiol Clin.* 1989; 7:265-297.

13. Fuster V, Driscoll DJ, McGoon DC. Congenital heart disease in adolescents and adults. In: Brandenburg RO, Fuster V, Giulani ER, McGoon DC, eds. *Cardiology: Fundamentals and Practice.* Chicago: Year Book Medical; 1987:1386-1458.

14. Bustamante-Labarta M, Perrone S, Leon de la Fuente R et al. Right atrial size and tricuspid regurgitation severity predict mortality

or transplantation in primary pulmonary hypertension. *J Am Soc Echocardiogr.* 2002; 15:1160-1164.

15. Kosturakis D, Goldberg SJ, Allen HD, et al. Doppler echocardiographic prediction of pulmonary arterial hypertension in congenital heart disease. *Am J Cardiol.* 1984; 53:1110-1114.

16. Marantz P, Capelli H, Ludomirsky A, et al. Echocardiographic assessment of balloon atrial septostomy in patients with transposition of the great arteries: prediction of the need for early surgery. *Echocardiography.* 1988; 5:99-104.

17. Weyman AE, Dillon JC, Feigenbaum H, et al. Echocardiographic patterns of pulmonic valve motion with pulmonary hypertension. *Circulation.* 1974; 50:905-910.

18. Stevenson JG. Comparison of several noninvasive methods for estimation of pulmonary artery pressure. *J Am Soc Echo.* 1989; 2:157-171.

19. Yock PG, Popp RL. Noninvasive estimation of right ventricular systolic pressure by Doppler ultrasound in patients with tricuspid regurgitation. *Circulation.* 1984; 70:657-662.

20. Beard JT, Byrd BF. Saline contrast enhancement of trivial Doppler tricuspid regurgitation signals for estimating pulmonary artery pressure. *Am J Cardiol.* 1988; 62:486-488.

21. Masuyama T, Kodama D, Kitabatake A, et al. Continuous wave Doppler echocardiographic detection of pulmonary regurgitation and its application to noninvasive estimation of pulmonary artery pressure. *Circulation.* 1986; 74:484-492.

22. Friedberg MK, Feinstein JA, Rosenthal DN. A novel echocardiographic Doppler method for estimation of pulmonary arterial pressures. *J Am Soc Echocardiogr.* 2006; 19:559-562.

23. Kitabatake A, Inoue M, Asao M, et al. Noninvasive evaluation of pulmonary hypertension by a pulse Doppler technique. *Circulation.* 1983; 68:302-309.

24. Fink, BW. *Congenital Heart Disease: A Deductive Approach to Its Diagnosis.* 2nd ed. Chicago: Year Book Medical; 1985.

25. Sahn DJ, Allen HD. Real-time cross-sectional echocardiographic imaging and measurement of the patent ductus arteriosus in infants and children. *Circulation.* 1978; 58:343-354.

26. Seward JB, Tajik AJ, Edwards WD, Hagler DJ. *Two-Dimensional Echocardiographic Atlas.* vol I: *Congenital Heart Disease.* New York: Springer; 1987.

27. Smallhorn JF. Patent ductus arteriosus—evaluation by echocardiography. *Echocardiography.* 1987; 4:101-118.

28. Smallhorn JF, Huhta JC, Anderson RH, et al. Suprasternal cross-sectional echocardiography in assessment of patent ductus arteriosus. *Br Heart J.* 1982; 48:321-330.

29. Kyo S. Congenital heart disease. In: Omoto R., ed. *Color Atlas of Real-Time Two-Dimensional Doppler Echocardiography.* 2nd ed. Philadelphia: Lea & Febiger; 1987:149-209.

30. Ritter SB. Application of Doppler color flow mapping in the assessment and the evaluation of congenital heart disease. *Echocardiography.* 1987; 4:543-556.

31. Snider AR. Doppler echocardiography in congenital heart disease. In: Berger M, ed. *Doppler Echocardiography in Heart Disease.* New York: Marcel Dekker; 1987.

32. Armstrong, WF. Congenital heart disease. In: Feigenbaum H, ed. *Echocardiography.* 4th ed. Philadelphia: Lea & Febiger; 1986:365-461.

33. Perry SB, Keane JF, Lock JE. Interventional catheterization in pediatric congenital and acquired heart disease. *Am J Cardiol.* 1988; 61:109G-117G.

34. NeSmith J, Philips J. The sonographer's beginning guide to surgery for congenital heart disease. *J Am Soc Echo.* 1988; 1:384-387.

35. Sanders SP. Echocardiography and related techniques in the diagnosis of congenital heart defects Part I: Veins, atria and interatrial septum. *Echocardiography.* 1984; 1:185-217.

36. Schmidt KG, Silverman NH. Cross-sectional and contrast echocardiography in the diagnosis of interatrial communications through the coronary sinus. *Int J Cardiol.* 1987; 16:193-199.

37. Lin F, Fu M, Yeh, S, et al. Doppler atrial shunt flow patterns in patients with secundum atrial septal defect: determinants, limitations and pitfalls. *J Am Soc Echo.* 1988; 1:141-149.

38. Fraker TD, Harris PJ, Behar VS, et al. Detection and exclusion of interatrial shunts by two-dimensional echocardiography and peripheral venous injection. *Circulation.* 1979; 59:379-384.

39. Valdez-Cruz LM, Sahn DJ. Ultrasonic contrast studies for the detection of cardiac shunts. *J Am Coll Cardiol.* 1984; 3:978-985.

40. Van Hare GF, Silverman NH. Contrast two-dimensional echocardiography in congenital heart disease: techniques, indications and clinical utility. *J Am Coll Cardiol.* 1989; 13:673-686.

41. Hsiao JF, Hsu LA, Chang CJ, et al. Late migration of septal occluder device for closure of atrial septal defect into the left atrium and mitral valve obstruction. *Am J Cardiol.* 2007; 99:1479-1480.

42. Meier B. Iatrogenic atrial septal defect, erosion of the septum primum after device closure of a patent foramen ovale as a new medical entity. *Catheter Cardiovasc Interv.* 2006 ;68:165-168.

43. Baykut D, Doerge SE, Grapow M, et al. Late perforation of the aortic root by an atrial septal defect occlusion device. *Ann Thorac Surg.* 2005; 79:e28.

44. Sanders SP. Echocardiography and related techniques in the diagnosis of congenital heart defects Part II: Atrioventricular valves and ventricles. *Echocardiography.* 1984; 1:333-391.

45. Goldfarb BL, Wanderman KL, Rovner M, et al. Ventricular septal defect with left ventricular to right atrial shunt: documentation by color flow Doppler and avoidance of the pitfall of the diagnosis of tricuspid regurgitation and pulmonary hypertension. *Echocardiography.* 1989; 6:521-525.

46. Ritter S, Rothe W, Kawai D, et al. Identification of ventricular septal defects by Doppler color flow mapping. *Clin Res.* 1988; 36:311A.

47. Stevenson JG, Kawabori I, Dooley T, et al. Diagnosis of ventricular septal defects by pulsed Doppler echocardiography. *Circulation.* 1978; 58:322-326.

48. Murphy DJ, Ludomirsky A, Huhta JC. Continuous-wave Doppler in children with ventricular septal defect: noninvasive estimation of interventricular pressure gradient. *Am J Cardiol.* 1986; 57:428-432.

49. Schmidt KG, Cassidy SC, Silverman, NH. Doubly committed subarterial ventricular septal defects: echocardiographic features and surgical implications. *Am Coll Cardiol.* 1988; 12:1538-1546.

50. Silverman NH, Zuberbuhler JR, Anderson RH. Atrioventricular septal defects: Cross-sectional echocardiographic and morphologic comparisons. *Int J Cardiol.* 1986; 13:309-331.

51. Cohen M. Common atrioventricular canal defects. In: Lai W, Mertens L, et al., eds. *Echocardiography in Pediatric and Congenital Heart Disease—from Fetus to Adult.* Wiley-Blackwell; 2009:230-248.

52. Chambers J. Low "gradient," low flow aortic stenosis. *Heart.* 2006; 92:554-558.

53. Brenner JI, Baker KR, Berman MA. Prediction of left ventricular pressure in infants with aortic stenosis. *Br Heart J.* 1980; 44:406-410.

54. Rakowski H, Sasson Z, Wigle ED. Echocardiographic and Doppler assessment of hypertrophic cardiomyopathy. *J Am Soc Echo.* 1988, 1:31-47.

55. McKay RG. Balloon valvuloplasty for treating pulmonic, mitral, and aortic valve stenosis. *Am J Cardiol.* 1988; 61:102G-108G.

56. Sweeney MS, Walker WE, Cooley DA, et al. Apicoaortic conduits for complex left ventricular outflow obstruction: 10-year experience. *Ann Thorac Surg.* 1986; 42:609-611.

57. Marek J, Fenton M, Khambadkone S. Aortic arch anomalies: Coarctation of the aorta and interrupted aortic arch. In: Lai W, Mertens L, et al., eds. *Echocardiography in Pediatric and Congenital Heart Disease—from Fetus to Adult.* Wiley-Blackwell; 2009:339-361.

58. Huhta JC, Gutgesell HP, Latson LA, et al. Two-dimensional echocardiographic assessment of the aorta in infants and children with congenital heart disease. *Circulation.* 1984; 70:417-424.

59. Nihoyannopoulos P, Karas S, Sapsford RN, et al. Accuracy of two-dimensional echocardiography in the diagnosis of aortic arch obstruction. *J Am Coll Cardiol.* 1987; 10:1072-1077.

60. George B, DiSessa TG, Williams R, et al. Coarctation repair without cardiac catheterization in infants. *Am Heart J.* 1987; 114:1421-1425.

61. Pfammatter JP, Ziemer G, Kaulitz R, et al. Isolated aortic coarctation in neonates and infants: results of resection and end to end anastomosis. *Ann Thorac Surg.* 1996; 62:778-782.

62. Redington AN, Booth P, Shore DF, Rigby ML. Primary balloon dilatation of coarctation of the aorta in neonates. *Br Heart J.* 1990; 64:277-281.

63. Bash SE, Huhta JC, Vick GW, et al. Hypoplastic left heart syndrome: is echocardiography accurate enough to guide surgical palliation? *J Am Coll Cardiol.* 1986; 7:610-616.

64. Cassidy SC, Van Hare GF, Silverman NH. The probability of detecting a subaortic ridge in children with ventricular septal defect or coarctation of the aorta. *Am J Cardiol.* 1990; 66:505-508.

65. Burrows PE, Freedom RM, Rabinovitch M, et al. The investigation of abnormal pulmonary arteries in congenital heart disease. *Radiol Clin North Am.* 1985; 23:689-717.

66. Smallhorn J. Right ventricular outflow tract obstruction. In: St. John Sutton M, Oldershaw P, eds. *Textbook of Adult and Pediatric Echocardiography and Doppler.* Boston: Blackwell Scientific; 1989:761-790.

67. Frantz EG, Silverman NH. Doppler ultrasound evaluation of valvar pulmonary stenosis from multiple transducer positions in children requiring pulmonary valvuloplasty. *Am J Cardiol.* 1988; 61:844-849.

68. Tynan M, Anderson RH. Pulmonary stenosis. In: Anderson RH, Baker EJ, MacCarthy FJ, et al., eds. *Pediatric Cardiology.* 2nd ed. London: Harcourt; 2002:1461-1479.

69. Levine J. Pulmonary atresia with intact ventricular septum. In: Lai W, Mertens L, et al., eds. *Echocardiography in Pediatric and Congenital Heart Disease—from Fetus to Adult.* Wiley-Blackwell; 2009:264-279.

70. Minich LL, Tani LY, Ritter S, et al. Usefulness of the preoperative tricuspid/mitral valve ratio for predicting outcome in pulmonary atresia with intact ventricular septum. *Am J Cardiol.* 2000; 85:1319-1324.

71. Hanley FL, Sade RM, Blackstone EH, et al. Outcomes in neonatal pulmonary atresia with intact ventricular septum. A multi-institutional study. *J Thorac Cardiovascular Surg.* 1993; 105:406-423.

72. Sullivan ID, Robinson PJ, DeLeval M, et al. Membranous supravalvular mitral stenosis: a treatable form of congenital heart disease. *J Am Coll Cardiol.* 1986; 8:159-164.

73. Lipshultz SE, Sanders SP, Mayer JE, et al. Are routine preoperative cardiac catheterization and angiography necessary before repair of ostium primum atrial septal defect? *J Am Coll Cardiol.* 1988; 11:373-378.

74. Geggel RL, Fyler DC. Mitral valve and left atrial lesions. In: Keane J, Lock J, Fyler D, eds. *Nadas' Pediatric Cardiology.* 2nd ed. St. Louis, MO: Saunders Elsevier 2006:697-714.

75. Keane JF, Fyler DC. Tricuspid atresia. In: Keane J, Lock J, Fyler D, eds. *Nadas' Pediatric Cardiology.* 2nd ed. St. Louis, MO: Saunders Elsevier 2006:753-758.

76. Zuberbuhler JR, Anderson RH. Ebstein's malformation of the tricuspid valve: morphology and natural history. In: Anderson RH, Neches WH, Park SC, Zuberbuhler JR, eds. *Perspectives in Pediatric Cardiology.* Mt. Kisco, NY: Futura Publishing; 1988:99-112.

77. Shiina A, Seward JB, Edwards WD, et al. Two-dimensional echocardiographic spectrum of Ebstein anomaly: detailed anatomic assessment. *J Am Coll Cardiol.* 1984; 3:356-370.

78. Silverman NS, Birk E. Ebstein's malformation of the tricuspid valve: cross-sectional echocardiography and Doppler. In: Anderson RH, Neches WH, Park SC, Zuberbuhler JR, eds. *Perspectives in Pediatric Cardiology.* Mt. Kisco, NY: Futura Publishing; 1988:113-125.

79. McIrvin DM, Murphy DJ, Ludomirsky A. Tetralogy of Fallot with absent pulmonary valve. *Echocardiography.* 1989; 6:363-367.

80. Caldwell RL, Ensing GJ. Coronary artery abnormalities in children. *J Am Soc Echo.* 1989; 2:259-268.

81. Smallhorn J. Complete transposition. In: St. John Sutton M, Oldershaw P, eds. *Textbook of Adult and Pediatric Echocardiography and Doppler.* Boston: Blackwell Scientific; 1989:791-808.

82. Yutani C, Go S, Kamiya T, et al. Cardiac biopsy of Kawasaki disease. *Arch Pathol Lab Med.* 1981; 105:470-473.

83. Neches WH. Kawasaki syndrome. In: Anderson RH, Neches WH, Park SC, Zuberbuhler JR, eds. *Perspectives in Pediatric Cardiology.* Mt. Kisco, NY: Futura Publishing; 1988:411-424.

84. Lloyd TR, Mahoney LT, Marvin WJ, et al. Identification of coronary artery to right ventricular fistulae by color flow mapping. *Echocardiography.* 1988; 5:115-120.

85. Meyer RA. Echocardiography in Kawasaki disease. *J Am Soc Echo.* 1989; 2:269-275.

86. Keane JF, Fyler DC. Vascular fistulae. In: Keane J, Lock J, Fyler D, eds. *Nadas' Pediatric Cardiology.* 2nd ed. St. Louis, MO: Saunders Elsevier; 2006:799-804.

87. Velvis H, Schmidt KG, Silverman NH, et al. Diagnosis of coronary artery fistula by two-dimensional echocardiography pulsed Doppler ultrasound and color flow imaging. *J Am Coll Cardiol.* 1989; 14:968-976.

88. Zellers TM, Hagler DJ, Julsrud PR. Accuracy of two-dimensional echocardiography in diagnosing left superior vena cava. *J Am Soc Echo.* 1989; 2:132-138.

89. Huhta, JC, Smallhorn JF, Macartney FJ, et al. Cross-sectional echocardiographic diagnosis of systemic venous return. *Br Heart J.* 1980; 44:718-723.

90. Van Hare GF, Schmidt KG, Cassidy SC, et al. Color Doppler flow mapping in the ultrasound diagnosis of total anomalous pulmonary venous connection. *J Am Soc Echo.* 1988; 1:341-347.

91. Keane JF, Fyler DC. Total anomalous pulmonary venous return. In: Keane J, Lock J, Fyler D, eds. *Nadas' Pediatric Cardiology.* 2nd ed. St. Louis, MO: Saunders Elsevier; 2006:773-781.

92. Randolph GR, Hagler DJ, Connoly HM, et al. Intraoperative transesophageal echocardiography during surgery for congenital heart defects. *J Thorac Cardiovasc Surg.* 2002; 124:1176.

93. van der Velde EA. Echocardiography in the catheterization laboratory. In: Lock JE, Keane JF, Perry SB, eds. *Diagnostic and Interventional Catheterization in Congenital Heart Disease.* Norwell, MA: Kluwer Academic Publishers; 2000:355.

94. Fyfe DA, Ritter SB, Snider AR, et al. Guidelines for transesophageal echocardiography in children. *J Am Soc Echocardiogr.* 1992; 5:640.

Questions

GENERAL INSTRUCTIONS: For each question, select the best answer. Select only one answer for each question unless otherwise specified.

1. What is the most common type of atrial septal defect?

   (A) primum
   (B) secundum
   (C) sinus venosus
   (D) single atrium

2. Which transducer position is most helpful in the 2-D visualization of atrial septal defects?

   (A) left parasternal
   (B) apical
   (C) subxiphoid
   (D) right parasternal

3. Partial anomalous pulmonary venous return is most commonly associated with which type of atrial septal defect?

   (A) secundum
   (B) primum
   (C) sinus venosus
   (D) coronary sinus

4. What is the most common congenital heart lesion in the pediatric population?

   (A) mitral stenosis
   (B) atrial septal defect
   (C) ventricular septal defect
   (D) pulmonary stenosis

5. A "T-sign" artifact demonstrated by _____ is useful in the detection of ventricular septal defects.

   (A) M-mode
   (B) 2-D
   (C) pulsed-wave Doppler
   (D) continuous-wave Doppler
   (E) color-flow Doppler

6. A small muscular ventricular septal defect may be most easily localized by which of the following?

   (A) M-mode
   (B) 2-D
   (C) pulsed-wave Doppler
   (D) continuous-wave Doppler
   (E) color-flow Doppler

7. Which of the following will *not* cause a reversal of flow in the descending aorta during diastole?

   (A) large patent ductus arteriosus with severe pulmonary hypertension (suprasystemic pulmonary pressures)
   (B) severe aortic insufficiency
   (C) surgically created systemic to pulmonary shunt with normal pulmonary artery pressures
   (D) large patent ductus arteriosus with normal pulmonary artery pressures

8. Which of the following may be associated with valvar aortic stenosis?

   (A) patent ductus arteriosus
   (B) coarctation of the aorta
   (C) ventricular septal defect
   (D) pulmonary stenosis
   (E) all of the above

9. Which of the following is the most commonly associated findings in patients with coarctation of the aorta?

   (A) ventricular septal defect
   (B) bicuspid aortic valve
   (C) patent ductus arteriosus
   (D) aortic stenosis
   (E) mitral stenosis

10. In the normally related heart, where does the aortic valve lie?

    (A) anterior and to the left of the pulmonary valve
    (B) anterior and to the right of the pulmonary valve
    (C) posterior and to the right of the pulmonary valve
    (D) posterior and to the left of the pulmonary valve

11. Which of the following surgical procedures is *not* frequently used to treat transposition of the great arteries?

    (A) Senning procedure

    (B) Mustard procedure

    (C) arterial switch procedure

    (D) Fontan procedure

12. Which of the following is also known as the arterial switch procedure?

    (A) Rashkind procedure

    (B) Mustard procedure

    (C) Jatene procedure

    (D) Senning procedure

13. When the aorta and pulmonary artery are transposed, they course _____ as they exit the heart.

    (A) parallel to each other

    (B) perpendicular to each other

    (C) wound around each other

    (D) in no particular relationship to each other

14. Balloon atrial septostomy is most commonly performed in infants who have which of the following?

    (A) Ebstein's anomaly of the tricuspid valve

    (B) transposition of the great arteries

    (C) truncus arteriosus

    (D) tetralogy of Fallot

15. Of all children who suffer from Kawasaki disease, what percentage will develop coronary artery aneurysms?

    (A) 2%

    (B) 15%

    (C) 50%

    (D) 75%

    (E) 100%

16. Which of the following groups is most likely to develop coronary artery aneurysms as a complication of Kawasaki disease?

    (A) toddlers

    (B) infants

    (C) adolescents

    (D) adults

17. Which of the following is useful in the assessment of pulmonary artery pressure?

    (A) peak Doppler gradient through a patent ductus arteriosus

    (B) peak Doppler gradient of tricuspid regurgitation

    (C) end-diastolic Doppler gradient of pulmonary insufficiency

    (D) acceleration time to ejection time ratio calculated from a right ventricular outflow tract velocity curve

    (E) all of the above are useful in estimating pulmonary artery pressure

18. A child with tetralogy of Fallot is upset and crying during the echocardiogram. The Doppler gradient through the right ventricular outflow tract will be _____ than if the child were sleeping peacefully.

    (A) greater

    (B) less

    (C) outflow obstruction in tetralogy of Fallot is not affected by the patient's activity

19. A 3-year old child with Kawasaki disease undergoes an echocardiogram. Which of the following views is *not* really necessary in the 2-D evaluation of the coronary arterial system?

    (A) subcostal transverse

    (B) parasternal short axis

    (C) apical five chamber

    (D) subcostal coronal

    (E) all views are helpful

20. Which of the following Doppler findings is *not* characteristic of coarctation of the aorta?

    (A) forward flow through the descending aorta extending throughout diastole

    (B) normal or slightly increased velocity of flow in the aorta proximal to the left subclavian artery

    (C) rapid acceleration and deceleration of the Doppler signal taken from the descending aorta

    (D) Doppler signal from the descending aorta does not return to baseline during diastole

    (E) high-velocity flow detected in the descending aorta distal to the left subclavian artery

21. Careful echocardiographic evaluation of a child with complex congenital heart disease reveals absence of the inferior vena cava above the level of the renal arteries. The aorta is to the left of the spine. What is this child's situs mostly likely to be?

(A) solitus

(B) inversus

(C) left atrial isomerism

(D) right atrial isomerism

22. Which of the following characteristics will be demonstrated on the aortic valve M-mode tracing from a patient with discrete membranous subaortic stenosis?

(A) an asymmetric closure line

(B) early closure and partial reopening

(C) gradual closure (drifting closed)

(D) prolonged ejection time

23. Which of the following should *not* be included in the differential diagnosis when a Doppler tracing such as that in Fig. 3–1 is obtained from the descending aorta?

(A) patent ductus arteriosus

(B) severe aortic regurgitation

(C) arteriovenous malformation

(D) aortic to pulmonary window

(E) coarctation of the aorta

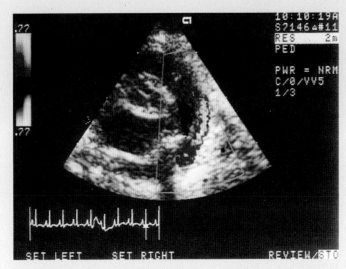

FIGURE 3–2. Color-flow Doppler image of a modified short-axis parasternal view, known as the "ductus view." The patient is a premature infant in congestive heart failure in whom a murmur is heard.

24. An echocardiogram was requested for a premature infant in the neonatal intensive care unit who appeared clinically to be in congestive failure and in whom a murmur was heard. The color-flow Doppler image in Fig. 3–2 was taken from the ductus view, which is a parasternal sagittal view. The closed aortic valve may be appreciated in the center of the image. What does this image demonstrate?

(A) a small patent ductus arteriosus

(B) a moderate patent ductus arteriosus

(C) a large patent ductus arteriosus

(D) no ductus arteriosus

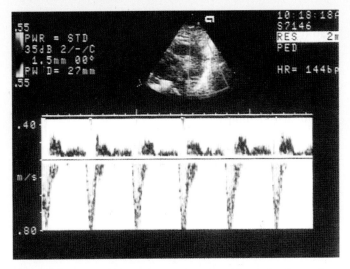

FIGURE 3–1. Pulsed Doppler spectral tracing of flow in the descending aorta as obtained from the suprasternal notch view.

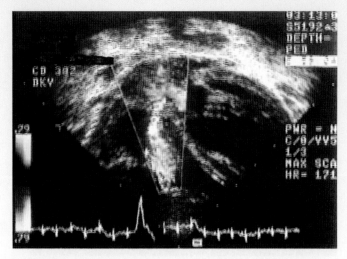

FIGURE 3–3. Color-flow Doppler image of a subcostal four-chamber view presented with the apex down (anatomically correct) presentation. The patient is an 8-month-old female with trisomy 21.

25. The image in Fig. 3–3 was taken from an 8-month-old female with trisomy 21. The color-flow Doppler image was taken from the subcostal four-chamber view. What does the image demonstrate?

(A) a left-to-right shunt through a primum atrial septal defect

(B) a right-to-left shunt through a primum atrial septal defect

(C) a left-to-right shunt through a secundum atrial septal defect

(D) a right-to-left shunt through a secundum atrial septal defect

(E) a normal heart

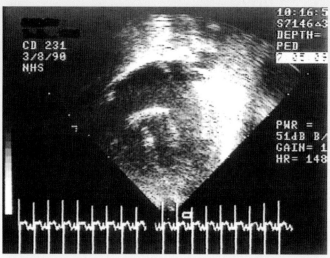

A

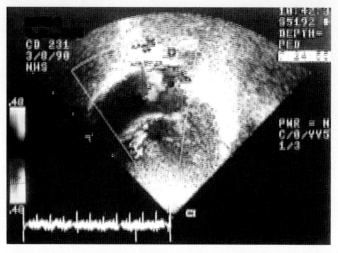

B

FIGURE 3–4. Apical four-chamber view presented with the apex down. (**A**) 2-D image. (**B**) Color-flow Doppler image. The patient is a cyanotic infant.

26. The images presented in Fig. 3–4 were taken from the cardiac apex of a cyanotic infant. What do these images demonstrate?

(A) a normal heart

(B) an isolated inflow ventricular septal defect

(C) single atrium

(D) tricuspid atresia with ventricular septal defect

(E) tricuspid atresia with intact ventricular septum

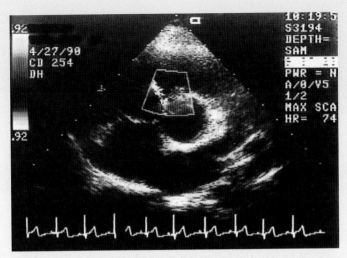

FIGURE 3–5. Color-flow Doppler image of the parasternal short-axis view at the level of the semilunar valves taken in early systole. The patient is an 8-year-old boy in whom a systolic murmur may be heard.

27. The color-flow Doppler image presented in Fig. 3–5 was taken from an 8-year-old boy with a systolic murmur. The image is of the parasternal short-axis view during early systole and demonstrates a left to right shunt through which of the following?

(A) inflow ventricular septal defect

(B) membranous ventricular septal defect

(C) muscular ventricular septal defect

(D) doubly committed subarterial ventricular septal defect

28. The 2-D image in Fig. 3–6 was taken from the cardiac apex. What does the image demonstrate?

(A) a normal apical four-chamber view

(B) tricuspid atresia

(C) Ebstein's anomaly of the tricuspid valve

(D) ventricular inversion

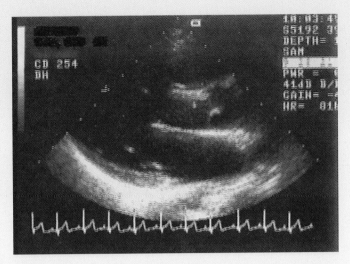

FIGURE 3–7. 2-D image of a parasternal long-axis view taken in diastole.

29. The 2-D image of the parasternal long-axis view presented in Fig. 3–7 was taken during diastole. What does the image demonstrate?

(A) a normal heart

(B) valvular aortic stenosis

(C) discrete membranous subaortic stenosis

(D) idiopathic hypertrophic subaortic stenosis

30. If the left ventricular outflow tract of the patient presented in Fig. 3–7 was interrogated by pulsed-wave Doppler, what is the most proximal location at which an increase in velocity would be detected?

(A) just proximal to the aortic valve

(B) at the aortic valve

(C) just distal to the aortic valve

(D) in the aortic root

(E) distal to the left subclavian artery

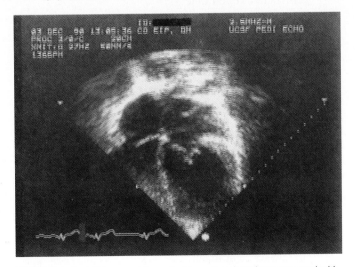

FIGURE 3–6. 2-D image of the apical four-chamber view presented with the apex down.

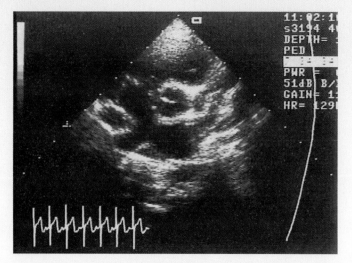

FIGURE 3–8. 2-D image of a parasternal short-axis view at the level of the semilunar valves. The patient is a young child who is in the convalescent phase of Kawasaki's disease.

31. The 2-D parasternal short-axis view image presented in Fig. 3–8 was taken from a young child who had recently had Kawasaki disease. What does this view demonstrate?

(A) left coronary artery involvement

(B) right coronary artery involvement

(C) both left and right coronary arteries are involved

(D) normal coronary arteries

32. The 2-D parasternal short-axis view image presented in Fig. 3–9 was taken from an infant who was diagnosed as having tetralogy of Fallot. What does this image demonstrate?

(A) a normal right ventricular outflow tract

(B) infundibular pulmonary stenosis only

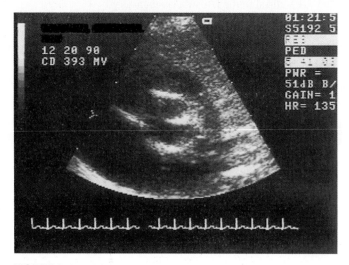

FIGURE 3–9. 2-D image of a parasternal short-axis view at the level of the semilunar valves. This infant has been diagnosed as having tetralogy of Fallot.

(C) infundibular and valvular pulmonary stenosis

(D) infundibular pulmonary stenosis with hypoplasia of the pulmonary valve and main pulmonary artery

33. Which of the following views would *not* be helpful in delineating the size of left and right pulmonary arteries in the patient imaged for Fig. 3–9?

(A) suprasternal coronal view

(B) apical outflow view

(C) subcostal short axis (sagittal) view

(D) high left parasternal view

(E) all of the above views would be useful

34. Which of the following methods is most reliable for estimating pulmonary artery pressures?

(A) thickness of the right ventricular free wall

(B) determination of the peak regurgitant gradient through the tricuspid valve

(C) determination of the peak regurgitant gradient through the pulmonic view

(D) dividing the acceleration time by the ejection time of flow as obtained from the main pulmonary artery

35. In which of the following surgically created shunts is the shunt originating from the innominate artery?

(A) central

(B) Glenn

(C) Waterston

(D) Blalock–Taussig

(E) Potts

36. What is needed to estimate Q_p:Q_s in a patient with a ventricular septal defect?

(A) diameters and peak flow velocities through the pulmonary and aortic valves

(B) peak pressure gradient through a tricuspid regurgitation jet

(C) diameters and peak flow velocities through the tricuspid and aortic valves

(D) diameters and peak flow velocities through the pulmonary and mitral valves

37. Which of the following is true about the shunt through the atrial septal defect of a patient with tricuspid atresia?

(A) always left to right

(B) always right to left

(C) may be bidirectional

(D) nonexistent

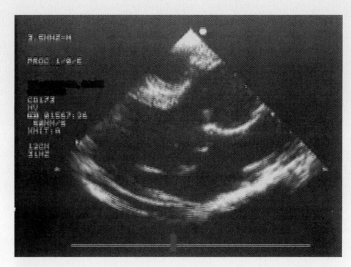

FIGURE 3–10. 2-D image of a parasternal long-axis view. The patient is an adolescent girl thought to have Marfan syndrome.

38. The 2-D image parasternal view presented in Fig. 3–10 was taken from an adolescent girl with Marfan syndrome. What abnormalities may be seen that are frequently associated with Marfan syndrome?

    (A) dilated aortic root and mitral valve prolapse

    (B) aortic aneurysm dissection

    (C) idiopathic hypertrophic subaortic stenosis

    (D) herniation of the sinus of Valsalva

39. The 2-D image presented in Fig. 3–11 was taken from the apex in a child who has had corrective surgery for transposition of the great arteries. What does the echogenic line in the left atrium represent?

    (A) cor triatriatum

    (B) supramitral ring

    (C) total anomalous pulmonary venous return

    (D) an interatrial baffle

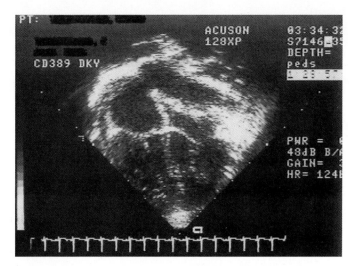

FIGURE 3–11. 2-D image of an apical four-chamber view presented with the apex down. This young child has had a previous repair for transposition of the great vessels.

40. If a patient has total anomalous pulmonary venous return, which of the following is descriptive of the right atrium?

    (A) atretic

    (B) small

    (C) normal in size

    (D) dilated

41. What is the most useful modality in the delineation of anatomy in total anomalous pulmonary venous return?

    (A) 2-D

    (B) M-mode

    (C) pulsed-wave Doppler

    (D) continuous-wave Doppler

    (E) color-flow Doppler

TRUE OR FALSE: Indicate whether each of the following statements is true or false.

42. Patent ductus arteriosus is more commonly seen in low-birth-weight premature infants than in term infants.

43. Patency of the ductus arteriosus may be desirable in some cases.

44. In cor triatriatum, the left atrial appendage is continuous with the anatomic left atrium and not with the proximal chamber that receives flow directly from the pulmonary veins.

45. Children with trisomy 21 frequently have partial atrioventricular septal defects.

46. Patients with truncus arteriosus are usually quite cyanotic in infancy.

47. Individuals with Ebstein's anomaly of the tricuspid valve are always symptomatic.

48. Distal coronary artery aneurysms are common in the absence of proximal aneurysm formation in patients who have had Kawasaki disease.

49. In patients with coarctation of the aorta, the gradient through the obstruction should approximate the difference in systolic blood pressures taken from the arm and leg of the patient.

50. Persistent left superior vena cava may exist in the absence of a dilated coronary sinus.

For each of the following transducer positions, indicate (true or false) whether the position could yield the highest pressure gradient estimate in a patient with valvular pulmonary stenosis.

51. parasternal

52. apical

53. subcostal

54. suprasternal

The 2-D image in Fig. 3–12 was obtained by placing the transducer at the cardiac apex of an infant. The infant was referred to echocardiology because of an enlarged heart on chest x-ray and cardiac failure. A systolic murmur may be heard at the apex. Indicate whether statements 55–60 are true or false for this image.

55. There is a secundum atrial septal defect.

56. There is a primum atrial septal defect.

57. The tricuspid valve appears normal.

58. The left ventricle is significantly smaller in size than the right ventricle.

59. The diagnosis for this patient is Ebstein's anomaly of the tricuspid valve.

60. The systolic murmur is probably caused by aortic stenosis.

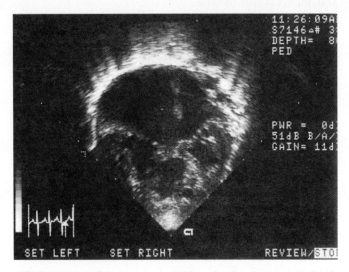

FIGURE 3–12. 2-D image of an apical four-chamber view presented with the apex down. This infant was in cardiac failure and reportedly had an enlarged heart on chest-x-ray. A systolic murmur may be heard at the apex.

Answers and Explanations

At the end of each explained answer, there is a number combination in parentheses. The first number identifies the reference source; the second number or set of numbers indicates the page or pages on which the relevant information can be found.

1. **(B)** Secundum. Sinus venosus is the rarest form, and the single atrium is not considered to be an atrial septal defect because there is complete absence of the atrial septum. *(13:1391)*

2. **(C)** In the subxiphoid position, the sound beam is perpendicular to the interatrial septum, thereby utilizing the axial resolution of the transducer. The atrial septum may also be visualized from the parasternal short-axis view, but it is more parallel to the sound beam and, therefore, may not be resolved optimally. In the apical position, the sound beam is parallel to the atrial septum, and the atrial septum is a great distance from the transducer, so echocardiographic dropout may be mistaken for an atrial communication. *(26:144–147)*

3. **(C)** Sinus venosus atrial septal defects are bordered posteriorly by the posterior atrial wall and superiorly by the entrance of the superior vena cava. Because of this, the upper right pulmonary vein may empty into the right atrium or superior vena cava. *(6:175)*

4. **(C)** Ventricular Septal Defect. Atrial septal defect and pulmonary stenosis are also common. Mitral stenosis is relatively uncommon in the pediatric population. *(6:190)*

5. **(B)** The "T" artifact is visualized on 2-D echocardiography as a prominence of echoes at the edges of the septal tissue. *(32:415)*

6. **(E)** Muscular ventricular septal defects may occur anywhere and be very small. Color-flow Doppler allows relatively rapid evaluation of the entire interventricular septum. Visualization of a jet of turbulent flow identifies a ventricular septal defect; pulsed-wave or continuous-wave Doppler interrogation can be tedious and may miss a small muscular defect in an unusual position. *(30:544–548)*

7. **(A)** When pulmonary pressures exceed systemic pressures, the flow through the patent ductus arteriosus will be right to left; therefore, there would be no reversal in the descending aorta. All of the other choices should cause a reversal of flow in the descending aorta. *(12:285–287)*

8. **(E)** Although patent ductus arteriosus and coarctation of the aorta are more commonly associated with valvar aortic stenosis, ventricular septal defect and pulmonary stenosis may also be associated. *(6:224)*

9. **(B)** Although all of the listed malformations may be associated findings, bicuspid aortic valve has been reported to be an associated finding in as much as 85% of cases. *(6:244)*

10. **(C)** The aortic view is posterior and to the right of the pulmonic valve in the normally related heart. The aortic valve is located centrally in the base of the heart, whereas the pulmonic valve is anterior and left. *(1:578–581)*

11. **(D)** The Fontan procedure was originally developed to treat patients with tricuspid atresia. Although it is now used in a modified form to treat other forms of complex congenital heart disease, it is not commonly used to treat patients with transposition of the great arteries. *(6:357–359, 402–417)*

12. **(C)** The Jantene procedure. The Rashkind procedure is an interventional catheterization technique that also is known as a balloon atrial septostomy. The Mustard and Senning procedures also are known as atrial switches. *(6:402–417)*

13. **(A)** Normally related great vessels course perpendicular to each other. Demonstration of this relationship rules out transposition of the great vessels. *(26:498)*

14. **(B)** The purpose of an atrial septostomy is to mix deoxygenated systemic venous return with oxygenated pulmonary venous return. In truncus arteriosus and tetralogy of Fallot, this mixing occurs through a large ventricular septal defect. In Ebstein's anomaly of the tricuspid valve, blood flow sequence is normal; therefore, mixing is not desirable. *(6:399–400)*

15. **(B)** There is about a 15–25% incidence of coronary artery aneurysm formation in children with untreated Kawasaki disease. *(85:269)*

16. **(B)** Kawasaki disease is a childhood disease. Infants seem to be more likely to develop aneurysms than other children. *(85:273)*

17. **(E)** All of the above that are available should be used. *(7:223; 18:157–171)*

18. **(A)** Greater. The right ventricular outflow obstruction of tetralogy of Fallot is a dynamic obstruction; therefore, it may increase when the patient is distressed. *(6:278)*

19. **(E)** Although the proximal portions are the most frequently involved, the coronary system should be evaluated from every available view because aneurysms may occur anywhere. *(85:269–273)*

20. **(C)** In coarctation of the aorta, the descending aortic flow pulsatility is blunted such that the Doppler signal shows a slow acceleration and deceleration. *(7:217–221)*

21. (D) Right atrial isomerism. *In situ* solitus, the aorta descends anterior and to the left of the spine and the inferior vena cava ascends to the right of the spine. *In situ* inversus, the opposite is true. In left atrial isomerism, the inferior vena cava is frequently interrupted. (2:35–56)

22. (B) Early closure and partial reopening. An asymmetric closure line is suggestive of a bicuspid aortic valve. Gradual closure is suggestive of depressed left ventricular contractility. Ejection time may be prolonged in severe valvular aortic stenosis. (32:380–386)

23. (E) Reversal of flow during diastole, as shown in Fig. 3–1, may be seen in any of the other conditions. The characteristic pulsed-wave Doppler pattern in the descending aorta is very different for coarctation of the aorta. (7:217–228; 12:279–295)

24. (B) From the ECG, we can see that this is an end-diastolic frame. The 2-D image shows closed aortic and pulmonary valves, confirming that this is an end-diastolic frame. Red color representing flow toward the transducer may be appreciated coming into the main pulmonary artery from the patent ductus arteriosus. (29:161, 162, 189, 190)

25. (C) The red jet seen traversing the interatrial septum represents flow coming toward the transducer, therefore, it is shunting from the left atrium to the right atrium. Portions of the superior and inferior interatrial septum may be seen in the 2-D image. (30:548–550)

26. (D) The mitral valve is open in Fig. 3–4A. A thick bank of tissue appears in place of a normal tricuspid valve. A ventricular septal defect may be appreciated at the top of the ventricular septum in this image. In Fig. 3–4B, flow through the ventricular septal defect into the right ventricle is demonstrated by color-flow Doppler during systole. (32:374–375)

27. (B) Flow through an inflow ventricular septal defect would be visualized at the level of the mitral annulus. Flow through a doubly committed subarterial ventricular septal defect would be visualized just proximal to the pulmonary valve in this view. Flow through a muscular ventricular septal defect would be visualized in the muscular portion of the ventricular septum. This portion of the ventricular septum is visible from the parasternal short axis at the level of the mitral valve and more apically. (32:155–161, 183–188)

28. (D) The mitral valve is always higher on the ventricular septum in the absence of an inflow ventricular septal defect. In this case, the atrioventricular valve of the right-sided ventricle inserts higher on the ventricular septum than the atrioventricular valve of the left-sided ventricle. (26:324, 325)

29. (C) Discrete membranous subaortic stenosis. The aortic valve is closed and does not appear thickened. There is an echogenic line that extends posteriorly from the ventricular septum just proximal to the aortic valve. This represents a discrete subaortic membrane. In idiopathic hypertrophic subaortic stenosis, the interventricular septum would be significantly thickened. (26:424–427)

30. (A) Valvular aortic stenosis would cause the velocity of flow to increase just distal to the valve. Supravalvular aortic stenosis would cause the velocity of flow to increase in the aortic root. Coarctation of the aorta would cause the velocity of flow to increase past the level of the left subclavian artery. (32:382)

31. (C) The left coronary artery appears mildly dilated, and the large circle noted in the right atrium is the right coronary artery (with aneurysmal dilatation) as it courses within the right atrioventricular groove. (85:268–273)

32. (D) The entire right ventricular outflow tract is small in caliber. (26:434)

33. (E) The pulmonary artery branches may be imaged from all of these views. (66:767–782)

34. (B) The thickness of the right ventricular free wall may not be proportionate to the increase in pulmonary artery pressure. The end-diastolic and not peak gradient of pulmonary regurgitation may be used. Acceleration and ejection time should be measured from the right ventricular outflow tract. (18:157–171)

35. (D) The modified Blalock–Taussig shunt is a Gore-Tex tube that provides pulmonary blood flow with its takeoff from the innominate artery (the classic Blalock–Taussig shunt connected the subclavian artery to the pulmonary artery—rarely in use these days). In a central shunt, the pulmonary artery is connected to the aorta directly or via a conduit. In the Waterston shunt, the ascending aorta is connected to the right pulmonary artery, and in the Potts anastomosis, the descending aorta is connected to the pulmonary artery. Both the Waterston and the Potts shunts are rarely used today but occasionally can be found in adult congenital patients. (34:384, 385)

36. (A) $Q_p:Q_s$ is a comparison of pulmonary flow to systemic flow used to estimate the amount of blood flow through a systemic to pulmonary shunt. Flow is calculated by multiplying area by velocity of flow. This calculation must be done for the systemic circulation and for the pulmonary circulation. When the shunt is at the level of the ventricles, pulmonary flow may be calculated using the pulmonary valve or the mitral valve (i.e., pulmonary venous return). The systemic flow may be calculated by using the aortic valve or tricuspid valve (i.e., systemic venous return). The calculation is done to determine how much more blood is going through the pulmonary vasculature than the systemic vasculature. (9:825–827; 11:339–344)

37. (B) Because the atrial septal defect is the only outlet for the blood in the right atrium, it is an obligatory right-to-left shunt. (32:375)

38. (A) Patients with Marfan syndrome are also at risk for aortic dissections, but only a limited amount of the aorta is visualized here. The other two abnormalities are not frequently associated with this syndrome. (6:792, 793)

39. (D) The echogenic line visualized in the left atrium in Fig. 3–11 is an interatrial baffle constructed to redirect blood flow in what is known as an "atrial switch." (26:552–557)

40. (D) Because pulmonary venous flow returns directly to the right atrium, it will be dilated. (32:368–371)

41. (E) Color flow aids tremendously in demonstrating the anomalous channels and connections. (90:341–347)

42. True. Constriction of the ductus is physiologically delayed in this group. (6:209–218)

43. True. Prostaglandin E may be administered to keep the ductus arteriosus patent in infants with severe right ventricular outflow obstruction or atresia or great vessel malformations. (6:221, 222)

44. True. The membrane inserts proximal to the left atrial appendage in cor triatriatum and distal to it in supravalvar mitral ring. (6:599–602)

45. False. These children more commonly have the complete form of atrioventricular defect. (6:176)

46. False. Significant cyanosis during infancy occurs only when there is associated pulmonary stenosis. (6:507)

47. False. There is a spectrum of severity in this malformation, and mild forms may remain asymptomatic. (24:142)

48. False. It is very rare to have distal involvement in the absence of proximal aneurysm formation. (85:275)

49. True. In severe cases, it may be difficult to obtain a reliable Doppler signal because of decreased flow through the area of obstruction. The Doppler derived gradient may be somewhat higher than the systolic pressure differences measured from the arm and thigh because peak systolic pressure occurs at slightly different times in these two areas; therefore, the blood pressure method yields a peak-to-peak pressure difference, whereas the Doppler method yields an instantaneous pressure difference. (7:217–219)

50. True. Suprasternal coronal evaluation of the extracardiac vessel should be included in patients in whom this may be a concern for planning of surgical procedures, as the left superior vena cava may drain into the roof of the right atrium. (88:137)

51. True. This has traditionally been the most common position for evaluation of pulmonary valve stenosis. (66:765)

52. True. The sound beam is angled anteriorly, and the transducer is moved to just below the left nipple. (67:844–848)

53. True. The sound beam is angled anteriorly and slightly to the left. (66:765)

54. True. In a few cases, this may be the only position from which a diagnostic Doppler signal can be obtained. (67:844–848)

55. False. The area of the fossa ovalis appears to be intact. (6:173, 174)

56. True. The portion of atrial septum just above the level of the atrioventricular valves is absent. (50:309–314)

57. False. There is a common atrioventricular valve with chordal insertions onto the ventricular septum. (50:315–319)

58. True. The left ventricle is about one-third the size of the right ventricle. The interventricular septum may be seen bowing into the left ventricle. (50:319–330)

59. False. The diagnosis is an unbalanced complete atrioventricular septal defect. In Ebstein's anomaly of the tricuspid valve, the tricuspid valve leaflets are adherent to the right ventricular walls. (26:293–305)

60. False. The systolic murmur is probably caused by atrioventricular valve insufficiency. (6:181–187)

4

Abdominal Sonography

*Charles S. Odwin and Arthur C. Fleischer**

Study Guide

VASCULAR ANATOMY

Major Vessel Landmarks. Major vessels are used as landmarks to identify normal anatomy and pathology. All vessels are anechoic and are tubular shaped when imaged along their long axis and round or oval shaped in their short axis. It is important to know the location of the organ to help determine the long axis of the vessel. Fig. 4–1 illustrates the major vessels of the abdomen.

Aorta. The aorta is the largest artery in the body, which enters into the abdominal cavity through the hiatus of the diaphragm at the level of the twelve thoracic vertebra (T12). At this level, it is called the abdominal aorta. It follows a vertical course anterior to the spine and slightly to the left of midline. The aorta distributes oxygenated blood to all parts of the body through systemic circulation. An increased distance between the aorta and spine may indicate retroperitoneal pathology such as adenopathy, fibrosis, or a hematoma.

The abdominal aorta bifurcates at the level of the fourth lumbar vertebra (L4) into the right and left common iliac arteries. The common iliac arteries bifurcate into the internal iliac arteries (hypogastrics), which supply blood to the internal organs in the pelvis and to the external iliac arteries, which supplies blood to the lower extremities.

Measurements. The abdominal aorta decreases in caliper as it courses inferiorly. The normal anteroposterior dimension of the aorta lumen should be <3 cm at the diaphragm narrowing to approximately 1.5 cm at bifurcation.

Thoracic:	2.5 cm
Diaphragm:	2.5–3 cm
Midabdomen:	2–2.5 cm

Renals:	1.8–2 cm
Bifurcation:	1.5–1.8 cm
Common iliac:	1–1.3 cm

Branches of the Aorta. Superior to inferior

Celiac. The celiac axis or trunk is the first visceral branch of the abdominal aorta. It is approximately 2–3 cm long and trifurcates into common hepatic artery, left gastric artery, and splenic artery.

1. *The common hepatic artery,* which follows a horizontal course to the right. The gastroduodenal artery is a branch of the common hepatic artery and follows a vertical course and is used as the landmark for the anterior lateral aspect of the head of the pancreas. After the gastroduodenal artery branch, the common hepatic artery becomes the proper hepatic artery and enters the liver at the level of the porta hepatis. The hepatic artery courses anteriorly to the portal vein and adjacent to the common bile duct. Once the hepatic artery is intrahepatic, it branches into the right, left, and middle hepatic arteries.

2. *The left gastric artery* is sometimes visualized on ultrasound.[1]

3. *The splenic artery* follows a tortuous horizontal course along the posterosuperior margin of the pancreatic body. It enters the spleen at the splenic helium.

Superior mesenteric artery (SMA) arises from the anterior border of the abdominal aorta about 1 cm inferior from the celiac trunk and follows a vertical and parallel course with the aorta. The SMA is posterior to the body of the pancreas.

Renal arteries branch from the posterior-lateral border of the aorta and course horizontally to the hilum of the kidneys. The right renal artery courses posteriorly to the inferior vena cava. The left renal artery courses directly into the renal hilum.

Gonadal arteries are small vessels that arise off the anterior border of the aorta and inferior to the renal arteries. They are not routinely visualized by ultrasound.

Kerry E. Weinberg wrote the previous-edition version of this chapter.

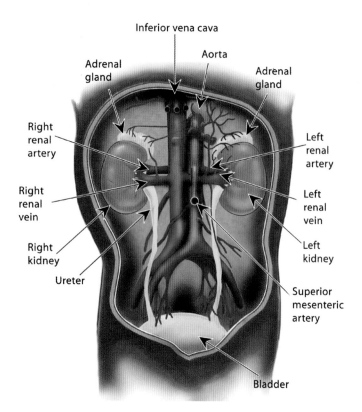

FIGURE 4–1. The abdominal viscera with major vessels.

The *inferior mesenteric artery* is a small artery that arises off the anterior aspect of the abdominal aorta. It follows a vertical course and is slightly to the left of midline. It is not routinely imaged on an ultrasound examination.

PATHOLOGY OF ARTERIES

Arteriosclerosis is primarily an arterial disease in which the vessel wall loses its elasticity and becomes hardened. Atherosclerosis is the most common form in which lipid deposits occur in the inner lining of the artery wall (tunica intima). These deposits may lead to fibrosis and calcifications.

Aneurysm is the dilatation of a segment of a vessel wall caused by a weakness of all three layers of the vessel wall. They are more common in arteries than veins. The most common cause of aneurysms is arteriosclerosis and associated hypertension. Other causes include congenital weakness of a vessel wall, trauma, untreated syphilis, or infections, especially those resulting from bacterial endocarditis. Marfan syndrome is associated with aneurysms in the ascending portion of the aorta extending up to the aortic valve.

Aortic abdominal aneurysm (AAA) is diagnosed when a focal or generalized dilatation is depicted with the aortic anteroposterior diameter >3 cm. The aorta is measured from outer border to outer border. In addition, the size of the lumen is also measured when plaque or calcifications are present. Any aneurysm >7 cm is at a great risk of rupturing. A ruptured aortic aneurysm is a surgical emergency with the majority of

rupture from the lateral wall below the level of the renal arteries. Untreated aortic aneurysm has a mortality rate of almost 100%. Aneurysms are classified as true, dissecting, or pseudo (false).

True aneurysm has dilatation of all three layers of the vessel wall (tunica intima, tunica media, tunica adventitia). Clinical findings include palpable pulsatile abdominal mass of physical examination and back or leg pain. The following lists the types of true aneurysms:

1. Fusiform: the most common type of aortic aneurysms characterized by an elongated spindle-shaped dilatation of the artery
2. Saccular: characterized by a focal outpouching of the vessel wall; primarily caused by trauma or infection
3. Berry: small round outpouchings 1–1.5 cm in diameter, typically found within the cerebral vascular system; rupture usually causes death

Dissecting aneurysm (not a true aneurysm) occurs when there is a tear of the intima layer of the vessel wall causing blood to collect between the intima layer and media layer. The artery will have two lumens, a true lumen and a false lumen. Dissecting aneurysms most frequently involve the ascending aorta and more commonly seen in people with hypertension or Marfan syndrome. Clinical findings include severe pain over the site of the aneurysm, and in cases where the dissection is at the level of the ascending aorta, the pain may mimic myocardial infarction (MI). Sonographic appearance may include the demonstration of two lumens with a pulsating intimal flap.

Pseudoaneurysm (false aneurysm) results from a tear in the vessel wall that permits blood to escape into the surrounding tissue. The blood becomes walled off from the vessel and presents as a mass adjacent to the vessel wall. Color Doppler is used to diagnose a pseudoaneurysm; the site of communication between the true lumen and false lumen may be demonstrated, and the blood flow in the false lumen is turbulent. The major causes are from either an arterial catheterization or trauma.

Inferior Vena Cava. The inferior vena cava (IVC) is a large vein formed at the confluence of the right and left common iliac veins at the level of the fourth lumbar (L4). The IVC lies slightly to the right of midline and courses anteriorly as it carries deoxygenated blood into the right atrium of the heart. The IVC varies in size with respiration, increases with exhalation and held inspiration, and decreases with a Valsalva maneuver.

Major Branches into the IVC

Hepatic Veins. See section under liver.

Renal Veins. The right renal vein is located anterior to the right renal artery and follows a short course from the hilum of the right kidney into the IVC. The left renal vein follows a course anterior to the aorta and posterior to the superior mesenteric artery (SMA) before entering into the IVC.[5]

Gonadal Veins. The right gonadal vein empties directly into the IVC. The left gonadal vein empties into the left renal vein, which drains into the IVC.

Pathology that Affects the Size of the IVC

The IVC is dilated with hepatomegaly, pulmonary hypertension, congestive heart failure (CHF), constrictive pericarditis, right atria myxoma, atherosclerotic heart disease, and right ventricular failure.

The most common tumor that involves the IVC is renal cell carcinoma. Renal cell carcinoma may invade the renal vein and the IVC. This is more common with the right kidney because of the short distance the right renal vein has to travel to enter into the IVC. Thrombus may also be identified as low-level echoes within the IVC. Thrombus in the IVC may cause Budd–Chiari disease.

Causes of IVC Displacement

Lymphadenopathy

Mass in posterior, caudate, or right hepatic lobe of the liver

Right renal mass

Right adrenal mass

Tortuous aorta

Retroperitoneal tumors: retroperitoneal liposarcoma, leiomyosarcoma, osteosarcoma, rhabdomyosarcoma

Portal System.   See liver section below.

LIVER

Gross Anatomy of the Liver

The liver is the second largest organ in the body. The right lobe is five to six times larger than the left lobe. The normal sonographic longitudinal measurement of the liver is <15 cm, >15.5 cm is considered hepatomegaly.[1] The mean anterior to posterior measurement taken at the midclavicular line is approximately 10.5 cm. A Riedel's lobe is a normal variant of the right lobe of the liver, which is more common in women than men. Riedel's lobe is a tongue-like projection extending downward from the right lobe of the liver. This can sometimes be mistaken for a hepatomegaly or a tumor.

The liver is completely covered by connective tissue known as Glisson's capsule. It is mostly an intraperitoneal organ except for the bare area posterior to the dome of the liver, porta hepatis region, and the gallbladder fossa region.

Standards for Describing Liver Anatomy: Lobes, Ligaments, and Fissures

A number of different standards are used for liver division: hepatic veins, fissures, ligaments, and portal veins. Ligaments and fissures are used as landmarks in the more caudad liver sections. (See Fig. 4–2.) Couinaud segment anatomy (used for hepatic lesion localization) divides the liver into eight segments and uses both hepatic veins and portal veins as landmarks.[5]

Traditional Anatomy of the Liver

Traditionally the liver is anatomically subdivided into four lobes: right, left, quadrate, and caudate lobes, which are based on external landmarks. (See Fig. 4–3.)

Couinaud Standard for Describing Liver Segments

This method of anatomy is widely used in Europe and now becoming the universal nomenclature for location of hepatic lesions.[1] Each segment has its own blood supply with a branch of the portal vein in the center bounded by a hepatic vein. The liver is divided into eight functionally segments with each segment having its own blood supply. (See Fig. 4–4.)

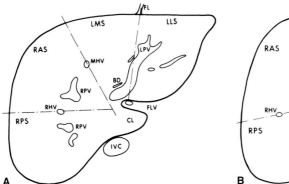
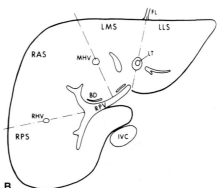

FIGURE 4–2. (A) Graphic representation. IVC = inferior vena cava; RPS, RAS = right lobe posterior and anterior segments; LMS, LLS = medial and lateral segments of left lobe; FLV = fissure of ligamentum venosum; RPV = right vein branch; RHV, MHV = right and middle hepatic veins; BD = bile duct. **(B)** LMS, LLS = medial and lateral segments of left lobe; FL = falciform ligament; LT = ligamentum teres. *(Reprinted with permission from Sexton CC, Zeman RK: Correlation of computed tomography, sonography and gross anatomy of the liver, AJR 1983; Oct;141(4):711–718.)*

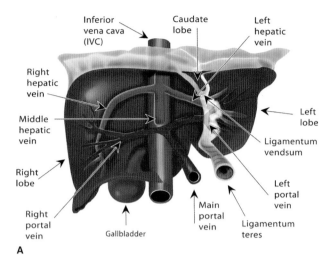

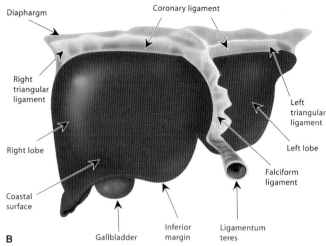

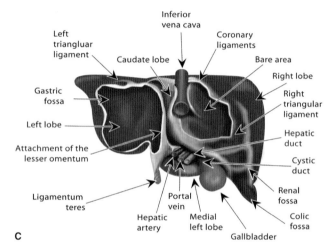

FIGURE 4–3. (**A**) Lobes, ligaments, and fissures. (**B**) Anterior projection of the liver. (**C**) Posterior view of the diaphragmatic surface of the liver. The caudate lobe is located on the posterosuperior surface of the right lobe, opposite the tenth and eleventh thoracic vertebrae.

Functional Anatomy of the Liver

Functionally, the liver is divided into three lobes: right, left, and caudate, which is based on vascular supply.

Parenchymal Architecture

The normal liver parenchyma is homogeneous in texture, and its echogenicity may be compared with other abdominal organs.

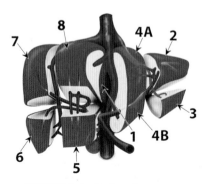

FIGURE 4–4. Couinaud's anatomy.

The following is going from the most echogenic to the least echogenic:

renal sinus > pancreas > liver ≥ spleen > renal cortex > renal medullary pyramids

Middle Hepatic Vein. Divides the liver into right and left lobes (Fig. 4–3A).

Right Hepatic Vein. Divides the right lobe of the liver into anterior and posterior segments (Fig. 4–3A).

Left Hepatic Vein. Divides the left lobe of the liver into medial and lateral segments (Fig. 4–3A).

Both the right and left hepatic veins drain blood from the caudate lobe.

Ligamentum Venosum. The ligamentum venosum is a remnant of the fetal ductus venosus. It divides the caudate lobe from the left lobe. It may be visualized sonographically on either a longitudinal or a transverse scan as an echogenic line extending transversely from the porta hepatis.

Ligamentum Teres (Round Ligament). (Fig. 4–3C). The ligamentum of teres is contained in the falciform ligament. It is a remnant of the fetal umbilical vein. It courses within the

TABLE 4–1 • Intersegmental Fissures

Fissures	Location	Landmark
Right intersegmental	Divides the right lobe into anterior and posterior segments	Right hepatic vein
Left intersegmental	Divides the left lobe into medial and lateral segments	Left hepatic vein Ligament of Teres Left portal vein Middle hepatic vein
Middle intersegmental (Main lobar fissure)	Divides the liver into right and left lobes	Oblique plane connecting gallbladder fossa and IVC

TABLE 4–2 • Couinaud's Anatomy

Segments	Location	Supplied by Branches of
1	Caudate lobe	Right and left portal veins
2	Lateral segment of left lobe–superior	Ascending segment of LPV
3	Lateral segment of left lobe–inferior	Descending segment of the LPV
4	Medial segment of the left lobe–quadrate	Horizontal segment of the LPV
5	Anterior segment of the right lobe	Anterior branch of the RPV
6	Posterior segment of the right lobe–inferior	Posterior branch of the RPV
7	Posterior segment of the right lobe–superior	Posterior branch of the RPV
8	Anterior segment of the right lobe–superior	Anterior branch of the RPV

left intersegmental fissure, dividing the left lobe into medial and lateral segments. Sonographically, it is best visualized on a transverse view as a round echogenic structure just to the left of midline.

Falciform Ligament. (Fig. 4–3B). The falciform ligament is a fold of peritoneum, which contains the ligamentum of teres. It extends from the umbilicus to the diaphragm and attaches the liver to the anterior abdominal wall and diaphragm. It divides the right and left lobe of the liver on the diaphragmatic surface. Sonographically it is seen as a round, hyperechoic area in the left lobe of the liver.

Coronary Ligament. The coronary ligament is contiguous with the falciform ligament. It connects the posterior surface of the liver to the diaphragm.

Main Lobar Fissure (Middle Intersegmental Fissure). The main lobar fissure separates the right and left lobes of the liver. It is visualized sonographically as an echogenic linear line extending from the portal vein to the neck of the gallbladder. Table 4–1 is a guide to the anatomic structures useful in defining segmental anatomy.

Liver Vessels—Hepatic Veins, Portal Vein, Hepatic Artery

The liver has a dual blood supply system. It receives blood from both the hepatic artery and the portal vein. The main portal vein blood carries nutrients from the gastrointestinal tract, gallbladder, pancreas, and spleen. The majority of the total blood supplied to the liver is from the main portal vein.

Hepatic Veins. There are three hepatic veins: right, middle, and left. They follow a superior posterior course and drain deoxygenated blood into the inferior vena cava. Hepatic veins are nonpulsatile, increase in size as they course superiorly toward the inferior vena cava, and the walls are less echogenic than the portal veins (Table 4–2) (Table 4–3).

Portal Vein. The portal vein is formed posterior to the pancreatic neck by the confluence of the splenic vein and superior mesenteric vein. It follows a cephalic right oblique course and enters into the liver at the porta hepatis also known as the portal triad. The portal triad contains (1) portal vein, (2) hepatic artery, and (3) bile duct. The main portal vein lies anterior to the inferior vena cava, cephalic to the head of the pancreas, and caudal to the caudate lobe. The main portal vein bifurcates in the liver into the right and left portal veins.

TABLE 4-3 • Differentiation between the Portal Vein and Hepatic Veins

Portal Veins	Hepatic Veins
Walls are more echogenic because of collagen within the wall	Caliper changes in size with respiration
Branches horizontally and orientates toward the portal hepatic	Branches vertically and orientates toward the IVC
Decreases in caliper as it courses away from the portal hepatis	Increases in caliper as it courses toward the IVC

Right Portal Vein. The right portal vein is larger than the left portal vein. It follows a posterior caudad course and further divides into anterior and posterior branches.

Left Portal Vein. The left portal vein follows a cephalic anterior course to supply blood to the left lobe of the liver. It is the umbilical portion of the portal vein.

Hepatic Artery. The hepatic artery originates from the celiac axis and courses transversely. The hepatic artery and the common bile duct are anterior to the portal vein as they enter the liver at the portal hepatis, with the common bile duct slightly more lateral. The hepatic artery is at the same level as the hepatoduodenal ligament and is superior to the head of the pancreas.

Common Bile Duct. The common bile duct is formed by the confluence of the common hepatic duct and the cystic duct. The superior portion of the biliary duct, which is anterior to the right portal vein is the common hepatic duct. The common bile duct follows an oblique postero-caudal course and travels along the dorsal aspect of the pancreatic head before it joins with the main pancreatic duct, and together they enter into the second portion of the duodenum.

Liver Function Tests

1. Aspartate aminotransferase (AST), formerly known as serum glutamic-oxaloacetic transaminase (SGOT): This is increased with hepatocellular disease and is useful in detecting acute hepatitis before jaundice occurs and following in the course of hepatitis. It is not increased in cases of such chronic liver disease as cirrhosis or obstructive jaundice. It is increased in liver cell necrosis due to viral hepatitis, toxic hepatitis, and other forms of acute hepatitis.

2. Alanine aminotransferase (ALT), formerly known as serum glutamic pyruvic transaminase (SGPT): This enzyme is increased with hepatocellular disease and is used to assess jaundice. It rises higher than AST in cases of hepatitis and takes 2–3 months to return a normal level.

3. Alkaline phosphatase (ALP): Normally found in serum. Its level rises in liver and biliary tract disorders when bile excretion is impaired. Obstruction of bile can be caused by either a biliary or liver disorder such as; obstructive jaundice, biliary cirrhosis, acute hepatitis, and granulomatous liver disease.

4. Ammonia: Normally metabolizes in the liver and is excreted as urea; increased in hepatocellular disease.

5. Alpha-fetal protein (α-AFP): A protein normally produced by the fetal liver and yolk sac, GI tract, scrotal and hepatocellular (hepatomas) germ cell neoplasms, and other cancers in adults. AFP level is used to monitor chemotherapy treatment and prenatal diagnosis neural tube defects in the fetus, rarely in other cases.

6. Bilirubin: Derived from the breakdown of red blood cells into hemoglobin. Excreted by the liver in bile (main pigment). When destruction of red blood cells increases greatly or when the liver is unable to excrete normal amounts, the bilirubin concentration in the serum increases. If it is increased too high, jaundice may occur. Levels of indirect and direct bilirubin may determine intrahepatic and extrahepatic obstruction.

   Direct bilirubin (conjugated bilirubin): It is elevated when there is an obstruction of the biliary system. obstructive jaundice.

   Indirect bilirubin (unconjugated bilirubin): Excessive destruction of red blood cells/hemolysis associated with anemias and liver disease; elevation of the total bilirubin occurs with hepatitis, hepatic metastasis.

7. Hematocrit: Volume percentage of erythrocytes in the whole body; a drop in hematocrit can indicate a hematoma due to liver trauma or bleeding elsewhere in the body.

8. Leukocytosis: A substantial increase in white blood cells above the normal range indicates an inflammatory process or abscess.

9. Prothrombin time (PT): Prothrombin is converted to thrombin in the clotting process by action of vitamin K that is absorbed in the intestines and stored in the liver. When liver function is compromised by liver disease, prothrombin is decreased and can cause uncontrolled hemorrhage.

10. Urinary bile and bilirubin: Bile and bilirubin are not normally found in the urine. There may be spillover into the blood when there is obstructive liver disease and excessive red cell destruction. Bile pigments are found in the blood when there is a biliary obstruction. Bilirubin is found alone when there is an excessive amount of red blood cell destruction.

11. Urinary urobilinogen: This test is used to differentiate between a complete obstruction of the biliary tract versus an incomplete obstruction of the biliary tract.

    Urobilinogen is a product of hemoglobin breakdown and can be elevated in cases of liver disease, hemolytic disease, or severe infections. Urobilinogen does not increase or there is no excess amount found in urine in cases of complete biliary obstruction.

12. Fecal urobilinogen: Traces of urobilinogen are normally found in fecal matter, but an increase or decrease in normal amounts may indicate hepatic digestive abnormalities. An increase may suggest an increase in hemolysis. A decrease is seen with complete obstruction of the biliary system.

Diffuse Hepatocellular Disease. There is a decrease in liver function with an increase in the liver enzymes; the increase in the liver enzymes is directly related to the amount of hepatocytic necrosis. Total bilirubin levels may be elevated with increase prothrombin time (blood clotting factor). Diffuse liver disease has a varied sonographic appearance depending on whether it is acute or chronic (Tables 4–4 and 4–5).

TABLE 4–4 • Diffuse Liver Disease

Diffuse Liver Disease	Clinical Findings/Etiology	Laboratory Data	Sonographic Appearance
Fatty liver—accumulation of fat within the hepatocytes	ETOH abuse, steroids, malignancy, diabetes mellitus, protein malnutrition, hepatitis	Increased LFTs because of hepatocellular disease	Progressive disease—enlarged left and caudate lobe, increase liver echogenicity with decrease through transmission as the disease progresses, decreases visualization of vessel walls
Acute viral hepatitis—diffuse inflammatory process of the liver, most common types HAV, HBV, and HCV	Malaise, nausea, fever, pain, may be jaundiced, enlarged tender liver	Increased bilirubin, ALT higher levels than AST, alkaline phosphatase	Hepatosplenomegaly, hypoechoic liver parenchyma, renal cortex more echogenic than the liver, increased echogenicity of portal vein walls, thickening gallbladder wall
Chronic viral hepatitis most common types HBV and HCV	Malaise, nausea, fever, pain, may be jaundiced, enlarged tender liver in the early stages	Increase—bilirubin, ALT, AST, alkaline phosphatase	Liver parenchyma is coarse and echogenic, the walls of the portal system blend with the liver echogenicity
Cirrhosis—diffuse fibrotic process that involves the entire liver, most commonly caused ETOH abuse, HBV or HBC	Fatigue, weight loss, diarrhea, dull RUQ pain, increased abdominal girth if ascites is present	LFTs depend upon the stage and function of the liver, the following values are increased: ALT, AST, alkaline phosphatase, serum and urine conjugated bilirubin values	Late features—small nodular echogenic liver with decrease through transmission, caudate lobe may be spared in severe cases—ascites, portal hypertension, collateral vessels, patent umbilical vein
Chronic (passive) hepatic congestion	History of heart failure, acute phase causes RUQ pain	Normal or slightly abnormal LFTs	Acute disorder—hepatomegaly, dilatation of IVC, hepatic veins—reverse flow during systole, slightly pulsatile portal vein
Glycogen storage disease—autosomal recessive disorder of carbohydrate metabolism, Von Gierke's disease is the most common type	Usually occurs in infancy or young childhood, hypoglycemia	Decreased glucose-6-phosphatase	Hepatomegaly, fatty liver infiltration with diffuse increased liver echogenicity

Causes of Jaundice

Medical Jaundice (Nonobstructive)

Hepatocellular Diseases—Disturbances within the liver cells that interfere with excretion of bilirubin:

    Hepatitis

    Drug-induced cholestasis

    Fatty liver (most common cause ETOH abuse)

    Cirrhosis

Hemolytic Disease—An increase in red blood cell destruction that results in the increase of indirect bilirubin (nonobstructive jaundice):

    Sickle-cell anemia

    Cooley's anemia

Surgical Jaundice (Obstructive)—Interference with the flow of bile caused by obstruction of the biliary tract. There are many causes of obstruction, some of the causes are:

    Choledocholithiasis

    Pancreatic pseudocyst

    Mass in the head of the pancreas

    Hepatoma

    Metastatic carcinoma

    Cholangiocarcinoma

    Mass in the porta hepatis

    Enlarged lymph nodes at the level of the porta hepatis

Vascular Abnormalities Within the Liver

Portal Hypertension

Etiology:

    Intrahepatic—Most common cause is cirrhosis, Budd–Chiari syndrome

    Extrahepatic—thrombosis, occlusion and compression of portal or splenic veins, congestive heart failure

TABLE 4–5 • Focal Disease of the Liver

Tumors	Clinical Findings	Laboratory Values	Sonographic Appearance
Cysts, congenital	Usually asymptomatic—if cysts become large hepatomegaly and jaundice may occur	Normal LFTs	Round, smooth thin walls, anechoic, increased through transmission
Polycystic disease	More than 50% associated with renal cystic disease	Normal LFTs	Multiple cysts of various sizes in the liver parenchyma
Acquired cysts Echinococcal cyst (hydatid)–caused by a parasite	Usually asymptomatic—may cause pain if cysts become large	Jaundice and increased alkaline phosphatase if cysts cause biliary obstruction	Depends on the level of maturity—solitary cysts which may have thick or calcified walls, mother-daughter cysts, honeycomb appearance or solid in appearance
Infection Abscess (pyogenic)	Fever, pain, nausea, vomiting, diarrhea, pleuritic pain	Leukocytosis, elevated LFTs, anemia	Usually found in the right lobe, solitary, variable size, anechoic to echogenic or complex may have calcifications or shadowing from gas
Fungal infection–Candidiasis	Immunocompromised; i.e., AIDS, organ transplant, malignancy; RUQ pain, fever	Varied–depending on the cause	Hepatomegaly, fatty infiltrations, focal lesions. "wheel within a wheel,"* becomes more hypoechoic
Hematoma	RUQ pain, hypotension	Decreased hematocrit, leukocytosis	Varied depending on age—mostly cystic (fresh blood), echogenic, mixed appearance, irregular shape
Benign solid tumors Cavernous hemangioma (most common)	Usually asymptomatic, more prevalent in women	Normal LFTs	Varied—usually small, round in the right lobe, subcapsular, usually homogeneous with increased through transmission
Focal nodular hyperplasia (FNH)	Usually asymptomatic, increased incidence in women on oral contraceptives	Normal LFTs	Varied—usually echogenic, usually found in the right lobe, similar in appearance as adenomas, hepatomas
Liver cell adenoma	Usually asymptomatic, or as a palpable mass, increased incidence in women on oral contraceptives or men on steroids.	Normal LFTs	Varied—most often found in the right lobe, subcapsular, hyperechoic may have areas of hemorrhage
Infantile hemangioendothelioma	Usually occurs before 6 months of age, abdominal mass, congestive heart failure secondary to arteriovenous shunting	Normal AFP excludes the mass being malignant	Varied—hyperechoic, hypoechoic or mixed echogenicity
Malignant tumors Hepatocelluar carcinoma (HCC) hepatoma-associated with longstanding cirrhosis Hepatic angiosarcoma (rarely seen in people 60–80 years of age)	Acute–palpable mass, rapid liver enlargement, jaundice, weight loss, Chronic–, portal hypertension, ascites, splenomegaly, Budd–Chiari syndrome	Increased AST, ALT, alkaline phosphatase, 70% of the time AFP will be present	Varied—hypoechoic in early stage and becomes hyperechoic, may be singular or multiple
Hepatoblastoma–usually found during infancy or childhood	Abdominal enlargement, hepatomegaly, weight loss, nausea, vomiting, precocious puberty	Abnormal LFTs, elevated AFP	Varied—heterogeneous, hyperechoic or cystic with internal septations
Metastatic lesions–more common than primary malignancies	Primary sites–gastrointestinal tract, breast, lungs Causes symptoms 50% of the time	LFTs usually abnormal, increase in total bilirubin, alkaline phosphatase	Varied—hyperechoic, hypoechoic, complex, target lesions, anechoic

*Jeffrey RB, Rallas PW: New York: Raven Press; 1995.

Clinical Findings:

Formation of collateral venous channels

Splenomegaly

Gastrointestinal tract bleeding caused by opening of low pressure vascular channels

Ascites

Sonographic Findings:

Dilatation of the portal vein (>13 mm)

Dilatation of SMV and splenic vein (>10 mm)

Formation of collaterals (portal vein, splenic vein, SMV can be normal size)

Varices—esophageal, splenorenal, gastrorenal, intestinal

Portafugal (reversal) blood flow

Splenomegaly

Recanalization of the umbilical vein >3 mm

Portal Vein Obstruction

Etiology:

Thrombosis, invasion of the portal vein by tumor

Clinical Findings:

Hepatocellular carcinoma, pancreatic or GI cancer or lymphoma

Sonographic Findings:

Nonvisualization of the portal vein

Echoes within the portal vein

Dilatation of the splenic and superior mesenteric vein (proximal to the level of obstruction)

Budd–Chiari Syndrome

Etiology:

Obstruction of the hepatic veins caused by thrombosis or compression from a liver mass

Clinical Findings:

Abdominal pain

Jaundice

Abnormal liver function tests

Hepatomegaly

Ascites

Sonographic Findings:

Reduced or nonvisualization of the hepatic veins

Hepatic veins proximal to the obstruction may be dilated

Large and hypoechoic caudate lobe

Ascites

Abnormal Doppler blood flow

Sonography of Transjugular Intrahepatic Portosystemic Shunt (TIPS)

Transjugular intrahepatic portosystemic shunt (TIPS) is a procedure performed on patients with portal hypertension or cirrhosis. The procedure consists of placement of a metallic shunt with fluoroscopic guidance using the internal jugular vein as an access site. Once the catheter with the preloaded shunt is directed into a major hepatic vein, usually the right, the catheter is directed toward the main portal vein and pushed through the liver. Once the shunt is deployed, there is flow from the portal vein directly into a hepatic vein.

Duplex color Doppler sonography is used to confirm patency of the TIPS and determines the relative velocity in the proximal, mid, and distal portion of the TIPS. In general, velocities within the TIPS can range from 90 to 190 cm/s. Intimal hyperplasia or thrombus can obstruct the shunt.

Sonography of Liver Transplant

Sonography has an important role in assessing the flow within liver transplants. It is also used for guided biopsy/aspiration of intrahepatic lesions or perihepatic collections. Sonography is also used for preoperative assessment of candidates for liver transplants to ensure patency of the main portal vein and to determine whether there are any intrahepatic masses.

Duplex color Doppler sonography of a patient with a liver transplant includes assessment of flow (spectral and color Doppler) of the main portal vein, right and left portal veins, main hepatic artery, right and left hepatic artery, right, middle, and left hepatic veins, inferior vena cava, and splenic artery and vein. Spectral waveforms obtained from these vessels determine direction and relative velocity of flow. Waveforms obtained from the hepatic veins correlate with "liver compliance," which is diminished in cirrhosis and passive liver congestion or rejection. Normal values for velocities of the blood flow in these vessels have been reported.

In addition, the shape of the waveforms suggests "downstream" resistance. For example, the waveform from the main hepatic artery can demonstrate a "spikey" appearance early after transplantation only to become less resistant as the anastomosis matures. The interested reader should consult the reference suggested in this study guide for further information regarding this topic.

GALLBLADDER

Gross Anatomy

The gallbladder is mostly intraperitoneal and is located in the gallbladder fossa, which is on the visceral surface of the liver. It lies between the right and left lobes of the liver and posterior and caudal to the main lobar fissure. The gallbladder is a pear-shaped structure with a thin wall that is <3 mm. It is approximately 8 cm in length, with a transverse diameter <5 cm. The gallbladder is divided into three main segments: fundus, body, and neck. The fundus is the most anterior segment, while the neck has a fixed anatomic relationship to the right portal vein and main lobar fissure. The neck tapers to form the cystic duct. The spiral valves of Heister are located in the cystic duct, and stones may collect here.

The right and left hepatic ducts join to form the common hepatic duct whose function is to transport bile to the gallbladder. Bile enters and exits the gallbladder via the cystic duct. The cystic duct unites with the common bile duct to transport concentrated bile to the second portion of the duodenum.

Function

The three main functions of the gallbladder are to concentrate bile, store the concentrated bile, and transport the bile to the duodenum. The release of the hormone cholecystokinin is stimulated when food enters into the stomach, especially fatty foods and dairy products. Cholecystokinin stimulates the gallbladder to contract and the sphincter of Oddi to relax and open. The intraductal pressure decreases with the contraction of the gallbladder and the opening of the sphincter of Oddi. The bile flows to the small intestine, which aids in the digestion of food by breaking down fatty foods and dairy products.

Gallbladder Variants and Anomalies

Junctional Fold. Is the most common variant, which is a fold or kinking located on the posterior gallbladder wall between the body and neck.

Phrygian Cap. A fold located in the fundal portion of the gallbladder (Fig. 4–5).

Hartmann's Pouch. A small sac located between the junctional fold and the neck of the gallbladder. It is an area where stones may collect (Fig. 4–5)

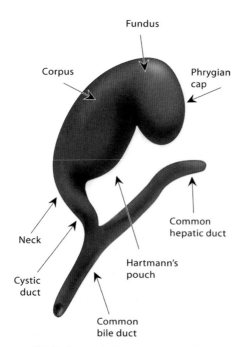

Fundus

Corpus

Phrygian cap

Neck

Cystic duct

Hartmann's pouch

Common hepatic duct

Common bile duct

FIGURE 4–5. Gallbladder with variants.

Septation. A thin wall or partition into the lumen of the gallbladder. This is seen as a thin linear hyperechoic structure within the gallbladder.

Congenital anomalies are rare; the gallbladder can have an ectopic location and be found intrahepatic.

Laboratory Values of Biliary Tract Disease

White Blood Count (WBC). Increases in cases of infection, acute cholecystitis, chronic cholecystitis, cholangitis

Serum Bilirubin. Increases in cases where the biliary system becomes obstructed, gallbladder carcinoma

Abnormal Liver Function Tests

Serum Alkaline Phosphatase (ALP). Increases in cases of posthepatic jaundice

Prothrombin Time (PT). The clotting time is longer in patients with acute cholecystitis, carcinoma of the gallbladder, and prolonged common bile duct obstruction.

Aspartate aminotransferase (AST) and alanine aminotransferase (AST) are abnormal in cases of cholecystitis, choledocholithiasis, and any injury to the bile ducts.

Sonographic Nonvisualization of the Gallbladder. The most common reason for not visualizing the gallbladder on a sonogram is normal physiological contraction of the gallbladder caused by the patient not being NPO. The gallbladder may not be identified in patients who have had a cholecystectomy, ectopic gallbladder, chronic cholecystitis with the gallbladder lumen filled with gallstones, solid mass obliterating the gallbladder, intrahepatic obstruction, or a porcelain gallbladder. Agenesis of the gallbladder is very rare. When the gallbladder in not identified on ultrasound, the gallbladder fossa should be documented. This can be accomplished by locating the right portal vein and following the main lobar fissure from the right portal vein to the gallbladder fossa region.

Causes of a Large Gallbladder (Hydrops). A large gallbladder can be caused by prolonged fasting, intravenous hyperalimentation, a cystic obstruction, or obstruction of the common bile duct. A Courvoisier gallbladder is a large gallbladder caused by an obstruction at the distal portion of the common bile duct. The patient has "painless" jaundice, elevated serum bilirubin, and abnormal liver function tests. The obstruction is usually caused by a malignancy in the area of the distal CBD (pancreatic head carcinoma, common duct carcinoma, duodenal carcinoma, ampulla of Vater carcinoma) or diabetes and postvagotomy.

Causes of a Small Gallbladder. A common cause of a small gallbladder is that the patient has eaten. Other causes include: intrahepatic biliary obstruction (bile is unable to enter into the gallbladder) chronic cholecystitis; liver disease that destroys the liver parenchyma and, therefore, decreases the production of bile; and in extremely rare cases, congenital hypoplasia of the gallbladder.

Causes of Low Level Echoes in the Gallbladder Lumen/with Mobility

Biliary Sludge. The most common cause of sludge is stasis of bile attributable to cholecystitis, extrahepatic obstruction, hyperalimentation, or in patients who have been NPO for a long period of time. Sludge is a common precursor to gallstones. Sludge appears as low-level nonshadowing echoes in the dependent portion of the gallbladder that moves with a change in the patient position. Other causes of mobile low level echoes within the gallbladder lumen include; blood, pus and viscous bile. Intraluminal echoes that do not shadow or are nonmobile include: polyps, cholesterosis, artifacts, septi (junctional fold), and gallbladder carcinoma.

Pathology of the Gallbladder

Reasons for Gallbladder Wall Thickening >3 mm (Table 4–6)

Cholelithiasis (Gallstones). Patients may present asymptomatic or with right upper quadrant (RUQ) pain and a history of nausea and vomiting after eating. Cholecystitis is sometimes present. The following sonographic characteristics need to be present in order to diagnose gallstones:

1. Echogenic foci—Echogenic due to the acoustic mismatch between the stones and bile

2. Posterior acoustic shadowing—Most of the sound is absorbed (attenuated), producing a shadow.

3. Gravity dependent—Stones are gravity dependent and move to the most dependent portion of the GB when the patient position is changed.

TABLE 4–6 • Reasons for Gallbladder Wall Thickening >3 mm

Diffuse Thickening	Focal Thickening	Pseudo Thickening
Physiological due to postprandial	Adenomyomatosis	Gain setting too high Time-gain compensation set inappropriate
Ascites	Polyps–cholesterol, papillary	Beam averaging artifact
Acute hepatitis	Gallbladder carcinoma–primary and secondary	Sludge
Congestive heart failure	Metastatic wall masses	
Cholecystitis		
Hypoalbuminemia		
AIDS		
Sepsis		

Structures That Can Mimic Gallstones

- Gas in the duodenum
- Surgical clips from post-cholecystectomy
- Valves of Heister and folds in gallbladder

Shadowing from the spiral valves of Heister—refraction artifact from the cystic duct

Bowel—usually not a clean shadow

Air in the biliary tree—from previous surgery or GB fistula

Low-level echoes in the gallbladder lumen—no shadowing

Polyps. Polyps are not gravity dependent and do not move with changing patient position.

Adenomyomatosis. Hyperplastic change in the gallbladder wall (Table 4–6).

Causes of gallstones in children include hemolysis; for example, sickle cell disease, cystic fibrosis, malabsorption syndrome (Crohn's disease), hepatitis, and congenital biliary anomalies (choledochal cyst, biliary atresia).

Mirizzi Syndrome. Refers to a common hepatic duct obstruction caused by a stone in the cystic duct with a normal common bile duct. Most patients present with clinical findings of RUQ pain, jaundice and fever.

Acute Cholecystitis. Acute cholecystitis is inflammation of the gallbladder wall with decreased gallbladder function. Acute cholecystitis is usually caused by an obstruction at the level of the cystic duct, bacterial infection in the biliary system, or pancreatic enzyme reflux. Clinically, the patient may present with acute RUQ pain that may radiate to the right scapular area. Patient may have a sonographic Murphy's sign which is a focal pain over the gallbladder when compressed by the transducer, this should not be confused with clinical Murphy's sign in which tenderness occur with a sudden stop in inspiratory effort when pressure is applied to the RUQ. Sonographic findings may include diffuse gallbladder wall thickening >3 mm; gallstones; "halo" sign suggestive of subserosal edema; cystic artery along the anterior gallbladder wall; transverse diameter >5 cm; sludge; and pericholecystic fluid. The laboratory findings in acute cholecystitis may include elevated serum bilirubin and abnormal liver function test results.

Complications of Acute Cholecystitis

Empyema—Pus in the Gallbladder. Clinically, the patient presents sicker than with acute cholecystitis, and sonographically, there will be low-level echoes in the gallbladder lumen with thickening gallbladder wall.

Emphysematous Cholecystitis—Rare occurrence caused by gas forming bacteria in the wall of the gallbladder

Gangrene of the Gallbladder—Caused by absence of blood supply to the gallbladder

Perforation of the Gallbladder—Caused by infection and gallstones

Pericholecystic Abscess—Usually caused by perforation of the gallbladder

Ascending Cholangitis—Caused by spreading of the inflammation of the gallbladder

Acalculous Cholecystitis—Less than 5% of patients with cholecystitis will not have gallstones. The cause of acalculous cholecystitis is a combination of bile stasis and direct vascular changes. The etiology of this combination: trauma, patients who are NPO for long period of time

Chronic Cholecystitis—Caused by recurrent or chronic inflammatory changes of the gallbladder. It is the most common cause of symptomatic gallbladder disease and is associated with gallstones in 90% of the cases. Clinically, the patient presents with intermittent RUQ pain and intolerance to fatty and fried foods. Laboratory findings can include elevated AST, ALT, alkaline phosphatase, and increase of direct serum bilirubin. The sonographic appearance includes small or normal size gallbladder, gallstones, sludge, and thicken echogenic gallbladder wall. A positive WES sign may be imaged: the double arc and shadowing are caused by W-echo from the gallbladder wall, E-echo from the gallstone, S-shadowing from gallstones.

Complications:

Bouveret's syndrome

Mirizzi's syndrome

Fistula between the gallbladder and duodenum

Causes of pericholecystic fluid include acute cholecystitis, pericholecystic abscess, ascites, pancreatitis, peritonitis, and acquired immunodeficiency syndrome (AIDS).

Porcelain Gallbladder—Porcelain gallbladder is defined as an intramural calcification of the gallbladder wall, which occurs in association with chronic cholecystitis in most cases. The etiology is unknown and has an increased incidence of gallbladder carcinoma. The sonographic appearance of porcelain gallbladder includes the following:

* Curvilinear echogenic structure in the gallbladder fossa with posterior acoustic shadowing. The gallbladder wall of porcelain gallbladder can be so calcific that the distal acoustic shadow obscures the visualization of the posterior wall.

* Hyperechoic anterior and posterior gallbladder wall with distal acoustical shadowing

* Convex or Irregular gallbladder wall with areas of echo densities and shadowing

Benign Tumors of the Gallbladder—Benign tumors of the gallbladder are rare. They represent overgrowth of the epithelial lining. Patients are usually asymptomatic.

Adenoma—The most common of the benign gallbladder tumors. They are frequently located in the fundus portion of the gallbladder and <1 cm in size. Sonographically they appear as low-level echo masses that do not shadow or move to the dependent portion of the gallbladder.

Adenomyomatosis (a form of hyperplastic cholecystosis)—Characterized by:

* Hyperplasia of the epithelial and muscular surfaces of the gallbladder wall

* Epithelial and intramural diverticula (Rokitansky–Aschoff sinuses)

There are various types and the most common type is usually located at the fundus. They may also be annular or they can be either diffuse or segmental

Sonographic appearance:

Diffuse or segmental wall thickening

Intraluminal diverticula (RS sinuses) may be filled with bile, sludge or stones and appear either as anechoic or echogenic with distal shadowing or comet tail artifact. The reverberations are the sonographic appearance that differentiates this disease from an adenoma.

Cholesterolosis (strawberry gallbladder)—A form of hyperplastic cholecystosis. The gallbladder usually appears normal on ultrasound.

Polyps—Small echo-densities attached to the gallbladder wall by a stalk; they do not shadow or move to the dependent portion of the gallbladder.

Carcinoma of the Gallbladder—The most common biliary malignancy. Pancreatic cancer is the most common malignant cause to obstruct the biliary tree. Most carcinomas of the gallbladder are adenomas. They usually do not occur until the sixth or seventh decade and are more common in women than men. Previous gallbladder disease; for example, inflammatory disease or gallstones are often precursors. Gallstones are usually present. Most patients have direct extension into the liver and surrounding structures (lymphatic). Signs and symptoms are similar to chronic cholecystitis (may be asymptomatic, loss of appetite, nausea, vomiting, intolerance to fatty foods and dairy products.) Sonographic appearance usually includes gallstones in addition to:

Solid mass filling the gallbladder lumen (most common type)

Localized thickened gallbladder wall with a small gallbladder lumen

Fungating mass projecting from the gallbladder wall into the lumen

Secondary findings:

Liver metastasis

Regional lymphadenopathy

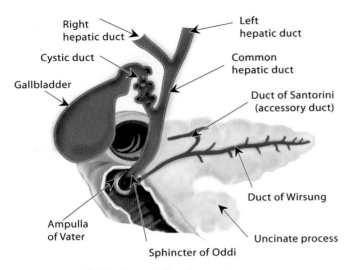

FIGURE 4–6. Gallbladder and biliary ducts anatomy.

BILE DUCTS

Gross Anatomy

The intrahepatic radicles converge to form the main right and left hepatic ducts at the porta hepatis. The right and left hepatic ducts unite to form the common hepatic duct.

The common hepatic duct joins the cystic duct to form the common bile duct. The common bile duct courses along the hepatoduodenal ligament (ligament that attaches the liver to the duodenum), behind the duodenal bulb and posterior aspect of the pancreatic head to enter the second portion of the duodenum. The common bile duct joins with the main pancreatic duct at the ampulla of Vater (see Fig. 4–6).

The common hepatic duct is always anterior the right portal vein, except in cases normal variant or congenital anomalies. The normal common bile duct lumen measures ≤6 mm; the walls are not included in the measurement. The normal diameter of the common bile duct may increase 1 mm per decade starting at the sixth decade. This is due to the common bile duct becoming ecstatic with age. An enlarged common bile duct after a cholecystectomy is normal; if a patient is symptomatic (jaundiced or RUQ pain), a retained stone or a postoperative stricture must be ruled out.

Bile Duct Measurements in a Fasting Patient

Common Hepatic Duct ≤ 4 or 5 mm

Common Bile Duct ≤ 6 mm

Sonographic Appearance of the Biliary System. The
cystic duct and intrahepatic ducts (right and left hepatic ducts) are not usually visualized on ultrasound unless they are dilated. The extrahepatic ducts (common hepatic duct and common bile duct, which are also known as the common ducts) are routinely visualized on ultrasound.

TABLE 4–7 • Types of Biliary Obstruction	
Biliary Obstruction without Dilatation	**Dilatation without Biliary Obstruction**
Obstruction occurred within 12–24 hours before exam–ducts may not be dilated yet	Postop cholecystectomy Stone in biliary tree has passed

Sonographic Criteria for Intrahepatic Dilatation

The bile duct courses anterior to the portal veins. When dilated, a "parallel channel sign" or "double-barrel shotgun sign" is imaged.

Increased numbers of tubular structures are imaged in the periphery of the liver.

Stellate formation of the tubes near the porta hepatis.

Posterior acoustic enhancement distal to the ducts.

The sonographic appearance of the biliary system varies depending on the level of obstruction. Ducts dilate proximal to the level of obstruction. Intrahepatic dilatation may be the only sonographic indication of an obstruction (Table 4–7). There may be intrahepatic dilatation with common bile duct dilatation with a normal gallbladder or intrahepatic and common bile duct dilatation with a small gallbladder (Table 4–8). The cause of the latter is chronic cholecystitis.

Biliary Atresia—The most common fatal liver disorder in children in the United States. There are two forms. In atresia of the intrahepatic radicles, there is nonvisualization of the biliary radicles and gallbladder. In atresia of the extrahepatic radicles, there is an anastomosis of the biliary tree to the jejunum (second part of the small intestine), there will be dilatation of the intrahepatic radicles, and occasionally, the gallbladder will also be imaged. It is difficult to differentiate between biliary atresia and neonatal hepatitis. A nuclear

TABLE 4–8 • Level of Obstruction Causing Intrahepatic Dilatation	
Common Bile Duct and Gallbladder Normal Size	**Common Bile Duct–Dilated with Enlarged Gallbladder**
Bile duct tumor (cholangiocarcinoma, Klatskin tumor)	Stones in the common bile duct
Sclerosing cholangitis	Chronic pancreatitis
Biliary atresia	Mass of the head of the pancreas (carcinoma)
Choledochal cyst	

medicine scan and hepatic biopsy may be needed to make a definite diagnosis.

Caroli's Disease—Caroli's disease is a genetic trait characterized by a segmental saccular dilatation of the intrahepatic ducts. Caroli's disease leads to bile stasis, bacterial growth, abscesses, cholangitis, formation of stones, and decreased liver function caused by the compression of the hepatocytes.

Sonographically, the liver will have multiple cystic structures that communicate with the intrahepatic ducts. Stones and echoes may appear within the bile ducts.

Choledochal Cyst—Choledochal cyst is characterized as a cystic dilatation and outpouching of the common duct wall. The signs and symptoms are intermittent jaundice, RUQ pain, RUQ mass, and failure to thrive. Sonographically, the dilated common bile duct is imaged entering into the cystic mass, and the gallbladder is imaged as a separate cystic structure. The intrahepatic radicles may be dilated.

Biliary System Pathology

Cholangitis—Inflammation of the biliary tract caused by bacterial infection of the biliary tract. Cholangitis is associated with biliary stasis caused by obstruction; for example, choledocholithiasis, biliary stricture, and neoplasm. The signs and symptoms are fever, jaundice, and upper abdominal pain. Abnormal laboratory tests include leukocytosis, increased serum bilirubin, and increased serum alkaline phosphatase. Sonographic appearance may include air in the biliary system, dilatation of the extrahepatic ducts, and the gallbladder may be enlarged.

Sclerosing cholangitis—Inflammation and fibrosis of bile duct commonly associated with intrahepatic calculi complications

Choledocholiths—Stones in the common bile duct, which may cause common bile duct obstruction. The stones usually originate in the gallbladder. The signs and symptoms are biliary colic and jaundice. Patients may also present with gallstones and cholangitis. Laboratory tests show an increased serum bilirubin, increased alkaline phosphatase, and bacteremia. Sonographically, stones in the common bile duct are difficult to image because of the deep position of the duct, overlying bowel gas and a very small amount of fluid surrounding the stone. A stone may be positioned more posterior than the focal zone of the transducer. The common bile duct may be dilated with an echogenic focus and posterior acoustic shadowing.

Primary Malignant Tumors of the Biliary Tree

Adenocarcinoma and Squamous Cell Carcinoma—All branches of the biliary tree may be affected, with the common bile duct being the most common site. Predisposing factors associated with carcinoma of the biliary tree are inflammation,

cholelithiasis, and chronic ulcerative colitis. Signs and symptoms are anorexia, weight loss, RUQ pain, and jaundice. Sonographically, intraluminal soft tissue echoes mark dilatation with a normal pancreatic head, focal biliary stricture, or abrupt termination of the duct.

Klatskin Tumor—A Klatskin tumor is a carcinoma that arises at the union of the right and left hepatic ducts. This type of tumor has the worst prognosis because the patient typically does not have any symptoms and, therefore, does not get diagnosed until the liver is involved. Sonographically, it presents as a solid mass at the junction of the right and left hepatic ducts. There is intrahepatic duct dilatation without extrahepatic duct dilatation.

PANCREAS

Gross Anatomy

The pancreas lies transversely in the retroperitoneal cavity. It extends from the C-loop of the duodenum to the splenic helium and is divided into four parts: head, neck (sometimes included with the head), body, and tail. The size and shape of the pancreas may vary in size depending on the age and body habitus of the patient. The anteroposterior measurements of the pancreas are approximately: head 3 cm, body 2 cm, and tail 2 cm. The pancreas has no capsule and is generally dumbbell or sausage shaped. Fig. 4–7 demonstrates the pancreas and its related landmarks.

The pancreas can sometimes be difficult to visualize on ultrasound, and vascular landmarks are used to identify the pancreas and the pancreatic region. The head of the pancreas

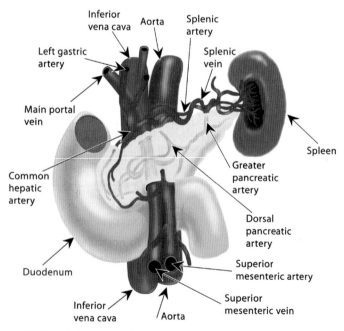

FIGURE 4–7. Anatomy of the pancreas.

is anterior to the inferior vena cava and right renal vein. The common bile duct can be seen at the posterior lateral margin of the pancreatic head. The gastroduodenal artery may be visualized at the anterior lateral margin. Both structures are imaged as anechoic round structures that appear to be within the head of the pancreas.

The uncinate process is a tongue-like extension of the pancreatic neck. A prominent uncinate process will displace the superior mesenteric artery and vein anterior to the pancreas.

The body of the pancreas is the largest portion of the gland. The splenic vein is the most reliable landmark used to visualize the pancreas. The splenic vein courses along the posterior margin of the pancreas and joins with the superior mesenteric vein to form the portal vein. The portal confluence is posterior to the neck of the pancreas. The body is anterior to the superior mesenteric artery, superior mesenteric vein, splenic vein, left renal vein, and aorta. The left renal vein is imaged posterior to the superior mesenteric artery and anterior to the aorta.

The tail of the pancreas lies anterior to the left kidney and medial to the splenic helium. The splenic artery courses along the superior anterior border, and the splenic vein courses along the posterior border.

The main pancreatic duct, also called the Wirsung's duct, courses the entire length of the pancreas. It extends from the tail of the pancreas and joins with the common bile duct at the ampulla of Vater before entering into the second portion of the duodenum. The accessory duct, or Santorini duct, courses diagonally through the head of the pancreas and enters into the duodenum separately.

Table 4–9 lists the landmarks used for visualizing the pancreas on a sonographic examination.

Sonographic Appearance. The pancreas is a homogeneous organ with either the same echogenicity as the liver or slightly more echogenic than the normal liver. In children, the pancreas is less echogenic and relatively larger than in the adult. The pancreas is more difficult to visualized with advance age. The pancreas, which has no true capsule and becomes more echogenic, tends to blend in with the surrounding retroperitoneal fat. The main pancreatic duct may be seen as a tubular structure coursing from the tail of the pancreas to the head. The normal caliber varies from 2 to 3 mm, the largest diameter being in the head of the pancreas.

Functions. The pancreas has endocrine and exocrine functions. The islets cells of Langerhans has three different types of cells, and each cell secretes a different type of hormone. The alpha cells secrete glucagon; beta cells secrete insulin; and delta cells secrete somatostatin.

The exocrine function of the pancreas secretes amylase, lipase, and trypsin. These enzymes aid in digestion and are produced in the pancreas and travel to the duodenum through the pancreatic duct.

TABLE 4–9 • Landmarks for Visualizing the Pancreas

Head	Neck	Body	Tail
Anterior to the inferior vena cava	Anterior to the superior mesenteric vein (SMV)	Anterior to the aorta	Anterior to the splenic vein
Medial to the second portion of the duodenum	Anterior to the confluence of the SMV and splenic vein (portal confluence)	Anterior to the SMA	Anterior to the left kidney
Right of the SMA		Anterior to the left renal vein	Posterior to the stomach
Medial and anterior to the common bile duct		Anterior to the splenic vein	Medial to the spleen
Medial and posterior to the gastroduodenal artery		Posterior to the antrum of the stomach	Posterior to the splenic artery

Pancreatic Diseases (Table 4–10)

Pancreatitis. Pancreatitis is a diffuse inflammatory process of the pancreas in which the pancreatic enzymes autodigest the pancreatic tissue. There are a number of mechanisms that cause the pancreatic enzymes to become activated within the pancreas. The most common causes in older adults include alcohol, biliary tract disease, trauma, surgery, perforated peptic ulcer disease, and drugs.

Causes of pancreatitis in younger patients include infectious agents—mumps and mononucleosis. Hereditary causes include cystic fibrosis and congenital pancreatitis (rare). Pancreatitis can be classified as either acute with or without complications or chronic.

Acute Pancreatitis. Patients present with abdominal pain characteristically in the epigastrium or periumbilical region with nausea and vomiting. The pain usually radiates to the back and commonly occurs following a large meal or alcohol binge. There is abdominal distention attributable to the decrease in gastric and intestinal motility and chemical peritonitis. The entire gland is usually affected, and sonographically, the pancreas may appear normal or is less echogenic.

Laboratory Values. Serum amylase will increase within the first 24 hours and remain elevated for 48–72 hours. Serum lipase will remain elevated for 5–14 days. There will also be an elevated white count, and if biliary obstruction occurs, an

TABLE 4–10 • Diseases of the Pancreas

Disease	Etiology	Signs and Symptoms	Laboratory Values	Sonographic Appearance	Complications
Acute pancreatitis	Alcohol abuse, biliary disease	Abdominal pain radiating to the back, nausea and vomiting, abdominal distention	Increased serum amylase and lipase	Enlarged, deceased echogenicity, extrapancreatic fluid, may have dilated pancreatic duct	Pseudocyst, abscess, hemorrhage, phlegmon, biliary and duodenal obstruction
Chronic pancreatitis	Alcohol abuse, biliary disease	Same as in acute pancreatitis, weight loss	Amylase and lipase level are not useful, fat in feces	Normal or smaller in size, heterogeneous, increased echogenicity, dilated pancreatic duct may have stones, dilated common bile duct	Pseudocyst, dilation of the biliary system, thrombosis of splenic and/or portal vein

elevation in serum bilirubin will also be present. Complications of pancreatitis may include: pseudocyst, abscess, hemorrhage, phlegmon, and biliary and duodenal obstruction.

Edematous form occurs when the pancreas goes through inflammatory changes and interstitial edema. The gland becomes enlarged and is less echogenic on ultrasound. Acute pancreatitis may also be associated with intraperitoneal or retroperitoneal fluid.

Hemorrhagic pancreatitis occurs when there is a rapid progression of the disease caused by autodigestion of the pancreatic tissue, which causes areas of fat necrosis. This leads to rupture of the vessels in the pancreas and hemorrhage. Sonographically, the appearance will vary depending on when the bleeding occurred. A mass may appear as homogeneous, cystic with debris, or heterogeneous. The pancreatic duct may be dilated.

Phlegmonous pancreatitis is a severe form of acute pancreatitis where the inflammation may extend to outside the pancreas. Sonographically, the pancreas is hypoechoic.

Pancreatic pseudocyst is the most common complication associated with acute pancreatitis. They are not true cysts because they do not have an epithelial covering. Pancreatic enzymes and blood escape from the pancreatic tissue and become encapsulated form pseudocysts. They are most commonly found in the lesser sac (anterior to the pancreas and posterior to the stomach) and may also be found in the pararenal space and transverse mesocolon. Sonographically, they are round, smooth thin-walled, and primarily anechoic and may be either singular or multiple. The fluid usually reabsorbs into the body; a small percentage may rupture.

Chronic pancreatitis occurs from continued destruction of the pancreatic parenchyma usually from repeated bouts of acute pancreatitis. Sonographically, the pancreas is either normal or small in size, with an irregular contour. The parenchyma is heterogeneous with increased echogenicity, and in 50% of cases, patients with malabsorption syndromes will have calcifications. With dilation of the pancreatic duct, stones may be imaged within the dilated duct. The common bile duct may also be dilated.

Benign neoplasms may originate from endocrine or exocrine tissue. These focal lesions include: islet cell tumors, cystadenoma, and papilloma of the duct. Pancreatic cysts, abscesses, metastatic diseases to the pancreas, and lymphomas have the same sonographic appearances as when they are visualized in other areas of the body (Table 4–11).

Malignant Tumors. Pancreatic carcinoma can be subdivided into adenocarcinoma, cystadenocarcinoma, and such endocrine tumors as islet cell carcinoma. Adenocarcinoma is the most common, and it is usually located within the head. Sonographically, the pancreas is enlarged with irregular borders, the parenchymal pattern changes and becomes less echogenic. Dilation of the pancreatic duct. Associated findings include: dilatation of the common bile duct secondary to enlargement of the pancreatic head; liver metastases; nodal metastases; portal vein involvement; compression on the inferior vena cava; and Courvoisier's sign (Table 4–11).

Cystadenocarcinoma is visualized sonographically as an irregular cystic lobulated mass with thick walls. It is more commonly seen in the body or tail.

Islet Cell Carcinomas are usually small and well circumscribed and found in the body and tail. One-third of all islet cell tumors are nonfunctioning tumors, and 92% of these are malignant.

With any type of pancreatic carcinoma, clinically, they are associated with an increase in alkaline phosphatase and bilirubin secondary to biliary obstruction. Metastasis to the liver, portal vein, and lymphadenopathy may also be seen.

TABLE 4–11 • Focal Lesions of the Pancreas

Growth	Signs and Symptoms	Laboratory Values	Clinical Pathology	Sonographic Appearance
Cysts True cysts	Usually asymptomatic		Have epithelial lining, may be continuous with the duct or arise from pancreatic tissue, most often found in the head	Smooth, thin wall, anechoic, increased through posterior transmission
Pseudocyst	Asymptomatic or may have the same symptoms as in acute pancreatitis. If pseudocyst is large may have pain	Increased serum amylase and lipase	Pancreatic enzymes that escape the pancreatic duct can tract anywhere, fluid may spontaneously reabsorb, or the pseudocyst may rupture	Round or takes the shape of the potential space; thick walls, usually anechoic, but may have debris; increased through posterior transmission
Benign Tumors Cystadenoma (microcytic adenoma)	No clinical symptoms	Increased serum amylase	More common in females	Found most commonly in the body and tail; anechoic masses with increased posterior enhancement; irregular margins, may have internal echoes
Islet cell tumor Insulinoma	Hypoglycemia	Elevated plasma insulin levels	Arises from the B cells of the islets of Langerhans; usually found in the tail and body	Small (1–2 cm) homogeneous solid masses; usually hypoechoic; may have areas of cystic degeneration
Malignant Tumors Adenocarcinoma	Symptoms occur late in the disease process, pain, weight loss, painless jaundice	Increased serum amylase, bilirubin; increased alkaline phosphatase (liver metastases); increased AST (SGOT)	Arises from the exocrine tissue; accounts for the majority of all malignant pancreatic tumors; usually found in the pancreatic head	Focal masses with irregular ill-defined borders; decreased echogenicity; Courvoisier's sign (enlarged gallbladder); ascites; metastases
Cystadenoma-carcinoma	Epigastric pain		Rare malignant tumor; usually found in the body or tail	Cystic masses with irregular borders; thick walls, and may have solid components

SPLEEN

Gross Anatomy

The spleen is the largest mass of reticuloendothelial tissue in the body. It normally measures approximately 12–14 cm in length, 7 cm in width, and 3 cm in anteroposterior dimension. It is located in the left upper quadrant, left hypochondriac region, inferior to the diaphragm, and posterolateral to the stomach. The tail of the pancreas is medial to the splenic hilum. The left kidney is medial and posterior to the spleen; the stomach and left colic flexure are both medial to the spleen.

The spleen is an intraperitoneal organ except for the hilum area. The capsule is fibroelastic and is composed of small fibrous bands that give the spleen its framework and permit it to expand in size. The splenic artery, which is a branch of the celiac axis, courses along the anterior superior border of the pancreas and enters into the spleen at the splenic hilum. The splenic artery divides into six branches once it enters into the spleen. The splenic vein exits at the splenic hilum and courses transversely across along the posterior aspect of the pancreas and joins with the superior mesenteric vein to form the portal vein.

The spleen is not essential to life, but it has important functions, especially during the fetal period. It is the main component of the reticuloendothelial system and its functions include the breakdown of hemoglobin and the formation of bile pigment; formation of antibodies, production of lymphocytes and plasma cells; a reservoir for blood; and blood formation in the fetus (erythrocytes) or when there is severe anemia.

The spleen is a homogeneous organ and is either slightly less echogenic or isoechoic to the normal liver. The spleen is crescent shaped with a convex superior lateral border and concave medially. The inferior portion is tapered.

Congenital Anomalies. The most common congenital anomaly is the accessory spleen. Splenic tissue separate from the spleen is usually found near the splenic hilum or adjacent to the tail of the pancreas. Accessory spleens are typically small and round and have the same echogenicity as the spleen. They are difficult to demonstrate on ultrasound and must be differentiated from lymphadenopathy.

A *wandering spleen* is a spleen in an ectopic location usually found in the pelvis. The patient usually presents with an abdominal or pelvic mass and intermittent pain. Splenic torsion may occur and color Doppler is used to document the vascularity.

Asplenia is rare and often associated with congenital heart disease and other anomalies.

Aplasia is failure of the spleen to develop.

Neoplasms of the Spleen

The spleen is seldom the site for primary disease but often the site for secondary disease. Benign and malignant tumors are rare.

Benign Neoplasms of the Spleen. These include congenital cysts, cysts associated with polycystic disease, hemangiomas (most common primary tumor of the spleen), and lymphangioma (Table 4–12).

Trauma. Blunt trauma (motor vehicle accident, sports injury) to the spleen is a common cause for trauma to the spleen. A subcapsular hematoma may form, grow, and cause the spleen to rupture. Spontaneous rupture of the spleen may also occur in certain disease states (i.e., leukemia), when the spleen is massively enlarged and soft.

Malignant Tumors of the Spleen

Primary malignant tumors arise from the capsule (sarcoma) the most common one being angiosarcoma or they may come from the splenic tissue (lymph), lymphoma. Secondary malignant tumors of the spleen are metastatic from the breast, malignant melanoma, or the ovaries (Table 4–12).

Pathologies of the Spleen

The pathological sonographic appearance of the spleen can be divided into two categories: focal and diffuse. Diffuse splenomegaly can be caused by congestive splenomegaly (i.e., cirrhosis, portal hypertension, and heart failure); infections (i.e., hepatitis, HIV/AIDS, tuberculosis); storage disease (i.e., Gaucher's disease, diabetes mellitus, and Niemann–Pick disease); and hemodialysis. It is important to remember that diseases go through different stages and the sonographic appearance will vary depending upon the stage of the disease (Table 4–13).

Some disease processes that affect the spleen will not produce any focal lesions or changes in the echogenicity of the spleen. They will affect the splenic size by either causing atrophy or enlargement of the spleen (Table 4–13).

Atrophy of the spleen is seen less commonly than splenomegaly. Myelofibrosis and sickle cell disease cause destruction of the splenic parenchyma. The spleen decreases in size and sonographically becomes echogenic. In many cases, an atrophic spleen is not visualized on ultrasound.

Splenic Size. The size of the spleen varies with energy and nutritional state of the person. It also varies at different states in life—at birth, it has the same proportion to the total body weight as in the adult. The relationship of the spleen to body size and nutritional state of the individual is important.

TABLE 4–12 • Focal and Diffuse Pathology of the Spleen

Sonolucent Focal Pathology
Splenic cysts
Abscess
Hematoma
Lymphoma
Metastases
Infarction
Cystic lymphangioma

Echogenic Focal Pathology
Metastases
Cavernous hemangioma
Hamartoma

Varied Focal Echogenicity
Infarction
Abscess

Diffuse Pathology–Decreased Echogenicity
Congestion
Multiple myeloma
Lymphopoiesis
Granulocytopoiesis (e.g., acute or chronic infection)
Erythropoiesis (e.g., sickle cell disease, hemolytic anemia, thalassemia)

Diffuse Pathology–Increased Echogenicity
Leukemia
Lymphoma

TABLE 4–13. Causes of Splenomegaly

Minimal	Moderate	Massive
Acute splenitis	Acute leukemia	Chronic leukemia
Acute splenic congestion (congestive heart failure, portal hypertension)	Infectious mononucleosis	Lymphoma
	Cirrhosis with portal hypertension	Hodgkin's disease
		Parasitic infections
		Primary tumors of the spleen
Acute febrile disorders (systemic toxemias, intra-abdominal infections)	Chronic splenitis	
	Storage diseases (e.g., Gaucher's disease, amyloidosis)	
	Tuberculosis	
	Chronic congestion	

KIDNEY

Gross Anatomy

The paired kidneys and ureters are retroperitoneal, lying anterior to the deep muscles of the back (psoas major muscle). The kidneys have three layers for protection and support. The true capsule or fibrous capsule is the most inner layer and is imaged sonographically as an echogenic reflector surrounding the renal cortex. Surrounding the true capsule is a layer of fat (adipose) called the perirenal fat. The adrenal gland is located anterior, superior, and medial to the each kidney and is separated from the kidney by the layer of perirenal fat. Gerota's fascia is a fibrous sheath that encloses both the adrenal gland and the kidney.

The kidney is divided into two regions, the renal sinus and the parenchyma. The renal parenchyma is measured from the margin of the renal sinus to the border of the kidney. The average adult kidney size is 11.5 cm in length, 6 cm in width, and 3.5 cm in thickness. In children, renal size varies with age.

Sonographically, the kidney parenchyma has two distinct areas: the outer cortex and the inner medullary pyramids, which surround the renal sinus. The cortex is homogeneous with relativity low-level echoes that are slightly less echogenic than the normal liver. The medullary pyramids are relatively hypoechoic round or triangular areas between the cortex and the renal sinus. These are separated from each other by bands of cortical tissue, called columns of Bertin, which also extend inward to the renal sinus. The intense specular echoes at the corticomedullary junction are from the arcuate arteries.

The inner echogenic portion of the kidney consists of the renal sinus. The renal sinus contains fat, calyces, infundibula, renal pelvis, connective tissue, renal vessels, and lymphatics. The renal hilum is where blood vessels, nerves, lymphatic vessels, and the ureter enter or exit the renal sinus.

The superior end of the ureter is expanded and forms a funnel-shaped sac called the renal pelvis, which is located within the renal sinus. The renal pelvis is divided into two or three tubes called major calyces, and they are divided into 8 or 18 minor calyces. The apex of the medullary pyramid, called the renal papilla, indents each minor calyx.

The infundibula (funnel portion of the calyces) are collapsed and not seen within the echogenic renal sinus in a subject that has restricted fluid intake. During diuresis, the narrow channels traversing the sinus can be identified. In patients with an extrarenal pelvis, a fluid-filled structure extending medially to the kidney can be identified. Placing the patient in a prone position will compress the extrarenal pelvis and assist in making the diagnosis.

Maternal pyelocaliectasis without mechanical obstruction is commonly observed during pregnancy and seen more frequently in the right kidney. Fetal pyelectasis is also common in utero, and there are measurements used to distinguish it from hydronephrosis. Structures adjacent to the kidneys (Table 4–14).

TABLE 4–14 • Structures Adjacent to the Kidneys

Anterior to the Right Kidney	Anterior to the Left Kidney	Posterior to the Kidneys
Right adrenal gland	Left adrenal gland	Diaphragm
Liver	Stomach	Quadratus lumborum muscles
Duodenum	Spleen	Psoas muscle
Right colic (hepatic flexure)	Pancreas	
Small intestine	Jejunum (2nd part of the small intestine)	

Functions of the Kidneys

The kidneys serve in the excretion of inorganic compounds; for example Na^+, K^+, Ca^{++}; excretion of organic compounds; for example, creatinine; blood pressure regulation; erythrocyte volume regulation; and vitamin D and Ca^{++} metabolism.

The ultimate goals of the kidney functions are to

1. Maintain salt and water balance
2. Regulate the fluid volume
3. Maintain acid and base balance

Laboratory Values

Blood and urine tests are performed to determine renal dysfunction. Renal function cannot be estimated by the use of ultrasound.

1. Serum creatinine is elevated with renal dysfunction. Renal dysfunction occurs when the functioning unit of the kidney (nephron) is destroyed.
2. Blood urea nitrogen (BUN) is elevated when there is acute or chronic renal disease or urinary obstruction. A decrease in BUN may occur with overhydration, liver failure, or pregnancy.

Renal Congenital Anomalies

Renal congenital anomalies include incorrect position, number, and shape. One of the most common anomalies is a duplex collecting system. There may be duplication of the ureters, which may enter into the bladder separately, or more commonly, they will join together and enter into the bladder as one ureter.

Position. Embryologically, the kidneys form in the pelvis in an anteroposterior orientation. They ascend and rotate to the adult position, so that the upper pole of each kidney is more medial than the lower pole. Kidneys located outside of the renal fossa are called ectopic kidneys.

Pelvic kidney occurs when the kidney fails to ascend out of the pelvis.

Horseshoe kidney is the most common form of fusion anomaly. The kidneys lie in an oblique transverse position in the lower abdomen. The kidneys are more commonly fused together at lower poles than at the middle or upper poles.

Number. Anomalies of kidney number would include a solitary kidney (single functioning kidney with the ipsilateral atrophied kidney), unilateral renal agenesis (absence of one kidney and ureter), and a supernumary kidney (duplication of the kidney, pelvis, and ureter).

Unilateral renal agenesis is frequently associated with other genital anomalies; for example, bicornuate uterus, unicornuate uterus, and uterine and vaginal septations.

Bilateral renal agenesis is fatal.

Shape. Congenital variations include hypertrophied columns of Bertin (prominent cortical tissue in the medulla <3 cm), fetal lobulation (lobulated renal surface), dromedary (splenic) hump (bulge of cortical tissue on the lateral aspect of the left kidney), renunculus, and fusion of the kidney (horseshoe kidney, cake kidney). All of the above, except the latter, may mimic a mass on ultrasound. Congenital cystic diseases that distort the reniform shape are also included in this category, infantile polycystic kidney disease, adult polycystic kidney disease and multicystic kidney disease.

Polycystic Disease. Polycystic disease may be present at birth or may not manifest until adulthood.

Infantile Polycystic Kidney Disease (IPKD) or autosomal recessive polycystic disease (ARPKD) or (Potter type I). This is the least common and most fatal of the three cystic diseases. It is an autosomal recessive trait and is more common in females (2:1). Sonographically, it presents as bilateral echogenic, enlarged kidneys with cysts (the cysts classically are too small to be resolved). If survival past infancy occurs, hepatic fibrosis becomes a complication, with death resulting from hepatic failure and/or bleeding from esophageal varices.

Adult Polycystic Kidney Disease (APKD) or autosomal dominant polycystic kidney disease (ADPKD) or Potter type III. This is an autosomal dominant disease and occurs relatively frequently. The disease may be latent for many years and not manifest itself until the fourth decade. Patients present with decreasing renal function, hypertension, and may have flank pain. Sonographically, APKD presents as bilateral large kidneys with randomly distributed cortical cysts of various sizes, and in the advanced stages, the kidneys loose the reniform shape. Associated finding include cysts in the liver, pancreas, and spleen. Destruction of the residual renal tissue in advance stages leads to renal failure.

Medullary Cystic Disease. It can be either dominant or recessive. Juvenile onset is autosomal recessive and adult onset is autosomal dominant. Clinically, patients present with renal failure. Sonographically, there are small cysts in the medullary portion of both kidneys with a decreased definition between the cortical/medulla junctions. Hydronephrosis is caused by an obstruction of the outflow of urine. The renal pelvis and calyces become dilated and compress the renal parenchyma causing renal insufficiency. The dilatation may be unilateral or bilateral depending upon the level of the obstruction. The amount of dilation determines whether it is mild (Grade 1), moderate (Grade 2), or severe (Grade 3). The absence of a renal jet and an RI of less than 0.70 will substantiate the diagnosis of renal obstruction.

Hydronephrosis. There are two major classifications of hydronephrosis: intrinsic and extrinsic.

Intrinsic Hydronephrosis. This may be the result of
  Stricture
  Renal calculi
  Bleeding or blood clot
  Ureterocele
  Pyelonephrosis
  Tuberculosis

Extrinsic Hydronephrosis. This may be the result of
  Pregnancy (usually involves the right kidney)
  Pelvic masses (e.g., ovarian or fibroids)
  Bladder neck obstruction
  Trauma
  Retroperitoneal fibrosis
  Prostatic hypertrophy
  Urethritis
  Inflammatory lesions—pelvis, gastrointestinal, retroperitoneal
  Neurogenic bladder

Congenital Hydronephrosis. This is present and existing from the time of birth. This may present as
  Ureteropelvic junction (UPJ) obstruction
  Ectopic ureterocele usually caused by a duplex collecting system
  Retrocaval ureter
  Posterior urethral valve (PUV)

False-Positive Hydronephrosis. This denotes a test result positive for hydronephrosis when there is no hydronephrosis present. Sonographically, the following may mimic hydronephrosis (dilatation of the collecting system).
  Normal diuresis
  Overdistended bladder
  Parapelvic cyst

Renal sinus lipomatosis

Extrarenal pelvis

Reflux–vesicoureteral

Diabetes insipidus

False-Negative Hydronephrosis. This denotes a test result that wrongly excludes the diagnosis of hydronephrosis. Patients suffering from severe dehydration or intermittent obstruction may have hydronephrosis without dilatation of the collecting system.

Severe dehydration

Nephrolithiasis with intermittent obstruction

Tables 4–15 and 4–16 outline the clinical and sonographic findings associated with cystic and solid renal masses.

Nephrolithiasis (Renal Calculi)

Nephrolithiasis are more commonly found in men than women and typically in people who have urinary stasis. Nephrolithiasis may be composed of uric acid, cystine, or calcium. Sonographically, renal calculi appear as highly reflective echogenic foci. A high-frequency transducer with proper settings of the focal zones is necessary to document posterior shadowing. Using tissue harmonics can also assist in seeing posterior acoustic shadowing. The "twinkle sign" is a color artifact that has been seen with urinary stones. The "twinkle sign" is described as rapidly changing colors that are seen posterior to an echogenic reflector, that is, stones). A Staghorn calculus is large stones located in the central portion of the kidney, the collecting system, and takes the shape of the calyces. Renal obstruction may be secondary to stones located in the collecting system.

Laboratory Values. In cases of chronic obstruction, there is an increase in serum creatinine and BUN levels. In acute obstruction, there are no specific lab values. Urine may show hematuria and/or bacteria.

Signs and Symptoms. Renal colic, flank pain, nausea, and vomiting.

Renal Failure

Renal failure is the kidneys' inability to filter metabolites from the blood resulting in decreased renal function, which may be either acute or chronic. Laboratory findings are increased serum BUN and serum creatinine levels.

Etiology

Prerenal Causes. Renal hypoperfusion secondary to a systemic cause can occur as a result of vascular disorders leading to renal failure and includes the following conditions.

Nephrosclerosis. Arteriosclerosis of the renal arteries, resulting in ischemia of the kidney. Nephrosclerosis develops rapidly in patients with severe hypertension.

Infarction. This may result from occlusion or stenosis of the renal artery.

Renal Artery Stenosis. Any narrowing of the renal artery will affect the blood flow to the kidney, resulting in atrophy of the kidney and decreased renal function.

Congestive Heart Failure. This may cause renal hypoperfusion secondary to heart failure.

Thrombosis. Thrombosis of the renal vein will increase the intravascular pressure and, thus, decrease blood flow to the kidney.

Sonography. Doppler of the renal artery is employed to detect arterial blood flow patterns either directly from the renal artery or indirectly from parenchyma flow patterns.

Renal Parenchymal Disease—Infection and Inflammatory Disease

Acute Tubular Necrosis. Of the acute renal medical diseases, this is the most common cause of acute renal failure. The destruction of the tubular epithelial cells of the proximal and distal convoluted tubules may occur as a result of ingestion or inhalation of toxic agents, ischemia caused by trauma, hemorrhage, acute interstitial nephritis, cortical necrosis, and diseases of the glomeruli.

Pyelonephritis. Infection is the most common disease of the urinary tract, and the combination of parenchymal, caliceal, and pelvic inflammation constitutes pyelonephritis. Bacteria ascending from the urinary bladder or adjacent lymph nodes to the kidney usually cause infection of the kidney.

Glomerulonephritis. Etiology is unknown, but it frequently follows other infections.

Metabolic Disorders. Diabetes mellitus, amyloidosis, gout, and nephrocalcinosis (deposit of calcium in the renal parenchyma) are metabolic disorders associated with renal failure.

Chronic Nephrotoxicity. This is caused by exposure to radiation, heavy metals, industrial solvents, and drugs.

Sonography. In acute renal failure, the kidney may be normal sized or enlarged. There may be decreased definition between the medullary/cortical junctions. As the case progresses from acute to chronic, the echogenicity will increase. There is no definite correlation between the echogenicity of the kidney, the kidney size, and degree of decreased renal function. Patients in end-stage renal failure will have small echogenic kidneys that are difficult to image sonographically.

Postrenal Causes. These include urinary tract obstruction, which cause hydronephrosis, and may be congenital or acquired intrinsically and extrinsically.

Sonography. There are varying degrees of the dilation of the renal sinus, calyces, infundibulum, and pelvis.

Renal Medical Diseases (Table 4–17)

Type I. There is increased cortical echogenicity with a decrease in corticomedullary differentiation. Type I diseases are those caused by glomerular infiltrate, such as acute and chronic glomerulonephritis, acute lupus nephritis, nephrosclerosis, any

TABLE 4–15 • Renal Cystic Masses

Cystic Masses	Clinical Findings	Sonographic Findings
Simple cyst	1. Seen in 50% of patients over the age of 55 2. Usually originates in the renal cortex 3. Asymptomatic unless they are large and obstruct the collecting system 4. Unilocular	1. Anechoic 2. Thin walls 3. Round 4. Increased through acoustical transmission
Atypical cyst	1. Septated or multilocular 2. Septations have no pathological significance	Fulfills all of the criteria for a simple cyst but, will have internal echogenic lines, i.e., septations
Parapelvic cyst	1. Originates from renal parenchyma and is seen in the renal hilum 2. May present with hypertension and pain	1. Fulfills the criteria for a simple cyst but located within the renal pelvis 2. Solitary and large 3. Does not communicate with the collecting system
Peripelvic cysts	1. Originates in the renal pelvis 2. May develop from the lymphatic system or obstruction	1. Small, multiple, and irregular shape 2. May appear as dilated renal pelvis 3. Does not communicate with the collecting system
Inflammatory cysts	1. Simple cysts that have become infected 2. An increase in leukocytosis 3. Pain	1. Complex pattern of internal echoes from inflammatory debris 2. Slightly thickens walls, not as thick as chronic abscess
Hemorrhagic cysts	1. 6% of all renal cysts will hemorrhage 2. Increases incidence in polycystic disease	Complex echo pattern dependent upon state of hemorrhage
Calcified cysts	2% of all cysts will calcify	1. Anechoic 2. Smooth round borders that are echogenic or have echogenic foci 3. Calcified walls attenuate sound making it difficult to visualize the complete cyst
Renal abscess (carbuncle)	1. Fever, chills, flank pain 2. Elevated white blood count	1. May appear solid early in the course 2. Complex echo pattern due to debris 3. Walls are thicken and irregular 4. Gas may produce a dirty shadow
Hydronephrosis	Obstruction a. Intrinsic–within the collecting system by a stone or stricture b. Extrinsic–a mass compresses the ureter or bladder outlet	The calices, infundibula and renal pelvis dilate due to the obstruction of urine flow. Minor dilatation (Grade 1)–slight splaying of the collecting system Moderate dilatation (Grade 2)–increased dilatation of the collecting system with thinning of the parenchyma Severe dilatation (Grade 3)–huge anechoic collecting system with lose of shape and very little parenchyma
Pyonephritis	Pus in the dilated collecting system complication of hydronephrosis that occurs secondary to urinary stasis and infection	Dilated pelvicaliceal system filled with internal echoes, shifting urine-debris level, may have shadowing caused by gas-forming organisms
Renal sinus disease Renal sinus lipomatosis	More common in older patients; may be secondary to chronic calculus disease and inflammation. The renal sinus is replaced by fatty tissue	In replacement lipomatosis, the kidney is enlarged, the renal sinus appears hypoechoic because of fat (one of the few times that fat appears hypoechoic instead of echogenic)

TABLE 4–16 • Solid Renal Masses

Tumors	Clinical Findings	Sonographic Findings
Benign Solid Tumors Angiomyolipoma, also called renal hamartoma (tumor composed of fat, muscle, and blood vessels)	More common in women than men (2:1). Symptoms are flank pain, hematuria, and hypertension	Discrete highly echogenic mass found in the cortex
Adenomas (benign counter part of renal cell carcinoma)	Asymptomatic or painless hematuria, usually found on autopsy	Small well-defined isoechoic or hypoechoic mass found in the cortex
Connective tissue tumors 1. Hemangiomas 2. Fibromas 3. Myomas 4. Lipomas	Gross hematuria	These tumors present as homogenous echogenic lesions relating to their vascularity and fat content
Malignant Solid Tumors Hypernephroma (also known as adenocarcinoma, renal cell carcinoma [RCC], and Grawitz tumor)	1. Affect males more than females (2:1) commonly after the age of 50 2. Hematuria 3. An arteriogram of the kidney demonstrates a mass with increased vascular supply with irregular branching 4. Metastases to bone, heart, and brain	1. Unilateral, solitary and encapsulated 2. Varied echogenicity from hypoechoic to echogenic 3. Look for metastases via the bloodstream infiltrating the renal vein and inferior vena cava 4. Look for metastases to the contralateral kidney, ureter, peritoneum, liver, and spleen
Transitional cell carcinoma (affects the urothelium and may be located anywhere within the urinary system)	1. Occurs in the renal pelvis 2. Usually asymptomatic, may have pain or palpable mass 3. Painless hematuria 4. Known to be invasive	1. Invasive tumor not well-defined or encapsulated within the renal pelvis 2. Occasionally appears as a bulky discrete mass 3. Hypoechoic or isoechoic
Renal lymphoma	1. Relatively common in patients with widely disseminated lymphomatous malignancy	1. Solid mass with low-level internal echoes 2. May appear similar to renal cysts but will not demonstrate increase through acoustic transmission
Wilms' tumor (nephroblastoma)	1. Most common malignancy of renal origin in children 2. Abdominal mass, hypertension, nausea 3. Hematuria	1. Early on encapsulated later on it may extend into the perirenal area 2. Varied sonographic appearance depending upon the amount of necrosis and/or hemorrhage

type of nephritis, and renal transplant rejection. All these disorders can cause the echogenicity of the renal cortex to be greater than the liver and spleen. As the disease progresses to the chronic state, the kidney becomes smaller, the cortex becomes more echogenic, and eventually the medulla will become equally echogenic.

Type II. There is distortion of normal anatomy involving cortex and medullary pyramids; sonographically, there is a decrease in the corticomedullary differentiation in either a focal or diffuse manner. The type II pattern is seen with such focal lesions as cysts, abscesses, hematomas, bacterial nephritis (lobar nephronia), infantile polycystic disease, adult polycystic disease, chronic pyelonephritis, and chronic glomerulonephritis.

Renal Transplants

The transplanted kidney is placed within the iliac fossa. A baseline sonogram is performed within 48 hours postoperatively to document the exact location, size, and sonographic appearance of the transplanted kidney. The most serious sign of transplant rejection is renal failure. Clinical signs of renal rejection include, fever, pain, and decreased urine output. The laboratory results are the same as renal failure, elevated BUN, and serum creatinine.

Acute rejection of the transplanted kidney may be caused by acute tubular necrosis or arterial obstruction. Differentiating between the different causes of renal failure is important to ensure proper treatment is administered.

In cases of acute rejection, the kidney appears sonographically as an enlarged kidney with increased cortical echogenicity, decreased renal sinus echogenicity, irregular sonolucent areas in the cortex, enlarged and decreased echogenicity of the pyramids, distortion of the renal outline, and indistinct corticomedullary junction.

Rejection caused by acute tubular necrosis usually results in a normal sonogram. In rejection caused by acute renal arterial occlusion, the sonographic appearance seems grossly normal.

TABLE 4–17 • Renal Medical Diseases

Disease	Clinical Findings	Sonographic Appearance
Acute pyelonephritis	Ninety percent are female, dysuria, urinary frequency, fever, leukocytosis, bacteriuria	Normal or enlarged kidneys, may have mild hydronephrosis; enlarged corticomedullary area with decreased echogenicity and loss of definition between the cortex and medulla; low level echoes may be produced by multiple small abscesses and areas of necrosis in the cortex and medulla
Chronic pyelonephritis	Affects male and females; usually caused by recurrent urinary tract infection or inadequately treated pyelonephritis; proteinuria	Normal or small kidneys; parenchymal thinning; increased echogenicity due to fibrosis
Acute lobar nephronia (acute focal bacterial nephritis)	Inflammatory mass without drainable pus results from gram-negative bacteria that ascends from ureteral reflux; fever, chills, flank pain	Poorly defined cystic mass containing echoes that may disrupt the corticomedullary junction; unable to differentiate from an abscess
Xanthogranulomatous pyelonephritis	Rare form of inflammatory disease found in patients with long-standing renal calculi	Enlarged kidneys with multiple anechoic or hypoechoic areas
Glomerulonephritis	Glomerular disease results from an immunological reaction in which antigen-antibody complexes in the circulation are trapped in the glomeruli. It is the most common cause of renal failure. In the acute stage–oliguria, edema, increased BUN, increased creatinine and increased serum K. In the chronic state–polyuria, proteinuria to such a high extent that 50% of patients develop nephritic syndrome.	Increased echogenicity of the renal cortex with a decrease of the renal size as the disease progresses
Acute tubular necrosis	Most common cause of acute renal failure may result from ischemia, decreased blood flow to and from the kidney, renal transplant. It may be toxin induced or result from trauma/surgery.	Enlarged kidney, especially in the anteroposterior diameter; normal renal parenchyma; renal medullary pyramids will appear more prominent and anechoic

However, duplex Doppler studies may reveal an absence of or decreased diastolic flow.

Perinephric fluid collections, commonly associated with the transplanted kidneys, are lymphocele, urinoma, abscess, and hematoma (Table 4–18).

URETERS

The ureters are located in the retroperitoneal cavity and course along the anterior surface of the psoas muscle along the medial side. The ureters are approximately 6 mm in diameter. The three most common places for obstruction to occur are: at the ureteropelvic junction (UPJ); as they cross over the pelvic brim; and at the junction into the bladder. In the pelvis, the ureters are anterior to the iliac vessels.

Urine can be imaged entering into the urinary bladder with the use of color Doppler. Color Doppler is used because the ureteral jet will cause a Doppler shift because of the continued changes in the turbulent flow in the urine. If the bladder has recently been overly distended, ureteral jets may not be imaged because of the specific gravity of the urine in the ureters and in the bladder being similar, thus causing no Doppler shift. Ureteral jets occur at regular intervals, approximately every 2–3 seconds. They appear as bursts of color entering from the base of the bladder flowing toward the center of the bladder and lasting for a fraction of a second. The absence or decrease of a ureteral jet indicates the presence of an obstruction.

Congenital Anomalies of the Ureters

These include double or bifid ureter, narrowing, strictures, diverticuli, and hydroureter caused by a congenital defect, as in a polycystic kidney, or acquired, as in a low ureteral obstruction.

Megaureter in Childhood (Primary-Nonobstructive, Nonrefluxing Megaureter)

This includes prune belly syndrome (Eagle–Barrett syndrome), deficiency of the abdominal musculature, and urinary tract abnormalities (large hypotonic bladder, undescended testes, hydroureter), and retroperitoneal fibrosis, which fixes the ureter and prevents peristalsis, leading to functional obstruction.

TABLE 4–18 • Perinephric Fluid Collections

Type	Clinical Findings	Sonographic Appearance
Abscess (renal carbuncle is a confluence of several small abscesses.)	Flank pain, high white blood count, fever	Usually echogenic with irregular thickened walls, may have shadowing within caused by gas
Hematoma	Drop in hematocrit	Same sonographic appearance as an abscess depending upon the age and amount of clot/liquification
Urinoma	An encapsulated collection of extravasated urine	Usually anechoic, may have low-level echoes if superimposed with infection
Lymphocele	Collection of lymphatic fluid	Usually anechoic, may have low-level echoes if superimposed with hemorrhage

Abscess, hematoma, urinoma, and lymphocele are commonly associated with renal transplant, although it is not exclusive.

Secondary Megaureter

This is caused by reflux of urine or obstruction. Ureteral abnormalities are viewed in Table 4–19.

URINARY BLADDER

Gross Anatomy

The urinary bladder is a thin-walled triangular structure that is located directly posterior to the pubic bone. The apex of the bladder points anteriorly and is connected to the umbilicus by the median umbilical ligament, the remains of the fetal urachus. The ureters enter at a posteroinferior angle, and the urethra extends from the bladder neck to the exterior of the body. The trigone is the area of the bladder between the neck and apex. It contains three orifices: two for the ureters and one for the urethra.

A normal distended urinary bladder on ultrasound is imaged as a midline symmetrical anechoic structure. The bladder wall is imaged as a thin, smooth, echogenic line that measures between 3 and 6 mm in thickness. The normal bladder volume varies and can usually reach 500 mL without any major discomfort.

Bladder stones can develop in the bladder or form in the kidney. Patients passing a urinary tract stone present with renal colic, flank pain, and hematuria. Sonographically, the bladder stone appears as an echogenic focus with posterior acoustic shadowing. Calculi are gravity dependent (calculi moves to the dependent portion of the bladder when the patient is placed in a decubitus position). Ureteral jets are usually normal; rarely do the calculi obstruct the ureter.

During a pelvic ultrasound examination, the bladder wall thickness, irregularities of the wall, bladder shape, and lumen should be evaluated. There may be an extrinsic mass; for example, a fibroid or enlarged prostate, compressing the bladder and causing bladder distortion. Table 4–20 reviews abnormalities that will distort the wall and shape of the bladder.

ADRENAL GLANDS

Gross Anatomy

The adrenal glands are part of the endocrine system and consist of two distinct regions: the medulla, which is surrounded by the cortex. The adrenal glands are triangle-shaped structures located superior and anteromedial to the upper pole of the kidney. They measure $5 \times 5 \times 1$ cm but at birth are proportionately much larger. Gerota's fascia encloses the kidneys, adrenals, and perinephric fat.

TABLE 4–19 • Ureteral Abnormalities

Abnormality	Clinical Finding	Sonographic Appearance
Posterior urethral valves syndrome (PUV): A flap of mucosal tissue covers the opening in the area of the prostatic urethra, causing a urinary outlet obstruction.	Most common cause of urinary obstruction in the male infant and are the second most common cause of hydronephrosis in the neonate. Decreased urine output, failure to thrive and severe cases renal failure in infants. Older patients will experience decreased urine output, dysuria, and urinary tract infections (UTIs).	Distended bladder with a thickened wall bilateral hydroureters seen medial and posterior to the bladder and in severe cases hydronephrosis. The bladder may have a "keyhole" appearance with dilation of the proximal portion of the urethra.
Ureterocele: A cystic dilation of the distal portion of the ureter with narrowing of the ureteric orifice; can be either congenital or acquired.	Patients are usually asymptomatic and the cysts are usually small. Ureteroceles may cause obstruction and infection of the upper urinary tract. If large they may cause bladder outlet obstruction.	An anechoic thin-walled structure of variable size and shape projecting into the bladder.

TABLE 4–20 • Urinary Bladder Abnormalities

Abnormality	Clinical Findings	Ultrasound Findings
Urachal cysts: The urachus connects the apex of the bladder with the allantois (an embryological structure with no function after birth) through the umbilical cord. Normally, it fibroses at birth, but it may, in part or in whole, remain patent. The urachus lies in the Retzius space (anterior to the urinary bladder)	A urachal cyst remains clinically asymptomatic until an infection develops, and then there is vague abdominal pain or urinary complaints.	An anechoic tubular structure in the lower mid-abdominal anterior wall. It may extend from the umbilicus to the bladder.
Diverticuli of the bladder: Pouchlike envaginations of the bladder wall. They can be either congenital or acquired.	The diverticula constitute a site of urinary stasis that tends to become infected	Diverticula vary greatly in size and may appear separate from the bladder. They are round, well-defined, thin-walled cystic masses. To help delineate it from an adnexal mass, have the patient void; it should disappear.
Reduplication: Complete reduplication of the bladder is rare	Unilateral reflex, obstruction or infection	Two bladders will be visualized separated by a peritoneal fold with two urethras and two external openings.
Reflux: Vesicoureteral reflux is a common urinary tract abnormality in children secondary to anomalies such as ectopic, posterior urethral valves, prune belly syndrome, neurogenic bladder, and primary congenital abnormalities of the bladder	Reflux may be a cause of chronic renal failure with scarring and atrophic changes in the kidney	Cysto-Conray (20%) is injected into the bladder. Each kidney is scanned while the contrast is injected. With each increasing grade of reflux, there is increasing renal collecting system dilation.
Bladder neck obstruction: The lower portion continuous with the urethra is called the neck.	In the male bladder, neck obstruction commonly is secondary to benign prostatic hypertrophy (BPH) or carcinoma. With prolonged obstruction the bladder wall will become thickened and trabeculated.	A thickened and irregular-walled bladder
Cystitis: Infection or inflammation of the bladder. More common in females because of the shorter urethra.	Secondary to diverticula, urethral obstruction, fistulas, cystocele, bladder neoplasm, pyelonephritis, neurogenic dysfunction, bladder calculi, trauma, pregnancy, rectal/vaginal fistula	In cases of long-standing infection or inflammation (chronic), the bladder walls may show inflammatory changes and thickening. In cases of a neurogenic bladder, low-level echoes may be seen in the bladder producing a pus–urine fluid level.
Primary benign tumor (uncommon): papilloma, epithelial, leiomyoma, neurofibroma, adenoma (associated with cystitis)	Patients present with painless hematuria, dysuria, frequent urination	Ultrasound cannot distinguish between a benign or malignant tumor. Small to massive solid tumors are seen projecting from the bladder wall, some may evaginate the bladder wall and may be smooth or irregular in contour. May mimic benign prostatic hypertrophy or cystitis. Outflow obstruction and hydronephrosis also need to be evaluated.
Primary malignant tumor: 95% are transitional cell carcinoma (TCC); 5% are squamous cell carcinoma	Invasive growths, with 40% having metastases to lymph nodes and invasion of the prostate and seminal vesicles. They are usually not detected until they have metastasized. Patients present with hematuria, urinary frequency, dysuria	Ultrasound cannot distinguish between a benign or malignant tumor. Small to massive solid tumors are seen projecting from the bladder wall, some may evaginate the bladder wall, and may be smooth or irregular in contour. May mimic benign prostatic hypertrophy or cystitis. Outflow obstruction and hydronephrosis also need to be evaluated.

The right adrenal gland lies posterior and lateral to the inferior vena cava, lateral to the right crus of the diaphragm, and medial to the right lobe of the liver. To image the right adrenal gland the patient is typically placed in a left lateral decubitus position (right side up). The right adrenal gland is located between the right lobe of liver, inferior vena cava, and right kidney.

The left adrenal gland lies medial to the spleen, lateral to the aorta, and posterior to the tail of the pancreas. Sonographically, the normal adrenal glands in adults are difficult to visualize because of their small size and the echo texture being similar to the surrounding retroperitoneal fat. To image the left adrenal gland, the patient lies in a right lateral decubitus position (left side up) the transducer is placed in a coronal position. The left adrenal glands lie- between the spleen, aorta, and left kidney, and these structures are used as sonographic landmarks. Computed tomography (CT) is the imaging modality of choice. Adrenal tumors may be identified on a sonogram usually by their displacement and/or compression of adjacent structures. See Table 4–21 for adrenal gland malfunctions.

TABLE 4–21 • Adrenal Gland Malfunctions

Malformations	Clinical Findings	Sonographic Findings
Adrenal Cortex Adrenocortical hyperfunction Cushing's syndrome	Increased corticosteroid production produces diabetes mellitus, protuberant abdomen from muscle weakening and loss of elastic tissue, rounded faces, mild hypertension, cardiac enlargement, and edema.	Varied—the adrenal glands may appear normal, diffusely enlarged, solid, cystic, or complex, with focal areas of necrosis or hemorrhage.
Conn's syndrome—benign	Hyperaldosteronism caused by an increase of aldosterone producing sodium retention, which leads to essential hypertension, increased thirst, and urination.	Varied—the adrenal glands may appear normal, diffusely enlarged, solid, cystic, or complex with focal areas of necrosis or hemorrhage.
Adenomas—may be functional or nonfunctional	Benign tumors associated with Cushing's and Conn's syndrome. May present with hypertension, diabetes, hyperthyroidism, and renal cell carcinoma.	Round or oval in shape usually larger than 1 cm, hypoechoic.
Adrenocortical hypofunction Addison's disease—rare condition	Decreased hormonal production causing hypotension, malaise, weight loss, changes in skin pigmentation, loss of body hair, and menstrual irregularity. 80% are attributable to idiopathic destruction, probably autoimmune in nature, and 20% are caused by tuberculosis.	Varied normal or hyperechoic may be small because of the destruction of cortical tissue.
Adrenal Medulla Pheochromocytoma—rare vascular tumors	Paroxysmal or sustained hypertension, angina, cardiac arrhythmias, anxiety, nausea, vomiting, and headaches. These features are caused by the concentration of catecholamines released into circulation. Large tumors may lead to heart failure and death.	Well-defined large, highly vascular masses that can be cystic, solid, or heterogeneous with calcifications.
Neuroblastoma	A highly malignant tumor that arises from the sympathetic nervous tissue or adrenal medulla. Children can be asymptomatic or have weight loss, fever episodes of tachycardia, sweats, and headaches with a palpable abdominal mass.	Varied presentation—large echogenic, heterogeneous mass with areas of cystic degeneration and focal calcifications. The kidney will be displaced posteriorly and inferiorly.
Adrenal Masses Adrenal metastases	Most commonly from bronchogenic CA, lung adenocarcinoma, breast or stomach carcinoma.	Metastases to the adrenals vary in size and echogenicity.
Adrenal cysts—rare	None—patients are usually asymptomatic	Round or oval in shape, anechoic with increased through acoustical transmission. Adrenal cysts tend to become calcified, which appear as an echo-free structure, with an echogenic back wall with posterior shadowing (no through acoustic transmission).
Adrenal hematomas	Most often seen in infants caused by trauma from birth, prematurity or hypoxia. In adults, it is caused by trauma or anticoagulant therapy.	Varies depending upon the age of the bleed initially the hematoma is echogenic, and then it becomes sonolucent to complex and then calcified.

Right Adrenal Pathology Will Displace

Anteriorly

The retroperitoneal fat line

The inferior vena cava

The right renal vein

Posteriorly

The right kidney

Left Adrenal Pathology Will Displace

Anteriorly

The splenic vein

Posteriorly

The left kidney

Adrenal Cortex

The adrenal cortex, which produces steroid hormones, is subdivided into three zones listed from outer to inner: (1) the zona glomerulosa, which produces mineralocorticoids (for the regulation of aldosterone to regulate electrolyte metabolism); (2) the zona fasciculata, which produces glucocorticoids (for the regulation of cortisol, which is an anti-stress and anti-inflammatory hormone); and (3) the zona reticularis, which produces gonadocorticoids (for regulation of the secretion of androgens and estrogens, which are the sex hormones of an individual).

The adrenal cortical hormones are regulated by the adrenocorticotropic hormones (ACTH) of the anterior pituitary gland. A *decrease* in adrenal cortical function leads to an increased ACTH, which then stimulates the adrenal cortex. An *increase* in concentration of adrenal hormones leads to a drop in ACTH secretion, which leads to a drop in the activity of adrenal cortex.

The adrenal cortex may be affected either by lesions that produce an excess of steroid hormones or by lesions that produce a deficiency. The adrenocortical hormone levels may be abnormal (increased or decreased production) as a result of a pituitary tumor, which can cause the overproduction or underproduction of ACTH.

Adrenal Medulla

The adrenal medulla produces epinephrine (adrenalin) and norepinephrine. These hormones have a wide range of effects.

Epinephrine dilates the coronary vessels and constricts the skin and kidney vessels. It increases coronary output, raises oxygen consumption, and causes hyperglycemia.

Norepinephrine constricts all arterial vessels except the coronary arteries (which dilate). It is the essential regulator of blood pressure.

Epinephrine, in particular, is responsible for the fight or-flight reaction. It stimulates the metabolic rate, allowing energy that is more available.

GASTROINTESTINAL TRACT

Sonography is not routinely used to image the gastrointestinal tract because of the air within the bowel lumen. Normal bowel patterns can be imaged and recognize bowel peristalsis on abdominal sonographic examination. Knowledge of the gastrointestinal (GI) tract is essential for identifying the location of the pathology.

Gross Anatomy

The GI tract is composed of the esophagus, the stomach, the small intestine, and the colon.

The esophagus is a tubular structure that extends from the pharynx to the stomach. Its main function is to bring food and water to the stomach. The gastroesophageal junction (GEJ) can be identified slightly to the left of midline on a sagittal scan. Sonographically, it appears round with an echogenic center with a hypoechoic rim also referred to as a "target sign" or "bull's eye" located posterior to the left lobe of the liver and anterior to the aorta.

The stomach lies between the esophagus and the duodenum. The opening between the stomach and the duodenum is called the pyloric orifice. The main function of the stomach is to break down food to chyme, which then passes through to the duodenum. Sonographically, the fluid-filled stomach is imaged as an anechoic structure with echogenic foci and thin walls. The small intestine lies between the stomach and the colon and is divided into three parts: duodenum, jejunum, and the ileum. The main function of the small intestine is to absorb food.

The ileocecal valve connects the distal portion of the ileum to the first section of the colon, the cecum. The appendix is located in the right lower quadrant as a tubular structure that extends from the cecum. The ascending colon ascends from the cecum along the right side of the body to the posterior inferior surface of the liver. The ascending colon bends to the left and forms the hepatic flexure. The transverse colon extends across the body from the hepatic flexure to the splenic flexure. The splenic flexure is located posterior and inferior to the spleen and bends inferiorly forming the descending colon, which courses along the left side to the body and terminates at the sigmoid colon.

The sigmoid is the narrowest portion of the colon, and the distal end forms the rectum. The anal canal is the distal end of the rectum, which expels solid waste products (feces) from the body.

DIAPHRAGM

Gross Anatomy

The diaphragm is a dome-shaped muscle separating the thorax from the abdominal cavity. The diaphragm covers the superior and lateral border of the liver on the right side and the spleen on the left side. Sonographically, the diaphragm is identified as a thin, echogenic, curvilinear interface between the lungs and liver (spleen).

The *subphrenic space* is between the liver (or spleen) and the diaphragm and is a common site for abscess.

CRURA OF THE DIAPHRAGM

The diaphragmatic crura are right and left fibromuscular bundles that attach to the lumbar vertebra at the level of L3 on the right and L1 on the left. They act as anchors to the diaphragm.

The left crus can be visualized anterior to the aorta above the level of the celiac artery. Below the celiac artery, the crura extend along the lateral aspects of the vertebral columns. The right crus is visualized posterior to the caudate lobe and the inferior vena cava.

FLUID COLLECTIONS

Ascites

Ascites is an abnormal accumulation of serous fluid in the peritoneum. The most common cause for ascites in the United States is cirrhosis and accounts for about 80 percent of causes.[3] Ascites are catogrized into:

- Transudative—anechoic/freely mobile usually benign, free-floating bowel in the abdomen
- Exudative—internal echoes/loculated—associated with infection and malignancy
- Bowel matted or fixed to posterior abdominal wall—associated with malignancy
- Nonmobile fluid associated with coagulated hematoma (trauma)

Pathology Associated with Ascites

- Congestive heart failure
- Infection (inflammatory process)
- Kidney failure
- Liver failure/disease—end-stage fatty liver, cirrhosis
- Malignancy
- Ruptured aneurysm
- Pyogenic peritonitis
- Tuberculosis
- Portal venous system obstruction
- Obstruction of lymph nodes
- Obstruction of vessels—Budd–Chiari syndrome
- Acute cholecystitis
- Ectopic pregnancy
- Postoperative

Clinical Presentation

The clinical presentation of ascites is a distended abdomen. In cases of massive ascites, respiratory distress will also be present.

Sonographic Findings

Accumulations occur (supine position) in the following order:

1. Inferior tip—right lobe liver
2. Superior portion—right flank
3. Pelvic cul de sac
4. Right and Left paracolic gutter
5. Morison's pouch
   - Ascites is found inferior to the diaphragm
   - Gross (massive) ascites—extrahepatic portion falciform ligament seen attaching the liver to anterior abdominal wall
   - Ascites may cause a downward displacement of the liver
   - May cause gallbladder wall to appear to thicken
   - Liver may appear more echogenic
   - May see patent umbilical vein
   - Changing patient's position to observe fluid movement may be useful
   - Disproportional accumulation in lesser sac suggestive of adjacent organ pathology (i.e., acute pancreatitis, pancreatic CA)

Abscess

An abscess is an encased collection of pus (acute/chronic). A cavity formed by liquefactive necrosis within solid tissue.

Pathology Associated with Abscesses

- Penetrating trauma (wounds)
- Postsurgical procedures
- Retained products of conception
- Pelvic inflammatory disease
- Chronic bladder disease
- Sepsis—blood-borne bacterial infection
- Long-standing hematomas
- Postcholecystectomy—site of the gallbladder fossa
- GI tract—peptic ulcer perforation; bowel spill during surgery (peritonitis)
- Urinary tract infection
- Infected ascites with septa/debris
- Amebic abscess—may be densely echogenic

Clinical Presentation. Pain, spiking fever, chills, elevated white blood cell count, solitary or multiple sites, tenderness

Hepatic Abscess Intrahepatic

Abscesses are most often associated in the Western hemisphere with cholangitis; also seen with sepsis and penetrating trauma to liver.

- Location: within liver parenchyma
- Differential diagnosis: solid tumor, usually round lesion with scattered internal echoes, variable through transmission

Subhepatic

Abscess associated with cholecystectomy
- Location: inferior to liver; fluid collection anterior to right kidney (Morison's pouch); gallbladder fossa (postcholecystectomy)

Subphrenic

Abscess associated with bacterial spill into peritoneum during surgical procedure; bowel rupture; peptic ulcer perforation; trauma

- Location: fluid collection superior to the liver, inferior to diaphragm; transmission variable; gas (dirty shadowing)

General Sonographic Findings. A variable, complex, solid, cystic lesion with septa, debris, and scattered echoes; through transmission may be good; mass/cyst with shaggy/thick irregular walls; mass displacing surrounding structures; complex mass with dirty shadowing from within. *Presence of gas within a mass suggests an abscess (may also be attributable to fistulous communication with bowel or airway or outside air).*

General Differential Diagnosis. Necrosing tumor with fluid center (these usually have thicker walls and *no gas*).

Ascites Versus Abscess

A localized area of ascites may be mistaken for an abscess. Place the patient in the erect or Trendelenburg position; ascites will shift to the dependent portion, but an abscess will not, unless it contains air; the air/fluid level will shift.

Pleural Effusion

Pleural effusions are nonspecific reactions to an underlying pulmonary or systemic disease such as cirrhosis. Obtaining fluid for analysis may allow a more specific diagnosis.

Sonographic appearance shows a pleural effusion usually as an echo-free (anechoic), wedge-shaped area that lies posteromedial to the liver and posterior to the diaphragm. Occa-sionally, pleural effusions contain internal echoes, sometimes indicating the presence of a neoplasm. These echoes may be caused by blood or pus (empyema), especially when the collection is loculated. Loculated effusions do not always lie adjacent to the diaphragm and may be loculated anywhere on the chest wall. Sometimes effusions lie between the lung and the diaphragm and are known as subpulmonic. Right-sided pleural effusions can be assessed easily on a view demonstrating the diaphragm and the liver. Effusions on the left side are more difficult to see in the supine position but can be seen more readily with the patient in an oblique position and imaging through the spleen.

RETROPERITONEUM

The retroperitoneum is the area between the posterior portion of the parietal peritoneum and the posterior abdominal wall, extending from the diaphragm to the pelvis.

Divisions

The retroperitoneum is divided into three areas by the renal fossa (Gerota's fascia). Fig. 4–8 demonstrates the division of the retroperitoneum into anterior perirenal and posterior perirenal spaces.

1. The anterior perirenal space contains the retroperitoneal portion of the intestines and the pancreas.
2. The perirenal space contains the kidneys, ureters, adrenal glands, aorta, IVC, and retroperitoneal nodes.
3. The posterior perirenal space contains the posterior abdominal wall, iliopsoas muscle, and quadratus muscle.

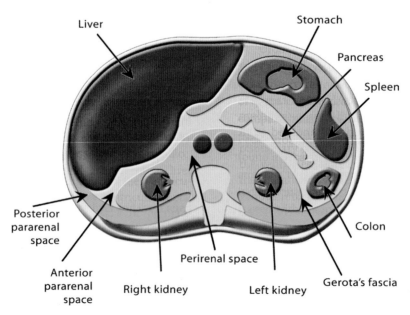

FIGURE 4–8. Cross-sectional anatomy of the retroperitoneal compartments.

Pathology

The retroperitoneal area is subject to infection, bleeding, inflammation, and tumors.

Anterior Perirenal Space. Pancreatic pathology, carcinoma of the duodenum, ascending and descending colon causing bowel thickening or infiltration resulting in a "bull's eye."

Perirenal Space. Kidney diseases, adrenal diseases, invasion or displacement of inferior vena cava, aortic aneurysms, ureteral abnormalities, sarcoma, liposarcoma, aortic, and retroperitoneal adenopathy.

Posterior Perirenal Space. Renal transplant is usually performed in this extraperitoneal space within the iliac fossa, using the iliac vessels for anastomosis.

Primary Retroperitoneal Tumors

Primary retroperitoneal tumors are mostly malignant; rapidly growing; and larger tumors are more likely to show evidence of necrosis and hemorrhage. Concurrence of mass with ascites indicates invasion of peritoneal surfaces.

Liposarcoma. Originates from fat. Liposarcoma has a complex echogenic pattern with thick walls.

Fibrosarcoma. Originates from connective tissue. Fibrosarcoma has a complex mostly sonolucent pattern, invading surrounding tissues.

Rhabdomyosarcoma. Originates from muscle. It occurs as a solid, complex, or homogeneous echogenic mass, invading surrounding tissue.

Leiomyosarcoma. Originates from smooth muscle. It occurs as a complex echo-dense mass that may have areas of necrosis and cystic degeneration.

Teratoma. Originates from all three germ cell layers. Most teratomas occur in the area of the upper pole of the left kidney. Ninety percent are benign. They are complex with echogenic and cystic areas. Fifty percent occur in children.

Neurogenic Tumors. Originate from nerve tissue and occur mostly in the paravertebral region. They are heterogeneous and echogenic.

Secondary Retroperitoneal Tumors

Secondary retroperitoneal tumors are primary recurrences from previously resected tumors or recurrent masses from previous renal carcinoma.

Ascitic fluid along with a retroperitoneal tumor usually indicates seeding or invasion of the peritoneal surface. Evaluation of the para-aortic region should be made for extension to the lymph nodes. The liver should also be evaluated for metastatic involvement.

Retroperitoneal Fibrosis

Retroperitoneal fibrosis is the formation of thick sheets of connective tissue extending from the perirenal space to the dome of the bladder. It encases, rather than displaces, the great vessels, ureters, and lymph channels, causing obstruction. Severe uropathy may ensue. The etiology of retroperitoneal fibrosis is usually idiopathic, but it may sometimes be associated with aortic aneurysm.

Clinical Findings. The clinical findings in retroperitoneal fibrosis include hydronephrosis, hypertension, anuria, fever, leukocytosis, anemia, nausea and vomiting, weight loss, malaise, palpable abdominal or rectal mass, and abdominal, back, or flank pain. It is more frequent in males than females, and it most common at age 50 through the 60s.

Sonographic Findings. Retroperitoneal fibrosis appears as thick masses anterior and lateral to the aorta and inferior vena cava, extending from renal vessels to the sacral promontory. The anterior to hypoechoic sheets have smooth, well-defined anterior margins and irregular, poorly defined posterior margins. The differential diagnosis includes lymphoma, nodal metastases, and retroperitoneal sarcoma or hematoma.

Retroperitoneal Fluid Collections. Collections of fluids in the retroperitoneum include abscesses, hematomas, urinomas, lymphoceles, and cysts.

LYMPHATIC SYSTEM

Gross Anatomy

The lymphatic system arises from veins in the developing embryo and is closely associated with veins throughout most parts of the body. Lymphatic vessels assist veins in their function by draining many of the body tissues and, thus, increasing the amount of fluid returning to the heart. The lymph vascular network does not form a closed-looped system such as the blood vascular system. Lymph vessels begin as tiny, colorless, unconnected capillaries in the connective tissues. These merge to form progressively larger vessels that are interrupted at various sites by small filtering stations called lymph nodes. The lymph fluid from the entire body ultimately drains into the inferior vena cava.

This lymphatic network has tremendous clinical significance. Interruption of lymph drainage in an area generally creates considerable swelling (edema) owing to the accumulation of fluids. In addition, the lymph vessels offer a variety of routes for cancer cells to move from one site to another (metastasis).

Lymph Nodes

Lymph nodes contain lymphocytes and reticulum cells, their function being one of filtration and production of lymphocytes and antibodies. All the lymph passes through nodes, which act as filters not only for bacteria but also for cancer cells. Enlargement of lymph nodes is a usual sign of an ongoing bacterial or carcinogenic process. Normal lymph nodes measure <1 cm in size. The parietal nodes follow the same course as the prevertebral vessels, while the visceral nodes are more superficial and generally follow the same course that the organ-specific vessels follow. Sonographically, we can evaluate lymph nodes in the pelvis, retroperitoneum, portahepatis, perirenal, and prevertebral vasculature.

Function. The functions of the lymph nodes are: (1) the formation of lymphocytes, (2) the production of antibodies, and (3) the filtration of lymph.

Sonographic Appearance. To visualize lymph nodes, they must be at least 2 cm in size. They are very homogeneous. Lymph nodes are typically hypoechoic, but there is no through transmission. Lymphomas have a nonspecific appearance but in general the following are true:

- Adenopathy secondary to lymphoma is usually sonolucent.
- Adenopathy secondary to metastatic disease is usually complex.
- Posttherapy enlarged nodes are usually very echogenic but may develop cystic areas secondary to necrosis.

Periaortic nodes have specific characteristics: They may drape the great vessels anteriorly (obscuring sharp anterior vascular border); may have a lobular, smooth, or scalloped appearance; and with mesenteric involvement, they may fill most of the abdomen in an irregular complex necrosis.

Para-aortic nodes may displace the celiac axis and superior mesenteric artery anteriorly. Enlarged nodes posterior to the aorta will displace the great vessels away from the spine; this is referred to as the floating aorta sign. The "sandwich" sign occurs when nodes surround the mesenteric vessels.

Sonographic Technique. Concentrates on prevertebral vessels, aorta, inferior vena cava; portahepatic (can produce *biliary obstruction*); spleen size; iliopsoas muscles; urinary bladder contour; perirenal; retroperitoneum; and pelvis.

Para-aortic lymph nodes are involved with lymphoma in 25% of cases and 40% with Hodgkin's disease. The sonographic appearance of these lymphomatous nodes varies from hypoechoic to anechoic with no increased through transmission. Occasionally, anechoic nodal masses may resemble cystic structures. Nodal enlargement secondary to other neoplasms or inflammatory processes, such as retroperitoneal fibrosis, may be indistinguishable from lymphomatous lymphadenopathy. Para-aortic or paracaval nodes frequently obscure the sharp anterior vascular border or compress the aorta or inferior vena cava. Placing a patient in a decubitus position

demonstrating the aorta and inferior vena cava facilitates sonographic imaging of the retroperitoneal area down to the aortic bifurcation.

Tumors of Lymphoid Tissue

Lymphomas (Tumors of Lymphoid Tissue). *Hodgkin's disease* (40%) is a malignant condition characterized by generalized lymphoid tissue enlargement (e.g., enlarged lymph nodes and spleen). Twice as many males as females are affected. It usually occurs between the ages of 15 and 34, or after 50. Histopathologic classification: Reed–Sternberg (RS) cells and multinucleated cells are present.

Non-Hodgkin's disease (60%) is further subdivided into nodular and diffuse histopathologies. It is a heterogeneous group of diseases that consists of neoplastic proliferation of lymphoid cells that usually disseminate throughout the body. It occurs in all age groups with the incidence increasing with age.

Mesenteric nodal involvement in <4% in patients with Hodgkin's disease but >50% in non-Hodgkin's patients. Lymphomatous cellular infiltration of the greater omentum may be seen as a uniformly thick, hypoechoic band-shaped structure. The appearance of mesenteric nodes can resemble that of retroperitoneal nodes.

Mesenteric masses may also appear as multiple cystic or separated masses that may resemble fluid-filled bowel loops. Perihepatic nodes, celiac axis nodes, splenic-hilar, and renal-hilar nodes may also be demonstrated sonographically. Although most are hypoechoic to anechoic, inhomogeneous areas of increased echogenicity can be found in areas of focal necrosis within large nodes. Nodes can encase or invade adjacent organs and produce significant organ displacement, whereas portal nodes produce biliary obstruction.

Extranodal Lymphoma. The liver, kidneys, GI tract, pancreas, and thyroid may show lymphomatous involvement.

Hepatic Lymphoma. Hepatic lymphomatous involvement presents as multiple hypoechoic or anechoic focal parenchymal defects. Although these anechoic lesions may resemble cystic structures, they rarely demonstrate enhanced posterior acoustic transmission or peripheral refractory shadowing. Hepatic abscesses, metastases from sarcomas or melanomas, focal areas of cholangitis, radiation fibrosis, and extensive hemosiderosis have presented with findings sonographically indistinguishable from hepatic lymphoma.

Renal Lymphomas. Less than 3% of all non-Hodgkin's lymphomas present with renal involvement, mainly Burkitt's lymphoma or diffuse histiocystic lymphomas.

Gastrointestinal Lymphoma. Fifteen percent of non-Hodgkin's lymphomas may present with gastrointestinal involvement. Sonographic features include a relatively hypoechoic mass with central echogenic foci. The sonographic appearance is nonspecific for lymphomatous involvement; gastric carcinoma or gastric wall edema may have the same sonographic appearance.

Pancreatic Lymphoma. Ten percent of non-Hodgkin's patients present with pancreatic involvement—portions of tissue represented by focal hypoechoic or anechoic masses.

Thyroid Lymphoma. Lymphomatous thyroid masses also present in the same manner.

Inflammatory Conditions

There are three inflammatory conditions of the lymphatic system: acute and chronic lymphadenitis and infectious mononucleosis.

Common primary tumors with metastases to lymph are those of the breast, lung, melanoma, prostate, cervix, and uterus.

Sonographic Pitfalls

1. Enlarged nodes can mimic aortic aneurysm at lower gain settings on longitudinal scans; transverse scans are needed to differentiate.
2. Aneurysms enlarge fairly symmetrically, whereas enlarged nodes tend to drape over prevertebral vessels.
3. Bowel can mimic enlarged nodes so check for peristalsis; nodes are reproducible, whereas bowel is not.

RETROPERITONEAL VERSUS INTRAPERITONEAL MASSES

The retroperitoneal location of a mass is confirmed when there is any of the following:

- Anterior renal displacement
- Anterior displacement of dilated ureters
- Anterior displacement of the retroperitoneal fat ventrally and often cranially, whereas hepatic and subhepatic lesions produce inferior and posterior displacement. The direction of displacement may permit diagnosis of the anatomical origin of right upper quadrant masses.
- Anterior vascular displacement—aorta, inferior vena cava, splenic vein, superior mesenteric vein

References

1. Crossin JD, Mauradali D, Wilson SR. US of Liver Transplants: Normal and Abnormal 1. *RadioGraphics.* 2003:1093-1114.
2. Kanterman RY, Darcy MD, Middleton WD, et al. Doppler sonography findings associated with transjugular intrahepatic portosystemic shunt malfunction. *AJR.* 1997; 168:467-472.
3. Runyon BA. Care of Patients with Ascitis. *N. Engl J Med* 1994; 330:337.
4. Rumack CM, Wilson SR, Charboneau JW. Diagnostic Ultrasound. 3rd ed. Elsevier Mosby. St. Louis. Missouri; 2005
5. Tortora GJ. Derrickson B. Principles of Anatomy and Physiology. 11th ed. John Wiley & Sons Inc. Hoboken, NJ; 2006

Questions

GENERAL INSTRUCTIONS: For each question, select the best answer. Select only one answer for each question unless otherwise instructed.

1. What three structures comprise the portal triad?

   (A) portal vein, portal artery and common bile duct
   (B) hepatic artery, portal vein and bile duct
   (C) hepatic vein, portal artery and cystic duct
   (D) hepatic artery, portal artery and bile duct
   (E) hepatic duct, hepatic vein and common bile duct

2. A 4-year-old boy presents with high blood pressure, hematuria, and a palpable left flank mass. An ultrasound examination is performed, and a solid renal mass is identified. This finding is most characteristic of which of the following?

   (A) hypernephroma
   (B) infantile polycystic kidney disease
   (C) neuroblastoma
   (D) nephroblastoma
   (E) acute lymphoblastic leukemia

3. A patient presents with ampulla of Vater obstruction, distention of the gallbladder, and painless jaundice. Which of the following is this presentation associated with?

   (A) hydropic gallbladder
   (B) choledochal cyst
   (C) Courvoisier's sign
   (D) Mirizzi's syndrome
   (E) Caroli's disease

4. Which of the following will long-standing cystic duct obstruction give rise to?

   (A) porcelain gallbladder
   (B) hydropic gallbladder
   (C) septated gallbladder
   (D) gallbladder septations
   (E) gallbladder contraction

5. While performing an ultrasound examination, the sonographer finds that both kidneys measure 5 cm in length. They are very echogenic. One should consider the possibility of all of the following *except*

   (A) chronic glomerulonephritis
   (B) chronic pyelonephritis
   (C) renal vascular disease
   (D) renal vein thrombosis
   (E) renal hypoplasia

6. Staghorn calculus refers to a large stone within which of the following?

   (A) pancreas
   (B) urinary bladder
   (C) renal pelvis of the kidney
   (D) neck of the gallbladder
   (E) hepatic duct

7. What gastrointestinal peptide hormone stimulates gallbladder contraction?

   (A) gastrin
   (B) cholecalciferol
   (C) cholestyramine
   (D) cholecystokinin
   (E) cholestasis

8. What is the name of the portion of the liver that is *not* covered by the peritoneum?

   (A) quadrate lobe
   (B) intraperitoneal
   (C) Riedel's lobe
   (D) bare area
   (E) hepatopetal

9. What is the normal thickness of the gallbladder wall?

   (A) 15 mm
   (B) 10 mm
   (C) 3 cm
   (D) 5 mm
   (E) 3 mm

10. **Where does the pancreatic head lie?**

    (A) caudad to the portal vein and medial to the superior mesenteric vein

    (B) cephalad to the portal vein and medial to the superior mesenteric vein

    (C) caudad to the portal vein and anterior to the inferior vena cava

    (D) cephalad to the portal vein and anterior to the inferior vena cava

11. **Identify the sonographic pattern that best describes hydronephrosis.**

    (A) distortion of the reniform shape

    (B) multiple cystic space masses throughout the kidneys

    (C) fluid-filled pelvocaliceal collecting system

    (D) fluid-filled pararenal space

    (E) echogenic renal cortex

12. **A patient presents with a dilated interhepatic duct, dilated gallbladder, and a dilated common bile duct. This is most characteristic of which one of the following levels of obstruction?**

    (A) proximal common bile duct

    (B) distal common bile duct

    (C) distal common hepatic duct

    (D) cystic duct

    (E) neck of the gallbladder

13. **What is the most common location of pancreatic pseudocyst?**

    (A) lesser sac

    (B) porta hepatis area

    (C) groin

    (D) splenic hilum

    (E) mediastinum

14. **Which of the following is true about the extrahepatic portion of the falciform ligament?**

    (A) courses between the inferior vena cava and the gallbladder

    (B) is visualized when massive ascites is present

    (C) connects the liver to the lesser sac

    (D) is visualized when peritonitis is present

    (E) is visualized when there is recanalization of the umbilical vein

15. **The superior mesenteric artery arises 1 cm below the celiac trunk and courses**

    (A) 1 cm before it bifurcates

    (B) inferiorly and lateral to the head of the pancreas

    (C) anterior and parallel to the aorta

    (D) transversely and caudad

    (E) posterior to the inferior vena cava

16. **The division by using Couinaud's sections into right and left lobes of the liver is**

    (A) main lobar fissure

    (B) ligamentum venosum

    (C) falciform ligament

    (D) hepatoduodenal ligament

    (E) hepatic arteries

17. **Which of the following is the portion of the pancreas that lies posterior to the superior mesenteric artery and vein?**

    (A) head

    (B) neck

    (C) uncinate process

    (D) body

    (E) tail

18. **Which vessel courses along the posterior surface of the body and tail of the pancreas?**

    (A) superior mesenteric artery

    (B) left renal vein

    (C) aorta

    (D) splenic artery

    (E) splenic vein

19. **Sonographically, where can the gastroesophageal junction be visualized?**

    (A) anterior to the inferior vena cava and posterior to the right lobe of the liver

    (B) anterior to the aorta and posterior to the left lobe of the liver

    (C) lateral to the head of the pancreas

    (D) anterior to the stomach and medial to the spleen

    (E) posterior to the left lobe of the liver and medial to the stomach

20. Which of the following describes adenomyomatosis of the gallbladder?

    (A) a congenital anomaly that presents itself in the fourth or fifth decade

    (B) an inflammation of the gallbladder and biliary ducts

    (C) associated with chronic hepatitis

    (D) proliferation of the mucosal layer, which extends into the muscle layer

    (E) a malignant process that involves the gallbladder wall and lumen

21. What is the most common cause of acute pyelonephritis?

    (A) hypertension

    (B) *Escherichia coli*

    (C) *Klebsiella*

    (D) hydronephrosis

    (E) enterococcus faecalis

22. A renal sonogram is performed and an echogenic well-defined mass is identified in the renal cortex. This is characteristic of which of the following?

    (A) angiomyolipoma

    (B) column of Bertin

    (C) adenocarcinoma

    (D) pyonephrosis

    (E) renal stone

23. The gastroduodenal artery is a branch of which of the following?

    (A) aorta

    (B) celiac axis

    (C) common hepatic artery

    (D) left gastric artery

    (E) duodenal artery

24. Identify the vessel that is seen anterior to the aorta and posterior to the superior mesenteric artery.

    (A) splenic vein

    (B) common hepatic artery

    (C) gonadal artery

    (D) left renal artery

    (E) left renal vein

25. The liver is covered by a thick membrane of collagenous fibers intermixed with elastic elements. What is this membrane called?

    (A) Glisson's capsule

    (B) Gerota's fascia

    (C) Bowman's capsule

    (D) adipose capsule

    (E) membrane capsule

26. Which of the following can cause anterior displacement of the splenic vein?

    (A) pancreatitis

    (B) pseudocysts

    (C) left adrenal hyperplasia

    (D) aneurysm

    (E) inferior vena cava thrombi

27. Which one of the following vessels originates from the celiac axis and is very tortuous?

    (A) splenic artery

    (B) hepatic artery

    (C) right gastric artery

    (D) gastroduodenal artery

    (E) coiled artery

28. When accessory spleens are present, where are they usually located?

    (A) at the superior margin of the spleen

    (B) on the posterior aspect of the spleen

    (C) near the kidney

    (D) near the splenic hilum

    (E) near the left diaphragm

29. What is a fold at the fundal portion of the gallbladder usually called?

    (A) Hartmann's pouch

    (B) junctional fold

    (C) valves of Heister

    (D) Phrygian cap

    (E) pouch of Douglas

30. The inferior vena cava forms at the confluence of which of the following vessels?

    (A) right and left carotid veins

    (B) right and left common iliac veins

    (C) right and left lumbar veins

    (D) right and left renal veins

    (E) right and left common iliac arteries

31. **Diffuse thickening of the gallbladder wall can be seen sonographically in all of the following *except***

    (A) acute cholecystitis

    (B) hepatitis

    (C) congestive heart failure

    (D) ascites

    (E) portal hypertension

32. **A gallbladder sonographic examination is performed, and a small gallbladder with intrahepatic dilatation is seen. This may indicate that the level of obstruction is at the level of which of the following?**

    (A) neck of the gallbladder

    (B) common bile duct

    (C) cystic duct

    (D) common hepatic duct

    (E) none of the above

33. **What is the maximum inner diameter of the main pancreatic duct in young adults?**

    (A) 10 mm

    (B) 5 mm

    (C) 2 cm

    (D) 3 cm

    (E) 2 mm

34. **Which of the following is produced by the endocrine function of the pancreas?**

    (A) insulin

    (B) lipase

    (C) amylase

    (D) trypsin

    (E) chymotrypsin

35. **Which laboratory test is used to assess renal function?**

    (A) serum creatinine

    (B) serum bilirubin

    (C) aspartate aminotransferase (AST)

    (D) alkaline phosphatase

    (E) serum amylase

36. **Adult polycystic disease may be characterized by all of the following *except***

    (A) it is autosomal dominant disease

    (B) it may be associated with cysts in the liver, pancreas, and spleen

    (C) bilateral small and echogenic kidneys

    (D) usually does not produce any symptoms until the third or fourth decade of life

    (E) the kidneys lose their reniform shape

37. **What is the best sonographic window to image the left hemidiaphragm?**

    (A) liver

    (B) spleen

    (C) stomach

    (D) left kidney

    (E) urinary bladder

38. **A patient in the late stages of sickle cell anemia will have a spleen that is which of the following?**

    (A) enlarged and lobulated

    (B) enlarged and echogenic

    (C) small and hypoechoic

    (D) small and echogenic

    (E) atrophic and isoechoic

39. **Bilateral hydronephrosis frequently occurs in all of the following *except***

    (A) urinoma

    (B) posterior urethral valve (PUV)

    (C) late pregnancy

    (D) fibroid uterus

    (E) benign prostate hypertrophy (BPH)

40. **In a patient with acute hepatitis, what is the appearance of the liver parenchyma sonographically?**

    (A) hypoechoic

    (B) echogenic

    (C) complex

    (D) normal

    (E) anechoic

41. **What is a hypertrophied column of Bertin?**

    (A) benign tumor of the kidney

    (B) malignant tumor of the lower urinary tract

    (C) renal variant

    (D) a common cause of hydronephrosis

    (E) complication of a renal transplant

42. **What is a ureterovesical junction?**

    (A) junction between the renal pelvis joins the proximal ureter

    (B) junction between the distal ureter and the base of the bladder

    (C) junction between the renal pyramids and the distal calyces

    (D) junction between the ejaculatory ducts and urethra

43. **What is the landmark for the posterolateral border of the thyroid?**

    (A) trachea

    (B) esophagus

    (C) strap muscle

    (D) common carotid artery

    (E) superior thyroid artery

44. **Which of the following is *not* a clinical sign of renal disease?**

    (A) oliguria

    (B) palpable flank mass

    (C) generalized edema

    (D) hypertension

    (E) jaundice

45. **Acute hydroceles may be caused by all of the following *except***

    (A) infarction

    (B) tumor

    (C) testicular torsion

    (D) trauma

    (E) infection of the testis or epididymis

46. **What is the most common malignancy of the adrenal gland in children?**

    (A) adrenal adenoma

    (B) neuroblastoma

    (C) nephroblastoma

    (D) pheochromocytoma

    (E) lymphoma

47. **If a mass in the area of the pancreatic head is found, what other structure should be examined sonographically?**

    (A) the liver

    (B) the inferior vena cava

    (C) the spleen

    (D) the kidney

    (E) the bowel

48. **What is the most common primary carcinoma of the pancreas?**

    (A) insulinoma

    (B) cystadenocarcinoma

    (C) adenocarcinoma

    (D) pancreatic pseudocyst

    (E) lymphoma

49. **The ligament of venosum separates which two lobes of the liver?**

    (A) right and left lobes

    (B) medial portion of the left lobe and the lateral portion of the left lobe

    (C) caudate lobe and left lobe of the liver

    (D) anterior portion of the right lobe and the posterior portion of the right lobe

    (E) quadrate lobe and the left lobe of the liver

50. **What is the most common benign neoplasm of the liver?**

    (A) hemangioma

    (B) angiomyolipoma

    (C) focal nodular hyperplasia

    (D) abscess

    (E) Wilms' tumor

51. **Which of the following may develop in patients with right-sided heart failure and elevated systemic venous pressure?**

    (A) fatty liver

    (B) portal-systemic anastomoses

    (C) focal liver lesions

    (D) dilatation of the intrahepatic veins

    (E) hematomas

52. **Which of the following separates the right and left lobes of the liver?**

    (A) coronary ligament

    (B) main lobar fissure

    (C) falciform ligament

    (D) ligament of venosum

    (E) interhemispheric fissure

53. Which of the following is *not* a retroperitoneal structure?

(A) kidney

(B) pancreas

(C) aorta

(D) spleen

(E) psoas muscle

54. Which of the following statements is *true* about the portal vein?

(A) It is formed by the union of the common hepatic duct and the cystic duct.

(B) It is only imaged sonographically when there is liver pathology.

(C) It is formed by the union of the splenic vein and superior mesenteric vein.

(D) It is very pulsatile.

(E) It is commonplace for stones to form.

55. The common bile duct is joined by the pancreatic duct as they enter the

(A) first portion of the duodenum

(B) second portion of the duodenum

(C) third portion of the duodenum

(D) fourth portion of the duodenum

(E) pylorus of the stomach

56. A patient presents with empyema of the gallbladder. What should the sonographer expect to find?

(A) pus within the gallbladder

(B) common bile duct obstruction

(C) stones within the gallbladder

(D) abscess surrounding the gallbladder

(E) duplication of the gallbladder

57. Identify the laboratory value that is specific for a hepatoma of the liver.

(A) alkaline phosphatase

(B) alpha-fetoprotein

(C) serum amylase

(D) bilirubin

(E) serum albumin

58. If the prostate is found to be enlarged, which of the following should the sonographer also check?

(A) spleen for enlargement

(B) scrotum for hydroceles

(C) kidneys for hydronephrosis

(D) liver for metastases

(E) gallbladder for stones

59. The body of the pancreas is bound on its anterior surface by which of the following?

(A) atrium of stomach

(B) greater sac

(C) splenic vein

(D) common bile duct

(E) duodenum

60. On a transverse scan, the portal vein is seen as a circular anechoic structure

(A) anterior to the inferior vena cava

(B) posterior to the aorta

(C) medial to the head of the pancreas

(D) inferior to the head of the pancreas

(E) anterior to the common bile duct

61. Hyperthyroidism associated with a diffuse goiter is associated with which of the following?

(A) papillary carcinoma

(B) Graves' disease

(C) Hashimoto's thyroiditis

(D) adenoma

62. Identify the part of the pancreas that lies anterior to the inferior vena cava and posterior to the superior mesenteric vein.

(A) head

(B) neck

(C) body

(D) uncinate process

(E) tail

63. In a dissecting aneurysm, the dissection is through which of the following?

(A) the adventitia

(B) the media

(C) the intima

(D) all three layers

(E) lumen

64. The adrenal gland can be divided into which of the following parts?

    (A) pelvis and sinus

    (B) cortex and medulla

    (C) major and minor calices

    (D) head and tail

    (E) fundus and body

65. Where can a patent umbilical vein be found?

    (A) ligamentum venosum

    (B) main lobar fissure

    (C) ligamentum teres

    (D) intersegmental ligament

    (E) gallbladder fossa

66. All of the following are characteristic for dilated intrahepatic bile ducts *except*

    (A) the parallel channel sign

    (B) irregular borders to dilated bile ducts

    (C) echo enhancement behind dilated ducts

    (D) decreasing size as they course toward the porta hepatis

    (E) they do not fill with color

67. A retroperitoneal abscess may be found within in all of the following *except*

    (A) the rectus abdominis muscle

    (B) the psoas muscle

    (C) the iliacus muscle

    (D) the quadratus lumborum muscle

68. Dilatation of the intrahepatic biliary ducts without dilatation of the extrahepatic ducts may be caused by all of the following *except*

    (A) a Klatskin tumor

    (B) enlarged portal lymph nodes

    (C) a cholangiocarcinoma

    (D) a pancreatic carcinoma

69. A 42-year-old woman presents postcholecystectomy with right-upper-quadrant pain, elevated serum bilirubin (mainly conjugated), and bilirubin in her urine. Which of the following is this best characteristic of?

    (A) hepatitis

    (B) stone, tumor, or stricture causing obstruction of the bile duct

    (C) small common duct stone <5 mm in diameter

    (D) alkaline phosphatase will be normal

    (E) pancreatic pseudocyst

70. What is a cause of a small gallbladder?

    (A) prolonged fasting

    (B) insulin-dependent diabetes

    (C) chronic cholecystitis

    (D) hydrops

    (E) ascites

71. Identify the vessel that is located superior to the pancreas.

    (A) inferior vena cava

    (B) superior mesenteric artery

    (C) splenic vein

    (D) celiac axis

    (E) left renal vein

72. A tumor in the retroperitoneal space will displace surrounding organs in what position?

    (A) anterior

    (B) posterior

    (C) medial

    (D) lateral

    (E) inferior

73. Which of the following can cause anterior displacement of the abdominal aorta?

    (A) enlarged adrenal gland

    (B) kidney mass

    (C) aortic aneurysm

    (D) enlarged lymph nodes

    (E) inferior vena cava thrombus

74. Sonographically, how do enlarged lymph nodes most commonly appear?

    (A) as solid masses

    (B) as complex masses

    (C) as cystic masses with increased through transmission

    (D) as hypoechoic masses with no increased through transmission

    (E) as irregular-shaped masses with small focal areas of calcification

75. Which of the following best describes hepatofugal blood flow?

    (A) blood flows away from the liver

    (B) turbulent blood flow

    (C) intermittent blood flow

    (D) blood flows toward the liver

    (E) blood fungi in the hepatic veins

76. What anatomic landmarks can be used to sonographically locate the left adrenal gland?

(A) aorta, stomach, and spleen

(B) aorta, spleen, and left kidney

(C) inferior vena cava, spleen, and left kidney

(D) inferior vena cava, stomach, and left kidney

(E) stomach, pancreas, and left kidney

77. Which of the following most likely appears as nonshadowing, nonmobile, echogenic foci imaged within the gallbladder lumen?

(A) polyps

(B) calculi

(C) biliary gravel

(D) sludge balls

(E) thin bile

78. What is hydrops of the gallbladder?

(A) a small contracted gallbladder

(B) a gallbladder with a thickened wall

(C) a thick walled gallbladder filled with stones

(D) congenital duplication of the gallbladder

(E) an enlarged gallbladder

79. Which of the following most likely causes jaundice in a pediatric patient?

(A) hepatitis

(B) fatty infiltration

(C) biliary atresia

(D) cirrhosis

(E) portal hypertension

80. The majority of primary retroperitoneal tumors are malignant. Which of the following is an example of a primary retroperitoneal tumor?

(A) hepatoma

(B) hypernephroma

(C) leiomyosarcoma

(D) adenocarcinoma

(E) hematoma

81. Compare the echogenicities of the following structures and place them in increasing echogenic order.

(A) renal sinus < pancreas < liver < spleen < renal parenchyma

(B) renal sinus < liver < spleen < pancreas < renal parenchyma

(C) pancreas < liver < spleen < renal sinus < renal parenchyma

(D) renal parenchyma < liver < spleen < pancreas < renal sinus

(E) renal parenchyma < pancreas < renal sinus < spleen < liver

82. In comparison to the normal echotexture in adults, the pancreas in children will be relatively

(A) more echogenic

(B) less echogenic

(C) the same echogenicity

(D) larger and less echogenic

(E) complex

83. The kidneys, the perinephric fat, and the adrenal glands are all covered by which of the following?

(A) a true capsule

(B) Gerota's fascia

(C) peritoneum

(D) Glisson's capsule

(E) quadratus lumborum muscle

84. What is the largest major visceral branch of the inferior vena cava?

(A) portal vein

(B) hepatic veins

(C) renal veins

(D) inferior mesenteric vein

(E) gonadal veins

85. The spleen is variable in size, but it is considered to be which of the following?

(A) concave superiorly and inferiorly

(B) convex superiorly and concave inferiorly

(C) concave superiorly and convex inferiorly

(D) convex superiorly and inferiorly

86. A malignant solid renal mass can be all of the following *except*

(A) renal cell carcinoma

(B) adenocarcinoma of the kidney

(C) oncocytoma

(D) transitional cell carcinoma

87. Which one of the following statements correctly describes the anatomic location of structures adjacent to the spleen?

    (A) the diaphragm is superior, lateral, and inferior to the spleen.

    (B) the fundus of the stomach and lesser sac are medial and posterior to the splenic helium.

    (C) the left kidney lies inferior and medial to the spleen.

    (D) the pancreas lies anterior and medial to the spleen.

    (E) the adrenal gland is anterior, superior, and lateral to the spleen.

88. Which of the following sonographic findings are associated with hematoceles?

    (A) a cyst along the course of the vas deferens

    (B) a blood-filled sac that surrounds the testicle, secondary to trauma or surgery

    (C) dilated veins caused by obstruction of the venous return

    (D) a condition in which the testicles have not descended

    (E) a solid mass outside the testes

89. When scanning a 22-year-old patient to rule out cholelithiasis, a single echogenic lesion is seen within the liver. What is this most characteristic of?

    (A) a cavernous hemangioma

    (B) a hematoma

    (C) a hepatic cyst

    (D) an abscess

    (E) lipoma

90. What are normal measurements of the thyroid gland?

    (A) 3–4 cm in anteroposterior and length dimensions

    (B) 2–3 cm in anteroposterior dimensions and 4–6 cm in length

    (C) 1–2 cm in anteroposterior dimensions and 4–6 cm in length

    (D) 3–5 cm in anteroposterior dimensions and 6–8 cm in length

    (E) 4–6 cm in anteroposterior dimensions and 8–10 cm in length

91. Ascites can be caused by all of the following *except*

    (A) malignancy

    (B) nephritic syndrome

    (C) congestive heart failure

    (D) tuberculosis

    (E) adenomyomatosis

92. What is the best way to delineate a dissecting aneurysm on sonography?

    (A) begin scanning in the transverse section and document serial scans.

    (B) show an intimal flap pulsating with the flow of blood.

    (C) scan the patient in a decubitus position to document the aorta and inferior vena cave simultaneously.

    (D) document the renal arteries.

    (E) have the patient perform a Valsalva maneuver to dilate the aorta.

93. Obstructive jaundice may be diagnosed sonographically by demonstrating which of the following?

    (A) a mass in the head of the pancreas with a dilated common bile duct

    (B) an enlarged liver

    (C) a fibrotic and atrophic liver

    (D) cholangitis

    (E) portal hypertension

94. Where would a subhepatic abscess be located?

    (A) superior to the liver

    (B) inferior to the liver, anterior to the right kidney

    (C) inferior to the liver, posterior to the right kidney

    (D) adjacent to the porta hepatis

    (E) inferior to the pleura and superior to the liver

95. Which of the following is *not* a remnant of the fetal circulation?

    (A) ligamentum teres

    (B) ligamentum venosum

    (C) falciform ligament

    (D) coronary ligament

96. Which of the following is a major branch of the common hepatic artery?

    (A) gastroduodenal artery

    (B) coronary artery

    (C) esophageal artery

    (D) left gastric artery

    (E) duodenal artery

97. A 44-year-old patient presents with painless jaundice and a palpable right-upper-quadrant mass, which is most characteristic of which of the following?

    (A) acute hepatitis

    (B) cirrhosis

    (C) porcelain gallbladder

    (D) Courvoisier's gallbladder

    (E) Klatskin tumor

98. A common anatomical variant is a bulge of the lateral border of the left kidney. What is this called?

    (A) junctional parenchymal defect

    (B) Phrygian cap

    (C) column of Bertin

    (D) Bowman's capsule

    (E) dromedary hump

99. Which of the following *cannot* be imaged in a case of end-stage liver disease?

    (A) ascites

    (B) small atrophied liver

    (C) biliary dilatation

    (D) portal hypertension

    (E) echogenic nodular liver

100. The head of the pancreas is located anterior to which of the following vessels?

    (A) inferior vena cava

    (B) aorta

    (C) superior mesenteric artery

    (D) splenic vein

    (E) portal vein

101. What is the lesser sac located between?

    (A) pancreas and the inferior vena cava

    (B) stomach and pancreas

    (C) abdominal wall and stomach

    (D) liver and right kidney

    (E) stomach and spleen

102. Where are the renal pyramids found?

    (A) cortex

    (B) medulla

    (C) renal pelvis

    (D) renal sinus

    (E) loop of Henle

103. Which of the following is chronic renal disease associated with?

    (A) an enlarged kidney with a small contralateral kidney

    (B) unilateral hydronephrosis

    (C) small echogenic kidneys

    (D) renal carbuncle

    (E) an ectopic kidney

104. A 50-year-old woman with a long history of alcoholism presents with increased abdominal girth. Which of the following is the most probable finding on a sonogram of the abdomen?

    (A) liver metastases

    (B) massive ascites with a small echogenic liver

    (C) hepatoma

    (D) gallstones with a mass in the lumen of the gallbladder

    (E) dilated intrahepatic biliary ducts

105. Chronic active hepatitis is a progressive destructive liver disease that eventually leads to which of the following?

    (A) liver cysts

    (B) hepatoma

    (C) cirrhosis

    (D) pancreatitis

    (E) liver metastases

106. A 6-year-old child presents with recurrent fever, right-upper-quadrant pain, and jaundice. An abdominal sonogram is performed. The liver and gallbladder appear normal, but a 2-cm cyst is seen communicating with the common bile duct. What does this cystic structure most likely represent?

    (A) a choledochal cyst

    (B) a pseudocyst

    (C) an aortic aneurysm

    (D) a mucocele

    (E) hydatid cyst

107. A 35-year-old woman presents with a tender neck, and on physical exam, an enlarged thyroid is found. An enlarged inhomogeneous thyroid with irregular borders is seen on the sonogram. What is this most characteristic of?

    (A) a malignant lesion

    (B) Graves' disease

    (C) cyst

    (D) adenomatous hyperplasia

    (E) Hashimoto's thyroiditis

108. What is calcification of the gallbladder wall called?

    (A) cholesterolosis

    (B) Courvoisier's gallbladder

    (C) hydropic gallbladder

    (D) porcelain gallbladder

109. A 60-year-old man presents with an abdominal pulsatile mass and high blood pressure. What is this most characteristic of?

    (A) an aneurysm

    (B) a mesenteric cyst

    (C) gallstones

    (D) Budd–Chiari syndrome

    (E) portal hypertension

110. Identify the vessel that may be imaged posterior to the inferior vena cava.

    (A) right renal vein

    (B) right renal artery

    (C) left renal vein

    (D) left renal artery

    (E) no vessels course posterior to the inferior vena cava

111. The retroperitoneal space is defined as the area between which of the following?

    (A) posterior portion of the parietal peritoneum and the posterior abdominal wall muscles

    (B) anterior portion of the parietal peritoneum and the posterior abdominal wall muscles

    (C) anterior portion of the parietal peritoneum and the posterior portion of the parietal peritoneum

    (D) anterior abdominal wall and the posterior parietal peritoneum

    (E) posterior to the great vessels and anterior to the lumbar spine

112. An abdominal sonogram is performed, and there is a suggestion of a mass in the head of the pancreas. Identify the other structures that should be evaluated.

    (A) the biliary system and gallbladder to evaluate biliary obstruction

    (B) the hepatic artery and splenic artery to document dilatation

    (C) the kidney to evaluate renal obstruction

    (D) liver to evaluate focal masses

    (E) spleen to document size

113. Identify the laboratory values that are most consistent for a patient with acute pancreatitis.

    (A) creatinine and BUN will both rise, but creatinine remains higher for a longer period of time.

    (B) amylase and alkaline phosphatase will both rise, but amylase remains higher for a longer period of time.

    (C) amylase and lipase rise at the same rate, but lipase remains higher for a longer period of time.

    (D) insulin and glucose will both rise, but glucose will remain higher for a longer period of time.

    (E) epinephrine and norepinephrine will both rise and stay elevated for the same period of time.

114. When hypertrophic pyloric stenosis is imaged in the short axis, what is the least measurement of the muscle wall?

    (A) 2 mm

    (B) 4 mm

    (C) 6 mm

    (D) 8 mm

    (E) 12 mm

115. What is a malignant tumor of the adrenal gland found in children called?

    (A) nephroblastoma

    (B) neuroblastoma

    (C) hepatoma

    (D) lymphoma

    (E) sarcoma

116. Lymph nodes may be confused sonographically with all of the following except

    (A) an abdominal aortic aneurysm

    (B) chronic pancreatitis

    (C) the crus of the diaphragm

    (D) the bowel

117. An abdominal sonogram is performed on a 35-year-old man with a history of primary cancer of the liver who now presents with abdominal pain and increasing abdominal girth. What is this most consistent with?

    (A) cholecystitis

    (B) pancreatitis

    (C) portal hypertension

    (D) Budd–Chiari syndrome

    (E) renal failure

118. During an abdominal sonogram, recanalization of the umbilical vein is identified. What could this be associated with?

    (A) ascites
    (B) an abscess
    (C) a hematoma
    (D) hepatoma
    (E) portal hypertension

119. Which of the following is characteristic of a pelvic kidney?

    (A) an abnormal appearance in a normal location
    (B) a normal appearance in an abnormal location
    (C) a normal appearance in a normal location
    (D) an irregular shape
    (E) twice the renal volume

120. The ureteropelvic junction is located between which of the following?

    (A) renal pelvis and the proximal portion of the ureter
    (B) distal ureter and base of the bladder
    (C) urethra and the bladder
    (D) medulla and the cortex
    (E) apex and the base of the bladder

121. One method to diagnosis renal obstruction is to document a resistive index (RI) of greater than

    (A) 0.07
    (B) 0.09
    (C) 0.30
    (D) 0.50
    (E) 0.70

122. Identify the syndrome that is associated with an adrenal mass.

    (A) Murphy's syndrome
    (B) Budd–Chiari syndrome
    (C) Cushing's syndrome
    (D) Frohlich's syndrome
    (E) Graves' syndrome

123. Islet cell tumors of the pancreas are *most* likely to be located in which portion of the pancreas?

    (A) head and neck
    (B) neck and tail
    (C) uncinate process
    (D) body and tail
    (E) head and body

124. What do the celiac axis branches consist of?

    (A) common hepatic, splenic, and right gastric arteries
    (B) common hepatic, gastroduodenal, and left gastric arteries
    (C) common hepatic, left gastric, and splenic arteries
    (D) common hepatic, coronary, and phrenic arteries
    (E) common hepatic, right, and left gastric arteries

125. What is the most common benign mass of the spleen?

    (A) cavernous hemangioma
    (B) angiosarcoma
    (C) congenital cyst
    (D) lymphoma
    (E) hematoma

126. Which of the following is the membrane that lines the abdominal cavity?

    (A) visceral peritoneum
    (B) parietal peritoneum
    (C) pleura
    (D) endometrial lining
    (E) serosal lining

127. A normal functioning transplanted kidney will appear sonographically as which of the following?

    (A) more echogenic than a normal kidney
    (B) with a thin renal cortex and prominent medullary pyramids
    (C) the same as a normal kidney
    (D) twice the size of a normal kidney
    (E) with the renal sinus and renal cortex being isoechoic

128. When performing a gallbladder examination, why is the patient asked to be NPO (nothing by mouth) for approximately 6 hours before the examination?

    (A) to eliminate any overlying bowel gas
    (B) to make the patient more cooperative
    (C) to bring about dehydration, which will make the patient easier to scan
    (D) causes bile to collect in the gallbladder
    (E) causes the bile ducts to dilate

129. Where are transplanted kidneys usually placed?

    (A) within the renal fossa
    (B) in the pelvis along the iliopsoas margin
    (C) in the pelvis anterior to the bladder
    (D) within the abdominal rectus sheath
    (E) in Morrison's pouch

130. **What do Klatskin tumors cause?**

   (A) dilatation of intrahepatic ducts
   (B) dilatation of extrahepatic ducts
   (C) gallstones
   (D) pancreatitis
   (E) porcelain gallbladder

131. **Which of the following is *not* located in the peritoneal cavity?**

   (A) gallbladder
   (B) liver
   (C) spleen
   (D) pancreas
   (E) hepatic veins

132. **The splenic artery**

   (A) originates from the anterior abdominal aorta
   (B) lies posterior to the inferior vena cava
   (C) is tortuous, and courses along the superior aspect of the body and tail of the pancreas
   (D) is the first branch of the abdominal aorta
   (E) courses along the posterior aspect of the body and tail of the pancreas

133. **Artifactual echoes may occur within cysts owing to each of the following *except***

   (A) slice thickness artifacts
   (B) side-lobe artifacts
   (C) edge artifacts
   (D) reverberation artifacts

134. **In which of the following ways does ascites sonographically affect the liver?**

   (A) there will be no effect.
   (B) the liver will appear more echogenic.
   (C) the ascites will attenuate the liver, resulting in decreased echoes.
   (D) the ascites will cause the liver to appear inhomogeneous.

135. **If the ultrasound beam passes through a fatty tumor within the liver, and we know that the speed of sound in fat is lower than in soft tissue, where will this fatty tumor be placed?**

   (A) farther away than it really is
   (B) closer than it really is
   (C) its true position
   (D) smaller is size than it really is
   (E) can be any of the above, depending on the frequency of the transducer

136. **Which of the following is representative of a post-trauma fluid collection located between the diaphragm and the spleen?**

   (A) ascites
   (B) a pleural effusion
   (C) a subcapsular hematoma
   (D) a subphrenic abscess
   (E) retroperitoneal fibrosis

137. **Which of the following can be displaced by a retroperitoneal sarcoma?**

   (A) kidney posteriorly
   (B) spleen anteriorly
   (C) pancreas posteriorly
   (D) diaphragm inferiorly
   (E) aorta posteriorly

138. **Splenomegaly may be caused by all of the following *except* which one?**

   (A) an inflammatory process
   (B) portal vein thrombus
   (C) a left subphrenic abscess
   (D) polycythemia vera
   (E) chronic leukemia and lymphoma

139. **The causes of a large gallbladder include all of the following *except***

   (A) adenomyomatosis
   (B) pancreatic carcinoma
   (C) diabetes mellitus
   (D) a fasting patient
   (E) common duct obstruction

140. **Where are the quadratus lumborum muscles located?**

   (A) medial to the lumbar spine
   (B) in the anterior abdominal wall
   (C) between the kidneys and the adrenal glands
   (D) posterior to the kidneys
   (E) perirenal

141. **All of the following are associated with cirrhosis *except***

   (A) ascites
   (B) splenomegaly
   (C) jaundice
   (D) hepatomegaly
   (E) collateral vessel development

142. **Which of the following is absence of a ureteral jet consistent with?**

    (A) pyelonephrosis

    (B) parapelvic renal cyst

    (C) obstructive hydronephrosis

    (D) posterior urethral values

    (E) renal cell carcinoma

143. **A cystic mass that extends from the renal pelvis to outside the renal capsule is**

    (A) a parapelvic cyst

    (B) an extrarenal pelvis

    (C) a renal artery aneurysm

    (D) a grade II hydronephrosis

    (E) duplex collecting system

144. **Fig. 4–9 is a longitudinal scan to the left of midline. The long narrow arrow points to which of the following structures?**

    (A) diaphragm

    (B) ascites

    (C) inferior vena cava

    (D) left pleural effusion

    (E) heart

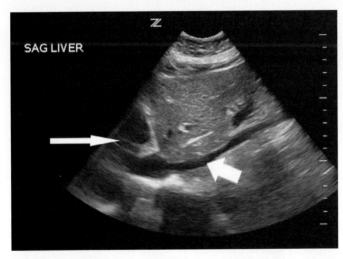

FIGURE 4-9. Longitudinal sonogram of the upper abdomen.

145. **Which of the following is the wide short arrow in Fig. 4–9 pointing to?**

    (A) an abdominal aneurysm

    (B) an esophagus

    (C) the inferior vena cava

    (D) an hepatic vein

    (E) the aorta

146. **Fig. 4–10 is a transverse view of the upper abdomen. What is the arrow pointing to?**

    (A) the aorta

    (B) the inferior vena cava

    (C) the portal vein

    (D) the spine

    (E) an enlarged lymph node

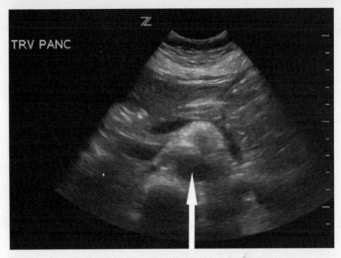

FIGURE 4-10. Transverse sonogram of the upper abdomen.

147. **A patient with normal renal function test results presents for a sonogram of the kidneys. Fig. 4–11 is a longitudinal image of the left kidney. What does this image most likely represent?**

    (A) polycystic kidneys

    (B) infected cysts

    (C) hydronephrosis

    (D) parapelvic renal cysts

    (E) two simple cysts

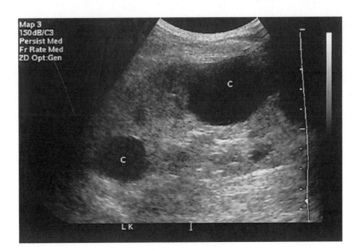

FIGURE 4-11. Longitudinal view of the left kidney.

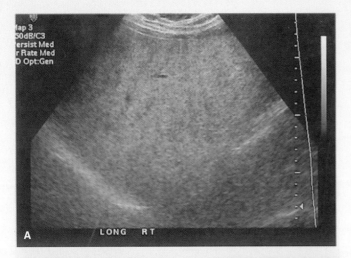

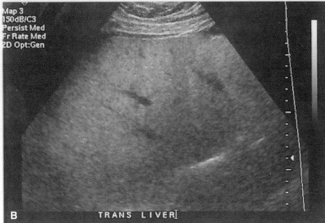

FIGURE 4–12. (A) Longitudinal sonogram through the liver. **(B)** Transverse sonogram through the liver.

148. A 35-year-old man with a history of diabetes presents with an increase of ALT and AST and vague abdominal pain. What do the longitudinal and transverse images shown in Fig. 4–12 most likely represent?

 (A) fatty liver

 (B) severe hepatitis

 (C) cirrhosis

 (D) metastases

 (E) Budd–Chiari syndrome

149. The arrow in Fig. 4–13 points to

 (A) aorta

 (B) superior mesenteric artery

 (C) portal vein

 (D) enlarged lymph node

 (E) inferior vena cava

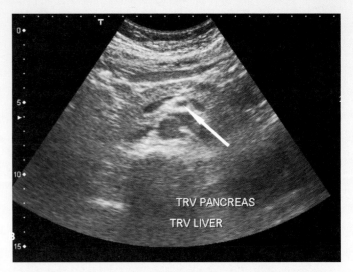

FIGURE 4–13. Transverse sonogram of the upper abdomen.

150. A 35-year-old woman presents with right-upper-quadrant pain, nausea, and vomiting. The findings in Fig. 4–14 are most consistent with which of the following?

 (A) acute cholecystitis

 (B) chronic cholecystitis

 (C) adenomyosis

 (D) a gallbladder of a patient who has just eaten

 (E) a normal gallbladder

151. What is the arrowhead in Fig. 4–14 pointing to?

 (A) pericholecystic fluid collection

 (B) loop of bowel

 (C) cystic artery

 (D) gastroduodenal artery

 (E) portal vein

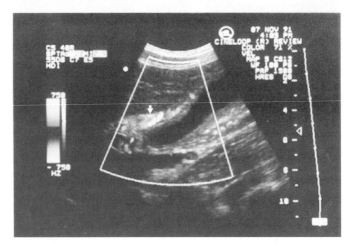

FIGURE 4–14. A longitudinal sonogram at the level of the gallbladder.

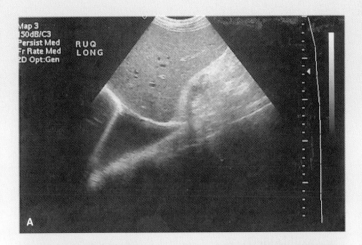

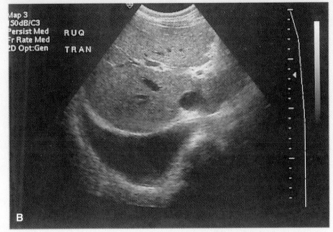

FIGURE 4-15. (A) Longitudinal sonogram through the upper abdomen. (B) Transverse sonogram through the upper abdomen.

152. What is the finding in Fig. 4–15A and B characteristic of?

(A) pleural effusion

(B) pleural abscess

(C) ascites

(D) dissecting aneurysm

(E) fatty liver

153. Fig. 4–16 is a transverse scan at the level of the liver and right kidney. What is this liver abnormality most consistent with?

(A) a hydatid cyst

(B) a hematoma

(C) metastatic lesions

(D) a cavernous hemangioma

(E) infected cysts

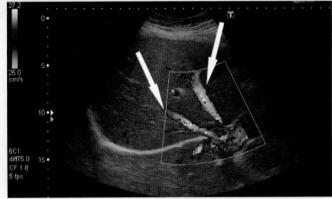

FIGURE 4-17. Transverse scan of the upper abdomen.

154. What are the arrows in Fig. 4–17 pointing to?

(A) main portal veins

(B) hepatic veins

(C) right and left portal vein

(D) phrenic veins

(E) hepatic ducts

155. What is the arrow in Fig. 4–18 pointing to?

(A) the right crus of the diaphragm

(B) the right renal artery

(C) the right adrenal gland

(D) the right renal vein

(E) the right portal vein

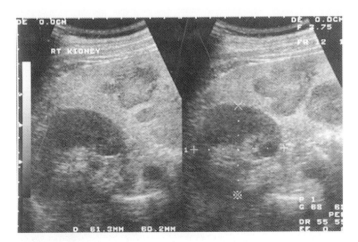

FIGURE 4-16. A transverse view of the right kidney.

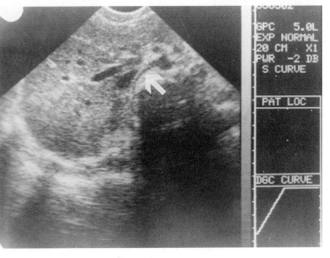

FIGURE 4-18. Transverse scan of the abdomen.

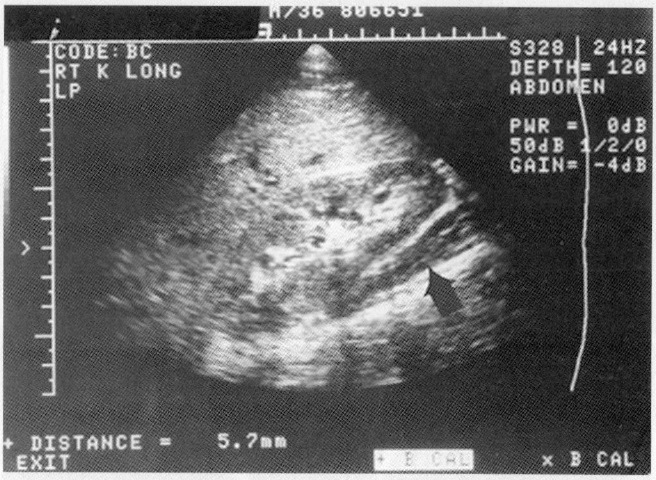

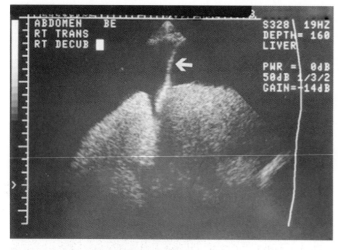

FIGURE 4–19. Longitudinal scan through the right kidney.

156. What is the arrow in Fig. 4–19 pointing to?

    (A) levator ani muscle

    (B) quadratus lumborum muscle

    (C) psoas muscle

    (D) internal oblique muscle

    (E) rectus abdominis muscle

157. The patient in Fig. 4–20 presented with massive ascites. What is the arrow pointing to?

    (A) ligamentum teres

    (B) ligamentum venosum

    (C) falciform ligament

    (D) coronary ligament

    (E) splenorenal ligament

FIGURE 4–20. Transverse scan through the liver.

158. A 1-week-old male infant presents with a left flank mass. An IVP demonstrates a normal right kidney, but there is no visualization of the left kidney. A sonogram is performed and numerous noncommunicating round cystic structures are demonstrated in the left renal fossa, the largest of which is located laterally. No renal parenchyma is identified. The right kidney is normal. This most probably represents which of the following?

    (A) severe hydronephrosis

    (B) polycystic kidneys

    (C) a multicystic kidney

    (D) nephroblastoma

    (E) unilateral renal agenesis

159. Which of the following is an echogenic linear line extending from the portal vein to the neck of the gallbladder?

    (A) cystic duct

    (B) right hepatic vein

    (C) left portal vein

    (D) main lobar fissure

    (E) round ligament

160. What is the most common primary neoplasm of the pancreas?

    (A) an adenocarcinoma

    (B) an insulinoma

    (C) a pseudocyst

    (D) a cystadenoma

    (E) a congenital cyst

161. A patient presents with epigastric tenderness, fever, and an increase in serum amylase and lipase. What is the arrowhead in Fig. 4–21 pointing to?

    (A) superior mesenteric artery

    (B) splenic vein

    (C) portal vein

    (D) hepatic artery

    (E) pancreatic duct

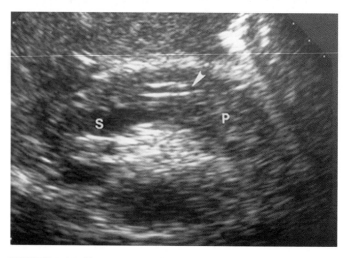

FIGURE 4–21. Transverse scan through the pancreas.

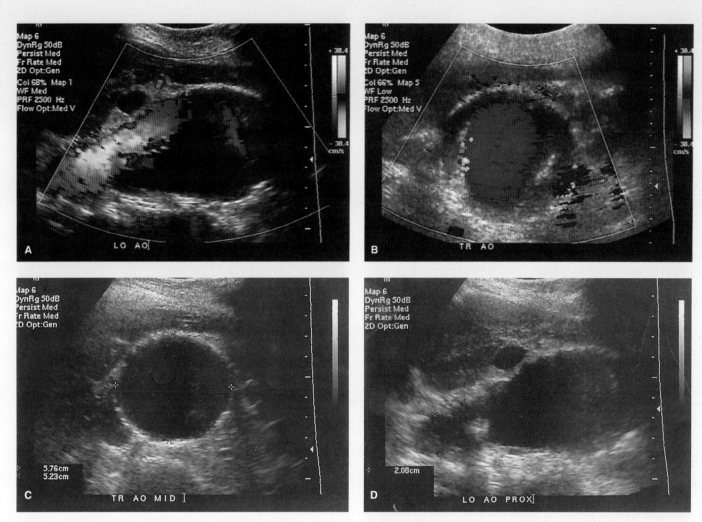

FIGURE 4–22. (**A**) Longitudinal scan through the aorta. (**B**) Transverse scan through the aorta. (**C**) Transverse sonogram through midabdomen aorta. (**D**) Longitudinal sonogram through the proximal section of the aorta.

162. Which of the following is the most likely diagnosis of the patient in Fig. 4–21?

   (A) acute pancreatitis

   (B) phlegmonous pancreatitis

   (C) hemorrhagic pancreatitis

   (D) chronic pancreatitis

   (E) normal pancreas

163. A 65-year-old patient presents with a history of hypertension and a palpable pulsatile mass on physical examination. What is the most likely finding in Fig. 4–22A–D?

   (A) cholecystitis with a gallstone

   (B) a hematoma

   (C) an aortic aneurysm

   (D) an abscess

   (E) a hemorrhagic pseudocyst

164. What is the arrow in Fig. 4–23 pointing to?

   (A) splenic vein

   (B) superior mesenteric artery

   (C) celiac artery

   (D) splenic artery

   (E) superior mesenteric vein

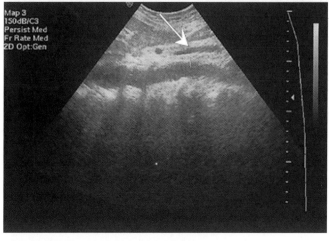

FIGURE 4–23. Longitudinal scan through the midline of the abdomen.

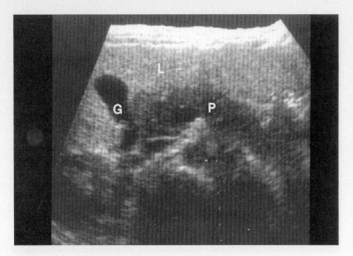

FIGURE 4–24. Transverse sonogram through the pancreas.

165. **What do the findings in Fig. 4–24 represent?**

   (A) acute pancreatitis

   (B) a pancreatic pseudocyst

   (C) chronic pancreatitis

   (D) adenocarcinoma of the pancreas

   (E) a normal pancreas

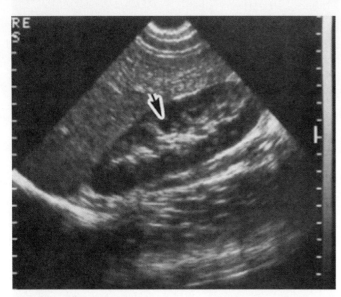

FIGURE 4–25. Sagittal sonogram through the right upper abdomen.

166. **What does the arrow in Fig. 4–25 point to?**

   (A) a medullary pyramid

   (B) a renal cyst

   (C) diverticula of the calyce

   (D) a parapelvic cyst

   (E) a renal artery aneurysm

167. **What is the arrow in Fig. 4–26 pointing to?**

   (A) a sludge ball in the gallbladder

   (B) a polyp in the gallbladder neck

   (C) calculi

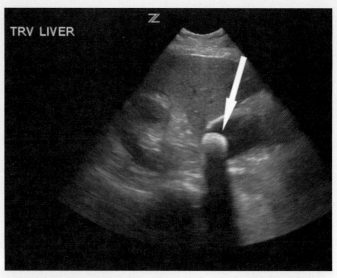

FIGURE 4–26. Longitudinal sonogram through the gallbladder.

   (D) a surgical clip with distal acoustic shadow

   (E) a normal gallbladder

168. **What is the artifact on Fig. 4–26 called?**

   (A) reverberation

   (B) a comet-tail artifact

   (C) scattering

   (D) acoustic shadowing

   (E) posterior acoustic enhancement

169. **What linear anechoic structure is being measured by the calipers in Fig. 4–27?**

   (A) left portal vein

   (B) main portal vein

   (C) middle hepatic vein

   (D) patient umbilical vein

   (E) common bile duct

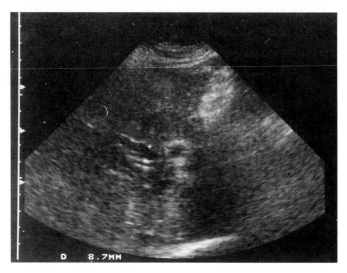

FIGURE 4–27. Transverse view through the right upper quadrant.

170. **What can be said about the structure being measured by the caliper in Fig. 4–27?**

    (A) normal in caliber

    (B) small in caliber

    (C) large in caliber

    (D) unable to determine

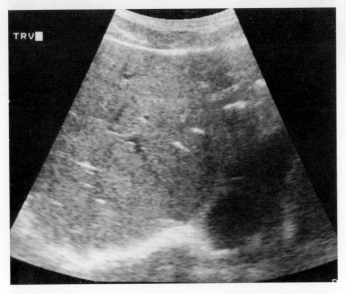

FIGURE 4–28. Transverse sonogram through the upper abdomen.

171. **What are the findings in Fig. 4–28 characteristic of?**

    (A) intrahepatic dilatation

    (B) pneumobilia

    (C) acute hepatitis

    (D) chronic hepatitis

    (E) hepatocellular carcinoma

172. **Which of the following abnormal findings is shown in Fig. 4–29?**

    (A) hydrated disease

    (B) fatty liver

    (C) cavernous hemangioma

    (D) multiple abscesses

    (E) liver metastasis

173. **Which of the following sonographic findings is shown in Fig. 4–30?**

    (A) splenomegaly

    (B) a subphrenic abscess

    (C) subcapsular hematoma

    (D) normal appearing spleen

    (E) metastasis within the spleen

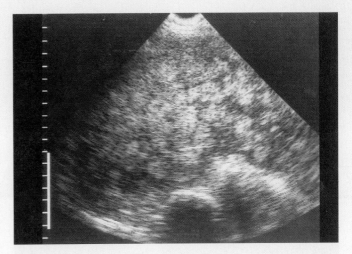

FIGURE 4–29. Transverse scan through the liver.

174. **The common bile duct is formed by which of the following?**

    (A) right and left hepatic ducts joining the cystic duct

    (B) cystic duct joining the right hepatic duct

    (C) common duct joining the cystic duct

    (D) common duct joining the neck of the gallbladder

    (E) common duct joining the pancreatic duct

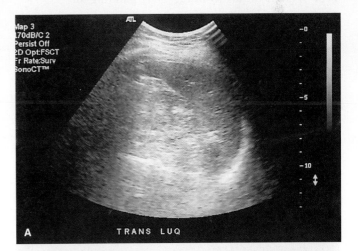

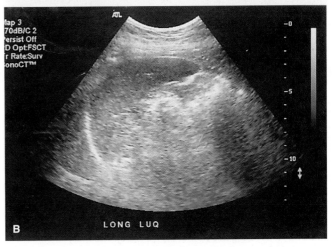

FIGURE 4–30. Coronal image through the left upper quadrant.

175. **Which of the following is usually the cause of an aneurysm?**

    (A) degenerative joint disease

    (B) atherosclerosis

    (C) hypertension

    (D) diabetes

    (E) cystic fibrosis

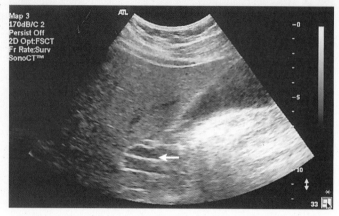

FIGURE 4–31. Magnified sagittal sonogram of the porta hepatis area.

176. **What is the arrow in Fig. 4–31 pointing to?**

    (A) common hepatic duct

    (B) hepatic artery

    (C) common bile duct

    (D) portal vein

    (E) hepatic vein

177. **What are the sonographic findings shown in Fig. 4–32 consistent with?**

    (A) column of Bertin

    (B) prominent renal pyramid

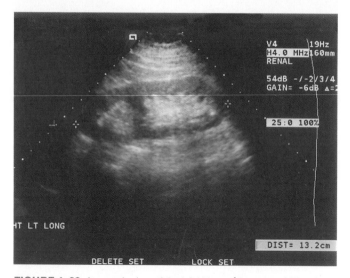

FIGURE 4–32. Long-axis view of the left kidney. *(Courtesy of Shpetim Telegrafi, MD, New York University.)*

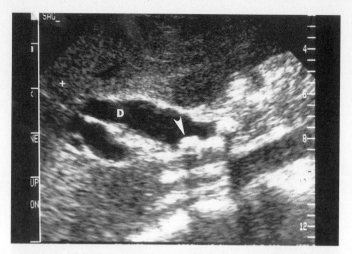

FIGURE 4–33. Magnified oblique sonogram of the porta hepatis area.

    (C) junctional parenchymal defect

    (D) duplex collecting system

    (E) sinus lipomatosis

178. **What is the arrowhead in Fig. 4–33 pointing to?**

    (A) calculi in the common bile duct

    (B) calculi in the neck of the gallbladder

    (C) air in the bile system

    (D) a Klatskin tumor

    (E) sludge

179. **A renal ultrasound is performed on a 30-year-old patient with right flank pain, elevated BUN, and creatinine. The findings in Fig. 4–34 are consistent with all of the following *except***

    (A) a stone in the ureter

    (B) an enlarged prostate

    (C) gallstones

    (D) the posterior urethra valve (PUV)

    (E) a bladder mass

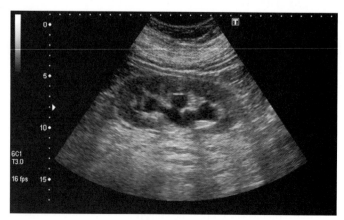

FIGURE 4–34. Long-axis scan through the left kidney. *(Courtesy of Shpetim Telegrafi, MD, New York University.)*

180. Sonographers are sometimes asked to assist in sonographic-guided needle thoracentesis. What is the recommended position for the patient?

(A) Trendelenburg position

(B) sitting upright

(C) Sims position

(D) recumbent position

(E) supine position

181. Patients with hyperthyroidism caused by Graves' disease is most likely to have which of the following biochemical markers?

(A) increased T3 and T4

(B) decreased T3 and T4

(C) high TSH

(D) no changes in T3 and T4

(E) hyponatremia

182. What is the sonographic characteristic of Hashimoto's thyroiditis?

(A) atrophic thyroid tissue with homogeneous echo-texture

(B) multiple hypoechoic micronodules

(C) bilateral enlargements of the thyroid with multiple small cyst

(D) hypertrophy of the thyroid gland with homogeneous echo-texture

(E) hyperplasia with fluid levels

183. Which of the following is associated with an increase with the biochemical marker CEA?

(A) postradioimmunotherapy

(B) bowel decompression surgery

(C) follicular cyst of the ovaries

(D) relapse of colorectal cancer

(E) colostomy

184. A 35-year-old man was found to have an abdominal mass, and a sonographically guided fine needle aspiration biopsy is required. What kind of anesthesia is normally used for this type of procedure?

(A) topical

(B) regional

(C) general

(D) local

(E) spinal

185. Pneumobilia is most likely seen after which of the following procedures?

(A) cholecystectomy

(B) barium enema

(C) gallstone lithotripsy

(D) endoscopic retrograde cholangiopancreatography (ERCP)

(E) radiographic oral contrast cholecystogram

186. Which of the following anatomical structures is *not* seen anterior to the inferior vena cava in the abdomen?

(A) main lobar fissure

(B) main portal vein

(C) left hepatic vein

(D) caudate lobe

(E) right renal artery

187. Hashimoto's disease is a chronic disease of which of the following glands?

(A) pancreas

(B) thyroid

(C) adrenal

(D) prostate

(E) thymus

188. What is the most common cause for acute pancreatitis in the United States?

(A) smoking and alcohol abuse

(B) cocaine and marijuana

(C) cholelithiasis and pancreatic tumor

(D) cholelithiasis and alcoholism

(E) peptic ulcer and abdominal trauma

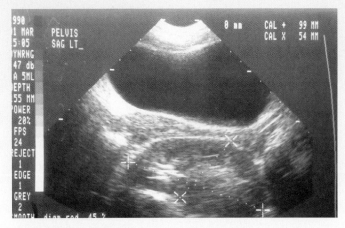

FIGURE 4–35. Sagittal sonogram through the pelvis.

189. Fig. 4–35 suggests that the patient has which of the following?

(A) horseshoe kidney
(B) unilateral renal agenesis
(C) three kidneys
(D) pelvic kidney
(E) cross ectopic kidney

190. A patient presents with a history of epigastric pain and elevated lipase. What does the arrows in Fig. 4–36 point to?

(A) lymph nodes
(B) mesenteric cysts
(C) pseudocyst
(D) abscesses
(E) normal vessels

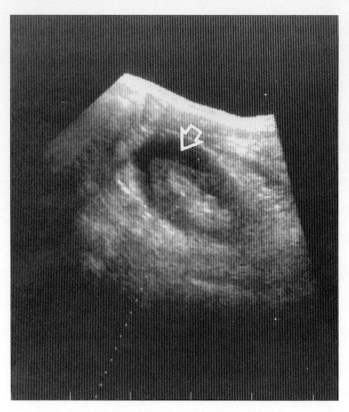

FIGURE 4–37. Longitudinal sonogram through the kidney.

191. What is the arrow in Fig. 4–37 pointing to?

(A) a pseudocyst
(B) perirenal fluid
(C) a dromedary hump
(D) pleural effusion
(E) a renal cyst

192. What are the findings in Fig. 4–38 most consistent with?

(A) patient who has just eaten
(B) porcelain gallbladder with gallstones

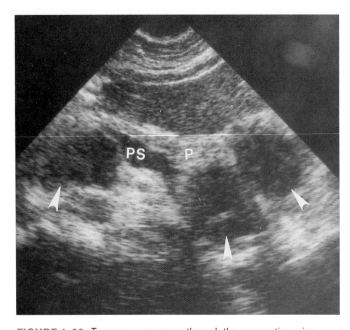

FIGURE 4–36. Transverse sonogram through the pancreatic region.

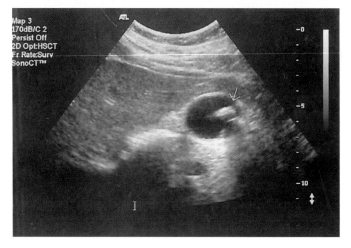

FIGURE 4–38. Left decubitus scan through the upper abdomen.

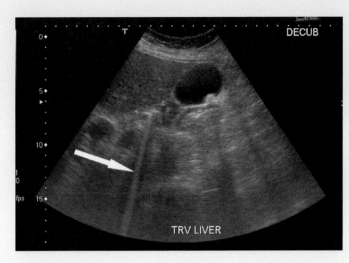

FIGURE 4–39. Left decubitus scan through the upper abdomen.

(C) gallbladder carcinoma

(D) adenomyomatosis

(E) acute cholecystitis with gallstones

193. Identify the artifact shown in Fig. 4–39 (arrow).

(A) comet tail

(B) noise

(C) distal acoustic shadow

(D) refraction

(E) side lobes

194. What is the arrowhead in Fig. 4–40 pointing to?

(A) the gallbladder

(B) an upper pole hydronephrosis

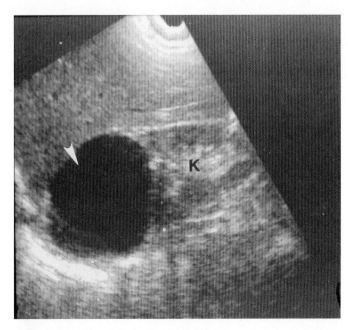

FIGURE 4–40. Long-axis view through a kidney.

(C) a renal cyst

(D) an aneurysm

(E) a dilated ureter

195. The patient in Fig. 4–40 will most likely present with which of the following?

(A) flank pain

(B) fever

(C) nausea and vomiting

(D) no symptoms

(E) jaundice

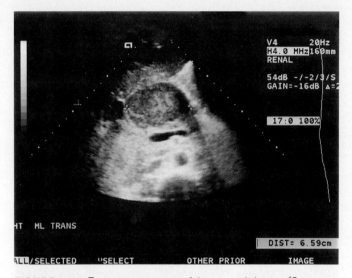

FIGURE 4–41. Transverse sonogram of the upper abdomen. *(Courtesy of Shpetim Telegrafi, MD, New York University.)*

196. What are the calipers in Fig. 4–41 measuring?

(A) antrum of stomach

(B) lymph node

(C) pancreatic pseudocyst

(D) body of pancreas

(E) aorta filled with thrombus

197. A 35-year-old man presents with right-upper-quadrant pain and recurrent attacks of pancreatitis. His laboratory results would be expected to indicate which of the following?

(A) increased blood urea nitrogen (BUN)

(B) decreased serum amylase

(C) increased lipase

(D) increased indirect bilirubin

(E) increased alkaline phosphatase

198. Sonographically, one can recognize fatty infiltration of the liver by all of the following *except*

    (A) hepatomegaly

    (B) parenchymal echoes are echogenic

    (C) decreased vascular structure

    (D) decreased through transmission

    (E) a focal mass

199. Obstruction of the common bile duct by a mass in the head of the pancreas will lead to which of the following?

    (A) a dilated gallbladder with dilated biliary radicles

    (B) a contracted gallbladder with dilated biliary radicles

    (C) dilated biliary radicles with normal or shrunken gallbladder

    (D) portal hypertension

    (E) cirrhosis

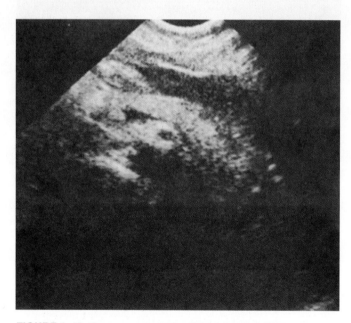

FIGURE 4–42. Transverse sonogram of the upper abdomen.

200. A 41-year-old man presents with epigastric pain and a history of alcoholism. The findings in Fig. 4–42 include which of the following?

    (A) fatty pancreas

    (B) adenocarcinoma

    (C) metastatic disease to the pancreas

    (D) chronic pancreatitis

    (E) normal results

201. A 50-year-old woman presents with painless hematuria. A longitudinal view of the left kidney is imaged in Fig. 4–43. What are the findings most consistent with?

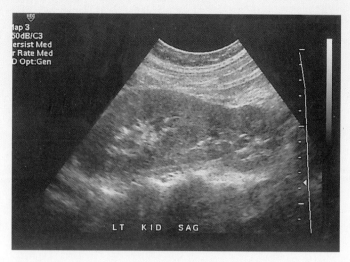

FIGURE 4–43. A longitudinal sonogram of the left kidney.

    (A) transitional cell carcinoma

    (B) renal cell carcinoma

    (C) adenoma

    (D) angiolipoma

    (E) oncocytoma

202. What is the most common medical disease that causes acute renal failure?

    (A) acute tubular necrosis

    (B) renal infarction

    (C) diabetes

    (D) hypertension

    (E) nephrocalcinosis

203. What is Fig. 4–44 consistent with?

    (A) adult polycystic kidneys

    (B) hydronephrosis

    (C) medullary sponge kidney

    (D) medullary cystic disease

    (E) acquired cystic disease found in dialysis

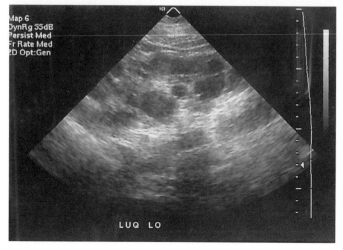

FIGURE 4–44. Longitudinal sonogram of the kidney.

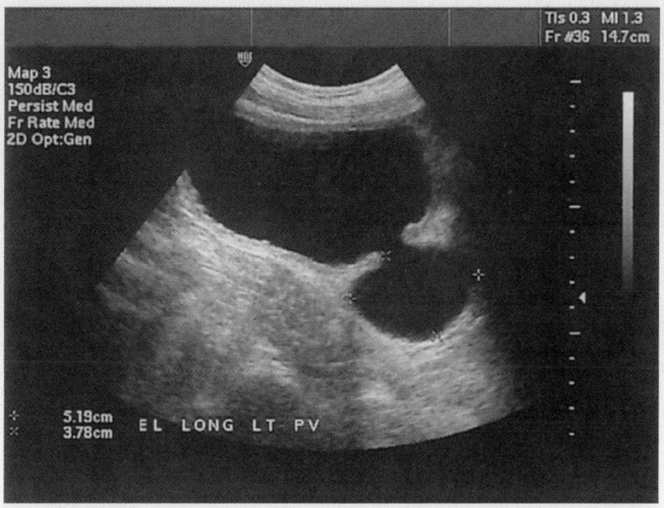

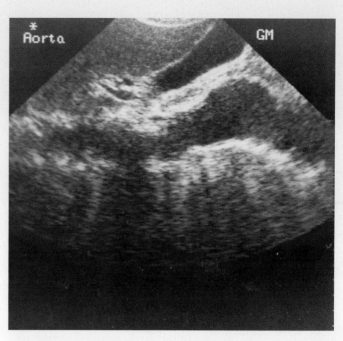

FIGURE 4–45. Left sagittal sonogram of the pelvis.

204. A pelvic sonogram is performed. What is Fig. 4–45 consistent with?

(A) an enlarged prostate

(B) a Foley catheter balloon

(C) a ureterocele

(D) a bladder cyst

(E) diverticula

205. What are the arrows in Fig. 4–46 pointing to?

(A) thrombus

(B) polyp

(C) bowel

(D) calculi

(E) parapelvic cyst

FIGURE 4–47. Midline longitudinal scan of the abdomen.

206. Fig. 4–47 is a midline longitudinal scan of the abdomen. What is the abnormality?

(A) an ectopic gallbladder

(B) aneurysmal dilatation of the distal abdominal aorta

(C) occlusion of abdominal aorta by thrombus

(D) a dissecting aneurysm

(E) an enlarged psoas muscle

207. What term is used to describe onset of pain while scanning over the gallbladder?

(A) Kehr's sign

(B) candle sign

(C) Murphy's sign

(D) Chandelier's sign

(E) Courvoisier's gallbladder

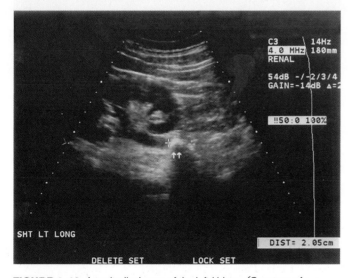

FIGURE 4–46. Longitudinal scan of the left kidney. *(Courtesy of Shpetim Telegrafi, MD, New York University.)*

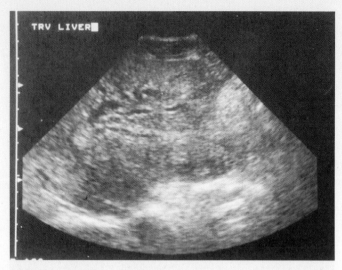

FIGURE 4–48. Transverse sonogram of the liver.

208. **What is the most likely diagnosis that can be made by the findings shown in Fig. 4–48?**

(A) biliary obstruction caused by cholelithiasis

(B) biliary obstruction caused by pancreatitis

(C) distended portal vein caused by portal hypertension

(D) distended hepatic vein caused by chronic congestive heart failure

(E) obstruction of the distal common duct caused by a pancreatic tumor

209. **Which one of the following statements concerning the sonographic patterns of periaortic lymph nodes is *not* correct?**

(A) they may drape or mantle the great vessels anteriorly.

(B) they may displace the superior mesenteric artery posteriorly.

(C) they may displace the great vessels anteriorly.

(D) they may have lobar, smooth, or scalloped appearance.

(E) as mesenteric involvement occurs, the adenopathy may fill most of the abdomen in an irregular complex pattern.

210. **Which of the following findings is *not* represented in Fig. 4–49?**

(A) diabetes

(B) hepatitis

(C) malignancy

(D) chronic pancreatitis

(E) portal caval shunts

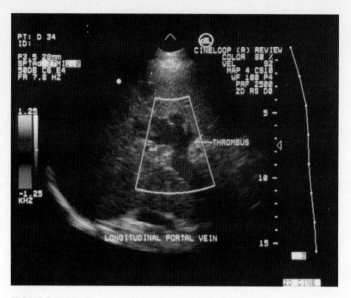

FIGURE 4–49. Longitudinal sonogram of the portal vein.

211. **What is the blood flow in Fig. 4–50 consistent with?**

(A) right-sided heart failure

(B) cirrhosis

(C) Budd–Chiari syndrome

(D) cavernous transformation of the portal vein

(E) normal blood flow in the hepatic and portal veins

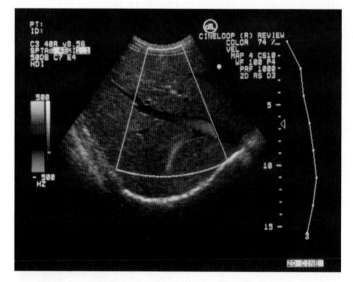

FIGURE 4–50. Transverse sonogram of the upper liver.

212. **What is the arrow in Fig. 4–51 pointing to?**

(A) a mass in the head of the pancreas

(B) c-loop of duodenum

(C) bowel mass

(D) calculi

(E) loculated fluid with debris

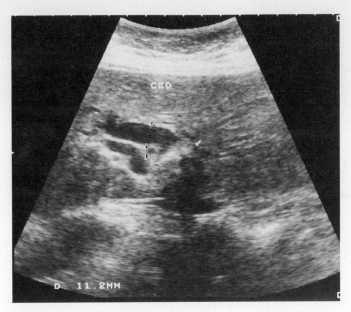

FIGURE 4–51. Oblique sonogram of the liver.

213. What are the calipers in Fig. 4–51 measuring?

(A) common hepatic duct

(B) common bile duct

(C) main portal vein

(D) hepatic vein

(E) inferior vena cava

214. What are the findings in Fig. 4–51 most consistent with?

(A) mass in the head of the pancreas

(B) intrahepatic obstruction

(C) choledocholithiasis

(D) liver trauma

(E) liver cell carcinoma

215. Fig. 4–52 is a transverse sonogram through the right lobe of the thyroid. What are the findings consistent with?

(A) Graves' disease

(B) thyroiditis

(C) papillary carcinoma

(D) primary hyperplasia

(E) adenoma

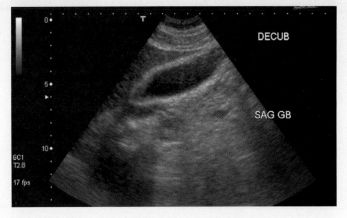

FIGURE 4–53. Sonogram of the right upper abdomen.

216. Which of the following findings is *least* likely to be associated with the disorder shown in Fig. 4–53?

(A) leukocytosis

(B) afebrile

(C) Murphy's sign

(D) elevation of serum total bilirubin

(E) nausea and vomiting

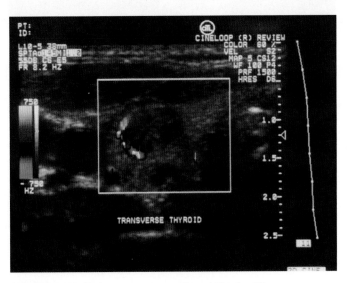

FIGURE 4–52. Transverse sonogram through the thyroid.

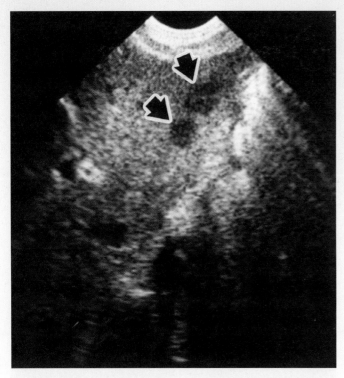

FIGURE 4–54. Transverse sonogram of the left lobe of the liver.

217. **Fig. 4–54 is a transverse sonogram of the left lobe of the liver. What do the arrows point to?**

    (A) hepatic vessels

    (B) hypoechoic lesions

    (C) portal sinuses

    (D) biliary radicles

    (E) none of the above

218. **Diagnostic possibilities in the findings in Fig. 4–54 include which one of the following?**

    (A) metastases

    (B) hemangiomas

    (C) infectious foci

    (D) abscesses

219. **What is the arrow in Fig. 4–55 pointing to?**

    (A) coronary ligament

    (B) ligamentum of Teres

    (C) gallstone

    (D) lesser omentum

    (E) main lobar fissure

220. **The findings in Fig. 4–56 are associated with all of the following** *except*

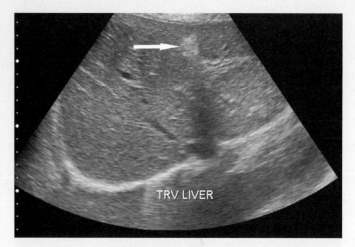

FIGURE 4–55. Transverse scan of the liver.

    (A) increase in alpha-fetoprotein level

    (B) increase in direct bilirubin

    (C) increase in alkaline phosphatase

    (D) jaundice

    (E) none of the above

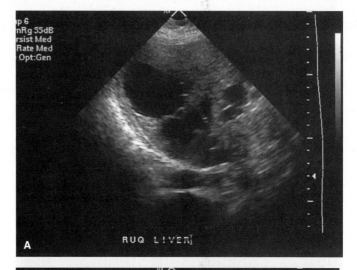

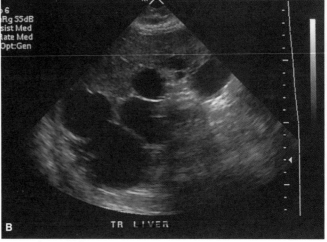

FIGURE 4–56. (A) Longitudinal **(B)** Transverse scans of the right lobe of the liver.

221. **What are the findings in Fig. 4–56 consistent with?**

    (A) Budd–Chiari syndrome
    (B) portal hypertension
    (C) right-sided heart failure
    (D) hepatic hydatid cysts
    (E) hemangioma

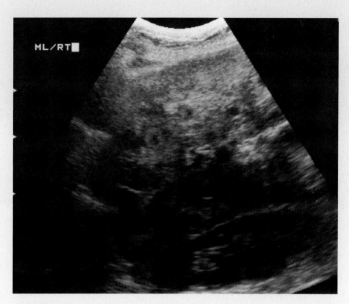

FIGURE 4–58. Longitudinal sonogram of the right lobe of the liver.

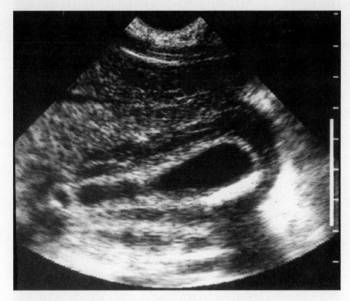

FIGURE 4–57. Longitudinal magnified sonogram of the gallbladder.

222. **The findings in Fig. 4–57 are associated with all of the following *except***

    (A) hypoproteinemia
    (B) congestive heart failure
    (C) acute hepatitis
    (D) cholecystitis
    (E) choledocholithiasis

223. **What are the findings in Fig. 4–58 suggestive of?**

    (A) acute hepatitis
    (B) fatty liver
    (C) metastatic disease of the liver
    (D) multiple hematomas
    (E) cirrhosis

224. **The laboratory findings of renal failure include which of the following?**

    (A) creatinine and alkaline phosphatase
    (B) creatinine and blood urea nitrogen
    (C) serum amylase and lipase
    (D) serum amylase and creatinine
    (E) alkaline phosphatase and alpha-fetoprotein

225. **The head of the pancreas is located to the right of which of the following?**

    (A) celiac axis
    (B) inferior vena cava
    (C) gastroduodenal artery
    (D) common bile duct
    (E) portal splenic confluence

226. **What is Crohn's disease?**

    (A) a mass in the stomach
    (B) a parasitic condition
    (C) an inflammation of the bowel
    (D) loculated fluid in the peritoneal cavity
    (E) a mass relating to the pancreas and biliary system

227. **A resistive index (RI) >0.70 in a kidney is consistent with early**

    (A) obstructive jaundice
    (B) obstructive hydronephrosis
    (C) renal cell carcinoma
    (D) benign renal cyst
    (E) polycystic renal disease

228. A postrenal transplant perirenal fluid collection can be all of the following *except*

    (A) parapelvic cyst

    (B) urinoma

    (C) lymphoma

    (D) hematoma

    (E) abscess

229. Which of the following describes the Doppler characteristic of the venous blood flow in a varicocele?

    (A) increased blood flow

    (B) irregular waveform

    (C) triphasic flow

    (D) no change in flow

    (E) no blood flow

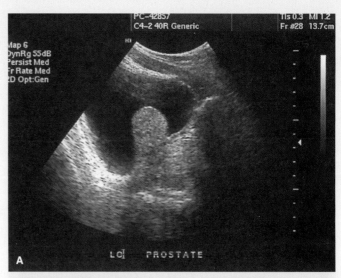

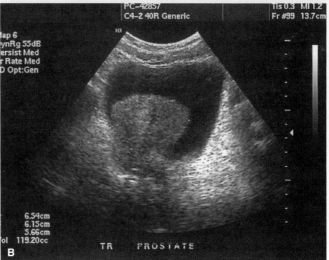

FIGURE 4–60 (**A**) Longitudinal transabdominal scan at the level of the bladder. (**B**) Transverse transabdominal scan of the bladder.

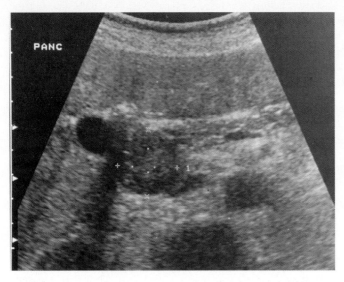

FIGURE 4–59. Transverse sonogram at the level of the pancreas.

230. A 40-year-old patient presents with epigastric pain and jaundice. Fig. 4–59 is a transverse scan through the mid-abdomen. The crossbars delineate the area of interest. This is consistent with which of the following?

    (A) bowel mass

    (B) liver mass

    (C) omental mass

    (D) pancreatic mass

    (E) normal finding

231. A 60-year-old man presents for a pelvic ultrasound. What are the findings in Fig. 4–60A and B consistent with?

    (A) Foley catheter

    (B) cystitis

    (C) bladder carcinoma

    (D) polyp

    (E) enlarged prostate

232. What is the arrow in Fig. 4–61 pointing to?

    (A) ascites

    (B) pleural effusion

    (C) an abscess

    (D) a hematoma

    (E) a cyst

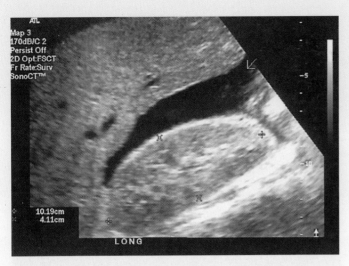

FIGURE 4–61. Sagittal sonogram obtained through the right upper abdomen.

233. Fatty infiltration of the liver can be assessed sonographically by visualizing which of the following?

(A) echogenic vessel walls seen throughout the liver

(B) hypoechoic diaphragm

(C) increased liver echogenicity

(D) multiple echogenic focal masses

(E) small nodular liver

234. What is the most likely diagnosis of the patient shown in Fig. 4–62?

(A) hematoma

(B) metastases

(C) abscess

(D) hemangioma

(E) hydrated cysts

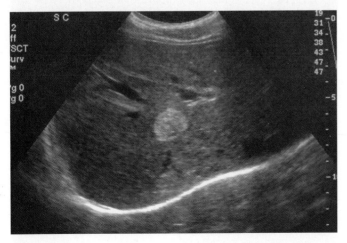

FIGURE 4–62. Transverse sonogram throughout the right hepatic lobe. (Courtesy of Dunstan Abraham, MPH, PA-C, RDMS.)

235. A patient who has blunt trauma to the abdomen earlier in the day presents with left-upper-quadrant pain and a decrease in hematocrit. An echogenic mass is seen in the spleen. What is this consistent with?

(A) abscess

(B) lymphoma

(C) infection

(D) hematoma

(E) leukemia

236. Which of the following tests can be used to diagnose hemangiomas?

(A) needle biopsy

(B) a tagged red blood cell liver scan

(C) a computed tomographic (CT) scan

(D) a magnetic resonance imaging (MRI) scan

(E) all of the above

237. What is the most likely diagnosis of the patient in Fig. 4–63?

(A) cirrhosis

(B) pyonephritis

(C) acute glomerulonephritis

(D) chronic renal disease

(E) renal agenesis

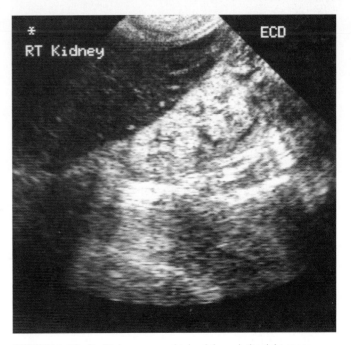

FIGURE 4–63. Sagittal sonogram obtained through the right upper quadrant.

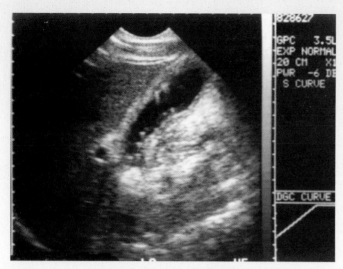

FIGURE 4-64. Longitudinal scan of the gallbladder.

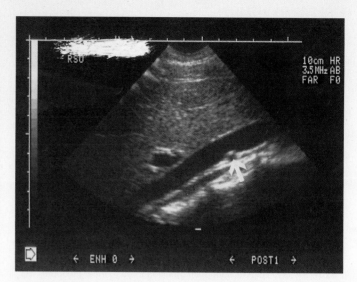

FIGURE 4-65. Longitudinal scan of the upper abdomen.

238. The findings in Fig. 4–64 are consistent with which of the following?

    (A) gallbladder carcinoma
    (B) adenomyomatosis
    (C) cholecystitis
    (D) gallbladder polyp
    (E) metastasizes to the gallbladder

239. Which of the following may a jaundiced male child with a hemolytic disorder be found to have?

    (A) increase in direct bilirubin
    (B) increase in indirect bilirubin
    (C) increase in alpha-fetoprotein
    (D) increase in prothrombin time
    (E) normal liver function test results

240. Which of the following statements are true?

    (A) Bowman's capsule is the fibrous capsule around the kidney.
    (B) a glomerulus, Bowman's capsule, and renal tubules together constitute a nephron.
    (C) nephrons are the only structures, in which active transport of substances through cell membrane does not occur.
    (D) the renal cortex secretes hormones called corticoids.
    (E) nephrons are not an important part of the production of urine.

241. Fig. 4–65 is a longitudinal scan through the abdomen. Which linear longitudinal vessel is being imaged?

    (A) aorta
    (B) inferior vena cava
    (C) main portal vein
    (D) none of the above

242. The arrow in Fig. 4–65 is pointing to which of the following?

    (A) psoas muscle
    (B) left renal vein
    (C) superior mesenteric artery
    (D) right renal artery
    (E) phrenic artery

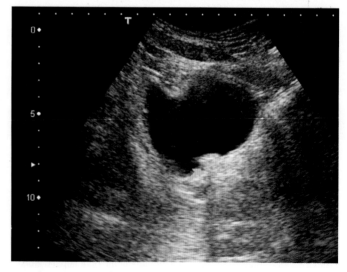

FIGURE 4-66. Transverse sonogram obtained through the urinary bladder.

243. Fig. 4–66 is a transverse sonogram obtained through the urinary bladder. This image is consistent with which of the following conditions?

    (A) a thickening of the posterior bladder wall
    (B) bladder calculi
    (C) cholelithiasis
    (D) ureterocele
    (E) urinary bladder diverticula

244. Which of the following is the most likely diagnosis in the patient in Fig. 4–66?

    (A) bladder tumor
    (B) overdistended bladder
    (C) cystitis
    (D) ureterocele
    (E) Foley catheter

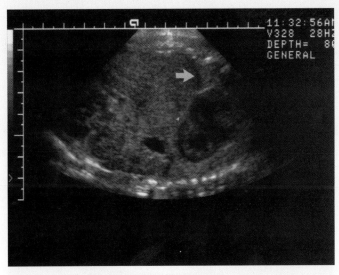

FIGURE 4–67. Longitudinal scan through the right upper abdomen.

245. A longitudinal scan is performed on the right side of the abdomen. The arrow in Fig. 4–67 is pointing to a small fluid collection in which of the following structures?

    (A) pleural cavity
    (B) lesser sac
    (C) right paracolic gutter
    (D) subhepatic space
    (E) right subphrenic space

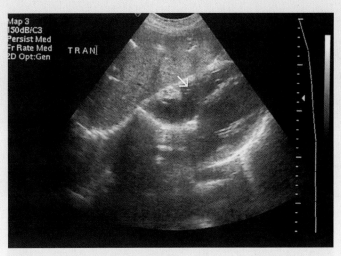

FIGURE 4–68. Transverse scan through the upper abdomen.

246. A transverse scan of the upper abdomen is performed. What is the arrow in Fig. 4–68 pointing to?

    (A) the heart
    (B) pleural effusion
    (C) pericardial effusion
    (D) hemangioma
    (E) hydatid cyst

247. The liver in Fig. 4–68 is consistent with which one of the following findings?

    (A) fatty infiltrations
    (B) hepatitis
    (C) hepatocellular carcinoma
    (D) diabetes mellitus
    (E) normal finding

248. Which of the following terms describes a normal variant of the liver in which the right lobe of the liver extends below the lower pole of the right kidney?

    (A) Murphy's lobe
    (B) caudate lobe
    (C) duplication of the right lobe
    (D) Riedel's lobe
    (E) extra lobe

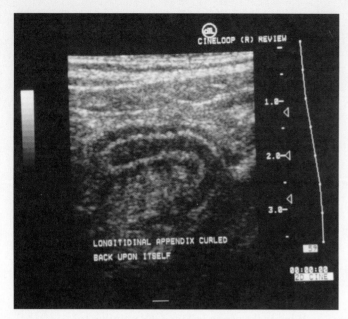

FIGURE 4–69. Longitudinal sonogram of the right lower quadrant.

249. Fig. 4–69 is a longitudinal scan through the right lower quadrant. This image is consistent with which one of the following diagnoses?

(A) appendicitis

(B) bowel obstruction

(C) Crohn's disease

(D) intussusception

(E) volvulus

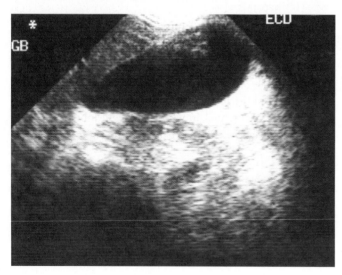

FIGURE 4–70. Long-axis image of the gallbladder.

250. Fig. 4–70 is a long-axis view of the gallbladder that shows which of the following abnormalities?

(A) a distended gallbladder with thickened walls

(B) a positive wall-echo-shadow (WES) sign

(C) multiple floating, low-level echoes

(D) an hydropic gallbladder

(E) porcelain gallbladder

251. What is the most likely diagnosis of the patient in Fig. 4–70?

(A) obstruction of the cystic duct

(B) Klatskin tumor

(C) acalculous cholecystitis

(D) gallbladder carcinoma

(E) adenoma of the gallbladder

252. Hydrops of the gallbladder may be secondary to all of the following *except* which one?

(A) sludge

(B) mass in the head of the pancreas

(C) obstruction of the distal common bile duct by a mass of the ampulla of Vater

(D) stones in Hartmann's pouch

(E) surgery

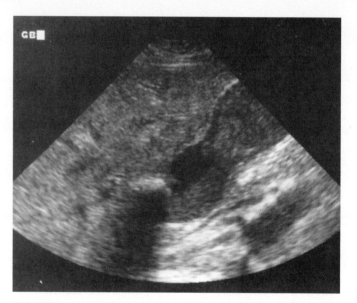

FIGURE 4–71. Longitudinal magnified sonogram through the right upper quadrant.

253. Fig. 4–71 is a longitudinal view of the gallbladder in a patient with a history of gallbladder disease. This image is most consistent with which of the following?

(A) chronic cholecystitis

(B) hepatitis

(C) metastasizes to the gallbladder

(D) gallbladder carcinoma

(E) a patient who just ate a fatty meat

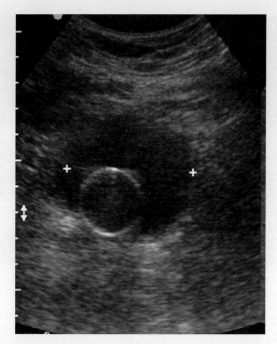

FIGURE 4–72. Sonogram of urinary bladder

254. Fig. 4–72 is a sonogram of the urinary bladder. What is the round anechoic structure in the bladder?

(A) a Foley catheter

(B) a bladder cyst

(C) an ureterocele

(D) a bladder stone

(E) an ureteral jet

255. A longitudinal scan of the right lobe of the liver is performed in a postoperative patient. What is the most likely diagnosis in the patient in Fig. 4–73?

(A) subphrenic collection

(B) subcapsular collection

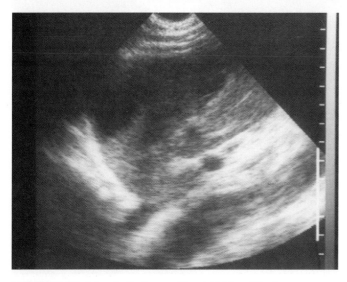

FIGURE 4–73. A longitudinal scan of the right lobe of the liver.

(C) subhepatic collection

(D) loculated ascites

(E) perigastric collection

256. The patient in Fig. 4–73 has a fever and a low hematocrit. The patient was placed in a decubitus position and the low-level echoes within the collection did not move. This is most diagnostic of which of the following?

(A) abscess

(B) hematoma

(C) infected cyst

(D) hemorrhagic cyst

(E) malignant fluid

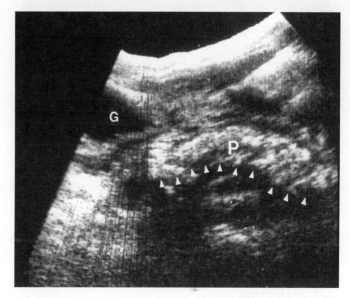

FIGURE 4–74. A transverse scan at the level of the pancreas.

257. Fig. 4–74 is a transverse scan at the level of the pancreas. What structure are the arrows pointing to?

(A) bowel

(B) stomach

(C) lesser sac

(D) duodenum

(E) pancreas

258. The patient in Fig. 4–74 presents with normal laboratory values and persistent epigastric pain. Which of the following pathologies is this image most consistent with?

(A) chronic pancreatitis

(B) acute pancreatitis

(C) complicated pancreatic pseudocyst

(D) bowel mass

(E) insulinoma

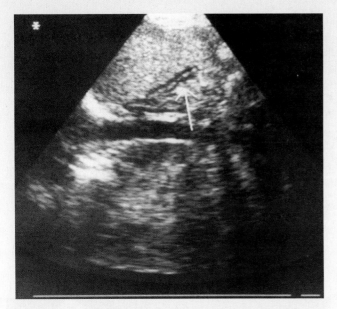

FIGURE 4–75. Coronal image through the left upper quadrant.

259. Fig. 4–75 is a coronal image through the left upper quadrant of the abdomen. What is the arrow pointing to?

(A) left kidney

(B) the normal left adrenal gland

(C) stomach

(D) the left crus of the diaphragm

(E) the splenic flexure

260. What is the longitudinal anechoic structure shown in Fig. 4–75?

(A) right renal vein

(B) left renal artery

(C) aorta

(D) inferior vena cava

(E) artifact

261. Which of the following conditions may affect the adrenal gland?

(A) neonatal hypotension

(B) severe fulminant tuberculosis infection

(C) malignant lung carcinoma

(D) breast carcinoma

(E) all of the above

262. Fig. 4–76 is a transverse scan obtained through the abdomen of a child with a palpable mass that is what?

(A) a complex mass with areas of septations and debris

(B) a cystic mass that appears to displace bowel and mesentery

(C) free-fluid within the abdomen

(D) loculated fluid collection

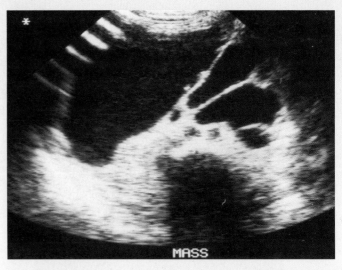

FIGURE 4–76. Transverse scan obtained through the abdomen of a child with a palpable mass.

263. What is the most likely diagnosis of the patient in Fig. 4–76?

(A) mesenteric cyst

(B) complicated ascites

(C) ovarian carcinoma

(D) abscess

264. Fig. 4–77A and B are long- and short-axis sonograms through the gastric antrum of a child. Which of the following best describes the image?

(A) atrophy of the antrum wall

(B) mass of the antrum wall

(C) thickened antrum wall and increase length

(D) shorten pyloric canal and shorten length

(E) normal

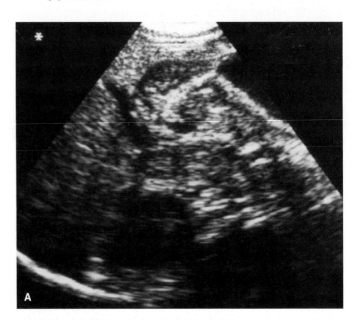

FIGURE 4–77 (A) Longitudinal image through the gastric antrum of a child.

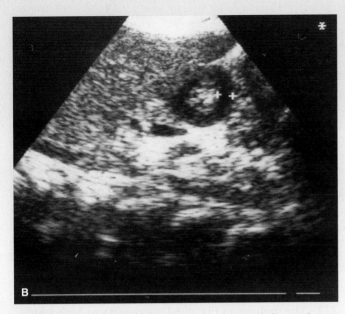

FIGURE 4–77. *(Continued)* **(B)** Transverse scan through the gastric antrum of a child.

265. **What is the most likely diagnosis of the patient in Fig. 4–77A and B?**

(A) normal stomach

(B) hypertrophic pyloric stenosis

(C) duodenal tumor

(D) mass in the lesser sac

(E) infected lymph nodes

266. **Fig. 4–78 is a transverse sonogram through the upper abdomen. This image is most consistent with which of the following diagnoses?**

(A) chronic pancreatitis

(B) gastric outlet obstruction

(C) insulinoma

(D) portal hypertension

(E) normal pancreas

267. **What portion of the pancreas is anterior to the formation of the portal vein?**

(A) head

(B) neck

(C) isthmus

(D) body

(E) tail

268. **What is the most common islet cell tumor?**

(A) adenocarcinoma

(B) pseudocyst

(C) true cyst

(D) insulinoma

(E) gastrinoma

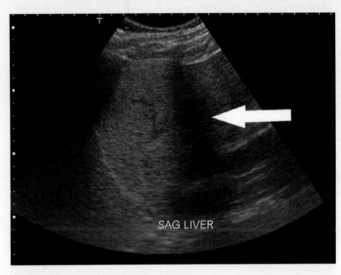

FIGURE 4–79. Longitudinal scan of the liver.

269. **Fig. 4–79 is a longitudinal image of the liver. What is the distal acoustic shadow in this image?**

(A) rib shadow

(B) comet tail artifact

(C) calculi

(D) bowel shadow

(E) shadow from falciform ligament of the liver

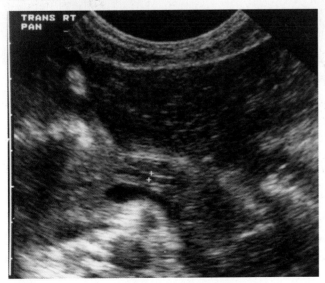

FIGURE 4–78. Transverse image obtained in the upper abdomen.

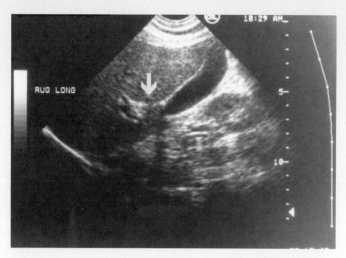

FIGURE 4–80. Longitudinal scan of the right upper quadrant.

270. What is the arrow in Fig. 4–80 pointing to?

(A) major lobar fissure

(B) ligamentum of Teres

(C) ligamentum of venosum

(D) air in bile duct

(E) cholecystectomy clip

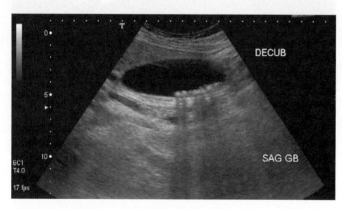

FIGURE 4–81. Longitudinal scan of the gallbladder.

271. The findings in Fig. 4–81 are associated with all of the following *except*

(A) an increase alkaline phosphatase

(B) an increase serum glutamic–oxaloacetic transaminase

(C) sickle cell disease

(D) an increase alpha-fetoprotein

(E) jaundice

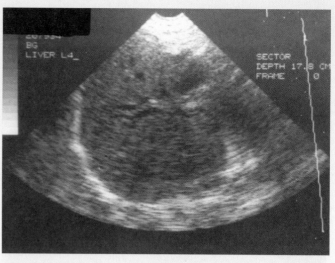

FIGURE 4–82. Longitudinal scan of the liver.

272. The findings in Fig. 4–82 are consistent with which of the following diagnoses?

(A) Budd–Chiari syndrome

(B) hepatitis

(C) dilated biliary radicles

(D) gallstones

(E) fatty infiltrations

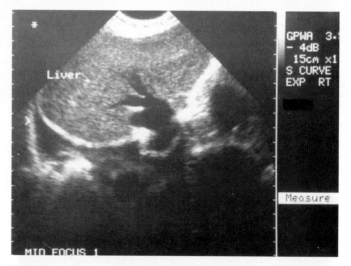

FIGURE 4–83. Transverse scan of the liver.

273. The findings in Fig. 4–83 are consistent with which of the following diagnoses?

(A) portal hypertension

(B) congestive heart failure

(C) fatty liver disease

(D) cirrhosis

(E) a normal scan

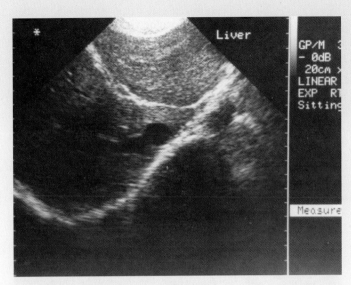

FIGURE 4–84. Transverse scan of the liver.

274. **Which of the following ligaments are visualized in Fig. 4–84?**

(A) middle lobar ligament

(B) ligament venosum

(C) coronary ligament

(D) round ligament

(E) gastroduodenal ligament

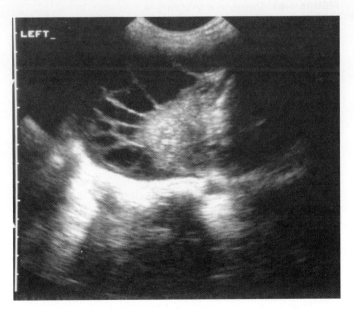

FIGURE 4–85. An upright coronal image of the lower left hemithorax of a 12-year-old child with a cough and fever.

275. **Fig. 4–85 is an upright coronal image of the lower left hemithorax of a 12-year-old child with a fever. Which of the following abnormalities can be seen?**

(A) loculated pleural effusion

(B) nonloculated pleural effusion

(C) hydronephrotic kidney

(D) herniated bowel

276. **Which of the following is the most likely diagnosis of the patient in Fig. 4–85?**

(A) simple effusion

(B) cystic lung mass

(C) obstructed bowel

(D) empyema

(E) obstructed kidney

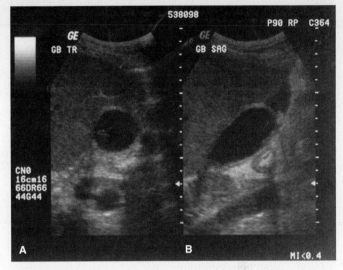

FIGURE 4–86. (**A**) Transverse image of the gallbladder. (**B**) Long-axis image of the gallbladder.

277. **A patient presents with right-upper-quadrant pain, fever, nausea, and leukocytosis. The findings in Fig. 4–86 are most consistent with which of the following diagnoses?**

(A) gallbladder carcinoma

(B) chronic cholecystitis

(C) adenomyomatosis

(D) acute cholecystitis

(E) postprandial gallbladder contraction

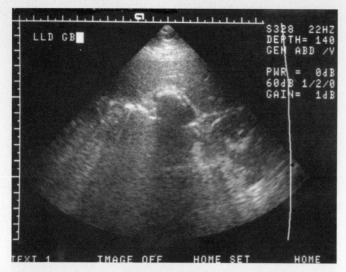

FIGURE 4–87. Longitudinal scan of the right upper quadrant.

278. The findings shown in Fig. 4–87 are consistent with which of the following diagnoses?

(A) chronic cholecystitis with cholelithiasis

(B) adenomatosis

(C) postprandial gallbladder contraction

(D) duodenal bulb

(E) postcholecystectomy clip

279. A patient presents with an increase in direct bilirubin, alanine aminotransferase (ALT), and alkaline phosphatase. What are the findings in Fig. 4–88 suggestive of?

(A) liver metastases

(B) hepatoma

(C) cirrhosis

(D) fatty infiltrations

(E) hematomas

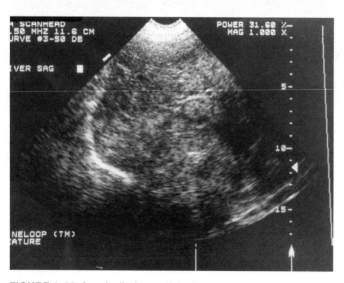

FIGURE 4–88. Longitudinal scan of the liver.

280. A patient presents with vague right-upper-quadrant pain and normal liver function laboratory test results. The echogenic mass in Fig. 4–89 is suggestive of a liver

(A) abscess

(B) hematoma

(C) hepatoma

(D) echinococcal cyst

(E) hemangioma

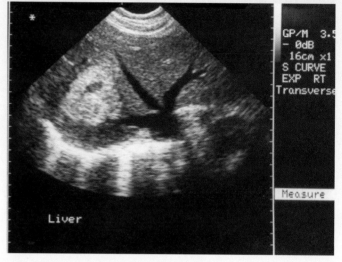

FIGURE 4–89. Transverse scan of the liver.

281. Where is the echogenic mass shown in Fig. 4–89 located?

(A) posterior segment of the right lobe

(B) anterior segment of the right lobe

(C) anterior segment of the left lobe

(D) medial segment of the right lobe

(E) medial segment of the left lobe

282. Which of the following terms describes the malformation variant in the gallbladder that involves an acutely angulated pouch of the fundus?

(A) Phrygian cap

(B) duplication of the gallbladder

(C) Hartmann's pouch

(D) junctional fold

(E) Murphy's cap

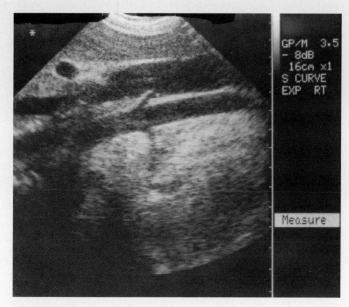

FIGURE 4–90. Coronal scan of the midabdomen.

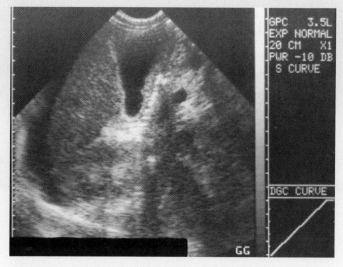

FIGURE 4–91. Longitudinal scan of the liver and gallbladder.

283. Identify the vessels being imaged in Fig. 4–90 in the order in which they appear (anterior to posterior).

(A) inferior vena cava, portal vein, left renal vein, right renal vein

(B) inferior vena cava, aorta, right hepatic artery, splenic artery

(C) inferior vena cava, aorta, left renal vein, right renal vein

(D) inferior vena cava, aorta, right renal artery, left renal artery

(E) inferior vena cava, portal vein, right hepatic vein, left hepatic vein

284. Which of the following statements does *not* differentiate the portal veins from the hepatic veins?

(A) portal veins become larger as they approach the diaphragm.

(B) portal veins have echogenic borders.

(C) portal veins bifurcate into the right and left branches.

(D) the main portal vein is part of the portal triad.

285. Horseshoe kidney may be confused sonographically with which of the following?

(A) carcinoma of the head of the pancreas

(B) lymphadenopathy

(C) hypernephroma

(D) gastric mass

(E) aortic aneurysm

286. A 53-year-old man with a history of liver cirrhosis presents with increased abdominal girth. Fig. 4–91 demonstrates a thickened gallbladder wall, which is most often associated with which of the following?

(A) calculous cholecystitis

(B) pancreatitis

(C) portal hypertension

(D) adjacent ascites

(E) loss of appetite

287. What is the arrow in Fig. 4–92 pointing to?

(A) inferior vena cava

(B) superior mesenteric artery

(C) celiac

(D) right crus of the diaphragm

(E) psoas muscle

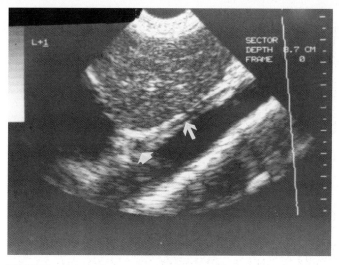

FIGURE 4–92. Longitudinal scan of the aorta.

288. The left crus of the diaphragm may be confused with which of the following?

    (A) left adrenal gland

    (B) aorta

    (C) splenic vein

    (D) superior mesenteric artery

    (E) accessory spleen

289. What is the long arrow in Fig. 4–93 pointing to?

    (A) inferior vena cava

    (B) psoas muscle

    (C) lumbar artery

    (D) right crus of diaphragm

    (E) right adrenal gland

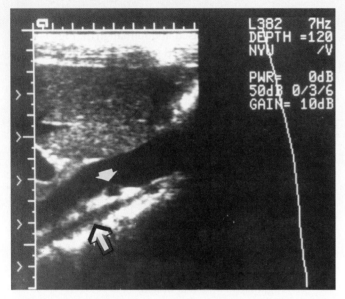

FIGURE 4–93. Longitudinal scan of the inferior vena cava.

290. What is the short arrow in Fig.4–93 pointing to?

    (A) right renal vein

    (B) right renal artery

    (C) left renal vein

    (D) left renal artery

    (E) celiac axis

291. What is the arrow in Fig. 4–94 pointing to?

    (A) hepatic artery

    (B) common duct

    (C) hepatic vein

    (D) portal vein

    (E) inferior vena cava

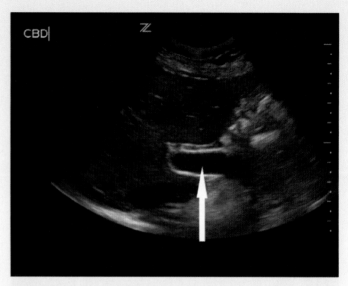

FIGURE 4–94. Longitudinal scan of the gallbladder.

292. What is the lumen seen anterior and parallel to the arrow in Fig. 4–94?

    (A) celiac axis

    (B) cystic duct

    (C) left renal vein

    (D) hepatic vein

    (E) common duct

293. There appear to be two echogenic masses in Fig. 4–95. One is anterior to the diaphragm (indicated by the calipers), and the other one is posterior to the diaphragm (indicated by the arrow). Which of the following usually causes this phenomenon?

    (A) slice-thickness artifact

    (B) reflection

    (C) mirror-image artifact

    (D) refraction

    (E) side lobe artifact

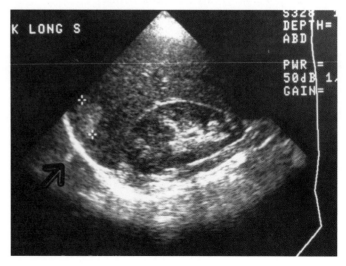

FIGURE 4–95. Longitudinal scan of the right upper quadrant.

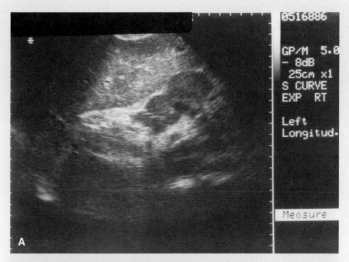

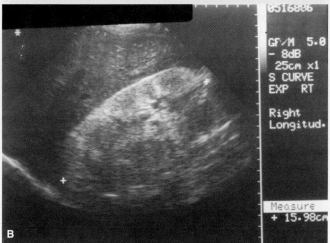

FIGURE 4–96. (**A**) Sagittal scan of the right upper quadrant. (**B**) Sagittal scan through the right kidney.

294. A 38-year-old man, who is an intravenous drug abuser, with a known mediastinal mass is seen in Fig. 4–96A and B. What does Fig. 4–96A show?

(A) a mass near the head of the pancreas

(B) periportal lymphadenopathy

(C) chronic cholecystitis

(D) Klatskin tumor

(E) liver mass

295. Which of the following is demonstrated in Fig. 4–96B?

(A) a normal kidney

(B) a kidney consistent with acute renal insufficiency

(C) a kidney consistent with chronic renal insufficiency

(D) renal cell carcinoma

(E) an adrenal gland in the renal fossa

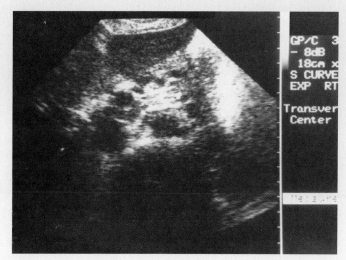

FIGURE 4–97. Transverse scan of the abdomen.

296. A sonogram is performed on a 32-year-old woman with a history of pancreatic carcinoma. Which of the following diagnoses is most likely represented in the scan in Fig. 4–97?

(A) celiac nodes

(B) an aortic aneurysm

(C) horseshoe kidney

(D) gastric lesion

(E) lesser sac mass

297. What type of aneurysm is demonstrated in Fig. 4–98?

(A) fusiform

(B) saccular

(C) cylindrical

(D) berry

(E) dissecting

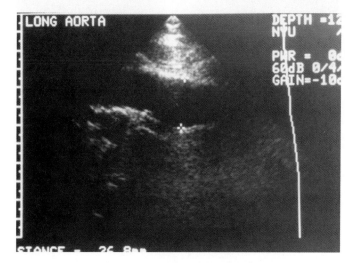

FIGURE 4–98. Longitudinal scan through the abdominal aorta.

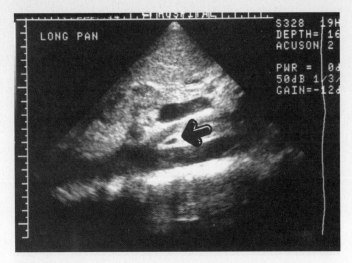

FIGURE 4–99. Longitudinal scan through the abdominal aorta.

298. What is the arrow in Fig. 4–99 pointing to?

    (A) right renal artery

    (B) right renal vein

    (C) left renal artery

    (D) left renal vein

    (E) gastroesophageal junction

299. What is the arrow in Fig. 4–100 pointing to?

    (A) head of the pancreas

    (B) body of the pancreas

    (C) caudate lobe of the liver

    (D) medial aspect of the left lobe

    (E) right lobe of the liver

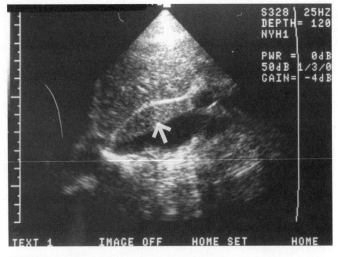

FIGURE 4–100. Sagittal scan through the right upper quadrant.

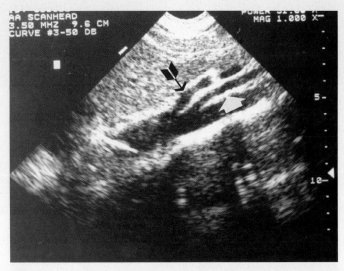

FIGURE 4–101. Sagittal scan through the right upper quadrant.

300. What is the thin black arrow in Fig. 4–101 pointing to?

    (A) celiac artery

    (B) superior mesenteric artery

    (C) portal vein

    (D) left gastric artery

    (E) hepatic artery

301. What is the white arrowhead in Fig. 4–101 pointing to?

    (A) celiac artery

    (B) superior mesenteric artery

    (C) portal vein

    (D) left gastric artery

    (E) hepatic artery

302. What is the name of the vessel that lies posterior to the pancreas in Fig. 4–101?

    (A) splenic vein

    (B) aorta

    (C) portal vein

    (D) left renal vein

    (E) hepatic vein

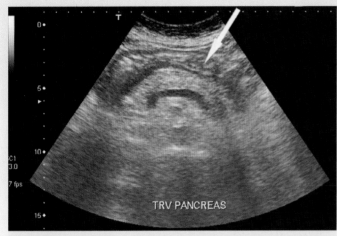

FIGURE 4–102. Transverse scan through the pancreas.

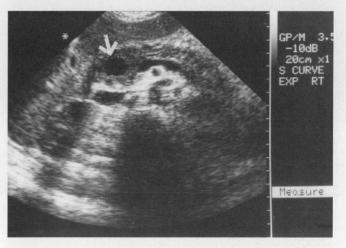

FIGURE 4–104. Transverse sonogram through the pancreas.

303. What is the arrow in Fig. 4–102 pointing to?

(A) stomach

(B) pancreas

(C) C-loop of the duodenum

(D) gastroduodenal artery

(E) spleen

306. Which of the following structures defines the anterolateral aspect of the head of the pancreas?

(A) superior mesenteric artery

(B) inferior vena cava

(C) splenic vein

(D) common bile duct

(E) gastroduodenal artery

307. What are the arrows in Fig. 4–105 pointing to?

(A) peripelvic cysts

(B) extrapelvic cysts

(C) parapelvic cysts

(D) renal pyramids

(E) dilated calyces

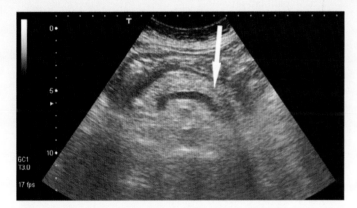

FIGURE 4–103. Transverse sonogram through the pancreas.

304. What is the arrow in Fig. 4–103 pointing to?

(A) normal head of pancreas

(B) normal stomach

(C) pancreatic duct

(D) superior mesenteric artery (SMA)

(E) normal tail of the pancreas

305. What is the arrow in Fig. 4–104 pointing to?

(A) gastroduodenal artery

(B) common bile duct

(C) portal vein

(D) superior mesenteric vein

(E) hepatic artery

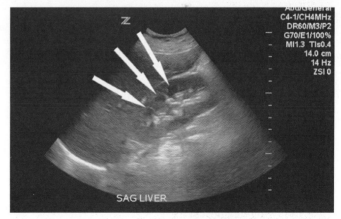

FIGURE 4–105. Long-axis image of the right kidney.

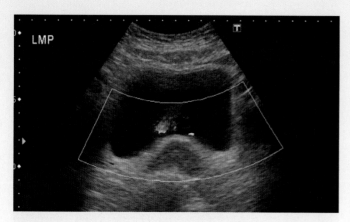

FIGURE 4–106. Short-axis sonogram through the urinary bladder.

308. What is demonstrated in this color Doppler image of the bladder in Fig. 4–106?

(A) acute obstructive uropathy

(B) ureteral dilatation

(C) diverticular jet effect

(D) color Doppler flow

309. What is the finding seen within the urinary bladder of the patient imaged in Fig. 4–106?

(A) ureteral jet

(B) thickened Foley catheter

(C) bladder aneurysm

(D) ureteral venous flow

(E) intraluminal arterial bladder flow

310. Ureteral jets will not be seen in which of the following?

(A) extrapelvic cyst

(B) obstructive hydronephrosis

(C) renal artery aneurysm

(D) parapelvic cyst

(E) transient diuresis

311. A 30-year-old patient with a history of biliary disease presents with fever, pain, and leukocytosis. An abdominal sonogram is performed. The areas labeled "A" in Fig. 4–107 are consistent with which of the following diagnoses?

(A) hematomas

(B) complicated cysts

(C) abscesses

(D) echinococcal disease

(E) metastatic lesions

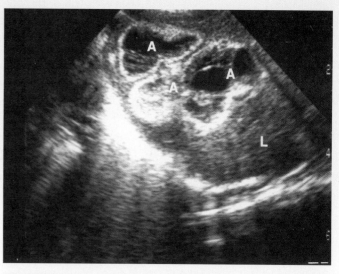

FIGURE 4–107. Sonogram of the urinary bladder.

312. A patient presents with polycystic liver disease. What other organ should also be evaluated by sonogram?

(A) spleen

(B) pancreas

(C) gallbladder

(D) adrenal glands

(E) kidneys

313. Identify the vessel with a postprandial low-resistive blood flow.

(A) celiac artery

(B) hepatic artery

(C) splenic artery

(D) superior mesenteric artery

(E) aorta

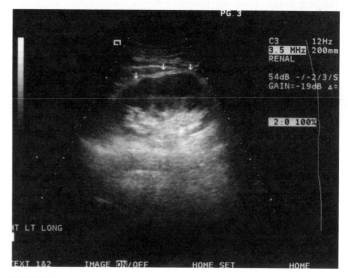

FIGURE 4–108. Longitudinal sonogram of the left kidney. (Courtesy of Shpetim Telegrafi, MD, New York University.)

314. **What are the arrows in Fig. 4–108 pointing to?**

   (A) ascites

   (B) perinephric fluid

   (C) pleura effusion

   (D) fluid in Morrison's pouch

   (E) normal renal cortex

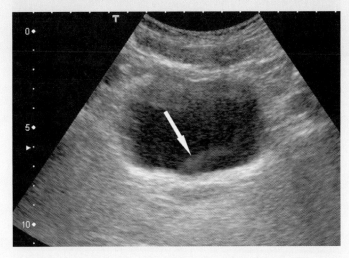

FIGURE 4–109. Transverse scan of the urinary bladder.

315. **Fig. 4–109 is a transverse view of the bladder. What is the arrow pointing to?**

   (A) bladder stone

   (B) bladder diverticula

   (C) bladder mass

   (D) Foley catheter

   (E) ureteral jet

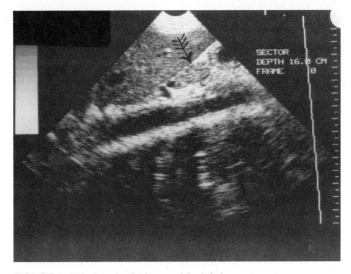

FIGURE 4–110. Longitudinal scan of the inferior vena cava.

316. **What is the arrow in Fig. 4–110 pointing to?**

   (A) antrum of the stomach

   (B) head of the pancreas

   (C) caudate lobe of the liver

   (D) body of the pancreas

   (E) adrenal gland

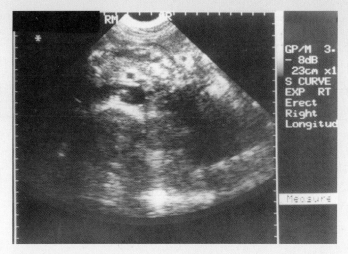

FIGURE 4–111. Transverse sonogram through the pancreas.

317. **Fig. 4–111 is consistent with which of the following findings?**

   (A) chronic pancreatitis

   (B) acute pancreatitis

   (C) adenocarcinoma

   (D) islet cell tumor

   (E) normal scan

318. **A 37-year-old man with a history of repeated episodes of pancreatitis due to alcoholism presents with an epigastric mass. What does Fig. 4–112 suggest?**

   (A) negative study

   (B) adenocarcinoma

   (C) pancreatic pseudocyst

   (D) acute pancreatitis

   (E) chronic pancreatitis

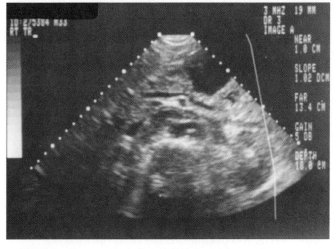

FIGURE 4–112. Transverse sonogram through the pancreas.

319. What is the most common complication of a pancreatic pseudocyst?

    (A) infection
    (B) reabsorption
    (C) calcification
    (D) hemorrhage
    (E) rupture

320. A sonogram of the abdominis rectus muscle is ordered. Which of the following is the most appropriate transducer to use to obtain optimal images?

    (A) 2.5 MHz curve linear
    (B) 5 MHz curve linear
    (C) 3.5 MHz mechanical sector
    (D) 5 MHz linear
    (E) 3.5 MHz vector array

321. What is the name of the area anterior to the right kidney and posterior to the right lobe of the liver?

    (A) pouch of Douglas
    (B) Morison's pouch
    (C) Hartmann's pouch
    (D) lesser sac
    (E) greater sac

322. A 34-year-old man presents with flank pain. The ureteral jets are normal. What finding does the image in Fig. 4–113 suggest?

    (A) renal cell carcinoma
    (B) pyonephrosis
    (C) pyelocaliectasis
    (D) pyelonephrosis
    (E) renal transplant

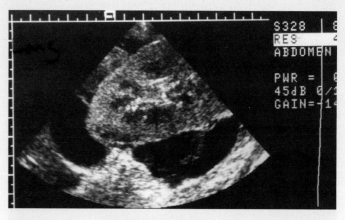

FIGURE 4–114. Longitudinal scan though the kidney.

323. The renal transplant patient shown in Fig. 4–114 was referred for a sonogram. The perirenal fluid collection may be associated with all of the following *except*

    (A) abscess
    (B) hematoma
    (C) ascites
    (D) urinoma
    (E) lymphocele

324. A post-renal-transplant patient presents with fever, flank pain, localized tenderness, and leukocytosis. A renal sonogram is performed, and a perinephric fluid collection is documented. This finding is most consistent with which of the following?

    (A) abscess
    (B) hematoma
    (C) lymphocele
    (D) renal cyst
    (E) urinoma

325. In Fig. 4–115, what are the anechoic structures visualized within the liver?

    (A) normal bile ducts
    (B) dilated bile ducts
    (C) hepatic arteries
    (D) hepatic veins
    (E) portal veins

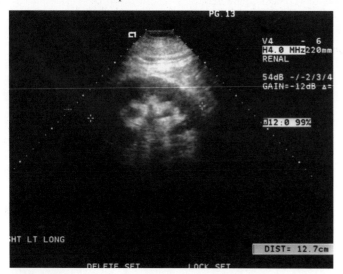

FIGURE 4–113. A longitudinal sonogram through the left kidney. (*Courtesy of Shpetim Telegrafi, MD, New York University.*)

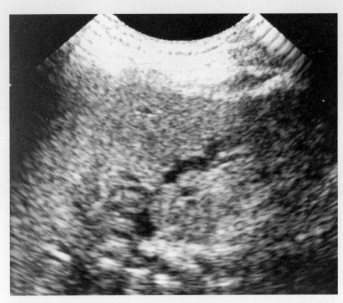

FIGURE 4–115. A magnified view through the liver.

326. In Fig. 4–116, the organ that the arrow is pointing to is consistent with which of the following diagnoses?

(A) normal pancreas

(B) acute pancreatitis

(C) chronic pancreatitis

(D) adenocarcinoma

(E) islet cell tumor

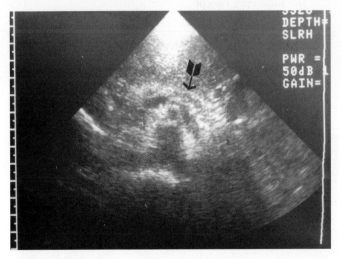

FIGURE 4–116. Transverse scan through the pancreas.

327. A 38-year-old man with a history of enuresis presents for a pelvic sonogram. Fig. 4–117 is most consistent with which of the following diagnoses?

(A) a normal pelvic sac

(B) an enlarged prostate

(C) diffuse bladder-wall thickening

(D) bladder outlet obstruction

(E) endometriosis of the bladder wall

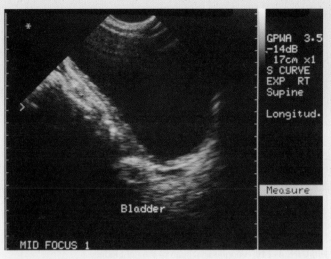

FIGURE 4–117. Longitudinal scan of a male pelvis.

328. Fig. 4–118 is most consistent with which of the following diagnoses?

(A) hepatitis

(B) cirrhosis

(C) pyelonephritis

(D) pyelocaliectasis

(E) chronic renal failure

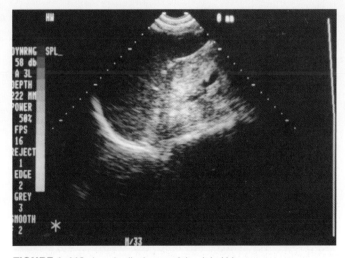

FIGURE 4–118. Longitudinal scan of the right kidney.

329. Identify the laboratory values that would most likely be elevated in the patient in Fig. 4–118.

(A) alanine aminotransferase (ALT) and aspartate aminotransferase (AST)

(B) alkaline phosphatase and bilirubin

(C) amylase and lipase

(D) creatinine and blood urea nitrogen (BUN)

(E) acid phosphatase and white blood cell (WBC) cell

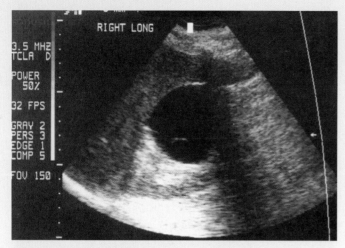

FIGURE 4–119. Longitudinal scan of the right kidney.

330. Internal echoes inside the renal cyst shown in Fig. 4–119 may be due to all of the following *except*

    (A) reverberation

    (B) beam width artifact

    (C) refraction

    (D) attenuation

    (E) side lobe artifact

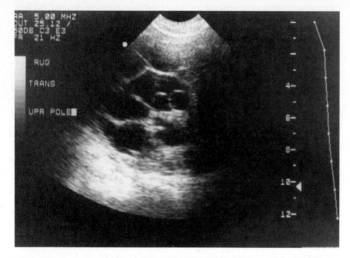

FIGURE 4–120. Transverse scan of the right kidney.

331. The findings in the transverse scan in Fig. 4–120 of the right kidney is most consistent with which of the following diagnoses?

    (A) parapelvic cyst

    (B) ureteropelvic junction (UPJ) obstruction

    (C) nonobstructive hydronephrosis

    (D) adult polycystic kidney disease

    (E) infantile polycystic kidney disease

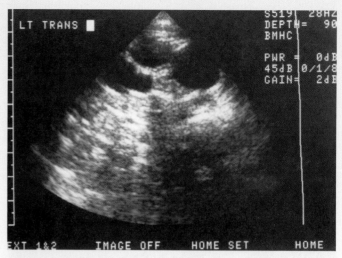

FIGURE 4–121. Transverse scan of the left kidney of a newborn.

332. The neonate in Fig. 4–121 presented with a palpable abdominal mass. What is the sonogram most suggestive of?

    (A) multicystic dysplastic kidney

    (B) pyonephrosis

    (C) infantile polycystic disease

    (D) peripelvic cysts

    (E) extrapelvic cysts

333. Fig. 4–122 suggests that this patient may have all of the following *except*

    (A) a normal kidney

    (B) benign prostate hyperplasia

    (C) prostatitis

    (D) calculi

    (E) retroperitoneal fibrosis

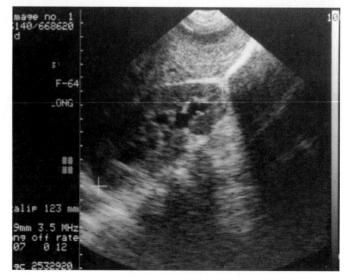

FIGURE 4–122. Longitudinal scan of the right kidney.

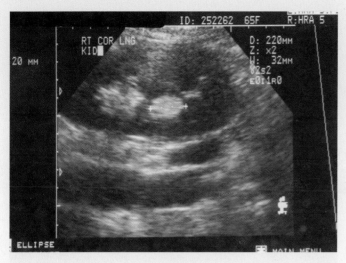

FIGURE 4–123. Coronal scan of the right kidney.

334. The longitudinal scan of the right kidney in Fig. 4–123 is consistent with which of the following diagnoses?

(A) acute pyelonephritis

(B) acute tubular necrosis

(C) tubular sclerosis

(D) acute focal bacteria nephritis

(E) duplex collecting system

335. A transverse scan of the upper abdomen is shown in Fig. 4–124. What is the arrow pointing to?

(A) hepatic vein

(B) splenic artery

(C) celiac axis

(D) hepatic artery

(E) portal confluence

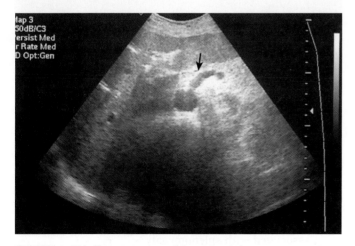

FIGURE 4–124. Transverse scan of the upper abdomen.

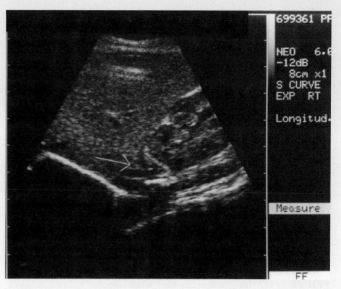

FIGURE 4–125. Longitudinal sonogram of a neonate through the area of the right kidney.

336. Fig. 4–125 is an abdominal longitudinal scan of a 14-day-old male infant born 2 weeks prematurely. What is the arrow pointing to?

(A) normal adrenal gland

(B) perirenal hemorrhage

(C) retroperitoneal fat

(D) neuroblastoma

(E) pheochromocytoma

337. The coronal scan of the left kidney shown in Fig. 4–126 is suggestive of which of the following diagnoses?

(A) an extrapelvic cyst

(B) hydronephrosis

(C) pyonephrosis

(D) urinoma

(E) renal infarct

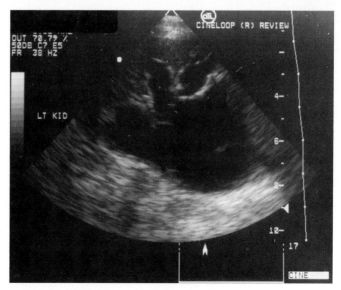

FIGURE 4–126. Coronal scan of the kidney.

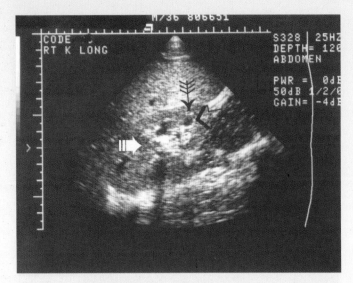

FIGURE 4–127. Longitudinal scan of the right kidney.

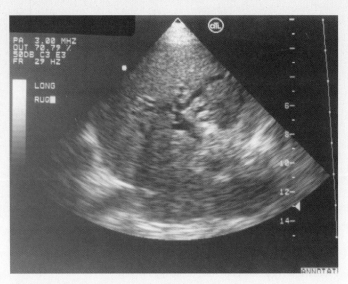

FIGURE 4–128. Longitudinal scan of the liver.

338. A longitudinal scan of the right kidney is performed. What is the thin black arrow in Fig. 4–127 pointing to?

   (A) the renal sinus

   (B) arcuate arteries

   (C) renal medullary pyramids

   (D) simple renal cysts

   (E) renal stone

339. What is the open arrowhead in Fig. 4–127 pointing to?

   (A) the renal sinus

   (B) arcuate arteries

   (C) renal medullary pyramids

   (D) simple renal cyst

   (E) renal stones

340. What is the white arrow in Fig. 4–127 pointing to?

   (A) renal column of Bertin

   (B) an angiomyolipoma

   (C) dromedary hump

   (D) bifid collecting system

   (E) the renal pelvis

341. A patient presents with vague abdominal pain and elevated bilirubin level and liver function test results. The finding in Fig. 4–128 may be initiated by all of the following *except*

   (A) stone in the common bile duct

   (B) mass in the head of the pancreas

   (C) mass in the ampulla of Vater

   (D) diffuse metastatic disease of the liver

   (E) cirrhosis

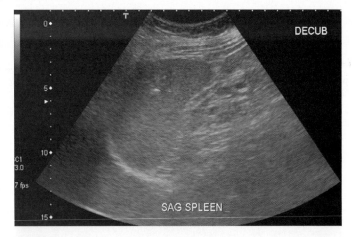

FIGURE 4–129. Longitudinal scan of the spleen.

342. A patient presents with a spleen that is palpable on physical examination. Fig. 4–129 is a longitudinal image of the spleen. Which of the following is not associated with splenomegaly?

   (A) lymphoma

   (B) portal hypertension

   (C) infectious disease

   (D) myeloproliferation

   (E) neuroblastoma

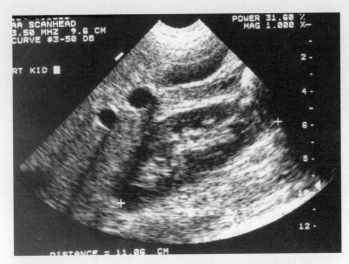

FIGURE 4–130. Longitudinal scan through the right upper quadrant.

343. A 25-year-old woman presents for an abdominal sonogram. A longitudinal scan of the liver is performed. What is the most likely diagnosis for the two cystic structures in Fig. 4–130?

   (A) liver metastases
   (B) hydatid cysts
   (C) simple benign cysts
   (D) lymphoma
   (E) polycystic liver disease

344. Fig. 4–131A–C is a scan of a 70-year-old man with a history of weight loss, abdominal pain, and anorexia. What does the scan suggest?

   (A) negative study
   (B) pancreatic pseudocyst
   (C) acute pancreatitis
   (D) chronic pancreatitis
   (E) pancreatic adenocarcinoma

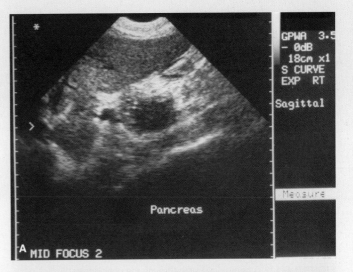

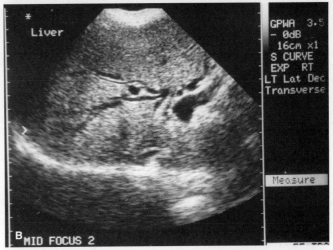

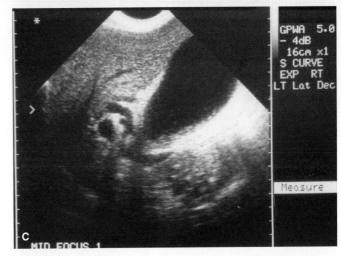

FIGURE 4–131. (**A**) Sagittal scan through the head of the pancreas. (**B**) Sagittal scan through the liver. (**C**) Sagittal scan through the gallbladder.

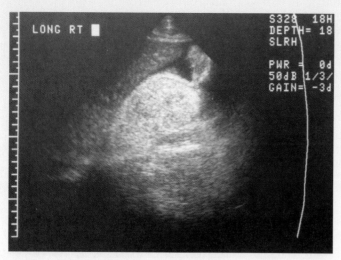

FIGURE 4-132. Longitudinal scan through the right kidney.

345. Fig. 4–132 is most consistent with which of the following diagnosis?

    (A) acute pyelonephritis

    (B) acute tubular necrosis

    (C) tubular sclerosis

    (D) chronic glomerulonephritis

    (E) medullary nephrocalcinosis

346. Fig. 4–133 is a transverse sonogram of the liver. What is the white arrow pointing to?

    (A) pancreas

    (B) spleen

    (C) abdominal aortic aneurysm

    (D) stomach

    (E) heart

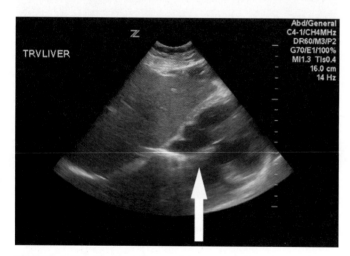

FIGURE 4-133. Transverse image of the upper abdomen.

347. Hashimoto's disease is a type of chronic

    (A) gastroenteritis

    (B) thyroiditis

    (C) orchitis

    (D) prostatitis

    (E) hepatitis

348. Which of the following is a type of a malignant adrenal mass?

    (A) adenoma

    (B) myelolipoma

    (C) cyst

    (D) pheochromocytoma

    (E) neuroblastoma

349. An enlarged right adrenal gland will displace the inferior vena cava in which of the following directions?

    (A) anteriorly

    (B) posteriorly

    (C) medially

    (D) laterally

    (E) no displacement

350. The findings in Fig. 4–134 is most-likely

    (A) normal liver parenchyma

    (B) dilated portal veins

    (C) dilated common bile ducts

    (D) dilated hepatic veins

    (E) dilated intrahepatic ducts

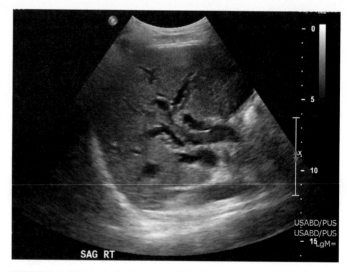

FIGURE 4-134. Longitudinal view of the liver.

351. Which of the following conditions is not associated with pneumobilia

    (A) emphysematous cholecystitis
    (B) cholecysto-enteric fistula
    (C) choledochojejunostomy
    (D) pancreatic carcinoma
    (E) prolonged acute cholecystitis

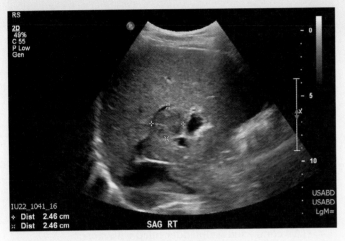

FIGURE 4–135. Longitudinal view of the liver.

352. Which of the following structures is most likely being measured in Fig. 4–135?

    (A) hypernephroma
    (B) peliosis hepatis
    (C) fungal infection of the liver
    (D) hemangioma
    (E) hydatid cyst

353. Which of the following will *not* increase the chance of documenting shadowing posterior to a small renal stone?

    (A) decreasing gain
    (B) focal zone set at the level of the calculi
    (C) increasing the transducer frequency
    (D) using a linear probe
    (E) use of tissue harmonics

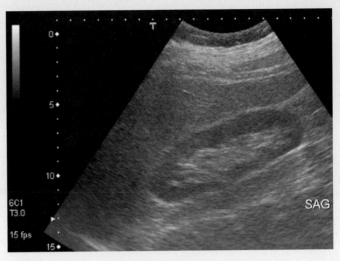

FIGURE 4–136. Longitudinal view of the liver and right kidney.

354. Fig. 4–136 of the kidney is consistent with which of the following diagnoses?

    (A) hydronephrosis
    (B) hydroureter
    (C) pyonephrosis
    (D) vesicoureteral obstruction
    (E) normal findings

355. Fig. 4–137 is a longitudinal scan of the right upper quadrant. What abnormality is seen?

    (A) a hypoechoic texture of the renal parenchyma
    (B) an echogenic liver texture
    (C) atrophy of the kidney
    (D) metastases
    (E) none—inappropriate technical settings

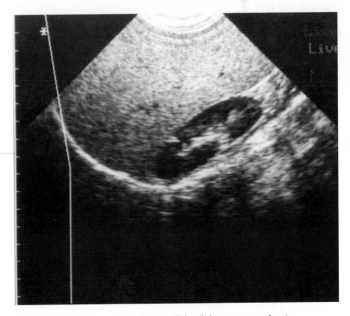

FIGURE 4-137. Longitudinal scan of the right upper quadrant.

356. Fig. 4–137 is *not* consistent with which of the following diagnoses?

(A) glycogen storage disease

(B) fatty metamorphosis

(C) echinococcal disease

(D) severe hepatitis

(E) hemochromatosis

357. To optimize a sonogram, all of the following must be taken into consideration *except*

(A) change overall gain

(B) time-gain compensation (TGC)

(C) depth and focus

(D) transducer frequency and type

(E) speed of sound

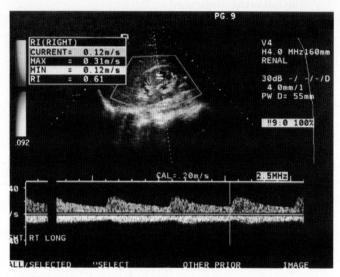

FIGURE 4–138. Long-axis view of the right kidney. *(Courtesy of Shpetim Telegrafi, MD, New York University.)*

358. Fig. 4–138 is a duplex color Doppler sonogram of the right kidney. Which of the following diagnoses is consistent with the Doppler findings?

(A) normal kidney

(B) obstructive uropathy

(C) pelviectasis

(D) renal artery stenosis

(E) hypertension

359. Splenomegaly is diagnosed when the spleen is greater than how many centimeters?

(A) 8 cm

(B) 11 cm

(C) 13 cm

(D) 15 cm

(E) 18 cm

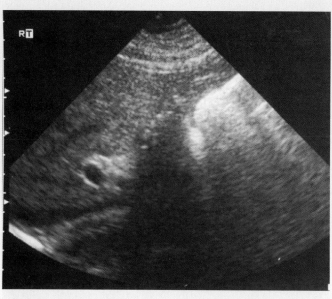

FIGURE 4–139. Long-axis sonogram of the upper abdomen.

360. Fig. 4–139 is a long-axis sonogram of the right upper quadrant of the abdomen. Which of the following best describes the image?

(A) contracted gallbladder filled with stones

(B) contracted gallbladder without stones

(C) postcholecystectomy

(D) heterogeneous liver

(E) echogenic focal mass

361. Which of the following is the most likely diagnosis of the patient in Fig. 4–139?

(A) cholecystectomy

(B) gastric mass

(C) acalculous cholecystitis

(D) calculous cholecystitis

(E) normal abdomen

362. The laboratory finding in the patient in Fig. 4–139 would most likely be consistent with which of the following?

(A) increase in amylase

(B) increase in creatinine

(C) decrease in prothrombin time

(D) decrease in indirect bilirubin

(E) increase in alkaline phosphatase

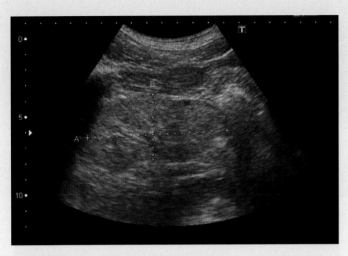

FIGURE 4-140. Longitudinal scan of the kidney.

363. The findings in Fig. 4–140 are most likely due to which of the following diagnoses?

    (A) medullary sponge kidney
    (B) renal parenchymal disease
    (C) renal cell carcinoma
    (D) medullary nephrocalcinosis
    (E) renal sinus lipomatosis

364. What is the most common congenital cause of urinary track obstruction in males?

    (A) ureteropelvic junction obstruction (UPJ)
    (B) posterior urethral valve (PUV)
    (C) infantile polycystic kidney disease
    (D) undescended testes
    (E) duplex collecting system

365. Where are the spiral values of Heister located?

    (A) ampulla of Vater
    (B) junction of the cystic duct and common duct
    (C) junction of the right and left common hepatic duct
    (D) proximal portion of the cystic duct
    (E) fundus of the gallbladder

366. Identify the pre-existing condition that occurs in patients with hepatomas.

    (A) hematomas
    (B) abscesses
    (C) gallstones
    (D) developmental cysts
    (E) cirrhosis

367. A 3-year-old child with a clinical history of intermittent pain, jaundice, and a palpable mass presents for an abdominal sonogram. A cystic dilatation of the common bile duct is seen in the liver. This is most characteristic of which of the following diagnoses?

    (A) biliary atresia
    (B) hepatitis
    (C) choledochal cyst
    (D) hypertrophy pyloric stenosis
    (E) normal liver finding

368. Which of the following describes how carcinoma of the gallbladder would most likely appear?

    (A) thin-walled gallbladder
    (B) small gallbladder with thickened walls
    (C) large gallbladder with a halo surrounding it
    (D) diffusely thickened gallbladder with gallstones
    (E) echogenic mass with no distinguishing features of a gallbladder

369. Where is a Baker's cyst usually located?

    (A) adjacent to the thyroid
    (B) behind the nipple in a breast
    (C) within the liver parenchyma
    (D) posterior to the uterus
    (E) behind the knee

370. What is Riedel's lobe?

    (A) elongation of the left lobe
    (B) a duplication of the caudate lobe
    (C) tongue-like extension of the right lobe
    (D) a small right lobe
    (E) transposition of the liver lobes

Case Studies

CASE 1

History: 56-year-old man presenting with jaundice. Sagittal gray scale (A) (C) (D) and color Doppler (B) images of liver and common bile duct and pancreatic head.

1-1. Which of the following are true statements concerning this sonogram?

    A. there are no dilated intrahepatic or extrahepatic bile ducts.

    B. only the extrahepatic bile ducts are dilated.

    C. only the intrahepatic bile ducts are dilated.

    D. both the intrahepatic and extrahepatic bile ducts are dilated.

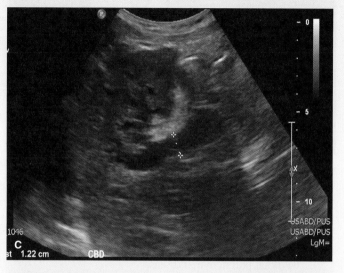

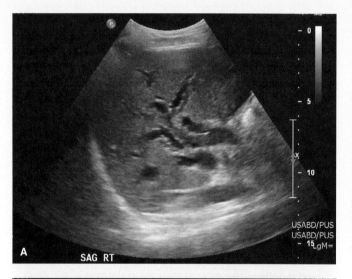

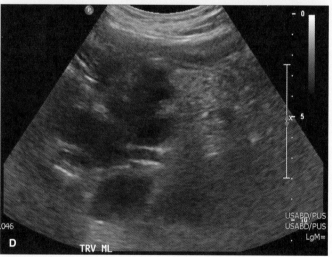

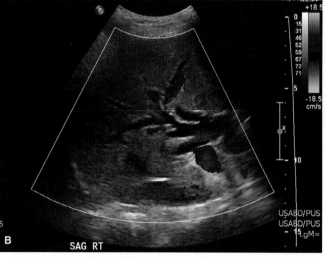

1-2. What is the possible cause of this finding?

    A. stenosis at the ampulla of Vater

    B. pancreatic head mass

    C. stones at the distal common bile duct

    D. all of the above

1-3. In this case, what is the most likely cause of dilated ducts?

    A. pancreatic cancer

    B. stones in the distal common bile duct

    C. cannot tell

    D. hepatoma

CASE 2

History: 36-year-old woman with chronic hepatitis C. Sagittal gray scale (A), color Doppler (B), and sonograms of liver (C).

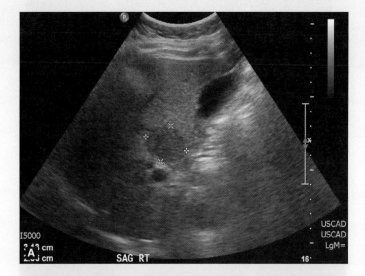

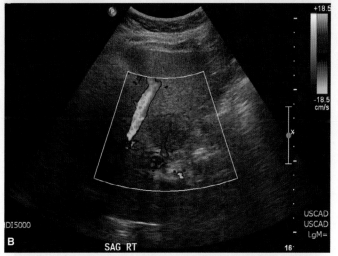

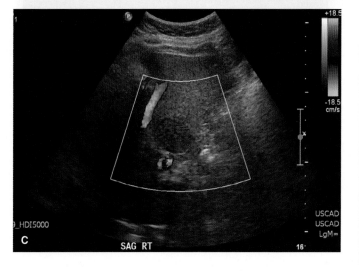

2-1. What is the most correct statement concerning this patient's sonogram?

A. there is a 2-cm hypoechoic mass with a central vessel.

B. there is an anechoic mass in the liver.

C. there is a vascular mass within the liver.

D. there is a focal area of normal liver surrounded by fatty liver.

2-2. What is the most likely diagnosis?

A. hepatocellular cancer

B. hemangioma

C. focal nodular hyperplasia

D. metastatic lesion

2-3. Which of the following modalities may be helpful to confirm this sonographic impression?

A. computed tomography

B. magnetic resonance

C. angiography

D. nuclear imaging

E. either A or B

CASE 3

History: 51-year-old man with elevated liver function tests. Sagittal and transverse gray scale (A, B, C) sonograms of the liver.

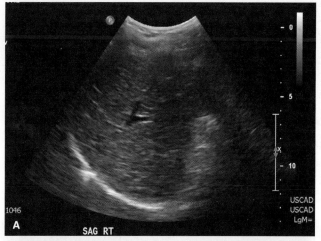

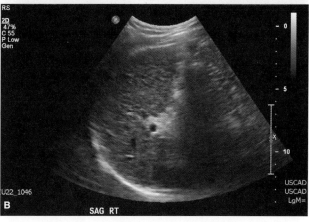

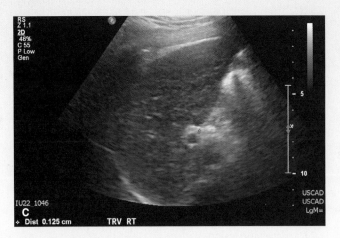

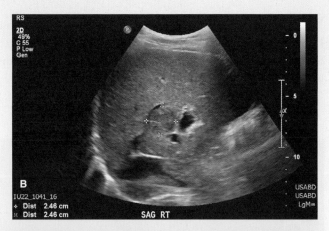

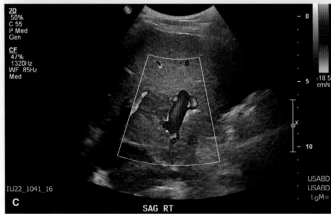

3-1. Which of the following are true statements concerning this patient's sonogram?

A. the liver texture is normal.

B. the liver texture is diffusely irregular.

C. the liver is fatty replaced.

D. there are innumerable metastatic lesions.

3-2. What do the calipers measure?

A. the hepatic artery

B. the portal vein

C. the common bile duct

D. the pancreatic duct

3-3. Which of the following can be included in the diagnostic possibilities?

A. normal liver

B. fatty change

C. hepatitis

D. metastatic disease

CASE 4

History: 51-year-old man with elevated liver function tests. Sagittal (B) and transverse gray scale (A) and color Doppler (C) sonography and arterial phase computed tomography (CT) scan (D).

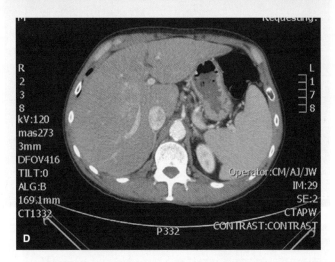

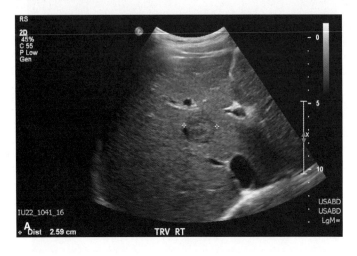

4-1. Which of the following statements are true concerning this patient's imaging studies?

A. there is a solid mass in the left lobe.

B. there is a solid mass in the anterior segment of the right lobe.

C. there is a solid mass in the posterior segment of the right lobe.

D. there are no masses within the liver.

4-2. Based on the imaging findings, what is the most likely diagnosis?

A. hepatocellular carcinoma

B. hemangioma

C. metastatic lesion

D. all of the above are possible

4-3. Which of the following are shown in the arterial-phase CT scan?

A. peripheral "cloud-like" enhancement

B. central vascularity

C. nothing

D. diffuse metastatic disease

CASE 5

History: 62-year-old man S/P liver transplant with elevated liver function tests. Transverse gray scale (A) and color Doppler (B, C) images of main and right portal veins.

5-1. Which of the following abnormal findings are shown in the images?

A. reversed flow in the main portal vein

B. abnormal liver texture

C. both A and B

D. none of the above

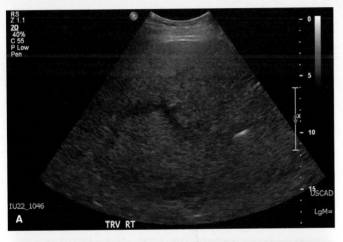

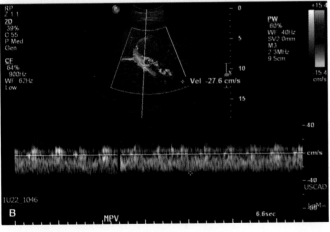

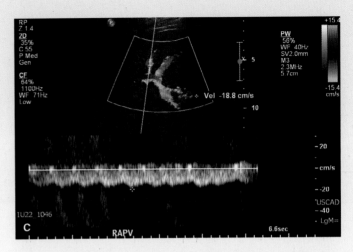

5-2. Which of the following are possible causes of this finding?

A. rejection

B. arterial thrombosis

C. diffuse infiltration by tumor

D. faulty anastomosis of portal vein

5-3. What is the most likely diagnosis?

A. portal hypertension

B. liver steatosis

C. both A and B

D. none of the above

CASE 6

History: 53-year-old with history of inflammatory bowel disease. Sagittal gray scale (A) (B) and color Doppler (C) of liver.

6-1. Which of the following abnormal findings are shown in the images?

A. thrombosis of main portal vein

B. multiple liver masses

C. dilated intrahepatic and extrahepatic bile ducts

D. none of the above

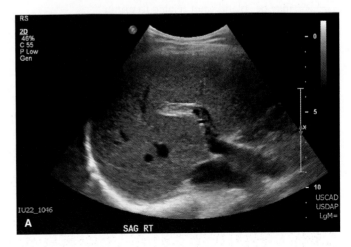

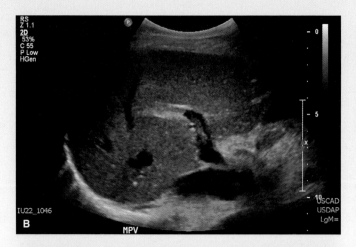

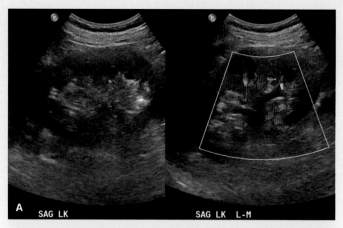

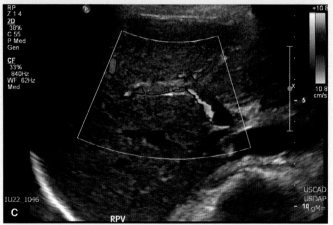

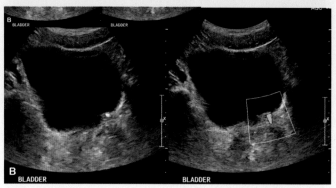

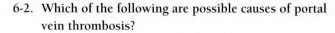

6-2. Which of the following are possible causes of portal vein thrombosis?

    A. extension of hepatic tumor into portal vein

    B. hematologic disorder

    C. gastrointestinal inflammatory disorders

    D. all of the above

6-3. What is the clinical importance of portal vein thrombosis?

    A. hepatic transplantation cannot occur

    B. increased risk of metastatic spread

    C. may be "bland"; not related to tumor

    D. must be removed by catheter technique

CASE 7

History: 19-year-old with left-lower-quadrant pain. Sagittal gray scale and color Doppler sonography of (A) left kidney and (B) bladder.

7-1. Which of the following are true statements concerning this sonogram?

    A. there is a nonobstructing stone in the left kidney.

    B. there is a stone at the left ureterovesicular junction.

    C. both A and B are true.

    D. neither A nor B is true.

7-2. Which of the following are true statements concerning the "twinkle" sign?

    A. It can overestimate size of stone.

    B. It can underestimate size of stone.

    C. It is only found with certain stones.

    D. It does not occur secondarily to vascular calcification.

7-3. Though not shown here, the presence of a ureteral jet indicates which of the following findings?

    A. no ureteric obstruction

    B. urinary sediment within the bladder

    C. cannot represent urine since all fluids are hypoechoic

    D. none of the above

CASE 8

History: 30-year-old woman with right upper quadrant pain. Sagittal (A) and transverse (B) gray scale and (C) color Doppler sonogram of the gallbladder.

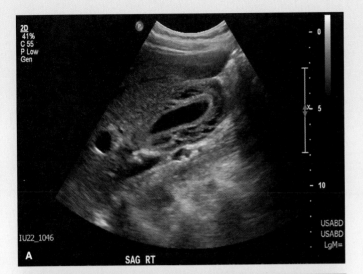

A SAG RT

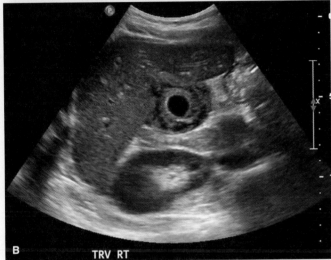

B TRV RT

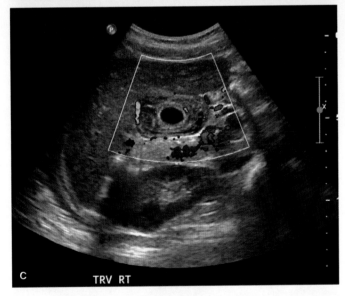

C TRV RT

8-1. Which of the following are true statements concerning this sonogram?

A. there is severe edema of the gallbladder wall.

B. there are multiple calculi within the lumen.

C. there is no diffuse cholesterosis of the wall.

D. there is focal thickening of the wall.

8-2. Which of the following are diagnostic possibilities?

A. cardiac causes

B. metastatic involvement

C. hepatitis

D. cirrhosis

E. all of the above

8-3. Which of the following is true if the patient experiences pain when the transducer is over the gallbladder?

A. there must be acute cholecystitis.

B. this is referred to as Murphy's sign.

C. you must stop with the examination.

D. none of the above are true.

CASE 9

History: 56-year-old man with chronic hepatitis C. Sagittal gray scale (A) and color Doppler (B) sonogram of liver.

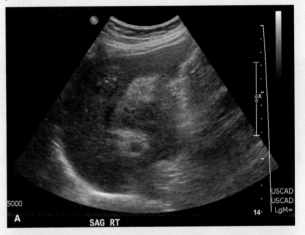

A SAG RT

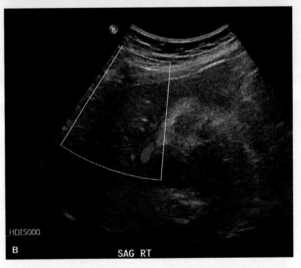

B SAG RT

9-1. Which of the following is a false statement concerning this sonogram?

A. there is a focal, well-defined mass.

B. the mass contains echogenic focus.

C. A or B

D. there is a well-defined hypoechoic halo surrounding the mass

9-2. Which of the following are diagnostic possibilities for this study?

    A. metastatic lesion

    B. hepatocellular carcinoma

    C. A or B

    D. hemangioma

9-3. Which of the following can be said about sonography-guided biopsy of this lesion?

    A. not possible

    B. can be performed

    C. requires CT scanning follow-up

    D. none of the above

CASE 10

History: 64-year-old man S/P TIPS procedure. Multiple color Doppler (A, B) sonograms of the liver with an accompanying hepatic venogram (C).

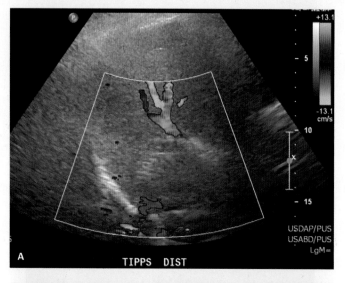

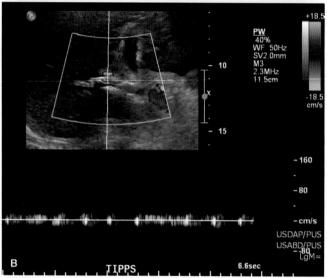

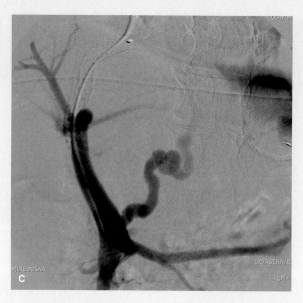

10-1. Which of the following statements are true concerning these images?

    A. the TIPS is perfect

    B. the TIPS is obstructed

    C. the main portal vein is occluded

    D. the left hepatic vein is occluded

10-2. What is the most likely diagnosis?

    A. occlusion of the TIPS

    B. main portal vein occlusion

    C. hepatic vein occlusion

    D. normal TIPS patency

10-3. On spectral Doppler, normal velocities in a TIPS:

    A. are between 50 and 150 cm/s

    B. are near 0 cm/s

    C. cannot be calculated, just due to the power

    D. do not vary with respiration

CASE 11

History: 28-year-old pregnant patient with right-lower-quadrant pain. Transverse gray scale (A, C) and color Doppler (B) images of right lower quadrant.

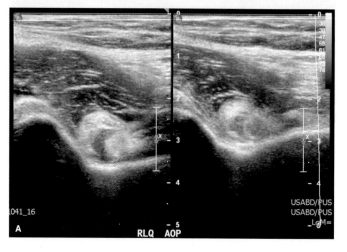

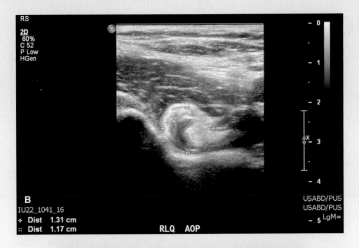

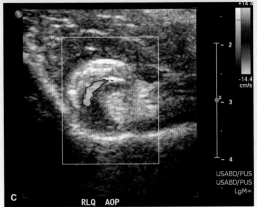

CASE 12

History: Sagittal gray scale (A) and color Doppler (B) sonogram of the right thyroid lobe.

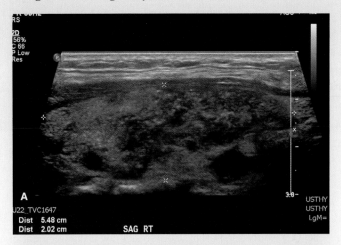

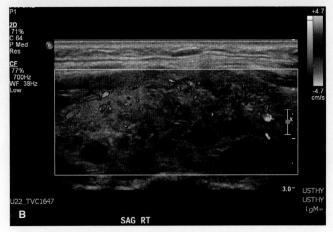

11-1. Positive findings include which of the following?

    A. an abnormal bowel segment

    B. an abnormal kidney

    C. an ectopic pregnancy

    D. renal calculi

11-2. Which of the following are diagnostic possibilities?

    A. appendicitis

    B. small bowel intussusception

    C. A or B

    D. none of the above

11-3. The normal thickness of a compressed appendix:

    A. cannot be measured accurately

    B. less than 3 mm

    C. less than 6 mm

    D. less than 9 mm

12-1. Which of the following statements are true concerning this patient?

    A. there are multiple nodules throughout the entire right lobe.

    B. the right lobe is markedly enlarged.

    C. there is diffuse textural inhomogeneity of the right lobe.

    D. the gain settings are not properly set.

12-2. Diagnostic consideration includes which of the following?

    A. chronic lymphocytic thyroiditis

    B. Hashimoto's thyroiditis

    C. cancer

    D. both A and B

12-3. You are asked to provide sonographic guidance for a biopsy of this patient. Which of the following should be included in your next steps?

    A. question whether a biopsy of this lesion is truly indicated

    B. use a needle guide

    C. refuse to help with the biopsy

    D. ask someone else to do it

Answers and Explanations

At the end of each explained answer, there is a number combination in parentheses. The first number identifies the reference source; the second number or set of numbers indicates the page or pages on which the relevant information can be found.

1. **(B)** The three structures that make up the portal triad are the hepatic artery, portal vein, and bile duct. (1:82)

2. **(D)** Wilms' tumor, also known as nephroblastoma, is the most common type of renal cancer in children between the ages of 2 and 4 years. The most common symptoms for Wilms' tumor are hematuria and hypertension. (1:1926)

3. **(C)** Courvoisier's sign. Courvoisier law is enlargement of the gallbladder caused by an obstruction of the common bile duct from outside the biliary system. The obstruction usually results from carcinoma of the head of the pancreas and not from a stone in the common duct. The latter produces little or no dilatation of the gallbladder because the gallbladder is usually scarred from infection. Classically, patients present with painless jaundice and a nontender and distended gallbladder. (1:213)

4. **(B)** Hydropic gallbladder. Complete obstruction of the neck of the gallbladder or the cystic duct leads to hydrops or mucocele of the gallbladder. In this condition, the bile within the gallbladder is absorbed and replaced by a mucoid secretion from the lining of the gallbladder. (6:130)

5. **(D)** Renal vein thrombosis in the acute stage is associated with enlarged kidneys with dilation of the renal vein proximal to the obstruction. There will be either a decreased or no blood flow on Doppler. Bilateral small kidneys are associated with end-stage renal disease. The normal adult kidneys range from 9 to 12 cm in length. The renal parenchyma is normally less echogenic when compared to the liver parenchyma. In cases of end-stage renal disease, the kidneys become more echogenic. End-stage renal disease may be caused by chronic glomerulonephritis, pyelonephritis, and renal vascular disease. (2:98, 99)

6. **(C)** A staghorn calculus is a large stone located within the renal pelvis of the kidney. (7:375)

7. **(D)** Cholecystokinin, a hormone released by the intestinal mucosa, stimulates the release of bile from the gallbladder and pancreatic enzymes from the pancreas. (2:164)

8. **(D)** The liver is an intraperitoneal structure. The portion of the liver that is not covered by peritoneum is termed the bare area. The bare area is located between the right and left triangular ligaments. (2:144–146)

9. **(E)** The normal thickness of the gallbladder wall is 3 mm. Thicker walls suggest a pathologic condition that may be biliary in nature. (2:175)

10. **(C)** The pancreatic head lies caudad to the portal vein and anterior to the inferior vena cava. (2:208)

11. **(C)** Hydronephrosis is a fluid-filled pelvocaliceal collecting system. Sonographically, hydronephrosis has varied appearances from a mildly distended pelvocaliceal collecting system to moderately distended fluid-filled pelvocaliceal collecting system, and in the most severe form, the kidneys appear cystic with very little renal cortical tissue. (2:284, 285)

12. **(B)** On a sonographic examination dilatation of the interhepatic ducts, common bile duct, and gallbladder (the gallbladder enlarges before the biliary tree because it has the greatest surface area) is imaged, one should expect the obstruction to be at the distal common bile duct. (2:189)

13. **(A)** The most common location of a pancreatic pseudocyst is in the lesser sac, which is located anterior to the pancreas and posterior to the stomach. (2:216)

14. **(B)** The extrahepatic portion of the falciform ligament can be visualized when there is massive ascites. The falciform ligament contains the ligamentum of teres and will appear sonographically as an echogenic linear band attaching the bare area of the liver to the anterior abdominal wall. (2:114)

15. **(C)** Anterior and parallel to the aorta. (7:55)

16. **(A)** The division by using Couinaud's sections into right and left lobes of the liver is by the imaginary plane, the main lobar fissure. (6:94)

17. **(C)** A prominent uncinate process of the pancreas lies posterior to the superior mesenteric artery and vein. (2:208; 7:55)

18. **(E)** The splenic vein courses transversely across the body along the posterior portion of the body and tail of the pancreas. (6:151)

19. **(B)** The gastroesophageal junction can sonographically be visualized anterior to the aorta and posterior to the left lobe of the liver. (2:231)

20. **(D)** Adenomyomatosis is a benign proliferation and thickening of the muscle layer and glandular layer of the gallbladder with formation of intramural diverticula called Rokitansky–Aschoff sinuses (RAS). There are three forms: diffuse, segmental, and localized. It is more common in women, with increasing incidence after the age 40 years. (6:134, 135)

21. **(B)** The most common cause for acute pyelonephritis is *Escherichia coli* a Gram-negative rod-shaped bacterium, which invades the renal tissue. It is more common in women than men. *(10:142)*

22. **(A)** Angiomyolipoma is an uncommon benign renal mass, which is composed of blood vessels, fat, and muscle. They appear on ultrasound as an echogenic well-defined mass located in the renal cortex. When the mass is small, the patient is usually asymptomatic. Symptoms usually do not appear until the mass enlarges and bleeds, which causes severe flank pain and hematuria. *(10:152)*

23. **(C)** The gastroduodenal artery is a branch of the common hepatic artery. It is a landmark for the anterior lateral aspect of the head of the pancreas. *(7:241)*

24. **(E)** The left renal vein courses transversely across the body to enter into the inferior vena cava. It may be identified sonographically as a tubular anechoic structure between the aorta and superior mesenteric artery. *(9:183)*

25. **(A)** Glisson's capsule is a dense fibroelastic membrane that completely surrounds the liver and encloses the portal vein, hepatic artery, and bile ducts within the liver. *(4:117)*

26. **(C)** Left adrenal hyperplasia may cause anterior displacement of the splenic vein and posterior or inferior displacement of the left kidney. *(7:489)*

27. **(A)** The celiac axis has three branches, the common hepatic artery, left gastric artery, and splenic artery. Sonographically, only a short section of the splenic artery can be seen because of its tortuous course. *(6:72, 73)*

28. **(D)** Accessory spleens are the most common congenital anomaly of the spleen. They are difficult to image sonographically, but when imaged, they are most often seen at the hilum of the spleen. *(2:312)*

29. **(D)** A congenital fold between the body and fundus of the gallbladder is called a Phrygian cap. *(6:126)*

30. **(B)** The inferior vein cava forms at the confluence of the right and left common iliac veins, and it empties into the right atrium of the heart. *(6:75)*

31. **(E)** Diffuse thickening of the gallbladder wall is a nonspecific finding frequently seen when there is no primary gallbladder disease. It can be seen with acute and chronic cholecystitis but may also be secondary to right-sided heart failure, hepatitis, and benign ascites. In a patient not being NPO, physiologic contraction of the gallbladder has occurred and is one of the most common causes of diffuse thickening of the gallbladder wall. *(7:217)*

32. **(D)** If on a sonographic examination, one finds dilated intrahepatic ducts and a small gallbladder, the obstruction will usually be at the level of the common hepatic duct above the entry of the cystic duct. Bile will not be able to pass through the level of obstruction to fill the gallbladder. *(7:220)*

33. **(E)** The maximum inner diameter of the main pancreatic duct in a young adult patient measures 2 mm. *(6:152)*

34. **(A)** The endocrine function of the pancreas is to produce insulin, glucagon, and somatostatin. The exocrine function of the pancreas is to produce lipase, amylase, trypsin, and chymotrypsinogen. *(6:149–159)*

35. **(A)** Creatinine and blood urea nitrogen (BUN) are commonly used to measure renal function. Creatinine is normally filtered out of the blood by the kidneys and removed from the body via the urine. *(2:296)*

36. **(C)** Adult polycystic renal disease is an autosomal dominate disease, which usually does not produce symptoms until the third or fourth decade of life. It is also associated with cysts in the liver, pancreas, spleen, and testes. Sonographically, the kidneys are enlarged with multiple cysts of varied size. The kidneys lose their reniform shape as the cysts enlarge. *(2:264)*

37. **(B)** The spleen is the best sonographic window to use to image the left hemidiaphragm. *(6:225)*

38. **(D)** Patients in the sickle cell crisis (early stages of the disease) will have an enlarged spleen. In the later stages, the spleen becomes fibrotic and atrophies. When the spleen is not imaged, it is referred to as autosplenectomy. *(6:233)*

39. **(A)** Urinoma. Bilateral hydronephrosis occurs because of obstruction in the lower urinary system, i.e., enlargement of the prostate from benign or malignant cause, uterine fibroids, late pregnancy, and posterior urethral valve syndrome. Urinoma is a collection of urine usually outside of the kidney due to a tear in the ureter or renal pelvis. *(6:186)*

40. **(D)** Normal. The amount of liver damage in patients with acute hepatitis varies from mild to severe. The liver parenchyma may appear normal in a patient with acute hepatitis. *(2:138, 139)*

41. **(C)** Renal variant. A hypertrophied column of Bertin is a normal variant of the kidney where there is an indentation of cortical tissue into the renal sinus. *(2:257)*

42. **(B)** The ureterovesical junction is the junction between the distal ureter and the base of the bladder. *(6:172)*

43. **(D)** Posterolateral to the thyroid is the common carotid artery, internal jugular vein, and the vagus nerve. *(2:397)*

44. **(E)** Jaundice. Signs of renal failure included: oliguria, palpable flank mass, generalized edema, pain, fever, hypertension, and muscle weakness are some of the clinical signs of acute renal failure. *(7:392, 393)*

45. **(C)** Testicular torsion. A hydrocele is a common cause of scrotal pain. It can be either congenital or caused by trauma, mass, infarction, inflammation, or trauma. *(2:418)*

46. **(B)** Adrenal neuroblastoma is the most common malignancy of the adrenal gland found in children. *(2:343)*

47. **(A)** When a mass is visualized in the area of the head of the pancreas, one should check the liver for metastasis and dilatation of the intrahepatic ducts. The common bile duct and main pancreatic duct may be dilated secondary to obstruction caused by enlargement of the mass. *(3:218, 219)*

48. **(C)** Adenocarcinoma is the most common primary carcinoma of the pancreas. It is most frequently found in the head of the pancreas. The clinical symptoms are weight loss, painless jaundice, nausea, and pain radiating to the back. *(2:218)*

49. **(C)** The ligamentum of venosum separates the anterior portion of the caudate lobe from the left lobe of the liver, and the ligament of teres (round ligament) is a cord-like ligament that is located in the free margin of the falciform ligament. The falciform ligament divides the left lobe of the liver into medial and lateral segments. The main lobar fissure divides the liver into right and left lobes. *(6:95)*

50. **(A)** The most common benign neoplasm of the liver is a hemangioma, which is also called a cavernous hemangioma. It can be either single or multiple and is more commonly found in women and in the right lobe of the liver. *(6:103, 104)*

51. **(D)** Blood from the hepatic veins drain into the inferior vena cava, which delivers deoxygenated blood to the right atrium of the heart. Right-side heart failure will produce venous congestion of the liver, which will lead to marked dilation of the intrahepatic veins. *(7:155)*

52. **(B)** The main lobar fissure separates the right and left lobes of the liver. The ligamentum of venosum separates the anterior portion of the caudate lobe from the left lobe of the liver, and the ligament of teres (round ligament) is a cord-like ligament that is located in the free margin of the falciform ligament. The falciform ligament divides the left lobe of the liver into medial and lateral segment. *(4:121)*

53. **(D)** The spleen is an intraperitoneal structure. Retroperitoneal structures include the kidney, pancreas, great vessels, adrenal glands, psoas muscles, and duodenum. *(7:507)*

54. **(C)** The splenic vein and superior mesenteric vein join together to form the portal vein. The junction of the splenic vein and superior mesenteric vein occurs posterior to the neck of the pancreas. *(6:78)*

55. **(B)** The common bile duct unites with the main pancreatic duct just before entering the second portion of the duodenum. *(2:197)*

56. **(A)** Empyema of the gallbladder is a complication of acute cholecystitis. The patient presents with high spiking fever, chills, and leukocytosis. The walls of the gallbladder are thickened, and the lumen is filled with pus and debris. There may be a "dirty" shadow caused by the gas, which is formed by the bacteria. *(7:216)*

57. **(B)** A cause of an increase in alpha-fetoprotein in a non-pregnant patient is a hepatoma of the liver. *(2:148)*

58. **(C)** If the prostate is found enlarged, one should check the kidneys for hydronephrosis. An enlarged prostate gland is a common cause of bladder neck obstruction in older men. *(7:419)*

59. **(A)** The anterior wall of the body of the pancreas is the posterior wall of the antrum of the stomach. *(2:196)*

60. **(A)** On a transverse scan, the portal vein is seen as a circular structure anterior to the inferior vena cava and superior to the head of the pancreas. *(2:87)*

61. **(B)** The most common cause of hyperthyroidism is Graves' disease that is an autoimmune disease where by the immune system attacks the thyroid and causes diffuse enlargement of the thyroid gland. *(6:277)*

62. **(D)** A prominent uncinate process is anterior to the inferior vena cava and posterior to the superior mesenteric vein. *(2:196)*

63. **(C)** A dissecting aortic aneurysm is when there is a tear through the intima layer and a blood-filled channel forms within the aortic wall. Patients are usually hypertensive males and have a known aneurysm. *(2:91, 92)*

64. **(B)** The adrenal glands can be divided into the cortex and medulla. The cortex has three zones, and each zone secretes a different type of steroid hormone, while the medulla secretes epinephrine and norepinephrine. *(2:336)*

65. **(C)** The ligament of teres is formed embryologically from the portal sinus branch of the umbilical vein. This canal closes after birth. Recanalization of the umbilical vein is associated with end-stage cirrhosis and portal hypertension. *(6:97, 111)*

66. **(D)** The parallel channel sign, irregular borders, and echo enhancement posterior to the dilated ducts are all characteristic of dilated intrahepatic bile ducts. It is common bile duct near the porta hepatis that is the first to dilate and is greatest in size. *(7:227–229)*

67. **(A)** The rectus abdominis muscle arises from the pelvis lines, but it lines the anterior abdominal wall; therefore, it is not located in the retroperitoneal cavity. *(7:19)*

68. **(D)** A Klatskin tumor originates at the junction of the right and left hepatic ducts. Cholangiocarcinoma is a primary adenocarcinoma located in the intrahepatic ducts. A Klatskin tumor, cholangiocarcinoma, and enlarged portal lymph nodes will only cause intrahepatic obstruction. Pancreatic carcinoma will initially obstruct the common bile duct before intrahepatic dilatation occurs. *(2:189)*

69. **(B)** Direct or conjugated bilirubin elevated levels are seen in cases of obstructive jaundice. The laboratory results suggest obstructive jaundice, and one must check for the causes of the obstruction. *(7:199)*

70. **(C)** Prolonged fasting and diabetes, especially in one who is insulin dependent, are causes of enlarged gallbladder. Ascites is a nonbiliary cause of diffuse thickening of the gallbladder wall. Chronic cholecystitis is a cause of a small gallbladder. (7:217, 220)

71. **(D)** The celiac axis originates within the first 2 cm of the abdominal aorta; therefore, it is located superior to the pancreas. All of the vessels listed are used as landmarks for locating and imaging the pancreas. (6:150, 151)

72. **(A)** Retroperitoneal masses tend to cause anterior and cranial displacement of surrounding organs. The direction of the displacement is one way to distinguish between a retroperitoneal versus a peritoneal mass. (2:343)

73. **(D)** Enlarged paraspinal lymph nodes may displace the aorta anteriorly, causing the aorta to appear to be "floating." (2:339)

74. **(D)** Sonographically, enlarged nodes appear as hypoechoic masses with no demonstration of through transmission, because of its composition. (2:340, 341)

75. **(A)** Hepatofugal (portafugal) blood flow is the reversal of blood flow, that is, blood flow away from the liver. This may be caused by portal hypertension or liver disease. (4:10, 11)

76. **(B)** Anatomical landmarks helpful in locating the left adrenal gland are the aorta, spleen, left kidney, and left crus of the diaphragm. (2:331)

77. **(A)** Gallbladder polyps can be distinguished from calculi by the absence of shadowing and mobility. (1:207–208)

78. **(E)** Hydrops is dilatation of the gallbladder, which may be caused by an obstruction in the cystic duct. The gallbladder is palpable, and the patient may be asymptomatic or may present with pain, nausea, and vomiting. The intrahepatic and extrahepatic ducts are not dilated. (5:130)

79. **(C)** The most common cause of jaundice in the pediatric patient is biliary atresia, a narrowing and obstruction of the intrahepatic bile duct. (7:204)

80. **(C)** Examples of primary retroperitoneal tumors imaged sonographically are leiomyosarcomas, neurogenic tumors, fibrosarcomas, rhabdomyosarcomas, and teratomatous tumors. (2:344)

81. **(D)** A series of relative echogenicity has been established. Going from least echogenic to most: renal parenchyma < liver < spleen < pancreas < renal sinus. (6:153; 7:328)

82. **(D)** The pancreas in children will be relatively less echogenic and larger in size relative to the body size. The echogenicity of the pancreas increases with age because there is an increase in body fat deposition, which increases the amount of body fat within the parenchyma of the pancreas. (2:248–249)

83. **(B)** The kidneys are covered by three layers: the true capsule is the most internal layer that covers only the kidney; the perinephric fat is the middle layer, which is between the kidney and adrenal gland; and Gerota's fascia surrounds the kidneys, perinephric fat, and the adrenal glands. (2:292)

84. **(B)** The middle, right, and left hepatic veins originate in the liver and drain directly into the inferior vena cava at the level of the diaphragm. They are the largest major visceral branches of the inferior vena cava. (6:76)

85. **(B)** The spleen is variable in size but it is considered to be convex superiorly and concave inferiorly. (2:258–359)

86. **(C)** Hypernephroma is a malignant solid renal tumor, which is also called renal cell carcinoma or adenocarcinoma of the kidney. Transitional cell carcinoma is the most common tumor to the collecting system. Oncocytoma is a rare benign renal tumor. (1:350–352; 2:322–327)

87. **(C)** The left kidney lies inferior and medial to the spleen. The diaphragm is superolateral, and posterior to the spleen, and the stomach, tail of the pancreas; splenic flexure is medial to the spleen. (1:322–323; 2:92)

88. **(B)** A hematocele is a condition in which blood fills the scrotal sac. Sonographically, an acute hematocele appears with thickened scrotal walls and fluid within the scrotal sac without increased through transmission. It is usually a result of trauma or surgery. (7:752, 753)

89. **(A)** A cavernous hemangioma is the most common benign hepatic neoplasm, and the most common sonographic appearance is an echogenic round or oval with well-defined borders. (2:147)

90. **(C)** The normal thyroid gland measures 1–2 cm in anteroposterior dimension and 4–6 cm in length. (2:396)

91. **(E)** Ascites in most cases is secondary to a primary disease process. Some of the causes of ascites include congestive heart failure, nephritic syndromes, and infections, e.g., tuberculosis, trauma, and malignancy. Adenomyomatosis is a benign gallbladder condition, where there proliferation of the mucosal lining of the gallbladder into the muscle layer. Diverticulum of the muscle layer occurs and bile may collect there and cause ring-down artifacts. (6:134, 135; 7:46)

92. **(B)** Sonographically, the best way to diagnosis a dissecting aneurysm is to document the intimal flap moving with the pulsations of blood through the aorta. (7:70, 71)

93. **(A)** A mass in the head of the pancreas with a dilated common bile duct is suggestive of obstructive jaundice. (2:189)

94. **(B)** A subhepatic abscess would be located inferior to the liver and anterior to the right kidney. This space is also referred to as Morrison's pouch. Other common sites for abscesses are the subphrenic, perinephric, intrarenal, intrahepatic, pelvic, and around lesions at the site of surgery. (6:255)

95. **(D)** The ligamentum venosum is a remnant of the fetal ductus venosus; the ligament of teres and the falciform ligament are remnants of the fetal umbilical vein. The coronary ligaments define the bare area of the liver. (2:114; 5:95)

96. **(A)** The gastroduodenal artery is a major branch of the common hepatic artery. (6:73)

97. **(D)** Patients with Courvoisier gallbladder present with painless jaundice and a palpable right-upper-quadrant mass. The obstruction of the common bile duct is usually caused by enlargement of the head of the pancreas. Patients with acute hepatitis and cirrhosis do have painless jaundice. The jaundice is not caused by obstruction of the biliary system. It is caused by destruction of the liver parenchyma. Porcelain gallbladder is calcification of the gallbladder wall. (6:109–111, 137)

98. **(E)** A dromedary hump is a cortical bulge of the lateral border of the left kidney. A junctional parenchymal defect is a distinct division between the upper and lower pole of the kidney. A column of Bertin is prominent indentations of the renal sinus. All of these variants have a mass effect on ultrasound. A Phrygian cap is a fold between the fundus and body of the gallbladder. (2:256, 257)

99. **(C)** Ascites, small liver, portal hypertension, and nodular liver borders may all be present with end-stage liver disease. The bile ducts will not be dilated because of the fibrotic liver parenchyma. (2:139)

100. **(A)** The head of the pancreas is located anterior to the inferior vena cava. (2:196)

101. **(B)** The lesser sacs are located between the stomach and pancreas. (2:216)

102. **(B)** The renal pyramids are located in the medulla of the kidney. (2:248)

103. **(C)** In chronic renal disease, both kidneys are small and echogenic. (2:268)

104. **(B)** A long history of alcoholism is a major cause of cirrhosis and ascites often is seen secondarily to cirrhosis. (7:149, 152)

105. **(C)** Chronic active hepatitis may progress to cirrhosis. The etiology of chronic active hepatitis is usually idiopathic but may be viral or immunological. (2:148)

106. **(A)** Choledochal cyst is a rare focal cystic dilatation of the common bile duct caused by an anomalous junction of the common bile duct with the main pancreatic duct. The reflux of the pancreatic enzymes causes a weakness of the common bile duct wall and an outpouching of the wall. Choledochal cysts may be associated with gallstones, cirrhosis, and pancreatitis. Clinically, the patient presents with pain, fever, abdominal mass, or jaundice. (2:177)

107. **(E)** Hashimoto's thyroiditis is chronic inflammation of the thyroid. It is a common cause of hypothyroidism in regions where there is a lack of iodine. The entire thyroid gland is involved, and sonographically, the thyroid is enlarged with irregular borders with decreased heterogeneous echoes. People with Graves' disease present with hyperthyroidism, bulging eyes, and skin thickening. The thyroid is enlarged with increased vascularity. Malignant tumors of the thyroid are rare and have varied appearance on ultrasound, from a single small solid nodule to hypoechoic to being isoechoic with the thyroid tissue. In 50% of cases, there will be calcification. (2:402)

108. **(D)** Calcification of part or the entire wall of the gallbladder is called a porcelain gallbladder. It is associated with chronic cholecystitis and gallstones. These patients have a higher risk of carcinoma of the gallbladder. (2:185)

109. **(A)** Patients typically are diagnosed with an aortic aneurysm by a pulsatile mass noted on physical examination. They usually have a history of smoking and vascular disease, such as hypertension. On ultrasound, it is important to measure the diameter of the lumen and the location of the aneurysm in reference to the renal arteries. (2:90, 91)

110. **(B)** The right renal artery courses posterior to the inferior vena cava and may be imaged as a round anechoic structure posterior to the inferior vena cava on a longitudinal scan. (2:84)

111. **(A)** The retroperitoneal space is the area between the posterior portion of the parietal peritoneum and the posterior abdominal wall muscle. (2:238)

112. **(A)** When there is extrinsic pressure and obstruction of the common bile duct (i.e., a mass in the head of the pancreas), the gallbladder and biliary tree will be enlarged. (6:159–162)

113. **(C)** The serum amylase and lipase both elevate upon the onset of pancreatitis, but amylase reaches its maximum value within 24 hours. Lipase remains elevated for a longer period of time. (7:249)

114. **(B)** Hypertrophic pyloric stenosis (HPS) is more commonly seen in males between the ages of 1 week and 6 months. The pylorus is the channel between the stomach and duodenum. When the muscle of the pylorus is thickened, it prevents food from entering the stomach. The child typically presents with projectile vomiting, dehydration, and a palpable olive-size mass in the epigastric region. The diagnosis of HPS is made if the length of the pylorus is greater than 18 mm, the anterior to posterior diameter is greater than 15 mm, or the muscle thickness is greater than 4 mm. (7:587, 588)

115. **(B)** Neuroblastoma is a malignant tumor of the adrenal medulla that is found in children. (7:503)

116. **(B)** Chronic pancreatitis. Enlarged lymph nodes are hypoechoic with no increase in through transmission. Aortic aneurysm, crus of the diaphragm, and bowel may all appear sonographically as hypoechoic. Chronic pancreatitis is imaged as echogenic. *(7:512)*

117. **(D)** Budd–Chiari syndrome is caused by thrombus in the hepatic veins or in the inferior vena cava causing obstruction of blood flow to the heart. The obstruction may be congenital or acquired. Budd–Chiari is associated with renal cell carcinoma, primary carcinoma of the liver, or prolonged usage of oral contraceptives. It is characterized by abdominal pain, massive ascites, and hepatomegaly. Sonographically, the right lobe of the liver may be small with normal or enlarged caudate lobe. There will either be absence of blood flow in the hepatic veins and inferior vena cava or abnormal blood flow pattern on Doppler. *(7:160, 161)*

118. **(E)** In response to the increased pressure in the portal vein, which is associated with portal hypertension, there may be recanalization of the umbilical vein, which is located within the ligamentum of teres. *(2:154, 155)*

119. **(B)** A pelvic kidney is a kidney that has failed to ascend to the renal fossa. It is located in the pelvis but has the same sonographic appearance as a kidney located in the renal fossa. *(6:173)*

120. **(A)** The ureteropelvic junction is where the renal pelvis narrows and joins the proximal portion of the ureter. *(6:172)*

121. **(E)** According to Platt et al. an RI of the renal artery greater than 0.70 is 90% accurate in diagnosing renal obstruction. *(6:211)*

122. **(C)** Cushing's syndrome is an adrenal disease where there is oversecretion of glucocorticoids. *(2:343)*

123. **(D)** Body and tail. Islet cell tumors of the pancreas are well-circumscribed solid masses with low-level echoes and are frequently found in the body and tail of the pancreas and rarely in the head of the pancreas. *(2:219, 223)*

124. **(C)** The celiac artery has three branches: the common hepatic artery, left gastric artery, and the splenic artery. *(6:72)*

125. **(A)** The most common benign mass of the spleen is a cavernous hemangioma. The most common malignant tumor of the spleen is an angiosarcoma. Congenital cysts of the spleen are rare, and lymphomas are not benign masses. *(6:234)*

126. **(B)** The parietal peritoneum lines the abdominal cavity. Organs are intraperitoneal if they are surrounded by peritoneum or retroperitoneal if only their anterior surface is covered. *(7:35–37)*

127. **(C)** A normally functioning transplanted kidney will have the same sonographic appearance as a normal kidney located in the renal fossa. *(7:400)*

128. **(D)** When food containing fat enters the small intestines, cholecystokinin is released into the bloodstream, which activates the contraction of the gallbladder and the relaxing of the sphincter of Oddi. *(7:198)*

129. **(B)** A transplanted kidney is usually placed in the pelvis along the iliopsoas margin and anterior to the psoas muscle. The ureter of the donor kidney is anastomosed to the bladder. The donor renal artery is anastomosed to the external iliac artery, while the renal vein is connected to the internal iliac vein. *(7:399)*

130. **(A)** Klatskin tumors arise at the junction of the right and left hepatic ducts and causes dilation of the intrahepatic ducts with no dilatation of the extrahepatic ducts. *(6:141, 142)*

131. **(D)** Pancreas. The liver, spleen, hepatic veins, and gallbladder are located in the peritoneal cavity. The great vessels, pancreas, adrenal glands, and kidneys are not surrounded by peritoneum; therefore, they are located in the retroperitoneal cavity. *(2:328)*

132. **(C)** The splenic artery originates from the celiac axis and courses along the superior aspect of the pancreas body and tail. *(6:72)*

133. **(C)** Artifacts result from a variety of sources including thickness and side-lobe artifacts, reverberation artifacts, electronic noise, and range in ambiguity effects. Edge effects cause acoustic shadowing owing to reflection and refraction of sound. *(6:12, 13)*

134. **(B)** When ascites is present, it acts as an acoustic window. Therefore, the liver will appear more echogenic. There is always posterior acoustic enhancement when the sound travels through fluid. *(6:11)*

135. **(A)** All ultrasound equipment is calibrated at 1,540 m/s, the speed of sound in soft tissue. When the ultrasound beam goes through a fatty tumor with a lower propagation speed, the tumor will appear *farther* away than its actual distance. *(6:13)*

136. **(D)** A fluid collection located between the diaphragm and the spleen may represent a subphrenic abscess. *(2:348)*

137. **(B)** If a mass is solid, displacement of adjacent organs will aid in helping to evaluate the origin of the mass. In a retroperitoneal sarcoma, the kidney, spleen, and pancreas would be displaced anteriorly. *(2:348, 349)*

138. **(C)** Splenomegaly may be caused by congestion, i.e., portal thrombosis, trauma, infection, Hodgkin's disease, lymphoma, neoplasms, storage diseases, and polycythemia vera. *(2:318, 319)*

139. **(A)** Adenomyomatosis is a benign infiltrative disease that causes a diffuse thickening of the gallbladder wall. It does not cause enlargement of the gallbladder. *(6:134, 135)*

140. **(D)** Posterior to the kidneys are the quadratus lumborum muscles, diaphragm, psoas muscle, and twelfth rib. *(6:248)*

141. **(D)** Patients with chronic cirrhosis will have a small nodular fibrotic liver, which impedes blood flow through the liver causing collateral vessel development and portal hypertension. Ascites, peripheral edema, and splenomegaly are usually secondary to the increase in pressure in the portal vein. Liver failure causes jaundice and an increase in the clotting time. Sonographically, the liver is small and echogenic. (7:151)

142. **(C)** Ureteral jets are not present if there is an obstructive hydronephrosis. A bladder tumor or posterior urethra valves may obstruct urine from exiting the body. In cases of severe obstruction, the increased pressure in the urinary bladder may cause the ureters and renal collecting system to dilate. A parapelvic cyst usually does not cause hydronephrosis. (2:285)

143. **(B)** An extrarenal pelvis extends from the renal pelvis to outside the renal capsule. One way to differentiate an extrarenal pelvis from hydronephrosis is to place the patient prone. The pressure will collapse the extrarenal pelvis. (6:285, 284)

144. **(E)** The long narrow arrow points to the heart. The aorta and the inferior vena cava enter the thoracic cavity to the heart. (2:104)

145. **(E)** The short wide arrow is pointing to the aorta, which enters the thoracic cavity to the heart. The aorta lies posterior to the left lobe of the liver. (2:104)

146. **(A)** The arrow is pointing to a round anechoic structure anterior and slightly to the left of the spine, which is the aorta. (2:108)

147. **(E)** Simple cysts are present in 50% of all adults older than 50 years. They are usually of no clinical significance and may be located anywhere in the kidney. Fig. 4–11 of the left kidney documents a small upper pole cyst with a larger cyst of the lower pole. (2:263)

148. **(A)** The most common causes of a fatty liver are alcohol abuse and obesity. Diabetes, chemotherapy, cystic fibrosis, and tuberculosis are other causes of fatty liver infiltration. The liver varies in appearance depending on the severity of the fatty changes. The liver parenchyma will have an increase in echogenicity with a decrease in acoustic penetration. In cases of severe fatty infiltration, there will be a decrease in the echogenicity of the portal vessel walls caused by the increase in the echogenicity of the liver parenchyma. There may be difficulty in visualization of the diaphragm because of the increase of the liver parenchyma. (7:145)

149. **(B)** Superior mesenteric artery (SMA) arises from the abdominal aorta. It is seen posterior to the pancreas (1:216)

150. **(A)** Acute cholecystitis is usually associated with gallstones. Sometimes there may be cholecystitis without gallstones, which is referred to as acalculous cholecysti-

tis. The sonographic appearance will be the same except for the presence of echogenic foci with posterior shadowing within the gallbladder lumen. (6:213)

151. **(C)** Cystic artery. The sonographic characteristics of acute cholecystitis include an enlarged gallbladder with a transverse diameter >5 cm, gallbladder wall >5 mm, pericholecystic fluid, a positive Murphy's sign, and an enlarged cystic artery. Not all of the sonographic criteria will be present in every case of cholecystitis. (6:213, 216)

152. **(A)** The pleural sac surrounds the lungs. The internal pleura (visceral pleura) line the lungs, while the external pleura (parietal pleura) line the inner surface of the chest wall. A pleural effusion is fluid superior to the diaphragm in the pleural sac. The diaphragm must be identified to differentiate fluid in the pleural space verses fluid in the abdominal cavity (ascites). (2:552)

153. **(C)** The liver is a common site for metastatic involvement. The most common primary sites include the colon, breast, and lungs. Metastatic lesions to the liver have varied sonographic appearances. They may be hypoechoic, echogenic, and well-defined or cause a diffuse echogenic hepatic pattern. (2:152, 153)

154. **(B)** The arrow is pointing to a normal hepatic vein, which drains into the inferior vena cava. (6:76)

155. **(B)** The arrow is pointing to the right renal artery, which lies posterior to the inferior vena cava. (6:74)

156. **(B)** The quadratus lumborum muscle is posterior to the kidney and courses lateral to the psoas muscle. It protects the posterior and lateral abdominal wall. (7:19, 324)

157. **(C)** The falciform ligament extends from the umbilicus to the diaphragm and can only be imaged sonographically when massive ascites is present. (2:114)

158. **(C)** A multicystic (dysplastic) kidney is a common cause of a palpable neonatal mass. It is usually unilateral. Bilateral multicystic pathology is not compatible with life. (2:270)

159. **(D)** The main lobar fissure is a landmark used to document the gallbladder fossa when there is nonvisualization of the gallbladder. It appears sonographically as an echogenic linear structure that extends from the portal vein to the neck of the gallbladder. (2:114)

160. **(A)** The most common primary neoplasm of the pancreas is an adenocarcinoma. (2:218)

161. **(E)** The arrowhead is pointing to an enlarged pancreatic duct. The normal measurement of the pancreatic duct is <2 mm. (7:244)

162. **(A)** Sonographically, acute pancreatitis may appear normal or diffusely enlarged with a decrease in echogenicity. The pancreatic duct may be enlarged. Hemorrhagic pancreatitis appearance depends upon the age of the

hemorrhage. Usually there will be a well-defined mass in the head of the pancreas. Phlegmonous pancreatitis typically has an ill-defined hypoechoic mass on ultrasound. Chronic pancreatitis on a sonogram is usually atrophied and is very echogenic. There may be dilatation of the main pancreatic duct secondary to a stone in the duct.

163. **(C)** Aortic aneurysm with a small thrombus in the proximal aorta and partial occlusion documented by color Doppler on both a transverse and a longitudinal view. *(7:66)*

164. **(B)** The superior mesenteric artery is a ventral branch of the aorta. It courses parallel and anterior to the abdominal aorta. *(9:44)*

165. **(A)** The sonographic appearance of acute pancreatitis varies depending on the severity of the inflammation. The echogenicity is hypoechoic and usually less than the liver. The pancreas may be enlarged with a dilated pancreatic duct. *(10:88–89)*

166. **(A)** The arrow is pointing to a medullary pyramid. *(2:255)*

167. **(C)** Gallstones (calculi) sonographically appear as mobile echogenic foci with posterior shadowing. *(10:59)*

168. **(D)** Acoustic shadowing. *(10:59)*

169. **(E)** The common bile duct is a sonolucent tubular structure that is imaged anterior to the portal vein. *(10:53)*

170. **(C)** The upper limits of the normal common bile duct (CBD) is 8 mm. The CBD diameter increases in size after the age of 50 years by approximately 1 mm/decade. *(10:53)*

171. **(B)** Pneumobilia is air in the biliary tract. Air in the biliary tract may be caused from chronic cholecystitis, biliary-enteric fistula, or a surgical complication. Sonographically, pneumobilia appears as echogenic foci usually found in the region of the porta hepatis. There may be motion and weak posterior acoustic shadowing of the foci. *(10:80)*

172. **(E)** Liver metastatic disease has various sonographic appearances. It may present as multiple echogenic masses of varying sizes. Malignant masses tend to have irregular borders and invade the surrounding tissue. Metastasis of the liver may present as a well-defined mass, hypoechoic mass, or a cystic lesion. Primary sites include the colon and breast. *(10:34)*

173. **(D)** The spleen appears normal. *(9:139)*

174. **(C)** The common bile duct is formed from the confluence of the common hepatic duct and the cystic duct. *(9:92)*

175. **(B)** Atherosclerosis is the most common cause of an aneurysm. *(2:90)*

176. **(C)** The arrow is pointing to the common bile duct, which is located anterior to the portal vein. The main portal vein, common bile duct, and hepatic artery form the porta hepatis. *(9:82)*

177. **(D)** A duplex collecting system is a common renal variant. The echogenic renal sinus is separated by renal parenchyma. A duplex collecting system can mimic a mass occupying part of the renal sinus. *(2:257)*

178. **(A)** An echogenic foci with posterior acoustic shadowing is the sonographic appearance of a calculi. A calculi in the common bile duct may cause dilatation of the duct. *(2:86)*

179. **(C)** Gallstones. Hydronephrosis may be unilateral or bilateral. An enlarged prostate, posterior urethra valve, pelvic mass, or a mass in the urinary bladder may cause bilateral renal obstruction. A stone in the ureter may cause unilateral hydronephrosis. Gallstones do not cause compression on the urinary system and have no effect on the urinary system. *(7:368, 369)*

180. **(B)** Sitting upright. The correct positioning for the patient undergoing needle thoracentesis is significant for successful procedure. *(12:118)*

181. **(A)** Graves' disease is an autoimmune disease that affects the thyroid gland, eyes, and the skin. The name derives from Robert Graves, MD, and Irish physician who was the first to describe this type of hyperthyroidism. The biochemical abnormality is decreased thyroid-stimulating hormone and increased T3 and T4. *(2:520; 7:665, 666)*

182. **(B)** Multiple hypoechoic micronodules. Hashimoto's thyroiditis is a chronic lymphocytic thyroiditis. The disease is autoimmune and most frequently caused by hypothyroidism. The typical sonographic appearance is enlargement of the thyroid glands with multiple hypoechoic micronodules. *(1:762)*

183. **(D)** CEA stands for carcinoembryonic antigen, a type of protein molecule found in tumor cells and the developing fetus. Both benign and malignant conditions can increase CEA. Types of cancer that can cause an increase in CEA are pancreas, liver, stomach, breast, and lungs. An increase in CEA-125 is associated with ovarian cancer. Increased levels are also seen in non-cancer conditions, such as inflammation, peptic ulcers, and ulcerative colitis. Smokers can have higher CEA values than nonsmokers. A consistent increase in CEA after surgical removal of a cancerous tumor is suggestive of relapse. *(13:490)*

184. **(D)** Fine needle biopsies are typically performed with local anesthesia. *(1:2072; 2:436–442)*

185. **(D)** Pneumobilia (air within the biliary tree) is commonly seen after previous biliary intervention: common bile duct stents, choledochoduodenal fistula, emphysematous cholecystitis, and gallstone ileus with endoscopic retrograde cholangiopancreatography (ERCP) are the most common. *(1:180; 4:30, 31)*

186. **(E)** The right artery arises from the anterolateral aorta and courses posterior to the inferior vena cava (IVC) to the right renal hilum. The pancreas, duodenum, hepatic veins, caudate lobe, and main lobar fissure are located anterior to the IVC. (2:111; 4:193)

187. **(B)** Hashimoto's disease is an autoimmune disease that affects the thyroid. It is also known as Hashimoto thyroiditis and is the most common cause for hypothyroidism. (2:522; 4:297)

188. **(D)** The most common cause for acute pancreatitis in the United States are gallstones (cholelithiasis) and alcohol abuse; other less common causes include abdominal trauma, peptic ulcer, pancreatic carcinoma, and use of certain medications. (2:255; 4:90)

189. **(D)** Pelvic Kidnet. Kidneys normally migrate to the renal fossa during the embryonic period. Any kidney not located in the renal fossa is an ectopic kidney. A pelvic kidney may mimic an adnexal mass and is associated with other abnormalities, vesicoureteral reflux, and genital. (2:258)

190. **(C)** Pancreatic pseudocysts are fluid-filled structures that may be a complication of acute pancreatitis. They are usually filled with pancreatic enzymes, but they may also consist of blood or pus. Pseudocysts have various sonographic appearances. They may appear cystic with or without debris, or they may appear solid. They are most often found in the region around the pancreas, lesser sac, or by the tail. (7:251)

191. **(B)** The retroperitoneum has three potential spaces where fluid collections and space-occupying lesions (abscesses and hematomas) can be found: the anterior pararenal space, the posterior pararenal space, and the perirenal space. The perirenal space is located within Gerota's fascia. The kidneys, adrenal glands, lymph nodes, blood vessels, and perirenal fat are located within Gerota's fascia. (2:40)

192. **(E)** In most cases with acute cholecystitis, there will also be gallstones. Symmetrical gallbladder wall thickening >3 mm is a nonspecific sign of acute cholecystitis. Gallbladder wall thickening is also seen in patients with ascites, hepatitis, hypoproteinemia, hypoalbuminemia, heart failure, renal disease, and systemic venous hypertension, as well as in patients who have eaten prior to imaging. (2:175)

193. **(A)** Ring-down artifact is also called comet-tail artifact. A ring-down artifact is a series of reverberations that appear as linear lines posterior to a strong interface. In Fig. 4–39, the gas in the bowel caused the reverberations. (7:226)

194. **(C)** Renal cysts are commonly seen in more than 50% of people older than 50 years. Cysts are anechoic, round, or oval in shape with increased through transmission. They can be either singular or multiple and located anywhere in the kidney. (2:263)

195. **(D)** Renal cysts usually affect renal function, and patients are typically asymptomatic unless the cyst is very large or compresses the collecting system causing hydronephrosis. (2:263)

196. **(B)** Lymph nodes are only visualized on a sonographic examination if they are enlarged >1 cm. Common sites to image for enlarged lymph nodes include around the great vessels (para-aortic and paracaval), peripancreatic, renal hilum, and mesenteric region. Sonographically, lymph nodes are seen round, echo poor, homogeneous masses with no increase in the posterior through transmission. (2:332, 338, 339)

197. **(C)** A rise in lipase level indicates acute pancreatitis or pancreatic carcinoma. Amylase levels will also rise with acute pancreatitis but do not stay as elevated as or as specific as lipase levels. (2:204, 205)

198. **(E)** Fatty infiltration of the liver usually causes a diffuse hyperechoic pattern, not a focal pattern. (7:145)

199. **(A)** Courvoisier's law states that obstruction of the common bile duct due to pressure from outside the biliary system will lead to an enlarged gallbladder with dilatation of the biliary radicles. (2:218)

200. **(D)** Chronic pancreatitis occurs after repeated bouts of acute pancreatitis, which is usually caused by biliary disease or alcoholism. The pancreatic tissue becomes fibrotic from chronic inflammation. The fibrotic and fatty changes cause the pancreas to appear more echogenic on a sonogram than normal. The borders may be irregular and dilatation of the pancreatic duct may be secondary to stone formation, causing dilatation of the pancreatic duct. As people get older, the pancreas becomes more echogenic; it is a normal part of the aging process. (2:214)

201. **(B)** Renal cell carcinoma is the most common renal tumor. It is more common in males, and there is an increased incidence of renal cell carcinoma in patients who are on long-term renal dialysis or have von Hippel–Lindau disease. The sonographic appearance varies depending on the stage of the mass. In stage one, the mass has not metastasized outside the true capsule of the kidney. Angiolipoma, adenoma, and oncocytoma are benign tumors of the kidney. (2:266, 272)

202. **(A)** Acute tubular necrosis is the most common medical cause of renal disease. Renal infarction is occlusion of a vessel caused by thrombus; it usually occurs in the periphery of the kidney. Patients with diabetes may have small echogenic kidneys, which is the sonographic appearance of chronic renal disease. Nephrocalcinosis disease sonographically appears as echogenic renal pyramids with or without shadowing. (2:289)

203. **(A)** Adult polycystic kidney disease is an inherited autosomal-dominant disease that most often manifests in the fourth decade. It manifests by cystic dilatation of the proximal convoluted tubules, Bowman's capsule, and the collecting tubules. It is mostly a bilateral process, with associated cysts in the liver, pancreas, lungs, spleen, thyroid, bladder, ovaries, and testes. The kidneys are enlarged with cysts in the renal cortex and the kidney may lose its reniform shape. (7:349, 350)

204. **(E)** A bladder diverticula is an outpouching of the bladder mucosa through the muscular layer. A diverticula may be congenital or acquired. An increase in the pressure within the bladder may be caused by a bladder outlet obstruction or a neurogenic bladder, which may lead to a weakening of the bladder wall leading to an outpouching of the wall. A small connection between the bladder and diverticula may be seen on ultrasound, even after the patient has emptied his or her bladder. A ureterocele is a saccular outpouching of the distal ureter into the urinary bladder. (2:352)

205. **(D)** A calculi in the proximal ureter. (2:301)

206. **(B)** A fusiform aneurysm is a uniform dilatation of a vessel. The majority of aneurysms occur below the level of the renal arteries. (7:65, 66)

207. **(C)** Sonographic Murphy's sign is pain over the gallbladder region upon palpation on physical examination. Kehr's sign is pain in the left upper quadrant radiating to the left shoulder. It is associated with a ruptured spleen. (6:127)

208. **(E)** This is an example of biliary duct obstruction of both the intrahepatic and extrahepatic ducts. A mass at the head of the pancreas may cause dilatation of both the intrahepatic and extrahepatic ducts in addition to an enlarged fluid filled gallbladder (Courvoisier's law). (10:94)

209. **(B)** Periaortic nodes will displace the superior mesenteric artery anteriorly, *not* posteriorly. (2:338, 339)

210. **(A)** Diabetes. Portal vein thrombus many be associated with various pathologies and conditions: hepatitis, chronic pancreatitis, trauma, malignancy, septicemia, pregnancy, portal caval shunts, and splenectomy. The development of collaterals is called cavernous transformation of the portal vein. (1:105)

211. **(E)** The image is of normal blood flow in the hepatic and portal veins. The color-flow map on the left of the image is used to decipher the direction of blood flow. According to the color-flow map, red is blood flow toward the transducer, and blue is blood flow away from the transducer. (1:28)

212. **(D)** The image is of calculi in the common bile duct causing dilatation of the duct. (1:186)

213. **(B)** The dilated common bile duct is located anterior to the portal vein. (1:186)

214. **(C)** Choledocholithiasis. Stones are usually produced in the gallbladder and the gallbladder should be evaluated for stones. Any obstruction of the common bile duct causes obstruction and dilatation of the duct. (2:181)

215. **(E)** An adenoma is a benign thyroid mass that compresses the surrounding tissue. Sonographically, it has varied appearances, from anechoic to echogenic. Commonly, a halo can be seen surrounding the adenoma.

When there is hyperfunction, an increase of blood flow may be demonstrated around the mass. Graves' disease is associated with hyperthyroidism with a diffuse homogeneous appearance on ultrasound. Papillary carcinoma has a hypoechoic appearance with microcalcification on ultrasound. (2:303)

216. **(B)** Afebrile. When inflammation of the gallbladder occurs without gallstones, it is referred to as acalculous cholecystitis. The clinical symptoms include right-upper-quadrant pain, Murphy's sign, fever, nausea, and vomiting. Laboratory findings include leukocytosis and elevation of serum total bilirubin (7:212, 213)

217. **(B)** The arrows point to hypoechoic lesions within the left lobe. Focal nodular hyperplasia can be either hypoechoic or hyperechoic focal masses. (7:168)

218. **(C)** Hypoechoic lesions may be the result of infectious foci. It is very unusual to have metastases with hypoechoic echogenicity. Occasionally, lymphomas may appear as hypoechoic liver metastases. Hemangiomas are echogenic. (7:168)

219. **(B)** The arrow is pointing to the ligamentum of Teres. The ligamentum of Teres is best visualized on a transverse scan of the liver. It divides the left lobe into medial and lateral segments. (2:111)

220. **(A)** Alpha-fetoprotein level is elevated in cases of hepatocellular carcinoma and in pregnant women. In cases of biliary obstruction, the patient may be jaundiced, have elevated direct bilirubin, alkaline phosphatase, and pruritus. (2:139, 148)

221. **(D)** This sonogram demonstrate multiple cystic masses of various size within the liver parenchyma, hepatic cyst or hepatic hydadid cyst could give such appearance (1:92–94)

222. **(E)** Choledocholithiasis appears as echogenic foci in the common bile duct with dilatation of the duct. Cholecystitis, right-sided heart failure, and hypoproteinemia are some causes of a thickened gallbladder wall. (3:38)

223. **(C)** Metastases are neoplastic involvement in the liver, causing liver enlargement with multiple nodules of varying sonographic patterns. Metastases have been described as hypoechoic, echogenic, bull's eye, anechoic, and diffusely inhomogeneous. The patient typically presents with weight loss, decreased appetite, abnormal liver function test results, and hepatomegaly. (2:152, 153)

224. **(B)** Increased levels of creatinine and blood urea nitrogen are seen in renal failure. (2:251)

225. **(E)** The head of the pancreas is to the right of the portal splenic confluence, anterior to the inferior vena cava, and medial to the c-loop of the duodenum. (2:196)

226. **(C)** Crohn's disease is chronic inflammation of the bowel. It usually affects the ileum but may affect both the small and the large intestines. It is most often seen in young adults. (7:296)

227. **(B)** An early sign of obstructive hydronephrosis is the intrarenal vessels having an RI >0.70. The RI returns to normal after 72 hours. *(2:285)*

228. **(A)** A parapelvic cyst is located in the renal hilum. A hematoma, lymphoma, abscess, and urinoma are perirenal fluid collections that can readily be identified on ultrasound. *(2:269, 292)*

229. **(A)** Increased blood flow within the dilated vessels can be seen with a Valsalva maneuver. Varicoceles are more common on the left side. *(4:750)*

230. **(D)** Mass in the head of the pancreas. *(10:94)*

231. **(E)** Enlarged prostate may be seen during a transabdominal pelvic examination indenting the base of the urinary bladder. An evaluation of the prostate gland can also be performed by transrectal sonography. *(1:424)*

232. **(A)** Ascites is free-fluid and appears anechoic on sonograms. *(2:38, 352)*

233. **(C)** In cases of moderate to severe fatty infiltration, the echogenicity of the liver will be increased. The diaphragm and intrahepatic vessel borders may be difficult to see because of the increased attenuation of the liver parenchyma. *(2:134, 135)*

234. **(D)** This is an echogenic focus within the liver most consistent with a hemangioma. Hemangiomas are the most common benign neoplasms of the liver. *(6:103)*

235. **(D)** The spleen is a common site of blunt abdominal trauma. The hematoma will be contained in the spleen if there is no rupture of the splenic capsule. A decrease in hematocrit is an indication that there is blood loss from the cardiovascular system. *(2:321)*

236. **(E)** A hemangioma has the same sonographic appearance as a live cell adenoma, focal nodular hyperplasia, hepatocellular carcinoma, and metastases to the liver. All of these are benign neoplasms that may appear echogenic on ultrasound. Other diagnostic tests can be used to make a definitive diagnosis. *(2:148)*

237. **(D)** Chronic renal disease is imaged as small echogenic kidneys. It may be unilateral or bilateral. Chronic renal disease has many causes such as parenchymal disease, hypertension, and renal artery stenosis. *(2:289)*

238. **(B)** This sonogram is a classic image of adenomyomatosis of the gallbladder. Sonographically, one should look for diffuse segmental thickening of the gallbladder wall with intramural diverticula protruding into the lumen. *(7:224)*

239. **(B)** In hemolytic disease associated with abrupt breakdown of large amounts of red blood cells, the reticuloendothelial cells receive more bilirubin than they can detoxify. Therefore, one would present with an elevated indirect or unconjugated bilirubin. *(2:154–155)*

240. **(B)** Bowman's capsule and the glomerulus together are termed the renal corpuscle. Extending from Bowman's capsule is a renal tubule. Each tubule has three sections: a proximal tubule, a distal convoluted tubule, and a loop of Henle. Together the Bowman's capsule, glomerulus, and renal tubules constitute a nephron. *(7:333–335)*

241. **(B)** The great vessel being imaged is the inferior vena cava. No vessel is imaged sonographically posterior to the aorta. *(9:171)*

242. **(D)** The right renal artery is the only vessel located posterior to the inferior vena cava. *(9:169)*

243. **(B)** Urinary bladder calculi. *(2:352–354)*

244. **(C)** A focal thickening of the bladder wall may be due to cystitis. There are many causes of inflammation of the bladder wall including catheterization, bladder stone, bladder mass, renal disease, poor hygiene, and any disease state that causes stasis of urine in the bladder. *(7:432)*

245. **(D)** The subhepatic space is located between the right lobe of the liver and the right kidney. *(7:39)*

246. **(A)** The arrow is pointing to the heart.

247. **(E)** The liver in the sonographic image is normal. The normal liver is homogeneous with midlevel echogenicity. *(9:85)*

248. **(D)** Riedel's lobe is a normal variant of the right lobe of the liver. There is a tongue-like inferior projection of the right lobe. It extends below the lower pole of the right kidney during normal respiration. *(9:86)*

249. **(A)** A patient with an acute appendicitis presents with right-lower-quadrant pain and rebound tenderness over McBurney's point, elevated white blood cell count, fever, nausea, and vomiting. Sonographically, the appendix wall will be thickened more than 2 mm, and the outer diameter will be >6 mm. The appendix will be noncompressible. *(2:237–240)*

250. **(D)** This sonogram documents an enlarged (hydropic) gallbladder. *(10:69)*

251. **(A)** Hydrops of the gallbladder may be related to obstruction at the level of the cystic or distal common bile duct. *(10:69)*

252. **(A)** Sludge in the gallbladder does not cause hydrops of the gallbladder. Same causes of hydrops include mucocutaneous lymph node syndrome (Kawasaki's disease), prolonged biliary status, hyperalimentation, and hepatitis. *(10:69)*

253. **(D)** Gallbladder carcinoma is rare. Patients who have had a history of gallbladder disease are at an increased risk of getting primary gallbladder carcinoma. Patients do not always have symptoms, and if they do, they are the same as those of other gallbladder diseases. Primary carcinoma of the gallbladder usually does not get diagnosed in the early stages; therefore, there is a high mortality rate. Gallbladder carcinomas have a number of different appearances on sonogram and are nonspecific. Gallstones with an interluminal mass are highly suggestive of gallbladder carcinoma. The sonographic appearance for

adenomyosis, acute or chronic cholecystitis, blood clot, cholesterolosis, and papillary adenoma may have the same sonographic appearance as gallbladder carcinoma. (10:71, 72)

254. **(A)** Foley catheter. The Foley catheter balloon has an anechoic appearance with an echogenic ring. Ureterocele is a submucosal cystic dilatation of the terminal segment of the ureter.(7:423)

255. **(B)** Subcapsular collections are located inferior to the diaphragm, and they conform to the shape of the organ. (2:34)

256. **(B)** Hematomas may be a complication from surgery. Most hematomas will resolve, but some will become infected and progress into an abscess. Patients may present with a decreased hematocrit and fever. One way to distinguish between a space-occupying lesion (hematoma, abscess) and ascites is to place the patient into a different position. A space-occupying lesion will not change its appearance, whereas free fluid will shift to the most dependent portion of the body. (2:445)

257. **(E)** The pancreas is echogenic with calcifications. (10:90)

258. **(A)** Patients with chronic pancreatitis may present with chronic epigastric pain or with right-upper-quadrant pain, which radiates to the back. The pain may be preceded by a large meal or alcohol consumption. Serum lipase, serum amylase, and bilirubin will be normal unless there is also acute inflammation of the pancreatic tissue. The sonographic appearance varies from a normal appearance to a heterogeneous echogenic pattern with areas of calcification. The main pancreatic duct may be dilated, and in some cases, there will be dilatation of the extrahepatic biliary ducts. (10:90, 91)

259. **(B)** Normal left adrenal gland. (2:337)

260. **(C)** Aorta. This sonogram demonstrates a normal left adrenal gland. The sonographic landmarks for imaging the left adrenal gland are the aorta and left kidney. (2:337)

261. **(E)** All of the above are conditions that may affect the adrenal gland. The primary malignancy that metastasize to the adrenal gland can be from the lungs, breast, liver, bones, lymphoma, melanoma, and the gastrointestinal tract. A decrease in oxygen during delivery may cause hemorrhage to the adrenal glands during the neonatal period. (7:489–491)

262. **(B)** A cystic mass appears to displace the bowel. (2:357)

263. **(A)** The image is most consistent with a mesenteric cyst. The mesenteric cyst displaces the bowel and mesentery posteriorly. An ovarian cyst and free fluid do not displace bowel posteriorly. (2:357)

264. **(C)** The longitudinal and transverse scan demonstrates marked thickening and lengthening of the antral muscle (pyloric canal and muscle). (2:462)

265. **(B)** This is consistent with hypertrophic pyloric stenosis. The criteria for this diagnosis include wall thickness >3.5 mm and pyloric length >16 mm. (2:463)

266. **(E)** The image is consistent with a normal pancreas. The main pancreatic duct may be visualized in a normal pancreas. The normal pancreatic duct measures <2 mm. (2:197)

267. **(B)** The main portal vein is formed posterior to the neck of the pancreas. (2:201)

268. **(D)** The most common functioning islet cell tumor is an insulinoma. Islet cell tumors can either be functional or nonfunctional, benign or malignant. (2:219)

269. **(A)** Distal acoustical shadow from the ribs. (7:144)

270. **(A)** The main lobar fissure is seen on a longitudinal scan as a linear echo coursing from the right portal vein to the neck of the gallbladder. It is also used as a landmark dividing the liver into right and left lobes. (4:121)

271. **(D)** In obstructive jaundice, alkaline phosphatase, and direct bilirubin will be very high, with aspartate aminotransferase (AST) also being increased. Patients with hepatitis will also have an increase in alanine aminotransferase (ALT). Alpha-fetoprotein is elevated in nonpregnant adults when there is carcinoma of the liver. Pigment gallstones are common in sickle cell disease. (4:9)

272. **(C)** The sonogram demonstrates dilated biliary radicles. Color Doppler may be used especially in the left lobe of the liver to distinguish the difference between dilated biliary radicles and portal veins. (7:29)

273. **(B)** This sonogram shows dilated hepatic veins and a dilated inferior vena cava. Congestive heart failure and hypertension are two of the most common causes of general dilatation of the inferior vena cava. (6:85)

274. **(B)** The ligament venosum is imaged on the sonogram. The fissure for the ligament venosum also contains the hepatogastric ligament, which is used as a landmark. It separates the caudate lobe from the left lobe of the liver. (6:95)

275. **(A)** This sonogram demonstrates a large amount of loculated fluid above the left hemidiaphragm. Pleural fluid is excess fluid that accumulates between the two pleural layers (visceral and parietal). (2:348)

276. **(D)** The sonogram demonstrates that the fluid density contains multiple septi causing loculations of the fluid, consistent with empyema. Empyema is a fluid collection filled with pus. (1:608)

277. **(D)** The clinical signs of acute cholecystitis are leukocytosis, fever, nausea, vomiting, and right-upper-quadrant pain that may be referred to the right shoulder if the inflammation irritates the diaphragm. Sonographically, the gallbladder is enlarged with a thickened wall >5 cm. There may be pericholecystic fluid, which is secondary to the inflammation. (7:212)

278. **(A)** In chronic cholecystitis, the gallbladder is usually contracted with thickened walls and cholelithiasis. The wall-echo-shadow (WES) sign, anterior wall of the gallbladder, echogenic foci, and shadowing caused by the stone are consistent findings in patients with chronic cholecystitis. In cases of acute cholecystitis, the gallbladder is usually enlarged with thickened walls and cholelithiasis. *(7:217, 220)*

279. **(A)** The liver is enlarged and heterogeneous consistent with metastatic disease. Metastatic patterns within the liver have various sonographic appearances anechoic, hypoechoic, echogenic, complex, or a bull's-eye appearance. *(77:176)*

280. **(E)** Hemangioma is a common benign neoplasm of the liver. They are usually incidental findings on a sonogram. Sonographically, they are usually echogenic and may be either singular or multiple in the liver. Clinically, the patients do not have any symptoms unless the hemangioma becomes very large and hemorrhages. *(7:168)*

281. **(B)** The hemangioma is located between the right and middle hepatic veins; therefore, it is in the anterior segment of the right lobe. The right hepatic vein separates the right lobe into anterior and posterior segments; the middle hepatic vein divides the liver into right and left lobes. *(7:121, 125)*

282. **(A)** A Phrygian cap is a normal variant of the gallbladder. It consists of a fold in the fundal end of the gallbladder. There are no associated problems with a Phrygian cap. *(2:126)*

283. **(D)** The patient is in a left lateral decubitus position (right side up) with the transducer placed along the longitudinal axis of the abdomen. The liver is used as a window to visualize the inferior vena cava anterior to the aorta. Sometimes the renal arteries may be visualized arising from the aorta. This view is used to rule out lymphadenopathy surrounding the great vessels. *(2:339)*

284. **(A)** The portal vein is the largest at the region of the porta hepatis, and the main portal vein branches into the right and left portal veins. The left portal vein follows a superior anterior course and supplies blood to the left lobe. The right portal vein is larger and follows a caudal posterior course supplying blood to the right lobe of the liver. The walls of the portal veins appear more echogenic than the walls of the hepatic veins. The hepatic veins course dorsomedial toward the inferior vena cava. The most accurate method to differentiate the portal veins from the hepatic veins is to follow the course of the vessels into the liver. *(2:117)*

285. **(B)** Lymphadenopathy. Horseshoe kidneys occur during fetal development with fusion usually of the lower poles of the kidneys. The fused poles and the isthmus drape over the spine and may be confused with lymphadenopathy. *(7:348)*

286. **(D)** Cirrhosis is a chronic progressive disease leading to liver cell failure, portal hypertension, hepatoma, and ascites. The thickened gallbladder wall is most likely related to hypoproteinemia and to the adjacent ascites that will make the gallbladder appear thickened. *(7:152)*

287. **(D)** The crura of the diaphragm are extensions (tendinous fibers) of the diaphragm that attach to the vertebral process of L3 on the right and L1 on the left. The right crus appears as a hypoechoic linear structure and can be visualized as it courses from posterior to the inferior vena cave to anterior to the aorta. *(2:331)*

288. **(A)** The left crus of the diaphragm is medial to the left adrenal gland. *(2:331)*

289. **(D)** The right crus of the diaphragm. The right crus is posteromedial to the inferior vena cava and anteromedial to the right adrenal gland. *(2:332)*

290. **(B)** The right renal artery courses posterior to the inferior cava and anterior to the right crus of the diaphragm. *(2:332)*

291. **(D)** Portal vein. *(7:132)*

292. **(E)** Common duct is located anterior and parallel to the portal vein. *(10:42)*

293. **(C)** The echogenic foci posterior to the diaphragm (arrow) is a mirror-image artifact. A mirror-image artifact is a duplication artifact secondary to the sound beam reflecting off a strong reflector in its path, i.e., the diaphragm. This strong reflector acts as a mirror, and the image will present as two reflected objects rather than one. The image farther from the transducer will be the artifact. *(6:13, 49)*

294. **(B)** The sonogram demonstrates periportal lymphadenopathy, which is characterized by enlarged lymph nodes that are secondarily involved in almost all infections and neoplastic disorders. Lymph nodes consist of lymphocytes and reticulum cells, their functions being filtration and production of lymphocytes. All lymph passes through these nodes that act as filters, not only for bacteria but also for cancer cells. Sonographically, we can evaluate lymph nodes in the pelvis, retroperitoneum, portal hepatis, and perirenal and prevertebral vasculature. The sonographic appearance of lymphomatous nodes varies from hypoechoic to anechoic with very good sound transmission. *(7:508)*

295. **(C)** There is no definite correlation between kidney size and echogenicity and the degree of renal function. As a general rule, if the renal parenchyma (cortex) is more echogenic than a normal liver, chronic renal insufficiency should be considered. *(7:388)*

296. **(A)** The sonogram demonstrates celiac nodes surrounding the celiac artery and its winglike configuration. Note the increased distance between the celiac artery and the aorta caused by these masses. *(7:508, 512)*

297. **(A)** This sonogram depicts a fusiform aneurysm. The fusiform aneurysm typically dilates and tapers at the ends. A saccular aneurysm is a discrete round structure, and the ectatic aneurysm is a dilatation longitudinally producing lengthening of the expanded vessel in a uniform diameter. The aorta is considered aneurismal if it exceeds 3 cm. Surgery is not required until the aorta becomes greater than 6 cm because the chance of rupturing is low. *(6:80)*

298. **(D)** The left renal vein courses between the aorta and the superior mesenteric artery. *(6:77)*

299. **(C)** The caudate lobe is anterior to the inferior vena cava and posterior to the caudate lobe. *(6:95)*

300. **(A)** The celiac artery is the first branch of the abdominal aorta. It arises off the anterior aspect of the aorta at the level thoracic vertebra. *(6:72)*

301. **(B)** The superior mesenteric artery is the second branch of the abdominal aorta. *(6:74)*

302. **(A)** The splenic vein is posterior to the body of the pancreas. *(6:78)*

303. **(A)** Stomach. The stomach is located anterior to the pancreas. *(2:251)*

304. **(E)** Normal tail, which lies anterior to the splenic vein. *(2:248, 249)*

305. **(B)** Common bile duct, which defines the posterolateral margin of the pancreas. *(6:150)*

306. **(E)** The gastroduodenal artery defines the anterolateral margin of the pancreas. *(6:150)*

307. **(D)** The renal medulla pyramids are hypoechoic. They are located between the echogenic renal sinus and the less echogenic renal cortex. *(1:255)*

308. **(D)** This sonogram demonstrate color Doppler flow with urine entering the urinary bladder, which is known as ureteric jet effect. *(2:334–335)*

309. **(A)** Color Doppler can be used to document ureteral jets. Obstruction of the ureter causes absence or decreased flow in the ureteral jet on the same side as the pathology. *(2:336)*

310. **(B)** The only time that ureteral jet is not present is when there is obstructive hydronephrosis or when the bladder is full. *(2:285)*

311. **(C)** The clinical symptoms of a patient with a liver abscess include pain, fever, right-upper-quadrant pain, and leukocytosis. Abscesses may appear sonographically as round, hypoechoic, with increased posterior acoustic enhancement, or they may be complex and irregular in shape. In pyogenic abscess, there may be gas present; and gas appears as hyperechoic with a dirty shadow. *(2:144, 145)*

312. **(E)** Polycystic renal disease is associated in 60% of patients with polycystic liver disease. *(2:144)*

313. **(D)** The blood flow in the superior mesenteric artery in a fasting patient has a high-resistive index. Post-prandially, the blood flow changes to a low resistive index with an increase in the diastolic flow. *(2:100)*

314. **(B)** The perinephric space is surrounded by Gerota's fascia. *(2:329)*

315. **(E)** The arrow is pointing to a normal ureteral jet. One reason for not documenting ureteral jets is obstructive hydronephrosis. *(2:285)*

316. **(B)** The head of the pancreas lies anterior to the inferior vena cava. *(6:150)*

317. **(A)** Chronic pancreatitis is associated with a normal or small pancreas, irregular borders, and increased echogenicity caused by fibrotic changes, and calcification. There may be ductal dilatation with or without a stone in the duct. The laboratory values for chronic pancreatitis are usually normal. *(2:259)*

318. **(C)** A pancreatic pseudocyst is a fluid collection that arises as a complication of acute pancreatitis. The obstructed pancreatic duct increases in size until it ruptures, which causes the pancreatic enzymes to escape outside of the pancreas. The fluid localizes and becomes walled-off forming a pseudocyst. The most common location is in the lesser sac, but a pseudocyst may also be found in the pararenal space or extending into the pelvis or superiorly into the mediastinum. *(2:216)*

319. **(E)** The most common complication of a pancreatic pseudocyst is spontaneous rupture, which occurs in 5% of the patients. The fluid will drain one-half of the time into the peritoneal cavity and one-half of the time into the gastrointestinal tract. The former has a 50% mortality rate. *(2:216)*

320. **(D)** 5 MHz linear transducer. The rectus abdominis muscle courses from the anterior aspect of the symphysis pubis and pubis crest to the 5th, 6th, and 7th costal cartilages and xiphoid process. It protects and covers the anterior abdominal wall; therefore, a high-frequency linear transducer is the best option because one does not need to penetrate deep to image the rectus abdominis muscle, and the linear array has a wide field of view. *(2:31; 5:15)*

321. **(B)** Morison's pouch is located anterior to the right kidney and posterior to the inferior right lobe of the liver. The lesser sac is anterior to the pancreas and posterior to the stomach. The pouch of Douglas is posterior to the uterus and anterior to the rectum. The greater sac extends from the diaphragm to the pelvis and contains most of the abdominal organs. Morison's pouch or hepatorenal ress was named after a British surgeon James Rutherford Morison. *(2:36, 51)*

322. **(C)** Pyelocaliectasis is dilatation of the collecting system. The collecting system may be dilated because of overhydration, and it is a common finding in post-renal transplant patients. *(2:301; 4:405)*

323. **(C)** Ascites. The perirenal fluid collection may be associated with lymphocele, a collection of lymph fluid caused by injury to the lymphatic channels during transplantation; hematoma, a collection of blood; and abscess, which are all associated with renal transplantation. It is difficult to differentiate one from the other. Urinoma is a collection of urine because of a urinary leak of a ureteropelvic or ureteroureter anastomosis. Abscess is a collection of pus caused by an inflammatory response. Ascites is not associated with a renal transplant. *(7:403, 404)*

324. **(A)** Perinephric fluid collections are common in postoperative renal transplant patients. Fever, flank pain, and leukocytosis best correlate with an abscess. Because many fluid collections have the same sonographic appearance, the patient's clinical symptoms will help differentiate between them. Abscesses and hematomas tend to be more complex in appearance than urinomas and lymphoceles. Hematomas, abscesses, and urinoma usually develop earlier than lymphoceles. Lymphoceles typically do not develop until 4–8 weeks postop. A renal cyst is not associated with a renal transplant. *(7:403, 404)*

325. **(B)** Several sonographic criteria are used to describe biliary dilatation. In this sonogram, we can recognize (1) tubular lucencies within the liver demonstrating posterior acoustic enhancement. Bile opposed to blood increases transmission; (2) the tubules are irregular with jagged walls as opposed to veins and arteries that are straight—normal ducts are not visualized within the liver. *(7:229)*

326. **(C)** The arrow is pointing to an example of chronic pancreatitis. With chronic pancreatitis, the pancreas generally is diffusely smaller and more fibrotic than usual with areas of calcification and ductal dilatation. In acute pancreatitis, the pancreas is generally diffusely larger and less echogenic than normal. In adenocarcinoma and islet cell tumors, the pancreas is generally focally enlarged in the pancreatic head with the former and the tail in the latter. *(2:211)*

327. **(C)** There is irregular diffuse thickening of the bladder wall of unknown origin. The prostate is not enlarged, and there is no evidence of a bladder outlet obstruction, which most commonly is secondary to benign prostatic hypertrophy or carcinoma. Enlarged endometrial tissue may be found penetrating the bladder wall and extending in the lumen in severe cases of endometriosis in premenopausal women. *(2:303)*

328. **(E)** Both kidneys in patients with chronic renal failure appear small and echogenic. It is a nonspecific finding and may result from hypertension, chronic inflammation, or chronic ischemia. *(2:289)*

329. **(D)** Serum creatinine and blood urea nitrogen are elevated in kidney disease. *(2:250)*

330. **(D)** Attenuation is the decrease in amplitude and intensity as a wave travels through a medium. One of the criteria for a cyst is the posterior acoustic enhancement. A characteristic of fluid is that it does not absorb (attenuate) sound waves. *(11:288)*

331. **(D)** Adult polycystic kidney disease is cystic dilatation of the proximal convoluted tubules, Bowman's capsule, and the collecting tubules. As the cysts grow, they compress the nephrons causing renal insufficiency, which usually manifests in the fourth decade of life. Cysts may also occur in the liver, spleen, pancreas, lungs, ovaries, or testes. Infantile polycystic disease in its most severe form is not compatible with life. In less severe forms, the kidney will appear enlarged and echogenic because of the small cystic interfaces that occur in the kidney. Parapelvic cysts are found around the renal pelvic region. They usually do not interfere with the renal function. The ureteropelvic junction is one of the most common congenital causes of hydronephrosis. Sonographically, it is seen as dilatation of the collecting system and proximal portion of the ureter. *(2:270)*

332. **(A)** Multicystic dysplastic kidney disease is the most common cause of an abdominal mass in the newborn. It is usually unilateral, occurring more often in the left kidney. The contralateral kidney is at an increased risk for such abnormalities as ureteropelvic junction obstruction. Sonographically, the cysts appear in varying sizes, with the largest cysts in the periphery, absence of the connections between the cysts, absence of an identifiable renal sinus, and absence of renal parenchyma surrounding the cysts. *(2:270)*

333. **(A)** This sonogram of the kidney is not normal. There is dilatation of the renal calyces. There are numerous causes for hydronephrosis; any pathology in the lower urinary system may cause bilateral hydronephrosis, while upper urinary pathology may cause unilateral hydronephrosis. Some of the causes of hydronephrosis include congenital anomalies, as in posterior urethral valves, bladder neck obstruction; acquired causes, such as calculi, prostate enlargement, inflammation, bladder tumor; intrinsic causes, such as calculi, pyelonephritis, stricture, inflammation; and extrinsic causes, such as neoplasm and retroperitoneal adenopathy. *(2:279)*

334. **(B)** Acute tuberous necrosis is the most common medical cause for renal failure. It is a reversible renal disease. Sonographically, the kidneys will appear enlarged with echogenic renal pyramids. Tuberous sclerosis involves numerous body systems. Sonographically, multiple cysts or angiomyolipomas are seen. *(2:289)*

335. **(C)** The celiac axis is the first major branch of the aorta. It arises off the anterior aspect of the aorta before it trifurcates into the proper hepatic artery, splenic artery, and left gastric artery. *(6:72)*

336. **(A)** The sonogram demonstrates a normal right adrenal gland. In utero and in the neonate, the adrenal glands are prominent, being one-third the size of the kidney. *(7:622)*

337. **(B)** This decubitus coronal sonogram documents a severe dilatation of the renal collecting system extending into the renal pelvis, with marked thinning of the renal parenchyma. The low-level internal echoes are caused by artifact. Pyonephrosis is a collection of pus within the dilated collecting system. The pus is caused by long-standing stasis of urine. Sonographically, the dilated calyces will have internal echoes without increased posterior acoustic enhancement. *(2:284, 289)*

338. **(B)** The arcuate arteries are arc-shaped vessels that separate the cortex from the medulla. They are imaged sonographically as a small echogenic line above the renal pyramids. *(2:247)*

339. **(C)** The open arrowhead is pointing to the renal medullary pyramids. *(2:254)*

340. **(A)** Renal column of Bertin is composed of cortical tissue that extends into the medullary area between the pyramids. *(2:257)*

341. **(E)** Cirrhosis. The sonogram documents dilated biliary radicles that are caused by obstructed biliary radicles. Dilatation of biliary radicle may be secondary to a stone, mass lesions in the area of the head of the pancreas, a neoplasm, or metastatic lesions within the liver. Cirrhosis is related to medical jaundice, and there will be no evidence of biliary dilatation. *(2:189)*

342. **(E)** A neuroblastoma is an adrenal mass found in children. It will not cause splenomegaly. *(1:1407)*

343. **(C)** The patient was asymptomatic; it is most likely a simple benign hepatic cyst. Symptoms usually do not develop unless the cyst is large. Patients who have lymphoma, metastases, hydatid cysts, or polycystic liver disease will present with symptoms and elevated laboratory results. *(2:142)*

344. **(E)** Adenocarcinoma is found most often in males, especially in black males. There is an increased incidence of adenocarcinoma in patients with a history of smoking, a high-fat diet, chronic pancreatitis, diabetes, or cirrhosis. Adenocarcinoma usually presents as a hypoechoic mass in the head of the pancreas (Fig. 4–131A) demonstrate a hypochoic mass in the head of the pancreas, (Fig. 4–131B), intrahepatic biliary dilatations (Fig. 131C), enlaged gallbladder (Courvoisier's gallbladder) *(7:255)*

345. **(D)** The sonogram documents a small echogenic kidney with a loss of distinction between cortex, medulla, and renal sinus. Chronic glomerulonephritis is the most common cause of chronic renal failure. *(2:289)*

346. **(E)** When the transducer is placed transversely in a upward sharp angle, the heart will be come visible on an abdominal scan. *(7:144)*

347. **(B)** There are different types of thyroiditis, and chronic thyroiditis is Hashimoto's disease. It is the most common cause of hypothyroidism. It usually occurs in young females. Sonographically, the thyroid is enlarged with either a heterogeneous or a hypoechoic echo pattern. *(6:279)*

348. **(E)** Neuroblastoma is a rare malignant mass found in children usually younger than 8 years. Adenoma, cyst, myelolipoma, and pheochromocytoma are benign adrenal masses. Infrequently, pheochromocytomas may be malignant. *(6:246)*

349. **(A)** The right adrenal gland is located posterior to the inferior vena cava. When the right adrenal gland enlarges, it may displace the inferior vena cava anteriorly. *(5:240)*

350. **(E)** Dilated Intrahepatic ducts. *(6:177)*

351. **(D)** Air within the biliary tree is known as pneumobilia. Pneumobilia is caused by; emphysematous cholecystitis, cholecysto-enteric fistula, choledochojejunostomy and prolonged acute choleystitis. Pancreatic carcinoma is not a known cause. *(1:180)*

352. **(D)** Hemangioma. Hepatic hemangiomas are the most common benign hepatic tumors and most are asymptomatic. *(7:375)*

353. **(D)** A linear transducer has a rectangular format, which allows a larger field of view. The large footprint of a linear transducer makes it difficult to scan intercostally because of the rib artifacts and does not increase resolution. The instrument settings of an ultrasound machine to produce the highest resolution are necessary to document posterior shadowing of small calculi. Factors that the sonographer can control to increase resolution include use of a high-frequency transducer, decreasing gain (decreases scattering), place the focal zone at the area of interest, and the use of tissue harmonics. *(5:15, 185)*

354. **(E)** Normal sonographic appearance of liver and right kidney. *(2:278)*

355. **(B)** This sonogram demonstrates a marked increased echogenicity of the liver as compared with the kidney. The echogenicity of the liver should be compared with the kidney. *(2:253)*

356. **(C)** In the adult, glycogen storage disease, fatty metamorphosis, chronic hepatitis, cirrhosis, and hemochromatosis all present with an echogenic liver and decrease through penetration. In a child, this is frequently a complication of glycogen storage disease. *(2:172)*

357. **(E)** The sonographer has no control over the speed of sound. To optimize a sonographic image, the sonographer is able to adjust and choose the overall gain, time-gain compensation, transducer type and frequency, and the depth and focus control. *(2:126)*

358. **(A)** A resistive index (RI) of less than 0.70 is considered normal. *(2:284)*

359. **(C)** Splenomegaly is diagnosed when the spleen measures greater than 13 cm in the long axis. Sonographically, the left kidney will be compressed and displaced posteriorly. *(2:314)*

360. **(A)** This image is of a gallbladder filled with stones. *(2:180)*

361. **(D)** This sonogram demonstrates calculus cholecystitis. When the gallbladder is filled with calculi, all that may be imaged on sonogram is the wall echo shadowing (WES) sign. *(2:180)*

362. **(E)** The laboratory findings in patients with cholelithiasis are consistent with an increase in alkaline phosphatase. Other liver function test results may be abnormal (AST, ALT). Serum amylase may be elevated in patients with pancreatitis; increased creatinine is consistent with renal insufficiency; serum indirect bilirubin is elevated in patients with hepatocellular disease. *(1:176)*

363. **(B)** Renal parenchymal disease. The sonographic hallmark of this disease is a bilateral increase in echogenicity throughout the renal parenchyma *(7:388)*

364. **(B)** Posterior urethral valves is the most common cause of urethral obstruction in boys. The valves are located in the posterior urethra and obstruct the urethra. Dilatation of the urethra, hydrouretera, and hydronephrosis may occur secondary to the obstruction. *(7:606)*

365. **(D)** The valves of Heister are tiny valves located in the proximal portion of the cystic duct. They prevent the duct from kinking. *(1:194; 2:204)*

366. **(E)** Patients with a history of cirrhosis have an increased incidence of developing hepatomas in the liver. *(2:139)*

367. **(C)** A choledochal cyst is usually diagnosed in childhood and is more common in Asians. The most common sonographic appearance of a choledochal cyst is a cyst communicating with the common bile. If choledochal cysts are not diagnosed and treated early, the patient is at an increased risk of developing gallbladder carcinoma and cholangiocarcinoma. *(6:137)*

368. **(D)** Primary gallbladder carcinoma is more commonly found in women, and there is an increased incidence in people working in the textile, rubber, and automotive industries. Gallstones are present in the majority of cases, and a percentage of cases will present with a porcelain gallbladder. Sonographically, the gallbladder may also have a thickened wall, and a mass may be seen within the gallbladder lumen. *(6:222)*

369. **(E)** A Baker's cyst is located in the bursa posterior to the distal femur. *(7:777)*

370. **(C)** A Riedel's lobe is an anatomic variation of the liver, where the right lobe of the liver has a tongue-like extension. It is more common in women, and on physical examination, the liver will give the impression of hepatomegaly. *(7:126)*

Case Studies Answer Sheet

Case 1

1-1. D
1-2. B
1-3. A

There is both intrahepatic and extrahepatic bile duct dilatation. The color Doppler sonogram shows the multiple tubular structures to be dilated with intrahepatic and extrahepatic bile ducts. The transverse midline image shows a hypoechoic mass in the pancreatic head.

Case 2

2-1. A
2-2. C
2-3. E

This is typical of focal nodular hyperplasia. These lesions typically have a central vessel. Computed tomography or magnetic resonance can confirm the diagnosis.

Case 3

3-1. B
3-2. C
3-3. C

This is an example of a diffusely irregular liver texture due to hepatitis. The common bile duct is of normal caliber.

Case 4

4-1. B
4-2. D
4-3. A

There is an hypoechoic mass that shows peripheral "cloud"-like arterial enhancement on arterial-phase computed tomography consistent with the diagnosis of a hemangioma.

Case 5

5-1. A
5-2. A
5-3. C

There is a revised flow in the portal vein secondary to portal hypertension. There is diffuse fatty change in the liver, which has a variety of causes including rejection, hepatitis, and vascular insult.

Case 6

6-1. A
6-2. D
6-3. A

Portal vein thrombosis may be associated with extension of tumor into the portal vein or "bland" due to hypercoagulability of blood or associated with gastrointestinal inflammatory disease. If present, hepatic transplantation cannot occur since this requires anastomosis of recipient portal vein to donor portal vein.

Case 7

7-1. C
7-2. A
7-3. D

This patient has a nonobstructing stone in the left kidney and one at the distal ureter. The "twinkle" is created on color Doppler due to reverberation within the stone and thus can overestimate its true size. The presence of a ureteral jet is seen even when there is near occlusion of the ureter by the stone.

Case 8

8-1. A
8-2. E
8-3. B

There is marked thickening of the gallbladder wall, which is a nonspecific finding. If there is localized pain when scanning directly over the gallbladder ("Murphy's sign"), acute cholecystitis may be present.

Case 9

9-1. C
9-2. C
9-3. B

This is a well-defined mass with a hypoechoic halo typical of a metastatic lesion. Sonography provided guidance for biopsy.

Case 10

10-1. A
10-2. A
10-3. A

Color Doppler and spectral Doppler are important in establishing flow within a TIPS shunt. Normal velocities range from 50 to 150 cm/s and may vary depending on respiration.

Case 11

11-1. A
11-2. C
11-3. C

There is a thickened loop of bowel in the right lower quadrant. Although this could also be seen in appendicitis, this was an intussuscepted Meckel's diverticulum.

Case 12

12-1. C
12-2. D
12-3. A

This is an example of chronic lymphocystic thyroiditis. There is diffuse irregularity of the mid and lower portion of the right lobe. Biopsy is not indicated.

References

1. Rumack CM, Wilson SR, Charboneau JW, Levine D. *Diagnostic Ultrasound*. 4th ed. Mosby; 2011.

2. Hagen-Ansert SL. *Textbook of Diagnostic Ultrasonography*. 6th ed. St. Louis: CV Mosby; 2006.

3. *Dorland's Illustrated Medical Dictionary*. 30th ed. Philadelphia: W.B Saunders; 2003.

4. *NCER National Certification Examination Review*. Dallas: Society of Diagnostic Medical Sonography; 2009.

5. Mc Gaham JP, Goldberg BB. *Diagnostic Ultrasound: A logical Approach*. Philadelphia PA: Lippincott-Raven Publishers. 1998.

6. Gill K. *Abdominal Ultrasound A Practitioner's Guide*. Philadelphia: WB Saunders; 2001.

7. Kawamura DM. Diagnostic Medical Sonography: A Guide to Clinical Practice: Abdomen and Superficial Structures. 2nd ed. Philadelphia: Lippincott; 1997.

8. Curry RA, Tempkin BB. *Sonography: Introduction to Normal Structure and Function*. 3rd ed. Saunders; 2011.

9. Krebs CA, Giyanani VL, Eisenberg RL. *Ultrasound Atlas of Disease Processes*. Norwalk, CT: Appleton & Lange; 1993.

10. Kremnau F. *Sonography: Principles and Instruments*. 8th ed. Saunders; 2011.

11. Criner GJ, Alonzo GE. *Critical Care Guide: Text and Review*. New York: Springer-Verlag; 2002.

12. Mc Catehey KD. Clinical Laboratory Medicine. 2nd ed. Philadelphia: Lippincott-Williams & Wilkins; 2002.

5

Sonography of the Thyroid and Scrotum

*Arthur C. Fleischer and Charles S. Odwin**

Study Guide

THYROID

Gross Anatomy

The thyroid is an endocrine gland that secretes three major hormones: thyroxine (T4), triiodothyronine (T3), and calcitonin. The thyroid is located in the neck and has two lobes connected anteriorly by a narrow band of tissue, referred to as the isthmus.

The common carotid artery and internal jugular vein lie posterior and lateral, defining the posterolateral margins of the thyroid. The "strap muscles" lie anterior to the lateral aspect of the thyroid defining the anterolateral margins of the thyroid.

Surrounding Musculature and Structures

Sternohyoid muscle—anterior and slightly lateral

Sternothyroid muscle—posterior to the sternohyoid

Longus colli muscle—adjacent to the trachea and is posterior to the thyroid and the common carotid arteries

Esophagus—slightly to the left of midline and posterior to the thyroid

Sonographically, the thyroid has a homogeneous echogenicity that is greater than the strap muscles.

Normal Measurements of the Thyroid

Lobes	Isthmus
Length: 4–6 cm	Length: 2 cm
Width: 1.5–2 cm	Width: 2 cm
Height: 2–3 cm	Height: 2–6 cm

Physiologically, there are two basic conditions that occur with the thyroid: hypothyroidism or hyperthyroidism. The anterior pituitary gland produces a thyroid-stimulating hormone (TSH), which regulates the hormones secreted by the thyroid gland. Table 5–1 outlines the pathologies of the thyroid that can be imaged sonographically.

SONOGRAPHY OF THYROID NODULES

Sonography provides important clinical information regarding the presence of a thyroid nodule, its internal consistency, and number of lesions. High-frequency transducers provide detailed depiction of the relative size, location, border, and vascularity with color Doppler sonography. There are certain parameters that the sonographer should document such as

- Size
- Location
- Borders
- Internal consistency
- Cervical lymphadenopathy

Sonographers should also be aware of certain "classic patterns" that allow characterization of thyroid nodules. These patterns can be divided with those that require fine needle aspiration (FNA) biopsy and those that usually do not need FNA. Findings usually requiring FNA include

- *Nodules containing microcalcifications*—These are usually papillary cancers.
- *Hyperechoic solid nodules with coarse calcification or echogenic foci*—These can also be seen in medullary and papillary

---

*Kerry E. Weinberg was the author of the previous-edition version of this chapter.

TABLE 5–1 • Thyroid Pathology

Pathology Imaged by Sonography	Sonographic Characteristics
Adenomas (benign): most common nodule occurring in the thyroid; may be singular or multiple; also commonly seen in the parathyroid glands	Well-defined round or oval mass that varies in size from small to very large; varied echogenicity from echogenic, isoechoic to a solid homogenous mass with few internal echoes, resembles a cystic structure; usually solid masses, which often have an anechoic halo, created by blood and edematous tissue compressing the surrounding parenchyma; a halo may also be seen with malignant masses.
Simple cyst: usually developmental, such as thyroglossal duct (located midline anterior to the trachea and brachial cleft (located more laterally)	Anechoic, no internal echoes, smooth, thin well-defined walls, increased acoustic through transmission
Hemorrhagic cysts: usually caused by trauma or degeneration of adenoma	Cystic mass with irregular borders that may have multiple septations or low-level internal echoes
Acute thyroiditis: thyroiditis usually found in middle-age women; clinically, the thyroid is enlarged, tender, and the patient has a fever	Diffuse enlargement with decreased echogenicity of the lobes; enlargement of the lobes is not symmetrical and the right lobe is usually larger
Subacute thyroiditis	Diffuse enlargement with decreased echogenicity of the gland
Hashimoto's thyroiditis: most common cause of hypothyroidism in young or middle-age women; characteristically, painless diffuse enlargement of the thyroid gland; treatment includes thyroid hormones	Inhomogeneous pattern with overall decreased echogenicity of the gland
Goiter: consists of multiple adenomas and is associated with hyperthyroidism	In its initial stages, the thyroid is enlarged and may have a normal sonographic pattern; in later stages, may have multiple discrete nodules or diffusely nodular with heterogeneous echo pattern and no normal tissue; nodes may have cystic degeneration and calcification within
Graves' disease: an autoimmune disease characterized by thyrotoxicosis and is the most common cause of hyperthyroidism.	The thyroid is diffusely enlarged and hypoechoic with an increased vascularity identified by color Doppler
Carcinoma–80% are papillary: usually grow slowly and are seen in adults; patients may present with difficulty breathing and swallowing with a palpable neck mass	Sonography cannot differentiate between a benign and a malignant lesion; malignancies tend to have irregular borders or are poorly defined; the sonographic appearance is varied; the mass may appear small or large, usually singular and hypoechoic; cystic degeneration and focal calcifications may be present.

cancers or rarely in benign lesions. These nodules should undergo FNA.

- *Solid nodule with peripheral calcifications*—These are usually benign follicular adenomas but may need resection for histologic evaluation.
- *Nodules with edge shadowing*—This may arise from a fibrous capsule of a thyroid cancer.

Findings that usually do not require FNA include:

- *Nodules containing echogenic foci with "ring-down" artifact*—These usually correspond to condensed colloid within a benign nodule.
- *Nodules containing "honeycomb" pattern*—These are typical of a benign colloid adenoma.

- Cystic nodules are typically benign.
- *Multiple hypoechoic foci*—These are typical of chronic lymphocytic (Hashimoto's) thyroiditis.

The sonographer should also document the size, shape, and morphology of cervical lymph nodes. Abnormal findings include enlargement (>6 mm height), hypoechoic areas, and microcalcification. Papillary thyroid cancers can be associated with spread to lymph nodes. "Reactive" lymph nodes can also be seen with neck inflammation.

Sonographers may also assist in guided FNA of one or more abnormal thyroid masses.

The interested reader is referred to the article below for further discussion of the various sonographic features of thyroid nodules.[1]

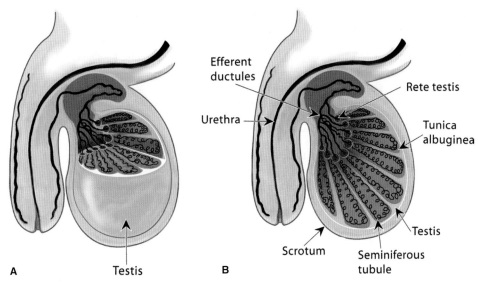

FIGURE 5–1. A and **B**. Section anatomy of the testis and epididymis.

SCROTUM

Gross Anatomy

The scrotum is a sac that is continuous with the abdomen and is divided by a septum, the medial raphe. Each space contains a testis, and epididymis, a portion of spermatic cord, and the ductus deferens (Fig. 5–1). A thin, double layer of peritoneum and the tunica vaginalis line the inner wall of the scrotum. This double layer of peritoneum normally contains a small amount of fluid.

The testicles are ovoid glands that measure approximately 4 × 2 × 3 cm. A dense white fibrous capsule, tunica albuginea, encases each testicle and then enters the gland, separating the testes into approximately 200 cone-shaped lobules. Within these lobules, two primary functions occur: spermatogenesis (the production of spermatozoa) and the secretion of testosterone by the interstitial cells (Leydig cells).

The secretions are carried through the lobules to the rete testis. A series of ducts, efferent ductules, drain the rete testis, piercing the tunica albuginea and entering the head of the epididymis.

The epididymis consists of a single tightly coiled duct that drapes the posterior aspect of the testis. The most superior aspect of the epididymis is the head, followed by the body and tail. This duct continues as the ductus deferens (vas deferens), leaving the pelvis via the inguinal canal with the testicular artery, the draining veins of the scrotum, nerves, and lymphatics to form the spermatic cord. Each spermatic cord now extends over the top and down the posterior surface of the bladder, coming together to join the duct from the seminal vesicle to form the ejaculatory ducts. The ejaculatory ducts pass through the prostate gland to terminate in the urethra.

Normal Sonographic Anatomy of the Scrotum

The normal testicle has a homogeneous echo pattern of medium-level echogenicity. The skin is a thin, smooth, echogenic, linear structure measuring <2 mm. Posteriorly and superiorly capping the testis, the epididymal head is clearly distinguished because of its coarser, more echogenic pattern. The body of the epididymis is more difficult to differentiate because of its posterior position, and the tail is rarely seen. A bright echogenic band, representing the mediastinum testis, is seen in the 9 o'clock position; on the left side, it is seen in the 3 o'clock position. Between the layers of the tunica vaginalis, a small amount of fluid is normally found.

The testicular artery and veins of the pampiniform plexus, which run along the posterior aspect of the testicle in the region of the epididymis, are not normally seen.

Scanning the testis transversely, comparing each testis and epididymis as to size, echogenicity, and vascularity, is the best guide for detecting lesions, enlargement, or torsion.

There are no specific laboratory tests that are used to identify scrotal pathology. A decrease in sperm count may occur in cases of male infertility. (Table 5–2 outlines scrotal pathology associated with clinical and sonographic findings.)

TABLE 5–2 • Scrotal Pathology

Pathology	Clinical Findings	Sonographic Findings
Epididymis		
Acute epididymitis	Specific epididymitis stemming from gonorrhea, syphilis, mumps, and/or tuberculosis. Nonspecific epididymitis is usually the result of a urinary tract infection. Traumatic epididymitis caused by strenuous exercise. Most common cause of acute scrotal pain that increases over a 1 to 2 day period, fever, and dysuria	The epididymis is enlarged and more hypoechoic.
Chronic epididymitis	Specific epididymitis stemming from gonorrhea, syphilis, mumps, and/or tuberculosis. Non-specific epididymitis is usually the result of a urinary tract infection. Traumatic epididymitis caused by strenuous exercise	The epididymis is thickened and very echogenic, and it may contain calcifications.
Scrotal abscess	Most commonly preceded by epididymitis or orchitis. Characterized by fever, scrotal pain, and scrotal swelling.	Sonolucent or complex mass with increased blood flow to the periphery and no blood flow in the mass.
Spermatocele	A cystic mass of the epididymis containing spermatozoa.	A cystic structure found superior to the testis, may be loculated and contain low-level echoes.
Testis		
Orchitis	Inflammation of a testis caused by trauma, metastasis, mumps, or infection (Chlamydia).	The testis is enlarged and is less echogenic than the normal testis. An abscess of the testis appears as localized heterogeneous areas.
Seminoma (malignant)	Most common but the least aggressive testicular malignant tumor found in men between the ages of 30 and 40. Usually found in the tunica albuginea. Patients have elevated follicle-stimulating hormone levels.	Usually a solid homogeneous hypoechoic mass that may have hyperechoic areas.
Teratoma	This tumor is usually benign, but may become malignant if not treated. Found in young men between the ages of 25 and 35.	Well-defined complex mass with areas of hemorrhage, necrosis, and calcifications.
Testicular torsion (spermatic cord torsion)	Usually occurs in prepubertal boys. There is torsion of the spermatic cord, which causes strangulation of the blood supply to the testis, which causes edema. Acute scrotal pain with nausea and vomiting.	Varied nonspecific appearance, initially the testicle and epididymal head are enlarged and hypoechoic because of edema. The scrotal wall may become thickened, and a hydrocele may be found. If the torsion is partial, there will be reduced blood flow with increased blood flow to the peritesticular soft tissue. If the torsion is complete, there will be no blood flow. In chronic torsion, the testicle is small and heterogeneous because of areas of infarcts and necrosis. Comparison of blood flow in the contralateral testicle is necessary for a diagnosis.
Intratesticular hemorrhage		Echogenic mass
Pampiniform plexus		
Varicocele	Enlargement of the veins of the spermatic cord, commonly occurring on the left side because of drainage into the left renal vein. A right side varicocele is associated with a renal tumor.	Numerous anechoic tortuous structures lying posterior to the testis and extending superiorly past the epididymis. Increasing the venous pressure by having the patient perform a Valsalva maneuver or having the patient stand will cause dilatation of the veins.
Scrotum hydrocele	Abnormal amount of serous fluid between the parietal and visceral layers of the tunica vaginalis of the scrotum. Usually caused by epididymitis but may also be caused by orchitis, torsion or trauma may also be congenital. Often found in male infants, and the fluid will reabsorb within the first year of life.	The testis and epididymis are surrounded by fluid.
Inguinal hernia	Herniation of the abdominal contents into the scrotal sac.	Peristalsis of the mass will be visualized sonographically. Echogenic foci with a dirty shadow representing air within the loops of bowel will be seen.
Undescended testicles (cryptorchidism)	The testicle or testis is not located in the scrotal sac. 80% are found in the inguinal canal and are palpable.	Difficult to identify testicles in the abdominal cavity.

Questions

GENERAL INSTRUCTIONS: For each question, select the best answer. Select only one answer for each question unless otherwise specified.

1. What is the most common location for a spermatocele?

   (A) head of the epididymis
   (B) body of the epididymis
   (C) tail of the epididymis
   (D) tunica vaginalis
   (E) mediastinum testis

2. A 15-year-old boy presents with sudden intense right scrotal pain, nausea, and vomiting. A sonogram is performed, and an enlarged hypoechoic right scrotum with decreased arterial flow is documented. The left scrotum is normal. This is most consistent with which of the following?

   (A) testicular rupture
   (B) varicocele
   (C) spermatocele
   (D) torsion
   (E) hydrocele

3. Which of the following statements is true in patients with uncomplicated acute epididymitis?

   (A) There is enlargement of the scrotum with focal or generalized thickening of the epididymis.
   (B) The epididymis is uniformly enlarged and more anechoic than usual.
   (C) The epididymis is small with areas of calcifications.
   (D) There is decreased blood flow to the epididymis.
   (E) The epididymis is too tender to be touched and cannot be scanned.

4. On a longitudinal scan of the scrotum, which of the following is the most superior portion?

   (A) ductus deferens
   (B) rete testis
   (C) head of the epididymis
   (D) tunica albuginea
   (E) spermatic cord

5. Which of the following is true concerning the seminal vesicles?

   (A) They produce sperm and are located within the prostate
   (B) They produce sperm and are located posterior to the urinary bladder
   (C) They are the reservoir for sperm and are located posterior to the urinary bladder
   (D) They are the reservoir for sperm and are located between the mediastinum testes and the pampiniform plexus
   (E) They are the reservoir for sperm and are located in the peripheral zone of the prostate

6. On a sonographic examination, which of the following describes the appearance of a seminoma of the testicle?

   (A) solid, homogeneous mass
   (B) large, multilocular cystic mass
   (C) small, simple cyst
   (D) diffuse enlargement of the testicle
   (E) small, complex mass

7. On a sonographic examination, which of the following describes the appearance of thyroiditis?

   (A) multiple cysts within the thyroid
   (B) a diffuse, enlarged thyroid with decreased echogenicity
   (C) a small, echogenic thyroid
   (D) multiple complex masses within the thyroid
   (E) fluid collection surrounding an enlarged thyroid

8. A pheochromocytoma is a benign hormone-producing tumor of which of the following?

   (A) thyroid
   (B) kidney
   (C) testicle
   (D) pancreas
   (E) adrenal gland

9. Which of the following is the most likely diagnosis shown in Fig. 5–2?

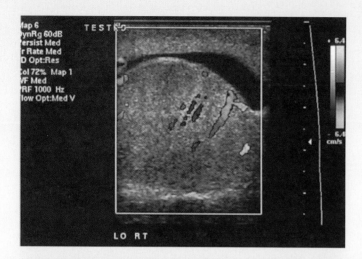

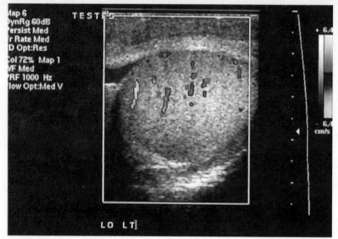

FIGURE 5–2. Longitudinal color Doppler sonograms of the right and left hemiscrotum.

(A) a testicular tumor
(B) testicular torsion
(C) epididymitis
(D) a cryptorchidism
(E) a normal testicle

10. Which of the following may be the presenting symptom of a testicular malignant tumor?

(A) para-aortic lymphadenopathy
(B) acute scrotal pain
(C) leukemia
(D) retroperitoneal lymphadenopathy
(E) all of the above

11. The left testicular vein drains into which of the following veins?

(A) inferior vena cava
(B) left internal iliac vein
(C) common internal iliac vein
(D) left renal vein
(E) prostatic vein

12. In the subacute phase of testicular torsion, which of the following describes the appearance of the testes?

(A) anechoic areas in testes with decreased blood flow
(B) small and echogenic
(C) enlarged with increased blood flow
(D) at normal size with a decrease in size of the epididymis

13. Fig. 5–3 is a transverse sonogram of the right and left hemiscrotum. Which of the following is this image most consistent with?

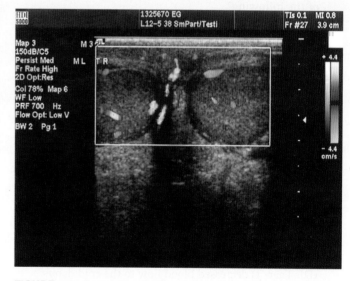

FIGURE 5–3. Transverse color Doppler sonogram of the right and left testicles.

(A) torsion
(B) orchiectomy
(C) cryptorchidism
(D) epididymitis
(E) normal testicles

14. Fig. 5–4 is a Duplex Doppler sonogram obtained in the upper hemiscrotum. What is the abnormality?

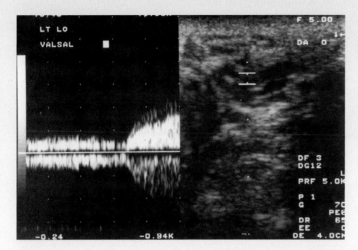

FIGURE 5–4. Duplex Doppler sonogram obtained in the right upper hemiscrotum.

(A) a dilated spermatic duct

(B) dilated vessels near the head of the epididymis

(C) an extratesticular vascular tumor

(D) a pampiniform venous plexus

(E) a dilated deferential artery

15. Based on the findings in Fig. 5–4, what is the most likely diagnosis?

(A) varicocele

(B) hydrocele

(C) testicular torsion

(D) spermatocele

(E) testicular infarct

16. A scrotal scan was performed on a 69-year-old man. The findings in Fig. 5–5 are consistent with which one of the following diagnoses?

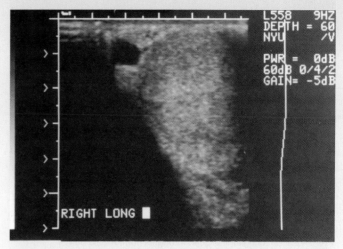

FIGURE 5–5. Longitudinal scan through the right testis.

(A) epididymitis

(B) hydrocele

(C) seminoma

(D) varicocele

(E) spermatocele

17. A scrotal scan was performed on a 78-year-old man. What is the arrow in Fig. 5–6 pointing to?

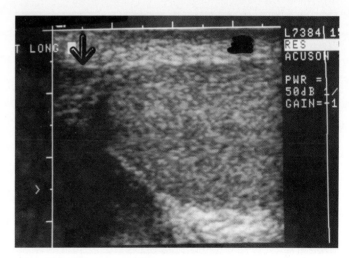

FIGURE 5–6. Magnified longitudinal scan of the right testis.

(A) a fractured testicle

(B) the normal head of the epididymis

(C) the mediastinum

(D) seminoma

(E) testicular torsion

18. Fig. 5–7 is a longitudinal scan through a male pelvis. What is the arrow pointing to in the image?

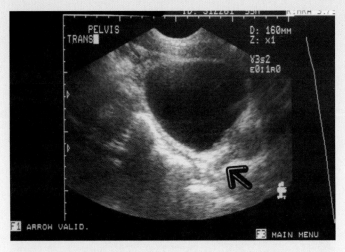

FIGURE 5–7. Longitudinal scan through a normal male pelvis.

(A) prostate

(B) seminal vesicle

(C) prostatic urethra

(D) membranous urethra

(E) urethra

19. A young male patient presents with left testicular pain. A scan of his testicles is performed. What is the arrow in Fig. 5–8 pointing to?

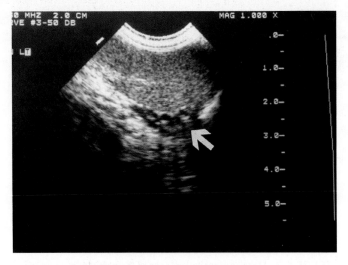

FIGURE 5–8. Longitudinal scan through the left testis.

(A) a spermatocele

(B) an epididymal cyst

(C) a cryptorchidism

(D) a varicocele

(E) the mediastinum

20. Which of the following connects the two lobes of the thyroid?

(A) sternothyroid muscle

(B) common carotid artery

(C) trachea

(D) isthmus

(E) lower poles

21. Parathyroid adenomas may be associated with which of the following?

(A) hypercalcemia

(B) hypertension

(C) bloating

(D) acne

(E) headaches

22. What is the most common congenital cause of urinary tract obstruction in males?

(A) ureteropelvic junction obstruction (UPJ)

(B) posterior urethral valve (PUV)

(C) infantile polycystic kidney disease

(D) undescended testis

(E) duplex collecting system

Case Studies

CASE 1

History: 65-year-old with bilateral a testicular mass. Sagittal gray scale (A) and transverse (B) sonograms of right testicle.

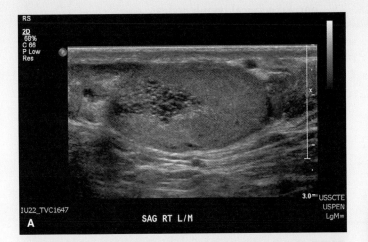

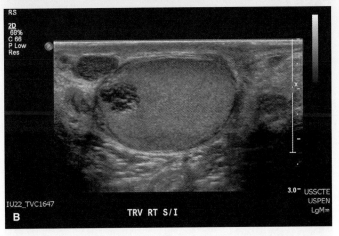

1-1. Which of the following statements is true concerning this scrotal sonogram?

A. There are bilateral masses in the mediastinum of both testes.

B. There is dilatation of the rete testes of the right testicle.

C. There is dilatation of both epididymides.

D. There is a bilateral testicular torsion.

1-2. What is the most likely diagnosis?

A. a normal variant

B. bilateral testicular tumor

C. chronic torsion

D. none of the above

1-3. What is the proper thing for sonographers to do if the patient states that he has a palpable scrotal mass?

A. Ignore anything a patient has to say about his scrotum.

B. Try to scan over the area of palpable abnormality to confirm presence of a mass.

C. Perform a scrotal sonogram while the patient performs a Valsalva maneuver.

D. Explain to the patient that most palpable scrotal masses are benign and you are sure his is.

CASE 2

History: 28-year-old man with acute right testicular pain. (A) Sagittal scan of right testicle (B) Sagittal gray scale and color Doppler scan of the right testicle.

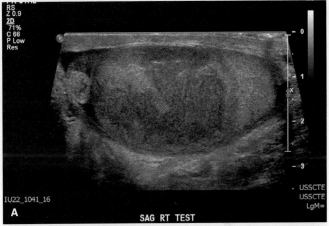

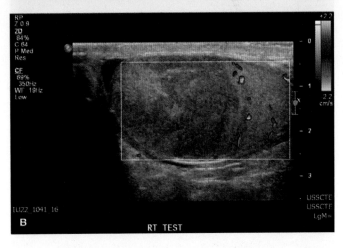

2-1. Which of the following can be included in the findings?

A. hypoechoic area in upper pole

B. hypovascular area in upper pole

C. diffuse abnormal texture

D. A and B

2-2. What is the most likely diagnosis?

A. testicular infarction

B. epididymitis

C. seminoma

D. none of the above

2-3. Why was power color Doppler used?

A. It is more sensitive to flow through frequency-based color Doppler sonography (CDS).

B. It has less exposure.

C. There is a possibility to hear the area and restore flow.

D. None of the above.

CASE 3

History: Sagittal images (A and B) at level III of the right side of the neck.

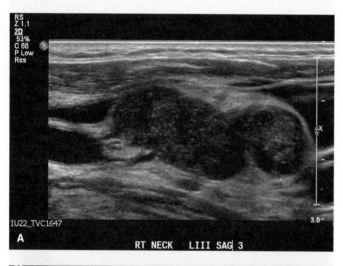

A   RT NECK   LIII SAG 3

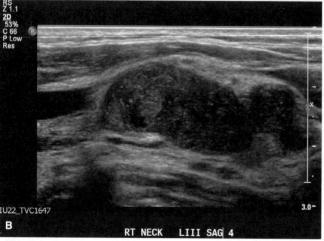

B   RT NECK   LIII SAG 4

3-1. Which of the following are true statements regarding this patient?

A. There are multiple thyroid nodules.

B. The lymph nodes are normal.

C. There is enlargement of the lymph nodes.

D. The lymph nodes have an abnormal morphology.

E. Both C and D are true.

3-2. Which of the following is a sonographic feature of normal cervical lymph nodes?

A. a central, echogenic hilum

B. oblong shape

C. <6 mm height

D. all of the above

3-3. If a sonographer finds a suspicious thyroid nodule, what is the most appropriate next step?

A. The cervical lymph nodes should be imaged.

B. A biopsy of the lesion must be performed.

C. A fine needle aspiration may be indicated.

D. Both A and C should be performed.

CASE 4

History: Sagittal gray scale (A) and transverse color Doppler (B) sonogram taken of the left lobe of thyroid.

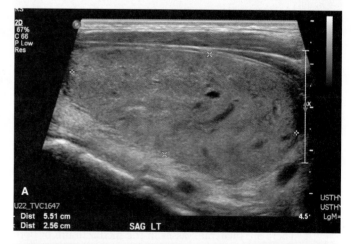

A   Dist 5.51 cm   Dist 2.56 cm   SAG LT

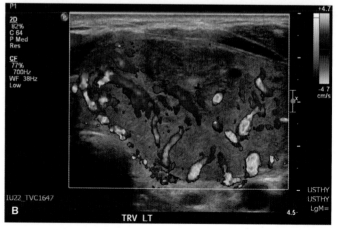

B   TRV LT

4-1. Which of the following statements is true concerning the role of color Doppler sonography (CDS) of thyroid nodules?

A. CDS is highly specific for thyroid cancers.

B. CDS should be performed when a thyroid nodule is seen on gray scale sonography.

C. Spectral tracings are needed to differentiate benign nodules from cancer.

D. CDS is of no clinical use for thyroid nodules.

4-2. What is the most likely diagnosis in this patient?

A. papillary thyroid cancer

B. benign nodule

C. hyperplastic nodule

D. metastatic lesion from colonic tumor

4-3. Sonographically guided fine needle aspiration (FNA) of this lesion:

A. would be contraindicated because of all the vessels

B. could be performed safely

C. most likely would result in extensive hemorrhage

D. This lesion requires biopsy, not FNA.

CASE 5

History: Sagittal (A) and color Doppler sonography (CDS) (B) of right thyroid lobe.

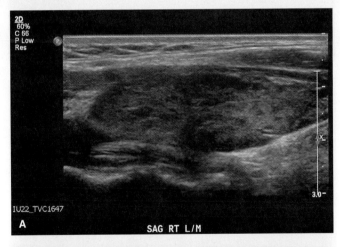

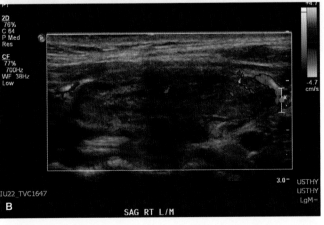

5-1. Which of the following statements is true concerning this patient's thyroid sonogram?

A. There is a large, hypoechoic nodule in the upper pole.

B. There is a hypoechoic, ill-defined nodule in the upper pole.

C. There is a hypervascular nodule in the upper pole.

D. There is a hypervascular nodule in the lower pole.

5-2. Which of the following statements is true concerning color Doppler sonogram of thyroid nodules?

A. Their relative vascularity reflects their functions.

B. Tumors have central vessels.

C. Benign lesions tend to have peripheral flow.

D. All of the above.

5-3. Which of the following statements are true regarding the sonographic findings in thyroiditis?

A. Focal hypoechoic areas may represent normal thyroid tumors.

B. Multiple hypoechoic punctate areas can be seen representing lymphocytic infiltrate.

C. Fine needle aspiration (FNA) is rarely indicated.

D. FNA is always indicated.

CASE 6

History: Sagittal gray scale (A) and color Doppler sonogram (B) obtained through left thyroid lobe.

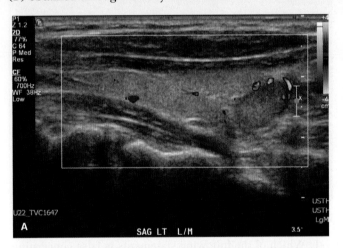

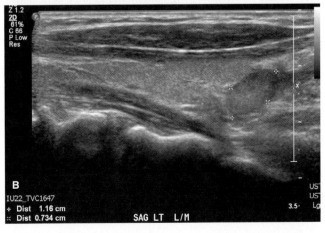

6-1. **Which of the following statements are true concerning this patient's thyroid sonogram?**

A. There is an enlarged lymph node obstructing the lower aspect of the lower pole.

B. There is a hypoechoic thyroid nodule within the lower pole.

C. There is an enlarged left parathyroid mass.

D. This is a normal thyroid sonogram.

6-2. **Which of the following is true regarding the sonographic appearance of normal parathyroid glands?**

A. They are typically posterior to thyroid.

B. They are seen in area of longus colli muscle.

C. They are approximately 3 × 5 mm.

D. All of the above.

6-3. **What is the most likely diagnosis?**

A. parathyroid adenoma

B. thyroid cancer

C. papillary thyroid cancer

D. follicular adenoma

CASE 7

History: A midline sagittal gray scale neck sonogram.

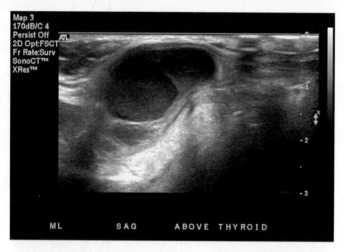

7-1. **Which of the following statements is false concerning this scan?**

A. There is enhanced through transmission suggesting a cystic internal consistency.

B. This mass has all the sonographic features of a thyroid tumor.

C. Since this mass is midline, it is possible to be a thyroglossal duct cyst.

D. Fine needle aspiration is required in this patient.

7-2. **What is the most likely diagnosis?**

A. thyroid neoplasm

B. multinodular cyst

C. thyroglossal duct cyst

D. enlarged lymph nodes

7-3. **Which of the following statements is true regarding thyroglossal duct cysts?**

A. They are typically midline.

B. They need to be aspirated.

C. They are malignant.

D. They should be biopsied to confirm the diagnosis.

CASE 8

History: Sagittal gray scale (A) and color Doppler sonogram (CDS) (B) of right thyroid lobe.

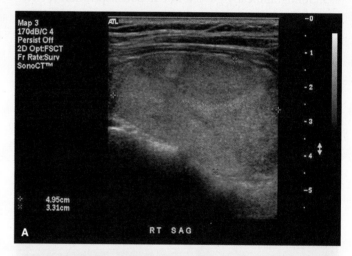

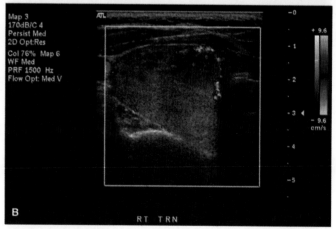

8-1. In this case, which of the following statements is true?

    A. CDS was helpful to confirm whether the nodule is benign.

    B. CDS was helpful to confirm whether the nodule is malignant.

    C. CDS was not helpful.

8-2. Which of the following should be included in the diagnostic considerations?

    A. benign adenoma

    B. follicular cancer

    C. metastatic nodule

    D. all of the above

8-3. Which of the following is true concerning metastases to the thyroid?

    A. never occurs

    B. rarely occurs

    C. not uncommonly occurs

    D. frequently occurs

Answers and Explanations

At the end of each explained answer, there is a number combination in parentheses. The first number identifies the reference source; the second number or set of numbers indicates the page or pages on which the relevant information can be found.

1. **(A)** The most common location of a spermatocele is the head of the epididymis. A spermatocele is a retention cyst that may occur following vasectomy, scrotal surgery, or epididymitis. (5:748)

2. **(D)** Torsion is more common in children or teenage boys. It is a weakening in the attachment of the mesentery from the spermatic cord to the testicle. Clinically, the patient presents with sudden extreme pain in the scrotum. Treatment must occur within 5 or 6 hours of onset to save the testicle. The sonographic appearance varies according to the length of time that diagnosis is made. Acute torsion occurs within the first 24 hours. In the early stages, there is a decrease in the arterial flow to the testis. An enlarged epididymis and an enlarged hypoechoic testis are imaged. There may be thickening of the scrotal skin or the formation of a hydrocele. (4:333)

3. **(B)** In patients with uncomplicated acute epididymitis, there will be enlargement of the epididymal head or the entire epididymis. The epididymis has a decrease in echogenicity, and there may be increased blood flow with a reactive hydrocele. (3:413–415)

4. **(C)** The head of the epididymis is located superior to the testes. The rest of the epididymis courses along the posterior margin of the testicle inferiorly. (5:721, 722)

5. **(C)** The seminal vesicles are reservoirs for sperm and are located posterior to the urinary bladder. (3:408)

6. **(A)** A seminoma is a solid malignant mass of the testicles that is usually unilateral and appears hypoechoic on a sonographic examination. (4:338)

7. **(B)** Thyroiditis appears sonographically as a diffuse enlargement of the thyroid with a decrease in echogenicity. (4:279)

8. **(E)** Pheochromocytoma is a benign adrenal tumor of the medulla. It secretes both epinephrine and norepinephrine. (5:502, 503)

9. **(A)** The image is of a testicular tumor. The epididymis is enlarged in cases of testicular torsion and epididymitis. In cases of varicocele, there will be enlarged vessels, and a spermatocele produces a sonolucent lesion usually in the region near the head of the epididymis. The epididymis is normal on the image. (3:415, 421)

10. **(E)** Lymphadenopathy, leukemia, or acute scrotal pain may be a presenting symptom associated with a testicular tumor. (3:421, 423)

11. **(D)** The left renal vein. (3:410)

12. **(A)** The testicle may have anechoic areas, and the epididymis has a complex appearance. Associated findings include an enlarged epididymis and a reactive hydrocele. Spectral Doppler and color Doppler are used to evaluate whether the torsion is complete or incomplete. In cases of complete torsion, there will be no blood flow to the affected testicle. (4:333)

13. **(E)** Normal testicles have a homogeneous appearance. When performing color Doppler, the setting should be set as low as possible on the unaffected side and be compared with the affected side. Cryptorchidism is an undescended testicle; orchiectomy is removal of the testicle; and epididymitis is inflammation of the scrotum. (3:323)

14. **(B)** This sonogram demonstrates dilated vessels near the head of the epididymis. (4:329)

15. **(A)** A varicocele appears as tortuous vessels near the head of the epididymis, mostly occurring on the left. The reason varicoceles occur more on the left side is that the left testicular vein courses into the left renal vein, whereas the right testicular vein drains into the right spermatic vein. (4:329)

16. **(E)** An extratesticular cyst is documented on the sonogram. This is consistent with a spermatocele, which is a cyst in the epididymis containing spermatozoa. An epididymis cyst would have the same sonographic appearance. A varicocele (enlargement of the veins of the spermatic cord) is also extratesticular, but it is located on the posterior surface, more common of the left; and sonographically, it has a tubular shape. Seminoma is a malignant germ cell tumor within the testicle. (4:331)

17. **(B)** Normal head of the epididymis. (3:410)

18. **(B)** The arrow is pointing to the seminal vesicle, which is posterior to the bladder and superior to the prostate. (3:424)

19. **(D)** Varicocele is an enlargement of the veins of the pampiniform plexus, which course along the posterior aspect of the testicle and is more prominent on the left testicle. Venous dilatation occurs with an increase of pressure either by having the patient perform a Valsalva maneuver or by having the patient stand. Spermatocele and epididymal cysts are found in the epididymis. Cryptorchidism is another name for undescended testes. Mediastinum testis is found within the testis and connects the rete testis with the epididymis. (3:415)

20. **(D)** The two lobes of the thyroid are connected by the isthmus, which is anterior to the trachea. The common carotid is located lateral to the thyroid and the sternothyroid muscle is anterolateral to the thyroid. (4:272)

21. **(A)** A patient with a parathyroid adenoma may present with hypercalcemia and low serum levels of phosphate. (2:405)

22. **(B)** Posterior urethra valves is the most common cause of urethral obstruction in boys. The valves located in the posterior urethra obstruct the urethra. Dilatation of the urethra, hydroureter, and hydronephrosis may occur secondary to the obstruction. (5:606)

Case Studies Answer Sheet

Case 1

1-1. A
1-2. B
1-3. B

This is a well-circumscribed hypoechoic area with decreased flow. This can occur as a sequela of infarction or tumor. The sonographer should scan an area of concern and endeavor an abnormality. This is a case of dilated rete testes, a normal variant in older men.

Case 2

2-1. D
2-2. A
2-3. A

This testicle contains a well-circumscribed hypoechoic, hypovascular area in the upper pole that is hypovascular. Though hypovascular, this could have a similar appearance to a testicular tumor such as a seminoma; this represented testicular infarction to lifting weights.

Case 3

3-1. C
3-2. D
3-3. D

This is an enlarged and distorted lymph node. This can be associated with metastatic spread of follicular papillary cancer or can be "reactive" due to inflammation.

Case 4

4-1. B
4-2. A
4-3. B

This is a large papillary thyroid cancer containing numerous vessels. A fine needle aspiration could be performed safely.

Case 5

5-1. B
5-2. D
5-3. B

There is an ill-defined group of hypervascular nodules in the upper pole. Fine needle aspiration would be indicated for further evaluation.

Case 6

6-1. C
6-2. D
6-3. A

This sonogram shows a parathyroid mass inferior to the left lobe.

Case 7

7-1. B
7-2. C
7-3. A

This is a typical thyroglossal duct cyst. They are usually found in the midline and can contain some low-level echoes.

Case 8

8-1. A
8-2. D
8-3. C

This is a solid nodule that was found to represent a metastatic lesion to the thyroid.

References

1. Reading CC, Charboneau JW, Hay ID, Sebo TJ. Sonography of thyroid nodules—A "classic pattern" diagnostic approach. *Ultrasound Q*. 205; 21(3).

2. Rumack CM, Wilson SR, Charboneau JW, Levine D. Diagnostic Ultrasound. 4th ed. Mosby; 2011.

3. Hagen-Ansert SL. *Textbook of Diagnostic Ultrasonography*. 6th ed. St. Louis: CV Mosby; 2006.

4. Gill K. *Abdominal Ultrasound A Practitioner's Guide*. Philadelphia: WB Saunders; 2001.

5. Kawamura DM. *Diagnostic Medical Sonography: A Guide to Clinical Practice: Abdomen and Superficial Structures*. 2nd ed. Philadelphia: Lippincott; 1997.

6

Endorectal Prostate Sonography

Dunstan Abraham

Study Guide

The prostate is a heterogeneous, oval-shaped organ that surrounds the proximal urethra. In the adult, the normal gland measures approximately 3.8 cm (cephalocaudal) by 3 cm (anteroposterior) by 4 cm (transverse).[1] It normally weighs about 20 g, but it can be slightly larger in men older than 40 years. The prostate is composed of glandular and fibromuscular tissue and is located in the retroperitoneum between the floor of the urinary bladder and the urogenital diaphragm. The base of the prostate, its superior margin, abuts the inferior aspect of the urinary bladder. The gland is bounded anteriorly by prostatic fat and fascia, laterally by the obturator internus and levator ani muscles, and posteriorly by areolar tissue and Denonvilliers' fascia, which separates it from the rectum.

The **seminal vesicles** are two sac-like lateral structures that outpouch from the vas deferens and are situated on the posterior-superior aspect of the prostate between the bladder and the rectum. The seminal vesicles join the vas deferens to form the **ejaculatory ducts,** which then enter the base of the prostate to join the urethra at the verumontanum. The **verumontanum** is a midpoint region between the prostatic base and apex and surrounds the urethra. The size and fluid content of the seminal vesicles are variable.

The **prostatic urethra** courses through the substance of the gland and is divided into a proximal and a distal segment. The proximal segment extends from the neck of the bladder to the base of the verumontanum; the distal segment begins at this point and extends to the apex of the gland.

Blood supply to the prostate is from the internal iliac arteries, which eventually give rise to urethral and capsular arteries. Venous return is via the prostatic plexus, which drains into the internal iliac vein.[2] The prostate produces seminal fluid, which is essential to the function of the spermatozoa.

NORMAL SECTIONAL ANATOMY

The earlier anatomic descriptions of the prostate divided the gland into five major lobes: **anterior, posterior, media,** and **two lateral.** More recent histological studies, however, have divided the prostate into three glandular zones: the **transitional, central,** and **peripheral zones.** There is also a nonglandular region called the **anterior fibromuscular stroma**[2] (Fig. 6–1A, B).

Transitional Zone

The transitional zone represents about 5% of the glandular prostate and is located in the central region on both sides of the proximal urethra.[2] The ducts of the transitional zone run parallel to the urethra and end in the proximal urethra at the level of the verumontanum.

Central Zone

The central zone constitutes approximately 25% of the prostatic glandular tissue and is located at the base of the gland.[2] It is wedge-like in shape, is oriented horizontally, and surrounds the ejaculatory ducts throughout their course. The zone narrows to an apex at the verumontanum. Ducts of the vas deferens and seminal vesicles come together to form the ejaculatory ducts, which pass through the central zone and join the urethra at the verumontanum.

Peripheral Zone

The peripheral zone constitutes about 70% of the glandular tissue.[2] This zone consists of the posterior, lateral, and apical parts of the prostate and also extends anteriorly. The ducts of the peripheral zone enter the urethra at, and distal to, the verumontanum.

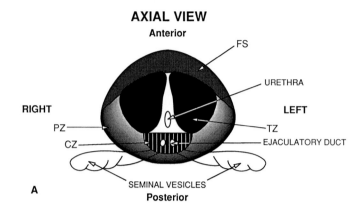

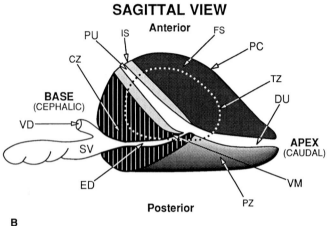

FIGURE 6–1. **(A)** An axial view of normal prostate anatomy: CZ is the central zone, FS is the fibromuscular stroma, TZ is the transition zone, and PZ is the peripheral zone. **(B)** Sagittal view of the normal prostate anatomy: SV is the seminal vesicle, ED is the ejaculatory duct, DU is the distal urethra, PC is the prostatic capsule, VD is the vas deferens, VM is the verumontanum, PU is the proximal urethra, CZ is the central zone, FS is the fibromuscular stroma, TZ is the transition zone, PS is the periurethral stroma, and PZ is the peripheral zone. *(Modified with permission from Dakin R., et al. Transrectal ultrasound of the prostate: Technique and sonographic findings. JDMS. 1989; 5(1):1-15.)*

Anterior Fibromuscular Stroma

The anterior fibromuscular stroma is a thick nonglandular sheath of tissue that covers the entire anterior surface of the prostate. This tissue is composed of smooth muscle and fibrous tissue.

NORMAL SONOGRAPHIC ANATOMY

Sonographically, the prostate is a homogeneous gland with low-level echoes. The periurethral glandular tissue that surrounds the proximal urethra is homogeneous and isoechoic. The central zone is normally more echogenic than the peripheral zone because it has a greater amount of **corpora amylacea** (calcified deposits) in the central zone. The fibromuscular capsule, located anteriorly, is smooth, hyperechoic, and sharply defined.

In sonography, the terms outer and inner gland are sometimes used to distinguish between the above zones. The outer gland consists of the peripheral and central zones, whereas the inner gland consists of the transitional zone, the inner anterior fibromuscular stroma, and the internal urethral sphincter. The surgical capsule separates the inner gland from the peripheral zone.

The seminal vesicles are visualized as symmetrically paired structures that are slightly less echoic than the prostate. The vas deferens can be depicted as tubular hypoechoic structures joining the seminal vesicles medially. On transverse imaging, they are round or oval and are located between the seminal vesicles. The ejaculatory duct, when empty, can be seen as a hyperechoic line joining the urethra. The empty urethra is identified by its echogenic walls coursing through the prostate. When filled with fluid, the urethra is recognized more easily. The surgical capsule is usually seen as a hypoechoic line but can also be echogenic due to calcification.

On longitudinal sections, the anterior space between the prostate and the seminal vesicles (**prostate–seminal vesicle angle**) is variable but is the same bilaterally. Similarly, the posterior space between the prostate and the seminal vesicle (or nipple) is symmetrical on both sides.[1]

INDICATIONS FOR SONOGRAPHY

Patients can be referred for endorectal prostate sonography for various reasons such as the following.[1,2]

- An abnormal digital rectal examination, as indicated by a palpable prostatic nodule or prostate with an asymmetrical size or shape
- Biopsy guidance of sonographically detected abnormal areas
- Clinical evidence of prostate cancer such as an elevated level of prostatic-specific antigen or radio-graphically detected bone metastasis
- Guide treatments for prostate cancer such as radiotherapy and cryotherapy
- Monitoring of a patient's response to therapy
- Inflammation leading to the formation of a prostatic abscess
- Infertility caused by the absence of the seminal vesicles or a bilateral obstruction of the ejaculatory ducts
- Difficulties in voiding caused by an obstruction of the prostatic urethra
- Calculation of prostatic volume prior to surgery

EQUIPMENT AND EXAMINATION TECHNIQUES

Technical innovations have led to the availability of several types of endorectal imaging systems. The original systems were **radial (axial) scanners** that produced transverse-oriented

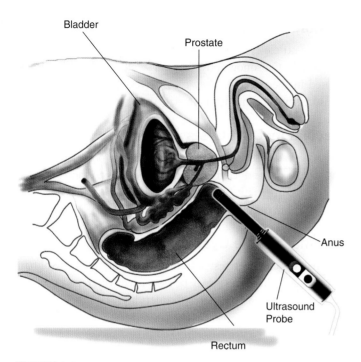

FIGURE 6–2. Drawing demonstrating the placement of the endorectal transducer and anatomy of the prostate.

slices of the prostate. Later, **linear array scanners** that imaged the gland in longitudinal sections were introduced. Today, **biplanar endorectal probes** that can produce both longitudinal and transverse sections of the gland are available, thus eliminating the need for two separate probes. The frequency of endorectal probes ranges from 5 to 8 MHz. A guide can be attached directly to the probe allows one to biopsy suspicious prostatic lesions safely and accurately. Fig. 6–2 demonstrates the placement of the endorectal transducer and anatomy of the prostate.

Preparation of the patient for endorectal sonography begins with a self-administered enema before the examination. This not only eliminates fecal material from the rectum that might adversely affect the quality of the image, but also reduces the risk of contamination of the prostate. If biopsy is to be performed, prophylactic antibiotics must be given before the procedure and continued for 24–48 hours afterward.[3]

The patient is generally examined in the left lateral decubitus position. The lithotomy position is sometimes used when other urological procedures are also being performed. The probe is previously sterilized and covered with a condom before insertion. A digital rectal examination is performed to exclude any obstructing lesions or rectal fissures and to correlate the exam with any palpable abnormalities. Axial scanning begins at the level of the seminal vesicles. The probe is then gradually withdrawn to image the gland sequentially down to the level of the apex.

Sagittal imaging begins in the midline and shows the gland from base to apex with portions of the seminal vesicles. The probe is then rotated clockwise and counterclockwise to demonstrate the right and left sides of the gland.

On color Doppler examination, moderate vascularity from the capsular and the urethral arteries and their branches can be visualized.

PATHOLOGY

Prostatic Carcinoma

In the United States 45,000 men die from prostate cancer each year. Men of African American descent and those with a family history of prostate cancer are at higher risk.[2] Although the etiology of prostatic cancer remains unclear, the factors implicated in its causation include age, genetic or racial makeup, hormonal influences and diet.

Screening tests for prostate cancer include annual digital rectal exam and prostate-specific antigen (PSA) blood test. Screening is recommended starting at age 50 years, or at age 40 years in men with a positive family history of prostate cancer. Normal PSA is less than 4 ng/mL. Elevated levels can be seen in patients with cancer, benign prostatic hyperplasia, prostatitis, and following procedures such as cystoscopy, prostate biopsy, and Foley catheter insertion. Artificially reduced levels of PSA are seen in patients taking medication such as Proscar (finasteride), which is used for treatment of benign prostatic hyperplasia.[2]

Anatomic studies have determined that 70% of prostate cancers originate *de novo* in the peripheral zone, 20% originate in the transitional zone, and 10% originate in the central zone.[1] Clinical symptoms include back pain and an obstruction of urinary outflow that may mimic benign prostatic hyperplasia.

Sonographically, prostate cancer varies in echogenicity. However, the most common appearance is a hypoechoic nodule on the peripheral zone. Hyperechoic cancers can rarely present as focal areas of calcification. Isoechoic cancers are difficult to detect, although secondary signs such as capsular bulging and asymmetry of the gland may aid in the diagnosis. Tumor invading the entire gland may have an inhomogeneous appearance.[2]

Invasion of the tumor into the seminal vesicles can be seen as solid material within this normally fluid-filled structure. Invasion may make the size, shape, and echogenicity of the seminal vesicles asymmetrical in appearance.

Obliteration of the nipple or the prostate–seminal vesicle angle is another diagnostic criterion for invasion by the tumor.[1] However, because the nipple is not imaged consistently, the criterion is of limited usefulness. Doppler ultrasound has not proven to be useful in the diagnosis of prostate cancer. Staging of prostatic cancer with ultrasound is also feasible but is limited by problems of resolution.

Benign Prostatic Hyperplasia and Hypertrophy

Benign prostatic hyperplasia affects 80–90% of adult men.[1] Its etiology is believed to be related to hormonal factors. The clinical symptoms of the disease may include decreased flow of urine, difficulty in initiating and terminating urination, nocturia, and urinary retention. Benign prostatic hyperplasia originates in the transitional zone and in periurethral glandular tissue.

The sonographic characteristics of hyperplasia nodules are variable. They can be hypoechoic, hyperechoic, or of mixed echogenicity. Enlargement of the central gland by benign prostatic hyperplasia causes lateral displacement of the peripheral zone. The prostatic calculi that are often encountered with benign prostatic hyperplasia are believed to be the result of stasis of prostatic secretions. Corpora amylacea are seen as echogenic foci similar to prostatic calculi. **Benign prostatic hyperplasia** causes the number of cells in the prostate to increase, whereas **benign prostatic hypertrophy** refers to an increase in the size of existing cells. Hyperplasia and hypertrophy often develop concurrently and result in the enlargement of the prostate gland. Transrectal ultrasound is not usually indicated in patients with benign prostatic hyperplasia unless prostate cancer is a clinical concern.

Prostatitis and Prostatic Abscess

Inflammation of the prostate can be the result of acute or chronic bacterial infections or of unknown nonbacterial factors. Clinical symptoms of prostatitis may include fever, pelvic and low back pain, urinary frequency and urgency, and dysuria. Although prostatitis usually involves the peripheral zone in its initial stages, it can originate in any area of the gland.

In acute prostatitis, the main sonographic finding is a hypoechoic gland with anechoic areas that may mimic carcinoma. Increased blood flow may be seen on color Doppler. In chronic prostatitis, sonographic findings may include focal masses of variable echogenicity, ejaculatory duct calcifications, thickening or irregularity of the prostatic capsule, dilatation of the periprostatic veins, and distention of the seminal vesicles.[2]

A prostatic abscess may develop secondarily to prostatitis. Endorectal sonography may show hypoechoic areas corresponding to liquefaction within the abscess. Sonography can be used to guide aspiration of an abscess if necessary.

Prostatic Utricle Cysts

Prostatic utricle cysts occur as a result of dilatation of the prostatic utricle. On sonography, they are small, anechoic structures located in the midline. They can, however, become large and measure several centimeters in size.

Ejaculatory Duct Cysts

Ejaculatory duct cysts occur secondarily to obstruction or a diverticular of the duct. They contain spermatozoa and are associated with infertility. On sonography, they are seen as anechoic masses within the ejaculatory ducts.

Seminal Vesicle Cysts

Seminal vesicle cysts result from an anomaly of the Wolffian duct. Large, solitary cysts may be associated with renal agenesis. They can also be associated with infertility when they obstruct the seminal vesicle.

Infertility

Patients with azoospermia (no sperm in the ejaculate) can be examined to exclude ejaculatory duct obstruction. This is diagnosed when the seminal vesicle measures more than 1.5 cm in anteroposterior diameter; presence of a dilated ejaculatory duct and a midline cyst. Additional ultrasound findings in infertility may include the following: bilateral absence of the vas deferens; bilateral occlusion of the vas deferens, seminal vesicles, and ejaculatory ducts by calcification or fibrosis; and obstructing cyst of the seminal vesicle, ejaculatory ducts, or prostate.

References

1. Rifkin M. *Ultrasound of the Prostate*. New York: Raven Press; 1988.

2. Toi A, Bree R. The prostate. In: Rumack C, Wilson S, Charboneau W, et al., eds. *Diagnostic Ultrasound*. 3rd ed, Vol. 1. St. Louis: Mosby; 2005.

3. Reiter R, Dekernion J. Epidemiology, etiology and prevention of prostate cancer. In: Walsh P, Ritik A, et al., eds. *Campbell's Urology*. 8th ed. Philadelphia: WB Saunders; 2001.

Questions

GENERAL INSTRUCTIONS: For each question, select the best answer. Select only one answer for each question unless otherwise specified.

1. Which of the following choices best describes the fibromuscular stroma?

   (A) covers the anterior surface of the prostate
   (B) is the major site of benign prostatic hypertrophy
   (C) is a nonglandular region
   (D) A and C

2. Which of the following is not an indication for endorectal prostate sonography?

   (A) a prostatic abscess
   (B) biopsy guidance of a palpable prostate nodule
   (C) an elevated prostatic-specific antigen
   (D) differentiation of a benign from a malignant nodule by imaging

3. Patients having endorectal prostate sonography are commonly examined in which of the following positions?

   (A) left lateral decubitus position
   (B) the erect position
   (C) the Trendelenburg position
   (D) Fowler's position

4. Which of the following statements about the transitional zone is false?

   (A) it is located centrally around the urethra.
   (B) it represents about 5% of the gland.
   (C) it is the primary site of benign prostatic hyperplasia.
   (D) it is the primary site of adenocarcinoma.

5. Which one of the following statements is false?

   (A) the central zone constitutes approximately 25% of the glandular tissue.
   (B) the central zone is located at the apex of the prostate.
   (C) the vas deferens joins the seminal vesicles in the central zone.
   (D) the central zone surrounds the ejaculatory ducts.

6. The peripheral zone accounts for what percentage of the prostatic glandular tissue?

   (A) 50%
   (B) 10%
   (C) 70%
   (D) 1%

7. Which of the following statements about the prostate is false?

   (A) its apex is located superiorly.
   (B) its base abuts the urinary bladder.
   (C) it has three zones.
   (D) the urethra runs through the gland.

8. Which of the following is a function of the prostate?

   (A) hormonal secretions
   (B) testosterone production
   (C) secretion of seminal fluid
   (D) spermatozoa production

9. The seminal vesicles join which of the following to form the ejaculatory duct?

   (A) the Denonvilliers' duct
   (B) the vas deferens
   (C) the verumontanum
   (D) the urethra

10. The ejaculatory duct joins which of the following structures at the verumontanum?

    (A) vas deferens
    (B) efferent ducts
    (C) epididymis
    (D) urethra

11. The seminal vesicles are located on which surface of the prostate?

    (A) the anterior-inferior surface
    (B) the posterior-inferior surface
    (C) the posterior-superior surface
    (D) the inferior-lateral surface

12. Which of the following statements about prostatic cancer is *not* true?

    (A) it originates mainly in the central zone.

    (B) it is commonly a hypoechoic lesion.

    (C) its associated factors include genetic and hormonal influence.

    (D) clinical presentation may include urinary obstruction.

13. Which of the following is commonly included in the sonographic features of acute prostatitis?

    (A) a hypoechoic gland with anechoic areas

    (B) a hypoechoic nodule on the peripheral zone

    (C) unilateral enlargement of the seminal vesicle

    (D) a midline anechoic mass

14. Benign prostatic hyperplasia originates in which of the following areas of the prostate?

    (A) the fibromuscular stroma

    (B) the peripheral zone

    (C) the ejaculatory ducts

    (D) the transitional zone

15. Which of the following statements is true about corpora amylacea?

    (A) they are part of the anterior fibromuscular capsule.

    (B) they are calcified deposits in the prostate.

    (C) they appear hypoechoic on endorectal ultrasound.

    (D) they are never seen on endorectal ultrasound.

16. Which of the following is *not* a common sonographic characteristic of prostatic cancer?

    (A) a hypoechoic nodule in the peripheral zone

    (B) distortion of the capsule

    (C) obliteration of the "nipple"

    (D) marked compression of the prostatic urethra

17. An endorectal examination of the prostate should begin with which of the following?

    (A) transverse scanning

    (B) longitudinal scanning

    (C) views of the seminal vesicles

    (D) a digital rectal examination

18. Which of the following best describes prostate cancer?

    (A) echogenic

    (B) anechoic

    (C) hypoechoic

    (D) sonographically variable

19. Which of the following best describes the verumontanum?

    (A) a midpoint region between the base and apex of the prostate

    (B) a congenital abnormality of the prostate

    (C) part of the peripheral zone

    (D) part of the seminal vesicle

20. An elevated prostatic-specific antigen may commonly indicate all of the following *except*

    (A) prostatic inflammation

    (B) prostatic cancer

    (C) benign prostatic hyperplasia

    (D) obstruction of the seminal vesicle

21. Which of the following narrows to an apex at the verumontanum?

    (A) the central zone

    (B) the peripheral zone

    (C) the transitional zone

    (D) the fibromuscular stroma

22. What does the normal adult prostate weigh?

    (A) 10 g

    (B) 20 g

    (C) 30 g

    (D) 40 g

23. Which of the following statements about the seminal vesicles is incorrect?

    (A) their absence does not usually affect fertility.

    (B) they are joined by the vas deferens.

    (C) they are normally less echoic than the prostate.

    (D) their sizes varies.

24. Fig. 6–3 represents a longitudinal scan taken to the right of midline. Which of the following structures is indicated by the arrow?

    (A) the proximal urethra

    (B) a seminal vesicle

    (C) the verumontanum

    (D) the ejaculatory duct

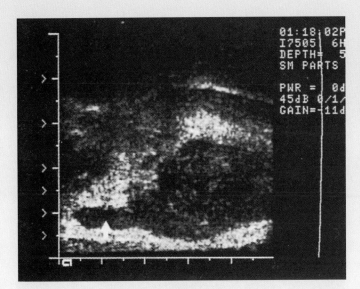

FIGURE 6–3. Longitudinal scan to the right of midline.

25. Fig. 6–4 represents a transverse scan. Which of the following structures are the arrows pointing to?

(A) a tumor in the peripheral zone

(B) prostatitis involving the periurethral areas

(C) central gland calcification

(D) distortion of the prostatic capsule

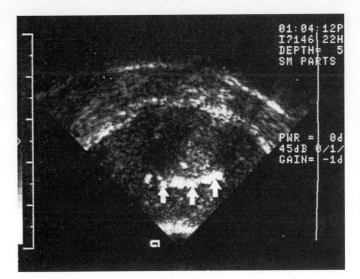

FIGURE 6–4. Transverse scan of the prostate.

26. Fig. 6–5 represents a longitudinal scan of a 60-year-old patient presenting with urinary frequency. He was referred for an endorectal prostate sonography examination. What area is outlined by the white arrow?

(A) obliteration of the "prostate-seminal vesicle angle"

(B) a hypoechoic mass in the central zone

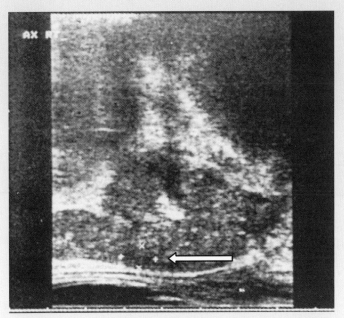

FIGURE 6–5. Longitudinal scan of the prostate.

(C) a tumor in the peripheral zone

(D) bulging of the prostatic capsule

27. Fig. 6–6 represents a longitudinal scan. What region is indicated by the white arrow?

(A) the fibromuscular stroma

(B) the seminal vesicle

(C) the peripheral zone

(D) the central zone

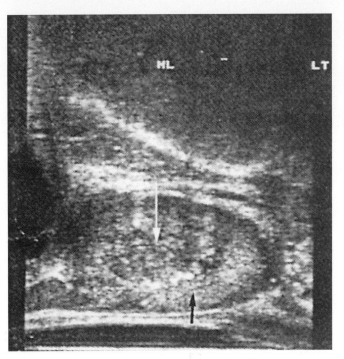

FIGURE 6–6. Longitudinal scan of the prostate.

28. Fig. 6–6 represents a longitudinal scan. What region is indicated by the black arrow?

    (A) the peripheral zone

    (B) the central zone

    (C) the prostatic capsule

    (D) the vas deferens

29. Fig. 6–7 represents a longitudinal scan taken from a patient presenting with a history of infertility. The white arrow most likely indicates which of the following findings?

    (A) benign prostatic hypertrophy

    (B) a cyst in the ejaculatory duct

    (C) extension of a tumor into the nipple region

    (D) central gland disease

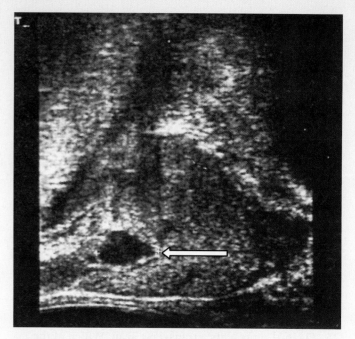

FIGURE 6–7. Longitudinal scan of the prostate.

Answers and Explanations

At the end of each explained answer, there is a number combination in parentheses. The first number identifies the reference source; the second number or set of numbers indicates the page or pages on which the relevant information can be found.

1. **(D)** Both A and C. The fibromuscular stroma is a nonglandular region that covers the anterior surface of the prostate. Therefore, both A and C are correct. *(1:396)*

2. **(D)** Differentiation of a benign from a malignant nodule by imaging. Ultrasound cannot make a specific diagnosis of prostatic diseases. Biopsy is required to establish the diagnosis. *(1:411)*

3. **(A)** The left lateral decubitus. Patients who are having endorectal prostate sonography are usually examined in the left lateral decubitus position. *(1:402)*

4. **(D)** It is the primary site of adenocarcinoma. The transitional zone is located on both sides of the proximal urethra and represents 5% of the gland. It also is the primary site of benign prostatic hyperplasia. *(1:397)*

5. **(B)** The central zone is located at the apex of the prostate. The central zone is a triangular structure located at the base of the prostate with its apex at the verumontanum. *(1:397)*

6. **(C)** 70%. The peripheral zone constitutes more than two-thirds of prostatic glandular tissue. *(1:396)*

7. **(A)** Its apex is located inferiorly and the base of the prostate is located superiorly. *(See Fig. 6–1B in the Study Guide.)*

8. **(C)** Secretion of seminal fluid. The prostate discharges this fluid into the urethra to enhance the motility of sperm. *(2:2)*

9. **(B)** The vas deferens. The seminal vesicles join the vas deferens to form the ejaculatory duct, which passes through the central zone. *(See Fig. 6–1B in the Study Guide.)*

10. **(D)** Urethra. The ejaculatory duct empties into the urethra at the verumontanum. *(See Fig. 6–1B in the Study Guide.)*

11. **(C)** The posterior-superior surface. *(See Fig. 6–1B in the Study Guide.)*

12. **(A)** It originates mainly in the central zone. Seventy percent of prostatic cancers originate *de novo* in the peripheral zone. *(1:411)*

13. **(A)** A hypoechoic gland with anechoic areas. *(1:403)*

14. **(D)** The transitional zone. *(1:403)*

15. **(B)** They are calcified deposits in the prostate. *(1:402)*

16. **(D)** Marked compression of the prostatic urethra. Early prostatic cancer can present as hypoechoic lesions on the peripheral zone. They can break through the prostatic capsule causing distortion, or they can invade the seminal vesicles. *(1:412)*

17. **(D)** A digital rectal examination. This examination should be done before the probe is inserted to exclude obstructing lesions and to correlate the imaging study with the digital rectal exam. *(1:402)*

18. **(D)** Sonographically variable. Prostate cancer can be hypoechoic, hyperechoic, or isoechoic. *(1:412)*

19. **(A)** A midpoint region between the base and apex of the prostate. *(See Fig. 6–1B in the Study Guide.)*

20. **(D)** Obstruction of the seminal vesicle. An elevated prostatic-specific antigen (PSA) may be indicated in prostate cancer, prostatitis, or benign prostatic hyperplasia (BPH). *(1:410)*

21. **(A)** The central zone. *(See Fig. 6–1B in the Study Guide.)*

22. **(B)** The normal postpubescent prostate weighs approximately 20 g. *(Study Guide:349)*

23. **(A)** Their absence does not usually affect fertility. In rare cases, infertility can be caused by absence of the seminal vesicles or by an obstruction in the ejaculatory ducts. *(1:405)*

24. **(B)** A seminal vesicle. The structure demonstrated in Fig. 6–1B is the right seminal vesicle, that joins the vas deferens (not shown) to form the ejaculatory duct. *(Study Guide: Fig. 6–1B)*

25. **(C)** Central gland calcification. Fig. 6–4 shows bright echoes representing prostatic calcification, which can be solitary or can occur in clusters. *(Study Guide:351)*

26. **(C)** A tumor in the peripheral zone. The hypoechoic mass seen on the peripheral zone in Fig. 6–4 is characteristic of prostatic cancer. *(Study Guide:351)*

27. **(D)** The central zone. The zone (white arrow) in Fig. 6–6 is clearly demarcated from the peripheral zone (black arrow) by a curved band of echoes. *(Study Guide:350)*

28. **(A)** The peripheral zone. *(Study Guide:350)*

29. **(B)** A cyst in the ejaculatory duct. The cystic structure shown in Fig. 6–7 is clearly located within the ejaculatory duct. *(Study Guide:350)*

References

1. Toi A, Bree R. The prostate. In: Rumack C, Wilson S, Charboneau W, et al. *Diagnostic Ultrasound.* 3rd ed., vol. 1. St. Louis, MO: Mosby; 2005.

2. Paulson D. Diseases of the prostate. *Clin Symposia.* 1989; 41.

7

Obstetrical and Gynecologic Sonography and Transvaginal Sonography

Charles S. Odwin, Cynthia A. Silkowski, and Arthur C. Fleischer

Study Guide

PATIENT CARE PREPARATION AND TECHNIQUES

Before starting an ultrasound examination, a thorough review of the patient's history is needed.

You should introduce yourself to the patient and explain the scanning techniques utilized for the procedure. Patients have the right to refuse the ultrasound. Menstrual history, abnormal vaginal bleeding, pain, and previous surgery should be obtained in the history.

The patient's referral diagnosis and clinical symptoms should be kept in mind as the history is reviewed. Often, the history will give clues as to the current abnormality. It is important to review the patient's reproductive history as well. Gravida (G) refers to the pregnancies. Primigravida is a first time pregnancy; multigravida is many pregnancies. Nulligravida is a patient that has never been pregnant. Parity (P) is the condition of a woman with respect to her having borne viable offspring. Typically, parity is displayed as a four-digit series. The first number being the term births, the second number being preterm births, the third number being abortions (spontaneous, elective, missed or ectopic pregnancy) as well as complications of pregnancy <20 weeks resulting in abortion, and the fourth number being the number of living children.[1] The duration of a pregnancy can be calculated from the first day of the last normal menstrual period and is referred to as menstrual age. The average duration of a pregnancy is approximately 280 days, 40 weeks, 9 calendar months, or 10 lunar months.[1] The expected date of delivery can be estimated by Nagele's rule, which is based on a 28-day menstrual cycle:

- Identify the date when the last menstrual period began
- Add 7 days
- Subtract 3 months
- Add 1 year

In addition to the medical history, laboratory tests should also be reviewed. For gynecologic sonograms, all blood work should be reviewed. An elevated white blood cell count could help diagnose an infectious mass, for example. Other tests might include pap smears, biopsies, and ovarian cancer screening tests (CA 125). For the obstetric patient, there are many laboratory tests that may be available at different stages in the pregnancy. Blood type should always be noted, as well as any antibody titers. In early pregnancy, serum hCG (human chorionic gonadotropin) titers may suggest failed pregnancy, ectopic pregnancy, or a normal intrauterine pregnancy depending on the levels.

Both gestational sac growth and hCG production relate to trophoblastic function. Any discrepancy between the two can suggest an abnormality in development. Markedly increased hCG may suggest twins or molar pregnancies. In the second trimester, all pregnant women may elect to have maternal serum alpha-fetoprotein (MSAF3) triple screen test, or alpha-fetoprotein 3 (AFP3). The number three refers to the markers tested, including AFP. These are unconjugated estriol and hCG. Assessment of MSAFP3 values is also related to such maternal factors as age, weight, diabetic status, multiple gestation, and race. Screening markers are used to calculate a woman's risk of having a child with Down syndrome or neural tube defects.

Proper documentation is pertinent to any medical examination. The images should be labeled with patient identification and the anatomy shown on the image. If any abnormalities are identified, the images should also be labeled according to location so that others reviewing the images can locate the abnormality. All exams should be documented in some form of hard copy, such as x-ray film, optic disc, thermal paper, hard drive, or DVD. In addition, a written report of the exam should be included with the hard copy. The picture archiving and communications systems (PACS) is a digital image storage device that is currently replacing the previously mentioned hard copy. The device enables images such as ultrasound, x-ray, computed tomography (CT), and magnetic resonance imaging (MRI) to be digitally stored and viewed on a screen without fading or distortion. The final report may contain varied information but should include any measurements, reason for exam, ultrasound findings, and the doctor's impression. For billing and coding purposes, all reports must contain a diagnosis derived from the exam or referral diagnosis that supports the billing code.

TRANSDUCER PREPARATION

Hand washing should be done before and after every sonographic procedure in order to reduce hospital-acquired infection. Based on American Institute of Ultrasound in Medicine (AIUM) guidelines, on completion of the exam, all transabdominal probes should have excess gel wiped off with a clean towel and cleaned with a disinfectant cleaner. Commercially available moist towelettes work well and are easy to use.

Transvaginal probes are reusable intracavity instruments. Therefore, precautionary measures should be addressed. The microorganisms that cause sexually transmitted disease, including the human immunodeficiency virus (HIV), are sometimes present in the vaginal secretions. Although these microorganisms are usually transmitted through sexual contact with an infected partner, they can be transmitted by contaminated reusable instruments. The current methods used to prevent transmission of infection with transvaginal transducers are as follows:

1. Chemical disinfectants
2. Disposable probe cover (condoms, latex gloves, and sheaths)

Both are required to prevent cross-infection from the transducer because although the probe is covered, a microscopic tear in the cover will expose the transducer to the vaginal membrane and the external cervical os. The transducer should be disinfected before it is returned to the manufacturer or technical support staff for maintenance or repair.

The first steps in preparing the transducer for an examination is disinfecting the probe from disease-causing organism bacteria, viruses, and fungi. Several methods of disinfecting agents are available; most are cold chemical disinfectants, which are glutaraldehyde based (e.g., Cidex, MetriCide, Wavicide). The piezoelectric crystal of the transducer is heat sensitive. Therefore, steam autoclaves should not be used because excessive heat could destroy the transducer. The transducer manufacturers normally recommend the type of chemical that is safe for their transducers, specifications, and the time limit for transducer chemical immersion.

Transvaginal transducers are composed of metals, plastic, crystal, and bonding materials, and all are not constructed in the same way. Thus, a disinfectant chemical may be safe for some transducers but destructive to others. Sonographers should not attempt to disinfect a transducer until they have carefully reviewed the manufacturer's instruction manual and consulted with the technical support staff regarding any changes that may have occurred since the manual was published. To avoid chemical spills and reduce chemical vapors to health care workers, a commercially available immersion station can be used but must comply with Occupational Safety and Health Administration (OSHA) and Joint Commission on Accreditation of Healthcare Organizations (JCAHO) regulatory requirements.

In addition to disinfectant requirements, a probe cover is employed. The probe covers are specially designed sheaths for covering the transducers; they are available in different sizes to fit all types of transducers. These covers are made of a variety of materials such as latex, polyethylene, and polyurethane and are approved by the U.S. Food and Drug Administration (FDA). Probe covers are also available in sterile or nonsterile packs. Patient and health care workers with latex hypersensitivity should use alternative covers and gloves. The used probe covers and gloves should be treated as potentially infectious waste and disposed of accordingly.

INTRODUCTION TO TRANSVAGINAL SONOGRAPHY

Transvaginal sonography (TVS) involves the insertion of a specifically designed transducer into the vagina for imaging pelvic structures. Numerous names have been applied to this type of scanning such as endovaginal, endocavity, endosonography, and transvaginal. The terms transvaginal and endovaginal are both descriptive of the technical approach to scanning and are not specific for imaging of the vagina. In fact, only a small area of the vagina is imaged; the images are predominantly of the uterus and its adnexa.

PHYSICAL CONCEPTS

The concept of using high-frequency transducers within the vaginal cavity to image the uterus and adnexa derived from the basic concept of ultrasound physics. Placing the transducer in close proximity to the pelvic organs or structures allows the use of higher frequencies, which in turn provide better resolution, both axial and lateral. The close proximity of the transducer also results in reduced attenuation and better focusing. As a result, transvaginal sonography allows for earlier and more definitive diagnosis than is possible with conventional transabdominal techniques.

Transvaginal sonography (TVS) has many clinical obstetrical and gynecologic applications because of its ability to delineate the uterus and its adnexa. These include:

- Evaluation of the endometrium in women with postmenopausal bleeding or dysfunctional uterine bleeding (DUB)
- Evaluation of pelvic masses
- Diagnosis of ectopic pregnancy and other complicated early pregnancy
- Evaluation of the cervix
- Monitoring the follicles of an infertile patient who is undergoing ovulation induction
- Guiding the placement of the needle during follicular inspiration or aspiration of fluid from the cul-de-sac
- Evaluation of the fallopian tube
- Evaluation of blood flow to the gestational sac and uterine artery with Doppler imaging
- Achieving additional diagnostic information in conjunction with transabdominal sonography
- Detecting the presence of placenta previa
- Evaluation of the fetal intracranial anatomy and prolapse of the umbilical cord during the second and third trimesters

CONTRAINDICATIONS TO TRANSVAGINAL SONOGRAPHY

- Patients who decline the procedure
- Infants and children
- Virgins
- Elderly patients with narrow introitus or atrophic vaginitis who experience pain or discomfort during probe insertion
- Unconscious patient (without informed consent)
- Mentally insane (without a health care proxy or an administrative consent)

ADVANTAGES OF TRANSVAGINAL SONOGRAPHY

- Higher resolution
- Earlier and more definitive diagnosis
- Does **not** require a full urinary bladder
- Faster medical management
- Additional information
- Eliminates the discomfort during bladder filling

DISADVANTAGES OF TRANSVAGINAL SONOGRAPHY

- Limited field of view
- Large masses may not be seen because they are beyond the focal zone of the transducer
- Unable to see both ovaries on the same image
- Documentation of uterine size may be difficult because of magnification in the near field
- The confined space of the vagina limits the mobility of the transducer; therefore, complete sequential images obtained with transabdominal sonography cannot be achieved with transvaginal sonography
- Only the presenting parts of the fetus and cervix can be seen in the second and third trimester pregnancy with the transvaginal approach

PATIENT PREPARATION

The patient should void before the examination begins, and the procedure should be explained to the patient. If a male examiner is to perform the examination, a female chaperone should be present during the entire examination. The staff in the room should be introduced to the patient. The chaperone should be a permanent staff member of the faculty who is familiar with the procedure. Volunteers and family members are not appropriate chaperones. The name of the chaperone and time of the procedure should be documented.

TRANSDUCERS

Transducers for transvaginal scanning have a specific size, shape, and frequency. Their diameter ranges from 12 to 16 mm; this smaller-than-usual diameter allows easy penetration within the vaginal lumen without patient discomfort. In addition, these transducers are twice as long when compared to transabdominal transducers.

Because the normal length of the vaginal lumen is approximately 7.5–9.5 cm, the transvaginal transducer must be longer so that part of it can be inserted and the other part can serve as a handle for the operator. The normal range of frequency used in transvaginal sonography is 5–10 MHz, with a sector field of view of 90°–115°. The larger the sector fields of view, the larger the portion of the organ or structure that can be visualized.

COLOR DOPPLER SONOGRAPHY (CDS)

Transvaginal color Doppler is a combination of B-mode image, pulse-wave Doppler, and a color-flow display (triplex imaging). The direction of blood flow is indicated by assigning color to the Doppler-shifted echoes that are superimposed on the gray-scale image.

The direction of flow toward and away from the transducer is presented in different colors on the image. For example, red represents flow toward the transducer, whereas blue represents flow away from the transducer, and a mixture of colors represents turbulent flow. Color Doppler has several advantages. First, because a network of blood vessels occasionally can mimic

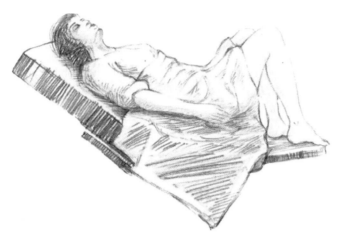

FIGURE 7–1. Examination table in a slight Fowler's position with a 20° elevation. The patient is in the lithotomy position.

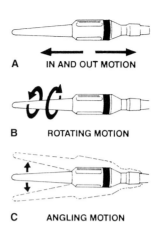

FIGURE 7–2. Scanning techniques: (**A**) in and out; (**B**) rotating motion; (**C**) angling motion. *(Reproduced with permission from Philips Healthcare.)*

follicles, color Doppler allows rapid differentiation between vascular structures and follicles. It also allows precise placement of the sample volume for Doppler waveform analysis.

POSITION OF THE PATIENT AND THE EXAMINATION TABLE

During the transvaginal examination, the patient is placed in the lithotomy position for insertion of the transducer and for scanning. The probe can be inserted by the patient, the physician, or the sonographer. When the patient does the insertion, the transducer cable should be held so that the patient cannot accidentally drop the transducer.

The ideal table is a gynecologic examination table that allows numerous degrees of pelvic tilt positions and has stirrups for the patient's heels. The table is placed in a slight Fowler's position (also called the reversed Trendelenburg position) (Fig. 7–1). Elevation of the thighs allows the transducer to be moved freely from side to side (horizontal plane). The gynecologic examination table allows free upward and downward movement of the transducer (vertical plane), and the slight Fowler's position of the table allows pooling of the small amount of peritoneal fluid normally found in the region of the cul-de-sac, which allows better delineation of pelvic structures. The Trendelenburg position should not be used because it drains away this fluid. If a gynecologic examination table is unavailable, a flat examination table can be prepared by placing a cushion or inverted bedpan under the patient's pelvis.

SCANNING TECHNIQUES

The commonly used transducer maneuvers for transvaginal sonography are:

a) In and out Fig. 7–2 (A)

b) Rotation Fig. 7–2 (B)

c) Anterior and posterior angulations Fig. 7–2 (C)

d) Right adnexal angulation Fig. 7–3 (D)

e) Left adnexal angulation Fig. 7–3 (E)

These maneuvers are limited by the size of the vaginal lumen. Fig. 7–2(A) illustrates the in-and-out motion of the transducer used to achieve variation in the depth of the imaging from the cervix to fundus. Imaging from cervix is optimized by gradual withdrawing the probe with up angulations. Fig. 7–2(B) illustrates the rotating motion of the transducer for obtaining various degrees of semiaxial to semicoronal planes. Fig. 7–2(C) illustrates the angling motion of the transducer within the vaginal canal to obtain images of the anterior and posterior cul-de-sac. The side-to-side movements used are to obtain images of the adnexa (Fig.7–3 D and E).

SONOHYSTEROGRAPHY

The recently developed technique for evaluation of the endometrium using saline infusion into the endometrial lumen during transvaginal sonography, termed sonohysterography is becoming more frequently used in the gynecologist's office or sonographic suites for the evaluation of suspected endometrial or certain myometrial disorders.[2] The technique provides a means to detect polypoid endometrial lesions, submucosal fibroids, adhesions, and uterine malformations that affect the lumen and can cause bleeding or infertility. Because the CPT code that is used for billing is listed as "sonohysterography," this is the preferred term.

Sonohysterography plays an important role in evaluation of the patient with unexplained postmenopausal bleeding and in those patients in whom the endometrium is thickened or indistinct on transvaginal sonography. Polyps are enigmatic tumors apparently caused by resistance to progesterone-induced apoptosis or exposure to excess endogenous or exogenous estrogen. They typically are associated with intermenstrual bleeding, cramping, or infertility. Carcinomas may also be polypoid or arise within polyps.[3] Sonohysterography affords clear detection

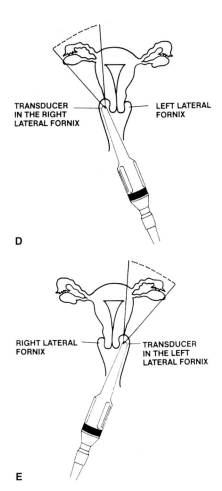

D

E

FIGURE 7–3. **(D)** Transducer in the right lateral fornix. **(E)** Transducer in the left lateral fornix. *(Reproduced with permission from Philips Healthcare.)*

of the polyp and its pedicle. This is in contrast to a thickened endometrium as a result of endometrial hyperplasia or carcinoma.

Intraluminal fluid collections are frequently seen on transvaginal sonography. Although they may be associated with endometrial cancer in some patients, they are more frequently associated with such benign conditions as cervical stenosis.[3] Sonohysterography can be used advantageously to outline endometrial surfaces. This review provides an overview to the clinical utility of sonohysterography, its limitations, as well as a discussion of the circumstances in which it should be ordered.

TECHNIQUE

With the more extensive use of transvaginal sonography and small flexible catheters, the possibility of improved delineation of the endometrial lumen with intraluminal fluid instillation became possible.[3] The technique uses sterile saline as a negative (anechoic) contrast media to outline the endometrial lumen under continuous transvaginal sonographic visualization.[4]

Sonohysterography is primarily used for evaluation of endometrial polyps, assessing the presence and extent of submucosal

fibroids, detection of uterine synechiae, and in selected cases of uterine malformations that involve the endometrial lumen. The reader is referred to several excellent descriptions of the spectrum of sonographic findings with this technique.[3,5]

Before saline instillation, the standard procedure for transvaginal sonography is followed, including covering the probe with a condom and placement of the transvaginal probe within the vaginal fornix and midvagina to optimally delineate the endometrial interfaces in both the long and short axes. The images should be recorded on hard-copy film, PACS, or DVD for later review.

Sonohysterography involves placement of a catheter into the uterine lumen through the endocervical canal. Catheter choices that can be used include insemination catheter, pediatric Foley, pediatric feeding tube, a plastic sonohysterography catheter, or a specially designed flexible catheter with an introducer (Akrad Co, Cranford, NJ). The Akrad catheter is preferred, because it can be introduced easily through the introducer into the cervix without much pain or discomfort (Fig. 7–4). The balloon catheter is recommended when trying to evaluate the uterine lumen for patency. Once the cervix is cleansed with a cleansing solution and stabilized with a speculum, the catheter can be advanced into the lumen, and 3–10 mL of sterile saline is injected during sonographic visualization. The slow instillation of saline, allowing reflux out of the cervix, also diminishes the possibility of pain during installation. The endometrium is imaged in both long and short axes, with specific attention to its regularity and thickness (Figs. 7–5, 7–6, and 7–7). Because of the dynamic nature of the examination, DVD recording of the procedure is recommended with a few representative frozen images recorded for interpretation.

The procedure is best performed in the early follicular phase. This avoids confusing images arising from mildly irregular interdigitating secretory endometrium or clot that may be encountered in the late secretory portion of the cycle and also decreases the possibility of dislodging an unsuspected early pregnancy. Because most endometrial polyps are echogenic,

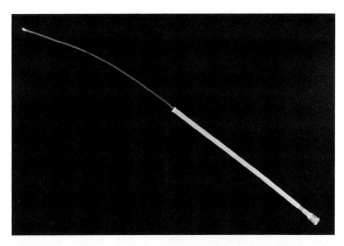

FIGURE 7–4. Tampa catheter consists of an introducer and flexible catheter.

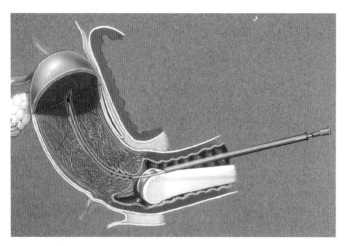

FIGURE 7–5. Diagram showing catheter in place. The catheter is advanced over the introducer and the tip is best positioned in the fundal position of the endometrial lumen.

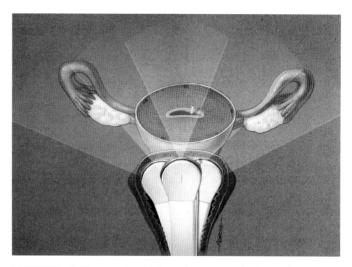

FIGURE 7–7. Diagram showing transducer sweep in short axis.

they can best be seen against the relatively hypoechoic proliferative phase endometrium.[5] Conversely, submucosal fibroids may best be imaged in the secretory phase because they are typically hypoechoic, and their relation to the displaced endometrium may be best delineated during this phase of the cycle.

Contraindications to sonohysterography include hematometra, extensive pelvic inflammatory disease, or significant cervical stenosis. Doxycycline (100 mg p.o. bid). can be given a few days before sonohysterography if pelvic inflammatory disease (PID) is suspected. Rarely an atrophic or stenotic vagina from aging or previous radiation therapy can produce significant discomfort, even with placement of the vaginal speculum.

Typically, the patient does not experience significant discomfort if the catheter is properly placed in the fundus, and only small amounts of fluid are gently infused and allowed to reflux out of the cervix. Prophylactic antibiotics are usually not needed, but preprocedural, nonsteroidal anti-inflammatory drugs (NSAIDs) are helpful to minimize uterine cramping.

TYPICAL SONOGRAPHIC FINDINGS

The intraluminal surface of the normal endometrium is usually delineated in its entirety after the introduction of intraluminal fluid. On short axis, the normal areas of endometrial invagination in both tubal ostia can be seen. In general, the endometrium measures up to 3 mm in thickness per single layer and should have a relatively regular and homogenous texture. The secretory phase endometrium is mildly irregular and may contain "endometrial wrinkles" a few millimeters in height, representing focal thickening in the interdigitated endometrial surface. The endometrium is typically similar in thickness and texture, but focal irregularities can be observed in some patients (Figs. 7–8 and 7–9).

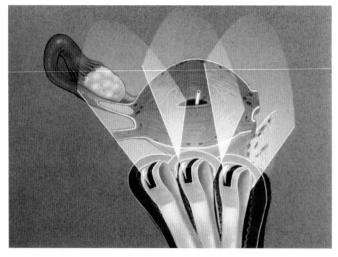

FIGURE 7–6. Diagram showing transducer sweep in long axis.

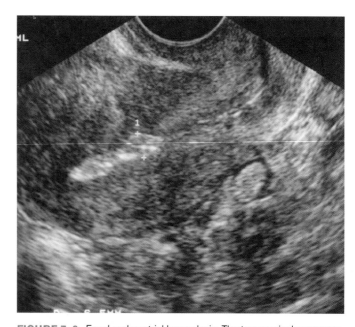

FIGURE 7–8. Focal endometrial hyperplasia. The transvaginal sonogram shows focal thickening (between cursors) in the corpus.

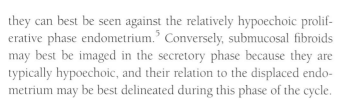

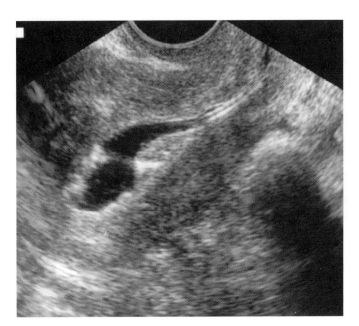

FIGURE 7–9. Focal endometrial hyperplasia. After saline is instilled, there is focal thickening of the endometrium, which was found to represent hyperplasia.

POLYPS

Endometrial polyps are typically echogenic and project into the endometrial lumen (Fig. 7–10). In the nondistended endometrium, they typically displace the median echo, which may represent refluxed cervical mucus, and are best seen just before ovulation. As they enlarge, they can distend the cavity and may be apparent without iatrogenic distention of the endometrial lumen. Some are outlined by trapped intraluminal fluid, mucus, or blood. The vascularity of the pedicle can be demonstrated in some cases with transvaginal color Doppler sonography.

SUBMUCOSAL FIBROIDS

Submucosal fibroids are typically hypoechoic and displace the basalis layer of the endometrium. Amount of extension into the myometrial layers is important to distinguish superficial

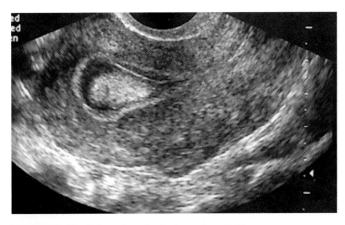

FIGURE 7–10. Echogenic polyp in the endometrial lumen.

submucosal fibroids from those that extend into the lumen may be treated with wire loop resections from the lumen, whereas submucosal or intramural fibroids require a transperitoneal approach. If a submucosal fibroid has a thin stalk, it may be removed by wire loop or alligator forceps, whereas those that extend beyond the endometrial–myometrial interface will not be amenable to wire loop resection.

SYNECHIAE

Synechiae typically occur as the sequelae of intrauterine instrumentation. They may be either echogenic or hypoechoic, depending on their fibrous content. The hypoechoic synechiae are best delineated in the background of the typically echogenic secretory phase endometrium.[6]

OTHER

Certain uterine malformations that affect the lumen, such as bicornuate or septated uteri, may be evaluated using 3D ultrasound and color doppler sonography (CDS). The presence or absence of a fundal cleft is important in distinguishing bicornuate uteri from septated uteri.

Color Doppler sonography may be helpful to identify the vascular pedicle of a polyp, as well as the vascular rim of certain leiomyomata. Sonohysterography is helpful in determining whether a polyp has a wide or narrow pedicle because those with a thin pedicle are more easily removed with a forceps in the office than those with a thick pedicle.

Sonohysterography is also particularly helpful in determining whether certain intraluminal cystic areas are within a polyp or the myometrium. Punctate cystic spaces are frequently seen within polyps as a result of glandular obstruction. They may also be seen within the myometrium in women who are on tamoxifen or a selective estrogen receptor modulator (SERM), possibly a result of reactivation of dormant adenomyosis.[2]

Sonohysterography affords detailed delineation of the endometrial surface. Polyps, submucosal fibroids, and synechiae are readily delineated using this technique.

This study guide provides a description of the major applications of TVS in obstetrics and gynecology. The reader is referred to the references listed at the end of this chapter for further information.

GYNECOLOGY (NORMAL PELVIC ANATOMY)

The female pelvic reproductive organs are divided into the external and internal genitalia.

The external genitalia is called vulva. The vulva or pudendum is a term for external genital organs that are visible on the skin. The internal genital organs are located in the true pelvis and are only visible during medical imaging or surgery.

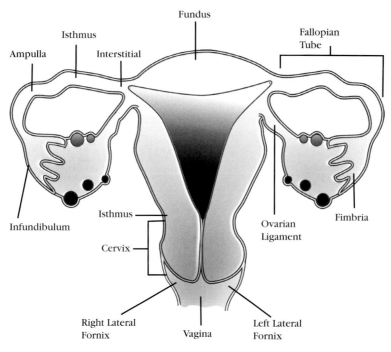

FIGURE 7–11. Diagram of the normal female internal reproductive organs.

Uterus

The uterus is situated medially in the pelvis and posteriorly to the urinary bladder and anteriorly to the rectum. The uterus can be divided into four different regions: (1) cervix, (2) isthmus, (3) corpus, and (4) fundus (Fig. 7–11). The uterus has three primary functions: (1) menstruation, (2) pregnancy, and (3) labor. The cervix is the inferior portion of the uterus and invaginates into the vagina. The isthmus is superior to the cervix and begins at the internal os of the cervix. The corpus or body of the uterus is larger than the cervix. The fundus is the uppermost portion of the uterus and is located superiorly to where the fallopian tubes arise from the uterus.

The uterus is composed of three layers of tissue:

1. Peritoneum (uterine covering)
2. Myometrium (uterine muscle)
3. Endometrium (uterine cavity)

The outer layer, or peritoneum, is the serosal layer. The muscular portion of the uterus is called the myometrium. The inner layer, where the two walls of the uterus meet, is called the endometrium. This layer varies in thickness and echogenicity with the menstrual cycle, and is described later in the chapter. The peritoneum is serous membrane that forms the lining of the abdominal and pelvic cavity. A fold of peritoneum forms three potential spaces in the female pelvic region, which are important to pelvic sonography. The peritoneum that covers the anterior surface of the uterus and the upper aspect of the bladder forms a cul-de-sac called anterior cul-de-sac or vesicouterine pouch. The peritoneum also covers the posterior surface of the uterus and

the anterior surface of the rectum called the posterior cul-de-sac or pouch of Douglas. This is the most dependent position of the potential space, thus allowing any blood or free-fluid collections to accumulate in this space. A small amount of fluid is sometimes identified in the pouch of Douglas due to follicular fluid secondary to ovulation. The third peritoneal space is anterior to the bladder and is termed the prevesical or retropubic space.[1]

The myometrium is homogeneous in echo texture except in cases of fibroids, which can cause multiple changes in the normal texture of the uterus. On occasion, a portion of the myometrium painlessly contracts causing a focal thickness lasting 20–30 minutes. This will spontaneously disappear with time. This finding is physiologic and should not be confused with a pathologic finding. Transvaginal sonography provides an objective means to evaluate the uterine cervical length and configuration. The normal cervix is between 2.0 and 2.5 cm in length and shows no funneling or dilatation of the endocervical canal. A thin echogenic stripe in the endocervical canal can be seen in most cases and is contiguous with the endometrial canal (Fig. 7–12). The endocervical canal opens into the vagina at the external os of the cervix. A single or multiple small cyst masses are sometimes seen in and around the cervical canal and represent nabothian cysts (mucinous retention cyst), which are caused by occlusion of the ducts of the cervical secreting glands (Fig. 7–13).

The size of the uterus varies and is dependent on the patient's age and gestational status. Before puberty and after menopause, the uterus is small in size. During reproductive years, an increase in gravida usually results in an increase in uterine size.[1] A prepubertal uterus is 2–4 cm in length, with the corpus (or body of uterus) half the length of the cervix. In an adult nulliparous

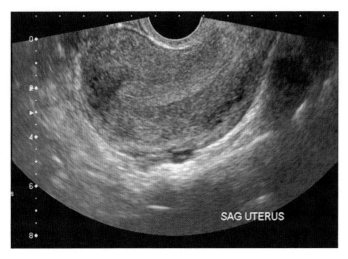

FIGURE 7–12. Transvaginal sonogram of the endometrium in long axis.

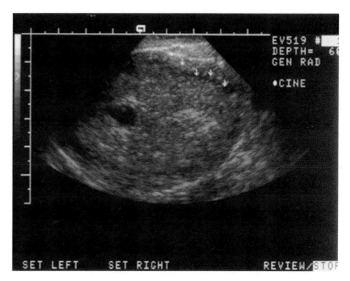

FIGURE 7–14. Transvaginal sonogram of the uterus in short axis. Small arrows points to the arcuate plexus.

woman, the uterine length is 6–8 cm, width 3–5 cm, and antero-posterior dimension 2–4 cm. The corpus and cervix are equal in length. An adult multiparous uterus is 8–9 cm × 4–5 cm × 3–5 cm with the corpus twice the length of the cervix. In post-menopausal women, the uterus atrophies, regardless of the gravida status premenopausally. The uterine measurements of a postmenopausal woman are 6.5–3.5 cm in length, 2–3 cm in width, and 2 cm anteroposterior dimensions.[3] Because of the magnification and the relatively small field of view provided by transvaginal sonography, measurements to indicate the size of the uterus are best obtained with transabdominal sonography. The uterus can vary slightly in position depending on the dis-tention of the bladder. The following descriptions refer to uter-ine position with an empty bladder. Ninety percent of the time, the uterus tilts forward in an anteverted position, meaning the uterus forms a 90° angle with the posterior vaginal wall. The uterus, however, may be in any of the following positions:

- Anteverted: The uterus tilts forward with a 90° angle to the posterior vaginal wall.

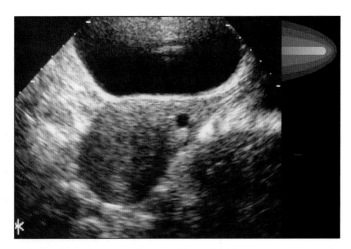

FIGURE 7–13. Retroverted uterus with a nabothian cyst.

- Anteflexed: The uterine corpus is flexed anteriorly on the cervix, forming a sharp angle at the cervix.
- Retroverted: The uterus tilts backward without a sharp angle between the corpus and cervix.
- Retroflexed: The uterine corpus is flexed posteriorly on the cervix, forming a sharp angle at the cervix.
- Medianus: Midline position.
- Dextroversion: Right lateral deviation.
- Levoversion: Left lateral deviation.

Blood Supply to the Uterus

The uterine and ovarian arteries are branches of the internal iliac (hypogastric) artery. The uterine artery travels superiorly from the cervix, running laterally to the uterus in the broad ligament. At the junction of the uterus and fallopian tubes, the uterine artery joins with the ovarian artery. The uterine artery gives rise to the arcuate arteries, which course within the outer myometrium (Fig. 7–14) identifying the arcuate venous plexus. Imaging of these vessels can be enhanced with color vaginal sonography. The arcuate arteries branch into the radial arteries, which supply the inner layers of the myometrium and endo-metrium. They then branch into the straight and spiral arteries, which supply the endometrium. The venous channels of the pelvis follow a course similar to the arteries.[1]

Congenital Abnormalities of the Uterus

Congenital abnormalities of the uterus result from improper fusion of the mullerian or paramesonephric ducts. As the ducts fuse, the septum that separates them breaks down, resulting in a single uterine cavity. The lack of fusion results in differ-ent uterine malformation, as shown in Fig. 7–15. Because of the close development of the corpus and cervix of the uterus, a uterine malformation may also affect the cervix and play a

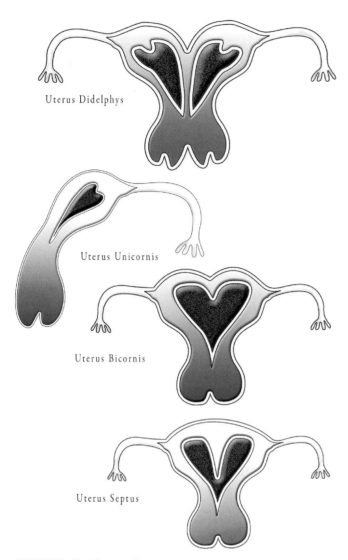

FIGURE 7-15. Diagram of common types of congenital uterine abnormalities.

part in its function during pregnancy. The uterus develops in synchronicity with the urinary system. When congenital uterine abnormalities are present, the kidneys should be evaluated sonographically.[3] In the absent of a kidney or an ectopic kidney, the uterus should be scanned for malformations. The bicornuate uterus is well recognized sonographically by two endometrial echoes in the cavities, which are widely separated.

Endometrium

The endometrial lining is the innermost layer of the uterus. It is greatly influenced by hormones and is responsible for accepting the embryo for implantation. Transvaginal sonography provides detailed delineation of the thickness and texture of the endometrium. The endometrium should be measured in its thickest anterior/posterior thickness as portrayed in its long axis (bilayer thickness).

Although the image and measurement are used to characterize the endometrium, they must be evaluated completely and characterized by scanning sweeps performed in the long and short axis of the uterus. In women of childbearing age, the endometrium measures between 3 and 6 mm in the proliferative phase (days 5–9 postmenstruation) and up to 14–16 mm in the secretory phase (days 14–28).

The texture changes from isoechoic to multilayered in midcycle to echogenic in the midsecretory phase. In postmenopausal women, the endometrial lining atrophies. Any uterine bleeding during this stage is considered abnormal.[3] A common cause of vaginal bleeding in postmenopausal women is endometrial hyperplasia.[5] In a postmenopausal woman, the endometrium should be 6 mm bilayer thickness and homogenous in texture. This is true for most women taking hormone replacement therapy. Punctate cysts can be seen in the inner myometrium in women taking tamoxifen. These are thought to represent reactivated adenomyomas. Polyps typically appear as echogenic endometrial masses that are insinuated between endometrial layers. They are especially seen when saline infusion SHG is performed.

Endometrial carcinoma typically causes asymmetry and irregularity of the endometrium. If there is invasion, the endometrial–myometrial junction is disrupted. Endometrial cancer is more commonly diagnosed in women 60–70 years of age but can occur at earlier ages. Symptoms may include metrorrhagia, menorrhagia, or both. Clinically, these symptoms are similar to endometrial hyperplasia and polyps. In woman not on hormone replacement therapy, the endometrial lining may be increased >5–6 mm on sonogram. An endometrial lining of > 5 mm is generally considered abnormal in postmenopausal patients on hormone replacement therapy.[2,3] The endometrial lining appears echogenic and may have irregular contours of the endometrium as the cancer invades into the myometrium. The diagnosis is made by endometrial biopsy.[2,3,5]

Ovaries

The ovaries are ellipsoid in shape, measuring approximately 3 cm in long axis and 2 cm in anteroposterior and transverse dimensions.[5] The ovaries are located lateral to the uterus in the ovarian fossa (also known as the fossa of Waldeyer). The ovarian fossa is bound laterally by the internal iliac artery and vein. The medial boundary is the uterus.[1] The normal ovaries are homogeneous in echo texture with the medulla appearing more echogenic. Multiple small follicular cysts may be seen peripherally in the cortex (Fig. 7–16). In most cases, transvaginal ultrasound gives a better visualization of the ovaries due to the close proximity of the transducer, which allows a higher frequency transducer to be used. This in turn provides better resolution. To image the right ovary using the transvaginal approach, the sonographer moves the transducer handle toward the patient's left thigh so that the tip of the transducer probe is in the right lateral fornix. To image the left ovary, the sonographer moves the handle toward the patient's right thigh so that the tip of the probe is in the left lateral fornix. Although the ovaries can be depicted from almost any parauterine position, they are usually depicted either lateral

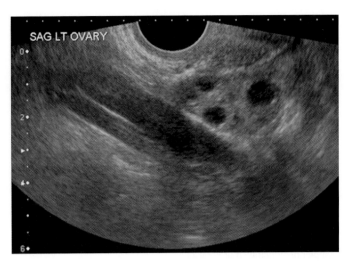

FIGURE 7–16. Transvaginal sagittal sonogram of the left ovary with normal follicles. The internal iliac vein and artery is seen posterior to the ovary.

to the uterus or in the cul-de-sac. Unlike transabdominal sonography, which allows the simultaneous imaging of both ovaries relatively often, transvaginal sonography can best image only one ovary at a time. Sonographically, the appearance of the ovaries varies with patient age, stage in menstrual cycle, pregnancy status, and body habitus. In reproductive years, the ovaries may be identified by follicles surrounding the outer edge of the ovaries. Follicular cysts are small (<3–5 mm), smooth, thin walled, and anechoic with good sound through transmission. Follicles will increase in size through the cycle with multiple follicles visible at days 5–7. At days 8–12, one or more dominant follicles (>10 mm) will begin to emerge. The dominant follicle reaches a mean diameter of 20 mm with a hypoechoic rim. After the ovum is released, bleeding may occur in the follicle, causing it to appear echogenic. The follicular cyst becomes a corpus luteal cyst with thick walls and appears anechoic to hypoechoic. The corpus luteal cyst will retain fluid for 4–5 days and measures approximately 2–3 cm. The corpus luteal cyst has a rich blood supply. Color-flow Doppler will reveal a ring of color around the periphery of the cyst. If no pregnancy occurs, the corpus luteal cyst will gradually atrophy. If pregnancy occurs, the corpus luteal cyst will remain and gradually regress by 12–14 weeks.[2] The follicular cyst and corpus luteal cysts are all functional cysts of the ovary.[1] In postmenopausal women, it is more difficult to identify the ovaries because of the absence of follicles and atrophy of the ovaries.[3,5] In patients who have had a hysterectomy, the ovaries can be difficult to depict because of the air-filled bowel occupying the space left by the removal of the uterus.

Fallopian Tubes

The fallopian tubes originate at the lateral aspect of the uterus, known as the cornua. Fallopian tubes vary in length from 7 to 12 cm. Each Fallopian tube is divided into five subdivisions: (1) interstitial, (2) isthmus, (3) ampulla, (4) infundibulum, and (5) fimbriae.[1] The interstitial portion of the tube sonographically appears as a fine echogenic line extending from the endometrial canal and traveling through the myometrium to cornua of the uterus.[7] The isthmus is the narrowest portion of the tube and is located adjacent to the interstitial segment at the uterine cornua. The tube continues laterally and widens to form the ampulla. The infundibulum is the most lateral portion of the tube and opens to the peritoneum at the fimbria.[1] The purpose of the fallopian tube is to aid in fertilization and to transport the ova from the ovary to the uterus. The normal fallopian tubes are difficult to identify by transabdominal or transvaginal sonography unless they are surrounded by fluid or filled with fluid.[5]

Ligaments

The uterus is loosely suspended in the center of the pelvic cavity by

- Round ligaments
- Uterosacral ligaments
- Cardinal ligaments

Although the uterus is suspended by ligaments, it has freedom of movement. During pregnancy, or in the presence of a uterine mass, the uterus moves upward, and during uterine prolapse, it moves downward. The upper portion of the uterus is supported by a series of ligaments. The cardinal ligaments or transverse cervical ligaments originate from the cervix and uterine corpus and insert on a broad portion of the lateral pelvic wall and sacrum. At the distal portion, this ligament is called the uterosacral ligament. This ligament anchors the cervix and is responsible for the uterine orientation.[1]

The two round ligaments originate from the uterine cornua and are located in a fold of the peritoneum and terminate in the upper portion of the labia majora.[1] This ligament is responsible for the anterior tilt of the uterus and aids in stabilizing the fundus of the uterus.

There are two ligaments that are not true ligaments, but are folds of the peritoneum. The first is the suspensory ligament. It arises from the pelvic sidewall and contains ovarian vessels. It aids in supporting both the fallopian tube and ovary within the broad ligament.[2] The broad ligament is also a double fold of the peritoneum. It fans over the adnexa and divides the anterior and posterior portions of the pelvis.[1] It does very little to actually support the uterus. The broad ligament is not usually seen on ultrasound except in cases of pelvic ascites or ruptured cyst or hemoperitoneum.[8]

Muscles

A series of different muscle bundles pass through the female pelvis. Some of these muscles are easily visualized by sonography and can often be confused for adnexal structures. The most commonly visualized muscle is the iliopsoas muscle. On sagittal views, it appears as a paired long hypoechoic stripe with echogenic linear lines. On transverse images, however, it appears ovoid and is visualized lateral and anterior to the iliac crests.[1] The iliopsoas muscle descends until it attaches on the lesser trochanter of the femur. This can often be confused for an ovary until the sagittal view is obtained. The pelvic muscles can be identified sonographically by their appearance. The muscles appear hypoechoic and exhibit linear internal echoes. The borders of the muscles are echogenic representing the fascia.[3,5] The rectus abdominis muscle is located in the anterior abdominal wall and extends from the xiphoid process to the symphysis pubis. The obturator internus muscles are bilateral muscles lining the lateral margin of the true pelvis; they lie lateral to the ovaries. The levator ani muscle is a hammock-like muscle that extends from the body of the pubis and ischial spine to the coccyx.

Bladder and Ureters

The urinary bladder is a thick-walled distendable muscle that lies anterior to the uterus. It is fixed in position inferiorly at the symphysis pubis. This lower region is described as the trigone, defined by the orifices of the two ureters and a urethra. The bladder is thicker and more rigid here than at any other location.[7] The ureter originates at the renal pelvis and descends anterior to the internal iliac artery and posterior to the ovary. The ureter travels from posterior to anterior and closely follows the uterine artery in its inferior portion. It then passes anteromedially to enter the trigone of the bladder.[1] During a transabdominal sonographic examination of the pelvis, the urinary bladder must be distended for a variety of reasons. This is because (1) the urine-filled bladder pushes the bowel cephalad out of the true pelvic cavity; (2) it pushes the uterus cephalad away from the symphysis pubis; (3) it permits rapid anatomic orientation; (4) it provides a low-attenuation pathway to which ultrasound can propagate; and (5) it helps to elevate the head of the fetus for easy measurements. Whereas a distended bladder is an extremely important prerequisite for a transabdominal study, an empty bladder is the most important prerequisite for a transvaginal study. The failure to fill the bladder adequately for transabdominal studies can result in serious diagnostic errors. On the other hand, an overdistended bladder can also result in errors. Sonographically, the position and shape of the uterus have an effect on the urinary bladder. If the uterus is anteverted, the normally distended bladder has a mild indentation on its posterocephalad region. If the uterus is surgically removed or absent, the bladder has a different contour. Therefore, bladder contour depends on the shape and position of its surrounding structures. When the bladder is being filled, urine can be observed entering the bladder on real-time and has been referred to as the "ureteral jets."[2] The jets begin at the ureteral orifices and flow toward the center of the bladder (Fig 7–17). Bladder diverticula may be acquired or congenital. Acquired diverticula result more commonly from bladder outlet obstruction. Congenital diverticula are located near the ureteral orifice and are known as Hutch diverticula.[3,5] Sonographically, bladder diverticula appear as outpouching sacs from the bladder wall with an opening in one end of the sac that communicates with the bladder.

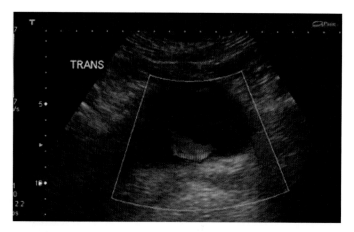

FIGURE 7–17. Transverse sonogram of the urinary bladder with color Doppler demonstrating ureteral jet.

Uterine Pathology

The most common uterine tumors are fibroids (also known as leiomyoma, myoma, and fibromyoma). They are present in 25% of the female population and occur at approximately 30–35 years of age, with a higher percentage in the African-American population and becoming more prevalent with advancing female age. Fibroids are thought to be estrogen stimulated, so they tend to increase in size during pregnancy and decrease in size after menopause. Fibroids are classified according to their location on the uterus (Fig. 7–18). If the fibroid is confined in the myometrium, it is called intramural. If is located in the uterine cavity, it is called submucosal, and if projecting from the peritoneal surface, it is called subserosal. Often, they are found on pelvic

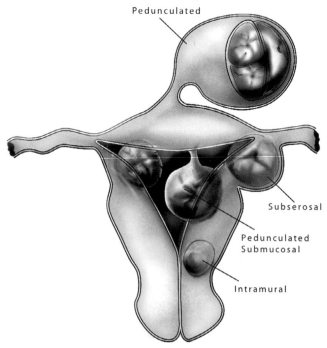

FIGURE 7–18. Diagram demonstrating various locations of fibroids.

examination without the patient having symptoms. When symptoms do occur, they can include abnormal bleeding, abdominal pressure, increased urinary frequency, and increased abdominal girth. The malignant form of the leiomyoma, a leiomyosarcoma, though rare, is believed to arise from a preexisting fibroid.[1] Leiomyosarcoma accounts for about 1.3% of uterine malignancies.[3] On sonogram, it appears similar to the leiomyoma and can be extremely difficult to diagnose preoperatively. Rapid accelerated growth may be the only clinical indication of a possible malignant process.[3,5] Fibroids has variable sonographic appearance:

- Inhomogeneous uterine texture
- Enlarged, irregular-shaped uterus
- Calcifications with distal acoustic shadowing
- Solid mass on the uterus that cannot be separated from the uterus
- Displacement of the endometrium
- Diffuse uterine enlargement

Fig. 7–19A shows an enlarged uterus with inhomogeneous echotexture. Fig. 7–19B demonstrates an intramural fibroid in the fundus of the uterus. Fig. 7–19C shows gross pathologic findings of the uterus with multiple fibroids.

Degeneration and necrosis of fibrous tissue can produce cystic spaces within the fibroids. Fibroids are the most common cause of uterine enlargement in the nonpregnant female. When the uterus is enlarged >14 cm in length, the kidneys should be scanned for hydronephrosis. A large fibroid uterus may compress the ureter as it enters the pelvis, resulting in obstruction in flow of urine. Fibroids in the uterine cavity can on some occasions cause heavy vaginal bleeding resulting in acute anemia.

Adenomyosis is defined as an invasion of endometrial tissue into the myometrium >2 mm. It occurs more often in multiparous women. Symptoms may include menorrhagia, dysmenorrhea, and pelvic tenderness.[9] Sonographically; the uterus is large with small cysts visible in the inner myome-

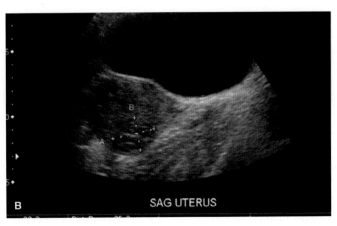

FIGURE 7–19B. Transabdominal sagittal sonogram of a fundal myoma.

trium. Often the myometrium of the uterus will appear inhomogeneous, similar to a fibroid, but distinct borders cannot be identified.[3,5]

Hematocolpos is an accumulation of blood within the vagina. This condition can be caused by an imperforate hymen or transverse vaginal septum.[3] On ultrasound, the vaginal cavity is distended with hypoechoic echoes and possible fluid/fluid levels, representing retained blood. Because the vagina can be distended to the same size of the uterine fundus, it may have an hourglass appearance.

Hematometra is an accumulation of blood within the uterine cavity secondary to atrophy of the endocervical canal or cervical stenosis. Sonographically, hematometra appears as marked distention of the uterus. Table 7–1 defines the terminology used to describe abnormal vaginal bleeding.

Ovarian Cyst

Benign cystic masses of the ovaries tend to be smooth walled, well-defined, and anechoic with increased posterior acoustic enhancement (Fig. 7–20). The normal ovaries in reproductive-age women have multiple follicles of various sizes

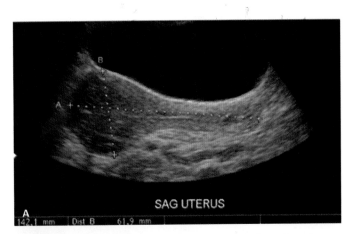

FIGURE 7–19A. Transabdominal sagittal sonogram of an enlarged uterus with fundal myoma.

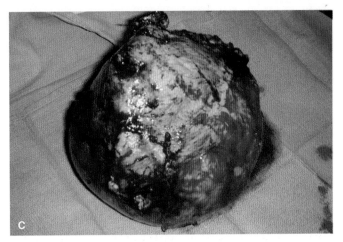

FIGURE 7–19C. Gross pathologic findings of the uterus with fibroids.

TABLE 7-1 • Abnormal Bleeding Terminology

Menorrhagia—prolonged bleeding occurring at the time of a menstrual period, either in duration or volume

Metrorrhagia—uterine bleeding occurring at irregular intervals

Metromenorrhagia—excessive and prolonged bleeding occurring at irregular, frequent intervals

(mature and immature). These follicles serve as anatomic sonographic markers to identify the ovaries. A follicular cyst occurs when a mature follicle fails to ovulate. The size of these follicles depends on the menstrual cycle.[3] The mature follicle measures approximately 20–25 mm.[3] A follicular cyst is a functional cyst. The three most common functional cysts of the ovaries are (1) follicular cysts, (2) corpus luteal cysts, and (3) theca-luteal cysts.[1,3,5] Sonographers should be aware of the normal cyclic changes of the ovaries and their normal multiple sonographic appearances. Fig. 7–21 shows normal ovaries with a follicular cyst.

Transvaginal sonography is an accurate means of evaluating the ovaries and adnexal structures for the presence or absence of a pelvic mass. Pelvic masses can be characterized according to their location (organ of origin) and internal consistency (cystic, solid, mixed, septated, multiloculated). Such physiologic cysts as the corpus luteum cyst can be characterized as arising from within or around the ovary, whereas such extra ovarian masses as endometriomas appear outside the ovary.

Cystic masses must be scrutinized with transvaginal sonography for the intactness of their walls and the presence of any papillary excrescence. Internal structures such as septate or solid areas need to be shown in a minimum of two imaging planes.

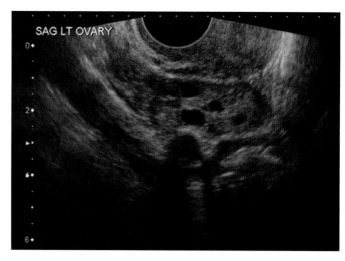

FIGURE 7–21. Left ovary with follicles.

Polycystic ovarian disease is an endocrinologic disorder characterized by excessive ovarian androgen production, which has spectrums of clinical manifestations[10]:

- Anovulation
- Amenorrhea
- Type 2 diabetes
- Obesity
- Acne
- Hirsutism
- Infertility

Polycystic ovaries are sonographically characterized by bilateral enlarged ovaries with an increased number of small immature follicles ranging in size from 3 to 5 mm and there are usually more than eight on each ovary (Fig. 7–22).

Ovarian Torsion

Ovarian torsion refers to the twisting of the ovary and its vessels resulting in occlusion of its blood supply. The twisting of

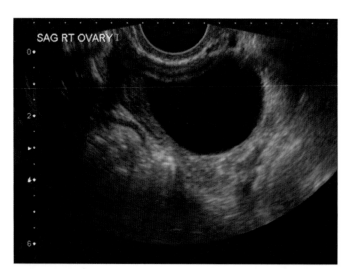

FIGURE 7–20. Right ovarian cyst.

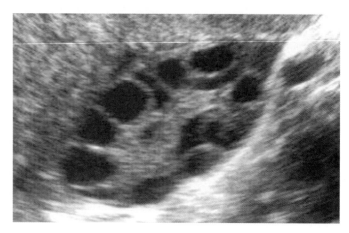

FIGURE 7–22. Polycystic ovary.

TABLE 7-2 • Doppler Findings for Ovarian Torsion

Doppler Study	Findings	Sonographic Findings
No venous or arterial Doppler flow	Complete obstruction	Torsion
No venous flow but arterial flow is present	Partial obstruction	Partial torsion
Venous and arterial flow are present	No obstruction	Decreased chances of torsion

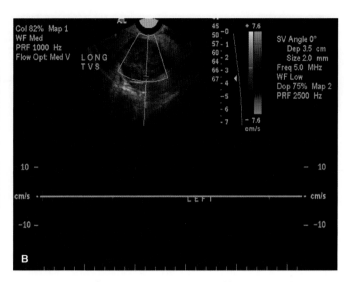

FIGURE 7-23B. Spectral and color Doppler with absence of flow.

the ovary with the vascular pedicle on its axis results in arterial, venous, and lymphatic obstruction causing necrosis of the ovary.[3,5] Approximately 95% of cases are associated with an adnexal mass. The right adnexa are more commonly involved due to the sigmoid colon occupying the left lower quadrant.[3,5,10] The most common mass associated with ovarian torsion is the dermoid cyst. The sonographic appearance of ovarian torsion will depend on whether the torsion is partial, intermittent, or complete. This type of mass is sonographically characterized by hyperechogenic areas, fluid/fluid layering, and calcifications within the mass. Color Doppler sonography is important in the evaluation of suspected torsion (Table 7-2).

Fig. 7-23A shows a left ovary and ovarian mass. Fig. 7-23B shows color and spectral Doppler with no flow. Fig. 7-23C shows gross pathologic findings of a necrotic ovary and ovarian mass surgically removed after an ovarian torsion.

Malignant ovarian disease has a peak incidence between the ages of 55 and 59 years. Other risk factors include family history (maternal or sibling), number of years of ovulation, and environmental (Tables 7-3, 7-4, 7-5).[2]

OBSTETRICS

Pregnancy Test

Human Chorionic Gonadotropin (hCG). hCG is a glycoprotein secreted by the syncytiotrophoblastic cells of the trophoblast.[1,11] The hCG is composed of two dissimilar subunits, alpha and beta. The antibodies against the beta subunit are used specifically to measure hCG.[1] The quantitative beta hCG is very helpful in the diagnosis of ectopic pregnancy, gestational trophoblastic disease, or abnormal pregnancy.

During the first trimester of pregnancy, the serum beta hCG normally doubles every 48 hours (2 days) or increases at least 66% every 48 hours before 8 weeks of gestation. In the presence of ectopic pregnancy, approximately 80% of serum beta hCG has abnormal doubling beta (low doubling time, remain the same, or decrease slightly). However, 10% of ectopic pregnancies may

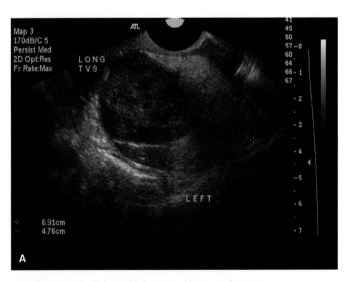

FIGURE 7-23A. Enlarged left ovary with an ovarian mass.

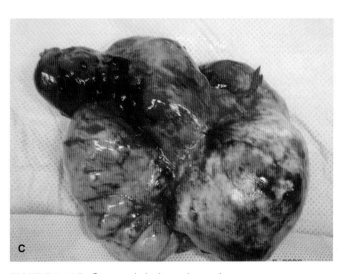

FIGURE 7-23C. Gross pathologic ovarian torsion.

TABLE 7–3 • Ovarian Cystic Masses

Mass	Clinical Findings	Sonographic Findings
Corpus luteum cyst	Associated with pregnancy	Unilocular: may contain low-level internal echoes; may appear as multiseptated cystic mass; normally regress after 14th week of pregnancy
Theca lutein cyst	Represents an exaggerated response to increased hCG Can be associated with ovarian hyperstimulation, molar pregnancy, chorioadenoma destruens, and choriocarcinoma	Bilateral enlarged ovaries; multiple small multilocular cysts
Polycystic ovaries (Stein–Leventhal syndrome)	A buildup of immature follicles with a thick outer covering preventing ovulation Associated with hirsutism, increased testosterone levels, irregular cycles	Bilaterally enlarged ovaries; multiple small cysts, appearing as "string of pearls"
Ovarian remnant syndrome	Residual ovarian tissue after oophorectomy	Can produce cysts, neoplasms; may cause symptoms; common with endometriosis and adhesions
Ovarian torsion	May be caused by a large cyst or tumor causing rotation of the ovary Dermoid cyst	In early phase, will have an enlarged ovary with intraovarian venous flow, but absent intraovarian arterial flow. In late stages, it will appear as a cystic or complex mass with thick walls and absent blood flow.

Source: Rumack et al.[3] and Mishell et al.[10]

TABLE 7–4 • Ovarian Solid Tumors

Mass	Clinical Findings	Sonographic Findings
Dysgerminoma	Uncommon malignant germ cell tumor. Occurs in second and third decades of life. One of the most common neoplasms in pregnancy. Historically similar to seminoma.	Predominately solid with hypoechoic internal echoes. Can grow rapidly.
Fibroma	Occurs in fifth and sixth decades. Part of stromal family, along with the other differentials: thecoma, granulosa cell, androblastoma. Meigs syndrome a triad of benign ovarian fibroma, ascites, and pleural effusion	Hypoechoic to echogenic with mixed heterogeneous pattern Solid ovarian mass with ascites and pleural effusion
Thecoma	84% occur postmenopausally	Similar sonographic features as in fibroma. Unilocular
Granulosa cell	95% occur postmenopausally	Similar sonographic features as in fibroma; small tumors are solid; large tumors are complex
Androblastoma (Sertoli–Leydig cell)	Occurs in second and third decades. May cause elevated testosterone and hirsutism.	Similar sonographic features as in fibroma.
Transitional cell (Brenner)	Occurs from fourth through eighth decades. Most are benign. Symptoms: abnormal uterine bleeding.	Small, hypoechoic tumors. Larger tumors are at greater risk for malignancy.

Source: Rumack et al.[3] and Mishell et al.[10]

TABLE 7–5 • Complex Ovarian Tumors

Mass	Clinical Findings	Sonographic Findings
Endometriosis	Ectopic endometrial tissue that may bleed during menses. Cysts are called endometriomas or chocolate cysts because of blood in the cysts. Symptoms: pain during menses and infertility.	Single or multiple cystic adnexal masses with thick walls and low-level internal echoes. Small echogenic lesions posterior to the uterus.
Benign cystic teratoma (dermoid)	Most common benign germ cell tumor. Composed of all three germ cell layers. Varies in composition with fat, bone, hair, skin, and teeth. More common in reproductive years.	Fluid–fluid levels. Distal acoustic shadow. Calcifications. Tip-of-the iceberg sign (no through sound transmission).
Serous cystadenoma	Benign. Usually unilateral. Accounts for 25% of benign ovarian tumors. Occurs in fourth and fifth decades.	Large cystic mass with thin-walled internal septations.
Serous cystadenocarcinoma	Accounts for 50% of malignant ovarian tumors in fourth through sixth decades.	Large, multilocular with papillary projections. Ascites is common.
Mucinous cystadenoma	Largest ovarian tumor. Accounts for 25% of benign ovarian tumors. Occurs in third through fifth decades.	Large cystic mass with thick-walled septations. May have debris layering due to thick internal components.
Mucinous cystadenocarcinoma	Malignant. Accounts for 5–10% of malignant ovarian tumors.	Papillary projections are not as common as with serous cystadenocarcinoma. Associated with ascites.
Endometrioid tumor	80% are malignant. Occurs in fifth through sixth decades. Arises from endometriosis.	Cystic mass with papillary projections. Can occasionally be solid.
Clear cell tumor	Invasive carcinoma occurring in fifth and sixth decades.	Complex, predominately cystic mass.
Tubo-ovarian abscess	Infectious process within the tubes and ovaries.	Fluid–fluid levels with hydrosalpinx. May be seen as complex or cystic mass with low-level echoes, irregular borders and internal septations.

Source: Rumack et al.[3] and Mishell et al.[10]

have a normal doubling in 48 hours but may eventually drop in titers or plateau.[11] A constant decreasing serial quantitative serum beta hCG in the first trimester is indicative of an abnormal pregnancy, regardless of the pregnancy location.

The serum levels for twins are twice as high as those for singleton pregnancies, and patients with a benign mole have higher levels than women with a normal pregnancy. Those with an invasive mole have higher ratios than those with noninvasive moles, and those with choriocarcinoma have even higher levels than those with invasive moles.[3]

There are various methods of reporting beta hCG. Some laboratories report serum quantitative beta hCG results in terms of International Reference Preparation (1st IRP), whereas others report the results in terms of Second International Standard (2nd IS). The most current is the Third International Standard (3rd IS). The 3rd IS is identical to the 1st IRP and 1.8 times those reported for the 2nd IS. Therefore, values in terms of the 3rd IS have been calculated by multiplying the 2nd IS by 1.88, which is the conversion factor.[11,12]

Rapid Qualitative Pregnancy Test. This small kit used for detection of hCG in urine or serum is readily available for immediate hospital or office use and is now available over the counter for private use. Beta hCG is a hormone that is normally produced by the placenta and present in the serum and urine of a pregnant woman. This rapid kit is an excellent marker on qualitative confirmation of pregnancy while awaiting the result of the more accurate quantitative serum beta hCG. The kit uses a color-coded result in a small result window, as the sample contains a detectable amount of hCG in 3–5 minutes. A minus (−) result in the result window means not pregnant or below the range of hCG sensitivity. A plus (+) in the result window indicates pregnancy or was recently pregnant. The first morning urine usually has a higher level of hCG present.

The sensitivity for urine varies from 20 to 25 mIU/mL as early as 7–10 days postconception with an accuracy of 99%. A false-negative result can occur with a urine sample that is too diluted. Therefore, to avoid a false-negative result, the test should be performed before high volume of fluid ingestion for sonography or high volume of intravenous fluid hydration. The test can also be false-negative if the sensitivity of the detectable hCG levels is below 20 mIU/mL. Fertility drugs containing hCG, such as Pergonal can alter the result.[1,10]

Serum Beta hCG Correlation with Ultrasound

The level of serum beta hCG to which a gestational sac should be seen on ultrasound is called the discriminatory zone. This concept was developed by Kadar et al., who correlated the ultrasound findings from patients with intrauterine pregnancy with serum beta hCG values using transabdominal scanning. This zone was between 6,000 and 6,500 mIU/mL of hCG using the First International Reference Preparation (1st IRP).[11,12] Later, Nyberg et al. reported a modification of the discriminatory zone at 1,800 mIU/mL Second International Standard (2nd IS), which is equivalent to 3,600 mIU/mL 1st IRP.[11]

The 2nd IS was released by the World Health Organization (WHO), which is approximately one-half of IRP values.[11] The most current beta hCG levels to which an intrauterine gestational sac can be seen with transvaginal ultrasound is now about 1,000–1,500 mIU/mL, depending on the frequency of the transvaginal probe used.[3] The increased sensitivity in the detectable amount of hCG in the urine and serum of pregnant women and the rapid advancement in computers, real-time ultrasound equipment are constantly changing. Therefore, the current level to which a gestational sac should be seen on ultrasound is expected to decrease as the technology advances. If the gestational sac is not seen at this level, the pregnancy may be either abnormal or ectopic. However, a repeated level may be needed to confirm. On some rare occasions, the serum beta hCG may be positive without evidence of pregnancy or disease; this is known as phantom beta hCG or false-positive hCG test. Antibodies generated in the body against other human antibodies may bind both human and animal antibodies (heterophilic antibodies). These may interfere with hCG tests, by causing phantom hCG or false-positive hCG results. Surgery and chemotherapy are sometimes performed for ectopic pregnancy, solely on the basis of phantom or false-positive hCG test data.[13] The interfering antibodies are present in serum but not urine samples. Phantom hCG can be confirmed by the demonstration of loss of the hCG in the urine samples.[13]

The Progesterone Level

Progesterone levels normally increase with gestational age. However, when an ectopic pregnancy is present, the corpus luteum does not secrete as much progesterone as occurs in normal pregnancy. Therefore, the concentration of the serum progesterone is usually lower in ectopic pregnancies. A value of 25 ng/mL or more is, 98% of the time, associated with a normal intrauterine pregnancy, whereas a value <5 ng/mL identifies a nonviable pregnancy, regardless of its location.[10]

The combination of serum beta hCG, progesterone level, and transvaginal sonography has resulted in great improvement in the diagnosis and management of ectopic pregnancy over the last 15–20 years.

ECTOPIC PREGNANCY

Any pregnancy outside the endometrial cavity is called ectopic pregnancy (Fig. 7–24). The incidence of this type of pregnancy has increased, but the rate of death from ectopic pregnancy has declined. This decrease is the result of earlier diagnosis.[3] Most ectopic pregnancies occur in the fallopian tube, approximately 90%. They account for approximately 12% of all maternal deaths.[1] They can occur in any anatomic segments of the fallopian tube but occur more frequently in the ampullary region. Other, less common sites for ectopic implantation are the uterine cervix, ovaries, and abdomen. If the pregnancy is in the abdomen with advanced gestational age, transabdominal scans should be performed first, and if necessary, transvaginal scans should be performed. Abdominal pregnancy is the only form of ectopic pregnancy that can go to term. The incidence of live-birth after an abdominal pregnancy is very rare. I have only seen two of these cases go to term in my 28 years of experience, and both were delivered by abdominal surgery. In both cases, the placenta was left in the abdomen after surgery. On occasion, the placenta in an abdominal pregnancy may be adherent to bowel and blood vessels; removal could result in massive hemorrhage. In such cases, the placenta is left *in situ* and ultimately resorbs.[1,10]

Pseudogestational sac is blood or decidual cast in the uterine cavity mimicking a gestational sac. The differentiation between the gestational sac at 5–6 weeks and the pseudogestational sac are as follows:

Gestational sac	*Pseudogestational sac*
Yolk sac	No yolk sac
Embryo	No embryo
Double decidual sac sign	No double decidual sac sign
Highly echogenic ring-choriodecidua	Thin wall
Grows 1 mm/day[3]	No increment in size
Lacunar structures with Doppler flow	No lacunar structures
Double-decidual sign	Single decidual layer
Peritrophoblastic flow	No peritrophoblastic flow

A coexistent intrauterine pregnancy and ectopic pregnancy, known as heterotopic, can occur. It was first reported at a rate of 1 in 30,000, then 1 in 16,000, and most currently 1 in 39,000.[1] This increase in heterotopic pregnancies may be attributable to increased ovulation induction.[3,10] Twin ectopic pregnancy in the same Fallopian tube can also occur (Fig. 7–25). On rare occasions, an ectopic pregnancy can also occur in a previous cesarean section scar (Fig. 7–26). This patient had multiple previous cesarean sections and presented with vaginal bleeding in pregnancy. Cornual ectopic pregnancies are often

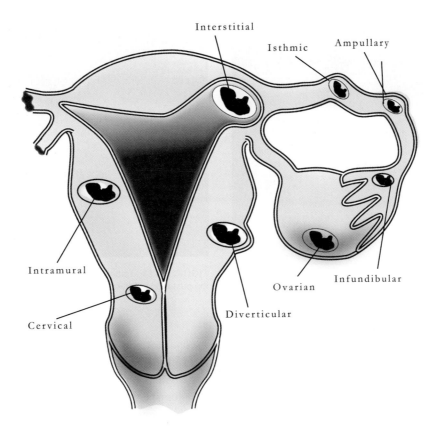

FIGURE 7–24. Diagram demonstrating various location of ectopic pregnancy.

misdiagnosed clinically and sonographically for multiple reasons. Its location allows clinical symptoms and rupture to occur late, approximately 12–16 weeks, and sonographically it can be misinterpreted as an intrauterine pregnancy with an eccentric implantation. Cornual ectopic pregnancy has a higher mortality when compared to other forms of ectopic pregnancies due to larger blood vessels at the implantation site and late rupture. Fig. 7–27 demonstrates a right cornual ectopic pregnancy.

Risk Factors for Ectopic Pregnancy

- Salpingitis from chlamydial infection or pelvic inflammatory disease
- Previous ectopic pregnancy
- Previous operations on the fallopian tube, bilateral tubal ligation, or tuboplasty surgery
- Cigarette smoking affects the ciliary action in the nasopharynx, respiratory tract, and fallopian tubes[10]

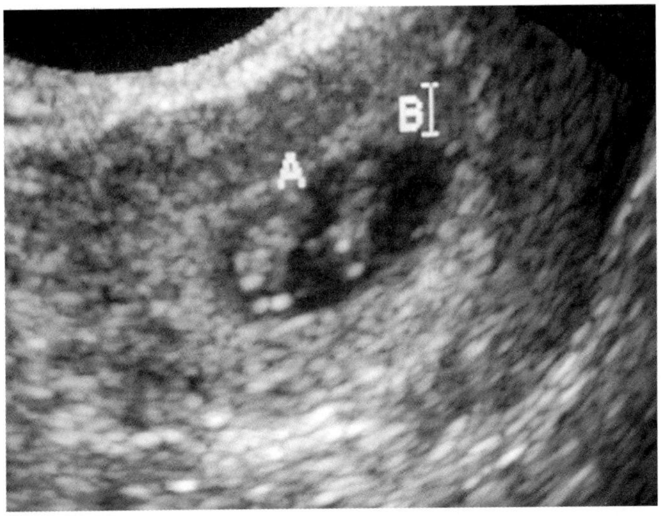

FIGURE 7–25. Transvaginal sonogram with twin ectopic pregnancy in the same fallopian tube.

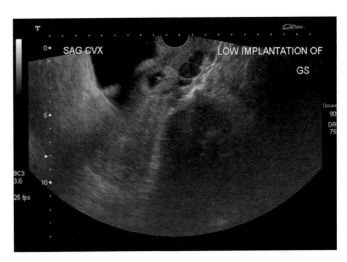

FIGURE 7–26. Transvaginal sagittal sonogram with an ectopic pregnancy in the cesarean section scar.

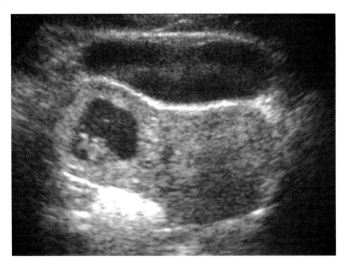

FIGURE 7–27. Transabdominal transverse scan with right cornual ectopic pregnancy.

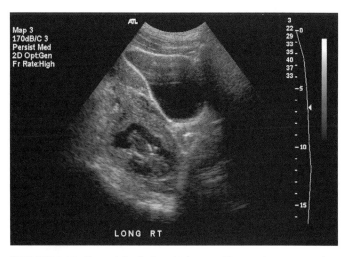

FIGURE 7–28. Transabdominal sagittal scan with ectopic pregnancy in the posterior cul-de-sac.

Clinical Signs and Symptoms of Unruptured Ectopic Pregnancy

- Unilateral pelvic pain, which increases in severity with time
- Vaginal spotting or bleeding
- Amenorrhea
- Adnexal mass
- Positive pregnancy test
- Nausea and vomiting

Clinical Signs and Symptoms of Ruptured Ectopic Pregnancy

- Generalized abdominal pain
- Rebound tenderness
- Cervical motion tenderness
- Bilateral adnexal tenderness
- Right shoulder pain
- Tachycardia and hypotension
- Decreased hematocrit
- Syncope
- Tachypnea

UNRUPTURED ECTOPIC PREGNANCY

Ectopic pregnancy should be suspected when there is no intrauterine gestational sac and the serum beta hCG is at a level in which a pregnancy should be seen (values 1,500 mIU/mL or greater). The sonographic appearance of ectopic pregnancy primarily depends on whether the pregnancy is ruptured, unruptured, its location, and size. The sonographic equipment, the frequency of the transvaginal transducer, as well as the skills of the operator play important roles. Advanced ultrasound equipment in the hands of a skilled operator can sometimes depict an ectopic pregnancy before the patient begins to have clinical symptoms. Early depiction of ectopic pregnancy before a tubal rupture occurs is imperative to avoid the potential risk of massive blood loss and tubal damage. However, some patients delay seeking medical treatment when the symptoms start, arriving at the emergency department after rupture.

The sonographic appearance of an unruptured ectopic pregnancy is an adnexal ring-like mass with increased color flow around its periphery ("ring of fire"). The center of this adnexal ring is anechoic, and its periphery echogenic, resembling a doughnut. It is imperative for the sonographer to identify and depict the ovary on the side of the adnexal ring. A hemorrhagic corpus luteum cyst could mimic this finding. Rarely, an extrauterine gestational sac is seen with a live embryo. Fig. 7–28 depicts a live ectopic pregnancy in the posterior cul-de-sac.

Fig. 7–29A is a sagittal view demonstrating the uterine cavity free of any intrauterine pregnancy. Fig. 7–29B is of the same patient in a transverse view with an extrauterine gestational sac with an embryo.

RUPTURED ECTOPIC PREGNANCY

An ectopic pregnancy in the fallopian tube grows linearly and circumferentially.[10] The growth occurs more parallel than circumferentially due to more space and less resistance to growth in the long axis of the tube. This gives the ectopic pregnancy a sausage-shape appearance (Fig. 7–30). Rupture of the fallopian tube is due to maximum stretching of the tube with ischemia and necroses.

After an ectopic pregnancy ruptures, blood accumulates in the abdomen and pelvis. It can readily be depicted with both transabdominal and transvaginal sonography. The blood may appear completely anechoic with some areas of echogenic

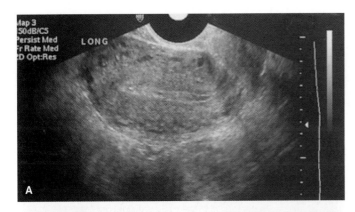

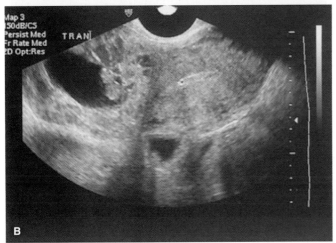

FIGURE 7–29. (A) Transvaginal sagittal scan of the uterus, free of any intrauterine pregnancy. **(B)** Transvaginal coronal scan with a right unruptured ectopic pregnancy.

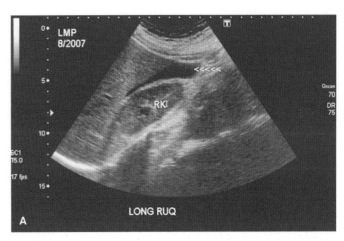

FIGURE 7–31A. Sagittal sonogram of the right upper quadrant with free-fluid in Morison's pouch.

out intraperitoneal collection is a cervical ectopic pregnancy. Patients with a large amount of blood in the abdomen may develop right shoulder pain because of diaphragmatic irritation, tachycardia, and hypotension secondary to vascular shock. There is no need to distend the urinary bladder in these cases because the intraperitoneal fluid is a good acoustic medium to view the abdominal and pelvic viscera. The ingestion of fluid to distend the urinary bladder for transabdominal scanning in a patient who is hemodynamically unstable may further delay immediate medical and surgical management and may further interfere with patients who need to be NPO for surgery. Sonographers should have experience in recognizing this emergency and call for assistance immediately. Fig. 7–31A shows free-fluid regions of Morison's pouches. Fig. 7–31B shows the uterus free of any pregnancy. Fig. 7–31C shows the adnexal ring next to the ovary. Fig. 7–31D shows the surgical findings of ectopic pregnancy via laparoscopic surgery.

fluid attributable to clotted blood. The patient is scanned in the supine position, allowing the free fluid to accumulate in a gravity-dependent position. The regions of Morison's pouch, paracolic gutters, and posterior cul-de-sac are the most common locations for intraperitoneal blood after rupture. A ruptured hemorrhagic corpus luteum cyst could mimic a ruptured ectopic pregnancy both clinically and sonographically. The only type of ectopic pregnancy that is known to rupture with-

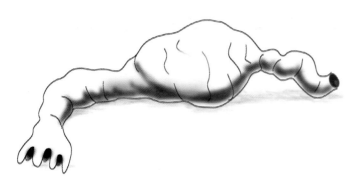

FIGURE 7–30. Diagram of a dilated fallopian tube due to an ectopic pregnancy.

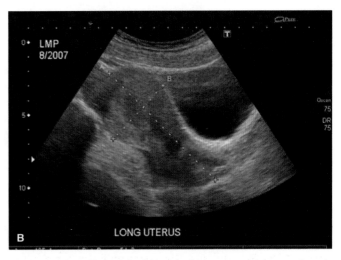

FIGURE 7–31B. Transabdominal sagittal sonogram of the uterus free of any intrauterine pregnancy.

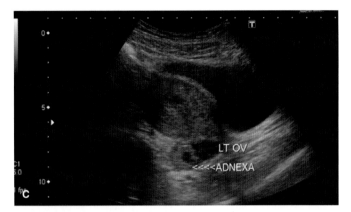

FIGURE 7–31C. Transabdominal sagittal scan of a left adnexa with an adnexal ring next to the left ovary.

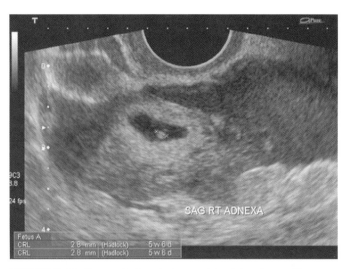

FIGURE 7–32. Transvaginal sagittal scan of the right adnexa with an ectopic gestational sac with a small embryo. Echogenic free-fluid is seen next to the gestational sac.

Treatment

The treatment for ectopic pregnancy depends on whether the pregnancy is ruptured or unruptured, size, location, and the patient's clinical condition. The use of methotrexate, which is a folic acid antagonist that inhibits DNA synthesis in the trophoblastic cells, has been successfully used in treatment of unruptured ectopic pregnancy.[10]

Medical treatment with methotrexate is very useful when the pregnancy is located in the cervix, tube, or ovary, or where surgical treatment carries a significant risk.[10] The purpose of medical treatment is to avoid potential risk of both anesthesia and surgery and spare the fallopian tube from surgical trauma or damage from spontaneous rupture. The success rate is high if the unruptured gestational sac is <4 cm and no sonographic evidence of fetal heart activity.[10] This medical treatment is not without failure. There is a possibility of rupture in 3–4% of medically treated cases.[3,5,10]

Patients with ruptured ectopic pregnancy usually present with severe pain, accompanied by hypotension, tachycardia, and rebound tenderness. Blood normally clots after rupture and is sonographically characterized as echogenic free-fluid. Fig. 7–32 demonstrates an ectopic gestational sac with a small embryo in the sac and echogenic free-fluid in the posterior

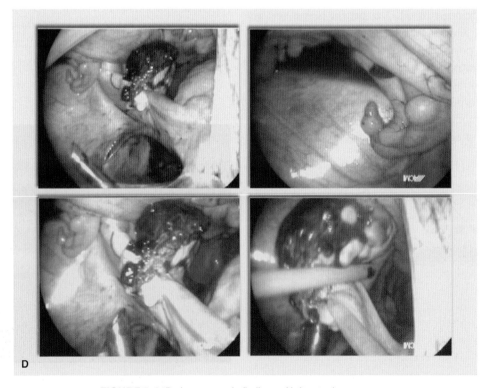

FIGURE 7–31D. Laparoscopic findings of left ectopic pregnancy.

cul-de-sac secondary to leaking hemorrhage. Sonographers should be aware that before rupture, the pain increases in severity and then decreases in its severity after rupture. The pain then recurs after rupture, as generalized abdominal pain or right-upper-quadrant (RUQ) pain with rebound tenderness secondary to hemoperitoneum. Sonographers must be informed before performing an ultrasound of any history of ectopic pregnancy that is currently or previously treated with methotrexate. In a patient in which methotrexate has failed and the patient is hemodynamically unstable, ultrasound scanning may not be helpful because a delay in surgical management could result in the patient going into shock.

Surgical Treatment

Laparoscopic salpingostomy or partial salpingectomy are currently the surgical procedures of choice for ectopic pregnancy when methotrexate is not advised, except for cornual ectopic pregnancy, which in most cases requires a cornual resection via laparotomy.[1,10] Laparotomy is indicated when patients are hemodynamically unstable or when laparoscopic surgery could be a significant risk.[14] Sonographers should obtain some past surgical history, if not included on the sonogram request form. Did you have an ectopic pregnancy before? Was your fallopian tube removed? On which side was your previous ectopic pregnancy? Sonographers should be alert for any abdominal and pelvic surgical scars, which may be a result of previous surgical removal of abdominal/pelvic viscera. Failure to be observant and to obtain patient history pertinent to scanning could result in misdiagnosis.

Salpingostomy: surgical incision of the fallopian tube for removal of tubal pregnancy. The incision is left open. The fallopian tube is not removed.

Salpingotomy: surgical incision of the fallopian tube for removal of tubal pregnancy. The incision is closed by suture. The fallopian tube is not removed.

Salpingectomy: surgical removal of tubal pregnancy by removing part or all of the fallopian tube.

FIRST TRIMESTER OBSTETRICS

Pregnancy is divided into three equal trimesters:

- First trimester: 0–13 weeks
- Second trimester: 13–28 weeks
- Third trimester: 28–42 weeks

Early Pregnancy

Documentation of intrauterine pregnancy can be made as early as 4 weeks with transvaginal sonography by the identification of a gestational sac within the uterus. The gestational sac at this time has an anechoic center that represents the chorionic fluid and a highly echogenic ring that represents the developing chorionic villi and decidual tissue (chorion-decidua capsularis). The gestational sac size is about 5 mm when first depicted and increases in size as pregnancy advances with a growth rate of 1 mm/day.[3] The gestational sac is empty and free of an embryo or yolk sac at this early stage. The gestational age at this time can be predicted by measuring the mean sac diameter.

These measurements are obtained by longitudinal sac diameter, the anteroposterior diameter, and the transverse diameter of the chorionic cavity, excluding the surrounding echogenic ring. All the dimensions are added then divided by 3 to obtain the mean sac diameter.

At approximately 5 weeks gestational age, the lacunae structures can be seen in a semicircle on one side of the gestational sac in the choriodecidua and represent the beginning of uteroplacental circulation (intervillous spaces).[8] Sonographically, they appear as small rounded hypoechoic structures that measure about 2–3 mm. Transvaginal color Doppler can demonstrate blood flow in these spaces. The yolk sac is the first anatomic structure seen within the gestational sac at 5 weeks and measures approximately 5–6 mm.

The yolk sac lies in the chorionic cavity (the extra-embryonic coelom) between the amnion and chorion (Fig. 7–33). The functions of the yolk sac are as follows:

1. Form blood cells (hematopoiesis)
2. Give rise to sex cell (sperm and egg)
3. Supply nutrients from the trophoblast to the embryo

Sonographically, the yolk sac can be depicted between 5 and 10 weeks of gestation. It is filled with vitelline fluid and appears anechoic on ultrasound. The sac is connected to the midgut by a narrow pedicle called the yolk stalk, vitelline duct, or the omphalomesenteric duct (Fig. 7–34). The yolk stalk detaches from the midgut by the end of the sixth week, and the dorsal part of the yolk sac is incorporated into the embryo as the primitive gut. As pregnancy advances, the yolk sac shrinks and becomes solid and its stalk becomes relatively longer.[1]

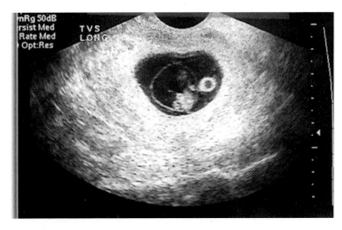

FIGURE 7–33. Yolk sac seen in the chorionic cavity and the embryo in the amniotic cavity.

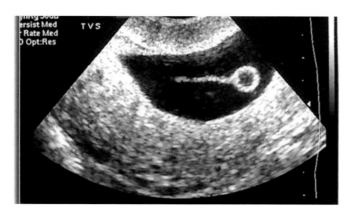

FIGURE 7–34. Yolk sac with its connecting yolk stalk.

Fig. 7–35 illustrates an early pregnancy, yolk sac, and its surrounding anatomic structures.

The yolk sac may prevail throughout the pregnancy and be recognized on the fetal surface of the placenta near the attachment of the umbilical cord; this situation is extremely rare and has no significance. In about 2% of adults, the proximal portion of the yolk stalk persists as a diverticulum of the ileum called Meckel's diverticulum.[1,3,10]

Yolk Sac-Embryo Complex. At approximately 6 weeks of gestation, the crown-rump length of the embryo measures 3–5 mm and abuts the yolk sac. The heartbeat can be depicted at this time. The upper limbs buds appear first at 7 weeks, followed by the lower limb buds.

At approximately 8 weeks of gestation, the physiologic herniation of the midgut can be seen sonographically as a hyper-

Gestational Age	Sonographic Observations
	TABLE 7–6 • Chronological Chart: Transvaginal Obstetrical Sonography
4 weeks	The gestational sac is first seen at this time. It measures 4–5 mm and is surrounded by decidua with an anechoic center. No embryo or yolk sac are depicted at this time.
5 weeks	The yolk sac is first seen and measures 3–5 mm. The lacunar structures can be seen on one side of the gestational sac, and blood flow from its spaces can be depicted with color Doppler.
6 weeks	The fetal pole can be seen measuring 4–5 mm and abutting the yolk sac (yolk sac/embryo complex). The heartbeats can be seen, and the crown-rump length can be measured.
7 weeks	The limb buds first appear, and the amnion membrane and chorionic cavity can be seen.
8 weeks	Sonolucent brain vesicles and midgut herniation are seen.
9 weeks	Choroid plexus is seen.
10 weeks	The intraventricular heart septum is seen.
11 weeks	The umbilical cord is visible. Nuchal translucency can be seen.
12 weeks	The extra-embryonic coelom is obliterated, and the midgut herniation disappears. The placenta can be seen.
13 weeks	The orbital structures are seen.
14 weeks	The four-chamber heart becomes visible.

echoic bulging of the cord near the point where the cord enters the fetal abdomen. The midgut returns to the abdomen, where it undergoes a second rotation, which is 180° counterclockwise.[1,10] Thus, the midgut undergoes a total rotation of 270°. If the bowel fails to return to the abdomen during this second stage of rotation, an omphalocele could be the result. Table 7–6 describes the chronological events of early pregnancy.

Nuchal Translucency

Nuchal translucency refers to the space between the back of the neck and the overlying fetal skin. This anechoic space is produced by a collection of fluid under the skin. This finding is observed in all fetuses between the gestational ages of 11 to 13 weeks and 6 days[15] (Fig. 7–36A). This should not be confused with a nuchal fold, which is measured from the outer edge of the occipital bone to the outer margin of the skin in the second

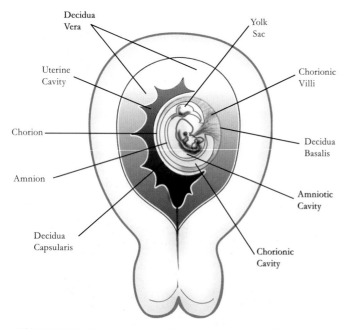

FIGURE 7–35. Early pregnancy with yolk sac and surrounding anatomic structures.

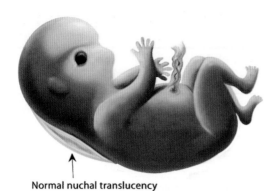

Normal nuchal translucency

FIGURE 7-36A. Normal nuchal translucency.

and third trimesters. There is a strong association between the size of the translucency and chromosome abnormality, particularly the risk for Down's syndrome (trisomy 21) and Turner's syndrome.[15]

FIRST TRIMESTER
CYSTIC HYGROMA

Cystic hygroma is congenital lymphatic obstruction between the lymphatic and venous pathway resulting in lymphatic fluid accumulation in the lymphatic sac within the nuchal region. The sonographic appearance of cystic hygroma in the first trimester is different from the sonographic appearance in the second trimester. The first trimester sonographic appearance of cystic hygroma is characterized by excessive enlargement of nuchal translucency (Fig. 7-36B), which extends along the entire long axis of the embryo with or without septations. First trimester cystic hygromas are associated with trisomies, whereas second trimester cystic hygromas are associated with monosomy x (Turner's syndrome).[15] After the 14th week of gestation the nuchal translucency measurements is no longer feasible and the sonographic appearance

of cystic hygroma is characterized by single or multiple septated masses of the fetal neck. Cystic hygromas occur in the neck in 80% of cases[15] and occur in the axilla, thorax, and abdominal wall.[16]

Sonographic measurements
of Nuchal Translucency

Approximately 90% of nuchal translucency (NT) measurements less than 3 mm at 12 weeks are normal at birth, while 10 % have abnormalities.[1] NT is a screening test and amniocentesis and chorionic villus sampling are diagnostic tests. This screening test is operator dependent, with the majority of errors occur because of incorrect digital calipers placement.[17] (Correct and incorrect placements for digital calipers Fig. 7-37.) In order to reduce this error, the following are recommendations.

Guidelines for measurements:

* Only use the "+" calipers, others are less accurate. Take three measurements and record the maximum measurement (do not average).
* The CRL should be 45–84 mm (11–14 weeks).
* Measurement can be performed either by transabdominal or transvaginal.
* The fetus should be in the mid-sagittal plane.
* The fetal neck should be in a neutral position.

Correct digital cursor placement

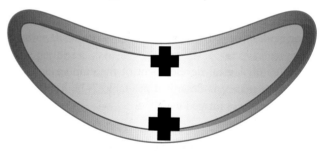

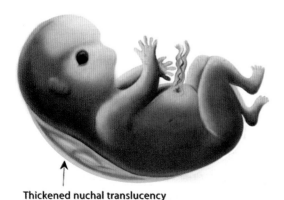

Thickened nuchal translucency

FIGURE 7-36B. Nuchal translucency enlargement.

Incorrect digital cursor placement

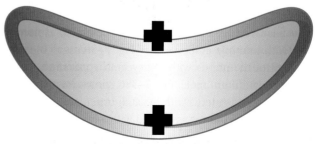

FIGURE 7-37. Correct and incorrect placements for digital calipers.

	TABLE 7-7 • Embryological Development	
Gestational Age	**Parameters**	**Sonographic Observations**
4–5 weeks	Avg. MSD 4–10 mm	Small gestational sac surrounded by echogenic rim of tissue "double decidual" sign (two echogenic lines surrounding portion of sac). Yolk sac is visible by the 5th week.
6 weeks	CRL 3–5 mm	CRL 3–5 mm with cardiac activity >100 bpm. All major internal and external structures beginning to form
7–8 weeks	CRL 6–16 mm	Limb buds evolving into upper/lower extremities, fetal trunk elongates. Herniation of midgut into UC begins, base of cord <7 mm. Heart rate >137 bpm
9 weeks	CRL 25 mm	Rhombencephalon visible as cystic structure in posterior cranium
10 to 11 weeks	CRL 45 mm	Bowel returns to abdomen. Cranium visualized with prominent choroid plexus. Fetal head large, comprising of half of CRL. Good fetal movement is present. All extremities are visualized. Anterior abdomen/thorax visualized. Can evaluate nuchal translucency (11–14 weeks). The fetal nasal bone can be visualized. Yolk sac begins to disappear.
12 weeks	CRL 55 mm	End of first trimester. Fusion of amnion/chorion begins. Can identify twins, encephaloceles, holoprosencephaly, ectopia cordis, and conjoined twins.
13–16 weeks	Multiple parameters	The femur length (FL), abdominal circumference (AC), head circumference (HC) and BPD can be measured. The HC > AC. Can identify cranium, abdominal wall, spine, and extremities.
16–20 weeks	Multiple parameters	Can fully evaluate fetal anatomy. Cardiac anatomy can usually be evaluated after 18 weeks.

Source: References[3,5,10]

- The calipers should be placed perpendicular to the long axis of the fetus.
- The calipers should be placed from inner-to-inner borders.
- Distinguish between fetal skin and amnion.

The chronological development of the embryo and fetus during a pregnancy is described in (Table 7–7). The first trimester findings are imaged with TVS.

FIRST TRIMESTER ABNORMALITIES

Hydatidiform Mole. This is the most common and benign component of gestational trophoblastic disease (abnormal proliferation of the trophoblastic elements) that may be partial or complete.

Complete—Sonographic findings are an enlarged uterine cavity filled with complex echoes often resembling placental tissue with multiple cystic vesicles Fig. 7–38A and B show a sonogram of the uterus with honeycomb appearance seen in cases of hydatidiform mole. Fig. 7–38C shows color and spectral Doppler of the uterus with hydatidiform mole.

Hydatidiform mole is associated with a markedly increased β-hCG and may have bilateral theca lutein cysts 18–30% of the time.[10] Fig. 7–38D shows a theca lutein cyst with multiple septations next to uterus. Fig. 7–38E shows a pathology specimen off hydropic villi following evacuation of the uterus. If hydatidiform mole is not treated, this can progress into malignant choriocarcinoma.[1,3,5,10]

Partial—The combination of a live or dead fetus and a localized area of placenta with molar degeneration. Ninety percent of partial moles are triploidy. On ultrasound, a partial mole presents as an enlarged hydropic placenta, with focal multicystic, anechoic spaces replacing the normal homogeneous appearance of placenta.[10]

Sonographic Appearance of Hydatidiform Mole

- Swiss cheese appearance
- Snowstorm appearance
- Vesicular sonographic texture
- Honeycomb appearance

Clinical Sign and Symptoms of Hydatidiform Mole

- Vaginal bleeding
- Uterus is larger than for expected gestational age
- Markedly elevated serum beta hCG
- Hyperthyroidism

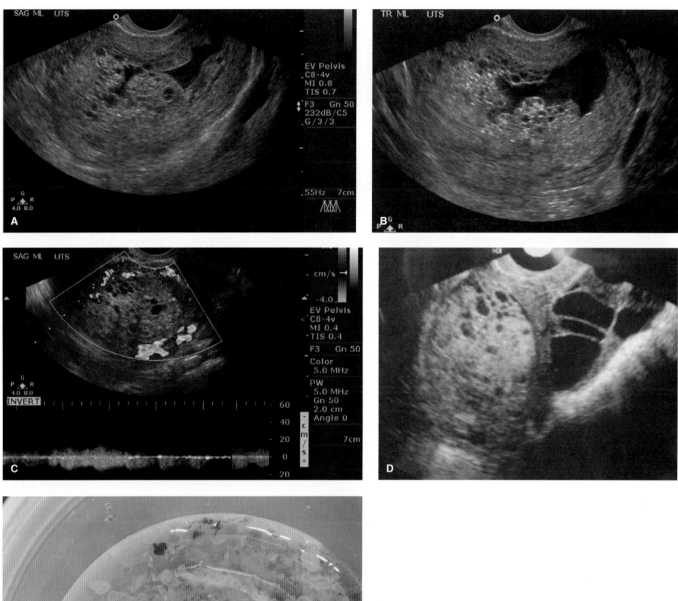

FIGURE 7-38. (**A** and **B**) Sagittal and transverse sonograms with the uterine cavity filled with tiny grapelike tissue, giving the sonographic characteristic of hydatidiform mole. (**C**) Color and spectral Doppler of the uterus with hydatidiform mole. (**D**) Hydatidiform mole with septated theca lutein cyst on the left adnexa. (**E**) Gross specimen findings after suction and curettage, numerous hydropic villi.

- Hyperemesis gravidarum
- Preeclampsia before 20 weeks of gestation

Blighted Ovum (Anembryonic Demise). This is a large (>2-cm) gestational sac without an embryo or yolk sac. The gestational sac is sometimes irregular in shape and fragmented with a thin choriodecidua. The serum β-hCG may fail to

double or decline. The gestational sac fails to grow at increasing increments of 1 mm/day.[3]

Missed Abortion. This is an embryo without fetal heart motion retained in the uterus before 20 weeks. Fetal demise after 20 weeks is called an intrauterine fetal demise (IUFD). The serum β-hCG will decline with time.

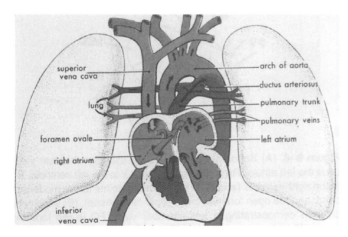

FIGURE 7–39. Schematic drawing demonstrating fetal cardiac circulatory system. *(Adapted with permission from Moore KL. The Developing Human: Clinically Oriented Embryology, 4, 8th ed, Philadelphia: WB Saunders, 2008.)*

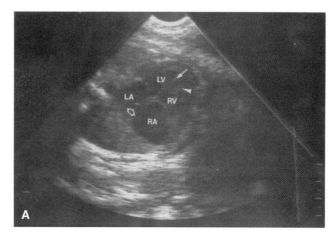

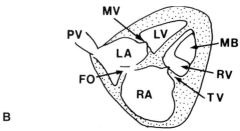

FIGURE 7–40. (**A**) Sonogram demonstrating the four-chamber view (**B**) Schematic diagrams demonstrating the four –chamber view. *(Reproduced with permission from Cyr DR, et al. A systematic approach to fetal echocardiography using real time two-dimensional sonography. J Ultrasound Med. 1986; Jun; 5(6):343–350.)*

SECOND AND THIRD TRIMESTER OBSTETRICS

Basic fetal cardiac evaluation has become an intricate component of obstetrical sonography. Fetal cardiac circulation is shown in Fig. 7–39. Note the three shunts present in fetal circulation that are not present after birth: (1) foramen ovale—between the left and right atria; (2) ductus arteriosus—between the pulmonary trunk and transverse aortic arch; and (3) ductus venosus—between the umbilical vein and inferior vena cava.[18]

The basic cardiac evaluation should include the four chamber view and views showing the outflow tracts origin and relationship to each other. The inferior vena cava should also be visualized and a fetal heart rate recorded. Sixty-five percent of cardiac abnormalities can be detected from the four-chamber view. Eighty-five percent of defects can be detected if the great vessels views are included (Fig. 7–40).[3,10]

Gestational Age and Growth

Estimation of gestational age can be calculated using multiple parameters listed in Table 7–8. The fetal weight may then be plotted on a normal growth curve to assess the size of the fetus. Macrosomia describes a fetus that weighs more than 4,000 g. Large for gestational age (LGA) is a clinical term and refers to the fundal height of the uterus. LGA has many causes, such as a large fetus (>90th percentile), excessive amniotic fluid, fibroids, twins, or a molar pregnancy. Macrosomia is often a manifestation of insulin-dependent diabetes mellitus (IDDM). It is associated with increased muscle mass and fat, leading to an increased AC and thickened shoulders. As well as a large fetus, there is often increased amniotic fluid volume (AFV) and a decreased HC/AC ratio because of the large AC. A macrosomic fetus is at risk for shoulder dystocia, humeral/ clavicle fractures,

meconium aspiration, prolonged labor, and asphyxial injury. Macrosomia carries an increased perinatal mortality, thus making its diagnosis by ultrasound important.[2]

Intrauterine growth restriction (IUGR), is defined by ultrasound as a weight <10th percentile. Other measurement findings with IUGR are an increased HC/AC and FL/AC ratios, oligohydramnios (a decrease in amniotic fluid), and advanced placental grade. Symmetrical IUGR refers to overall growth restriction, whereas asymmetrical IUGR refers to the abdomen measuring smaller than normal for the gestational age and increasing the HC/AC and FL/AC ratios. In asymmetrical IUGR, blood is shunted to the brain in a brain-sparing effort and taken away from the bowel. Early onset IUGR with oligohydramnios

TABLE 7–8 • Gestational Age and Range of Error		
Gestational Age	**Measurements**	**Range of Error**
First trimester	CRL	± 3–5 days, most accurate
14–20 weeks	BPD, HC, AC, FL	± 10 days
20–30 weeks	BPD, HC, AC, FL	± 14 days
30–40 weeks	BPD, HC, AC, FL	± 21 days

With multiple measurements, the more parameters used, the more accurate the estimated due date. At least two parameters must be used. *Sources:* [3,10]

is suggestive of a chromosomal abnormality or infection. Other causes of IUGR may be related to placental insufficiency. Maternal conditions that can be associated with IUGR include hypertension, vascular disease, autoimmune disease, and poor nutrition. Pulsed Doppler sonography may aid in assessing fetal well-being in addition to serial scans, AFV assessment, biophysical profile (BPP), and nonstress testing. When there is good umbilical cord blood flow, the waveform (systolic/diastolic ratio) demonstrates continuous diastolic flow.[3,10] An increased systolic/diastolic ratio of the umbilical artery suggests an increased resistance in the placenta, leading to a decrease in blood velocity and volume.[3] The compromised fetus may demonstrate pulsatile or reversed flow in the umbilical vein, another sign of increased resistance to forward blood flow from the placenta to the fetus and a sign of cardiac compromise. Color Doppler sonography (CDS) may be used to sample the middle cerebral artery and the ductus venosus. Doppler interrogation of these sites is crucial in identifying the fetus that is at high risk of severe compromise. In the severely compromised fetus, the increased flow to the brain is evidenced by increased diastolic flow in the middle cerebral artery. In addition, flow may be shunted away from the liver resulting in ductus venosus flow.[10]

Color Doppler sonography (CDS) can be used to assess flow in the maternal uterine artery as it branches from the internal iliac artery. Sampling at this point typically reveals a waveform with a diastolic notch. This notch should not be present after 26 weeks, and when it is, it may indicate faulty placentation and a tendency to have pregnancy-induced hypertension (PIH) or IUGR.[3,10]

Biophysical Profile

Real-time sonography is vital to determine fetal condition, as evidenced by physiologic activities seen in fetal "breathing" and body movements. The compromised fetus may exhibit decreased or absent body movement and "breathing." Hypoxia affects certain neurologic autonomic centers in reversed order to their maturation. For example, the central nervous center for body movement and "tone" develops early in fetal maturation followed by centers for cardiac rate variation and "breathing." However, one of the first abnormalities to develop in the hypoxic fetus is lack of fetal heart rate acceleration followed by decreased fetal breathing and body motion.

The standard nonstress test (NST) evaluates changes in heart rate when the fetus moves. A negative (reactive) NST has high negative predictive value, but false positives arise and are distressing for the new mother and her physician.

The biophysical profile incorporates the NST, amniotic fluid, fetal breathing, and body movements (both gross and tone). Each component is given a score of 2 if present, 0 if absent, with 10 being the highest score. Some biophysical profiles do not include the NST, with 8 being the highest score.

The Doppler techniques mentioned above may also be included in assessing fetal well-being. Thus, there are several sonographic techniques to monitor fetal well-being.[3]

Fetal Demise

Fetal demise is defined as death of the developing fetus after 20 weeks of gestation. The clinical and sonographic signs for fetal demise are numerous. The sonographic signs can be divided into specific and nonspecific. The specific signs are: (1) the failure to find the fetal heart tones on Doppler examination, (2) no fetal cardiac motion on M-mode, and (3) no movements or fetal heart pulsation seen on real-time sonography. The nonspecific signs are:

- Overlapping of the fetal sutures (Spalding's sign)
- Hydramnios or oligohydramnios
- Flattened (oblong) fetal head
- Absence of the falx cerebri
- Distorted fetal anatomy
- Decrease in the biparietal diameter when measurements are repeated from 1 week to the next
- Decrease in the size of the uterus
- Edematous soft tissue around the head (the "halo" sign or Druel's sign)
- Fragmentation of the fetal skin
- Diffuse edema of the entire fetus (anasarca)
- Separation of the amnion from the chorion after 20 weeks
- Gas in the fetal circulatory system (Robert's sign)
- Hydropic swelling of the placenta

The clinical and laboratory findings of fetal demise are the failure of the uterus to grow, two negative pregnancy test results (serum β-hCG), no fetal movement, no heart sounds on auscultation, and red or brown amniotic fluid.[14] Fig. 7–41 illustrates the overlapping of the fetal cranial bones at the skull sutures and scalp edema.

Amniotic Fluid

Amniotic fluid has many functions. It protects the fetus from trauma, allows for growth, controls temperature, allows for respiration, allows for normal gastrointestinal and musculoskeletal development, and prevents infection by its antibacterial properties. In the first trimester, amniotic fluid is made by the

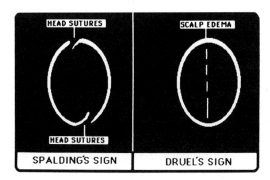

FIGURE 7–41. Spalding's and Druel's signs.

placenta. After 12 weeks, the primary sources of amniotic fluid are the fetal kidneys, lungs, and skin. Fluid is re-accumulated in the body through fetal swallowing. Amniotic fluid volume (AFV) normally increases until 33 weeks of gestation. It peaks and then begins to decline for the remainder of the pregnancy.[1,3,10] An exact volume of AFV cannot be obtained with ultrasound; however, the amniotic fluid index (AFI) is an indirect means of quantifying the amount of amniotic fluid. The maternal abdomen is divided into four quadrants. In each quadrant, an anteroposterior measurement of amniotic fluid is taken that does not contain body parts or umbilical cord. The four quadrant values are totaled, with the sum representing the AFI. The AFI can be compared to a normal AFI curve to assess AFV. Another means of measuring amniotic fluid is the single pocket measurement. The largest pocket of AF that does not contain body parts or umbilical cord is measured in an antero-posterior dimension. If a single deepest pocket of amniotic fluid measures between 0 to 2 cm, then the diagnosis of oligo-hydramnios can be made.[3,14] The single pocket measurement is less reliable than the AFI, but it can be useful in such situations as multiple gestations and pre-decompression and post-decompression amniocentesis.

Oligohydramnios is the decrease of AFV below the 2.5th percentile. It may be caused by a renal abnormality or obstruction, placental insufficiency, premature rupture of membranes, or post dates. Oligohydramnios with placental insufficiency is caused by a decreased blood flow to the uterus, which in turn, causes decreased renal perfusion.[5] A lack of AFV can contribute to pulmonary hypoplasia and extremity contractures. The mnemonic DRIPP serves as a key for memorizing the five more common conditions associated with oligohydramnios:

- D demise (polyhydramnios immediately after death due to absence of fetal swallowing, followed by oligohydramnios due to fetal absorption of fluid)
- R renal agenesis
- I intrauterine growth restriction (IUGR)
- P premature rupture of membranes (PROM)
- P postmaturity

Polyhydramnios is the excessive accumulation of AFV, measuring more than 95th percentile. Sixty percent of polyhydramnios are idiopathic, 20% are structural, and 20% are maternal (IDDM).[1,3]

Placenta and Umbilical Cord

The *placenta* is responsible for the maternal/fetal exchange of nutrients, oxygen, and waste. The placenta can attach anywhere in the uterus. The fetal side consists of a fused layer of amnion and chorion, with underlying vessels being located in the chorionic villi. The maternal component consists of cotyledons, composed of maternal sinusoids and chorionic villous structures. Oxygenated maternal blood enters the intervillous spaces

that bathe the chorionic villi. Gases and nutrients are exchanged across the walls of the villi, with waste crossing from inside the villi to the intervillous space for the maternal vessels to transport away from the placenta. Maternal blood flow increases in pregnancy to accommodate the increased demand of the placenta. The placenta is a low resistive organ that allows a decrease in resistance to the fetus as the fetus grows.[1] This results in progressively increasing blood flow as the pregnancy advances. Placental insufficiency is related to increased resistance in the vascular bed and results in decreased blood flow to the fetus. Placental insufficiency may be indirectly monitored by umbilical cord pulsed Doppler. The ratio of systolic flow to diastolic flow will show the amount of resistance in the placental bed. A lower ratio is less resistive; a higher ratio is more resistive. Normal ratios vary with gestational age and tables are available listing the normal ranges.

Placenta previa is the condition in which the placenta crosses the internal os of the cervix. Placenta previa is the primary cause of third trimester bleeding, although bleeding may occur from previa at any time in pregnancy.[1] Placenta previa may be further subcategorized into (1) complete—placenta totally covers the internal os; (2) partial—placenta is over the edge but does not cross the internal os; (3) marginal—placenta touches the edge of the internal os; and (4) low lying—the placenta is within 2 cm of the internal os. The clinical finding in placenta previa is painless vaginal bleeding. Bladder distention and myometrial contraction can distort the lower uterine segment and give a false image of placenta previa. Post void images helps to avoid this technical error. Placentas may have a succenturiate or accessory lobe that is connected to the main lobe of the placenta by blood vessels within a membrane. If these vessels cross the internal os it is considered a vasa previa.[1,3]

Placental abruption is the premature separation of the placenta from the uterine wall after 20 weeks of gestation. Symptoms may include painful vaginal bleeding and abdominal pain or cramping. Although the diagnosis is usually made clinically, sonographic findings are a retroplacental, hypoechoic area composed mainly of veins >2 cm, and large periplacental hematomas. Hematoma appearances vary with acute being from hyperechoic, becoming isoechoic, and finally becoming hypoechoic to anechoic. Placental abruption is one of the leading causes of perinatal mortality and accounts for 15–20% of all perinatal deaths.[1] It can be associated with maternal vascular disease, hypertension, abdominal trauma, cocaine abuse, cigarette smoking, advanced maternal age, and unexplained increased MSAFP.[1]

Placenta accreta is the abnormal adherence of placental tissue to the uterus. It is divided into (1) placenta accreta placental attachment to the myometrium without invasion; (2) placenta increta—invasion of the placenta into the myometrium; and (3) placenta percreta—invasion of the placenta through the uterus and often invasion into the bladder or rectum. Risk factors include uterine scarring from cesarean sections and advanced maternal age.[1] Implantation sites at risk are uterine scars, submucous fibroid, lower uterine segment, rudimentary horn, and uterine cornua. With placenta accreta, the normal hypoechoic 1–2 cm myometrial band is absent or thinned (<2 mm) with loss of placental/myometrial interface.[5,10] There may be large hypoechoic to anechoic spaces in the placenta, termed "Swiss cheese appearance." Placental vascularity is also increased.[5] Doppler ultrasound is used to aid in the sonographic diagnosis.

Chorioangioma is the most common benign tumor of the placenta. It is a vascular malformation arising from the chorionic tissue that appears as a well-defined, hypoechoic mass near the chorionic surface and often near the cord insertion site.[3] Color and pulsed Doppler will confirm the increased vascularity of this lesion.

The umbilical cord consists of two arteries and one vein. The vein enters the fetus and drains into the ductus venosum and left portal vein in the liver. The umbilical vein carries oxygenated blood. The umbilical arteries, carrying deoxygenated blood, are seen coursing laterally around the bladder as they leave the fetal body. The vessels in the cord are surrounded by Wharton's jelly for protection. The umbilical cord normally inserts into the central portion of the placenta. It can, however, insert eccentrically or near the membranes. It can also be a velamentous insertion when it inserts into the membranes and courses through the membrane to the placenta.[3,5] Both of these insertions can play a part in placental insufficiency and fetal growth. Occasionally, only one artery will be present resulting in a two vessel umbilical cord. It may be associated with other abnormalities and could possibly affect fetal growth, although not common. Color Doppler Sonography can help identify absence of the umbilical artery, as well as nuchal cord and cord knots.[5]

Fetal Head, Neck, and Spine

Neural Tube Defect. This is a spectrum of malformations of the neural tube including: (1) anencephaly, (2) spina bifida, and (3) cephalocele. Folic acid taken daily before and during pregnancy is known to reduce the risk of neural tube defect.[1]

Anencephaly. This is the most severe form of neural tube defect. It is characterized by absence of the upper portion of the cranial vault and underlying cerebral hemispheres. The fetal face and brainstem are normally present in anencephaly. It may be diagnosed as early as 12 weeks by transvaginal sonography and is associated with a markedly increased MSAFP, polyhydramnios, spinal defects, and bulging of the fetal orbits, giving the fetus a frog-like appearance.[19]

Spina Bifida. This is a defect in the lateral processes of the vertebrae allowing the spinal canal to be exposed, which in turn disrupts the muscle and skin covering. Herniation can be limited to meninges (meningocele) or involve the neural tissue as well (myelomeningocele). The most common sites of spina bifida are lumbar, lumbosacral, and thoracolumbar. Cranial findings associated with spina bifida are (1) "banana sign," consistently present with a defect (99%), and (2) "lemon sign." The banana sign is the displacement of the cerebrum inferiorly and the cisterna magna is usually obliterated. On the transverse view, the cerebellum resembles a banana instead of its characteristic view. The lemon sign includes bilateral depression of the frontal bone and gives the sonographic impression of a "lemon"-shaped head (Fig. 7–42 A and B). Spina bifida is often associated with increased MSAFP, ventriculomegaly, and clubfeet.[1,3,19]

Cephalocele. This is a protrusion of the cranial contents through a bony defect in the skull. An encephalocele contains brain tissue. The majority are occipital (75%).[3,19] They often cause blockage of cerebrospinal fluid and ventriculomegaly results. Very large defects may be associated with microcephaly. Both types have a poor prognosis.[3,19]

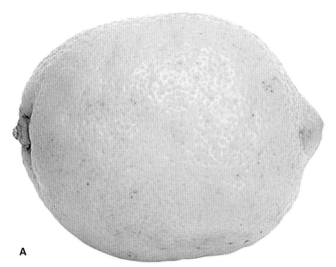

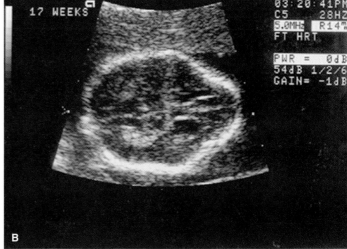

A **B**

FIGURE 7–42 (A) Lemon. **(B)** Sonogram of a "lemon"-shaped head.

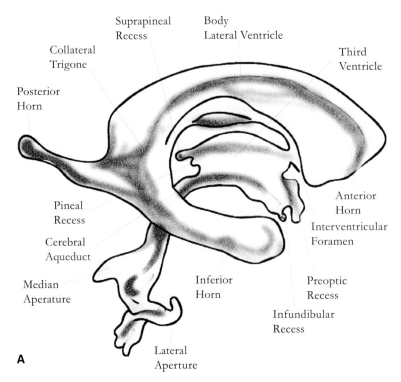

FIGURE 7–43A. Diagram of the ventricular system in the lateral view.

Ventriculomegaly. The anatomy of the ventricular system is imperative in order to recognize the normal and abnormal sonographic appearance (Figs. 7–43A and B). This is enlargement of the lateral ventricles, more than 10 mm in the atrial diameter. In the absence of a spinal defect, pronounced ventriculomegaly (>15 mm) is most commonly associated with an obstruction of the ventricular system. In order of occurrence, these obstructions are aqueductal stenosis, communicating hydrocephalus, and Dandy–Walker malformation. Congenital hydrocephaly is an X-linked abnormality with only males affected and females being carriers. If there is a strong family history, DNA testing is available.[3,19] Ventriculomegaly is often associated with other abnormalities.

Dandy–Walker Malformation. This consists of a splaying of the cerebellar vermis, dilated fourth ventricle, increased cisterna magna (>10 mm), and ventriculomegaly. It can be associated with chromosomal abnormalities and is frequently associated with such other cranial midline defects as agenesis of the corpus callosum. It is often associated with other system abnormalities as well.[3]

Holoprosencephaly. This is a group of midline defects resulting from incomplete cleavage of the prosencephalon. The three major varieties are (1) alobar—single rudimentary ventricle, absent cerebral falx, fused thalamus, absent third ventricle. Facial findings may range from cyclopia to severe hypotelorism. A medial cleft lip/palate is common. A proboscis may replace the nose or the nose may be very flattened; (2) semilobar—the

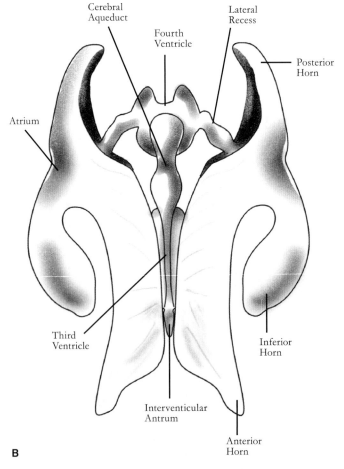

FIGURE 7–43B. Diagram of the ventricular system in the superior view.

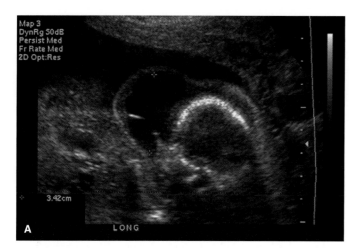

FIGURE 7–44A. Longitudinal sonogram of the fetus with cystic hygroma in the posterior region of the fetal neck.

cerebral hemispheres are partially separated posteriorly, with partial separation of the lateral ventricles. Both alobar and semilobar holoprosencephaly are associated with microcephaly; (3) lobar—almost complete separation of cerebellum and ventricles except for the fused anterior horns of the lateral ventricles. Other sonographic findings are absent cavum septum pellucidum. Facial findings are less severe than those found with alobar or semilobar holoprosencephaly.[3]

Cystic Hygroma. This most often occurs at the posterior neck. A hygroma is a sac filled with lymphatic fluid caused by an obstruction of the lymphatic system. It may be multiloculated or contain a midline septum and is often associated with Turner's syndrome or Down's syndrome.[19]

Fig. 7–44A shows a longitudinal sonogram of fetal neck with cystic hygroma. Fig. 7–44B shows a transverse sonogram of the same case demonstrating multiple septations in the mass.

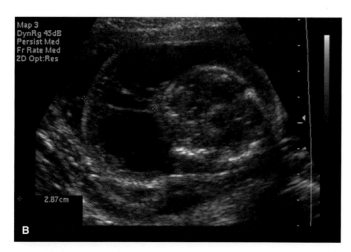

FIGURE 7–44B. Transverse sonogram of the same case demonstrating the multiple septations in the mass.

Choroid Plexus Cyst. This is a cyst in the choroid plexus of the lateral ventricles. With other sonographic findings, it may be associated with trisomy 18 or 21. Alone, many investigators consider this a normal anatomic variant.[3,10]

Iniencephaly. This is a defect in the occiput involving the foramen magnum characterized by marked retroflexion of the fetal head and frequently shortened spine. This is a rare finding and has a strong association with other abnormalities.[3]

Agenesis of the Corpus Callosum. The corpus callosum begins to develop at 12 weeks of gestation and its development is complete at approximately 20 weeks.[19] This abnormality cannot be diagnosed until after 18 weeks of gestation. Findings to aid in diagnosis include: (1) absence of the cavum septum pellucidum (2) enlargement of the posterior horn of the lateral ventricle (3) Extremely narrow frontal horns (4) enlargement and upward displacement of the third ventricle. Agenesis of the corpus callosum has a strong association with other abnormalities.[3,10,19]

Hydranencephaly. This is a severe destructive process, believed to result from occlusion of the internal carotid arteries. The cerebral cortex is replaced by fluid, causing macrocephaly. The thalamus, brainstem, and cerebellum are spared.[3,10]

Vein of Galen Aneurysm. This is an arteriovenous malformation in vein of Galen located posterior to the third ventricle in the midline. Color and pulsed Doppler will demonstrate high-velocity arterial and venous blood flow. This is associated with congestive heart failure and hydrops.[10]

Cleft Lip/Palate. Isolated cleft lip and/or palate is the most common congenital facial anomaly. Lateral cleft lip is commonly isolated. Medial cleft lip is associated with chromosomal abnormalities.[10]

Heart

Atrial/Ventricular Septal Defect. This is a congenital malformation of the septum that appears as an opening between the chambers. It is the most common cardiac defect, accounting for 26% of defects.[20]

Atrioventricular Canal Defect. This is also known as atrioventricular septal defect, or endocardial cushion defect. A complete defect has a single ventricle, a single atrium, and a single atrioventricular valve. This appearance may vary with partial defects of the atrial or ventricular septums. This is the most common cardiac defect in trisomy 21.[20]

Hypoplastic Left Heart Syndrome. This is hypoplasia of the left ventricle, atrium, mitral valve, and aortic outflow. The right side of the heart will be enlarged.[20] The appearance may vary with different degrees of severity.

Coarctation of the Aorta. This is a narrowed segment of aorta along the aortic arch. It is difficult to see the narrowing but may present as a milder form of hypoplastic left heart syndrome later in pregnancy. Pulsed Doppler studies may also show a decrease in blood flow in the proximal portion of the aorta.[20]

Tetralogy of Fallot. This presents with the following defects: (1) ventricular septal defect, (2) overriding aorta, (3) pulmonary stenosis or atresia, and (4) right ventricular hypertrophy. It has a strong association with chromosomal abnormalities.[19,20]

Ebstein's Anomaly. This is the inferior displacement of the tricuspid valve. The right atrium is enlarged, and the valve, which is commonly abnormal, may appear thick and irregular in motion. Tricuspid valve regurgitation is often appreciated.[20]

Double Outlet Right Ventricle. The pulmonary artery and aorta both originate from the right ventricle, giving the appearance of the great vessels running parallel. Often a ventricular septal defect is present.[20]

Transposition of the Great Vessels. The aorta arises from the right ventricle, and the pulmonary artery arises from the left ventricle. The great vessels appear parallel on ultrasound. The pulmonary bifurcation and brachiocephalic vessels must be identified to correctly diagnosis this entity. Atrial septal defect and ventricular septal defect are often present.[3,20]

Truncus Arteriosus. This is a single large ventricular outflow tract overriding a ventricular septal defect. Right ventricular outflow tract will not be visualized, and pulmonary artery branches as well as aortic branches will be seen arising from the truncus.[20]

Rhabdomyoma. This is the most common intracardiac tumor. It can be multiple and appears as an echogenic mass located anywhere within the cardiac system. It is not visualized <22 weeks and has a strong association with tuberous sclerosis.[20]

Supraventricular Tachycardia. The fetal heartbeat is more than 200 bpm. Both supraventricular tachycardia and atrial flutter can lead to cardiac failure because of increased cardiac output.[20]

Thorax

Congenital Diaphragmatic Hernia. This is a congenital defect in the diaphragm allowing abdominal contents to herniate into the thorax. It may be left sided (75–90%), right sided (10%), or bilateral (<5%). Sonographically, (1) the fetal heart may be deviated, (2) stomach or bowel may be visualized in the thorax, (3) the area adjacent to the heart may appear inhomogeneous, and (4) polyhydramnios may be present. The intrathoracic abdominal contents can cause pulmonary hypoplasia, a significant factor in the high perinatal mortality (50–80%) of this disorder. If the liver is intrathoracic, congenital diaphragmatic hernia has a poorer prognosis (43% survival) versus an intra-abdominal liver (80% survival). Associated anomalies (15–45%) and chromosomal abnormalities (5–15%) will also affect perinatal survival.[19,20]

Congenital Cystic Adenomatoid Malformation. This is the most frequently identified mass in the fetal chest. It is typically unilateral and has three types: (1) type I, macrocystic—multiple large cysts measuring 2–10 cm, (2) type II—multiple medium-sized cysts <2 cm, and (3) type III, microcystic—sonographically appearing as a solid, homogenous echogenic lung mass. Many congenital cystic adenomatoid malformations spontaneously regress in size during the third trimester. Prognosis is dependent on size, degree of mediastinal shift, and presence or absence of hydrops and polyhydramnios. Types I and II typically have a better prognosis.[20]

Pulmonary Sequestration. This is a solid, nonfunctioning mass of lung tissue that lacks communication with the tracheobronchial tree. It has its own blood supply commonly arising directly from the aorta and is fed by a single vessel. The majority are visualized as well circumscribed masses in the left lower lung base. They may cause mediastinal shift and hydrops. Ten percent can be found below the diaphragm and should be considered with any suprarenal mass in the left abdomen. Fifty percent to seventy-five percent of sequestrations regress spontaneously.[20]

Pleural Effusion. This is an abnormal accumulation of fluid in the pleural lining of the fetal thorax. The etiologies are hydrops fetalis, chromosomal, and fetal infection. Fig. 7–45

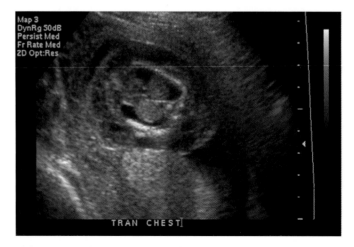

FIGURE 7–45. Transverse sonogram of a fetus with bilateral pleural effusions.

shows a transverse sonogram of the fetal thorax with bilateral pleural effusions.

Gastrointestinal

Esophageal Atresia. This is an incomplete formation of the esophagus. There are five types of atresia, with 90% of those having a tracheoesophageal fistula that communicates with the fetal stomach. Sonographically, the exam may be normal or there may be a small to absent stomach bubble and polyhydramnios. Even with a stomach bubble visualized, this must be considered normal with unexplained polyhydramnios. This has a strong association with other anomalies and chromosomal abnormalities.[20]

Duodenal Atresia. This is a partial to complete obstruction caused by the failure of recanalization of the duodenum. It is the most common perinatal intestinal obstruction. The stomach and duodenum fill with fluid proximal to the site of the obstruction creating the classic "double-bubble" sign. Fifty percent are associated with other findings including growth restriction, polyhydramnios, gastrointestinal, and cardiac anomalies. Duodenal atresia has a strong association with trisomy 21.[3,10]

Gastroschisis. This is an anterior abdominal wall defect, most commonly to the right side of the umbilicus, which allows herniation of abdominal contents into the amniotic cavity. The most common finding is free-floating bowel in the amniotic fluid, but stomach and bladder may also herniate into the amniotic fluid. Exposure to amniotic fluid and compression at an abdominal wall can lead to dilation and edema of the bowel. Overall, this has a good prognosis and does not have a strong association with chromosomal defects or other anomalies. It is associated with an elevated MSAFP.[3]

Omphalocele. This is a midline defect in the anterior abdominal wall with herniation of abdominal contents into the base of the umbilical cord. The mass is covered by a membrane and may not always have an elevated MSAFP, or may not elevate the MSAFP as significantly as gastroschisis. The umbilical cord can be seen inserting into the abdominal mass. Omphaloceles commonly contain liver but may contain other abdominal organs such as bowel. They have a strong association with other anomalies (50–80%), particularly cardiac, as well as chromosomal abnormalities (40–60%). If the omphalocele is small and contains only small bowel, the risk of aneuploidy increases.[2]

Pentalogy of Cantrell. This is an extensive defect of the thoraco-abdominal wall characterized by (1) ectopia cordis, (2) omphalocele, (3) ventricular septal defect, (4) defect of the sternum, and (5) diaphragmatic hernia. This anomaly is sonographically distinctive because of an omphalocele and ectopia cordis. There are many other associated craniofacial abnormalities, and it often is associated with chromosomal abnormalities.[19,20]

Beckwith–Wiedemann Syndrome. This is a group of disorders including omphalocele, macroglossia, organomegaly, hypoglycemia, and hemihypertrophy.[20]

Cloacal Exstrophy. This is an association of anomalies including omphalocele, herniated, fluid filled structure inferior to omphalocele in place of urinary bladder, imperforate anus, and neural tube defect. This defect has a marked increased MSAFP.[20]

Meconium Ileus. This is the third most common cause of neonatal bowel obstruction. Sonographic findings include echogenic small bowel, dilated fluid-filled loops of bowel, and echogenic dilated bowel. It has a strong association with cystic fibrosis. If the internal diameter of the small bowel is more than 7 mm, it is suggestive of obstruction.[1,3]

Meconium Peritonitis. This is a reaction to bowel perforation. Meconium causes a peritoneal reaction that forms a membrane, which seals the perforation and may be seen as a thick-walled cyst. Other findings are ascites and meconium calcifications.[1,3,19]

Limb–Body Wall Complex (LBWC). This is a complex set of abnormalities caused by failure of the anterior abdominal wall to close. Findings include complete body wall defects, absence of umbilical cord, severe scoliosis, and lower limb abnormalities. Abnormalities are widespread and appearance may be a mass of tissue with few distinctive features.[3,19]

Amniotic Band Syndrome. Rupture of the amnion early in pregnancy resulting in formation of amniotic strands that stick and entangle fetal parts resulting in amputation of digits, arms, and legs. Fetal movement restriction due to amniotic bands is helpful for the sonographic diagnosis.[3,19]

Hydrops. There are two types: (1) non-immune—accumulation of fluid in body cavities (pleural, pericardial, and peritoneal) and soft tissue. There are many causes for this entity, but major causes are cardiac failure, anemia, arteriovenous shunts, mediastinal compression, metabolic diseases, fetal infections, fetal tumors, congenital fetal defects, chromosomal and placental anomalies; (2) immune—sonographic findings are the same. These are caused by maternal antibodies destroying fetal red blood cells, which ultimately leads to erythroblastosis fetalis or congestive heart failure.[2]

Fig. 7–46 A, B, and C are sonograms demonstrating fetal hydrops, bilateral pleural effusions, and polyhydramnios, respectively.

Ascites. This is free fluid within the abdominal cavity. It may be part of the hydrops complex or isolated because of bowel perforation or bladder perforation.

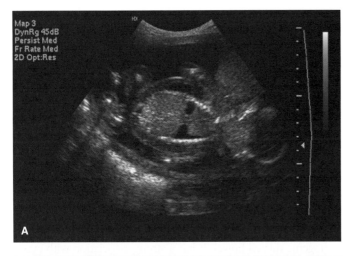

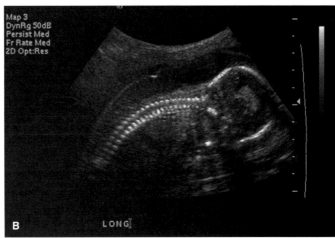

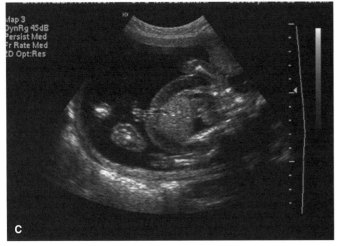

FIGURE 7-46. (A,B,C) Sonograms demonstrating fetal hydrops, bilateral effusions, and polyhydramnios.

Situs Inversus Totalis. This is complete thoracic and abdominal organ reversal. Partial situs involves the abdominal organs only. Often associated with polysplenia and congenital heart defects.[2]

Abdominal Cyst. The differential for an isolated abdominal cyst not related to the GI or GU tract include ovarian cyst, mesenteric cyst, omental cyst, or urachal cyst as the most common listings.

Genitourinary

Ureteropelvic Junction Obstruction. This is an obstruction at the junction of the renal pelvis and ureter. It is the most common cause of hydronephrosis. A complete obstruction will lead to massive hydronephrosis eventually causing dysplasia.

Ureterovesical Junction Obstruction. This is an obstruction at the junction of the ureter and bladder. Sonographic findings include mild hydronephrosis and hydroureter. Often associated with duplicated renal anomalies including the ureter. The abnormal ureter commonly has a stenotic opening into the bladder and forms an ureterocele, which appears as a cystic structure within or adjacent to the bladder.

Posterior Urethral Valve Bladder Outlet Obstruction. This is an obstruction of the posterior urethral valves. Overwhelming found in males, the bladder is massively dilated with hydroureters and hydronephrosis. The massive hydronephrosis may lead to atrophy of the kidneys. Anhydramnios is present with complete obstruction. On ultrasound, the bladder has the characteristic "keyhole" appearance as urine fills the proximal urethra. The abdominal wall becomes overly distended, which results in prune belly syndrome (abnormal development of abdominal musculature leading to a lax abdominal wall in newborns). The lack of amniotic fluid causes Potter facies (flattened facies, low set ears) and flexion contractures of the extremities. Pulmonary hypoplasia, caused by anhydramnios, is the primary cause of neonatal death in this syndrome.

Renal Agenesis. Diagnosis is made by the following findings: anhydramnios to severe oligohydramnios, nonvisualized bladder, and absent kidneys without evidence of renal blood flow. The adrenal glands appear flattened and elongated, which may aid in the diagnosis.

Multicystic Dysplastic Kidney. This is an obstruction in the first trimester that leads to atretic kidneys and formation of randomly positioned and varying sized cysts in the parenchyma of the kidney. The parenchyma is usually increased in echogenicity as well.

Autosomal Dominant Polycystic Kidney Disease.
There must be one affected parent for this disorder to occur. Findings are not always seen in pregnancy and if so, typically do not appear until third trimester. Kidneys may appear enlarged and echogenic with multiple large cysts.

Autosomal Recessive Polycystic Kidney Disease.
This is also known as infantile polycystic kidney disease. Multiple microscopic cysts give the appearance of very large, echogenic kidneys with decreased AFV after 20 weeks. Findings may be normal <20 weeks.

Congenital Mesoblastic Nephroma. This is a rare renal tumor that sonographically appears as a large, solid, well-circumscribed, highly vascular mass. The increased vascularity can cause cardiac overload and polyhydramnios.

Neuroblastoma. This malignant tumor is commonly found in the adrenal gland. Sonographically, it appears as an echogenic, heterogeneous, suprarenal mass.[19,20]

Skeletal

Limb shortening may be described as: (1) rhizomelic—shortening of the proximal limb, (2) mesomelic—shortening of the forearm bones or lower leg bones, (3) micromelia—shortening of all portions of the limbs, both severe and mild. There are many types of short limb syndromes, and the more common lethal and nonlethal varieties are discussed in this review.

Short limb syndromes are considered lethal if the thoracic circumference is less than fifth percentile for the gestational age, suggesting pulmonary hypoplasia. Other findings are: (1) severe micromelia, less than four standard deviations of mean, and (2) identification of such specific features as severe fractures.

Lethal
Thanatophoric Dysplasia. This is the most common skeletal dysplasia and is uniformly lethal.
Findings are:
- Cranium—macrocrania, hydrocephaly, frontal bossing, cloverleaf shaped skull, depressed nasal bridge
- Thorax—severely hypoplastic giving the "bell-shaped" appearance, short ribs
- Bones—severe rhizomelia with bowing ("telephone receiver"); hypomineralization; spinal column appears narrow; polyhydramnios

Achondrogenesis—Type I, Most Severe. This exhibits severe micromelia, protruding abdomen, poor skull, and vertebral ossification. Type II, accounts for 80%.
- Cranium—macrocrania
- Thorax—shortened trunk

- Bones—severe micromelia with bowing and decreased mineralization

Osteogenesis Imperfecta Type II—Lethal. OI type II is subcategorized into three types, but all three are discussed in general terms for this text.

- Thorax—bell shaped, with small thorax; ribs have multiple fractures, may appear thin and flared
- Bones—micromelia; may see fractures or bones may appear thickened, irregular, and bowed because of fractures folding on themselves
- Decreased fetal movement and polyhydramnios

Nonlethal
Heterozygous Achondroplasia. This is the most common form of genetic skeletal dysplasia. It may not always be identified before <27 weeks.

- Cranium—increased HC, frontal bossing, depressed nasal bridge
- Bones—mild to moderate rhizomelic shortening, "trident" hand

Osteogenesis Imperfecta—Types I, III, IV
- Type I—may not identify <24 weeks; mild micromelia and bowing; may see isolated fractures
- Type III—will show lagging long bone growth early with mild to moderate shortening and bowing
- Type IV—similar to type I

Asphyxiating Thoracic Dysplasia (Jeune Thoracic Dystrophy)
- Thorax—may appear bell shaped
- Bones—mild to moderate micromelia (rhizomelic) with possible bowing, possible polydactyly polyhydramnios.[2]

MULTIPLE GESTATIONS

Multiple pregnancies account for 3.3% of live births. Dizygotic, or fraternal, twins occur when two separate ova are fertilized. Monozygotic, or identical, twins occur when a single ovum divides. Seventy-five percent of twins are dizygotic, and 25% are monozygotic. The frequency of monozygotic twinning is constant and occurs in 1:250 births. Dizygotic twinning varies widely and is dependent on race, maternal age, parity (increased risk with increased parity), maternal family history, and infertility medication.[1]

It is very important to determine the number of chorionic and amniotic sacs in twin pregnancies. The best and most accurate time to assess this is in the first trimester. All dizygotic twins are dichorionic, diamniotic. Monozygotic twins, on the other hand, may have a variety of presentations depending on the day the zygote divides.[2]

Day of Division   **Appearance**

Day of Division	Appearance
<4 days	Dichorionic/diamniotic, same gender, occurs 24% of time
4–8 days	Monochorionic, diamniotic, occurs 75% of time
8–12 days	Monochorionic, monoamniotic, 1%
>13 days	Conjoined, monochorionic, monoamniotic

Sonography cannot distinguish between dizygotic and monozygotic twins unless they are different genders. There are sonographic clues to aid in the identification of chorionicity and amniocity.

First trimester sonographic findings are:

Dichorionic—sacs will be divided by a thick echogenic rim, counting the sacs determines the chorionicity.

Monochorionic—will appear similar to a single gestation with a thick echogenic gestational sac surrounding both fetuses.

Diamniotic—each sac will have its own yolk sac (> 8 weeks). The amniotic sac is very thin and can be difficult to identify in the first trimester.[2]

Second trimester—Dichorionic findings:

1) Different gender

2) Two separate placentas

3) Twin peak sign—triangular projection of chorion into dividing membrane appears as a "peak" on ultrasound; strong predictor <28 weeks

4) Thickness of membrane—thick membrane, more than 1 mm, is suggestive of dichorionicity. This finding is more accurate less than 26 weeks but is still a weak predictor.[2]

Twin pregnancies carry a four to six times higher perinatal mortality, and a two times higher morbidity rate for a variety of reasons. The most common complication of twins is preterm labor. Other complications are growth restriction, anomalies (two to three times more than a singleton), and such maternal conditions as hypertension and preeclampsia.[3,4]

Twin Abnormalities

Twin-to-Twin Transfusion Syndrome (TTTS). This condition can occur with monochorionic twins. Arteriovenous communications within the placenta can result in TTTS. One fetus will have blood shunted away and is labeled the donor, while the other fetus will receive the shunted blood and is labeled the recipient. This syndrome presents with a series of sonographic findings related to the shunting of blood. The donor twin is commonly growth restricted with a discordance between the twins of more than 20%. There is often oligohydramnios with the donor and polyhydramnios with the recipient. The donor fetus will appear "stuck" in the sac. This appearance is characteristic of TTTS. The donor will become hypovolemic and anemic. Umbilical cord Doppler images often show an increased systolic/diastolic ratio, demonstrating the increased resistance in the umbilical cord.

The recipient will become larger, hypervolemic, and plethoric. Hydrops may occur as the fetus enters into congestive heart failure. The ventricular walls of the heart may thicken, and the contractility of the heart may be decreased as the heart failure becomes worse. As the blood flow increases to the recipient, the S/D ratio decreases, and the overall blood velocity is high. Both fetuses are at a significantly increased risk for intrauterine and perinatal mortality.[1,20]

Monoamniotic Twins. This entity carries a 50% mortality risk because of cord entanglement that obstructs blood flow to the fetus. Sonographically, color Doppler may be helpful to look for a mass of cord with areas of increased velocity, suggesting stenotic flow.

Conjoined Twins. This is rare. Most conjoined twins are born prematurely, and 40% are stillborn. The most common presentation is fusion of the anterior wall. They may share organs, and those organs can often have abnormalities. Polyhydramnios is present 50% of the time. The most common types are: thoraco-omphalopagus (conjoined chest and abdomen), thoracopagus (conjoined chest), and omphalopagus (conjoined abdomen). They account for 56% of the types of conjoined twins.[1,20]

Acardiac Twin. This is rare. All cases have an arterial-to-arterial shunt and a venous-to-venous shunt allowing for perfusion of the acardiac twin.[20] The acardiac twin either has a rudimentary heart or is completely acardiac. It has a poorly underdeveloped upper body with a small or absent cranium and brain. If it does develop, there are often significant abnormalities. The lungs and abdominal organs may also be abnormal or absent. The lower extremities are slightly more developed.[1] The normal, or pump twin is at a great risk for congestive heart failure, which will present on ultrasound as polyhydramnios and fetal hydrops. Chromosomes have been reported to be abnormal in up to 50% of the cases. Doppler can verify the reversed flow in the umbilical cord of the acardiac twin.[20]

CHROMOSOMAL ABNORMALITIES AND TESTING

Trisomy 21. This is the most common chromosome disorder. Trisomy 21 occurs when there are three copies of chromosome 21. The Down's syndrome frequency increases with advanced maternal age. At this time, the only definitive test to determine Down's syndrome is amniocentesis. Noninvasive testing includes blood tests and ultrasound.[1]

First-trimester screening combines biochemistry markers, maternal age (MA), and fetal nuchal translucency. Nuchal translucency is a measurement made at the back of the fetal neck on the CRL image. It is applicable from 11 to 14 weeks. The nuchal translucency increases with gestational age and normal tables are available for comparison; however, any measurement less than 3 mm is normal. Screening for Down's syndrome by maternal age and nuchal translucency has been shown to identify 80% of fetuses with Down's syndrome (with a 5% false-positive rate). Other chromosomal defects (trisomy 18, 13, triploidy, and Turner's syndrome), cardiac defects, skeletal dysplasias, and genetic syndromes can also present with increased nuchal translucency.[3,19,20]

For the nuchal translucency to be accurate, very strict rules should be followed. The fetus is measured in the sagittal plane, the same used for the CRL. Careful consideration should be taken to bisect the fetus exactly in the midline, evidenced by the umbilical cord insertion. The image should be magnified so that the fetus occupies at least three-fourths of the image. The imager should be able to distinguish between the fetal skin and the amnion, both appearing as a thin membrane. This is accomplished by waiting for the fetus to spontaneously move away from the amnion. The first caliper should be placed so that the horizontal bar of the caliper is on the outside edge of the inner membrane in the nuchal region. The second caliper should be placed so that the horizontal bar is on the inside edge of the fetal skin. The placement of the caliper is very important for the predictability and accuracy of the nuchal translucency. Great care should be taken to achieve the correct image and caliper placement (Fig. 7–47).[3,19,20]

First-trimester biochemistry includes the analysis of hCG and PAPP-A (pregnancy associated plasma protein A).[6] The higher the hCG and the lower the PAPP-A, the higher the trisomy 21 risk. The detection rate of trisomy 21, combining MA, nuchal translucency, and biochemistry is 90%, with a 5% false-positive rate.[20]

Second-trimester ultrasound markers can be divided into major and minor findings. Major findings warrant offering invasive testing alone; whereas, minor markers require two or more findings to warrant offering invasive testing. Major sonographic markers include: increased nuchal skinfold (>6 mm), cardiac defect, diaphragmatic hernia, omphalocele,

facial cleft, and atresia (esophageal or duodenal).[3,20] Minor markers include abnormal ratio of observed/expected femur and humeral lengths, hypoplasia of midphalanx of fifth digit, echogenic foci of the heart, pyelectasis, echogenic bowel, sandal gap toe, choroid plexus cysts, small ears and, most recently, nasal bone.[6,20]

Second-trimester biochemistry or maternal serum AFP3 (MSAFP3), consists of hCG, AFP, and estriol. A risk of trisomy 21 is calculated based on these values. The risk increases with a higher hCG, lower AFP, and lower estriol. Combining the ultrasound with the biochemistry markers will detect approximately 60% of trisomy 21 fetuses.[20]

Trisomy 18. In this disorder, there are three copies of chromosome 18. Ninety-five percent are an intrauterine demise or stillborn.[1] It is commonly, but not always, associated with multiple defects. Sonographically, these major findings may be seen with trisomy 18; growth restriction, increased nuchal translucency, neural tube defect, strawberry-shaped head, choroid plexus cysts, ACC, enlarged cisterna magnum, decreased extremity lengths, cardiac defects, diaphragmatic hernia, esophageal atresia, omphalocele, and renal agenesis. Minor ultrasound findings include clenched hands, echogenic bowel, rocker-bottom feet, micrognathia, and single umbilical artery.[6,20] MSAFP3 shows all three markers decreased.[1]

Trisomy 13. In this disorder, there is an extra copy of chromosome 13. It may be associated with multiple abnormalities; however, the most common sonographic findings are holoprosencephaly (including the facial spectrums), cardiac defects, postaxial polydactyly, echogenic or polycystic kidneys, omphalocele, and microcephaly.[1,20]

Triploidy. In this disorder, there are three complete sets of chromosomes. If paternally derived, the typical finding is a large placenta with multiple cystic areas (partial mole). If maternally derived, multiple findings include severe IUGR with an abnormally large head and small abdomen, hypertelorism, micrognathia, ventriculomegaly, cardiac defects, neural tube defect, holoprosencephaly, Dandy–Walker malformation, cystic hygroma, renal anomalies, clubbed feet, single umbilical artery, and oligohydramnios.[1,20]

Sex Chromosome Abnormalities. The main sex chromosome abnormalities are Turner's syndrome, 47, XXX; 47, XXY; and 47, XYY.[20] Sonographically, Turner's syndrome findings are cystic hygroma, lymphangiectasia, cardiac defects, renal abnormalities, and hydrops.[1,20] The other sex chromosome abnormalities do not typically have prenatal sonographic findings.

INVASIVE TESTING

Amniocentesis. This is an invasive procedure in which a needle is inserted into the amniotic cavity and amniotic fluid

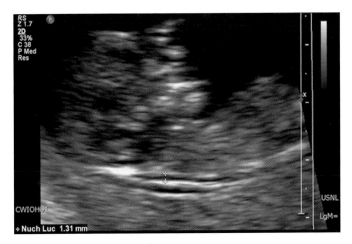

FIGURE 7–47. Fetus with electronic callipers measuring the nuchal translucency.

is withdrawn. The amniotic fluid is typically assessed for karyotype, levels of amniotic fluid bilirubin associated with Rh disease, amniotic fluid alpha-fetoprotein, acetylcholinesterase for spinal defects, infection, fetal lung maturity, and specific DNA studies. Our institution quotes a 1:300 risk of miscarriage with amniocentesis based on the national average. The standard amniocentesis is offered after 14 weeks.

Fluorescence *in Situ* Hybridization (FISH). This is currently an adjunct to amniocentesis. It is considered experimental at this time, so all findings from this test must be confirmed by amniocentesis results. "Tags," or markers, that attach to certain chromosomes (currently testing 13, 18, 21, X and Y) fluorescence. This allows the geneticist to count the chromosomes for extra or deleted chromosomes. Results are available in 24–48 hours.[21]

Early amniocentesis is performed the same as amniocentesis but during the 11th to 14th weeks of gestation. It has been associated with many problems. The loss rate is higher, 1:100, and is technically more difficult to perform because of the lack of fusion of the amnion and chorion. The unfused membranes are difficult to penetrate and often cause the need for multiple sticks, which in turn, increases the loss risk. Early amniocentesis has also been associated with talipes equinovarus.[20]

Chorionic Villus Sampling (CVS). This is a procedure in which a catheter is inserted into the placenta and chorionic villi are aspirated for karyotyping. This procedure may be done transabdominally or transvaginally, depending on placental location. CVS is performed between 10 and 12 weeks and results are obtained in 3–8 days versus 10–14 days for amniocentesis. CVS does not test for amniotic fluid alpha-fetoprotein and cannot rule out spinal defects. Although the loss rate is 1:100. Although the loss rate is slightly higher than amniocentesis, the CVS loss rate is comparable to early amniocentesis. CVS performed <10 weeks has an association with severe limb defects and is not typically performed at that time.[2,20,21]

Percutaneous Umbilical Blood Sampling (PUBS). This is similar to an amniocentesis except that the needle is advanced through the amniotic fluid to the cord insertion site into the placenta. The needle is then inserted into the base of the umbilical cord. CDS can aid in locating the umbilical cord insertion into the placenta.[5] This procedure has a higher loss rate, 1–2%, and is technically more difficult to perform. It allows for rapid karyotyping (48–72 hours). PUBS most common application is with Rh isoimmunization testing. The fetal blood is tested for the amount of bilirubin pigment and allows the perinatologist to perform a blood transfusion if necessary.[21]

References

1. Leveno K, Bloom S, Hauth J, et al. *Williams Obstetrics.* 23rd ed. New York, NY: McGraw-Hill Companies; 2009.

2. Fleischer AC. Sonohysterography combined with sonosalpingography: correlation with endoscopic findings in infertility patients. *J Ultrasound Med.* 1997; 16:381-384.

3. Rumack CM, Wilson SR, Charboneau JW, et al. *Diagnostic Ultrasound.* 3rd ed. St. Louis, MO: Elsevier Mosby; 2005.

4. Callen PW. *Ultrasonography in Obstetrics and Gynecology.* 5th ed. Philadelphia, PA: Sanders, Elsevier; 2008.

5. Fleischer A, Toy E, Manning F, et al. Sonography. In: *Obstetrics & Gynecology: Principles and Practice.* 7th ed. New York, NY: McGraw-Hill Companies; 2011.

6. Pardo J, Kaplan B, Nitke S, Ovadia J, Segal J, Neri A. Postmenopausal intrauterine fluid collection: correlation between ultrasound and hysteroscopy. *Ultrasound Obstet Gynecol.* 1994; 4:224-226.

7. Nyberg DA, Filly RA, Filho DD, et al. Abdominal pregnancy: early diagnosis by US and serum chorionic gonadotropin levels. *Radiology.* 1986; 158:393-396.

8. Timor-Tritsch IE, Rottem S. *Transvaginal Sonography.* 2nd ed. New York: Elsevier; 1991.

9. Lyons EA. Abnormal premenopausal vaginal bleeding. *Gynecological Causes. Lecture and Paper,* SDMS 17th annual conference; 2000.

10. Mishell DR, Stenchever MA, Droegemueller W, et al. *Comprehensive Gynecology.* 3rd ed. St. Louis, MO: Mosby–Year Book; 1997.

11. Braunstein GD. *hCG Testing: Volume I: A Clinical Guide for the Testing of Human Chorionic Gonadotropin.* Abbott Park, IL: Abbott Diagnostics Educational Services; 1993.

12. Braunstein GD. *hCG Testing: Volume II: Answers to Frequently Asked Questions about hCG Testing.* Abbott Park, IL: Abbott Diagnostics Educational Services; 1991.

13. Soderstrom RM. *Serum Pregnancy Test—The Dangers of False Positives.* OB Management. 2001; 86-89.

14. Mishell DR, Stenchever MA, Droegemueller W, Herbst A. *Comprehensive Gynecology.* 3rd ed. St. Louis, MO: Mosby Year Book; 1997.

15. Simpson LL, Levine D, et al. *First Trimester Cystic Hygroma and Enlarged Nuchal Translucency.* Waltham, MA: Up to Date; 2010.

16. Bianchi DW, Crombleholme TM, et al. *Fetology Diagnosis and Management of Fetal Patient.* New York: McGraw-Hill; 2000.

17. Thilaganathan B, Sairam S, Michailidis G, et al. First trimester *nuchal translucency: effective routine screening for Down's syndrome.* Br J Radiol. 1999; 72.

18. Tortora GJ, Derrickson B. *Principles of Anatomy and Physiology.* 11th ed. Hoboken, NJ: John Wiley & Sons. Inc; 2006.

19. Hagen-Ansert SL. *Textbook of Diagnostic Ultrasonography.* 7th ed. St. Louis, MO: Mosby; 2012.

20. Creasy RK, Resnik, R. *Maternal-Fetal Medicine.* 6th ed. Philadelphia, PA: WB Saunders Company; 2009.

21. Bianchi DW, Crombleholme TM, D'Alton ME. *Fetology: Diagnosis and Management of the Fetal Patient.* New York: McGraw-Hill; 2000.

Questions

GENERAL INSTRUCTIONS: For each question, select the best answer. Select only one answer for each question unless otherwise specified.

1. The sonographic finding in Fig. 7–48 is

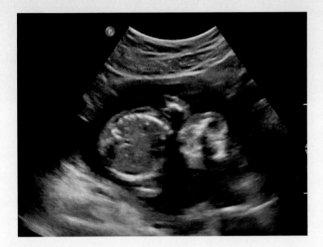

FIGURE 7–48.

   (A) normal fetal face

   (B) cleft lip

   (C) anencephaly

   (D) hypertelorism

   (E) epignathus

2. Fig. 7–49 demonstrates

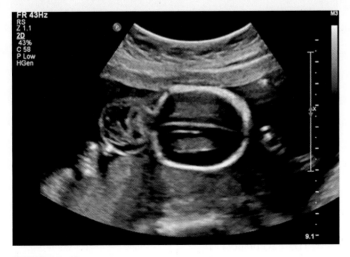

FIGURE 7–49.

   (A) omphalocele

   (B) encephalocele

   (C) cystic hygroma

   (D) craniosynostosis

   (E) arachnoid cyst

3. The sonographic finding in Fig. 7–50 include

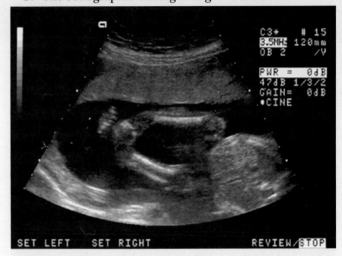

FIGURE 7–50.

   (A) equinovarus

   (B) normal foot posture

   (C) an association with spina bifida

   (D) both A and C

   (E) all of the above

4. Fig. 7–51 demonstrates

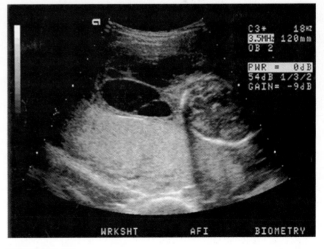

FIGURE 7–51.

   (A) cystic hygroma

   (B) spina bifida

   (C) encephalocele

   (D) nonimmune hydrops

   (E) scalp edema

5. Fig. 7–51 is a sonographic marker for

   (A) Turner's syndrome

   (B) Down's syndrome

   (C) trisomy 18

   (D) fetal infection

   (E) Potter's syndrome

6. The most likely diagnosis for Fig. 7–52 includes

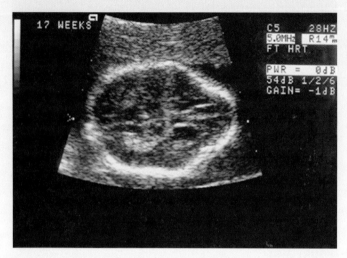

FIGURE 7–52.

   (A) spalding's sign

   (B) Down's syndrome

   (C) "lemon"-shaped skull

   (D) microcephaly

   (E) both A and D

   (F) both C and D

7. The sonographic finding in Fig. 7–53 is

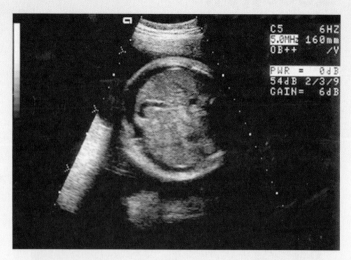

FIGURE 7–53.

   (A) fetal abdominal ascites

   (B) meconium peritonitis

   (C) Spalding's sign

   (D) nonimmune hydrops

   (E) scalp edema

8. Fig. 7–54 demonstrates

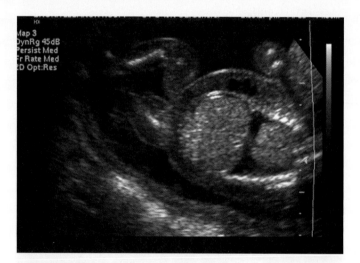

FIGURE 7–54.

   (A) bilateral pleural effusions and edema

   (B) cystic hygroma and scalp edema

   (C) increased nuchal sonolucency and fetal ascites

   (D) encephalocele

   (E) normal findings

9. Fig. 7–55 is an example of

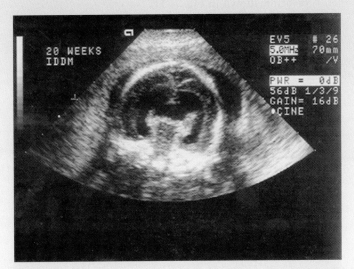

FIGURE 7–55.

(A) sonographic artifact

(B) severe ventriculomegaly

(C) holoprosencephaly

(D) scalp edema

(E) none of the above

10. Which of the following sonographic findings is not associated with trisomy 18?

(A) intrauterine growth retardation

(B) clenched hands

(C) holoprosencephaly

(D) cystic hygroma

11. Paternally derived triploidy has the following sonographic markers

(A) complete mole

(B) severe asymmetrical intrauterine growth retardation

(C) large placenta with multiple cystic areas

(D) oligohydramnios

(E) both A and D

(F) both B and D

12. Which of the following sonographic findings are seen in maternally derived triploidy?

(A) complete mole

(B) severe asymmetrical intrauterine growth retardation

(C) large placenta with multiple cystic areas

(D) oligohydramnios

(E) both A and D

(F) both B and D

13. Oligohydramnios is most likely associated with which one of the following?

(A) Potter's syndrome

(B) duodenal atresia

(C) hydrocephalus

(D) maternal diabetes

(E) fetal hydrops

14. Which one of the following is within the normal range of the fetal heart rate when documented on M-mode at 6 weeks gestation?

(A) 40–80 beats per minutes

(B) 80–100 beats per minutes

(C) 112–136 beats per minutes

(D) 136–200 beats per minutes

(E) 200–250 beats per minutes

15. A 60-year-old woman with primary adenocarcinoma of the stomach now presents with a large complex right ovarian mass and ascites. What is the most likely diagnosis?

(A) neurofibromatosis

(B) Sertoli–Leydig tumor

(C) Krukenberg's tumor

(D) Meigs' syndrome

(E) cystadenofibroma

16. A 25-year-old patient presents for ultrasound with a history of hyperemesis gravidarum and preeclampsia. Fig. 7–56 is a sonogram of the uterus that demonstrates which of the following?

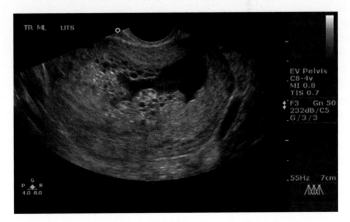

FIGURE 7–56.

(A) blighted ovum

(B) leiomyosarcoma

(C) missed abortion

(D) hydatidiform mole

(E) theca lutein cyst

17. When the sole of the foot is visualized in the same anatomical plane as the tibia and fibula, what is this findings most likely to be?

    (A) talipes

    (B) dwarfism

    (C) polydactyly

    (D) osteogenesis imperfecta

    (E) achondrogenesis

18. What is the most common twin zygosity?

    (A) conjoined twins

    (B) monochorionic/diamniotic

    (C) dichorionic/diamniotic

    (D) monochorionic/monoamniotic

19. Which of the following best describes the "twin peak" sign?

    (A) also known as the beta sign

    (B) a triangular projection of chorion into the dividing membrane

    (C) a sonographic predictor for dizygotic twins

    (D) both B and C

    (E) all of the above

20. Which of the following statements about conjoined twins is *not* true?

    (A) Sixty percent are born alive.

    (B) Fifty-six percent of conjoined twins are fused on the ventral wall.

    (C) Polyhydramnios is commonly present.

    (D) The largest risk of fetal demise is because of cord entanglement.

21. Which of the following best describes the uterine position shown in Fig. 7–57?

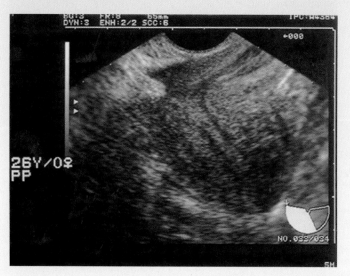

FIGURE 7–57.

    (A) retroverted

    (B) retroflexed

    (C) anteverted

    (D) anteflexed

22. What is the most reliable indicator for fetal demise in the second and third trimester?

    (A) oligohydramnios

    (B) polyhydramnios

    (C) mother stating she has not detected any fetal movement

    (D) the sonographic presence of fetal scalp edema, ascites and hydrops

    (E) absence of cardiac motion

23. Fluid in the endometrial cavity in a post-menopausal patient may be associated with which of the following?

    (A) increased in estrogen

    (B) vaginal atrophy

    (C) endometriosis

    (D) ectopic pregnancy

    (E) cervical stenosis

24. **Which one of the following signs/symptoms is usually not associated with placenta abruption?**

    (A) bloody amniotic fluid

    (B) painless bright red blood

    (C) sudden onset of pain and increase uterine tone

    (D) fetal distress

    (E) maternal shock

25. **Which of the following is not a midline structure?**

    (A) cavum septum pellucidum

    (B) third ventricle

    (C) foramen of Monro

    (D) pituitary gland

    (E) hippocampus

26. **Which of the following is the most common short limb syndrome?**

    (A) achondrogenesis

    (B) thanatophoric dysplasia

    (C) osteogenesis imperfecta

    (D) Jeune thoracic dystrophy

    (E) none of the above

27. **What sonographic findings would be identified in a fetus with heterozygous achondroplasia?**

    (A) hydrocephaly

    (B) frontal bossing

    (C) "bell-shaped" thorax

    (D) "trident hand"

    (E) both A and C

    (F) both B and D

    (G) all of the above

28. **Fig. 7–58 is a transverse plane of view through the uterus. What do the two-echogenic lines represent?**

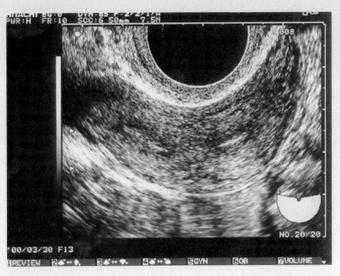

FIGURE 7–58.

    (A) the interstitial portion of the fallopian tube

    (B) two endometrial linings of a septate uterus

    (C) single endometrial lining

    (D) two endometrial linings of a bicornuate uterus

    (E) none of the above

29. **Fig. 7–59 demonstrates what fetal anomaly?**

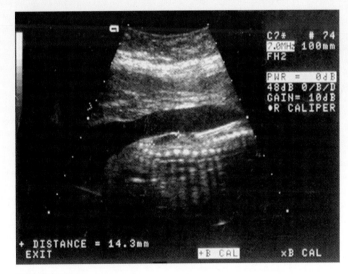

FIGURE 7–59.

    (A) sacral agenesis

    (B) meningocele

    (C) myelomeningocele

    (D) sacrococcygeal teratoma

    (E) pelvic cyst

30. Fig. 7–60 is a sonographic example of which of the following?

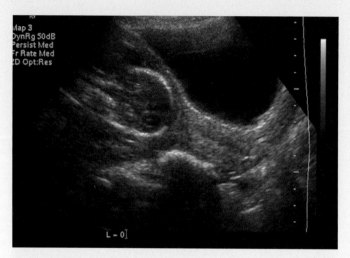

FIGURE 7–60.

(A) placenta accreta

(B) placental abruption

(C) marginal placenta previa

(D) placenta vasa previa

(E) normal findings

31. Fig. 7–61 is a transverse plane of view in the fetal nuchal region. Which of the following is the sonographic finding?

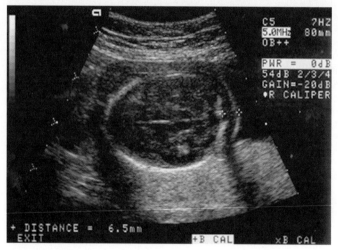

FIGURE 7–61.

(A) cystic hygroma

(B) increased nuchal skin fold

(C) fetal scalp edema

(D) increased nuchal translucency

(E) nuchal cord

32. Fig. 7–62 is a longitudinal plane of view through the midline of the uterus. The echogenic foci represent which of the following?

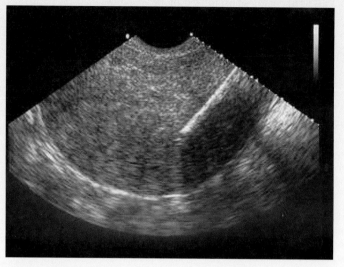

FIGURE 7–62.

(A) endometrial polyp

(B) IUD *in situ*

(C) endometrial hyperplasia

(D) endometrial cancer

(E) eccentric IUD

33. Fig. 7–63 demonstrates what ovarian abnormality?

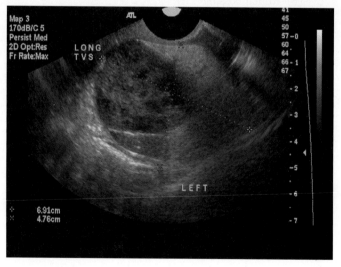

FIGURE 7–63.

(A) hemorrhagic corpus luteum cyst

(B) tubo-ovarian abscess

(C) benign cystic teratoma

(D) septated ovarian cyst

(E) polycystic ovaries

34. Fig. 7–64 demonstrates which of the following findings?

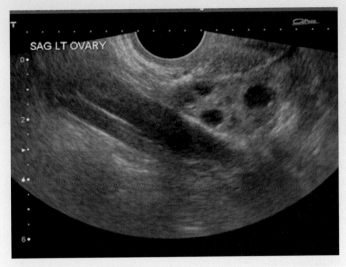

FIGURE 7–64.

(A) left ectopic pregnancy

(B) corpus luteal cyst

(C) polycystic ovarian disease

(D) left hydrosalpinx posterior to the left ovary

(E) normal ovary with iliac vessels

35. Fig. 7–65 is an image of a fetus at 8 weeks gestational age. What is the cystic structure within the fetus?

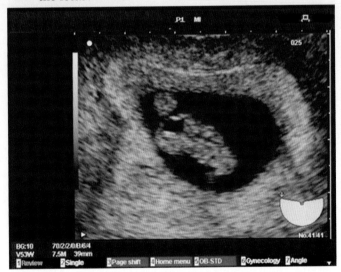

FIGURE 7–65.

(A) rhombencephalon

(B) cystic hygroma

(C) increased nuchal translucency

(D) hydrocephalus

(E) Dandy–Walker malformation

36. Fig. 7–66 shows transverse scans of the uterus. What is the mass measured in this figure?

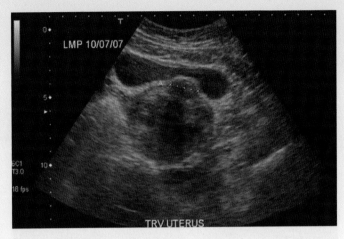

FIGURE 7–66.

(A) intramural fibroid

(B) calcified fibroid

(C) submucosal fibroid

(D) pedunculated fibroid

(E) subserosal fibroid

37. A 27-year-old female G5P4 with complaints of menorrhagia and pelvic pain. The serum β-hCG was 4,500 mIU/mL, no intrauterine pregnancy (IUP) was seen on the first sonogram, and a dilation and curettage (D&C) was performed. The serum β-hCG was repeated 48 hours after the D&C with findings of 4,900 mIU/mL. Fig. 7–67 is a longitudinal sonogram repeated after the D&C. What is the most likely diagnosis?

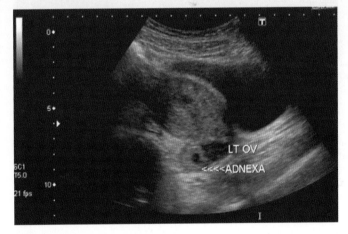

FIGURE 7–67.

(A) complete abortion

(B) hydatidiform mole

(C) missed abortion

(D) incomplete abortion

(E) ectopic pregnancy

38. What is the most likely diagnosis for the image of the adnexa Fig. 7–68?

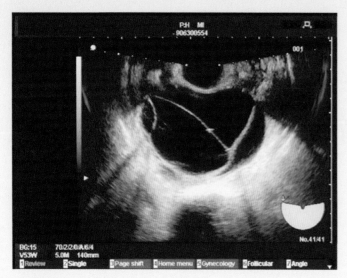

FIGURE 7–68.

   (A) serous cystadenoma

   (B) dermoid

   (C) septated ovarian cyst

   (D) tubo-ovarian abscess

   (E) paratubal cyst

   (F) all of the above

39. What is the abnormality in Fig. 7–69?

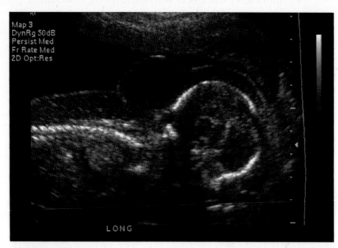

FIGURE 7–69.

   (A) abdominal ascites

   (B) encephalocele

   (C) anasarca with cystic hygroma

   (D) prune-belly syndrome

   (E) two fetuses next to each other

40. Fig. 7–70 demonstrates which one of the following sonographic abnormalities?

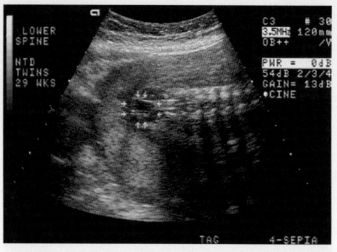

FIGURE 7–70.

   (A) hemivertebra

   (B) rachischisis

   (C) sacral agenesis

   (D) none of the above

41. The sonographic image in Fig. 7–71 is consistent with what findings?

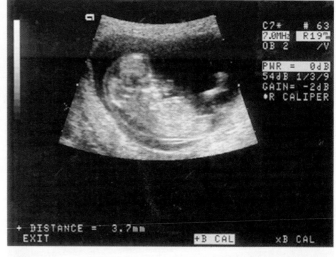

FIGURE 7–71.

   (A) 60% positive predictive value for trisomy 21

   (B) increased nuchal translucency

   (C) 80% positive predictive value for trisomy 21

   (D) both A and B

   (E) both B and C

42. **The findings in Fig. 7–71 are associated with which of the following?**

    (A) cardiac defects

    (B) skeletal dysplasia

    (C) Down syndrome

    (D) both A and C

    (E) all of the above

43. **Fig. 7–72 demonstrates what fetal bladder abnormality?**

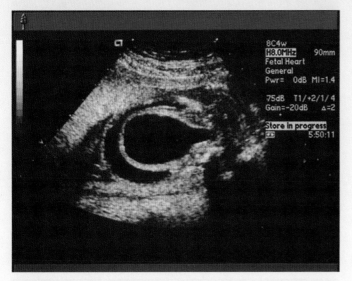

FIGURE 7–72.

    (A) ureterocele

    (B) posterior urethral valve obstruction

    (C) cloacal exstrophy

    (D) normal full bladder

44. **Fig. 7–73 is a sonographic image of what cardiac defect?**

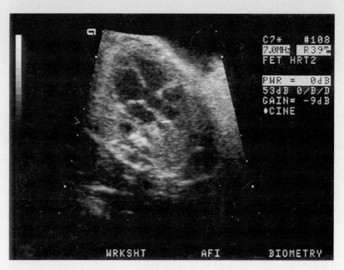

FIGURE 7–73.

    (A) ventricular septal defect

    (B) overriding aorta

    (C) tetralogy of Fallot

    (D) both A and C

    (E) all of the above

45. **Which of the following is demonstrated in the sonographic image of Fig. 7–74?**

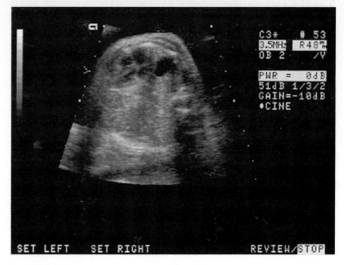

FIGURE 7–74.

    (A) normal fetal thorax and heart

    (B) congenital cystic adenomatoid malformation of the lung, type III

    (C) pulmonary sequestration

    (D) congenital left diaphragmatic hernia

    (E) none of the above

46. Fig. 7–75 demonstrates what sonographic finding?

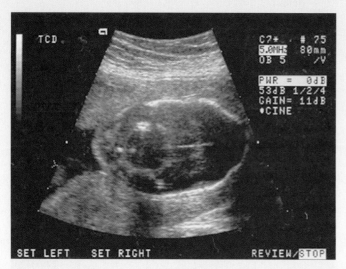

FIGURE 7–75.

- (A) Dandy–Walker malformation
- (B) normal cerebellum
- (C) arachnoid cyst
- (D) Arnold–Chiari malformation
- (E) holoprosencephaly

47. Fig. 7–76 is a sonographic example of which of the following?

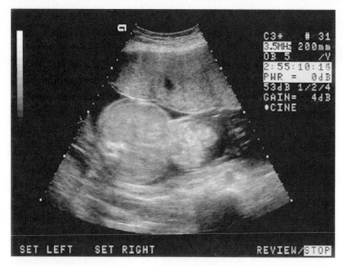

FIGURE 7–76.

- (A) gastroschisis
- (B) omphalocele
- (C) normal physiological herniation of midgut
- (D) duodenal atresia
- (E) encephalocele

48. Fig. 7–77 demonstrates what sonographic finding?

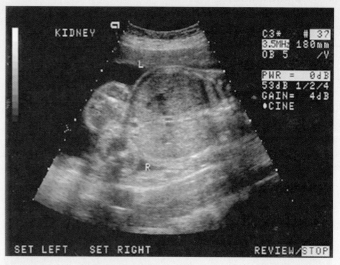

FIGURE 7–77.

- (A) normal kidneys
- (B) dysplastic kidneys
- (C) infantile polycystic kidney disease
- (D) enlarged kidneys
- (E) agenesis of the fetal kidneys

49. Fig. 7–78 demonstrates what fetal abnormality?

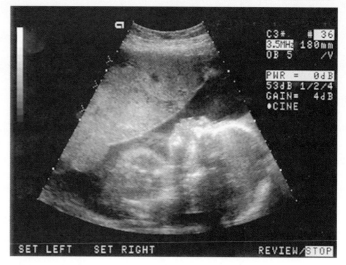

FIGURE 7–78.

- (A) micrognathia
- (B) macroglossia
- (C) frontal bossing
- (D) normal fetal profile
- (E) none of the above

50. What is the most likely diagnosis if Figs. 7–76, 7–77, and 7–78 are found in the same fetus?

   (A) trisomy 18

   (B) trisomy 13

   (C) Beckwith–Wiedemann syndrome

   (D) Finnish nephrosis

   (E) fetal alcohol syndrome

51. Fig. 7–79 is a sonographic example of which of the following?

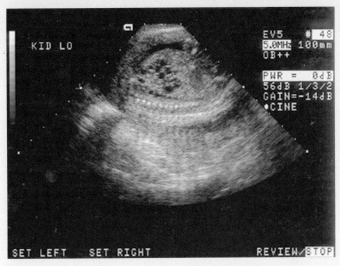

FIGURE 7–79.

   (A) multicystic dysplastic kidney disease

   (B) infantile polycystic kidney disease

   (C) UPJ obstruction

   (D) both A and B

   (E) both B and C

52. What is the most common congenital facial anomaly?

   (A) proboscis

   (B) hypotelorism

   (C) isolated cleft lip/palate

   (D) low set ears

   (E) midface hypoplasia

53. Three-dimensional surface rendering is used to do which of the following?

   (A) obtain volume measurements

   (B) obtain technically difficult images

   (C) image fetal spine

   (D) image fetal face

   (E) exclusion of artifact

54. What is the earliest age at which a gestational sac may be visualized by transvaginal sonography?

   (A) 2 weeks

   (B) 4 weeks

   (C) 6 weeks

   (D) 8 weeks

   (E) 10 weeks

55. What is the optimal time for performing a fetal echocardiogram ?

   (A) 14–18 weeks

   (B) 18–24 weeks

   (C) 24–28 weeks

   (D) 28–32 weeks

   (E) 38–40 weeks

56. Three-dimensional volumetric reconstructions are used to show all of the following except

   (A) fetal face

   (B) fetal limbs

   (C) kidneys

   (D) digits

   (E) heart

57. By 12 weeks of gestational age, the sonographer can identify what abnormalities?

   (A) conjoined twins

   (B) anencephaly

   (C) duodenal atresia

   (D) both A and B

   (E) all of the above

58. An unexplained increased in maternal serum triple screen (MSAFP3) can cause what third-trimester complications?

   (A) premature rupture of membranes

   (B) placental abruption

   (C) preterm labor

   (D) both A and B

   (E) all of the above

59. A markedly increased maternal serum alpha-fetoprotein (MSAFP) would be associated with which of the following findings?

   (A) amniotic sheets

   (B) cloacal exstrophy

   (C) congenital diaphragmatic hernia

   (D) Smith–Lemli–Opitz syndrome

   (E) Down's syndrome

60. **If the triple screen marker shows a decreased alpha-fetoprotein, a decreased estriol, and a decreased hCG, the fetus is at risk for which of the following?**

    (A) trisomy 21

    (B) Smith–Lemli–Opitz syndrome

    (C) trisomy 18

    (D) trisomy 13

    (E) trisomy 9

61. **Which of the following is not a direct sonographic finding of posterior urethral valve obstruction?**

    (A) "keyhole" sign

    (B) oligohydramnios

    (C) hydronephrosis

    (D) pulmonary hypoplasia

    (E) bilateral hydroureter

62. **What cranial finding can cause congestive heart failure and hydrops?**

    (A) vein of Galen aneurysm

    (B) periventricular leukomalacia

    (C) Dandy–Walker malformation

    (D) iniencephaly

    (E) corpus callosum

63. **What is the name of the cardiac abnormality with one outflow tract giving rise to both the pulmonary and aortic branches and associated with a ventricular septal defect?**

    (A) truncus arteriosus

    (B) double outlet right ventricle

    (C) tetralogy of Fallot

    (D) transposition of the great vessels

    (E) Ebstein's anomaly

64. **The cardiac abnormality consisting of a ventricular septal defect (VSD), an overriding aorta, a small or atretic pulmonary trunk, and right ventricular hypertrophy describes**

    (A) double outlet right ventricle

    (B) hypoplastic left heart syndrome

    (C) transposition of the great vessels

    (D) tetralogy of Fallot

    (E) Ebstein's anomaly

65. **All of the following are associated with infantile polycystic kidney disease except**

    (A) autosomal-recessive disorder

    (B) bilateral enlarged kidneys

    (C) oligohydramnios

    (D) echogenic kidneys

    (E) visible cysts greater than 20 mm in diameter are often seen on the kidneys

66. **Which of the following statements regarding congenital diaphragmatic hernia are true?**

    (A) more commonly right sided than left sided

    (B) carries a poor prognosis

    (C) may be associated with chromosomal abnormalities

    (D) all of the above

    (E) both A and C

    (F) both B and C

67. **Esophageal atresia is**

    (A) diagnosed by ultrasound 90% of the time

    (B) associated with oligohydramnios

    (C) a component of the VACTERL complex

    (D) easily diagnosed in the second and third trimester

    (E) all of the above

68. **An increased MSAFP is associated with all of the following *except***

    (A) trisomy 21

    (B) neural tube defect

    (C) maternal preeclampsia

    (D) gastroschisis

    (E) incorrect dating

69. **Which uterine ligament is responsible for uterine orientation?**

    (A) transversali ligament

    (B) broad ligament

    (C) uterosacral ligament

    (D) round ligament

    (E) ovarian ligament

70. **Which two ligaments are not true ligaments?**

    (A) uterosacral and broad ligaments

    (B) suspensory and broad ligaments

    (C) uterosacral and round ligaments

    (D) cardinal and suspensory ligaments

    (E) ovarian and round ligaments

71. **What is the most commonly visualized pelvic muscle that is often mistaken for an ovary?**

    (A) piriformis muscle

    (B) levator ani muscle

    (C) coccygeus muscle

    (D) iliopsoas muscle

    (E) gluteus maximus muscle

72. **What is the most dependent portion of the peritoneum called?**

    (A) pouch of Douglas

    (B) vesicouterine pouch

    (C) retropubic space

    (D) Morrison's pouch

    (E) none of the above

73. **What are the three peritoneal spaces in the pelvic cavity?**

    (A) posterior cul-de-sac, anterior cul-de-sac, and vesico-uterine pouch

    (B) posterior cul-de-sac, pouch of Douglas, and anterior cul-de-sac

    (C) posterior cul-de-sac, anterior cul-de-sac, and prevesical space

    (D) posterior cul-de-sac, anterior cul-de-sac, and interstitial space

    (E) Morrison's, retropubic space, and sac of Douglas

74. **What are the AIUM guidelines for cleaning and preparing a transvaginal probe?**

    (A) pre-clean with mild non-abrasive liquid soap and water

    (B) immerse in high-level disinfecting solution

    (C) clean with moist novelettes at the end of the day

    (D) disposable probe covers

    (E) lubricated or medicated condoms

    (F) all of the above

    (G) A, B, and D

75. **An invasive mole is also known as**

    (A) hydatidiform mole

    (B) triploid molar pregnancy

    (C) endometrioma

    (D) chorioadenoma destruens

    (E) lipomyosarcoma

76. **Which of the following is true regarding a hydatidiform mole and coexistent fetus?**

    (A) consistent with maternally derived trisomy 13

    (B) consistent with paternally derived trisomy 13

    (C) 2% will have a fetus

    (D) both A and C

    (E) both B and C

77. **In what portion of the fallopian tube does fertilization usually occur?**

    (A) interstitial

    (B) isthmus

    (C) ampulla

    (D) infundibulum

    (E) fimbria

78. **A patient informs you before her sonogram that she was previously diagnosed with an extrauterine pregnancy 10 days ago and was given the drug methotrexate. This indicates that previously she most likely had which of the following?**

    (A) ruptured ectopic pregnancy

    (B) unruptured ectopic pregnancy

    (C) intrauterine pregnancy greater than 12 weeks with no fetal heart motion

    (D) β-hCG greater than 10,000 mIU/mL

    (E) a ruptured ovarian cyst

79. **A patient informs you, before her sonogram that she fainted several times just prior to her being diagnosed with an ectopic pregnancy. She had a salpingectomy. This indicates that she most likely had which of the following?**

    (A) unruptured ectopic pregnancy

    (B) early intrauterine pregnancy (IUP) with a ruptured cyst

    (C) voluntary termination of pregnancy

    (D) missed abortion or spontaneous abortion

    (E) ruptured ectopic pregnancy

80. **Which of the following best defines intrauterine fetal demise?**

    (A) blighted ovum

    (B) absent fetal heart tone after 20 weeks of gestation

    (C) no fetal movement

    (D) missed abortion

    (E) all of the above

81. Which of the following is not true of dysgerminoma?

    (A) It is a solid malignant germ cell tumor of the ovary.

    (B) It is a counterpart of seminoma of the testis.

    (C) It is a relatively uncommon tumor accounting for about 2% of all ovarian cancers.

    (D) It is predominantly echogenic.

    (E) It is a solid benign tumor.

82. Which of the following is least likely to be true of dermoid tumors?

    (A) may cast an acoustic shadow

    (B) encountered more in women over 40 years

    (C) also called benign cystic teratoma

    (D) most common benign germ cell tumor in the female

    (E) unilateral in about 80% of cases

83. What is the measurement of the normal adult ovaries?

    (A) 3 × 2 × 2 cm

    (B) 3 × 2 × 2 mm

    (C) 4 × 4 × 2 cm

    (D) 4 × 2 × 2 mm

    (E) 7 × 4 × 3 mm

84. What is the first definitive sonographic sign of an intrauterine pregnancy?

    (A) gestational sac

    (B) yolk sac

    (C) fetal pole

    (D) double decidua sign

    (E) thickened endometrium

85. What percentage of cardiac defects can be detected from the four-chamber view?

    (A) 50

    (B) 65

    (C) 80

    (D) 85

    (E) 95

86. What percentage of cardiac defects can be detected from the four-chamber view and outflow tracts?

    (A) 50

    (B) 65

    (C) 80

    (D) 85

    (E) none of the above

87. A simple cyst may exhibit all of the following *except*

    (A) anechoic interior

    (B) posterior enhancement

    (C) thin walled

    (D) distal acoustic shadows

    (E) sonolucent

88. Which of the following types of ovarian cyst is commonly associated with hydatidiform mole?

    (A) dermoid

    (B) paraovarian

    (C) theca lutein

    (D) corpus luteal

    (E) hydropic villi

89. What is the most accurate method for establishing estimated date of confinement (EDC)?

    (A) first-trimester ultrasound

    (B) second-trimester ultrasound

    (C) last menstrual period (LMP)

    (D) Angele's rule

    (E) fundal height

90. What is the accuracy of crown rump length (CRL) in the first trimester?

    (A) 3–5 days

    (B) ± 10 days

    (C) ± 14 days

    (D) ± 21 days

    (E) has never been predicted

91. What is the accuracy of gestational age from 13 to 20 weeks?

    (A) 3–5 days

    (B) ± 10 days

    (C) ± 14 days

    (D) ± 21 days

    (E) has never been predicted

92. What is the accuracy of gestational age from 20 to 30 weeks?

    (A) 3–5 days

    (B) ± 10 days

    (C) ± 14 days

    (D) ± 21 days

    (E) has never been predicted

93. What is the accuracy of gestational age in the third trimester?

    (A) 3–4 days

    (B) ± 10 days

    (C) ± 14 days

    (D) ± 21 days

    (E) has never been predicted

94. The normal rise of hCG in a viable pregnancy should

    (A) double in 24 hours

    (B) double in 48 hours

    (C) double in 72 hours

    (D) double in 1 week

    (E) decrease in 2 days

95. Conditions associated with a poorly rising or decreasing hCG include all of the following except

    (A) twin pregnancy

    (B) ectopic pregnancy

    (C) anembryonic demise

    (D) incorrect dates

    (E) missed abortion

96. An ovarian mass identified on sonogram is complex, predominately hypoechoic with septations. The patient complains of severe pain during menses. What is the most likely diagnosis?

    (A) corpus luteal cyst

    (B) granulosa cell

    (C) thecoma

    (D) endometrioma

    (E) follicular cyst

97. If a patient's last menstrual period is 8/10/2011, by Nagele's rule, what is the estimated date of confinement?

    (A) 8/10/2012

    (B) 4/30/2012

    (C) 5/17/2012

    (D) 6/30/2012

    (E) 5/2/2012

98. Which of the following best describes Krukenberg tumors?

    (A) secondary metastatic ovarian neoplasms

    (B) usually of gastric or colonic primary origin

    (C) usually bilateral solid masses

    (D) all of the above

99. Which of the following is not a true characteristic of a serous cystadenoma?

    (A) usually large, thin-walled

    (B) thick septations

    (C) papillary projections are seen occasionally

    (D) most common benign ovarian neoplasm

    (E) peak incidence is in the fourth and fifth decade

100. What is another name for polycystic ovarian syndrome?

    (A) Stein–Leventhal syndrome

    (B) Sertoli–Leydig cell

    (C) Brenner's tumor

    (D) chocolate cyst

    (E) Mittelschmerz

101. What is the etiology of complete hydatidiform mole?

    (A) trophoblastic changes in a blighted ovum

    (B) hydatid swelling of the retained placenta in a missed abortion

    (C) fertilization of an empty ovum with normal diploid karyotype and no embryo

    (D) both A and B

    (E) all of the above

102. Which of the following characteristics of color Doppler energy (CDE) is true?

    (A) CDE can determine the direction of blood flow.

    (B) CDE can determine the velocity of blood flow.

    (C) the different colors represent flow toward or away from the transducer.

    (D) CDE is based on the amplitude of the sound wave.

103. Which of the following does the term trophoblast denote?

    (A) the extra-embryonic peripheral cells of the blastocyst

    (B) a rigid state of the flagellate microorganism

    (C) the gestation sac

    (D) the characteristics of a disease

    (E) multiplication of similar tissue

104. What is the mean diameter of a dominant follicular cyst at the time of ovulation?

    (A) 5 mm

    (B) 10 mm

    (C) 15 mm

    (D) 25 mm

    (E) 25 cm

105. What is the most common neoplasm of the uterus?

    (A) leiomyoma

    (B) adenomyosis

    (C) leiomyosarcoma

    (D) endometrial hyperplasia

    (E) endometrioma

106. A complex adnexal mass is identified in a patient with tenderness and elevated temperature and white blood cell count (cbc). What is the most likely diagnosis?

    (A) tubo-ovarian abscess

    (B) corpus luteal cyst

    (C) serous cystadenoma

    (D) Brenner's tumor

    (E) endometritis

107. Which of the following is true of mucinous cystadenocarcinoma?

    (A) composed of germ layers, ectoderm, mesoderm, and endoderm

    (B) when ruptured can result in pseudomyxoma peritonei

    (C) occurs more frequently in women 40 to 70 years old

    (D) contains fatty, sebaceous material, bone, teeth, and hair

    (E) gives a sonographic appearance called "tip–of-the-iceberg"

108. The endometrial lining in postmenopausal women *not* on hormone replacement therapy should be less than

    (A) 10 mm

    (B) 8 mm

    (C) 3 mm

    (D) 2 mm

    (E) 3 cm

109. The endometrial lining in postmenopausal women on hormone replacement therapy (HRT) should less than

    (A) vary, depending on the type and dosing of hormone replacement therapy used

    (B) 5 mm

    (C) 5 cm

    (D) 3 cm

    (E) 3 mm

110. In what stage of the menstrual cycle would be an ideal time to evaluate the endometrium for a polyp?

    (A) menstruation phase

    (B) follicular phase

    (C) proliferative phase

    (D) secretory phase

    (E) all of the above

111. The date of the last menstrual period is counted from

    (A) the date when fertilization occurred

    (B) the date when menstrual bleeding ended

    (C) the date when ovulation occurred

    (D) the date when menstrual bleeding began

    (E) 48 hours after the menstrual bleeding began

112. Which of the following diagnoses does not mimic the sonographic characteristic of hydatidiform mole?

    (A) endometriosis

    (B) incomplete abortion

    (C) degenerative uterine leiomyoma

    (D) trophoblastic changes in a blighted ovum

    (E) missed abortion

113. What percentage of patients diagnosed with hydatidiform mole will usually follow a benign course?

    (A) 20%

    (B) 10%

    (C) 50%

    (D) 80%

    (E) 2%

114. The uterus can be divided into regions. Which of the following choices lists them from inferior to superior?

(A) cervix, isthmus, corpus, fundus

(B) serosal, myometrial, endometrial

(C) fundus, isthmus, corpus, cervix

(D) cervix, corpus, isthmus, fundus

(E) vagina, cervix, body, fundus

115. What are the uterine layers?

(A) vagina, endometrium, endocervical

(B) serosal, myometrial, endometrial

(C) fundus, isthmus, corpus, cervix

(D) peritoneum, serosal, and myometrial

(E) vagina, uterus, tubes, ovaries

Questions 116–118. Match the structures numbered in Fig. 7–80 with the list of terms in Column B.

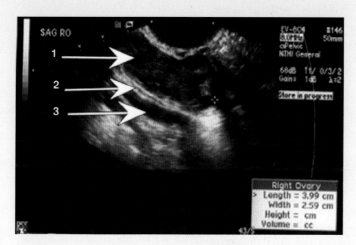

FIGURE 7-80.

COLUMN A

116. Arrow number 1: _____

117. Arrow number 2: _____

118. Arrow number 3: _____

COLUMN B

(A) internal iliac vein

(B) ovary

(C) internal iliac artery

(D) ureter

119. What is the normal size of a multiparous uterus,

(A) 5 × 4 × 3 cm

(B) 7 × 5 × 4 cm

(C) 9 × 6 × 5 cm

(D) 6 × 4 × 3 cm

120. What is the name of the anatomic opening between the third and fourth ventricle?

(A) aqueduct of Sylvius (cerebral aqueduct)

(B) interventricular foramina (foramen of Monro)

(C) Magendie's foramen (foramen of Magendie)

(D) foramen of Luschka

(E) choroid plexus

121. Congenital abnormalities of the uterus result from improper fusion of which of the following structures?

(A) mesonephric ducts

(B) paramesonephric ducts

(C) Gartner's duct

(D) Wolffian ducts

(E) Bartholin duct

122. During the early proliferative phase, the endometrium appears

(A) thin, echogenic line, 4–8 mm

(B) thin, hypoechoic line, 4–8 mm

(C) thickened and hypoechoic medially with an echogenic basal layer

(D) thickened and echogenic throughout

(E) thin, echogenic line, 4–8 cm

123. During the periovulatory phase, the endometrium appears

(A) thin, echogenic line, 4–8 mm

(B) thin, hypoechoic line, 4–8 mm

(C) thickened and hypoechoic medially with an echogenic basal layer

(D) thickened and echogenic throughout

(E) less than 2 mm

124. During the secretory phase, the endometrium appears

(A) thin, echogenic line, 4–8 mm

(B) thin, hypoechoic line, 4–8 mm

(C) thickened and hypoechoic medially with an echogenic basal layer

(D) thickened and echogenic

(E) less than 2 mm

125. Women with endometriosis may have

(A) dyspareunia

(B) metromenorrhagia

(C) dysmenorrhea

(D) all of the above

(E) both D and C

126. Which of the following best describes endometriosis?

(A) functional endometrial tissue outside the uterine cavity

(B) benign invasion of endometrial tissue into the myometrium

(C) endomyosarcoma with chocolate tissue

(D) inflammation of the endometrium

(E) a malignant invasion of endometrial tissue into the myometrium

127. What is the most common anatomical location for a dermoid cyst?

(A) posterior cul-de-sac

(B) right adnexa

(C) left adnexa

(D) superior to the uterine fundus

(E) right upper quadrant

128. Macrosomia is

(A) fetus weighing > 4,000 g

(B) fetus > 90% for gestational age

(C) fetus with a shoulder thickness > 10 mm

(D) large-for-gestational-age (LGA) fetus

(E) a fetus with a head size larger than 10 cm

129. What does the term LGA refer to?

(A) a fetus weighing > 4,000 g

(B) fetus > 90%

(C) a clinical assessment of an increased fundal height

(D) polyhydramnios

(E) an increase in head size

130. A macrosomic fetus is at risk for which of the following?

(A) shoulder dystocia

(B) increased perinatal morality

(C) prolonged labor

(D) all of the above

(E) none of the above

131. Which of the following is usually not a cause of oligohydramnios?

(A) cystic hygroma

(B) posterior urethral valve obstruction

(C) intrauterine growth retardation (IUGR)

(D) post maturity

(E) premature rupture of the membranes (PROM)

132. An increased fundal height may be caused by which of the following?

(A) macrosomic fetus

(B) polyhydramnios

(C) twins

(D) pregnancy with fundal fibroids

(E) all of the above

133. Intrauterine growth restriction (IUGR) is

(A) estimated fetal weight (EFW) below 10% for a given gestational age

(B) decreased AFV

(C) increased umbilical cord size

(D) abnormal growth ratios

(E) fetal weight at or below 3% for a given gestational age

134. An increased HC/AC is a suggestion of

(A) late onset of IUGR

(B) brain sparing effort

(C) placental insufficiency

(D) anasarca

(E) all of the above

135. Causes of asymmetric IUGR include

(A) fetal infection

(B) chromosomal abnormality

(C) placental insufficiency

(D) all of the above

(E) none of the above

136. Which of the following is the most sensitive indicator for assessment of IUGR

(A) BPD to OFD ratio

(B) FL to AC ratio

(C) HC to AC ratio

(D) AC

(E) none of the above

137. Doppler testing of vessels that may aid in the diagnosis of IUGR is

   (A) umbilical cord
   (B) straight sinus
   (C) celiac axis
   (D) jugular vein
   (E) both A and C
   (F) all of the above

138. Doppler sampling of the maternal uterine artery < 26 weeks shows a diastolic notch. This notch is indicative of

   (A) IUGR
   (B) maternal hypertension
   (C) normal
   (D) both A and B
   (E) none of the above

139. In Fig. 7–81, what is the most likely diagnosis?

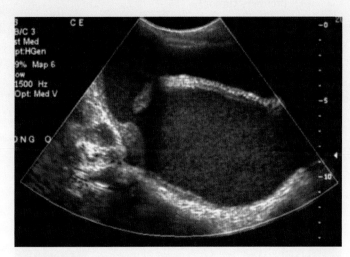

FIGURE 7–81.

   (A) hydrometra
   (B) hematometra
   (C) partial mole
   (D) myoma
   (E) hematometrocolpos

140. When a patient being treated for infertility demonstrated bilaterally enlarged multicystic ovaries and ascites, the diagnosis of ovarian hyperstimulation syndrome (OHSS) was made. Patients who are at risk of developing OHSS are

   (A) patients on Clomid or Pergonal
   (B) patients with Stein–Leventhal syndrome
   (C) patients with a history of OHSS
   (D) all of the above

141. In Fig. 7–82, the endovaginal image was taken at the level of the uterine corpus. The patient is a 55-year-old woman on hormone replacement therapy (HRT). Which of the following should not be included in the differential diagnosis?

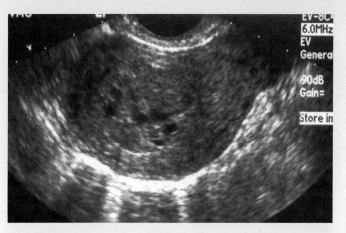

FIGURE 7–82.

   (A) endometrial hyperplasia
   (B) endometrial carcinoma
   (C) endometriosis
   (D) endometrial polyp
   (E) hydatidiform mole

142. In Fig. 7–83, what is the arrow pointing to?

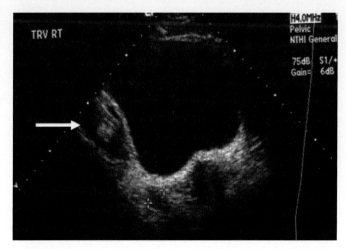

FIGURE 7–83.

   (A) iliopsoas muscle
   (B) right ovary
   (C) bowel mass
   (D) piriformis muscle

143. A pseudo-gestational sac will normally demonstrate

    (A) a secondary yolk sac within the pseudo-gestational sac

    (B) high-amplitude chorio-decidua

    (C) anechoic center with a thin ring

    (D) one mm increase in size each day

    (E) a small embryo

144. In Fig. 7–84, the endovaginal image of a 32-year-old woman with abnormal vaginal bleeding is most suggestive of which of the diagnoses?

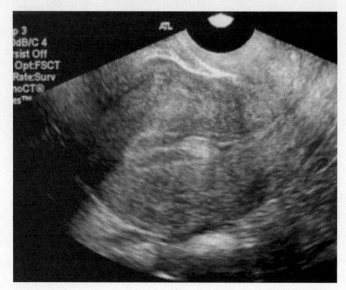

FIGURE 7–84.

    (A) endometrioma

    (B) adenoma

    (C) endometrial polyp

    (D) myoma

    (E) leiomyoma sarcoma

145. In Fig. 7–85, this 29-year-old patient presents with a history of chronic pelvic pain especially during menses, back pain, and dyspareunia. What is the most likely diagnosis?

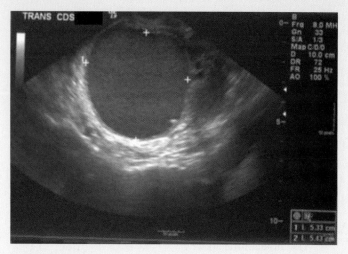

FIGURE 7–85.

    (A) Brenner's tumor

    (B) fibroma

    (C) thecoma

    (D) endometrioma

    (E) cystadenocarcinoma

146. Fig. 7–86 is of a 38-year-old black female patient who presented with an enlarged palpated uterus, pain, and abnormal vaginal bleeding. What is the most likely diagnosis?

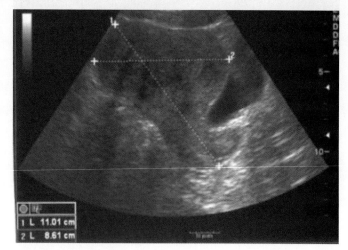

FIGURE 7–86.

    (A) intramural myoma

    (B) subserosal myoma

    (C) submucosal myoma

    (D) leiomyosarcoma

    (E) pedunculated fibroid

147. Fig. 7–87 is an endovaginal sonogram of the right adnexa of a 24-year-old patient that presented with an acute onset of pelvic pain. What does this most likely represent?

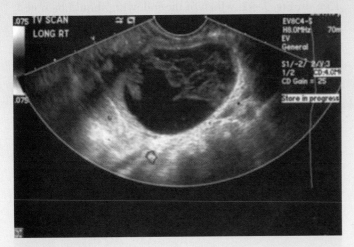

FIGURE 7–87.

(A) hemorrhagic cyst

(B) hyperstimulated ovarian syndrome

(C) endometrioma

(D) serous cystadenocarcinoma

(F) follicular cyst

148. Fig. 7–88 is suggestive of which of the following diagnoses?

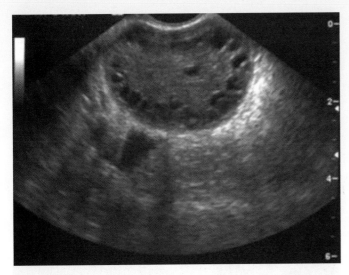

FIGURE 7–88.

(A) hyperstimulated ovary

(B) corpus luteal cyst

(C) cystadenoma

(D) polycystic ovary

(E) normal appearing ovary

149. The patient described in the previous question may present with any of the following except

(A) ovarian agenesis

(B) amenorrhea

(C) infertility

(D) hirsutism

(E) obesity

150. A 35-year-old patient presented with vaginal discharge and pelvic tenderness. The clinical information together with the endovaginal sonogram in Fig. 7–89 is most suggestive of which of the following diagnoses?

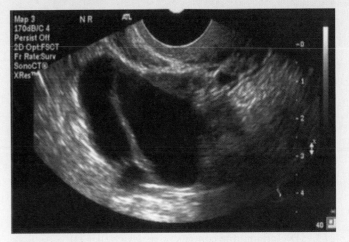

FIGURE 7–89.

(A) hydrosalpinx

(B) endometrioma

(C) ascites

(D) ectopic pregnancy

(E) dermoid

151. A 29-year-old patient presented with menorrhagia and dysmenorrhea. On physical examination an enlarged uterus was palpated. The sonogram Fig. 7–90 is suggestive of which of the following diagnoses?

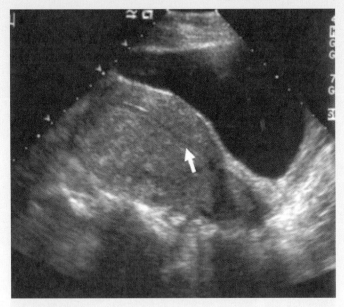

FIGURE 7–90.

(A) a myomatous uterus

(B) adenomyosis

(C) endometriosis

(D) intrauterine contraceptive device (IUCD)

(E) hematometra

152. In Fig. 7–91, the endovaginal sonogram of a post-menopausal female being treated with tamoxifen for breast cancer is suggestive of which of the following diagnoses?

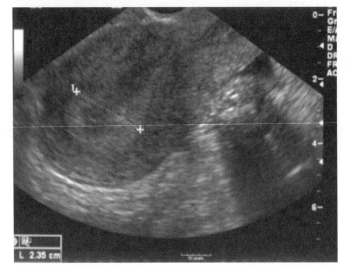

FIGURE 7–91.

(A) endometrial hyperplasia

(B) normal endometrium

(C) poor quality image and cannot make a diagnosis

(D) endometriosis

(E) none of the above

153. In Fig. 7–92, which of the following should be noted while performing the sonogram?

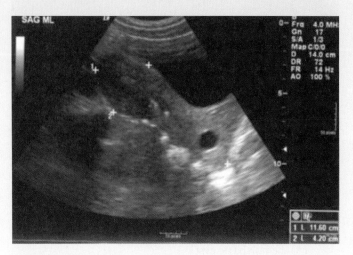

FIGURE 7–92.

(A) Gartner's duct cyst

(B) Nabothian cyst

(C) Bartholin's cyst

(D) cervical myoma

(E) intrauterine gestational sac

154. The endovaginal sonogram in Fig. 7–93 of a 28-year-old patient with a history of chlamydia, pelvic pain, and fever. Serum β-hCG is negative. This sonogram is suggestive of which of the following diagnoses?

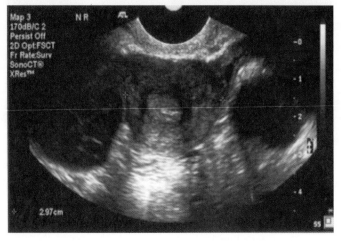

FIGURE 7–93.

(A) bilaterally enlarged ovaries

(B) right corpus luteal cyst

(C) bilateral dermoids

(D) tubo-ovarian abscesses

(E) bilateral ectopic pregnancy

155. The uterus in Fig. 7–94 is poorly visualized. What can be done to improve the visualization of the uterus?

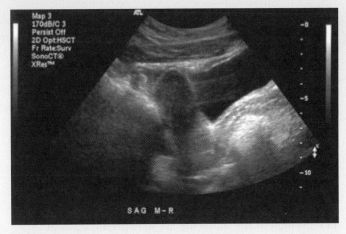

FIGURE 7–94.

(A) increase the near gain

(B) increase the far gain

(C) change transabdominal transducers

(D) distend the urinary bladder more

(E) have the patient post void

156. In Fig. 7–95, the echoes on the anterior aspect of the urinary bladder are an example of which artifact normally seen?

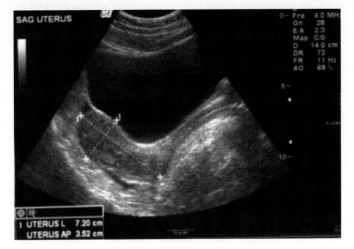

FIGURE 7–95.

(A) edge

(B) comet tail

(C) attenuation

(D) reverberation

(E) distal acoustic enhancement

Questions 157–160: Rank the following in order of their neurologic development, earliest to latest.

COLUMN A   COLUMN B

157. _____   (A) body motion

158. _____   (B) fetal tone

159. _____   (C) breathing

160. _____   (D) fetal heart rate acceleration

161. The pathological condition characterized by a solid ovarian tumor, right pleural effusions, and ascites is

(A) Meigs syndrome

(B) dysgerminoma

(C) Stein–Leventhal syndrome

(D) mucinous cystadenoma

(E) leiomyoma sarcoma

162. The components of biophysical profile (BPP) are

(A) fetal breathing, Doppler, non-stress test (NST), gross body movement, and amniotic fluid volume (AFV)

(B) placental grading, non-stress test (NST), gross body movement, and amniotic fluid volume (AFV)

(C) non-stress test (NST), Doppler, gross body movement, amniotic fluid volume (AFV), and fetal flexion/extension

(D) amniotic fluid volume (AFV), gross body movement, fetal flexion/ extension, fetal breathing, and non-stress test (NST)

(E) BPD, AC, FL, and non-stress test (NST)

163. Fetal breathing must last how long to be counted in the biophysical profile (BPP)?

(A) 20 seconds

(B) 30 seconds

(C) 1 minute

(D) 2 minutes

(E) 5 minutes

164. In a normal fetus, if the middle cerebral artery were sampled, one would expect to find which of the following?

(A) an increased S/D ratio

(B) a decreased S/D ratio

(C) retrograde flow

(D) absent flow

(E) has no change in S/D ratio

165. A 27-year-old female presented to the emergency department complaining of heavy vaginal bleeding and pain in pregnancy. What is the finding in the sonogram in Fig. 7–96?

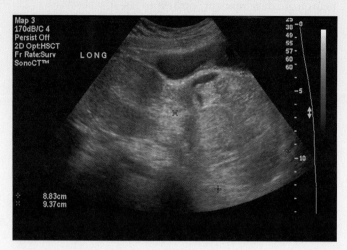

FIGURE 7–96.

  (A) ruptured ectopic pregnancy

  (B) fundal fibroid uterus

  (C) unruptured ectopic pregnancy

  (D) cervical phase of an impending abortion

  (E) none of the above

166. The fetus starts swallowing the amniotic fluid at what gestational age in pregnancy?

  (A) 8 weeks

  (B) 12 weeks

  (C) 20 weeks

  (D) 33 weeks

167. Which of the following is not a cause for pelvic inflammatory disease and its contribution to infertility?

  (A) chlamydia

  (B) actinomycetes

  (C) gonorrhea

  (D) genital herpes

  (E) mycobacterium tuberculosis

168. Which one of the following is not part of the adnexa?

  (A) urinary bladder

  (B) fimbria

  (C) follicular cyst

  (D) broad ligaments

  (E) internal iliac arteries

169. Using the single pocket technique for assessment of amniotic fluid, oligohydramnios is suggested when the amniotic fluid is?

  (A) a single pocket of 2 cm

  (B) a single pocket of 20 cm

  (C) a single pocket of 5 cm

  (D) a single pocket of 8 cm

170. In the amniotic fluid index method of measuring four quadrants, when is the diagnosis of oligohydramnios made?

  (A) when the amniotic volume is < 300 mL

  (B) when the amniotic volume is < 200 mL

  (C) when the amniotic fluid index is < the 10th percentile

  (D) when the amniotic fluid index is < the 2.5th percentile

  (E) none of the above

171. Which of the following are nonspecific signs of fetal death: (1) echoes in the amniotic fluid, (2) the absence of the falx cerebri, (3) a decrease in the biparietal diameter (BPD) measurements, (4) a double contour of the fetal head (sonographic halo sign), (5) no fetal heart motion?

  (A) both 3 and 4

  (B) only 4

  (C) only 1, 2, 3, and 4

  (D) only 5

  (E) 1, 2, 3, 4, and 5

172. How long after fetal death can scalp edema be first seen?

  (A) 2–3 days

  (B) 5–10 days

  (C) 10–20 days

  (D) 20–30 days

  (E) 2–3 weeks

173. The term decidua denotes the transformed endometrium of pregnancy. What are the different regions of the decidua?

  (A) two regions called decidua basalis and chorionic villi

  (B) one region called decidual reaction

  (C) three regions called decidua basalis, decidua parietalis, and decidua capsularis

  (D) three regions called endoderm, mesoderm, and ectoderm

  (E) amnion, chorion, and extraembryonic coelom

174. **Which of the following cannot be included in the category of cystic masses of the vagina?**

    (A) Gartner's duct cyst
    (B) Nabothian cyst
    (C) hematocolpos
    (D) Bartholin cyst
    (E) all of the above

175. **What are the functions of the secondary yolk sac?**

    (A) nutrients for the embryo
    (B) hematopoiesis
    (C) contributing to the development of the reproductive system
    (D) give rise to cells that later becomes sex cells
    (E) all of the above

176. **In about 2% of adults, the yolk sac persists as a diverticulum of the ileum. What is this known as?**

    (A) Michael's diverticulum
    (B) Meckel's diverticulum
    (C) Turner's diverticulum
    (D) Smith's diverticulum
    (E) diverticular coelom

177. **The location of the yolk sac is**

    (A) inside the umbilical cord
    (B) inside the amniotic sac
    (C) in the chorionic cavity between the amnion and the chorion
    (D) outside the chorionic cavity between the chorion and the endometrial wall
    (E) with the stomach of the embryo

178. **On transvaginal sonography, the yolk sac is visible as early as how many weeks?**

    (A) 4 weeks
    (B) 5 weeks
    (C) 6 weeks
    (D) 7 weeks
    (E) 8 weeks

Questions 179–182: Arrange in sequence in Column A the embryologic stages following fertilization listed in Column B.

COLUMN A   COLUMN B

179. _____   (A) morula

180. _____   (B) cleavage

181. _____   (C) zygote

182. _____   (D) blastocyst

183. **Which of the following is not a complication associated with oligohydramnios?**

    (A) premature rupture of membranes (PROM)
    (B) Intrauterine growth restriction (IUGR)
    (C) post date pregnancy (>42 weeks)
    (D) urethral stenosis
    (E) posterior urethral valve syndrome

184. **The umbilical cord S/D ratio normally**

    (A) increases throughout the pregnancy
    (B) decreases throughout the pregnancy
    (C) remains the same throughout pregnancy
    (D) is controlled by the fetal cerebellum
    (E) no change in S/D ratio

185. **Placental insufficiency is indirectly monitored by**

    (A) an increasing umbilical cord S/D ratio
    (B) a decreasing umbilical cord S/D ratio
    (C) Doppler of placental intervillous spaces
    (D) Doppler of maternal arcuate arteries
    (E) none of the above

186. **The terminology vasa previa best describes**

    (A) placenta near the internal os
    (B) placenta touching the internal os
    (C) placenta crossing the internal os
    (D) placenta vessels crossing the internal os
    (E) premature separation of the placenta

187. **What is the primary cause of third-trimester painless vaginal bleeding?**

    (A) placenta previa
    (B) ruptured ovarian cyst
    (C) placentomegaly
    (D) placenta abruption
    (E) malpresentation

188. **Which of the following is true concerning pseudogestational sac?**

    (A) It is located in the ampullary segment of the fallopian tube.

    (B) It is located in the uterine cavity.

    (C) It has two layers of decidua called double decidual sign.

    (D) It has a yolk sac.

    (E) Its growth rate is approximately 1mm per day.

189. **Which of the following statements *is not true* concerning the yolk sac?**

    (A) The yolk sac should be included in measurements of CRL.

    (B) The yolk sac shrinks as pregnancy advances.

    (C) The yolk sac plays a role in blood development and transfer of nutrients.

    (D) The yolk sac is attached to the body stalk and is located between the amnion and chorion.

    (E) The yolk sac contains vitelline fluid

190. **The vessels of the normal umbilical cord consist of**

    (A) two arteries, one vein

    (B) two veins, one artery

    (C) one artery, one iliac vein, and the iliac artery

    (D) one artery, one vein

    (E) two arteries, two veins

191. **The term "neural tube defect" refers to**

    (A) spinal defect

    (B) open tube defect

    (C) anencephaly

    (D) cephalocele

    (E) all of the above

192. **Myelomeningocele refers to**

    (A) neural tube defect characterized by absent of the cerebellum

    (B) protrusion of meninges and neural tissue though a defect

    (C) fat tumor and meninges at the lumbar region

    (D) meninges and brain herniate through a defect in the calvarium

    (E) muscle tumor of the fetal spine

193. **What is the estimated gestational age for a CRL of 28 mm**

    (A) 9.3 weeks

    (B) 6.5 weeks

    (C) 5.5 weeks

    (D) 12 weeks

    (E) 14 weeks

194. **The "lemon" sign of the fetal cranium in diagnosing spina bifida refers to**

    (A) the narrowing of the vertebral process at the area of the defect

    (B) the overall appearance of the fetal spine in the presence of a defect

    (C) the appearance of the cerebellum in the presence of a spinal defect

    (D) the appearance of the fetal skull in the presence of a spinal defect

    (E) lemon shape of the cerebellum

195. **The "banana" sign of the fetal cranium in diagnosing spina bifida refers to**

    (A) the narrowing of the vertebral process at the area of the defect

    (B) the overall appearance of the fetal spine in the presence of a defect

    (C) the appearance of the cerebellum in the presence of a spinal defect

    (D) the appearance of the fetal skull in the presence of a spinal defect

    (E) banana shape of the fetal skull bones

196. **The "banana" sign is present with spinal defects**

    (A) 50% of the time

    (B) 75% of the time

    (C) 85% of the time

    (D) 95% of the time

    (E) 25 % of the time

197. **Which of the following is true about the "lemon" sign and neural tube defects?**

    (A) The "lemon" sign is not as accurate as the "banana" sign.

    (B) The "lemon" sign may be present in the normal fetus in the third trimester.

    (C) The "lemon" sign can be artificially produced at the level of the ventricles.

    (D) The "lemon" sign is a predictor for spina bifida.

    (E) All of the above statements are true.

198. The diagnosis of placenta previa is most accurately made

    (A) transabdominally with a full maternal bladder
    (B) transabdominally with an empty maternal bladder
    (C) transrectally
    (D) transvaginally
    (E) all of the above

199. The definition of "low lying placenta" in the third trimester is

    (A) placental edge >3 cm from the internal os
    (B) placental edge <2 cm from the internal os
    (C) placental edge <3 cm from the internal os
    (D) placental edge in lower uterine segment
    (E) placenta edge >20 cm from the internal os

200. The rotation of the heart in the fetal chest should be

    (A) 45° with apex pointed to the right
    (B) 45° with apex pointed to the left
    (C) 60° with apex pointed to the right
    (D) the heart should not be rotated in fetal chest
    (E) parallel with apex pointed to the median plain

201. The fetal heart is horizontal in the chest because of

    (A) large spleen
    (B) flat diaphragm
    (C) large liver
    (D) large thorax
    (E) large bowel

202. The type of hydrops defined as absence of a detectable circulating antibody against red blood cells in the mother is

    (A) immune
    (B) nonimmune
    (C) erythroblastosis fetalis
    (D) isoimmunization fetalis
    (E) all of the above

203. What percentage of cephaloceles are occipital?

    (A) 50
    (B) 60
    (C) 75
    (D) 99
    (E) 25

204. The diagnosis of ventriculomegaly may be made when the ventricle measures

    (A) greater than 10 mm in the atrium of the occipital horn
    (B) greater than 15 mm in the posterior horn
    (C) when the third ventricle may be visualized
    (D) when the choroid does not touch the medial wall of the lateral ventricle
    (E) greater than 10 cm in the posterior horn

205. A patient states she was given a medication called RhoGAM after she had vaginal spotting in pregnancy. This was most likely due to

    (A) ectopic pregnancy
    (B) abortion
    (C) Rh-negative status of the mother
    (D) pelvic infection
    (E) human immunodeficiency virus

206. Congenital hydrocephalus is

    (A) genetically linked affecting both male and females
    (B) able to be detected in both male and females by DNA testing
    (C) expressed in males only
    (D) both A and C
    (E) both B and C
    (F) all of the above

207. Intracranial calcifications and microcephaly of the fetus are associated with

    (A) Dandy–Walker cyst
    (B) vein of Galen aneurysm
    (C) gestational diabetes
    (D) TORCH infections
    (E) agenesis of corpus callosum

208. Which of the following is a type of ectopic pregnancy that when ruptured is less likely to have internal hemorrhage?

    (A) cervical ectopic
    (B) cornual ectopic
    (C) abdominal ectopic
    (D) ampullary ectopic
    (E) ovarian

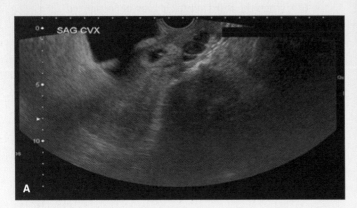

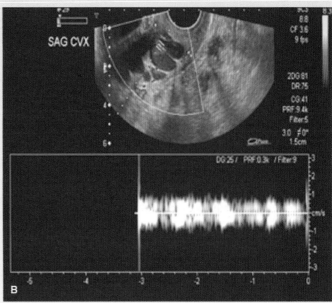

FIGURE 7-97.

209. A 29-year-old female presented to the emergency department with painless vaginal bleeding in pregnancy. The serum β-hCG taken was 3,500 mIU/mL. What is the finding in the transvaginal sonograms shown in Fig. 7–97A and B?

   (A) cervical scar implantation
   (B) pseudo-gestational sac
   (C) abdominal pregnancy
   (D) tubal pregnancy
   (E) complete abortion

210. What does the arrow in the sonogram shown in Fig. 7–98 point to?

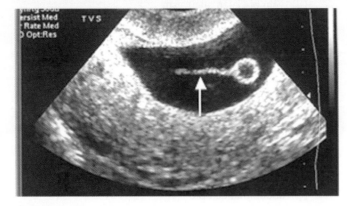

FIGURE 7-98.

   (A) yolk sac
   (B) amnion
   (C) chorion
   (D) vitelline duct
   (E) Wharton's duct

211. Fig 7–99 is a transvaginal sonogram after placement of an intrauterine device (IUD). What does this image demonstrate?

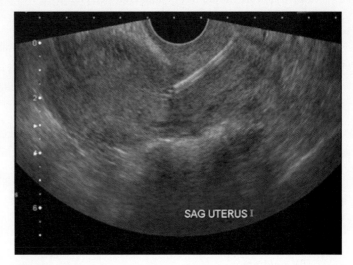

FIGURE 7-99.

   (A) IUD *in situ*
   (B) IUD in the uterine fundus
   (C) IUD in the vagina
   (D) none visualization of the IUD
   (E) IUD in the cervix

212. The cisterna magna is considered increased when

    (A) The measurement is >5 mm.
    (B) The cerebellum may be seen outlined by fluid.
    (C) The cerebellar vermis is splayed.
    (D) The measurement is >11 mm.
    (E) None of the above is true.

213. Findings on ultrasound include an increased cisterna magna, agenesis of the cerebellar vermis with communication to the fourth ventricle and ventriculomegaly. What is the most likely diagnosis?

    (A) Dandy–Walker malformation
    (B) Dandy–Walker malformation variant
    (C) arachnoid cyst
    (D) communicating hydrocephaly
    (E) agenesis of the corpus callosum

214. Findings on ultrasound include hydrocephaly, an enlarged cisterna magna, and an intact cerebellar vermis elevated by a cyst in the posterior fossa. What is the most likely diagnosis?

    (A) Dandy–Walker malformation
    (B) Dandy–Walker malformation variant
    (C) arachnoid cyst
    (D) communicating hydrocephaly
    (E) agenesis of the corpus callosum

215. What other findings are associated with Dandy–Walker malformation?

    (A) holoprosencephaly
    (B) facial clefting
    (C) cardiac defects
    (D) only B and C
    (E) all of the above

216. A patient who presented for pelvic ultrasound informs you that she has secondary infertility and is currently on a medication to stimulate ovulation induction. This drug is most likely

    (A) folic acid
    (B) clomiphene citrate
    (C) methotrexate
    (D) lupron
    (E) vitamin B12

217. Complications associated with Dandy–Walker malformation include

    (A) chromosomal abnormalities
    (B) subnormal intelligence after birth
    (C) increased neonatal death
    (D) only A and B
    (E) all of the above

218. The most common cause of hypotelorism is

    (A) Dandy–Walker malformation
    (B) Arnold–Chiari type II
    (C) Goldenhar syndrome
    (D) holoprosencephaly
    (E) arachnoid cyst

219. Cyclopia, hypotelorism, proboscis, cebocephaly, and cleft lip/palate are

    (A) abnormal intracranial findings
    (B) abnormal facial findings
    (C) associated with hydrocephaly
    (D) all of the above
    (E) none of the above

220. The most common chromosomal abnormality associated with holoprosencephaly is

    (A) trisomy 21
    (B) trisomy 18
    (C) trisomy 13
    (D) Turner's syndrome
    (E) trisomy 9

221. The most common cause of hypertelorism is

    (A) anterior cephalocele
    (B) holoprosencephaly
    (C) hydranencephaly
    (D) craniosynostosis
    (E) none of the above

222. Teratomas in pregnancy are located in

    (A) the sacrococcygeal region
    (B) intracranial
    (C) cervical
    (D) lumbar
    (E) all of the above

223. Maternal Graves' disease and Hashimoto thyroiditis may cause what finding in the fetus?

    (A) fetal ascites
    (B) fetal goiter
    (C) oligohydramnios
    (D) there is no effect on the fetus
    (E) all of the above

224. The most common cause of macroglossia is

    (A) micrognathia
    (B) trisomy 18
    (C) Beckwith–Wiedemann syndrome
    (D) obstruction of the fetal airway
    (E) Dandy–Walker malformation

225. The arrow is pointing to what anatomical structure Fig. 7–100.

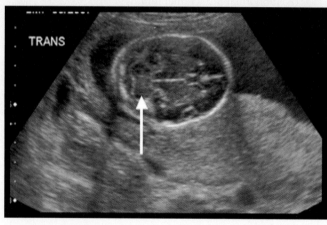

FIGURE 7–100.

    (A) cerebrum
    (B) cerebellum
    (C) cisterna magna
    (D) cerebral peduncle
    (E) cavum septum pellucidum

226. Macroglossia is present how often in Beckwith–Wiedemann syndrome?

    (A) 15% of the time
    (B) 25% of the time
    (C) 50% of the time
    (D) 97% of the time
    (E) 76% of the time

227. What is the most common type of isolated cleft lip/palate?

    (A) unilateral cleft lip
    (B) unilateral cleft lip and palate
    (C) bilateral cleft lip
    (D) bilateral cleft lip and palate
    (E) none of the above

228. The arrow in Fig. 7–101 is pointing to what anatomic structure?

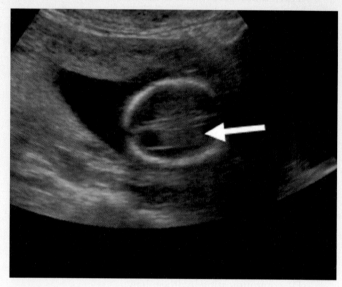

FIGURE 7–101.

    (A) falx cerebri
    (B) choroid plexus
    (C) cavum septum pellucidum
    (D) third ventricle
    (E) cerebellum

229. A medial cleft lip has a strong association with what abnormality?

    (A) hydrocephaly
    (B) Turner's syndrome
    (C) holoprosencephaly
    (D) hydranencephaly
    (E) all of the above

230. Micrognathia may be associated with which of the following syndromes?

    (A) Pierre Robin syndrome
    (B) trisomy 18
    (C) campomelic dysplasia
    (D) all of the above
    (E) none of the above

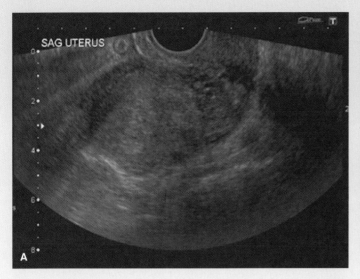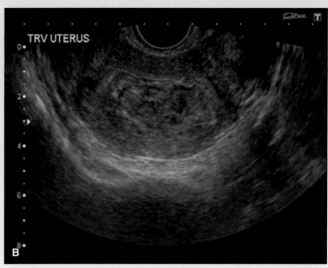

FIGURE 7–102.

231. A 32-year-old female is complaining of lower abdominal cramping and vaginal bleeding with clots. Her serum β-hCG 2 days ago was 5,200 mIU/mL and a repeated serum β-hCG taken 48 hours after the first β-hCG is now 1,200 mIU/mL. Figs. 7–102A and B are her sonograms. What are the most likely findings?

    (A) ruptured ectopic pregnancy

    (B) unruptured ectopic pregnancy

    (C) hydatidiform mole

    (D) complete abortion

    (E) incomplete abortion

232. If a fetal nasal bone is not visualized, which of the following should one look for?

    (A) increase nuchal fold

    (B) protruding tongue

    (C) cardiac defects

    (D) Down's syndrome

    (E) both A and D

    (F) all of the above

233. Which of the following is true in reference to focal myometrial contraction?

    (A) It is physiologic.

    (B) It increases the risk of spontaneous abortion.

    (C) It increases the risk of premature labor.

    (D) It is pathologic.

    (E) It is likely to resolve spontaneously.

    (F) Both B and D are true.

    (G) Both A and E are true.

234. Agenesis of the corpus callosum cannot be diagnosed by ultrasound before

    (A) 10 weeks

    (B) 14 weeks

    (C) 18 weeks

    (D) 28 weeks

    (E) 34 weeks

235. In 90% of cases with agenesis of the corpus callosum, what other sonographic finding is present?

    (A) polyhydramnios

    (B) omphalocele

    (C) polydactyly

    (D) teardrop ventricles

    (E) double bubble sign

236. Absent cerebral cortex is found in what cranial abnormality?

    (A) holoprosencephaly

    (B) hydrocephaly

    (C) hydranencephaly

    (D) agenesis of the corpus callosum

    (E) Dandy–Walker malformation

237. Microcephaly is defined as

    (A) HC ≤ 2 SD of mean

    (B) HC ≤ 3 SD of mean

    (C) 2-week lag in HC

    (D) both A and B

    (E) all of the above

238. A fetus presents with an anechoic midline lesion in the brain, fetal hydrops, and congestive heart failure. What is the most likely diagnosis for the lesion?

    (A) agenesis of the corpus callosum

    (B) dilation of the third ventricle

    (C) arachnoid cyst

    (D) atrioventricular malformation

    (E) hydranencephaly

239. Choroid plexus cysts, when found with other associated abnormalities, have a strong association with which of the following conditions?

    (A) Noonan's syndrome

    (B) trisomy 18

    (C) trisomy 13

    (D) X-linked hydrocephaly

    (E) none of the above

240. Which of the following is not a known cause for ectopic pregnancy

    (A) cigarette smoking

    (B) sterilization by bilateral tubal ligation

    (C) chlamydia trachomatis

    (D) pelvic inflammatory disease

    (E) herpes genitalis

241. The nuchal skin fold in the second trimester should be measured at what level?

    (A) the level of the cerebral peduncle

    (B) the same image as the circle of Willis, falx cerebri and 4th ventricle

    (C) the level of the cavum septi pellucidi, cerebellum and cisterna magna

    (D) the level of the ventricles

    (E) all of the above

242. Where are the ovaries normally located?

    (A) fallopian tubes

    (B) pouch of Douglas

    (C) Morrison's pouch

    (D) ovarian fossa

    (E) sacrouterine ligament

243. Abnormal accumulation of intraperitoneal fluid that becomes trapped by adhesions in a patient with a history of previous surgery is most likely caused by which of the following?

    (A) inclusion cyst

    (B) ovarian torsion

    (C) dermoid cyst

    (D) follicular cyst

    (E) leiomyosarcoma

244. If the cephalic index is > 85, it is an indication of what condition?

    (A) brachycephaly

    (B) dolichocephaly

    (C) microcephaly

    (D) macrocephaly

    (E) normal cephalic

245. If the cephalic index is < 75, it is an indication of what condition?

    (A) brachycephaly

    (B) dolichocephaly

    (C) microcephaly

    (D) macrocephaly

    (E) normal cephalic

246. When a sonographic procedure is to be performed that requires a needle insertion. The sonographer should use which one of the following types of gel?

    (A) warm ultrasound gel

    (B) sterile gel

    (C) hypoallergenic gel

    (D) transmission gel only

    (E) mineral oil

247. Which one of the following lubricants should *not* be used on latex probe covers?

    (A) K-Y jelly

    (B) coupling gel

    (C) water-based gel

    (D) oil-based products

    (E) hypoallergenic gel

248. Dolichocephaly is often associated with what conditions?

    (A) breech fetus

    (B) oligohydramnios

    (C) large-for-gestational-age fetus

    (D) both A and B

    (E) both A and C

    (F) all of the above

249. Brachycephaly is associated with what conditions?

    (A) trisomy 21

    (B) normal variant

    (C) myelomeningocele

    (D) both A and B

    (E) both A and C

    (F) all of the above

Questions 250–252: The ratio of head circumference to body circumference normally changes as pregnancy progresses. Match the weeks of gestation in Column A with the head and body ratio in Column B.

COLUMN A   COLUMN B

250. 12–24 _____   (A) abdomen larger than head

251. 32–36 _____   (B) head and body are equal

252. 36–40 _____   (C) head larger than abdomen

253. If performing a biparietal diameter (BPD) measurement and the midline echo is continuous and unbroken, this would indicate what about the scanning plane?

    (A) normal

    (B) too high

    (C) through the fetal neck

    (D) correct

    (E) too low

254. Which of the following is true regarding the fluid within a cystic hygroma?

    (A) serous fluid

    (B) amniotic fluid

    (C) ascites

    (D) lymphatic fluid

    (E) hemorrhagic

255. Cystic hygromas are caused by which of the following?

    (A) obstruction of the lymph system at the level of the jugular veins

    (B) obstruction of the lymph system at the level of the iliac veins

    (C) obstruction of the venous system at the level of the jugular veins

    (D) carotid artery obstruction

    (E) obstruction of the circle of Willis

256. Which of the following is *not* true of hydatidiform mole?

    (A) preeclampsia before 24 weeks of gestation

    (B) may have a clinical symptoms of hyperemesis gravidarum

    (C) patient may show signs of toxemia or hyperthyroidism

    (D) passing of small swollen villus via vagina

    (E) the uterus is frequently smaller for dates

257. Eighty percent of cystic hygromas occur in what region?

    (A) the axilla

    (B) the mediastinum

    (C) the cervical region

    (D) the lumbar region

    (E) the sacral region

258. Cystic hygromas are associated with which of the following?

    (A) Potter's syndrome

    (B) Beckwith–Wiedemann syndrome

    (C) elevated levels of alpha-fetoprotein

    (D) Turner's syndrome

    (E) both C and D

    (F) both B and D

    (G) all of the above

259. Which of the following best describes the sonographic appearance of molar pregnancy?

    (A) "snowstorm"

    (B) vesicular sonographic texture

    (C) Swiss cheese appearance

    (D) "tip of the iceberg" appearance

    (E) all of the above

    (F) A, B, and C only

Questions 260–269: Match the structures in Fig. 7–103 with the list of terms in Column B.

Early Pregnancy

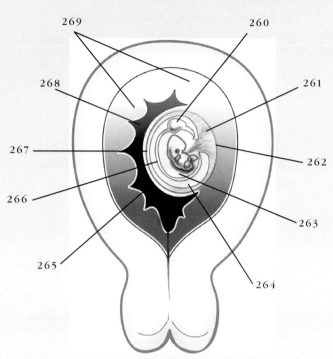

FIGURE 7–103.

COLUMN A	COLUMN B
260. _____	(A) amnion
261. _____	(B) chorion
262. _____	(C) decidua parietalis (vera)
263. _____	(D) decidua capsularis
264. _____	(E) yolk sac
265. _____	(F) amniotic cavity
266. _____	(G) uterine cavity
267. _____	(H) chorionic cavity
268. _____	(I) chorionic villi
269. _____	(J) decidua basalis

Questions 270–272: Match the structures in Fig. 7–104 with the list of terms in Column B.

Fibroids

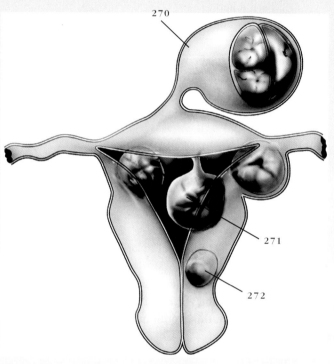

FIGURE 7–104.

COLUMN A	COLUMN B
270. _____	(A) submucous
271. _____	(B) pedunculated
272. _____	(C) intracavitary

Questions 273–281: Match the structures in Fig. 7–105 with the list of terms in Column B.

COLUMN A	COLUMN B
273. _____	(A) third ventricle
274. _____	(B) atrium
275. _____	(C) inferior horn
276. _____	(D) posterior horn
277. _____	(E) interventricular antrum
278. _____	(F) cerebral aqueduct
279. _____	(G) lateral recess
280. _____	(H) anterior horn
281. _____	(I) third ventricle

Ventricular System

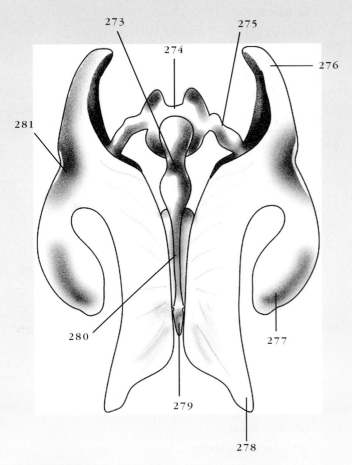

FIGURE 7–105.

282. The fetal shunt between the left and right atria is

(A) ductus venosum

(B) ductus arteriosus

(C) foramen ovale

(D) pulmonary ductus

(E) all of the above

283. The fetal shunt connecting the transverse aortic trunk and the main pulmonary trunk is

(A) ductus venosum

(B) ductus arteriosus

(C) foramen ovale

(D) pulmonary ductus

(E) all of the above

284. Hydranencephaly is thought to result from

(A) chromosomal abnormalities

(B) a vascular accident of the jugular veins

(C) a vascular accident of the internal carotid arteries

(D) calcification of the circle of Willis

(E) none of the above

285. The differential diagnosis for hydranencephaly may be

(A) semilobar holoprosencephaly

(B) alobar holoprosencephaly

(C) severe hydrocephaly

(D) both A and C

(E) both B and C

(F) all of the above

286. Hemivertebrae may be identified on sonogram

(A) as a narrowing of the individual vertebrae in the coronal plane of view

(B) as a narrowing of the individual vertebrae in the sagittal plane of view

(C) as a narrowing of the individual vertebrae in the axial plane of view

(D) all of the above

(E) none of the above

287. The downward displacement of the cerebellar vermis, the fourth ventricle, and medulla oblongata through the foramen magna is termed

(A) "lemon" sign

(B) Dandy–Walker malformation

(C) arachnoid cyst

(D) Arnold–Chiari malformation

(E) agenesis of the corpus callosum

288. Large encephaloceles may be associated with

(A) hydranencephaly

(B) hypotelorism

(C) microcephaly

(D) macrocephaly

(E) all of the above

289. A patient presents for an anatomy scan. The fetal head shows a single ventricle, single choroid, two cerebellar hemispheres, and fused thalamus. The abnormality is most likely

(A) semilobar holoprosencephaly

(B) alobar holoprosencephaly

(C) hydranencephaly

(D) hydrocephaly

(E) arachnoid cyst

290. A patient presents for an anatomy scan. The fetal head shows a single large cystic cavity with a rim of cerebral cortex. A fused thalamus is also identified. What is the most likely diagnosis?

    (A) alobar holoprosencephaly

    (B) semilobar holoprosencephaly

    (C) hydranencephaly

    (D) hydrocephaly

    (E) arachnoid cyst

291. A patient presents for an anatomy scan. The fetal head shows the cranium filled with anechoic fluid, and no cerebral cortex is identified. The brainstem is identified. What is the most likely diagnosis?

    (A) semilobar holoprosencephaly

    (B) alobar holoprosencephaly

    (C) hydranencephaly

    (D) hydrocephaly

    (E) Dandy–Walker malformation

292. How early can anencephaly be detected on ultrasound?

    (A) 10 weeks

    (B) 14 weeks

    (C) 16 weeks

    (D) 20 weeks

    (E) 24 weeks

293. Which of the following best describes acrania?

    (A) abnormal brain tissue with absent calvarium

    (B) the first stage of anencephaly before prolonged exposure to amniotic fluid

    (C) normal brain tissue with abnormal facies

    (D) both A and B

    (E) all of the above

For questions 294–298, which numbers in the term "parity G7 P3214" correspond to the following?

294. The number of living children: _____

295. The number of preterm infants: _____

296. The number of pregnancies total: _____

297. The number of abortions: _____

298. The number of full-term pregnancies: _____

299. A patient has had six pregnancies: three full term, one preterm delivery of twins, one spontaneous abortion, one fetal loss at 22 weeks. How would this be listed?

    (A) G6P3215

    (B) G6P3124

    (C) G7P5411

    (D) G7P2135

    (E) G6P3132

300. Adenomyosis is

    (A) benign penetration and growth of endometrial glands and stroma into the myometrium

    (B) malignant penetration and growth of endometrial glands and stroma into the myometrium

    (C) endometrial stroma and glands located outside of the uterus

    (D) inflammation of the endometrium

    (E) both B and C

301. An increased MSAFP3 may be associated with which of the following?

    (A) anencephaly

    (B) spina bifida occulta

    (C) skin covered spina bifida

    (D) both A and C

    (E) none of the above

302. An embryo is identified within a gestational sac with an estimated gestational age of 8 weeks. What is the approximate CRL measurement?

    (A) 4 mm

    (B) 1.5 cm

    (C) 2.7 cm

    (D) 80 mm

    (E) 0.8 mm

303. CRL is the appropriate dating measurement until what gestational age?

    (A) 8 weeks

    (B) 10 weeks

    (C) 12 weeks

    (D) 15 weeks

    (E) 40 weeks

304. **In a fetus without abnormalities in the second and early third trimester, what are the best parameters to use for estimated fetal weight (EFW)?**

    (A) CRL

    (B) FL/AC

    (C) BPD, HC, AC, FL

    (D) BPD/FL

    (E) orbital measurement and cerebellar measurement

305. **When measuring the femur, where should the calipers be placed?**

    (A) the outermost edge of the bone

    (B) include epiphyseal plate

    (C) the diaphysis of the shaft of the fetal femur

    (D) the edges of the entire bone, including the head and neck of the femur

    (E) all of the above

306. **Polyhydramnios is most commonly associated with what finding?**

    (A) insulin-dependent diabetes mellitus

    (B) duodenal atresia

    (C) idiopathic

    (D) micrognathia

    (E) fetal demise

307. **Polyhydramnios may be associated with which of the following?**

    (A) osteogenesis imperfecta

    (B) cleft lip

    (C) maternal diabetes

    (D) twin–twin transfusion

    (E) both A and B

    (F) all of the above

308. **At what gestational age should the amnion and chorion be fused?**

    (A) 8 weeks

    (B) 10 weeks

    (C) 16 weeks

    (D) 20 weeks

309. **The placenta is *not* responsible for which one of the following?**

    (A) exchange of nutrients

    (B) hematopoiesis

    (C) oxygen exchange

    (D) barrier to some medications

    (E) hormone production

310. **Which of the following is least likely to cause placental abruption?**

    (A) maternal hypertension

    (B) fibroids

    (C) cocaine

    (D) auto accident

    (E) focal myometrial contraction

311. **Which of the following best describes placental abruption?**

    (A) the premature separation of placenta before 20 weeks of gestation

    (B) the premature separation of placenta after 20 weeks of gestation

    (C) the premature separation of placenta at any gestational age week

    (D) the same as a retrochorionic clot

    (E) the implantation of the placenta in the lower uterine segment

312. **Sonographic signs of placental abruption include which of the following?**

    (A) retroplacental veins > 2 cm

    (B) intervillous lakes

    (C) hypoechoic periplacental hematomas

    (D) both A and C

    (E) all of the above

313. **Risks for placenta accreta include**

    (A) maternal hypertension

    (B) isoimmunization

    (C) previous cesarean section

    (D) infertility

    (E) all of the above

314. **Placenta percreta refers to**

    (A) invasion of placental tissue through the uterus into bladder

    (B) invasion of placental tissue into myometrium

    (C) invasion of placenta up to the serosal layer

    (D) placental attachment to the myometrium without invasion

    (E) the premature separation of placenta before 20 weeks of gestation

315. What is the placental vascular malformation that appears as a hypoechoic mass near the cord insertion?

(A) fetal vascular anastomosis

(B) placental lake

(C) placental aneurysm

(D) chorioangioma

(E) allantoic cyst

316. The vessels in the umbilical cord are protected by which of the following?

(A) Wharton's jelly

(B) amniotic fluid

(C) serosal fluid

(D) myometrium

(E) placenta

317. What is a cyst in the umbilical cord called?

(A) allantoic cyst

(B) yolk sac cyst

(C) Meckel's cyst

(D) ectodermal cyst

(E) chorioangioma

318. Which of the following terms denotes the umbilical cord inserting in the membranes and coursing to the placenta?

(A) normal cord insertion

(B) succenturiate cord insertion

(C) eccentric cord insertion

(D) velamentous cord insertion

(E) nuchal cord

319. Which of the following terms best describes the umbilical cord inserting into the edge of the placenta?

(A) normal cord insertion

(B) marginal cord insertion

(C) eccentric cord insertion

(D) velamentous cord insertion

(E) nuchal cord

320. Which of the following is the most common cardiac defect?

(A) hypoplastic left heart syndrome

(B) atrial/ventricular septal defect

(C) tetralogy of Fallot

(D) transposition of the great arteries

(E) Ebstein's abnormally of the tricuspid valve

321. The left side of the heart is responsible for perfusing

(A) cranial aspects of the fetus

(B) systemic aspects of the fetus

(C) placenta

(D) lower limbs of the fetus

(E) none of the above

322. The right side of the heart is responsible for perfusing

(A) cranial aspects of the fetus

(B) systemic aspects of the fetus

(C) placenta

(D) umbilical cord only

(E) none of the above

323. The heart should occupy what percentage of the fetal thorax?

(A) 25%

(B) 30%

(C) 60%

(D) 75%

(E) 90%

324. If the axis of the heart is pointed to the right, which of the following should the sonographer look for?

(A) an interrupted inferior vena cava

(B) other heart abnormalities

(C) abdominal organ orientation

(D) dextrocardia

(E) all of the above

325. What is the most common cardiac defect associated with trisomy 21?

(A) atrial/ventricular septal defect

(B) hypoplastic left heart syndrome

(C) atrioventricular canal defect

(D) transposition of the great vessels

(E) dextrocardia

326. From the four-chamber view, the transducer is tilted toward the fetal left shoulder. This will obtain what cardiac view?

(A) five-chamber view

(B) short-axis view

(C) long-axis view

(D) aortic arch

(E) none of the above

327. **What anatomy should be evaluated in the four-chamber view?**

    (A) junction of the atrioventricular valves with the atrial and ventricular septum intact

    (B) equally sized ventricular chambers

    (C) contractility of the heart

    (D) both A and B

    (E) all of the above

328. **Which of the following best describes the "banana" sign?**

    (A) concave formation of the frontal bones

    (B) flattening of the cerebellum

    (C) dumbbell-shaped cerebellum

    (D) dilatation of the third ventricle

    (E) absence of the corpus callosum

329. **A patient presents for ultrasound and informs you that she had a ruptured ectopic pregnancy one year ago in which she fainted. Which of the following most likely was her treatment for her ectopic pregnancy?**

    (A) methotrexate

    (B) hysterectomy

    (C) salpingectomy

    (D) dilation and curettage

    (E) folic acid

330. **Which of the following heart abnormalities is difficult or impossible to identify on fetal echocardiography?**

    (A) coarctation of the aorta

    (B) Ebstein's anomaly

    (C) double outlet right ventricle

    (D) atrial/ventricular septal defect

    (E) none of the above

331. **The majority of congenital diaphragmatic hernias are**

    (A) left sided

    (B) right sided

    (C) bilateral

    (D) midline

    (E) none of the above

332. **On fetal sonogram, the fetal heart is deviated to the right with apex pointed to the left. The sonographer should consider what possible abnormalities?**

    (A) congenital diaphragmatic hernia

    (B) congenital cystic adenomatoid malformation

    (C) teratoma

    (D) both A and B

    (E) all of the above

333. **In the identification of congenital diaphragmatic hernia, which of the following is the most important organ the sonographer should also assess?**

    (A) the location of the fetal liver

    (B) fetal kidneys

    (C) fetal bladder

    (D) placenta

    (E) all of the above

334. **The significant perinatal mortality of fetuses with congenital diaphragmatic hernia is caused by**

    (A) chromosomal abnormalities

    (B) oligohydramnios

    (C) associated cardiac defects

    (D) pulmonary hypoplasia

    (E) polyhydramnios

335. **Congenital diaphragmatic hernia has a poorer prognosis if**

    (A) it is a left-sided defect

    (B) the stomach is located on the left and anterior

    (C) if bowel is identified in the chest

    (D) if liver is identified in the chest

    (E) none of the above

336. **The most frequently identified chest mass is**

    (A) right-sided diaphragmatic hernia

    (B) left-sided diaphragmatic hernia

    (C) congenital cystic adenomatoid malformation

    (D) pulmonary sequestration

    (E) omphalocele

337. **Congenital cystic adenomatoid malformation is divided into three types. Type I is**

    (A) microcystic

    (B) medium-sized cysts

    (C) macrocystic

    (D) mixed-size cysts

    (E) megacystis

338. Type II congenital cystic adenomatoid malformation is

(A) microcystic

(B) medium-sized cysts

(C) macrocystic

(D) mixed-size cysts

(E) megacystis

339. Type III congenital cystic adenomatoid malformation is

(A) microcystic

(B) medium-sized cysts

(C) macrocystic

(D) mixed-size cysts

(E) megacystis

340. What type of tumor is most likely to produce hCG and AFP?

(A) dermoid cyst

(B) fibroid uterus

(C) Meigs syndrome

(D) dysgerminoma

(E) endometrioma

341. Where are the majority of pulmonary sequestrations found?

(A) inferior to the diaphragm

(B) in the lower left lung base

(C) in the lower right lung base

(D) in the upper left pulmonary lobe

(E) apex of the lungs

342. Methotrexate usually is *not* given in which of the following situations?

(A) unruptured ectopic pregnancy is present

(B) if the β-hCG is <1,500 U/L

(C) ectopic embryo heart motion not seen

(D) ectopic gestational sac >4 cm

(F) all of the above

343. What percentage of esophageal atresia has a tracheoesophageal fistula?

(A) 25%

(B) 50%

(C) 75%

(D) 90%

(E) 10%

344. Eighty percent of fetuses with esophageal atresia have what associated condition in the third trimester?

(A) intrauterine growth retardation

(B) macrosomia

(C) polyhydramnios

(D) decreased abdominal circumference

(E) oligohydramnios

345. Esophageal atresia has a strong association with what chromosomal abnormality?

(A) trisomy 21

(B) trisomy 18

(C) trisomy 13

(D) translocation

(E) none of the above

346. Which of the following does the "double-bubble" sign refer to?

(A) two-vessel umbilical cord

(B) duodenal atresia

(C) ureterocele

(D) hypotelorism

(E) two air-filled structures

347. Fifty percent of fetuses with duodenal atresia also have which of the following abnormalities?

(A) spinal defects

(B) cardiac defects

(C) macrosomia

(D) both A and B

(E) all of the above

348. Duodenal atresia has a strong association with what chromosomal abnormality?

(A) trisomy 21

(B) trisomy 18

(C) trisomy 13

(D) unbalanced translocation

(E) none of the above

349. The physiological herniation of bowel into the umbilical cord is complete by what gestational age?

(A) 8 weeks

(B) 9 weeks

(C) 10 weeks

(D) 13 weeks

(E) 40 week

350. **A pseudogestational sac does not have which one of the following characteristics?**

    (A) anechoic center

    (B) yolk sac

    (C) fail to grow from one week to the next

    (D) sac-like structure

    (E) sloughing decidua

351. **Which of the following is a sign/symptoms for ruptured ectopic pregnancy?**

    (A) unilateral adnexal pain which increase with time

    (B) heavy vaginal bleeding with clots

    (C) right shoulder pain and fainting

    (D) nausea and vomiting

    (E) vaginal discharge and urinary frequency

352. **Which of the following about gastroschisis is true?**

    (A) more common with advanced maternal age

    (B) often associated with other abnormalities

    (C) has a very good prognosis with 80–90% survival rate

    (D) has an autosomal recessive inheritance

    (E) has herniation covered by a membrane consisting of amnion and peritoneum

353. **Sonographic signs of bowel perforation do *not* include which one of the following?**

    (A) thickened bowel loops

    (B) abdominal calcifications

    (C) meconium cysts

    (D) oligohydramnios

    (E) polyhydramnios

354. **Which of the following can cause intrauterine complications of gastroschisis**

    (A) intrauterine growth retardation

    (B) edematous bowel wall

    (C) intestinal obstruction

    (D) dilated fetal stomach

    (E) all of the above

355. **Gastroschisis is a break in the anterior abdominal wall at what level**

    (A) right side of the umbilical cord

    (B) left side of the umbilical cord

    (C) at the umbilical cord insertion with cord attaching to the gastroschisis

    (D) medially and inferior to the umbilical cord

    (E) none of the above

356. **Physiological herniation of the midgut does not include**

    (A) small intestines

    (B) cecum and variform appendix

    (C) liver

    (D) superior mesenteric artery

    (E) vitelline artery

357. **A 24-year-old woman presents with c/o right-lower-quadrant pain, nausea with vomiting, and vaginal bleeding for 2 days, as well as serum β-hCG 1,500 mIU/mL. What is the finding in the sonogram shown in Fig. 7–106?**

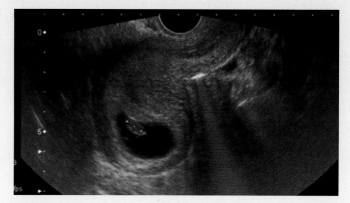

FIGURE 7–106.

    (A) ectopic pregnancy with free fluid

    (B) complete abortion

    (C) appendicitis with a ruptured ectopic pregnancy

    (D) early intrauterine pregnancy in a retroverted uterus

    (E) missed abortion

358. **A midline defect in the anterior abdominal wall with herniation of abdominal contents into the base of the umbilical cord is called which of the following?**

    (A) gastroschisis

    (B) omphalocele

    (C) cloacal exstrophy

    (D) pentalogy of Cantrell

    (E) double bobble

359. Omphaloceles are *not* associated with which one of the following?

    (A) advanced maternal age
    (B) chromosomal abnormalities
    (C) maternal smoking
    (D) cardiac abnormalities
    (E) has herniation covered by a membrane consisting of amnion and peritoneum

360. Which of the following terms best describes a midline defect of the chest with the heart herniated to the outside of the chest?

    (A) rachischisis
    (B) ectopia cordis
    (C) cloacal exstrophy
    (D) limb–body wall complex
    (E) tetralogy of Fallot

361. An omphalocele and ectopia cordis are identified on sonogram. What condition should be included in the differential?

    (A) pentalogy of Cantrell
    (B) trisomy 18
    (C) Beckwith–Wiedemann syndrome
    (D) both A and B
    (E) all of the above

362. Beckwith–Wiedemann syndrome is a group of which of the following disorders?

    (A) omphalocele
    (B) shortening of limbs unilaterally
    (C) macroglossia
    (D) polyhydramnios
    (E) both A and C
    (F) all of the above

363. If the bladder is herniated through the ventral wall and a spinal defect is identified, what condition should be considered?

    (A) bladder exstrophy
    (B) cloacal exstrophy
    (C) pentalogy of Cantrell
    (D) limb–body wall complex
    (E) omphalocele

364. A condition in which no umbilical cord may be identified, along with ventral wall defects, and scoliosis is most likely

    (A) cloacal exstrophy
    (B) amniotic synechiae
    (C) limb–body wall complex
    (D) complete ventral wall defect
    (E) pentalogy of Cantrell

365. Amniotic bands syndrome differs from amniotic sheets (synechiae) because

    (A) amniotic bands are attached to the uterus at both ends
    (B) amniotic sheets often cause disruption in the first trimester
    (C) amniotic bands can cause amputation or limb deformities
    (D) there is no difference between amniotic bands and sheets
    (E) none of the above

366. Rh isoimmunization results from which of the following combinations?

    (A) mother Rh– and father Rh–
    (B) mother Rh+ and father Rh–
    (C) mother Rh+ and fetus Rh–
    (D) mother Rh– and fetus Rh+
    (E) none of the above

367. What is the name of the drug given to Rh-negative mothers to prevent hemolytic disease of the newborn?

    (A) folic acid
    (B) Clomid
    (C) methotrexate
    (D) RhoGAM
    (E) lupron

368. The hemolytic process of destruction of the fetal red blood cells by the maternal antibodies is termed

    (A) hypercoagulation
    (B) erythroblastosis fetalis
    (C) thrombocytopenia
    (D) nonimmune hydrops
    (E) microcytic-hypochromic anemia

369. **Which of the following is not characteristic of a blighted ovum?**

    (A) gestational sac fails to grow from one week to the next

    (B) large empty gestational sac

    (C) dead embryo

    (D) thin trophoblastic reaction

    (E) irregularly shaped gestational sac

370. **Signs of congestive heart failure in the fetus are**

    (A) serous effusions

    (B) enlarged fetal liver

    (C) fetal ascites

    (D) pericardial effusions

    (E) all of the above

371. **How is the diagnosis of fetal hydrops made by sonography?**

    (A) two fetal sites of fluid accumulation

    (B) fetal ascites and one site of accumulated fluid

    (C) one site of fluid accumulation and oligohydramnios

    (D) both A and B

    (E) both A and C

    (F) all of the above

372. **In cases of fetal distress in diabetic mothers, the fetal heart may**

    (A) have thickened ventricular walls

    (B) have decreased contractility

    (C) have increased cardiac output

    (D) both A and B

    (E) all of the above

373. **The main causes for nonimmune hydrops include**

    (A) fetal abnormalities

    (B) parvovirus

    (C) anti-Kell antibodies

    (D) both A and B

    (E) both A and C

    (F) all of the above

374. **Ultrasound confirmation that an intrauterine device (IUD) is *in situ* is**

    (A) highly echogenic linear echo in the endometrial cavity with distal acoustic shadowing

    (B) depiction of the IUD string on ultrasound in the endometrial cavity

    (C) depiction of the IUD in the myometrium with distal acoustic shadow

    (D) demonstration of the endometrial stripe

    (E) eccentric position of the IUD with entrance–exit reflections

375. **Pain in the right upper quadrant (RUQ) due to adhesions and inflammation between the liver and the diaphragm secondary to ascending pelvic infection is known as**

    (A) Fitz–Hugh–Curtis syndrome

    (B) Mittelschmerz

    (C) Stein–Leventhal syndrome

    (D) ectopic pregnancy

    (E) right-sided salpingitis

376. **In cases of partial situs inversus, which of the following should the sonographer consider?**

    (A) cardiac defects

    (B) polysplenia

    (C) asplenia

    (D) interrupted inferior vena cava

    (E) both B and C

    (F) all of the above

377. **On a sonogram, the fetus has unilateral hydronephrosis, nonvisualized ureters, normal bladder, and normal amniotic fluid volume. What does this most likely represent?**

    (A) unilateral ureterovesical junction (UVJ) obstruction

    (B) unilateral ureteropelvic junction (UPJ) obstruction

    (C) posterior urethral valves (PUV)

    (D) all of the above

    (E) none of the above

378. **A ureterovesical junction (UVJ) obstruction is associated with what other findings?**

    (A) ureterocele

    (B) unilateral hydronephrosis

    (C) pelvic kidney

    (D) both A and C

    (E) none of the above

379. **What is the sonographic appearance of the fetal ureters on ultrasound**

    (A) the fetal ureters are dilated on most sonograms due to the fetal bladder

    (B) the fetal ureters are dilated on most sonograms due to the fetal kidneys

    (C) it is normally seen next to the iliac vessels on ultrasound

    (D) only one ureter is dilated due to the position of the fetal liver

    (E) the ureters are 1 to 2 mm in diameter and are rarely depicted on ultrasound

380. **The trigone refers to**

    (A) the point at which the ureter enters the kidney

    (B) the region where the urethra exits the body

    (C) the base of the bladder containing the orifices of the ureters and urethra

    (D) the region of the bladder containing the orifice of the urethra

    (E) the anterior wall of the bladder near the urethra

381. **A 35 year old with complaint of lower abdominal cramping, which comes and goes. She also complains of heavy vaginal bleeding with clots. Beta-hCG done on Monday was 8,200 mIU/mL and a second serum β-hCG done on Wednesday (48 hours later) was 20 mIU/mL. The patient now states the cramping and vaginal bleeding have stop. Transvaginal and transabdominal sonogram done demonstrate no intrauterine pregnancy (IUP), no adnexal mass, and no free fluid. The endometrial thickness is 2 mm. What is the most likely diagnosis?**

    (A) ruptured ectopic pregnancy

    (B) unruptured ectopic pregnancy

    (C) abdominal pregnancy

    (D) incomplete abortion

    (E) complete abortion

382. **Which of the following is not an ultrasound characteristic of complete posterior ureteral valve obstruction?**

    (A) hydramnios

    (B) hydronephrosis

    (C) hydroureter

    (D) "keyhole" urethra

    (E) abnormally distended urinary bladder

383. **Potter's facies refers to**

    (A) flattened facial features caused by the lack of amniotic fluid

    (B) abnormal development of the abdominal muscles caused by overdistention of the urinary bladder

    (C) cleft lip and palate

    (D) bulging orbits with assent of the cranial bones

    (E) small mouth with protruding tongue and small ears

384. **That is the primary cause of death in posterior urethral valve (PUV) outlet syndrome?**

    (A) renal failure

    (B) sepsis

    (C) cardiac overload

    (D) pulmonary hypoplasia

    (E) polyhydramnios

385. **Sonographic features of renal agenesis do not include which one of the following?**

    (A) inability to demonstrate blood flow in renal arteries

    (B) elongated adrenal glands in the renal fossa

    (C) polyhydramnios

    (D) unable to visualize fetal bladder

    (E) low amniotic fluid

386. **How often does the fetal urinary bladder empty?**

    (A) every 5 minutes

    (B) every 30 to 45 minutes

    (C) every 1 to 2 hours

    (D) every 4 hours

    (E) every 1 minute

387 **Causes for abnormal vaginal bleeding do not include which one of the following?**

    (A) endometrial carcinoma

    (B) polycystic ovarian syndrome

    (C) ovarian torsion

    (D) submucosal fibroids

    (E) hyperthyroidism

388. **In the early stages of organogenesis, how many kidneys form?**

    (A) 2

    (B) 3

    (C) 4

    (D) 6

    (E) two pairs

389. What other organ system has a strong correlation with renal abnormalities?

    (A) cardiac
    (B) uterine
    (C) ovarian
    (D) muscular
    (E) brain

390. Which of the following statements about multicystic dysplastic kidney disease is false?

    (A) caused by a first-trimester obstruction
    (B) caused by a second-trimester obstruction
    (C) multiple, varying sized cysts in the parenchyma
    (D) echogenic parenchyma
    (E) caused by a third-trimester obstruction

391. In the case of unilateral, multicystic, dysplastic kidney disease, the contralateral kidney will often

    (A) enlarge
    (B) become obstructed
    (C) have decreased function
    (D) remain the same
    (E) small

392. If one parent has autosomal-dominant polycystic kidney disease, the risk for the fetus having the same disease is

    (A) 25%
    (B) 50%
    (C) 75%
    (D) 90%
    (E) 100%

393. A 26-week fetus presents with large echogenic kidneys that contain some small cysts. The amniotic fluid volume is normal. Differential diagnosis includes

    (A) autosomal-recessive polycystic kidney disease
    (B) autosomal-dominant polycystic kidney disease
    (C) Meckel's syndrome
    (D) both A and C
    (E) all of the above

394. The kidneys should occupy how much of the fetal abdomen in an axial plane of view?

    (A) 1/4
    (B) 1/3
    (C) 1/2
    (D) 2/3
    (E) 3/4

395. Anechoic cysts that surround the periphery of the kidney in a "string of pearls" appearance most likely represent

    (A) multicystic dysplastic kidney disease
    (B) autosomal dominant polycystic kidney disease
    (C) normal renal pyramids
    (D) early stage obstructed renal pyramids
    (E) Stein–Leventhal syndrome

396. The fetus begins to produce urine at what gestational age?

    (A) 10 weeks
    (B) 12 weeks
    (C) 17 weeks
    (D) 20 weeks
    (E) 24 weeks

397. Ectopic pregnancy is defined as

    (A) pregnancy in the fallopian tubes
    (B) pregnancy in the peritoneal space
    (C) pregnancy outside of the uterus
    (D) pregnancy in the uterine cavity
    (E) pregnancy outside the endometrial cavity

398. In the second trimester, what is the normal renal pelvis size?

    (A) less than 20 mm
    (B) less than 15 mm
    (C) less than 8 mm
    (D) less than 6 mm
    (E) 4–6 cm

Questions 399–403: Match the renal grading system in Column A to the description in Column B.

COLUMN A

399. Grade 0 _____

400. Grade I _____

401. Grade II _____

402. Grade III _____

403. Grade IV _____

COLUMN B

(A) renal pelvis and calices dilated

(B) no dilation

(C) renal pelvic dilation with or without infundibula visible

(D) renal pelvis and calices dilated with parenchymal thinning

(E) renal pelvic dilation with calices visible

404. A rare renal tumor that is large, solid, and highly vascular is

(A) neuroblastoma

(B) renal teratoma

(C) congenital mesoblastic nephroma

(D) none of the above

(E) polycystic kidney

405. A malignant adrenal gland tumor that appears as an echogenic, heterogeneous mass is

(A) neuroblastoma

(B) teratoma

(C) Wilms' tumor

(D) nephroblastoma

(E) none of the above

406. A congenital mesoblastic nephroma is also known as a

(A) neuroblastoma

(B) teratoma

(C) Wilms' tumor

(D) William's tumor

(E) angiomyolipomas

Questions 407–409: Match the structures in Fig. 7–107 with one of the following muscles.

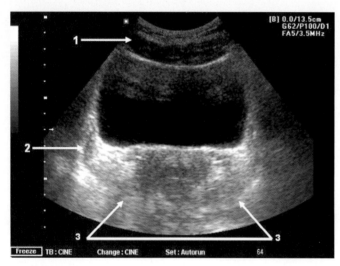

FIGURE 7–107.

407. Arrow no. 1 is pointing to _____   (A) obturator internus

408. Arrow no. 2 is pointing to _____   (B) rectus abdominis

409. Arrow no. 3 is pointing to _____   (C) piriformis

410. In Fig. 7–108, the bilateral hypoechoic regions visualized posterior and lateral to the vagina represent which of the following?

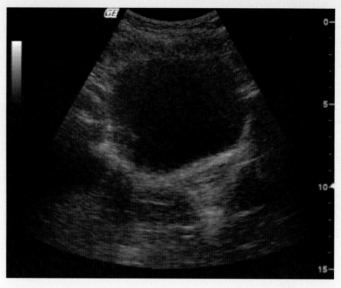

FIGURE 7–108.

(A) ovaries

(B) obturator internus muscles

(C) bilateral masses

(D) levator ani muscle group

411. The degree to which the head shapes may affect biparietal diameter (BPD) can be estimated by which of the following formulas?

(A) HC = BPD2 + OFD

(B) Index = HC/OFD × 1.54

(C) CI = BPD/OFD × 100

(D) BPD = BPD × OFD/1.256

(E) CI = BPD/OFD × 1.54

412. What is the most common cause for ovarian torsion?

(A) ovarian tumors

(B) hyperstimulation of the ovary

(C) adhesions

(D) hypervascularity to the ovary

(E) pelvic inflammatory disease

413. The blood supply to the ovaries comes from which of the following?

(A) ovarian artery

(B) aorta

(C) uterine artery

(D) both A and B

(E) both A and C

414. Ovaries that have been overstimulated by infertility medication are at risk for which of the following?

(A) producing grossly enlarged cysts

(B) torsion

(C) endometriosis

(D) both A and B

(E) all of the above

415. Which of the following is not a characteristic of ovarian torsion in adults?

(A) enlarged ovary with a large dermoid cyst

(B) Whirlpool sign

(C) no venous flow but arterial flow present

(D) variable sonographic appearances

(E) bilateral normal size ovary with follicular cyst and Doppler flow present

(F) bilateral salpingo-oophorectomy

416. Which of the following is an early sign/symptom of endometrial cancer?

(A) postmenopausal vaginal bleeding

(B) abdominal and pelvic pain

(C) ascites seen on ultrasound

(D) massive weight loss

(E) headache

417. A rapidly growing fibroid in the first trimester of pregnancy is not as worrisome as a rapidly growing fibroid in a postmenopausal woman because

(A) of the rapid rise of progesterone in the first trimester

(B) of the decrease of estrogen in postmenopausal women

(C) rapid fibroid growth is not worrisome

(D) both cases are cause for concern

(E) fibroids are not dependent on hormones

418. A rapidly growing fibroid in a postmenopausal woman not on hormone replacement therapy is suggestive of which of the following?

(A) leiomyosarcoma

(B) fibrous degeneration

(C) hemorrhagic infiltration

(D) calcific changes

(E) pregnancy

419. In the first and second trimesters, the fetal lung is

(A) of greater echogenicity than the fetal liver

(B) of decreased echogenicity compared to the fetal liver

(C) isoechoic to the fetal liver

(D) variable in appearance

(E) not visible sonographically

420. In the third trimester, the fetal lung is

(A) of greater echogenicity than the fetal liver

(B) of decreased echogenicity compared to the fetal liver

(C) isoechoic to the fetal liver

(D) variable in appearance

(E) fluid filled

421. The femoral epiphyseal plates are visualized on sonogram after

(A) 8 weeks

(B) 12 weeks

(C) 15 weeks

(D) 24 weeks

(E) 32 weeks

422. Postaxial polydactyly is

(A) an extra digit on the ulnar aspect of the fetal hand

(B) an extra digit on the radial aspect of the fetal hand

(C) curvature of the last digit on the ulnar aspect

(D) an extra digit on the fetal foot

(E) absent of the fetal hand

423. Preaxial polydactyly is

(A) an extra digit on the ulnar aspect of the fetal hand

(B) an extra digit on the radial aspect of the fetal hand

(C) curvature of the last digit on the ulnar aspect

(D) an extra digit on the fetal foot

(E) absence of the foot

424. Concordant growth in twins refers to

(A) <10% difference in estimated fetal weight (EFW) between the twins

(B) <20% difference in estimated fetal weight (EFW) between the twins

(C) both fetus within normal range on a normal growth curve

(D) fetus remaining at the same estimated fetal weight (EFW) percentile from exam to exam

(E) all of the above

425. **A 27-year-old woman presented for an anatomy ultrasound at 38 weeks of gestation. After 20 minutes of scanning, the patient complains of nausea, dizziness, and lightheadedness. She became pale and sweaty. What is this most likely due to?**

    (A) supine hypotensive syndrome

    (B) ectopic pregnancy

    (C) hyperemesis gravidarum

    (D) supine hypertensive syndrome

    (E) Fitz–Hugh–Curtis syndrome

426. **The formula for determining EFW discordance in twins is?**

    (A) smallest EFW + largest EFW/smallest EFW

    (B) smallest EFW × 2 − largest EFW/largest EFW

    (C) largest EFW − smallest EFW/largest EFW × 100

    (D) largest EFW × 100 − smallest EFW/largest EFW

    (E) none of the above

427. **What is frank breech?**

    (A) when both feet are prolapsed into the lower uterine segment

    (B) when one foot is prolapsed into the vagina

    (C) when the fetal head is to the maternal right and the buttocks are to the maternal left

    (D) when the buttocks descend first, the thighs and legs are extended upward along the anterior fetal trunk

    (E) when one foot is prolapsed in the lower uterine segment the other leg is above the head

428. **What is complete breech?**

    (A) when both feet are prolapsed into the lower uterine segment

    (B) when both feet are prolapsed into the vagina

    (C) when the buttocks descend first, the knees are flexed, baby sitting cross-legged

    (D) when the thighs and legs are extended upward along the anterior fetal trunk

    (E) when one foot is prolapsed in the lower uterine segment the other leg is above the head

429. **What is footling breech?**

    (A) when one or both feet are prolapsed into the lower uterine segment

    (B) when one foot is prolapsed into the fundus

    (C) when the buttocks descend first, the knees are flexed, fetus sitting cross-legged

    (D) when the thighs and legs are extended upward along the anterior fetal trunk

    (E) when the fetal head is toward the maternal left and the feet are toward the right

430. **Which site of ectopic pregnancy has the highest maternal morbidity or mortality?**

    (A) abdominal pregnancy

    (B) cornual

    (C) ampullary

    (D) ovarian

    (E) isthmic

431. **A fetal karyotype of 47X indicates which of the following about the fetus?**

    (A) affected with Down's syndrome

    (B) affected with Turner's syndrome

    (C) a boy

    (D) a girl

432. **When performing sonographic examination, the sonographer is expected to do all of the following except?**

    (A) explain the procedure that will be performed to the patient

    (B) input the patient's name and medical number in the ultrasound equipment

    (C) review any previous imaging

    (D) briefly explain the sonographic finding with her/his family members who are observing the procedure in the room

    (E) briefly examine the patient's chart for relevant laboratory values

433. **When labeling twins, fetus A should be**

    (A) the first fetus identified

    (B) the fetus closest to the fundus

    (C) the fetus closest to the internal os

    (D) any of the above methods is appropriate

    (E) the fetus seen first on the sonogram

434. **The fetus is vertex with the spine on the maternal right. The fetal left side should be**

    (A) anterior

    (B) posterior

    (C) inferior

    (D) superior

    (E) none of the above

435. **The fetus is transverse with head on the maternal left. The fetal spine is inferior. The fetal left side should be**

(A) anterior

(B) posterior

(C) inferior

(D) superior

(E) none of the above

436. **The fetus is breech with the spine on the maternal left. The fetal left side should be**

(A) anterior

(B) posterior

(C) inferior

(D) superior

(E) none of the above

437. **Subchorionic placental lakes are**

(A) associated with intrauterine growth retardation

(B) associated with oligohydramnios

(C) also known as subchorionic fibrin deposition

(D) are sonographic findings of abruptio placenta

(E) all of the above

438. **Early placental maturation may be associated with**

(A) hypertension

(B) gestational diabetes mellitus

(C) maternal smoking

(D) both A and C

(E) all of the above

439. **A thin placenta (<1.5 cm) is not associated with which one of the following?**

(A) preeclampsia

(B) intrauterine growth retardation

(C) insulin dependent diabetes mellitus

(D) triploidy

(E) intrauterine infection

440. **A thick placenta (>5 cm) is not associated with which one of the following?**

(A) gestational diabetes mellitus

(B) infection

(C) multiple gestations

(D) hypertension

(E) hydrops

441. **Maternal causes of intrauterine growth retardation do not include which one of the following?**

(A) maternal infection

(B) diabetic mothers with vasculopathy

(C) maternal smoking

(D) gestational diabetes mellitus

(E) previous history of fetus with intrauterine growth retardation

442. **A patient presents for amniocentesis, which of the following is most imperative before performing the procedure?**

(A) briefly examine the patient's chart for relevant laboratory values

(B) confirm that an informed consent was obtained

(C) input the patient's name and medical number into the ultrasound equipment

(D) obtain previous imaging

(E) ensure the room and the transducer are clean

443. **Caudal regression syndrome is associated with**

(A) insulin-dependent diabetes mellitus

(B) chromosomal abnormalities

(C) Noonan's syndrome

(D) hypertension

(E) all of the above

444. **Which organ or tissue has the furthermost concern with respect to biological effects when utilizing ultrasound on humans?**

(A) skin

(B) embryo

(C) spleen

(D) bone

(E) adult red blood cells

445. **What is the highest amount of output intensity typically utilized in diagnostic ultrasound?**

(A) pulse-wave Doppler with real-time imaging

(B) color power Doppler

(C) fetal Doppler monitor

(D) real-time

(E) none of the above

446. Turner's syndrome affects males and females

    (A) equally
    (B) males more than females
    (C) females more than males
    (D) males only
    (E) females only

447. In order to reduce the acoustic exposure to the obstetrical patient, which of the following should the sonographer do?

    (A) decrease the power output controls and increase the receiver gains
    (B) decrease the near gain and increase the far gain and power output
    (C) increase the overall receiver gain and the output power at the same time
    (D) decrease the scanning time and increase the power output
    (E) increase the power output and receiver gains in order to increase attenuation, which will decrease the patient exposure

448. Which of the following might be fetal complications caused by maternal diabetes?

    (A) caudal regression syndrome
    (B) cardiac defects
    (C) shoulder dystocia
    (D) both A and B
    (E) all of the above

449. Lung maturity amniocentesis is used in what cases?

    (A) intrauterine growth retardation fetus with decreasing estimated fetal weight (EFW)
    (B) insulin-dependent diabetes mellitus
    (C) complete premature rupture of membranes
    (D) both A and B
    (E) all of the above

450. Which of the following sonographic markers may *not* be used to assess macrosomia?

    (A) humeral shoulder thickness
    (B) cheek-to-cheek diameter
    (C) HC/AC ratio
    (D) amniotic fluid volume
    (E) abdominal subcutaneous tissue thickness

451. In the case of anhydramnios, how can karyotype be obtained?

    (A) percutaneous umbilical blood sampling
    (B) chorionic villus sampling
    (C) cystocentesis
    (D) all of the above
    (E) none of the above

452. Amniocentesis may *not* be used to test for which one of the following?

    (A) sickle cell disease
    (B) fetal bilirubin
    (C) specific short limb syndromes
    (D) cystic fibrosis
    (E) cleft palate

453. Maternal hypertension may have what effect on pregnancy?

    (A) polyhydramnios
    (B) placentomegaly
    (C) intrauterine growth retardation
    (D) chromosomal abnormalities
    (E) macrosomia

454. An excessively accelerated calcific placenta in the second trimester is associated with which of the following risk factors?

    (A) excessive maternal smoking
    (B) chromosomal abnormality
    (C) precursor to third-trimester intrauterine growth retardation
    (D) hydrops
    (E) all of the above

455. The abbreviation BBOW refers to

    (A) baby below outer water
    (B) brachycephalic baby on way
    (C) bulging bag of water
    (D) baby below occipital wing
    (E) baby below obstetrical weight

456. The abbreviation PROM refers to

    (A) partially ruptured outer membrane
    (B) previous rip of mucus plug
    (C) partial range of motion
    (D) premature rupture of membranes
    (E) postpartum removal of membrane

457. Overdistension of the urinary bladder may cause

(A) anterior placenta to appear previa

(B) closure of an incompetent cervix

(C) distortion or closure of the gestational sac

(D) obscured visualization of the internal iliac vein

(E) both A and B

(F) all of the above

458. Ovulation is assume to occurs

(A) during intercourse

(B) on the 7th day of the menstrual cycle

(C) on the 14th day of the menstrual cycle

(D) on the 2nd day of the menstrual cycle

(E) on the first day of menstruation

Questions 459–467: Match the terms in Column A to the correct description in Column B.

COLUMN A	COLUMN B
459. Gravida _____	(A) a woman who has given birth two or more times
460. Multipara _____	(B) one who has never been pregnant
461. Nullipara _____	(C) a woman who is pregnant
462. Primipara _____	(D) a woman who has never given birth to a viable infant
463. Nulligravida _____	(E) pregnant for the first time
464. Primigravida _____	(F) one who has been pregnant several times
465. Multigravida _____	(G) the number of pregnancies that have continued to viability
466. Para _____	(H) a woman who has given birth one time to a viable infant
467. Trimester _____	(I) a 3-month period during gestation

468. Puerperium refers to the period

(A) surrounding conception time

(B) after death

(C) 6–8 weeks before delivery

(D) beginning with the expulsion of the placenta

(E) the area of anatomy between the anus and vagina

469. A postpartum gynecologic sonogram may be needed for which of the following assessments?

(A) assessing maternal hydronephrosis

(B) examining the uterus for retained placenta

(C) checking for maternal bowel obstruction

(D) maternal gallstones

(E) all of the above

470. Which of the following components of the ultrasound system exposes a patient to greater potential risk?

(A) a cracked transducer face

(B) a transducer cable that is wet with ultrasound gel

(C) a hot TV monitor

(D) ultrasound equipment that need calibration

(E) cold transducer gel

471. Which of the following structures is most likely not seen in a postpartum pelvic sonogram?

(A) uterus

(B) endometrial echo

(C) vagina

(D) ovaries

(E) all of the above

472. Approximately what level is the fundus of the gravid uterus at 20 weeks of gestation?

(A) umbilicus

(B) xiphoid process

(C) half way between the umbilicus and the symphysis pubic

(D) at the level of the symphysis pubic

(E) below the symphysis pubic

473. What is the most common complication during the postpartum period?

(A) hemorrhage

(B) thromboembolism

(C) infection

(D) both A and B

(E) all of the above

474. **Which of the following is a least likely cause for abdominal and pelvic ascites?**

    (A) heart failure

    (B) nephrotic syndrome

    (C) pancreatitis

    (D) cancer

    (E) fibroid uterus

475. **What percentage of fetuses is in the breech presentation at term?**

    (A) 25%

    (B) 50%

    (C) 75%

    (D) 5%

    (E) 1%

476. **Which of the following characteristic is most suspicious of malignant ascites?**

    (A) free intraperitoneal fluid in paracolic gutters and Morison' s pouch

    (B) loculated fluid with loops of bowel adherent and fixed to the abdominal wall

    (C) free echogenic fluid in the peritoneal cavity with floating bowel loops

    (D) anechoic free fluid in the in the gravity-dependent position of the abdomen

    (E) homogeneous echogenic free fluid in the paracolic gutters and Morison's pouch

477. **The abbreviation VBAC refers to**

    (A) vaginal blockage and closure

    (B) vaginal blockage after cesarean

    (C) vaginal birth after cesarean

    (D) none of the above

    (E) vaginal bacteria at cesarean

478. **Which of the following anatomical sites is where the normal implantation of pregnancy occurs?**

    (A) ampullary region of the fallopian tube

    (B) endometrial cavity

    (C) myometrium

    (D) abdomen

    (E) ovaries

Questions 479–484: Match the terms in Column A to the correct description in Column B.

COLUMN A

479. placenta previa _____

480. placenta accreta _____

481. placenta succenturiata _____

482. abruptio placentae _____

483. placenta increta _____

484. placenta percreta _____

COLUMN B

(A) abnormal adherence of part or all of the placenta to the uterine wall

(B) premature separation of the placenta after 20 weeks of gestation

(C) accessory lobe of placenta

(D) implantation of the placenta in the lower uterine segment

(E) abnormal adherence of part or all of the placenta in which the chorionic villi invade the myometrium

(F) abnormal adherence of part or all of the placenta in which chorionic villi invade the uterine wall

485. **The chorion frondosum progressively develops to become**

    (A) fetal component of the placenta

    (B) maternal component of the placenta

    (C) the amniotic cavity

    (D) the yolk sac and stalk

    (E) fetus

486. **The decidua basalis progressively develops to become**

    (A) fetal component of the placenta

    (B) maternal component of the placenta

    (C) the amniotic cavity

    (D) the yolk sac and stalk

    (E) embryo

487. Which of the following choices is true about HELLP syndrome?

(A) abbreviation for hemolysis elevated liver enzymes, and low platelets

(B) abbreviation for hemivertebrae elevated liver enzymes, and low-lying placenta

(C) treated similar to severe preeclampsia

(D) Doppler may help in assessing HELLP syndrome

(E) acronym for help evaluation of lungs, liver and preeclampsia

488. A large fibroid uterus is seen on the ultrasound. The sonographer should scan what organ?

(A) kidneys

(B) liver

(C) posterior cul-de-sac

(D) pancreas

(E) spleen

489. What is the primary infection that causes varicella-zoster virus (VZV)?

(A) 5ths disease

(B) chicken pox

(C) human papilloma virus (HPV)

(D) herpes simplex

(E) cytomegalovirus

490. What is the most common congenital intrauterine viral infection?

(A) toxoplasmosis

(B) HIV

(C) parvovirus

(D) cytomegalovirus

(E) rubella

491. Which of the following statements about the secondary yolk sac is false?

(A) located in amniotic cavity

(B) disappears at approximately 12 weeks of gestation

(C) is depicted before the embryo is seen

(D) contains vitelline fluid

(E) is essential in blood development

492. What is the most common cause for hematocolpos?

(A) bicornuate uterus

(B) endometritis

(C) pelvic inflammatory disease

(D) imperforate hymen

(E) ectopic pregnancy

493. Sampling of the middle cerebral artery is helpful in determining

(A) IUGR and related complications

(B) prediction of fetal anemia

(C) the need for a fetal transfusion

(D) all of the above

494. Which of the following statements regarding leiomyoma is *false*?

(A) calcifies and attenuates the ultrasound beam

(B) may mimic a myometrial contraction

(C) normally increases in size after menopause

(D) distorts the endometrial cavity

(E) derives from the muscle of the uterus

495. A 24-year-old presents for an ultrasound with a markedly elevated serum β-hCG. Her sonogram demonstrates multiple small anechoic spaces about 3–5 mm in the uterine cavity. What is this finding most likely to be?

(A) theca lutein cyst

(B) corpus lutein cyst

(C) follicular cyst

(D) hydropic villi

(E) pseudogestational sac

496. Which of the following statements about stromal tumors is false?

(A) All have a similar sonographic appearance and can't be differentiated from one another.

(B) solid, hypoechoic ovarian tumors

(C) types include: fibromas, thecomas, Sertoli–Leydig cell tumors.

(D) types include: fibromas, thecomas, and Brenner tumors.

(E) all of the above

497. Endometrioma may appear sonographically similar to

(A) benign cystic teratoma

(B) polycystic ovaries

(C) hemorrhagic cyst

(D) hydrosalpinx

(E) follicular cyst

498. Hydrosalpinx may be differentiated from a multi-cystic ovarian mass on sonogram by

    (A) following the cystic spaces to ensure that they all communicate

    (B) using color Doppler to follow the ovarian artery to the ovary

    (C) having the patient roll to lengthen out the fallopian tube

    (D) the two cannot be differentiated

    (E) using power Doppler

499. An anechoic, smooth-walled cyst is identified in a patient who has had a hysterectomy/oophorectomy. Which of the following should be included in the differential diagnosis?

    (A) paraovarian cyst

    (B) ovarian remnant cyst

    (C) mesonephric cyst

    (D) inclusion cyst

    (E) all of the above

500. The hydatid cyst of Morgagni is

    (A) a complex ovarian mass

    (B) an hydatidiform mole cyst

    (C) paramesonephric cyst

    (D) another name for ovarian remnant syndrome

    (E) an hydatid cyst of the ovaries

501. The formula for determining ovarian volume is

    (A) $D1 \times D2 \times D3 \times 0.523$

    (B) $D1 + D2 + D3 \times 3.14$

    (C) $D1 \times D2 \times D3 \times 3.14$

    (D) $D1 + D2 \times 100$

    (E) $D1 + D2 \times 1.57$

502. The image in Fig. 7–109 represents

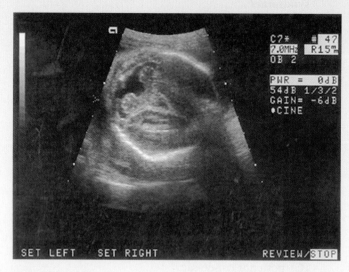

FIGURE 7–109.

    (A) arachnoid cyst

    (B) communicating hydrocephaly

    (C) "banana" sign

    (D) Dandy–Walker malformation

    (E) choroid plexus cyst

503. Fig. 7–110 demonstrates a

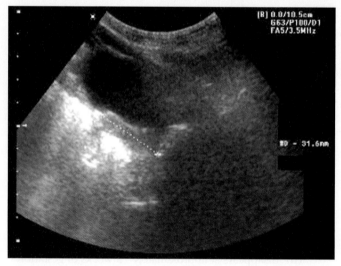

FIGURE 7–110.

    (A) normal adult uterus

    (B) multiparous uterus

    (C) prepubertal uterus

    (D) nulliparous uterus

    (E) enlarged fibroid uterus

504. Fig. 7–111 is of a 25-year-old patient referred for a sonogram because a right adnexal mass was palpated. What is the most likely diagnosis?

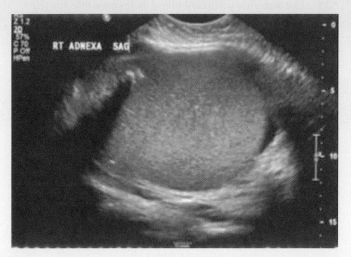

FIGURE 7–111.

(A) cystadenoma

(B) fibroma

(C) cystic teratoma

(D) dysgerminoma

(E) endometrioma

505. In Fig. 7–112, what are the arrows pointing to?

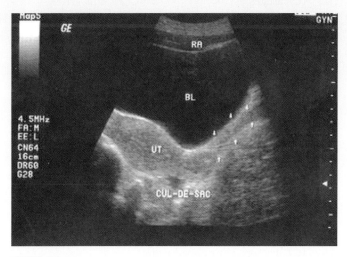

FIGURE 7–112.

(A) ovarian ligament

(B) broad ligament

(C) obturator internus muscle

(D) vagina

(E) cervix

506. In Fig. 7–113, the markers are placed on the endocervical canal; what do the markers represent?

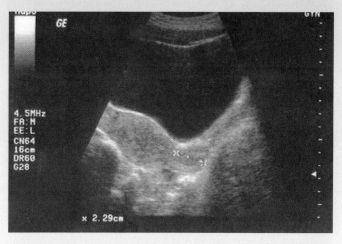

FIGURE 7–113.

(A) isthmus to corpus

(B) anterior cul-de-sac and internal os

(C) internal os to external os

(D) the vaginal fornices

(E) vaginal canal

Questions 507–510. Match the structures numbered in Fig. 7–114 with the list of terms in Column B.

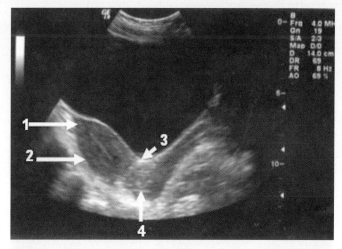

FIGURE 7–114.

507. Arrow no. 1 is pointing to _____

508. Arrow no. 2 is pointing to _____

509. Arrow no. 3 is pointing to _____

510. Arrow no. 4 is pointing to _____

(A) cervix

(B) fundus

(C) corpus

(D) isthmus

(E) endometrium

511. In Fig. 7–115, identify the potential space that is marked by the asterisk.

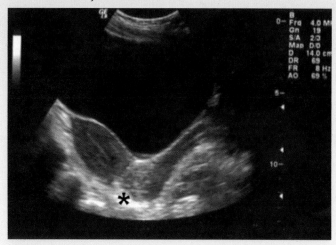

FIGURE 7–115.

(A) space of Retzius

(B) pouch of Douglas

(C) anterior cul-de-sac

(D) Morrison's pouch

(E) vesicouterine pouch

512. Female infertility may be caused by which of the following?

(A) uterine synechiae

(B) polycystic ovarian syndrome (PCOS)

(C) Asherman's syndrome

(D) adenomyosis

(E) all of the above may cause infertility

513. In Fig. 7–116, the endometrium is in what phase of the menstrual cycle?

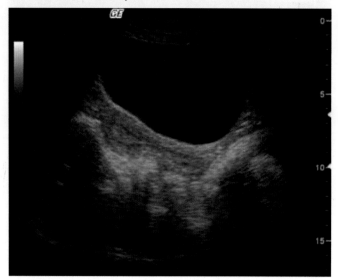

FIGURE 7–116.

(A) menstrual

(B) secretory

(C) proliferative

(D) luteal

514. The anterior pituitary gland is responsible for the production of which of the following?

(A) FSH (follicle-stimulating hormone)

(B) GnRH (gonadotropin releasing hormone)

(C) LH (luteinizing hormone)

(D) oxytocin

(E) both B and D

(F) both A and C

515. When performing a spectral Doppler evaluation of the ovary during the pre-ovulatory phase, which of the following is *false*?

(A) the waveform has a decreased diastolic flow

(B) decreased resistance index (RI)

(C) increased vasculature of the follicular wall

(D) high amount of flow during diastole

(E) no change in waveform

516. Meigs' syndrome consists of all of the following except?

(A) pleural effusion

(B) uterine tumor

(C) ascites

(D) fibrous ovarian tumor

517. The onset of menstruation is also referred to as?

(A) parity

(B) menarche

(C) climacteric

(D) Mittelschmerz

(E) puberty

518. Sonographically normal bowel can present as

(A) echogenic

(B) having peristaltic motion

(C) having acoustic shadowing

(D) fluid-filed

(E) all of the above

519. An 18-year-old female presents with amenorrhea. The sonogram demonstrates a cystic dilated uterine and vaginal cavity containing low-level echoes. The diagnosis of hematometrocolpos was made. This may have resulted from all of the following except

(A) obstruction at the vaginal level

(B) secondary to an imperforate hymen

(C) vaginal septum

(D) stenotic or atretic vagina

(E) cervical stenosis

520. The incidence of ovarian carcinoma is relatively low (1.4% lifetime risk, or 1 in 70). Women with at least a 2.0% lifetime risk include all of the following except

(A) infertility patients

(B) perineal talc exposure

(C) high-fat diet

(D) multiparity

(E) family history

521. There are various methods of assisted reproductive technology. Which of the following is not a method of assisted reproductive technology?

(A) in vitro fertilization

(B) GIFT

(C) FIFT

(D) ZIFT

(E) none of the above

522. In Fig. 7–117, the endometrium is in what phase of the menstrual cycle?

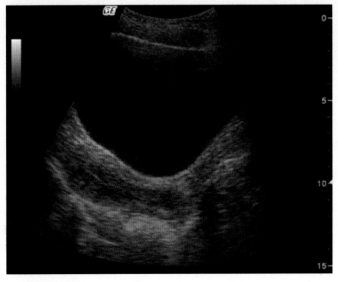

FIGURE 7–117.

(A) menstrual

(B) secretory

(C) proliferative

(D) luteal

(E) none of the above

523. What is the congenital uterine anomaly that is demonstrated in Fig. 7–118?

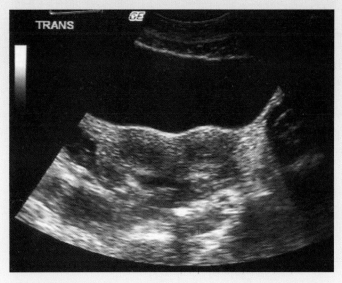

FIGURE 7–118.

(A) didelphys uterus

(B) septate uterus

(C) bicornuate uterus

(D) unicornis

(E) no congenital anomaly is visualized

524. This patient might present with a history of

(A) spontaneous abortions

(B) vaginal bleeding

(C) pelvic pain

(D) infertility

(E) vaginal discharge

525. Fig. 7–119 is a sagittal midline image of the pelvis demonstrating a mass superior to the fundus of the uterus, which most-likely represents a (an)

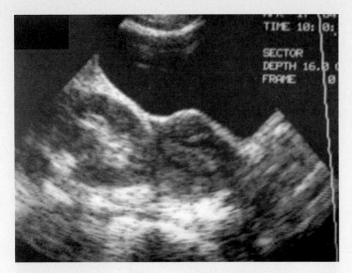

FIGURE 7–119.

(A) endometrioma

(B) ectopic kidney

(C) bowel

(D) thecoma

(E) ovary

526. Which of the following muscles is not located within the true pelvis?

(A) obturator internus

(B) levator ani

(C) piriformis

(D) iliopsoas

(E) coccygeus

527. Which of the following ligaments does not provide structural support for the uterus and cervix?

(A) round

(B) cardinal and uterosacral

(C) infundibulopelvic

(D) uterosacral

(E) cardinal

528. What sonographic study requires a catheter inserted into the endometrial cavity with the insertion of normal saline solution as contrast medium for the purpose of demonstrating abnormalities of the uterine cavity?

(A) in vitro fertilization

(B) hysterosalpingogram

(C) computerized tomography

(D) sonohysterography

(E) magnetic resonance imaging

529. In the presence of ascites, Fig. 7–120 is most suggestive of

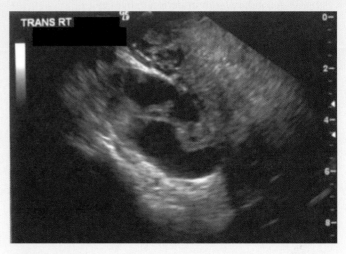

FIGURE 7–120.

(A) cystadenoma

(B) serous cystadenocarcinoma

(C) endometriosis

(D) paraovarian cyst

530. Which of the following patients will require an informed consent for transvaginal ultrasound?

(A) a comatosed intensive care unit patient on mechanical ventilation with possible small ovarian cyst

(B) a patient with history of bipolar disorder and schizophrenia to r/o ectopic pregnancy

(C) patient with ovarian torsion, who refuses transvaginal sonogram, which is warranted to confirmed the diagnosis

(D) a patient with morphine overdose and other control drugs including alcohol

(E) A, B, and D only

(F) all of the above

531. A sonographer working in a hospital ultrasound department was approach by a 22-year-old hospital employee who is requesting an ultrasound and a DVD of her baby. This is her first pregnancy and she is very excited about her pregnancy. She states that the DVD is to show her husband and family her unborn baby in 3D. What is the most appropriate next step for the sonographer to take?

   (A) do the ultrasound in 3D and charge her only for the cost of the DVD

   (B) do the ultrasound only

   (C) do the ultrasound and give her the DVD for free; DVD is part of her medical records, and therefore, she has a legal right to have it

   (D) refuse to do the ultrasound study, but do the 3D ultrasound on DVD for her

   (E) none of the above

532. A patient informs you prior to her sonogram that she is 30 weeks pregnant. She had prenatal care in Puerto Rico and came to the United States two weeks ago. She is now complaining of uterine contractions. She came to the hospital via ambulance because she is unable to tolerate the contractions. The sonogram performed today fails to demonstrate any pregnancy. The uterus is small, 6 cm in size. The urine and serum β-hCG test results are negative. What is the most likely finding?

   (A) abdominal pregnancy

   (B) fetal demise

   (C) pseudocyesis

   (D) ectopic pregnancy

   (E) missed abortion

533. Precocious puberty is

   (A) premature development of secondary sexual characteristics before 8 years

   (B) infants born with an atypical enlarged genitals with undetermined sex type

   (C) a rare and abnormal separation of the symphysis pubis and piriformis muscle

   (D) a congenital abnormality of the pubic bone

   (E) preventative measure before teenage reproductive years

534. What is the most common cause for requesting pelvic ultrasound in the pediatric age-group?

   (A) fibroid uterus

   (B) vaginal foreign body

   (C) ovarian cancer and ascites

   (D) precocious puberty and sexual ambiguity

   (E) endometrial polyps

535. The gold standard for predicting fetal lung maturity is

   (A) lecithin-sphingomyelin (L/S) ratio

   (B) grade III placenta

   (C) demonstration of the proximal humeral epiphyses

   (D) alpha-fetoprotein (AFP)

   (E) ultrasound utilizing all three parameters BPD, AC, and FL

536. An infection acquired via a medical instrument or a medical procedure is called

   (A) nosocomial

   (B) iatrogenic

   (C) mortality

   (D) mobility

   (E) autoclave

537. A 22-year-old presented to the emergency department complaining of vaginal bleeding and lower abdominal cramping for 7 days after a suction dilatation and curettage for an unwanted pregnancy at 8 weeks. Her serum β-hCG is currently 3,500 mIU/mL. What is the sonographic finding shown in Fig. 7–121?

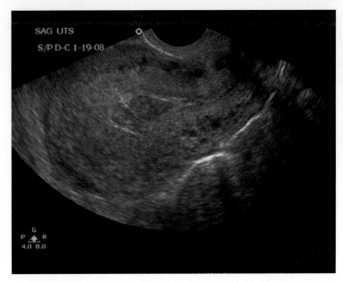

FIGURE 7–121.

   (A) ectopic pregnancy

   (B) abdominal pregnancy

   (C) complete abortion

   (D) pseudo-gestational sac

   (E) retained products

538. The fetal head should be in what position for a more precise nuchal translucency measurements

(A) neutral position

(B) brow presentation

(C) occiput transverse

(D) hyperflexion

(E) hyperextended

539. Sonographic measurements taken between the outer edge of the occipital bone to the outer margin of the skin is called

(A) nuchal fold

(B) nuchal translucency

(C) cisterna magna

(D) orbital distance

(E) cerebellar measurement

540. Enlarged nuchal translucency is often associated with all of the following except

(A) aneuploidy

(B) Down's syndrome and cystic hygroma

(C) Turner's syndrome

(D) congenital heart disease

(E) rhombencephalon

541. The optimal time to assess measurements for nuchal translucency is

(A) 6–12 weeks

(B) 4–5 weeks

(C) 14–16 weeks

(D) 11–14 weeks

(E) 6–14 weeks

542. The mean measurement for nuchal translucency is

(A) 30 cm

(B) 30 mm

(C) 1 mm

(D) 7 mm

(E) 3 mm

543. Which of the following terms is used in association with cystic hygroma and enlarged nuchal translucency?

(A) nuchal fold

(B) ventriculomegaly

(C) hydrops fetalis

(D) mesenchymal edema

(E) spina bifida

Answers and Explanations

At the end of each explained answer, there is a number combination in parentheses. The first number identifies the reference source; the second number or set of numbers indicates the page or pages on which the relevant information can be found.

1. **(C)** The fetal calvarium is absent superior to the eyes. This finding is consistent with anencephaly. *(1:19)*

2. **(B)** The image shows a defect in the posterior cranial vault. Because brain tissue is herniated through the defect, this would be an occipital encephalocele. This fetus also demonstrates microcephaly caused by the large defect. *(1:19)*

3. **(D)** Equinovarus, or clubfoot, may be isolated or associated with other defects, most commonly neural tube defects. *(2:363)*

4. **(A)** The image represents a cystic hygroma. The multiple septations seen are characteristic of second-trimester cystic hygroma. The intact cranium differentiates it from an encephalocele. *(2:992)*

5. **(A)** Seventy-five percent of fetuses with cystic hygromas have a chromosomal abnormality, most commonly Turner's syndrome. *(2:56)*

6. **(C)** The image is an example of a "lemon"-shaped skull. It is most commonly associated with spinal defects, but can be present with encephaloceles and in normal fetuses 1–2% of the time. *(2:286)*

7. **(A)** Abdominal ascites outlines the abdominal viscera. Ascites associated with meconium peritonitis may have particles of debris within it, and echogenic foci are often present in the fetal liver. Nonimmune hydrops must have two fluid collections or one fluid collection with anasarca. *(2:470, 471)*

8. **(A)** Bilateral pleural effusions and edema. *(14:1460–1461)*

9. **(C)** Alobar holoprosencephaly is characterized by a single ventricle, single choroid, and fused thalamus. *(1:20)*

10. **(D)** Cystic hygroma is associated with Turner's syndrome, not trisomy 18. *(3:499–502)*

11. **(C)** Paternally derived triploidy is associated with a relatively normally grown fetus that has a proportionate head size. The placenta is large with multiple cystic spaces resembling a molar pregnancy. This accounts for 90% of triploidy. *(2:850)*

12. **(F)** Maternally derived triploidy is associated with a small placenta. The fetus has severe asymmetric growth restriction and oligohydramnios. *(2:851; 3:506)*

13. **(A)** Potter's syndrome is associated with renal agenesis, oligohydramnios, pulmonary hypoplasia and malformation of the hands and feet. *(20:1282)*

14. **(C)** The embryo cardiac activity can be seen at 6 weeks gestation and on some occasion at 5 and half weeks with higher frequency transducers. The embryo heart rate at 6 weeks range from 112 to 136 bpm, which increases to a rate of 140 to 160 bpm at 9 weeks. A heart rate of less than 80 bpm is associated with pregnancy failure. *(20:994; 14:1094)*

15. **(C)** Krukenberg's tumor is a malignant tumor of the ovary that metastasizes from a primary in the gastrointestinal tract. Meigs' syndrome is a benign tumor of the ovaries associated with ascites and pleural effusion. *(20:920; 943)*

16. **(D)** Hydatidiform mole. This sonogram demonstrates multiple tiny cystic spaces representing vesicles. This gives a sonographic appearance of honeycomb or snow-storm appearance, which is characteristic of hydatidiform mole. *(20:1012;14:1578)*

17. **(A)** Talipes equinovarus or clubfoot is a developmental deformity in which the foot is inverted and planter flexed so that the metatarsal long axis is in the same plane as the tibia and fibula. The deformity affects the muscles and tendons of the foot. Clubfoot can also occur from restriction of movement due to oligohydramnios. *(20:1309;14:1453)*

18. **(C)** Seventy-five percent of twins are dizygotic. *(1:27)*

19. **(D)** The twin peak is formed when the placental tissue migrates between the chorionic layers. This is 94–100% predictive of dizygotic twins. *(2:182, 183)*

20. **(D)** Forty percent of conjoined twins are born stillborn. Fifty-six percent of conjoined twins are thoraco-omphalopagus, thoracopagus, and omphalopagus. Polyhydramnios is present 50% of the time. Commonly, there is one umbilical cord that may have an abnormal number of vessels and is shared by the conjoined fetuses. *(1:29)*

21. **(A)** Ninety percent of the time, the uterus tilts forward in anteverted position, meaning the uterus forms a 90° angle with the posterior vaginal wall. The uterus, however, may be in any of the following positions:
    - Anteverted: The uterus tilts forward with a 90° angle to the posterior vaginal wall.
    - Anteflexed: The uterine corpus is flexed anteriorly on the cervix, forming a sharp angle at the cervix.
    - Retroverted: The uterus tilts backward without a sharp angle between the corpus and cervix.
    - Retroflexed: The uterine corpus is flexed posteriorly on the cervix, forming a sharp angle at the cervix.

    This sonogram demonstrate a retroverted uterus *(2:531)*

22. **(E)** Absence of cardiac motion. (*Study Guide*)

23. **(E)** Fluid in the endometrial cavity in a post-menopausal patient may be associated with cervical stenosis or malignancy. (*14:544*)

24. **(B)** Painless bright red blood is associated with placenta previa. (*20:1149*)

25. **(E)** The hippocampus is a horseshoe shaped paired structure located in the left and right brain hemisphere. It is not a midline structure. (*10:853*)

26. **(B)** The occurrence rate for thanatophoric dysplasia is 1/6000–1/17,000 births. Sonographic findings are polyhydramnios, severe rhizomelia, and micromelia with bowing. The thorax is bell-shaped, and the cranium is cloverleaf-shaped with hydrocephaly and frontal bossing. (*1:28; 2:343*)

27. **(F)** Heterozygous achondroplasia accounts for 80% of achondroplasias. It is the most common form of genetic skeletal dysplasia. It is often not identified before 26–27 weeks. (*1:27*)

28. **(B)** The outline of a septate uterus is relatively normal and contains two endometrial cavities separated by a thin fibrous septum. A bicornuate uterus contains two endometrial cavities, but there is a deep indentation on the fundal contour. (*19:534–538*)

29. **(B)** A meningocele is a spina bifida with herniation of the meninges only. (*1:19*)

30. **(E)** Normal cephalic presentation, with the fetal head close to the internal os of the cervix. The placenta is not identified in this image. (*20:1148–1153*)

31. **(B)** This is an image of an increased nuchal skinfold (> 6 mm). Nuchal fold measurements are obtained between 15 to 20 weeks gestation. Nuchal translucency is performed between 11 to 14 weeks gestation. Both nuchal fold and nuchal translucency are used for screening Down's syndrome (*14:1233–1234; 20:1027*)

32. **(E)** This sonogram demonstrate an intrauterine contraceptive devices (IUD) that is eccentric in position. (*20:915–916*)

33. **(C)** The image represents a benign cystic teratoma (BCT). A differential for this mass could be an endometrioma. (*1:Table 9–4*)

34. **(E)** Normal left ovary with iliac vessels. (*20:885*)

35. **(A)** The cystic structure in the posterior aspect of the embryonic head represents the rhombencephalon. It is a normal structure seen between 7–9 weeks which later forms the fourth ventricle. (*2:139: 14:1113*)

36. **(E)** Subserosal fibroid. (*20:903*)

37. **(E)** The serum β-hCG normally decreases significantly after a dilation and curettage (D&C). An increase after the procedure is highly suggestive of an ectopic pregnancy. This image after a D&C is a transabdominal sagittal sonogram with a left unruptured ectopic pregnancy next to the left ovary. (*14:1102, 1113*)

38. **(A)** Serous cystadenomas are the most common ovarian neoplasm accounting for 20–25% of all benign ovarian neoplasms. They usually present as large, thin-walled, unilocular cystic masses that may contain thin echogenic septations. (*14:566–568*)

39. **(C)** Hydrops fetalis is an accumulation of fluid in body cavities and soft tissue. This image shows cystic hygroma with body anasarca. (*14:1137*)

40. **(D)** The abnormality is spina bifida of the lumbar spine. The differential may include a sacrococcygeal teratoma based on the image alone; however, this fetus had a positive lemon/banana sign. (*1:19*)

41. **(E)** The image is an increased nuchal translucency. It has an 80% positive predictive value for trisomy 21. If combined with the first trimester biochemistry, it has a 90% positive predictive value for trisomy 21. (*1:30*)

42. **(E)** An increased nuchal translucency is associated with specific chromosomal abnormalities, genetic syndromes, and structural defects. (*1:30*)

43. **(B)** The dilation of the proximal urethra gives the fetal bladder the classic "keyhole" appearance associated with posterior urethral valve obstruction. (*1:25*)

44. **(E)** Tetralogy of Fallot is comprised of a VSD, overriding aorta, pulmonary stenosis, and right ventricular hypertrophy. The hypertrophy is not always present, particularly in the early to midsecond trimester. This image shows the VSD and overriding aorta. (*1:21*)

45. **(D)** The stomach is located posterior to the fetal heart, which is deviated to the right side of the chest. The solid appearance on the left side of the thorax is consistent with the liver. (*1:22*)

46. **(D)** This image demonstrates a displaced and irregular shape cerebellum, which is curved like a banana and known as the "banana sign." It is characterized by the inferior displacement of the cerebellum and has a strong association with spinal defects and Arnold–Chiari malformation. (*2:73*)

47. **(B)** The image is an example of an omphalocele. Atypically, the bowel is herniated instead of the liver. Notice the membrane around the bowel and the umbilical cord inserting into the membrane. (*1:23*)

48. **(D)** The image is consistent with enlarged kidneys. Dysplastic kidneys would have multiple cysts. Infantile polycystic kidney disease is associated with large kidneys; however, they are echogenic and oligohydramnios is present. (*2:543*)

49. **(B)** The tongue can be seen protruding from the mouth, consistent with macroglossia. The chin, forehead, and profile are normal. (*4:225*)

50. **(C)** Beckwith–Wiedemann syndrome is a group of disorders including omphalocele, macroglossia, organomegaly, and hemihypertrophy. *(1:24)*

51. **(A)** Multicystic, dysplastic kidneys have multiple cysts of various sizes. The cysts occur randomly and do not follow any pattern, as with dilated renal pyramids. The parenchyma is usually echogenic. *(1:25)*

52. **(C)** It has a variable prevalence, with Native American being the highest at 3.6/1000 births. *(2:322)*

53. **(D)** Three-dimensional imaging of the internal organs is termed volume imaging. Three-dimensional images of surface structures, such as the fetal face, is surface rendering. *(1:1020)*

54. **(B)** There is a limitation on what can be visualized by the human eye using medical imaging. A 7 to 10 MHz transvaginal transducer can depict a 5mm gestational sac as early as 4 weeks. *(14:1081)*

55. **(B)** Fetal echocardiogram can be done earlier than 18 weeks, but is dependent on maternal habitus. After 24 weeks, the fetal bones become denser and more calcified and begin to limit the sonographic windows that allow visualization of the cardiac structures. *(2:378, 379)*

56. **(A)** Three-dimensional imaging of surface structures, such as the fetal face, is termed surface rendering. *(1:1020)*

57. **(D)** Although duodenal atresia has been detected in the first trimester, the classic "double bubble" sign is not usually present until the late second and early third trimesters. *(2:466)*

58. **(E)** When the increased AFP is unexplained, it is thought to be because of an increased placental transfer of AFP. The placental dysfunction can occur with various placental abnormalities that may be associated with certain third trimester complications. *(2:30)*

59. **(B)** Cloacal exstrophy is characterized by an abdominal wall defect inferior to the umbilical cord insertion with exstrophy of a cloacal sac and a neural tube defect. It is associated with a markedly increased MSAFP. Amniotic sheets and congenital diaphragmatic hernia do not increase MSAFP. Smith–Lemli–Opitz syndrome is associated with a low level of maternal uE3 and normal MSAFP. *(2:29, 503)*

60. **(C)** If AFP (<0.6 MoM), uE3 (<0.5 MoM), and hCG (<0.3 MoM) are all decreased, the triple screen will show an increased risk for trisomy 18. *(2:29)*

61. **(D)** Pulmonary hypoplasia can be assumed by the small thoracic circumference and anhydramnios, but underdeveloped fetal lungs are not visible by sonography. *(1:25)*

62. **(A)** Vein of Galen aneurysm is an AV malformation located posterior to the third ventricle in the midline of the brain. *(1:21)*

63. **(A)** Truncus arteriosus consists of one outflow tract overriding a VSD. The right ventricular outflow tract is absent. Differential diagnosis includes tetralogy of Fallot with pulmonary atresia. Identifying the pulmonary arteries branching from the main trunk would differentiate the defect. *(4:390)*

64. **(D)** The most predictive sonographic findings are the overriding aorta and VSD. If the VSD is perimembranous, it will not appear on the four-chamber view. The right ventricle may appear larger than the left, but this is not a consistent finding and is dependent of the degree of pulmonary stenosis. Differential diagnosis would include truncus arteriosus. *(4:426)*

65. **(A)** Congenital cystic adenomatoid malformation (CCAM) is divided into three subsets; macro, medium, and microcystic. Survival rate combines all types and sizes and is 75–80%. Studies have shown that CCAM regresses 55–69% of the time. *(2:439–441)*

66. **(F)** Congenital diaphragmatic hernia is left sided 75–90% of the time. Prognosis is poor, particularly if the liver is herniated into the chest. Five to fifteen percent of congenital diaphragmatic hernias are associated with chromosomal abnormalities, commonly trisomy 18. *(2:433–438)*

67. **(D)** Ninety percent of esophageal atresia have a tracheoesophageal fistula. This allows amniotic fluid to reach the stomach, but at a slower rate. The stomach will be visualized, but may be smaller than usual. Polyhydramnios occurs in the mid to late second trimester. The VACTERL complex is: vertebral anomalies, anal atresia, cardiac abnormalities, tracheoesophageal atresia, renal anomalies, and limb anomalies. At least three of the anomalies listed must be present to diagnosis the VACTERL condition. *(2:103, 460)*

68. **(A)** Trisomy 21 is associated with a decreased MSAFP and an increased hCG. *(5:71)*

69. **(C)** The uterosacral ligament is the distal portion of the cardinal ligament. It anchors the cervix and is responsible for uterine orientation. *(1:5)*

70. **(B)** Both the suspensory and broad ligaments are folds of peritoneum. *(1:5)*

71. **(A)** The piriformis muscles lie more posteriorly and are ovoid and symmetrical. *(16:292)*

72. **(A)** The most dependent portion is the pouch of Douglas, or the posterior cul-de-sac. It is located posterior to the cervix and anterior to the rectum. *(1:6)*

73. **(C)** The posterior cul-de-sac (pouch of Douglas) is located posterior to the uterus. The anterior cul-de-sac (vesicouterine pouch) is located anterior to the uterus. The prevesical space (retropubic space) is anterior to the bladder. They form the peritoneal spaces of the pelvic cavity. *(1:6)*

74. **(G)** Transvaginal probes need to be pre-cleaned with soap and water as well as soaked in a disinfecting solution and covered by a disposable probe cover. The probes should be cleaned after each examination. *(1:4)*

75. **(D)** An invasive mole and a hydatidiform mole are excessive trophoblastic proliferation. Unlike the hydatidiform mole, chorioadenoma destruens is malignant and invades into the myometrium. *(3:734)*

76. **(E)** Paternally derived trisomy 13 presents with a large placenta sometimes termed a partial mole. Less commonly, a dizygotic pregnancy may occur. One fetus results from normal fertilization of one egg and a complete molar pregnancy results from the fertilization of the other egg. In those cases, it is possible for the hydatidiform mole to advance to choriocarcinoma. *(3:734)*

77. **(C)** The ovum enters the fallopian tube at the fimbriated ends. It courses to the ampulla where fertilization occurs 24–36 hours after ovulation. *(6:211, 212)*

78. **(B)** Methotrexate (MTX) is a folic acid antagonist used as a medical treatment for a unruptured ectopic pregnancy. The recommended candidates for medical treatment are; hemodynamically stable, hCG of less than 5,000 mIU/mL, no fetal cardiac activity and the ectopic mass size should be less than 4 cm. The is the current recommendation at the time of writing. Previously the recommended was a serum beta hCG of less than 10,000 mIU/mL(24:25)

79. **(E)** This patient most-likely had a ruptured ectopic pregnancy. Medical treatment is the first option if the patient is hemodynamically stable and with an unruptured pregnancy. However, this patient stated that she had a syncope episode followed by a salpingectomy in which case a ruptured ectopic pregnancy is most-likely. *(14:1102-1113)*

80. **(B)** Intrauterine fetal demise (IUFD) is defined as an absence of fetal heart tones after 20 weeks. A blighted ovum does not have an embryo (anembryonic pregnancy). Missed abortion is a demise embryo that has not aborted in the first trimester. A fetus can be in a resting mode without movement but demonstrate a fetal heart tone. *(1:14)*

81. **(E)** Dysgerminoma is a malignant tumor. *(14:570)*

82. **(B)** Dermoid cysts are more common in younger women and they have a variable sonographic appearance ranging from completely anechoic to hyperechoic. *(14:569, 570)*

83. **(A)** Normal adult ovarian size is 3 × 2 × 2 cm. *(17:104)*

84. **(B)** The first finding is a gestational sac, however ectopic pregnancies may also present with a pseudo-sac. A yolk sac is the earliest definitive sonographic sign of an intrauterine pregnancy. *(6:198)*

85. **(B)** The detection rate is 65%, but may vary among patients depending on the maternal habitus, fetal position, AFV, ultrasound scanner, and expertise of the sonographer and physician. *(6:325)*

86. **(D)** The detection rate is 85%, but may vary among patients depending on the maternal habitus, fetal position, AFV, ultrasound scanner, and expertise of the sonographer and physician. *(6:325)*

87. **(D)** Distal acoustic shadowing is associated with a solid mass. *(6:124)*

88. **(C)** Theca lutein cysts are present in 18–37% of hydatidiform moles. *(20:1153)*

89. **(A)** The crown rump length (CRL) is the most accurate because fetal growth is very uniform and is rarely affected by pathological disorders. The choices C and D are based on human memory of the maternal LMP, which assumes ovulation on day 14. *(3:138)*

90. **(A)** Fetal growth in the first trimester is very uniform, thus allowing for accurate dating if the total of three crown rump length (CRL) measurements are taking and then averaged. *(1:Table 9–6)*

91. **(B)** Fetal growth is starting to show variation and multiple parameters are used to calculate the EDC. Both of these factors allow for an increased range of error. *(1:Table 9–6)*

92. **(C)** Fetal growth is showing a moderate amount of variation, which allows for an increasing range of error. *(1:Table 9–6)*

93. **(D)** Fetal growth has a large amount of variation in the third trimester and obtaining the images for EFW can be challenging depending on fetal position and size. This allows for the largest range of error in the pregnancy. *(1:Table 9–6)*

94. **(B)** The hCG doubles in approximately 48 hours until 10 weeks or a minimum of 66 percent in 48 hours. *(6:195)*

95. **(A)** Twin pregnancy is associated with an elevated hCG. *(6:225)*

96. **(D)** The internal component of an endometrioma is typically blood from bleeding ectopic endometrial tissue during menstruation. Differential diagnosis may include a dermoid tumor; however, most women tend to be asymptomatic with dermoids. *(Table 9–4)*

97. **(C)** Nagele's rule is: (1) identify the LMP, (2) add 7 days, (3) subtract 3 months, and (4) add one year. *(1:397)*

98. **(D)** Krubenberg tumor is a metastatic adenocarcinoma of the ovary. The stomach is the primary site in most cases. The mass is usually bilateral. *(14:571–572)*

99. **(B)** Cystadenomas may have thin septations. Cystadenocarcinomas may contain thickened septations. *(14:566)*

100. **(A)** Sertoli–Leydig cell tumor is an androblastoma and Brenner's cell tumor is a transitional cell tumor. Chocolate cyst is another name for endometrioma. Stein-Leventhal syndrome is a subgroup of a more encompassing disease

called polycystic ovarian syndrome (PCOS). (*1:Table 9–9, 3, 4*)

101. **(C)** The etiology of hydatidiform mole is fertilization of an ovum without any active chromosomal material. (*7:357*)

102. **(D)** Blood flow direction and velocity is characteristics of color Doppler imaging. (*1:1–2*)

103. **(A)** The extra-embryonic peripheral cells of the blastocyst. The trophoblast forms these cells, which form the wall of the blastocyst. (*7:357*)

104. **(D)** At the time of ovulation, a dominant follicle grows to approximately 20 to 25 mm. (*15:404*)

105. **(A)** Leiomyomas are present in 20–30% of the female population, with a higher percentage in black women. (*14:538*)

106. **(A)** Acute or chronic pelvic inflammatory disease (PID) is most commonly caused by gonorrhea or chlamydia. If left untreated, the infection can progress to a tubo-ovarian abscess, where pus is surrounded by tubal and ovarian tissue. (*16:399*)

107. **(B)** Mucinous cystadenocarcinomas when ruptures are associated with pseudomyxoma peritonei. All the other choices are related to dermoid cyst. (*20:937–939*)

108. **(C)** Normal endometrial lining in postmenopausal women not on hormone replacement therapy should be less than 3 mm. Endometrial thickness of less than 3 mm is associated with low risk of endometrial disease. (*14:543*)

109. **(B)** Women on tamoxifen for treatment or prevention of breast cancer and women on estrogen therapy are known to have thickened endometrium. An endometrial thickness of 5 mm is taken as the cutoff normal range for women on hormone replacement therapy (HRT). (*2:841*)

110. **(C)** In the proliferative phase, the lining is thick, but the internal component is hypoechoic. This allows for the echogenic polyp to be seen. In the secretory phase, the entire endometrial lining is echogenic and will mask a polyp. (*1:10*)

111. **(D)** LMP refers to the first day of menses. (*1:11*)

112. **(A)** The differential diagnoses that may mimic hydatidiform moles are missed abortions, cystic degenerative leiomyomas, blighted ovum, and incomplete abortion. Endometriosis is endometrial tissue outside of the endometrial lining. (*20:1012*)

113. **(D)** 80%. (*7:424*)

114. **(A)** The cervix is the most inferior portion of the uterus and invaginates into the vagina. Moving superiorly, the next section is the isthmus beginning at the internal os. The body, or corpus, of the uterus is the largest section of the uterus. The most superior portion is the fundus. (*1:4*)

115. **(B)** The outer layer is the serosal, or peritoneal layer. The large muscular middle layer is the myometrium, and the inner layer is the endometrium. (*1:4–5*)

116–118. **(B) (D) (A)** In a sagittal plane, the ovaries can be identified as a hypoechoic structure containing small anechoic follicles that undergo cyclic changes. The landmarks for the ovaries include the anechoic internal iliac vessels posteriorly. The ureters when visualized are tubular anechoic structures. As they enter the pelvis, they course along the psoas muscles, between the ovaries and internal iliac vessels and enter the urinary bladder posteriorly. (*18:180, 283–285*)

119. **(C)** A nulliparous uterus is 7 × 5 × 4 cm. Multiparous increases the normal size by more than 1 cm per dimension. A post-menopausal uterus becomes atrophic and decreases in size. (*14:532*)

120. **(A)** The aqueduct of Sylvius (cerebral aqueduct) is a narrow channel that connects the 3rd ventricle to the 4th ventricle. (*20:1224*)

121. **(B)** Congenital abnormalities result from improper fusion of the mullerian (paramesonephric) ducts. (*14:534*)

122. **(A)** The proliferative phases are days 5–9 post-menstruation. (*1:8*)

123. **(C)** The periovulatory, or late proliferative, phase is days 10–14 post-menstruation. (*1:8*)

124. **(D)** The secretory phase is day 15–28 post-menstruation. The echogenicity is a result of edema of the functional zone of the endometrium. (*1:8*)

125. **(D)** Symptoms of endometriosis caused by adhesions include dysmenorrhea, low back pain, dyspareunia (painful sexual intercourse), irregular bleeding and infertility. (*2:868*)

126. **(A)** Endometriosis is defined as the presence of endometrial glands in stroma outside of the uterine cavity. The endometrial tissue commonly involves structures within the pelvis, ovaries and broad ligament. However, endometrial ectopic tissue can be found in the abdomen, thorax or brain. (*14:522; 21-517–528*)

127. **(D)** Dermoid tumors are most commonly located superior to the uterine fundus. (*7:436*)

128. **(A)** A fetus greater than the 90th percentile for estimated fetal weight is termed large for gestational age (LGA). A fetus greater than 4,000 g is macrosomic. (*3:544; 2:215*)

129. **(B)** LGA refers to a fetus measuring greater than the 90th percentile for gestational age. (*3:544; 2:215*)

130. **(D)** All of the above. Identification of a macrosomic fetus can alert the obstetrician to watch for complications of macrosomia during delivery. (*2:215*)

131. **(A)** Cystic Hygroma is associated with polyhydramnios (*Study Guide*)

132. **(E)** Other causes for an increased fundal height include incorrect dates, and molar pregnancy. *(2:215; 6:465)*

133. **(A)** Although the other features, such as oligohydramnios, do often coexist and interact with IUGR, the diagnosis of IUGR is a fetus < 10% for gestational age. *(2:206)*

134. **(B)** An increased HC/AC ratio is the result of redistribution of fetal blood away from the bowel and directed to the fetal head. *(3:522)*

135. **(D)** All of the above. IUGR may be found in chromosomal abnormalities, infection early in pregnancy, and placental insufficiency. *(2:207)*

136. **(D)** The abdominal circumference (AC) is the single most sensitive indicator for IUGR. *(20:1076)*

137. **(A)** Doppler ultrasound has shown that in fetus with asymmetric IUGR, vascular resistant increases in the umbilical artery and decreases in the middle cerebral artery. *(20:1081)*

138. **(C)** The diastolic notch is normal before 26 weeks and is related to trophoblastic invasion. *(2:685)*

139. **(E)** Hematometrocolpos is an accumulation of secretions and blood due to an obstruction at the level of the vagina. The vagina and endometrial cavity become distended with echogenic material. If scanned prior to puberty, the secretions appear anechoic. *(14:544)*

140. **(D)** Patients receiving ovulation induction or follicle-stimulating hormones for assisted reproduction are at risk for OHSS. *(2:866)*

141. **(B)** Endometrial carcinoma is the most common gynecologic malignancy in North America with 75–80% occurring in post-menopausal women. There is a strong association for patients on hormone replacement therapy. The endometrium has a heterogeneous echo texture with irregular or poorly defined borders. Cystic changes in the endometrium are also seen in patients with endometrial hyperplasia and polyps. Endometriosis is ectopic endometrial tissue outside the uterus. *(14:548)*

142. **(A)** The sonographic appearance of the iliopsoas muscles are hypoechoic, bilateral mass-like structures with a bright central echo. In a transverse plane, the paired muscles are located on the anterolateral aspect of the urinary bladder. *(18:274)*

143. **(C)** Pseudo-gestational sac is seen in 20% of ectopic pregnancy. It does not have an embryo or a yolk sac. It does not grow with the same incline as a real gestational sac. *(20:1006)*

144. **(C)** Endometrial polyps can present either as a focal homogeneously echogenic or complex lesion within the endometrial cavity. They may contain one or more small cysts. *(17:293)*

145. **(D)** Given the clinical history, an endometrioma is the most likely diagnosis. The characteristic appearance is an adnexal cyst filled with homogeneously low-level echoes. This has been referred to as the "ground glass" appearance. Endometriomas are also referred to as chocolate cysts. They may also present as cysts with fine septations or similar to a hemorrhagic cyst. The may contain fluid-fluid levels. *(17:313)*

146. **(B)** Fibroids (myomas, leiomyomas) are common occurring benign tumors of the uterus. This subserosal myoma can be seen projecting from the serosal surface of the uterus. *(17:284)*

147. **(A)** Hemorrhagic cysts have a variable sonographic appearance dependent on the amount of hemorrhage and the time of the hemorrhage relative to the examination. Acute hemorrhagic cysts are generally hyperechoic and may mimic a solid mass. Diffuse low-level internal echoes are more commonly see in endometriosis. The more complex pattern of the mass represents clot hemolysis. Serous cystadenocarcinoma most frequently occurs in perimenopausal and postmenopausal women. *(14:557; 566)*

148. **(D)** Polycystic ovaries present with a more echogenic center with small anechoic immature follicles lining the periphery. *(16:289)*

149. **(A)** Patients with polycystic ovarian syndrome (Stein–Leventhal syndrome) usually present with amenorrhea, infertility, hirsutism and with multiple small immature follicles of the ovaries. Ovarian agenesis is an imperfect development or absent of the ovaries. *(16:289)*

150. **(A)** The typical sonographic appearance is that of a tubular or ovoid cystic structure. Visible folds, which appear echogenic, may be seen. *(14:560, 572, 573)*

151. **(B)** Adenomyosis results when endometrial glands invade the myometrium and may be diffuse or localized. These glands respond to hormone stimulation. There are various sonographic characteristics. The sonographic characteristics in this image include small cysts within the myometrium and enlargement of the posterior myometrium. Note the eccentrically situated endometrial cavity. *(17:287–289)*

152. **(A)** Tamoxifen has an estrogenic effect on the uterus. Patients treated with tamoxifen are at an increased risk for endometrial hyperplasia, endometrial carcinoma, and endometrial polyps. *(14:549)*

153. **(B)** Nabothian cysts, also referred to as inclusion cysts, are commonly seen in the cervix. They can be multiple and vary in size and may contain internal echoes due to hemorrhage or infection. *(14:551)*

154. **(D)** Tubo-ovarian abscess (TOA) usually results from chronic pelvic inflammatory disease. Patients usually have a history of a sexually transmitted disease. It is a progressive process and as the infection worsens,

peri-ovarian adhesions may form resulting in fusion of inflamed dilated tubes and ovaries (tubo-ovarian complex). With progression of the disease, a TOA may form and appear as a complex multiloculated masses with septations, irregular borders, internal echoes, and posterior acoustic enhancement. *(14:572, 573)*

155. **(D)** The urinary bladder should be distended to the point where it covers the entire fundus of the uterus. The distended bladder provides an acoustic window to view pelvic organs. It also serves as a reference standard for evaluating cystic structures. *(14:529)*

156. **(D)** Reverberation artifact occurs when the ultrasound beam bounces between two or more interfaces in a repetitious fashion. This is commonly seen on the anterior aspect of the urinary bladder due to reverberation between the fascial planes of the abdominal wall and the transducer and appears as echoes within the urinary bladder. *(16:631, 632)*

157. **(B)** The central nervous center that regulates fetal tone functions first at 7.5–8.5 weeks. *(2:663)*

158. **(A)** The central nervous center that regulates body movements starts functioning at 9 weeks. *(2:663)*

159. **(C)** The central nervous center that regulates fetal breathing starts at 21 weeks. *(2:663)*

160. **(D)** The central nervous center for fetal heart rate reactivity functions by the end of the second trimester or beginning of the third trimester. *(2:663)*

161. **(A)** Meigs' syndrome is define as a triad of a benign ovarian fibroma, ascites, and pleural effusion with the effusion is most frequently on the right. *(2:882)*

162. **(D)** Biophysical profile (PPP) is a test used to evaluate fetal well-being using a scoring system. This involves a combination of ultrasound and non-stress test with five variables. Each of these five variables is given a score of 0 or 2, depending if the specific criteria are met. *(14:1513)*

163. **(B)** Fetal breathing must last at least 30 seconds in a 30-minute time period in order to score a 2 in the biophysical profile. *(2:663)*

164. **(A)** In response to hypoxia, the fetus reroutes blood to the brain in a brain-sparing effort. The middle cerebral artery is normally of higher resistance, but it will decrease to compensate for the increased blood flow and brain-sparing effort. *(2:690, 691)*

165. **(D)** Cervical phase of an impending abortion. The uterus has an hourglass appearance because the cervix is dilated to the size of the fundus. Heavy vaginal bleeding and lower abdominal cramping are clinical sign and symptoms of an abortion in progress. The pain is due to uterine contraction. *(14:1092)*

166. **(B)** The amniotic fluid is produced by the fetal kidneys, umbilical cord, fetal skin, and lungs. The removal of the fluid is by the gastrointestinal tract, lungs, and umbilical cord. The maximum amniotic fluid volume peaks at approximately 33 weeks and then begins to decline. The fetus starts swallowing the amniotic fluid at 12 weeks of gestation. *(20:1169)*

167. **(D)** Pelvic inflammatory disease (PID) is an ascending infection. The most common causes of PID are chlamydia and gonorrhea. Other bacterial causes are *Actinomyces israelii*, mycoplasma, and tuberculosis. The disease causes inflammation of the pelvic organs as it ascends, causing occlusion of the fallopian tubes and thereby resulting in infertility. Genital herpes is a viral sexually transmitted disease that causes blisters on the genitals. The virus travels to the nerve cells and remains in the body for life. *(20:947)*

168. **(A)** The adnexa is any accessory part, organ, structures, or mass that is located lateral to the uterus. The fallopian tubes, ovaries, broad ligaments, ovarian cyst, and ovarian artery are all adnexal. The urinary bladder, uterus, and vagina are midline structures and are not adnexal structures. *(20:873)*

169. **(A)** The single deepest pocket (SDP) is a vertical dimension of the largest pocket of amniotic fluid. Measurements of less then 2 cm are suggestive of oligohydramnios. *(2:642)*

170. **(D)** All four quadrants are added and compared to an expected amniotic fluid volume for that fetus' gestational age. The normal range extends from 2.5% to 97.5%. *(8:1168)*

171. **(C)** Nonspecific signs of fetal death are double contour of the fetal head caused by scalp edema, absence of the falx cerebri because of liquefaction of the brain, echoes in the amniotic fluid because of fragmentation of the fetal skin, and a decrease in biparietal diameter measurements because of collapse of the cranial sutures after death. No fetal heart movement is a specific sign of fetal death. *(7:429)*

172. **(A)** Scalp edema can be seen 2–3 days, or 48–72 hours, after fetal death. *(7:429)*

173. **(C)** The decidua of early intrauterine pregnancy is divided into decidua basalis, decidua parietalis (vera), and decidua capsularis. This marked hypertrophic change in the endometrium occurs no matter where the pregnancy is located. The uterine mucosa responds by a decidual reaction caused by hormonal stimuli. However, when an ectopic pregnancy occurs, the uterine decidua responds by a cast-off called a decidual cast. This should not be confused with the normal decidua in an early pregnancy. *(7:431)*

174. **(B)** Nabothian cyst is located in the cervix. Gartner's duct cysts and Bartholin cysts are vaginal masses. Hematocolpos is also a vaginal mass in which the vagina is filled with menstrual blood. *(14:550)*

175. **(E)** All of the above. The functions of the yolk sac are: nutrition transfer of nutrients to the embryo; hemopoiesis-blood cell development; and development of sex cells that later become spermatogonia or oogonia. *(7:431)*

176. **(B)** The yolk sac reduces in size as pregnancy advances. However, it may persist throughout pregnancy and continue to persist into adulthood. In about 2% of adults, the proximal intra-abdominal part of the yolk sac is presented as a diverticulum of the ilium, called Meckel's diverticulum. *(7:431)*

177. **(C)** The yolk sac is located adjacent to the embryonic plate in early pregnancy and is located within the chorionic cavity. *(2:113)*

178. **(B)** The yolk sac may be visible as early as 5 weeks on transvaginal ultrasound, and 6 weeks on transabdominal ultrasound. *(20:788)*

179. **(C)** Zygote. *(7:433)*

180. **(B)** Cleavage. *(7:433)*

181. **(A)** Morula. *(7:433)*

182. **(D)** Blastocyst. *(7:433)*

183. **(D)** The most common abnormal conditions associated with oligohydramnios are (1) fetal demise, (2) renal agenesis, (3) intrauterine growth restriction, (4) premature rupture of membranes, (5) post-date pregnancy, and (6) posterior urethral valve syndrome. The mnemonic DRIPPP serves as a key for memorizing the six conditions most commonly associated with oligohydramnios. Urethral stenosis is associated with polyhydramnios. *(20:1174)*

184. **(B)** As the pregnancy advances, the placenta becomes less resistive. This allows for more blood and oxygen to reach the growing fetus. *(2:687)*

185. **(A)** An increasing S/D ratio of the umbilical cord is a sign of vascular resistance within the placenta, which ultimately leads to a decrease in oxygen to the fetus. *(2:268)*

186. **(D)** Vasa previa is condition in which the umbilical cord is the presenting part. This condition may also be associated with succenturiate placenta or a velamentous cord insertion. The rare condition has an increase risk of hemorrhage and cord compression. *(20:1093)*

187. **(A)** The incidence of placenta previa at term is 0.5–1%, with 90% of previa bleeding before 38 weeks. Clinically the patient may present with painless vaginal bleeding. *(9:403;20;1148)*

188. **(B)** Pseudogestational sac is a decidual cast (fluid) located in the uterine cavity that may mimic the sonographic appearance of an intrauterine pregnancy and is seen in approximately 20% of ectopic pregnancies. A pseudogestational sac does not contain an embryo or yolk sac and does not have an incline in growth size. *(20:999)*

189. **(A)** The yolk sac is located in the chorionic cavity between the amnion and chorionic sac. It measures 5 mm to 6 mm. The yolk sac shrinks as pregnancy advances. It should not be measured in the CRL. *(7:427)*

190. **(A)** The umbilical cord normally consists of two arteries and one vein. *(1:17)*

191. **(E)** Open tube defect, anencephaly, and cephalocele are part of the neural tube defect spectrum. *(1:19)*

192. **(B)** Herniation of meninges alone is termed a meningocele. *(1:19)*

193. **(A)** To calculate the gestational age using the rule of thumb, first convert 28 mm to centimeters by moving the decimal point one space to the left; 28 mm is now 2.8 cm. Then add 6.5 to the CRL to estimate the gestational age, which in this case is 9.3 weeks *(7:Table 8–4)*

194. **(D)** The "lemon" refers to the narrowing of the parietal bones giving the appearance of a lemon-shaped cranium in the axial view. *(1:19)*

195. **(C)** The "banana" refers to the displacement of the cerebellum inferiorly into the upper cervical canal. On transverse view, the cerebellum is small and resembles a banana. *(1:19)*

196. **(D)** 95% of the time. *(1:19)*

197. **(E)** The lemon sign is found in 1–2% of normal fetuses. *(2:286)*

198. **(D)** There is no contraindication to scanning a placenta previa transvaginally, and it provides the most accurate diagnosis. Transabdominal scanning may give a false-positive caused by a full maternal bladder compressing the internal os or an inadequate view of the internal os. *(2:591)*

199. **(B)** If the placenta is greater than 2 cm from the internal os, a vaginal delivery is considered safe. *(2:591)*

200. **(B)** The normally positioned heart should be rotated approximately 45° with the apex pointed to the left. *(2:384)*

201. **(C)** The horizontal position of the fetal heart is largely due to a large liver size. *(7:432)*

202. **(B)** Nonimmune hydrops is defined by the absence of detectible circulating antibiotic against red blood cells (RBCs) in the mother. Before the discovery of RhoGAM (anti-D immunoglobulin, most cases of hydrops were immune, which causes a hemolytic disorder known as erythroblastosis fetalis. *(14:1459)*

203. **(C)** 75% of cephaloceles are occipital. *(1:19)*

204. **(A)** In the absence of a spinal defect, if the lateral ventricles measure greater than 10 mm in the atrium of the occipital horn, it is commonly associated with an obstruction of the ventricular system. *(14:1242)*

205. **(C)** RhoGAM Rh (D) immune globulin is made from human plasma. The drug is an injection given intramuscularly to prevent hemolytic disease of the newborn. It is given at 28 weeks of pregnancy and another dose within 72 hours after childbirth if the child has Rh-positive blood. RhoGAM is not given to Rh-positive mothers with bleeding episodes. *(20:1087)*

206. **(E)** Congenital hydrocephaly is an X-linked abnormality, with the expression in males and the females being carriers. It is able to be detected through DNA testing. *(1:19)*

207. **(D)** TORCH represents a group of infections (toxoplasmosis, others, rubella, cytomegalovirus, and herpes simplex (HSV), which can cross the placenta barrier and cause microcephaly, ventriculomegaly, and calcifications. *(14:1262)*

208. **(A)** Cervical ectopic pregnancy is close to the vagina with the external os of the cervix positioned in the vagina; with rupture, the bleeding is external. When ruptured, all of the others results in hemoperitoneum. *(21:441)*

209. **(A)** Transvaginal sonogram demonstrates a gestational sac implanted in the lower uterine segment in the scar of a previous caesarian section. Note the close proximity of the ectopic sac to the posterior urinary bladder wall. There is prominent vascularity at the implantation site, and the multiple small cystic structures are multiple nabothian cyst. *(14:1109)*

210. **(D)** The arrow points to the vitelline duct, also known as omphalomesenteric duct or yolk stalk. *(14:1080)*

211. **(E)** The normal placement of an intrauterine device (IUD) is in the uterine cavity. Ultrasound can demonstrate malposition of an IUD. This IUD is seen in the cervix with double parallel echogenic lines (entrance–exit reflections). *(14:550)*

212. **(D)** The cisterna magna is enlarged if the measurement is greater than 11 mm. The normal cisterna magna measures 3–11 mm, with an average size 5–6 mm. *(20:1027)*

213. **(A)** A true Dandy–Walker malformation is associated with agenesis of the cerebellar vermis with communication to the fourth ventricle. A Dandy–Walker malformation variant is described as having some degree of cerebellar vermis agenesis, but not complete agenesis. An arachnoid cyst will push the cerebellum superiorly without splaying the cerebellum. *(2:292)*

214. **(C)** An arachnoid cyst will not cause splaying of the cerebellum and the cerebellar vermis will be intact. *(2:292)*

215. **(A)** Dandy–Walker malformation is associated with other midline defects including agenesis of the corpus callosum and cephaloceles, as well as holoprosencephaly, clefting, and cardiac defects. Dandy–Walker malformation has a 50–70% risk of associated abnormalities. *(2:292)*

216. **(B)** Clomiphene citrate (Clomid) is one of the first-line drugs used for ovulation induction. Folic acid is a B vitamin helpful in preventing neural tube defects. Methotrexate is a drug used in treating rheumatoid arthritis and ectopic pregnancy. *(20:963)*

217. **(E)** Subnormal intelligence is reported in 40–70% of cases. Morbidity rates are 24% but are improving with increased anesthesia and surgical techniques. *(2:295)*

218. **(D)** The most common cause of hypotelorism is holoprosencephaly. Hypotelorism is found in many different syndromes and chromosomal abnormalities and is strongly associated with abnormalities of the brain. *(2:309; 4:223)*

219. **(B)** Cyclopia—absent nose with protrusion of tissue at level of eye sockets; hypotelorism—close set orbits; cebocephaly—single nostril nose; and cleft lip/palate are all abnormal facial findings strongly associated with holoprosencephaly. *(2:309–311)*

220. **(C)** Thirty to fifty percent of fetuses with holoprosencephaly have chromosomal abnormalities, the most common being trisomy 13. *(4:119)*

221. **(A)** The most common cause of hypertelorism is a defect that prevents the migration of the eyes to their normal position. An anterior cephalocele is the most common blockage of that migration. *(2:311)*

222. **(E)** Teratomas can occur in many different locations. The most common region is sacrococcygeal accounting for 50% of fetal teratomas. The second most common location is orofacial (including intracranial) and cervical, accounting for 5% of fetal teratomas. *(2:317)*

223. **(B)** Maternal Graves' disease and Hashimoto thyroiditis produce antibodies that cross the placenta and may affect fetal thyroid production. *(2:318)*

224. **(C)** Macroglossia is present in 97.5% of Beckwith–Wiedemann syndrome. *(2:320)*

225. **(B)** The arrow points to the cerebellum. *(20:585)*

226. **(D)** Other findings of Beckwith–Wiedemann syndrome include omphalocele, organomegaly, hemi-hypertrophy, and hypoglycemia. Macroglossia is present in 97% of Beckwith-Wiedemann syndrome. *(1:24)*

227. **(B)** Of the isolated cleft lip and palate cases, 40% are unilateral cleft lip and palate, 29% are unilateral cleft lip, 27% are bilateral cleft lip and palate, and 5% are bilateral cleft lip. *(2:324)*

228. **(B)** The arrow is pointing to the choroid plexus. *(20:999)*

229. **(C)** Medial cleft lip is associated with a spectrum of midline defects, the most common being holoprosencephaly. *(2:314)*

230. **(D)** Pierre Robin syndrome, trisomy 18, and campomelic dysplasia are all associated with micrognathia and poly-hydramnios. Micrognathia commonly causes difficulty swallowing resulting in polyhydramnios. (2:56, 327, 352)

231. **(E)** Sonograms A and B demonstrate disorganized echoes in the lower uterine segment, suggestive of incomplete abortion (retained products). No intrauterine pregnancy or free-fluid is seen. The patient's complaint of lower abdominal cramping is a common clinical symptom in spontaneous abortion due to uterine contractions. The serum β-hCG has decreased greater than half in 48 hours, which is also suggestive of abortion. (14:577; 21:403)

232. **(F)** Absence of the fetal nasal bone is associated with trisomy 21 (Down's syndrome). The sonographer should look for other associated physical features: small ears, protruding tongue, spinal and heart defects, and increased nuchal fold. (2:327; 14:1135; 20:1116)

233. **(G)** Focal myometrial contraction is physiologic and should disappear within 20–30 minutes. (16:450)

234. **(C)** Development of the corpus callosum occurs between 12 and 18 weeks; therefore, visualization is not possible less than 18 weeks. (2:290)

235. **(D)** The "teardrop" appearance (enlargement of the atria and occipital horns and lateral displacement of the anterior horns) is present 90% of the time. (2:290; 6:255)

236. **(C)** Hydranencephaly exists when the cerebral hemispheres are replaced by fluid. The brain stem is usually spared. Causes are thought to be infection or obstruction of the internal carotid artery. (2:297)

237. **(D)** Microcephaly has been described as an HC between –2 and –3 standard deviations (SD) of the mean. (2:298)

238. **(D)** A vein of Galen aneurysm is a type of arteriovenous (AV) malformation. Agenesis of the corpus callosum, third ventricular dilation, and an arachnoid cyst are cystic midline lesions, but they will not have the high, turbulent blood flow of an AV malformation. (2:301)

239. **(B)** Isolated choroid plexus cyst has a small risk for trisomy 18. If other abnormalities are identified along with the choroid plexus cyst, the risk for trisomy 18 increases. (2:301)

240. **(E)** Cigarette smoking is known to affect the ciliary action in the nasopharynx, respiratory tract, and the fallopian tubes. Bilateral tubal ligation also is a risk factor. *Chlamydia trachomatis* and PID are among the most common risk factors. Herpes genitalis is a viral STD infection that causes painful lesions on the skin and hides within the nerve cells. Herpes virus is not known to cause PID or a risk factor for ectopic pregnancy. (21:434)

241. **(C)** The image should also show the cavum septi pellucidi, cerebellum and cisterna magna. The measurements should be taken from the outer edge of the cranium to the outer edge of the skin. The skin fold should be less than 5 mm. (6:245)

242. **(D)** The ovaries are normally located in the ovarian fossa, medial to the external iliac vessels, and anterior to the internal iliac vessels and ureter. (20:865)

243. **(A)** Inclusion cyst is when fluid produced by the ovaries is not absorbed and becomes trapped between the adhesions. This occurs more frequently in patients with a history of previous surgery or pelvic inflammatory disease. (14:507)

244. **(A)** A cephalic index of more than 85 describes an increased BPD when compared to a shorter OFD. The head has a rounded appearance on ultrasound. (6:244)

245. **(B)** Dolichocephaly is a long, narrow head with a small biparietal diameter when compared with a longer OFD. (6:381)

246. **(B)** Sterile procedure requires a sterile field. A sterile gel is required. (7:322–324)

247. **(D)** Oil-based lubricants such as petroleum jell, cold creams, baby oil, or mineral oils should be avoided because they cause deterioration of the latex, resulting in breakage. (7:323)

248. **(D)** Dolichocephaly is associated with breech fetuses and oligohydramnios. (2:991)

249. **(F)** Brachycephaly with a flat occiput is a feature of trisomy 21. Brachycephaly may also be present with a spina bifida due to ventricular enlargement. Most commonly, brachycephaly is a normal variant. (4:1009)

250. **(C)** The head is larger than the abdomen at 12–24 weeks. (7:434)

251. **(B)** At 32–36 weeks, the head and body are about the same size. (7:434)

252. **(A)** After 36 weeks, the abdomen is larger than the head. (7:434)

253. **(B)** The scanning plane is too high. When performing a biparietal diameter (BPD) measurement, the fetal head should be ovoid and the measurement obtained at the level of the thalami and cavum septum pellucidum. (7:440)

254. **(D)** The fluid within a cystic hygroma is lymphatic fluid from an obstructed lymph system. (6:263)

255. **(A)** A cystic hygroma occurs when the jugular lymph sacs fail to communicate with the venous system. The obstructed lymphatic fluid fills the sacs and forms the cystic hygroma. (6:263)

256. **(E)** The uterus is frequently larger for dates. (21:998)

257. **(C)** The cervical region. (7:426)

258. **(E)** C and D. Cystic hygromas are associated with elevated MSAFP and Turner's syndrome. (7:365)

259. **(F)** The sonographic appearance of hydatidiform mole are multiple, snowstorm, Swiss cheese, honeycomb, vesicular sonographic texture. (14:1577)

260–269. See Fig. 7–103.

270–272. See Fig. 7–104.

273–281. See Fig. 7–105.

282. **(C)** The foramen ovale allows for oxygenated blood to pass from the right atrium to the left atrium. (6:323)

283. **(B)** The ductus arteriosus allows for approximately 70% of the blood to bypass the nonfunctioning lungs. (6:323)

284. **(C)** It is a destructive process that obliterates the cerebral cortex. The brainstem is usually spared. Other causes include infection and intrauterine strangulation. (3:385)

285. **(E)** Alobar holoprosencephaly and severe hydrocephaly may sonographically present similar to hydranencephaly. Lobar holoprosencephaly sonographically presents with an interhemispheric fissure anterior and posterior, thus being excluded in the differential. (2:299)

286. **(D)** Hemivertebrae is easiest to view in the sagittal plane of view because the other vertebrae may be used as a reference of normal. It is visible in the other planes of view also, but requires more meticulous scanning. (3:456)

287. **(D)** Arnold–Chiari malformation is most commonly associated with myelomeningocele and hydrocephaly. (2:73)

288. **(C)** Microcephaly is a result of a large portion of the brain tissue being herniated out of the cranium. (1:19)

289. **(A)** Semilobar holoprosencephaly is a single anterior ventricle with partial separation of the posterior cerebellar hemispheres. (1:20)

290. **(A)** The most likely diagnosis would be alobar holoprosencephaly. Differential diagnosis would include hydranencephaly and hydrocephaly. Hydranencephaly would not show any cerebral cortex and only brainstem would be spared. Hydrocephaly would show a bi-lobed thalamus with a dilated third ventricle. (1:20)

291. **(C)** Hydranencephaly will present with no visible cerebral cortex. The differential includes alobar holoprosencephaly (fused thalamus) and severe hydrocephaly (bilobed thalamus with dilated third ventricle). (1:20)

292. **(B)** It may be possible to diagnose anencephaly as early as 12 weeks, but it should be definitely diagnosed by 14 weeks. (1:19)

293. **(D)** Acrania is theorized to be the first trimester finding of anencephaly. With prolonged exposure to the amniotic fluid, the abnormal brain tissue is eroded, and the second trimester finding of anencephaly is appreciated. (3:379, 380)

294. **(4)** The last number stands for the number of living children. (1:3)

295. **(2)** The number of preterm births is the second number after parity. (1:3)

296. **(7)** G refers to the gravida or number of pregnancies. (1:3)

297. **(1)** The third number after parity represents the number of abortions (spontaneous and elective). (1:3)

298. **(3)** The first number after parity represents the number of full term pregnancies. (1:3)

299. **(A)** The number of pregnancies is listed after gravida (G). The first number after parity (P) is the number of full term pregnancies (3), the second number is the number of preterm pregnancies (one set of twins, single pregnancy, and one preterm fetal death >20 weeks = 2), the third number is the number of abortions (1), and the final number is the number of living children (5). (1:3)

300. **(A)** Benign penetration and growth of endometrial glands and stroma into the myometrium. (21:898)

301. **(A)** AFP is produced by the fetus. An abnormal concentration occurs whenever there is an abnormal opening in the fetus allowing an increased amount of the protein in the amniotic fluid. (2:25)

302. **(B)** Using the rule of thumb, subtract 6.5 from 8, which equals 1.5 cm. (7:Table 8–4)

303. **(C)** After 12 weeks, the fetus has a curvilinear shape making it technically more difficult to obtain accurate linear measurement. (21:995)

304. **(C)** Multiple parameters help to increase the accuracy of estimated fetal weight. (3:146)

305. **(C)** Only the shaft of the femur should be measured in femur length, excluding the femoral neck and other epiphyseal calcification centers. (7:442)

306. **(C)** Of the cases with polyhydramnios, 60% are idiopathic, 20% are structural, and 20% are maternal insulin dependent diabetes mellitus. (1:16)

307. **(F)** Polyhydramnios has many causes that may include increased urine production or decreased fetal swallowing. (1:29; 2:348, 651)

308. **(C)** Amnion begins to fuse with the chorion at 12 weeks and is routinely complete by 14–16 weeks. (2:124)

309. **(B)** Hematopoiesis, or red blood cell production, is done by the fetus and by the yolk sac in early pregnancy. The placenta is responsible for the exchange of nutrients, oxygen, and waste. The placenta also acts as a barrier although some medication can cross through the placenta. (1:16)

310. **(E)** Maternal hypertension is seen in approximately 50% of cases of severe abruption. Other causes are cocaine abuse, trauma, fibroids, short cord, and placenta previa. Focal myometrial contraction is physiologic and temporary and is least likely to cause abruption. *(21:1152)*

311. **(B)** Placental abruption is defined as premature separation of the placenta after 20 weeks of gestation. If the placenta premature separate before 20 weeks, it is called spontaneous abortion. *(2:612 :20;1152)*

312. **(D)** The hypoechoic region behind the placenta should measure 1–2 cm in thickness. Any increase in thickness of this area should alert the sonographer to a possible hematoma. *(2:611)*

313. **(C)** Implantation sites at risk for placenta accreta are uterine scars, submucosal fibroids, lower uterine segment, rudimentary horn, and uterine cornua. *(2:613, 614)*

314. **(A)** Placenta accreta may be divided into (1) placenta accreta—placental attachment to the myometrium without invasion, (2) placenta increta—invasion of placenta into the myometrium and (3) placenta percreta—invasion of placenta through the uterus and into other organs. *(1:17)*

315. **(D)** Chorioangioma is a vascular mass arising from chorionic tissue and is similar to a hemangioma. *(2:612)*

316. **(A)** Wharton's jelly is a mucoid connective tissue that surrounds the umbilical vein and artery. *(6:440)*

317. **(A)** A true cord cyst is attributable to allantoic duct remnants and is thought to be more common in the first trimester. *(2:621; 3:212)*

318. **(D)** A velamentous cord insertion is associated with IUGR, particularly in monochorionic twins. *(2:620)*

319. **(C)** An eccentric cord insertion is considered a normal variant and is of no clinical significance. *(3:206; 2:620)*

320. **(B)** Atrial and ventricular septal defects are the most common defects accounting for 26% of the cardiac abnormalities. *(1:21)*

321. **(A)** Generally, the left side of the heart perfuses the fetal cranium. *(7:449)*

322. **(B)** Generally, the right side of the heart perfuses the systemic circulation of the fetus. *(7:449)*

323. **(B)** The ratio of the heart circumference to the thoracic circumference should be 30–50%. *(2:384)*

324. **(E)** This condition is called situs inversus (partial or total), dextrocardia and heterotaxy syndrome. Along with dextrocardia, there may be significant intracardiac anomalies, anomalies of the great vessels, an interrupted inferior vena cava, an anomalous venous return system, asplenia or polysplenia, and possible heterotaxy of the abdominal organs depending on whether it is complete or partial. *(4:385)*

325. **(C)** 50% of trisomy 21 cases have a cardiac defect, with the majority being atrioventricular canal defects. *(2:45)*

326. **(C)** This view allows for visualization of the right ventricular outflow tract, the left ventricular outflow tract and the crossing of the outflow tracts. *(2:385)*

327. **(E)** Other structures to evaluate include atrial sizes, foramen ovale, coronary vessels, and thickness of the ventricular walls, cardiac orientation, and size. *(2:385)*

328. **(B)** The banana sign is an abnormal flattening of the cerebellum giving it a banana shape. The normal cerebellum should have a dumbbell shape. The banana and lemon signs are both associated with spina bifida. *(20:1072)*

329. **(C)** The treatment for ectopic pregnancy depends on whether the ectopic pregnancy is ruptured or unruptured and if the patient is hemodynamically stable. This patient stated she had a ruptured ectopic pregnancy and fainted. Fainting is not a good sign with an ectopic pregnancy; this indicates a temporary loss of consciousness possibly secondary to blood loss from ruptured ectopic pregnancy. A salpingectomy via laparotomy is most likely this patient's previous surgery. Methotrexate is a drug given for unruptured ectopic pregnancies that are hemodynamically stable. *(21:452)*

330. **(A)** Coarctation of the aorta is a narrowing of the aorta, usually near the ductus arteriosus. It may be very difficult to image depending on the degree of stenosis. Often diagnosis relies on the ventricular discrepancy indicating that a stenosis is present. *(4:366)*

331. **(A)** Eighty percent of congenital diaphragmatic hernia is left sided. *(14:1304)*

332. **(E)** Whenever the heart is deviated with the correct apex orientation, the sonographer should consider a thoracic mass. *(2:429, 433, 440; 6:290)*

333. **(A)** It is important to identify the location of the fetal liver. If the liver is intrathoracic, the prognosis for survival is 43%. If the liver is intra-abdominal, the prognosis is 80% survival. *(1:22)*

334. **(D)** Although chromosomal abnormalities and associated anomalies are prevalent in congenital diaphragmatic hernia, the significant factor in mortality is pulmonary hypoplasia. *(1:22)*

335. **(D)** If the liver is intrathoracic, the survival rate is 43%, if the liver is intra-abdominal, the survival rate is 80%. *(1:22)*

336. **(C)** CCAM accounts for 75–80% of congenital lung malformations with over 95% of those being unilateral. *(2:439)*

337. (C) Macrocystic is defined as multiple large cysts measuring 2–10 cm. *(1:22)*

338. (B) Type II cysts are less than 2 cm, but still visible. *(1:22)*

339. (A) Sonographically, these appear as a solid, homogenous, echogenic lung mass. *(1:22)*

340. (D) Dysgerminoma is the most common type of malignant germ cell tumor and is associated with elevation of alpha-fetoprotein (AFP) and human chorionic gonadotropin (hCG). *(21:931)*

341. (B) The most common appearance detected prenatally is a well-circumscribed echogenic mass in the left lower lung base. *(2:441)*

342. (D) Methotrexate is a folic acid antagonist. It inhibits DNA synthesis and kills the rapidly dividing trophoblastic cells. The drug is a medical treatment for ectopic pregnancy and has a protocol for safe and effective use. The patient must be clinically stable, the ectopic should not be ruptured, the serum β-hCG should be less than 5,000 mIU/mL, and the ectopic sac should be less than 3.5 cm. *(14:1112; 21:455)*

343. (D) There are five types of TE fistulas. They make up 90% of the cases of esophageal atresia. *(2:460)*

344. (C) Regardless of the presence of a TE fistula, 80% of fetuses derive polyhydramnios by the third trimester. *(2:457)*

345. (B) Esophageal atresia is a very strong marker for trisomy 18. *(2:4547)*

346. (B) Amniotic fluid fills the stomach and duodenum proximal to the site of obstruction. The ultrasound appearance resembles a "double bubble." *(2:466)*

347. (D) Thirty-three percent will have spinal defects, 36% will have cardiac defects. *(2:466)*

348. (A) Thirty percent of fetuses with duodenal atresia have trisomy 21. *(2:466)*

349. (C) The bowel begins to herniate at 7 weeks and becomes most visible at 9–10 weeks on ultrasound. The bowel then returns to the abdomen by the end of the twelfth week. *(22:248)*

350. (B) Pseudo-gestational sac is seen in approximately 20% of ectopic pregnancies. It is anechoic and is the result of sloughing decidua. This is not a true gestational sac; therefore, it does not contain an embryo or yolk sac. It also does not have the normal incline of growth of 1 mm/day like a true gestational sac. *(14:1105; 20:1005)*

351. (C) The sign/symptoms of ectopic pregnancy vary depending on whether the pregnancy is ruptured or unruptured. A symptom of unruptured ectopic pregnancy is unilateral pain that increases in its intensity with time. After rupture, the symptoms change due to

hemoperitoneum, which is associated with generalized abdominal pain, rebound tenderness, fainting, tachycardia, hypotension, and right shoulder pain due to blood that irritates the diaphragmatic nerves. *(4:474)*

352. (C) Gastroschisis is rarely associated with chromosomal or non-gastrointestinal disorders and has an excellent survival rate. *(2:492)*

353. (D) When the bowel perforates, meconium enters the peritoneal space. A membrane forms that seals off the intestine at the site of the perforation. The meconium that entered the peritoneum may cause calcium deposits. Other findings are polyhydramnios, ascites with echogenic debris, and bowel dilation. *(2:470, 471)*

354. (E) All of the above. They may all cause a complication in gastroschisis and should be monitored with ultrasound throughout the pregnancy. *(2:497)*

355. (A) Although left-sided gastroschisis have been reported, it is typically to the right of the umbilical cord. *(4:473, 474)*

356. (C) The physiological hernia is the outpouching of the umbilical cord due to small and large bowel as they rotate around the superior mesenteric artery (SMA). It occurs at the beginning of the seventh week and is a normal migration of the midgut into the umbilical cord. This migration occurs because there is not enough room in the abdomen for the rapidly growing midgut. The midgut returns to the abdomen at about the tenth week. The fetal liver does not migrate in the umbilical cord. *(22:248)*

357. (D) This sonogram demonstrates an early intrauterine pregnancy with a small embryo in a retroverted uterus. Although this patient presented with clinical symptoms of an ectopic, her pregnancy is *in situ* confirmed by this sonogram. *(14:1102)*

358. (B) Small omphaloceles may be mistaken for a cord hematoma. If the defect at the base of the cord insertion is more than 7 mm, it is most likely an omphalocele. *(4:484)*

359. (C) Omphaloceles are not associated with teratogens, such as maternal smoking. *(4:484)*

360. (B) Ectopia cordis results from underdevelopment or agenesis of the fetal sternum. It is rarely isolated and is most commonly part of the pentalogy of Cantrell. *(4:467)*

361. (D) Pentalogy of Cantrell involves defects of the lower sternum, diaphragm, diaphragmatic pericardium, abdominal wall, and intracardiac defects. It is associated with trisomy 13 and trisomy 18. *(2:501; 4:493)*

362. (F) Beckwith–Wiedemann syndrome is due to a dysfunction of the placenta excreting increased levels of growth hormone. This causes organomegaly, macroglossia, omphalocele, hemi hypertrophy, and cardiac abnormalities. *(2:501)*

363. **(B)** Cloacal exstrophy is believed to arise from irregular development of the cloacal membrane. Neural tube defects are present 50% of the time. *(2:508)*

364. **(C)** Limb–body wall complex (LBWC) is the most severe abdominal wall defect with the entire ventral wall disrupted. If the umbilical cord is visualized at all, it is very short and severe scoliosis is present. *(2:508; 4:453–455, 762)*

365. **(C)** Amniotic band syndrome is a rupture of the amnion early in pregnancy. That rupture allows bands of amniotic tissue to float freely in the amniotic fluid. If these bands come in contact with the fetus, they can cause strictures, amputations, and adhesions to the band itself. Amniotic sheets, also known as uterine synechiae, are caused by scars or adhesions in the uterus. The amnion and chorion grow around the synechiae and form a thick membrane with two layers of amnion and chorion on either side of the membrane. It is attached to the uterus at both ends and does not impede the fetus in any way. *(2:502–504, 511; 4:762–766)*

366. **(D)** If a mother is Rh–, she will produce antibodies against an Rh+ fetus. The mother's antibodies will perceive the fetal blood as foreign and attack the fetal red blood cells resulting in erythroblastosis fetalis. *(9:413)*

367. **(D)** RhoGAM is an anti-D immune globulin used in preventing Rh immunization. Folic acid is a vitamin B used in preventing neural tube defect and Clomid is an infertility drug. The drug methotrexate is a chemotherapy drug and used for other medical conditions such as ectopic pregnancy and rheumatoid arthritis. *(20:1087)*

368. **(B)** This condition will cause immune hydrops in the fetus. *(9:413)*

369. **(C)** A blighted ovum is also known as anembryonic pregnancy. Sonographically, this is a large gestational sac that does not contain a yolk sac or an embryo. A missed abortion is defined as a dead embryo. Both blighted ovum and missed abortion are fail pregnancies. The difference is a blighted ovum is without an embryo and missed abortion is with an embryo but does not have heart activity. *(20:1011)*

370. **(E)** Findings of heart failure include pericardial effusions, decreased contractility, increased ventricular thickness, abnormal umbilical cord, and middle cerebral artery Doppler. *(2:567; 3:276; 6:492)*

371. **(D)** Fetal hydrops is defined as two sites of fluid accumulation or one site of fluid accumulation and fetal ascites. *(2:551)*

372. **(D)** The cardiac ventricular walls will thicken and contractility decreases. This causes the cardiac output to decrease. This may lead to acidosis, increased hematocrit, and increased neonatal morbidity. *(3:339)*

373. **(D)** The list of causes for nonimmune hydrops fetalis (NIHF) is more than 120 conditions, some of which are rare. Major causes are: cardiac arrhythmias and tumors, abnormal chromosomes, cardiac failure, anemia, arteriovenous shunts, mediastinal compression, metabolic disease, fetal infection, fetal tumors, congenital fetal defects, and placental defects. *(1:24)*

374. **(A)** *In situ* is defined as follows: in the correct place or position. The correct placement of an IUD is in the uterine cavity and the IUD string is placed in the vagina. The IUD string cannot be seen on ultrasound. Eccentric denotes "away from the center" and is a descriptive term for an IUD not in the correct position. Today's IUDs are made of flexible plastic with or without copper. When *in situ*, the IUD sonographically appears as high-amplitude linear echoes with a distal acoustic shadow. *(14:550)*

375. **(A)** Fitz–Hugh–Curtis syndrome is inflammation of the liver capsule and diaphragm secondary to bacterial spread, from the pelvis to the right upper quadrant. These findings are seen in cases of pelvic inflammatory disease. *(14:2002)*

376. **(F)** Partial situs inversus, divided into asplenia and polysplenia, has a 40% incidence of anomalies. They include complex heart disease, absent gallbladder, interrupted inferior vena cava with an azygous venous return and splenic abnormalities. *(2:480; 6:274)*

377. **(B)** A ureteropelvic junction (UPJ) obstruction is an obstruction at the junction of the ureter and renal pelvis. Therefore, the fetal urine is obstructed within the kidney causing hydronephrosis, but not hydroureter. As long as the contralateral kidney is functioning normally, the amniotic fluid should remain normal. *(1:25)*

378. **(A)** A ureterovesical junction (UVJ) obstruction is an obstruction at the junction of the ureter and fetal bladder. It is associated with ureter anomalies, such as duplication and abnormal insertion sites. There is often an ureterocele caused by the abnormal insertion of the ureter. Hydroureter and mild hydronephrosis are commonly present. *(1:25; 2:527)*

379. **(E)** The ureters is about 1 to 2 mm in diameter and not normally visible on ultrasound. *(20:1045;14:1396)*

380. **(C)** The trigone is located at the inferior portion of the posterior bladder wall. *(16:194, 195)*

381. **(E)** Spontaneous abortion is characterized by lower abdominal cramping and vaginal bleeding due to uterine contraction. When the abortion is complete, the contractions and vaginal bleeding stop. The serum β-hCG will usually decrease greater than half in 48 hours. Sonographically, the uterus will be free of any retain products. *(2:529)*

382. **(A)** Complete posterior urethral valves (PUV) obstruction does not allow for any fetal urination; therefore, severe oligohydramnios occurs. *(2:535)*

383. **(A)** Potter's facies is characterized by low set ears, flat nose and chin. Potters syndrome is predominately a male disorder and is associated with bilateral renal agenesis, oligohydramnios, and clubfoot. Small mouth with protruding tongue and small ears are facial features of Down's syndrome *(2:536)*

384. **(D)** The primary cause of neonatal death in posterior urethral valves (PUV) syndrome is pulmonary hypoplasia, although the other entities are also serious complications. *(1:25)*

385. **(C)** In cases of renal agenesis, particularly after 16 weeks, anhydramnios is present. *(2:537)*

386. **(B)** A normal fetal bladder should empty every 30–45 minutes. *(6:281)*

387. **(C)** Ovarian torsion can cause internal bleeding but not related to vaginal bleeding. All the others given choices are associated with abnormal vaginal bleeding. Hyperthyroidism and hypothyroidism can also cause abnormal vaginal bleeding. *(21:1025–1039)*

388. **(D)** Three pairs of kidneys form in successive stages: pronephros, mesonephros, and metanephros, with metanephros remaining as the functioning kidney. *(10:687)*

389. **(B)** The urinary system develops closely with the uterine development. Twenty to thirty percent of patients with uterine anomalies also have renal ectopia or agenesis. *(2:828)*

390. **(B)** Multicystic dysplastic kidney disease is caused by a first trimester obstruction. The kidney is nonfunctioning with ureteral atresia. *(2:541)*

391. **(A)** In cases of a unilateral nonfunctioning kidney, the contralateral kidney will often enlarge to compensate. The unilateral kidney usually provides enough function to be sufficient for the individual. *(2:5440)*

392. **(B)** The risk to the fetus in an autosomal dominant disease with one parent affected is 50%. *(2:542)*

393. **(B)** Autosomal dominant polycystic kidney disease does not typically cause renal disease prenatally therefore the amniotic fluid is normal. The kidneys may appear large and echogenic. Autosomal recessive polycystic kidney disease does affect renal function and is associated with oligohydramnios. Meckel's syndrome is associated with encephaloceles and post-axial polydactyly. *(2:545)*

394. **(B)** Although kidneys grow throughout gestation, the ratio of kidneys to abdomen remains constant at 0.27–0.30. *(2:519)*

395. **(C)** Unless the kidney is echogenic or obstructed, the anechoic cysts in the periphery represent normal renal pyramids. *(3:518, 534)*

396. **(B)** Fetal urine production begins at 12 weeks, but the fetal kidneys do not produce the majority of the fetal urine until 16 weeks. *(2:517; 6:296)*

397. **(E)** Ectopic pregnancy is defined as any pregnancy outside of the endometrial cavity. Although approximately 90% of ectopic pregnancies occur in the fallopian tube, it can occur in other locations such as the abdomen and ovaries. Ectopic pregnancy can occur in the uterus such as a cervical or a hysterotomy scar from a previous cesarean section. *(21:439: 14:1109)*

398. **(D)** Although this is somewhat debated, many sources quote a number from 4 to 6 mm as the upper limit of normal in the second trimester. *(2:520; 3:496)*

399. **(B)** Grade 0—no dilation. *(2:521)*

400. **(C)** Grade I—renal pelvic dilation with or without infundibula visible. *(2:521)*

401. **(E)** Grade II—renal pelvic dilation with calices visible. *(2:521)*

402. **(A)** Grade III—renal pelvis and calices dilated. *(2:521)*

403. **(D)** Grade IV—renal pelvis and calices dilated with parenchymal thinning. *(2:521)*

404. **(C)** Because of its vascularity, the fetus may experience heart failure and polyhydramnios. On ultrasound, a congenital mesoblastic nephroma will resemble a Wilms' tumor. *(2:548)*

405. **(A)** A neuroblastoma appears as a suprarenal mass and should be considered when a mass is identified superior to the kidney. Nephroblastoma (Wilms' tumor) is a malignant renal tumor that effect children. *(2:549)*

406. **(C)** Nephroblastoma, also known as Wilm's tumor, is a malignant renal tumor that sonographically appears similar to a mesoblastic nephroma. *(4:880, 881)*

407–409. **(B)** Rectus abdominis. **(A)** Obturator internus. **(C)** Piriformis. In a transverse plane, the rectus abdominis muscles appear as low-level hypoechoic echoes on the most midline anterior portion of the abdomina-pelvic wall. The obturator internus muscles are posterior and medial to the iliopsoas muscles and appear as thin, bi-linear, low-level echoes on the posterolateral aspect of the urinary bladder. The piriformis muscles are bilateral hypoechoic structures seen posterior to the uterus and anterior to the sacrum. *(18:275, 276)*

410. **(D)** The levator ani muscles make up the pelvic diaphragm and are easily visualized in a transabdominal transverse plane. These bilateral muscles appear hypoechoic and are seen medial to the obturator internus muscles and posterior to the cervix and vagina. *(18:275)*

411. **(C)** A change in head shape, such as brachycephaly or dolicocephaly, affects accurate measurement in predicting gestational age. The degree to which fetal head shape affects BPD can be estimated with the formula: CI = BPD/OFD × 100. *(7:438)*

412. **(A)** Ovarian tumors account for 50–81% of torsion. Hyperstimulated ovaries produce large cysts that may get a torsion but less common than ovarian tumors. *(2:872)*

413. (E) The ovary has a dual blood supply: the ovarian and uterine arteries. The ovarian arteries originate from the aorta just below the renal vessels, with each coursing into the retroperitoneal space. It enters the broad ligament and then enters through the hilum of the ovary. The left ovarian vein drains into the left renal vein. The right ovarian vein connects directly into the inferior vena cava. The uterine artery arises from the anterior division of the hypogastric (internal iliac artery). *(20:52; 21:866)*

414. (D) Hyperstimulated ovaries produce large cysts that may be torsed, as well as cause fullness and nausea to the patient. Rarely, more severe complications can occur because of the shift in fluid resulting in ascites and effusions. *(2:866)*

415. (F) The presentation of ovarian torsion varies, depending on the duration and degree of vascular compromise. Ovarian torsion is twisting of the ovary and its vessels resulting in occlusion of its blood supply. Approximately 95% of cases are associated with an adnexal mass. Although torsion of a normal ovary can occur, this is more frequent in children than adults. Doppler ultrasound is very helpful in confirming the presence of blood flow. However, on rare occasions, ultrasound may demonstrate bilateral flow in a patient who has an ovarian torsion. This is due to twisting and untwisting of the ovary. The clinical symptoms of unilateral pain with nausea and vomiting are usually present even in a false-positive sonogram. Ovarian torsion does not occur if the ovaries and fallopian tubes are removed. *(14:562, 563; 20:931; 21:507)*

416. (A) Endometrial cancer is one of the most common gynecologic malignancies, after cervical cancer. Postmenopausal bleeding is an early sign. Abdominal/pelvic ascites, intra-abdominal mass, and pelvic pain are late signs. Most cancers are painless in early stages. *(21:873)*

417. (B) Fibroids are estrogen dependent and commonly increase in pregnancy and decrease post-menopausally. The only sonographic difference between a leiomyoma and a leiomyosarcoma is a rapid increase in growth. *(2:841)*

418. (A) On sonography, a leiomyoma and a leiomyosarcoma appear the same. Clinically, the only difference is a rapid increase in growth in postmenopausal women. *(2:841)*

419. (C) The fetal lung is isoechoic to the fetal liver in the second trimester. *(2:634)*

420. (A) Although the lung increases in echogenicity throughout the pregnancy, researchers have not been able to correlate the increase with lung maturity. *(2:634; 6:272)*

421. (E) Visualization of the femoral epiphyseal plate is seen on fetuses with a gestational age greater than 33 weeks with 95% accuracy. *(2:632)*

422. (A) Polydactyly may be isolated or occur as part of a syndrome. The extra digit may have a bone or may be

soft tissue only. Postaxial refers to the ulnar aspect of the hand. *(2:362)*

423. (B) Polydactyly may be isolated or occur as part of a syndrome. The extra digit may have a bone or be soft tissue only. Preaxial refers to the radial aspect of the hand. *(2:362)*

424. (B) Discordance in dichorionic/diamniotic twins is more acceptable because of their different genetic makeup, provided that the smaller twin is not less than the 10th percentile in EFW. In monochorionic twins, EFW should be concordant and not differ by more than 20%. *(2:184)*

425. (A) Supine hypotensive syndrome is due to obstruction by the gravid uterus on the inferior vena cava, resulting in decreased venous return to the heart. The patient should be turned on the left side and the symptoms will disappear. Sitting up will also help. *(7:362)*

426. (C) Twin fetal discordance is determined by subtracting the largest twin from the smallest twin and dividing by the largest twin. This number is multiplied by 100 to determine the percentage. *(2:184)*

427. (D) Frank breech is described as the buttocks descending first with the thighs and legs extending upward along the anterior fetal trunk. *(7:445)*

428. (C) Complete breech is described as the buttocks descending first with the knees flexed, and the fetus sitting cross-legged. *(7:445)*

429. (A) A footling breech is when one or both feet are prolapsed into the lower uterine segment. *(7:445)*

430. (B) Ectopic pregnancy in the interstitial (cornual) region of the fallopian tube increases the risk for maternal mobility or mortality. This is due to its location giving the ectopic more room to grow. It ruptures at a larger size with a close proximity to the uterine artery, making this type of ectopic most potentially life-threatening. *(20:1009; 21:433)*

431. (B) XY karyotype indicates a male fetus. XX karyotype indicates a female fetus. Down's syndrome is labeled 47,+21, and Turner's syndrome in labeled 45X. *(2:20, 21)*

432. (D) HIPAA, is a federal laws, which forbid healthcare workers from giving out patient information without consent, even to other family members. Sonographers must comply with this legislation. If the sonographer is not compliant, he or she can face up to $250,000 in fines and/or jail time up to 10 years. *(23:77)*

433. (C) The fetus (regardless of the body part), as well as the sac, closest to the internal os is labeled fetus A. *(6:467)*

434. (A) The fetus would be lying on its right side, with left side closest to the maternal abdominal wall. *(7:432)*

435. (A) The fetus would be laying on its right side, with the left side closest to the maternal abdominal wall. *(7:432)*

436. **(A)** The fetus would be laying on its right side, with the left side closest to the maternal abdominal wall. (7:432)

437. **(C)** Placental lakes are areas of fibrin under the chorion, on the fetal side of the placenta. They carry no clinical significance. (2:603)

438. **(D)** Hypertension and maternal smoking can cause the placenta to undergo early maturation. Smoking can cause an increase in calcifications in the placenta. Unfortunately, placenta maturation has not proved to be a reliable tool in assessing placental function or fetal well-being. (2:604)

439. **(D)** Triploidy from the paternal component, presents with a large cystic placenta. (2:599; 6:421)

440. **(D)** Maternal hypertension can cause a restrictive flow in the uterine vessels, which in turn, may decrease the placental perfusion. (2:599; 6:421)

441. **(D)** Gestational diabetes mellitus is a cause for macrosomia because of the increased maternal blood sugars. (2:215)

442. **(B)** Although it is important to make sure the exam room and the transducer are sterilized prior to any procedure. The informed consent is most imperative prior to the procedure. An informed consent is an agreement by the patient to undergo a specific medical intervention. This agreement includes risks, benefits, and alternatives to the procedure. The form should be signed by the patient and physician and include a witness. The patient must be of legal age and mentally competent. (22:181)

443. **(A)** Caudal regression syndrome is associated with insulin-dependent diabetes mellitus in up to 16% of the cases. It is thought to occur with poor glucose control in the first trimester. Findings include sacral agenesis, spinal, and lower limb abnormalities, femoral hypoplasia, gastrointestinal and genitourinary abnormalities. (2:364–366)

444. **(B)** Adult tissue is more tolerant of temperature increases than embryo tissue or ossifying fetal bones. (24:306–334)

445. **(A)** Duplex pulse Doppler studies (pulse-wave Doppler with real time) are of significantly higher output intensities than power Doppler or fetal Doppler monitor. (24:306–334)

446. **(E)** The phenotype for Turner's syndrome is 45X, indicating only one single X, or female, chromosome. (2:21)

447. **(A)** The ALARA principle (as low as reasonably achievable) employs keeping the power output as low as possible and increasing the receiver gain in order to change the quality of the image. This principle also employs reducing the scanning time in order to minimize the patient's ultrasound exposure. (24:322)

448. **(E)** Caudal regression syndrome and cardiac defects are first-trimester insults and a risk of occurrence increases with increasing blood sugar levels in the first trimester. Shoulder dystocia can occur with delivery of macrosomic fetuses. (3:544)

449. **(D)** Depending on the fetal gestational age, lung maturity amniocentesis may be performed to assure lung maturation before delivery. In cases of complete PROM, often there is not an adequate sample of amniotic fluid available for maturity testing. (2:628)

450. **(D)** Although an increased amniotic fluid volume is associated with macrosomia, it is not a direct assessment of macrosomia. (3:544)

451. **(D)** CVS and PUBS may be performed provided the placenta or umbilical cord is accessible. If the fetal bladder is full, as in cases of PUV syndrome, fetal urine may be tested for karyotype. (2:32)

452. **(E)** Amniocentesis is a prenatal test to analyze the amniotic fluid. It can be used to detect multiple potential abnormalities such as Down's syndrome, cystic fibrosis, sickle cell disease, neural tube detect, and fetal lungs maturity. It also can be used to test the level of fetal bilirubin, infection, and for a limited amount of short-limb syndromes. However, amniocentesis is not useful in detecting cleft palate or cleft lips. (2:33, 566; 14:1602–1604)

453. **(C)** Hypertension can affect the vascular bed of the placenta resulting in intrauterine growth retardation. (2:214)

454. **(A)** Excessive maternal smoking has been linked to accelerated maturation of the placenta. It is not predictive, however, in actual placenta perfusion to the fetus. (6:420)

455. **(C)** BBOW, bulging bag of water, refers to the amniotic membrane bulging into the vagina. (13:156)

456. **(D)** PROM, premature rupture of membranes, is the rupture of membranes before 37 weeks. (2:588)

457. **(F)** All of the above. Overdistension of the urinary bladder can result in serious diagnostic error. Overdistension of the urinary bladder may result in closure of an incompetent cervix due to bladder compression on the cervix; placenta previa caused by bladder compression on the lower uterine segment; closure of the gestational sac caused by bladder compression that causes both sides of the sac walls to meet resulting in a loss of the anechoic center or a change in sac shape (distortion); nonvisualization of the internal iliac vein because of displacement. (7:432)

458. **(C)** Ovulation occurs approximately 14 days after the first day of the last menstrual period. (2:105)

459. **(C)** Gravida is a woman who is pregnant. (7:435)

460. **(A)** Multipara is a woman who has given birth two or more times. (7:435)

461. **(D)** Nullipara is a woman who has never given birth to a viable infant. (7:435)

462. **(H)** Primipara is woman who has given birth one time to a viable infant, regardless of whether the child was living at birth and regardless of whether the birth was single or multiple. (7:435)

463. **(B)** Nulligravida is a woman who has never been pregnant. (7:435)

464. **(E)** Primigravida is a woman who is pregnant for the first time. (7:435)

465. **(F)** Multigravida is a woman who has been pregnant several times. (7:435)

466. **(G)** Para is the number of pregnancies that have continued to viability. (7:435)

467. **(I)** Trimester is a 3-month period during gestation. (7:435)

468. **(D)** The puerperium period begins with the expulsion of the placenta and continues until maternal physiology and anatomy return to a prepregnancy level, approximately 6–8 weeks. (6:533)

469. **(B)** Sonographic assessment of the maternal kidneys and bowel would not be considered a gynecological sonogram. (6:533)

470. **(A)** When the transducer is in direct contact with the patient, it exposes the patient to the greatest risk of electrical shock from a cracked transducer. Water and metals are conductors of electricity. (24:330)

471. **(D)** The ovaries are least likely to be seen on a postpartum pelvic sonogram. This may be because of extrapelvic position of the ovaries caused by the large uterus. (7:438)

472. **(A)** At approximately 20–22 weeks of gestation, the fundus of the gravid uterus is at the level of the umbilicus, and at 12 weeks of gestation, it is at the symphysis pubic. This is known as fundal height. (7:347)

473. **(E)** Hemorrhage, thromboembolism, and infection are the most common complications during the postpartum period. Placenta previa is an antepartum complication. (7:438)

474. **(E)** Ascites is an abnormal accumulation of fluid in the abdominal (peritoneal) cavity. There are multiple causes, heart failure, nephrotic syndrome pancreatitis, cancer alcoholic hepatitis, and tuberculosis. Fibroid uterus is a benign tumor and generally does not cause ascites. (16:133)

475. **(D)** 25% of fetuses are breech at 28 weeks, 7% at 32 weeks, and 3–4% at term. (9:451)

476. **(B)** Malignant ascites is characterized by loculated intraperitoneal fluid collection with loops of bowel adherent to the abdominal wall. (16:143)

477. **(C)** VBAC is a commonly used abbreviation for vaginal birth after cesarean section. (12:370)

478. **(B)** The normal anatomical site for implantation of pregnancy is the endometrial (uterine) cavity, and the normal location for fertilization of the ovum is the ampullary region of the fallopian tube. (20:984)

479. **(D)** Placenta previa is the implantation of the placenta in the lower uterine segment. (7:438)

480. **(A)** Placenta accreta is the abnormal adherence of part or the all of placenta to the uterine wall. (7:439)

481. **(C)** Placenta succenturiata is an accessory lobe of placenta. (7:439)

482. **(B)** Abruptio placentae is the premature separation of the placenta after 20 weeks of gestation. (7:439)

483. **(E)** Placenta increta is the abnormal adherence of part or all of the placenta in which the chorionic villi invade the myometrium. (7:439)

484. **(F)** Placenta percreta is the abnormal adherence of part or all of the placenta in which the chorionic villi invade the uterine wall. (7:439)

485. **(A)** The fetal component of the placenta. (7:447)

486. **(B)** The maternal component of the placenta. (7:447)

487. **(A)** Sonographic fetal HELLP findings include IUGR, oligohydramnios, and possible signs of fetal distress (poor BPP, abnormal UC Doppler's, for example). Clinically, HELLP is an acronym for hemolysis, elevated liver enzyme, and low platelet count. It is a variant of preeclampsia but can occur on its own. (2:86)

488. **(A)** The kidneys should be scanned to look for hydronephrosis. An enlarged fibroid greater than 14 cm in size can compress the distal ureter and cause hydronephrosis. These findings can also be due to the gravid uterus in pregnancy. A pseudohydronephrosis can occur with overdistended urinary bladder but disappears after postvoid. (20:331)

489. **(B)** The primary infection that cause varicella-zoster virus (VZV) result from chicken pox. Herpes zoster, also known as shingles results from reactivation of varicella-zoster virus (VZV). (3:676)

490. **(D)** Cytomegalovirus (CMV) is the most common intrauterine congenital fetal viral infection. The maternal risk of transmission to the fetus is 40–50%, regardless of gestational age. (2:567)

491. **(A)** The secondary yolk sac is located in the chorionic cavity (extraembryonic coelom). The primitive yolk sac is not seen on ultrasound. The yolk sac contains vitelline fluid and has many functions including transfer of nutrients and development of blood (hematopoiesis). At approximately 12 weeks, the amnion and chorion begin to fuse and the yolk is no longer seen. (20:988, 989; 22:130, 131)

492. (D) Hematocolpos is blood in the vagina and is caused more commonly by imperforate hymen. Cervical stenosis is an acquired condition with obstruction at the cervical os, which can also result in hematometra but is less common. Hematometrocolpos is blood in the vagina and uterus. *(14:544)*

493. (D) In the case of IUGR, the fetus will direct more blood flow to the brain. This will lower the PI and S/D ratio of the middle cerebral artery (MCA). More recently, multiple studies have been conducted showing that the peak velocity of the MCA is a good predictor of fetal anemia. The peak velocity is measured and plotted of a curve to determine whether the fetus is in need of a fetal blood transfusion because of fetal anemia. *(2:689, 690; 11:13)*

494. (C) Leiomyomas (fibroids) are benign tumors of the muscle of the uterus, which are stimulated by estrogen. After menopause, the fibroid normally decreased in size due to the decrease in estrogen. An increase in size of fibroids after menopause is suggestive of leiomyosarcoma. *(20:902–905)*

495. (D) Multiple fluid-filled spaces in the uterine cavity with markedly elevated serum β-hCG are highly suggestive of hydatidiform mole, which is characterized by hydropic villi. The most common cyst associated with hydatidiform mole is theca lutein cyst, which is located on the ovary. Corpus lutein cyst is associated with an intrauterine pregnancy. Pseudo-gestational sac is associated with an ectopic pregnancy. *(14:1576)*

496. (D) Sex cord-stromal tumors include fibroma, thecoma, granulosa cell, and androblastoma (Sertoli–Leydig cell). They appear hypoechoic to echogenic with a mixed heterogeneous pattern and appear similar to each other on ultrasound. *(2:874, 877)*

497. (C) Endometriomas have a variety of sonographic appearances. Hemorrhagic cyst and ovarian abscesses is known to mimic its appearances. *(2:868-869)*

498. (A) A hydrosalpinx may initially look like a cystic mass with septations. On closer examination, the septations are not complete. The sonographer is able to follow the connection of the cystic spaces. This assumes that the structure is tubular and communicates as with hydrosalpinx. *(2:870)*

499. (E) A paraovarian, or mesonephric cyst originates from the mesonephric duct. A paraovarian cyst may form, regardless of uterine or ovarian status. Ovarian tissue does occasionally remain after an oophorectomy, especially if adhesions were present. The remaining ovarian tissue can still function and produce a cyst. It is called ovarian remnant syndrome and should be considered with any cystic mass identified in a post-oophorectomy patient. Peritoneal inclusion cyst is sometimes seen after oophorectomy due to fluid trapped between the adhesions. *(2:867, 868)*

500. (C) Hydatid cyst of Morgagni also known as a paratubal cyst is the most common paramesonephric cyst. It measures 2–10 mm and appears similar to ovarian cysts. *(2:868;21:492)*

501. (A) D1 × D2 × D3 × 0.523. *(14:554)*

502. (D) The image is a Dandy–Walker malformation. The cerebellum is splayed, and the vermis is absent. There is communication with the fourth ventricle. *(1:20)*

503. (C) Before puberty, the uterus is approximately 3 cm in length. *(16:281)*

504. (C) Cystic teratomas (dermoids) more frequently occur in females 10–30 years of age. They have a variable sonographic appearance. They can be cystic to complex, highly echogenic, and can contain echogenic foci with posterior shadowing. Fluid may be noted on the peripheral aspect of the mass. *(16:298, 299)*

505. (D) The vagina courses from the cervix to the external genitalia between the bladder and the rectum. It appears as a collapsed hypoechoic tubular structure with a highly reflective central echo representing the interface between the anterior and posterior walls of the vagina. The uterus forms a 90° angle with the posterior vaginal wall. *(14:551)*

506. (C) The endocervical canal extends from the internal os, which is approximately at the level of the isthmus where it joins the endocervical canal, to the external os, which projects into the vagina. *(18:259)*

507–510. (B) Fundus; **(C)** Corpus (body); **(D)** Isthmus; **(A)** Cervix. The uterus has four components. The fundus is the widest and most superior segment. The corpus (body), which is the largest segment, is continuous with the fundus. There is a normal constrictor where the cervical segment starts, which is called the isthmus. The cervix is cylindrical in shape and projects into the vagina. *(18:259)*

511. (B) Fluid can accumulate in several potential spaces in the pelvis. The pouch of Douglas (posterior cul-de-sac, rectouterine pouch) is situated posterior to the uterus and anterior to the wall of the rectum. The space of Retzius is between the symphysis pubis and the anterior wall of the urinary bladder. The anterior cul-de-sac (vesicouterine pouch) is situated between the uterus and the posterior wall of the urinary bladder. Morrison's pouch is located in the abdomen between the right lobe of the liver and the right kidney. *(18:257)*

512. (E) Synechiae are adhesions that occur within the uterus due to a mechanical trauma. In Asherman's syndrome, there are so many adhesions that the uterine cavity is completely closed. Adenomyosis is characterized by invasion of the endometrium into the myometrium. This condition is usually asymptomatic but may also present with uterine bleeding, pain, and infertility. Other possible causes of infertility include intracavity endometrial masses, submucosal myomas, endometrial polyps, and polycystic ovarian syndrome. *(19:1085–1101)*

513. **(B)** The sonographic appearance and thickness of the endometrium change cyclically with the menstrual cycle. During the secretory phase (days 15–28), the functional zone of the endometrium reaches its full thickness and becomes edematous. The sonographic appearance is more echogenic when compared to the adjacent myometrium and measures 7–14 mm. *(18:278, 279)*

514. **(F)** The hypothalamus secretes gonadotropin-releasing hormone (GnRH). Oxytocin is secreted by the posterior pituitary gland. *(18:265, 266).*

515. **(A)** A waveform with decreased diastolic flow would indicate a high-resistance pattern resulting in an increased RI. *(19:1078, 1079)*

516. **(B)** Fibromas are benign tumors of the ovary. When this tumor is associated with pleural effusion and ascites, it is referred to as Meigs' syndrome. *(14:571)*

517. **(B)** Parity refers to the number of viable offspring, climacteric is a term for menopause, and Mittelschmerz refers to the middle pain preceding ovulation. Puberty is physical development after which sexual reproduction first becomes possible. *(2:841, 861; 19:260)*

518. **(E)** Bowel can have a variable echogenic appearance depending on the internal contents. *(16:51)*

519. **(E)** Cervical stenosis frequently involves the internal os and may cause secondary obstruction to the uterine cavity but not the vaginal cavity. This may result from radiation therapy, neoplasia, and infection. The characteristic appearance is a dilated, fluid-filled endometrial cavity. Internal echoes may be visualized due to debris or clot. *(2:836, 827; 14:1998, 1999)*

520. **(D)** Women who have not given birth (nulliparous) have a 2% lifetime risk. *(19:1004, 1005)*

521. **(C)** In vitro fertilization (IVF) and embryo transfer are used in patients with absent or significantly diseased tubes. Gamete intrafallopian tube transfer (GIFT) and zygote intrafallopian tube transfer (ZIFT) both involve transferring sperm and ova directly into the fallopian tube. *(19:1048, 1049)*

522. **(C)** The sonographic appearance and thickness of the endometrium change cyclically with the menstrual cycle. In the proliferative phase (days 5–14), the endometrium starts to thicken (4–8 mm) and appears linear and hypoechoic relative to the adjacent myometrium. During the menstrual phase (days 1–4), the endometrium is thin with a bright central echo representing the interface between the two endometrial layers. *(18:278, 279)*

523. **(C)** A bicornuate uterus has 2 widely separated endometrial cavities and there is an indentation on the fundal contour. *(14:537)*

524. **(A)** Congenital uterine anomalies are associated with an increased incidence of spontaneous abortions. *(14:534)*

525. **(B)** A pelvic (ectopic) kidney occurs during embryologic development, and the kidney fails to ascend into the abdomen. The kidney is usually small and abnormally rotated. The normal echogenic renal sinus can be noted. *(14:328)*

526. **(D)** The iliopsoas muscles together with the rectus abdominis muscles and transverse abdominis muscles are located within the false pelvis. *(18:253)*

527. **(C)** The infundibulopelvic ligaments together with the ovarian ligaments provide support to the ovaries and help maintain their position in the adnexal region. *(18:255)*

528. **(D)** Sonohysterography involves the insertion of normal saline into the uterine cavity to visualize the endometrium. *(20:1134, 1135)*

529. **(B)** Serous cystadenocarcinoma accounts for 40–50% of all malignant ovarian neoplasms. Sonographically, they usually appear as large multilocular complex cystic masses with papillary projections arising from the walls. They may contain thickened septa and echogenic solid material. The walls may be thickened. The greater the amount of internal solid material or irregular septa, the more likely tumors are malignant. The presence of ascites may indicate tumor extension beyond its capsule. *(14:566; 19:906)*

530. **(E)** Under normal circumstances, transvaginal ultrasound are performed with verbal consent only. However, patients who are mentally incompetent, drug impaired, or unconscious are not in the capacity to consent. In most cases, these patients require an administrative informed consent, court order consent, or informed consent from a healthcare proxy or family member. If a patient who is coherent refuses a procedure that is performed without her consent even if the procedure is warranted to save her life, the sonographer could be liable for assault and battery. An implied consent, which is used when an unconscious patient is at risk or if an emergency exists, cannot be utilized in non-emergency situations. An emergency is defined as a situation wherein the procedure is immediately or imminently necessary and any delay occasioned by an attempt to obtain consent would reasonably jeopardize life. *(23:180, 181)*

531. **(E)** Although 3D ultrasound DVD may be a kind gesture to family bonding. The Food and Drug Administration and other professional medical organizations discourage the use of ultrasound for non-medical reasons. Sonograms should be requested by a physician with just medical cause. *(23:194)*

532. **(C)** Pseudocyesis (false pregnancy) is a condition in which a non-pregnant woman believes that she is pregnant. This patient will sometimes give convincing stories of pregnancy. The patient may actually exhibit morning

sickness, breast enlargement, and cessation of menstruation. However, in pseudocyesis, there is no physical, sonographic, or laboratory evidence of pregnancy. In missed abortion, ectopic, and abdominal pregnancy, the pregnancy test result is positive and will have some sonographic evidence. In fetal demise, the serum β-hCG is positive for several weeks depending on the gestational age at the time of death. *(25:32)*

533. **(A)** Precocious puberty is premature onset of secondary sexual characteristics before 8 years for girls and before 9 for boys. When a child's gender is in question at birth due to its atypical appearance, it is referred to as ambiguous genitalia. *(20:656; 21:271–278)*

534. **(D)** Precocious puberty and ambiguous genitalia are the most commonly requested pediatric ultrasound. Accidental ingestion of foreign body is very common but best demonstrated by x-ray. Vaginal foreign body is less requested. Fibroids uterus are rarely seen before puberty. *(21:268–275)*

535. **(A)** The gold standard for predicting fetal lungs maturity is lecithin-sphingomyelin ratio from the amniotic fluid. Ultrasound cannot predict fetal lung maturity, however, some sonographic findings increase the likelihood. *(25:969)*

536. **(B)** An infection acquired via a medical instrument or a medical procedure is called iatrogenic. An infection contracted while under medical care is called nosocomial. *(23:108)*

537. **(E)** Retained products of conception (RPOC). This transvaginal sonogram demonstrates disorganize echoes in the uterine cavity after a dilation and curettage, which is highly suggestive of RPOC. The serum β-hCG is positive after an abortion or after a normal delivery and can remain positive for several weeks depending on the gestational age. *(14:1578)*

538. **(A)** The scan should be obtained with the fetus in the sagittal section with a neutral position of the fetal head. *(28:90)*

539. **(A)** Nuchal fold measurements are preformed in the second trimester and are measured from the outer edge of the occipital bone to the outer margin of the skin. *(26:1)*

540. **(E)** Thickened nuchal translucency is associated with cystic hygroma, nuchal edema, aneuploidy, and congenital heart disease. The most common syndromes associated with thickened translucency are Turner's and Down's syndromes. Rhombencephalon (hindbrain) is a normal brain vesicle seen in the early developing embryo. *(26:1; 27:26)*

541. **(D)** The optimal time to assess measurements for nuchal translucency is between 11 to 14 weeks. *(26:1)*

542. **(E)** Nuchal translucency thickness increases with crown-rump-length (CRL). The measurements increase from 1.2 mm at 11 weeks to 3 mm at 14 weeks. *(26:1; 28:90)*

543. **(D)** Mesenchymal edema is a term used to describe excessive enlarged nuchal translucency in association with cystic hygroma. *(26:1)*

References

1. Krebs C. *Appleton & Lange's Review for the Ultra-sonography Examination.* 3rd ed. New York: Appleton & Lange; 2001.

2. Callen PW. *Ultrasonography in Obstetrics and Gynecology.* 4th ed. Philadelphia: WB Saunders; 2000.

3. Fleischer A, Manning F, Jeanty P, Romero R. *Sonography in Obstetrics and Gynecology: Principles and Practice.* 5th ed. Stanford, CT: Appleton & Lange; 1996.

4. Bianchi DW, Cromblelholme TM, D'Alton ME. *Fetalogy: Diagnosis and Management of the Fetal Patient.* New York: McGraw-Hill; 2000.

5. Nyberg D, Mahony B, Pretorius D. *Diagnostic Ultrasound of Fetal Anomalies.* St. Louis, MO: Mosby-Year Book; 1990.

6. Berman MC, Cohen HL. *Obstetrics and Gynecology.* 2nd ed. Philadelphia: Lippincott; 1997.

7. Odwin CS, Dubinsky T, Fleischer AC. *Appleton & Lange's Review for the Ultrasonography Examination.* 2nd ed. Norwalk, CT: Appleton & Lange; 1993.

8. Moore TR, Cayle JE. The amniotic fluid index in normal human pregnancy. *Am J Obstet Gynecol.* 1990; 162:1168-1173.

9. Zuspan F, Quilligan E, Blumenfeld M. *Handbook of Obstetrics, Gynecology, and Primary Care.* St. Louis, MO: Mosby-Year Book; 1998.

10. Tortora GJ, Derrickson B: *Principles of Anatomy and Physiology.* 11th ed. New York: John Wiley & Sons, Inc; 2006.

11. Mari G et al. *Proceedings SMFM.* Miami Beach, FL; January 2000.

12. Gabbe S, Niebyl J, Simpson JL. *Obstetrics: Normal and Problem Pregnancies.* New York: Churchill Livingstone; 1996.

13. Thomas C. *Taber's Cyclopedic Medical Dictionary.* Philadelphia: F.A. Davis; 1982.

14. Rumack C et al. *Diagnostic Ultrasound.* 3rd ed. St. Louis, MO: Elsevier Mosby; 2005.

15. Schmidt G. *Differential Diagnosis in Ultrasound Imaging.* Stuttgart, Germany: Thieme; 2006.

16. Sanders R et al. *Clinical Sonography A Practical Guide.* 4th ed. Maryland: Lippincott, Williams & Wilkins; 2007.

17. Doubilet P et al. *Atlas of Ultrasound in Obstetrics and Gynecology: A Multimedia Reference.* Philadelphia, PA: Lippincott, Williams & Wilkins; 2003.

18. Curry RA et al. *Sonography: Introduction to Normal Structure and Function.* 2nd ed. St. Louis, MO: Saunders; 2004.

19. Fleischer AC et al. *Sonography in Obstetrics and Gynecology: Principles and Practice.* 6th ed. New York: McGraw-Hill; 2001.

20. Hangen-Ansert S. *Textbook of Diagnostic Ultrasonography.* 6th ed. St. Louis, MO: Mosby; 2006.

21. Mishell DR, Stenchever MA, Droegemueller W, et al. *Comprehensive Gynecology.* 3rd ed. St. Louis, MO: Mosby–Year Book, Inc; 1997.

22. Moore KL, Persaud TVN. *The Developing Human: Clinically Oriented Embryology.* 5th ed. Philadelphia, PA: 1993.

23. Craig M. *Essentials of Sonography and Patient Care.* 2nd ed. St. Louis, MO; 1993.

24. Kremkau FW. *Diagnostic Ultrasound: Principles and Instruments.* 6th ed. St. Louis, MO; 2006.

25. Cunningham G, MacDonald, Grant NF, et al. *Williams Obstetrics.* 20th ed. New York: Appleton & Lange; 1997.

26. Simpson LL, Levine D, et al. *First Trimester Cystic Hygroma and Enlarged Nuchal Translucency.* Waltham, MA: Up to Date; 2010.

27. Bianchi DW, Crombleholme TM, et al. *Fetology Diagnosis and Management of Fetal Patient.* New York, NY: McGraw-Hill; 2000.

28. Goldberg BB, Mc Gaham JP. *Atlas of Ultrasound Measurements.* Elsevier Health Sciences; 2006.

29. Thilaganathan B, Sairam S, Michailidis G, et al. First trimester nuchal translucency: effective routine screening for Down's syndrome. *Br J Radiol.* 1999;72.

30. Lipscomb GH. Medical Therapy for ectopic pregnancy. *Semin Reprod Med Memphis.* TN; 25:93. 2007.

8

3D Obstetric and Gynecologic Sonography: An Illustrative Overview

Arthur C. Fleischer

Study Guide

Three-dimensional (3D) sonography has become a clinically useful problem-solving technique that can also expedite sonographic examinations in certain obstetric and gynecologic disorders. Improved instrumentation has afforded its incorporation into clinical practice and provides interesting new areas for future applications. This is an illustrative overview of the important points of 3D sonography for the sonographer and sonologist. The reader is encouraged to read the articles that describe new, ever-expanding applications of this technique.[1-5]

INSTRUMENTATION/TECHNIQUE

Three-dimensional acquisitions can be obtained with freehand sweeps of an area of interest or with automated transducers that interrogate a specified area of interest. Three-dimensional automated transducers consist of an imaging array mounted on a gimbal. These transducers can be as small as the transvaginal probe or as large as a large handheld probe. The scanning section axis can be selected from 30° to more than 120° (Figs. 8–1 and 8–2). The patient must suspend respiration and remain motionless when the images are obtained in order to avoid scan artefacts.

For freehand scanning, the scanner memory is filled with two-dimensional (2D) images that are reprocessed into a 3D volume. Although adequate 3D sonography can be obtained this way, its resolution is not as great as with images obtained with an automatically sectored probe.

Automated 3D transducer probes contain an array of transducer elements that are swept in a selectable arc through an area

of interest. The images are displayed in a multiplanar format with the long-axis, short-axis, and coronal planes, as well as the volumetric image. The multiplanar images are usually displayed with the long-axis view on the top left, followed by the short-axis images obtained at 90° or orthogonal to the long axis displayed in top right, followed by the coronal image scan plane (Fig. 8–3, bottom left). The combined volume is shown, within which (Fig. 8–3 bottom right) the scan plane can be maneuvered.

This layout of multiplanar reconstructed images can be varied to emphasize the volumetric images as the largest one displayed. Three-dimensional images can be manipulated to emphasize the surface (surface rendering) or the entire volume (volume rendering). The ability to visualize the structure from a selectable scan plane is particularly helpful when such planes cannot be readily obtainable from a 2D image. This is particularly true in the evaluation of the fetal heart when obtaining an optimal image of the outflow tracts, this may not be possible on 2D acquisition but quite possible with 3D. Another new feature is the ability to display multiple tomographic images (Philips' iSlice) obtained in selectable intervals and slice thicknesses.

OBSTETRICAL 3D SONOGRAPHY

Three-dimensional sonography offers a detailed depiction of the fetal face, extremities, outer contours, and certain organs such as the fetal heart, brain, liver, kidneys, and spine (Figs. 8–4 through 8–27). Depiction of the fetus with 3D sonography has gained widespread and universal demand. However, there should be clinical indication for such studies since any unnecessary

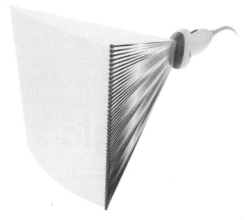

FIGURE 8-1. Three-dimensional obstetrical probe showing sectored volume. *(Courtesy of Philips Healthcare.)*

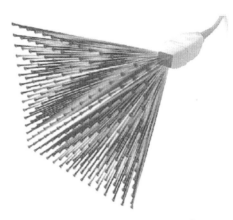

FIGURE 8-2. Four-dimensional matrix array probe. *(Courtesy of Philips Healthcare.)*

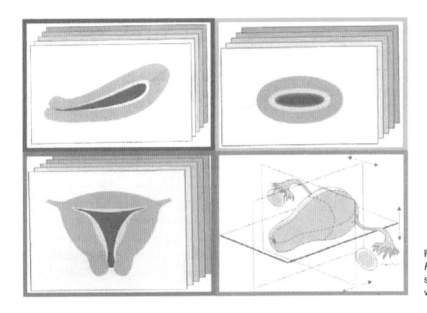

FIGURE 8-3. Multiplanar imaging format. *(Courtesy of Philips Healthcare.)*: Top left: long-axis plane; Top right: short-axis plane; Bottom left: coronal plane; Bottom right: 3D volume.

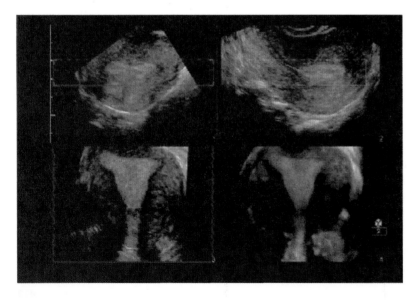

FIGURE 8-4. Normal uterus and endometrium as shown in multiplanar images. *(Courtesy of Philips Healthcare.)*: Top left: short-axis uterus; Top right: long-axis uterus; Bottom left: coronal; Bottom right: surface rendered volume.

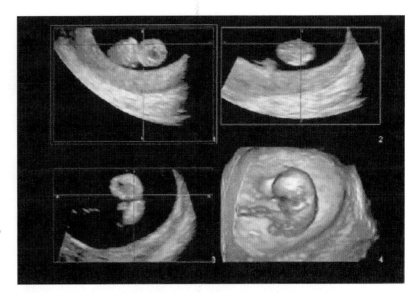

FIGURE 8–5. Three-dimensional sonogram of 10-week intrauterine pregnancy. *(Courtesy of Philips Healthcare.)*: Top left: long axis showing fetal heart and trunk; Top right: short axis through bottom of left hand; Bottom left: coronal plane; Bottom right: 3D volume with surface rendering showing the entire fetus and umbilical cord.

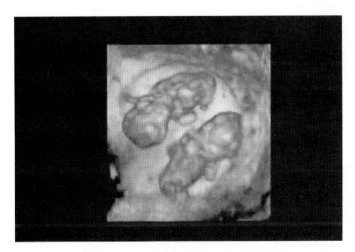

FIGURE 8–6. Three-dimensional image of twins at 11-weeks' gestation. *(Courtesy of Philips Healthcare.)*

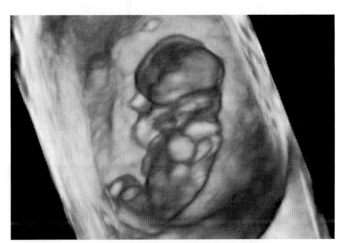

FIGURE 8–7. Three-dimensional sonogram of 12-week fetus showing normal umbilical cord fetal abdominal insertion. The physiologic herniation of bowel into the base of the cord that can be seen between 8 and 12 weeks should be completed by 12 weeks. *(Courtesy of Philips Healthcare.)*

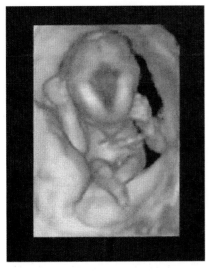

FIGURE 8–8. Three-dimensional sonogram of a 17-week fetus showing unfused cranial sutures. *(Courtesy of Philips Healthcare.)*

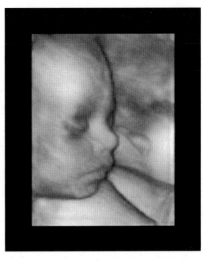

FIGURE 8–9. Three-dimensional sonogram of face of 20-week fetus. *(Courtesy of Philips Healthcare.)*

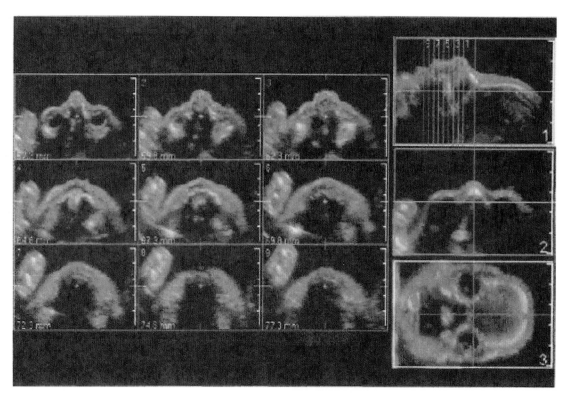

FIGURE 8-10. iSlice 3D showing normal fetal palate. *(Courtesy of Philips Healthcare.)*

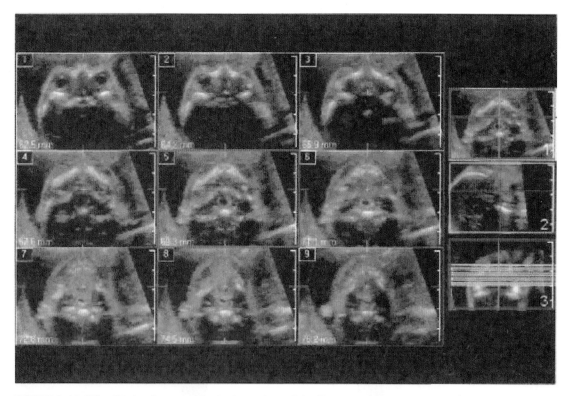

FIGURE 8-11. iSlice 3D showing normal fetal palate and mandible. *(Courtesy of Philips Healthcare.)*

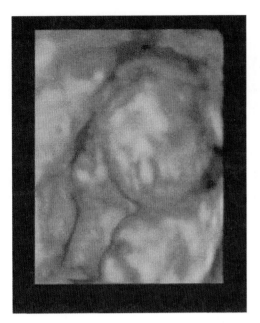

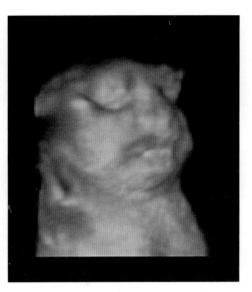

FIGURE 8–14. 3D sonogram of an encephalic fetus. *(Courtesy of Philips Healthcare.)*

FIGURE 8–12. Three-dimensional sonogram showing bilateral cleft palate. *(Courtesy of Philips Healthcare.)*

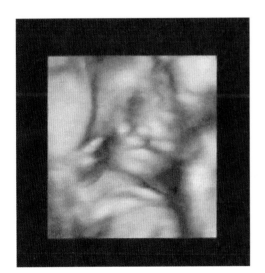

FIGURE 8–13. Three-dimensional sonogram of cleft lip and palate. *(Courtesy of Philips Healthcare.)*

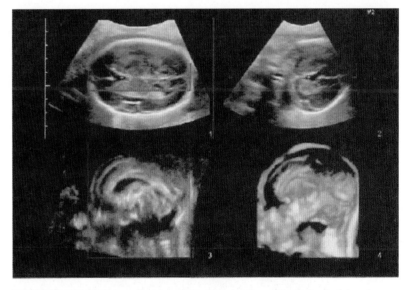

FIGURE 8–15. Multiplanar image and 3D reconstruction of the brain of a fetus at 25-weeks' gestation. The corpus callosum is clearly depicted on the volumetric image (4). *(Courtesy of Philips Healthcare.)*

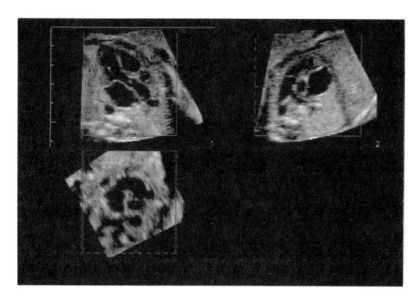

FIGURE 8–16. Spatial, temporal image correlation (STIC) of normal fetal ventricles/atria and outflow tracts. *(Courtesy of Philips Healthcare.)*

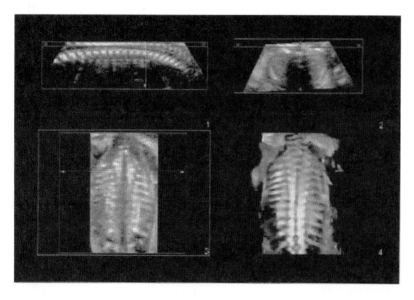

FIGURE 8–17. Multiplanar image of normal fetal spine. *(Courtesy of Philips Healthcare.)*

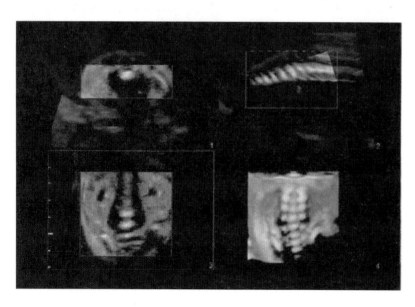

FIGURE 8–18. Multiplanar image of normal sacrum of a fetus at 26-weeks' gestation. *(Courtesy of Philips Healthcare.)*

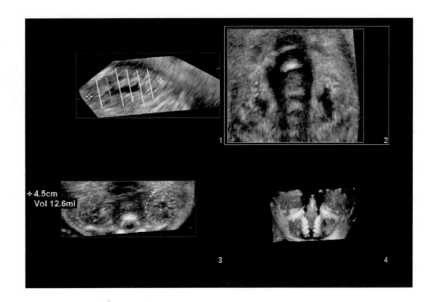

FIGURE 8–19. Multiplanar reconstructed image of normal kidneys. *(Courtesy of Philips Healthcare.)*

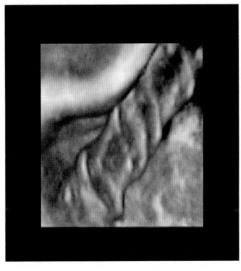

FIGURE 8–20. Three dimensional sonogram of normal umbilical cord showing two (paired) arteries coiled around umbilical vein. *(Courtesy of Philips Healthcare.)*

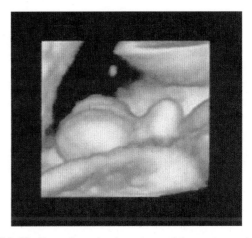

FIGURE 8–22. Three-dimensional sonogram of the scrotum and penis of a fetus at 31-weeks' gestation. *(Courtesy of Philips Healthcare.)*

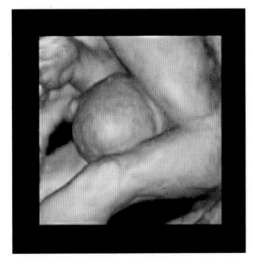

FIGURE 8–21. Three-dimensional sonogram of a fetus 26-weeks' gestation with a large omphalocele. *(Courtesy of Philips Healthcare.)*

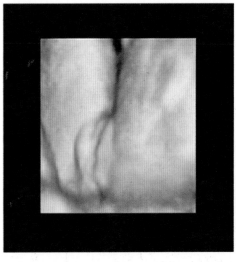

FIGURE 8–23. Three-dimensional sonogram of labia majora of a female fetus at 30-weeks' gestation. *(Courtesy of Philips Healthcare.)*

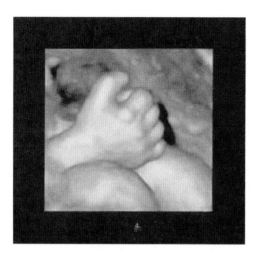

FIGURE 8–24. Three-dimensional sonogram of hand of a fetus at 29-weeks' gestation. *(Courtesy of Philips Healthcare.)*

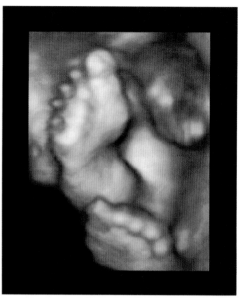

FIGURE 8–26. Three-dimensional sonogram of fetal feet and toes. *(Courtesy of Philips Healthcare.)*

exposure to ultrasound (see the American Institute of Ultrasound in Medicine statement regarding use of 3D ultrasound for "entertainment") should be avoided.

Fetal facial malformations such as cleft lip or cleft palate are readily seen on 3D. It is important to determine whether a cleft lip defect extends into the hard palate. Fetal facial anomalies have a higher association with brain malformations and 3D may be used to evaluate intracranial anomalies.

Three-dimensional sonography is particularly useful in the evaluation of the fetal heart. This is due to the ability to depict selected scan planes that may not be obtainable on 2D. The heart volume can be obtained with special software that affords spatial, temporal image correlation (STIC). This technique allows for systematic evaluation of cardiac structures regardless of fetal position.

Three-dimensional sonography may be useful in depicting complete anomalies involving an abnormal abdominal wall such as omphalocele or internal disruptions such as congenital diaphragmatic hernia. Using 3D, the actual volume of the remaining lungs of a fetus with congenital diaphragmatic hernia can be estimated.

Other applications of 3D in obstetrics include evaluation of placental vascular bed or umbilical cord insertion or coiling anomalies. Umbilical cord knots and nuchal cords are readily depicted on 3D.

Three-dimensional color Doppler sonography can provide the arrangement of intraplacental vessels as well as focal areas

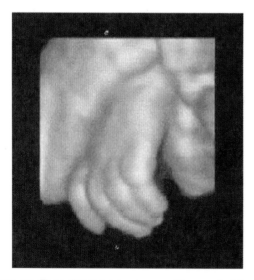

FIGURE 8–25. Three-dimensional sonogram of fingers of a fetus at 30-weeks' gestation. *(Courtesy of Philips Healthcare.)*

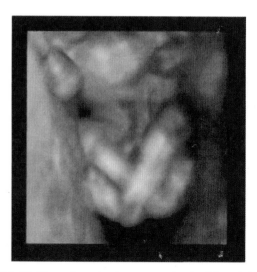

FIGURE 8–27. Three-dimensional sonogram showing bilateral club feet. *(Courtesy of Philips Healthcare.)*

of retroplacental hemorrhage. Three-dimensional sonography can depict abnormal umbilical cord placental insertion such as velamentous cord insertions onto the membrane rather than the placental surface chorionic plate.

Other applications may include using 3D sonography to depict ectopic pregnancies and their spatial relationship to the ovary, as well as to assess internal organ malformations. As 3D sonography is used more, sonographers will undoubtedly discover new and expanded clinical applications of this technique.

GYNECOLOGIC 3D SONOGRAPHY

Three-dimensional sonography has many clinical applications in gynecologic disorders (Figs. 8–28 through 8–37). As in obstetrical 3D, gynecologic 3D affords depiction of the uterus and ovaries in any selectable scan plane, including those not readily obtained with 2D. These include improved depiction of endometrial masses such as polyps or submucosal fibroids, improved localization and calculation of changes in fibroid volume, enhanced depiction of tubal masses, intrauterine device localization, and uterine malformations. Three-dimensional depiction of tumor morphology and vascularity within ovarian masses has important implications in distinguishing benign from malignant masses.

Three-dimensional sonography affords depiction of the configuration of the uterine fundus. With a septated uterus, the fundal contour is smooth, whereas with bicornuate and didelphys, a sharp cleft is seen.

Fibroids have a peripheral rim of vascularity and this is seen readily with 3D color Doppler sonography. Any collaterals such as those arising from the ovarian vessels can be seen. Marked changes in the vascularity fibroids such as that occurring post-uterine artery embolization can be documented accurately with 3D sonography.

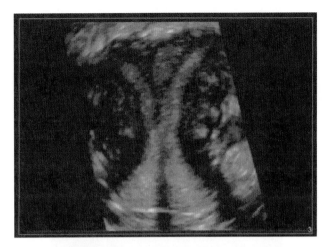

FIGURE 8–29. Two separate endometrial cavities and uterine horns. *(Courtesy of Philips Healthcare.)*

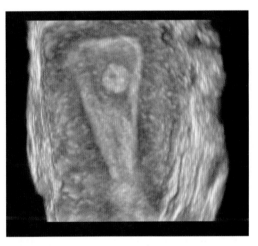

FIGURE 8–30. Endometrial polyp as shown in coronal plane 3D surface rendering pedunculated. *(Courtesy of Philips Healthcare.)*

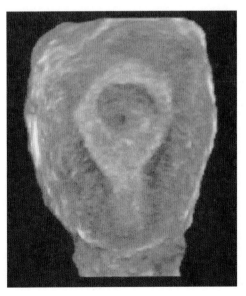

FIGURE 8–31. Submucosal fibroid that is intraluminal as depicted in coronal 3D. *(Courtesy of Philips Healthcare.)*

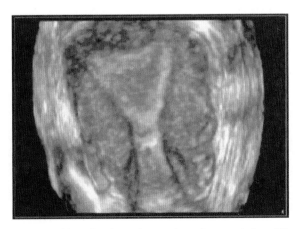

FIGURE 8–28. Normal endometrium as shown in coronal plane 3D. *(Courtesy of Philips Healthcare.)*

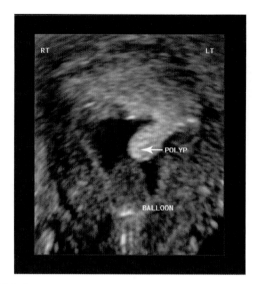

FIGURE 8–32. Three-dimensional surface-rendered image obtained during sonohysterography showing polyp (arrow). *(Courtesy of Philips Healthcare.)*

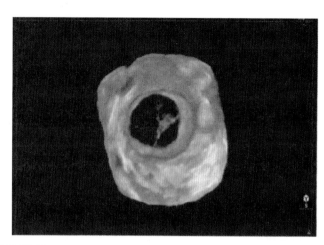

FIGURE 8–34. Three-dimensional image of ovarian cyst containing fibrin strands. *(Courtesy of Philips Healthcare.)*

Because of its ability to display in the coronal plane, 3D sonography is accurate in depicting intraluminal masses such as polyps or fibroids. The location of an intrauterine contraceptive device (IUCD) within the endometrium is readily depicted with 3D sonography. Three-dimensional sonography obtained in the transverse plane of the uterus fundus is also useful in identifying tubal masses since their origins can be traced to the cornual area of the uterus.

Three-dimensional sonography can depict focal wall irregularities within mostly cystic adnexal lesions. Three-dimensional color Doppler sonography can depict vessel density and

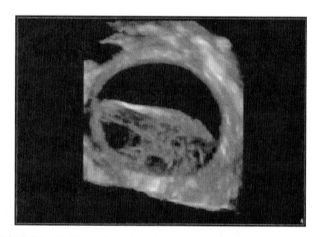

FIGURE 8–35. Three-dimensional image of hemorrhagic ovarian mass containing formed clot. *(Courtesy of Philips Healthcare.)*

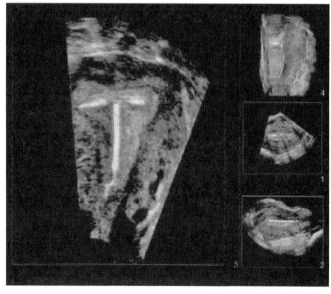

FIGURE 8–33. Multiplanar image showing centrally located intrauterine contraceptive device. *(Courtesy of Philips Healthcare.)*

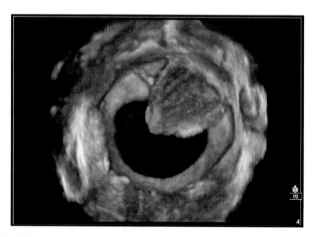

FIGURE 8–36. Three-dimensional image of ovarian tumor containing a papillary excrescence. *(Courtesy of Philips Healthcare.)*

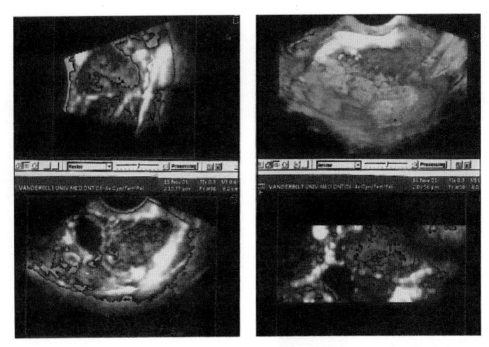

FIGURE 8–37. Three-dimensional images of ovarian cancer showing clusters of abnormal vessel (top right) in area of papillary excrescence. *(Courtesy of Philips Healthcare.)*

branching pattern. The vessels within a tumor typically are clustered and show differences in their caliber.

VOLUMETRIC SONOGRAPHY

Acquisition of large sample volumes affords later evaluation of organs in selected scan planes. Some advocate that volumetric acquisition in obstetrics and gynecology can expedite the examinations, making them quicker to obtain and complete.[3] Additional time is needed to obtain the required scan plans from the 3D volume set.

FUTURE APPLICATIONS

It is clear that 3D sonography has a role in the evaluation of certain obstetric and gynecologic disorders. Live 3D or "4D" can depict fetal behavior and also will have many applications for guided procedures.[4] Undoubtedly, future applications of this technique will evolve within its greater use.[5]

References

1. Merz E. *3D Ultrasound in Obstetrics/Gynecology.* New York: Lippincott Publishers; 1998.

2. Fleischer AC, Black AS, Grippo RJ, Pham T. 3D pelvic sonography: current use and potential applications. *J Women's Imaging.* 2003; 5(2):52-59.

3. Benacerraf BR. Tomographic sonography of the fetus: is it accurate enough to be a frontline screen for fetal malformation? *J Ultrasound Med.* 2006; 25:687-689.

4. Goncalves LF, Espinoza J, Kusanovic JP, et al. Applications of 2-dimensional matrix array for 3- and 4-dimensional examination of the fetus: a pictorial essay. *J Ultrasound Med.* 2006; 25:745-755.

5. Goncalves LF, Nien JK, Espinoza J, et al. What does 2-dimensional imaging add to 3- and 4-dimensional obstetric ultrasonography? *J Ultrasound Med.* 2006; 25:691-699.

Questions

GENERAL INSTRUCTIONS: For each question, select the best answer. Select only one answer for each question unless otherwise instructed.

1. The 3D sonogram in Fig. 8–38 is shown as which of the following?

   (A) surface-rendered image

   (B) multiplanar image

   (C) "see-through" or transparent mode image

   (D) has too many artifacts to be considered of diagnostic quality

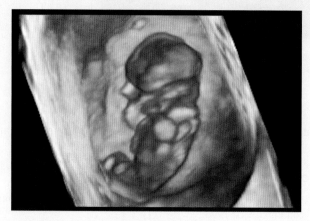

FIGURE 8–38. 3D sonogram of a 12-week fetus.

2. Which of the following statements is true concerning Fig. 8–38?

   (A) Cleft lip and palate are seen.

   (B) A large cranial structure defect is seen.

   (C) Numerous fetal limb abnormalities are seen.

   (D) None of the above

3. Which of the following statements is also true regarding Fig. 8–38?

   (A) There is a large diaphragmatic hernia.

   (B) There is a large abdominal wall hernia.

   (C) There is absence of an umbilical cord.

   (D) None of the above

4. Which of the following is a false statement concerning the image in Fig. 8–38?

   (A) There is an amniotic band.

   (B) There is anencephaly.

   (C) A and B

   (D) None of the above

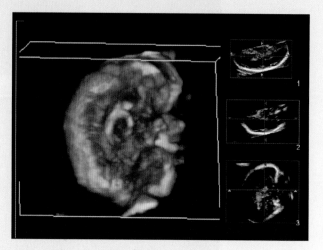

FIGURE 8–39. Long axis (1); short axis (2); and (3) coronal planes and 3D volume of the fetal brain in midline.

5. Which of the following is true concerning the 3D image in Fig. 8–39?

   (A) surface rendered

   (B) volume rendered

   (C) misleading

   (D) obtained through a lateral ventricle

6. The upside down U-shaped structure in the center of the 3D image in Fig. 8–39 is which of the following?

   (A) The corpus callosum

   (B) A large intraventricular clot

   (C) The choroid plexus

   (D) None of the above

7. Which of the following is shown in the 3D sonogram in Fig. 8–39?

   (A) marked ventricular dilation

   (B) agenesis of the corpus callosum

   (C) a vein of Galen aneurysm

   (D) none of the above

8. Which of the following statements is true concerning Fig. 8–39?

   (A) The fetus is brow down.

   (B) The fetus is in breech position.

   (C) The position of the fetus cannot be determined.

   (D) The fetus is anencephalic.

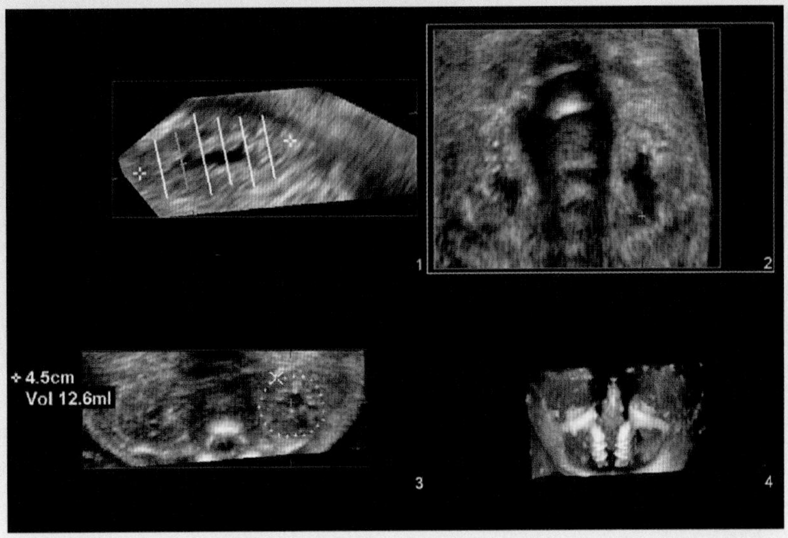

FIGURE 8-40. 3D sonogram of the kidneys of a second-trimester fetus.

9. In Fig. 8–40, image number 2 is taken through which of the following scan planes?

(A) long-axis

(B) short-axis

(C) coronal

(D) cannot be determined

10. In Fig. 8–40, which of the following best describes the appearance of the kidneys?

(A) normal

(B) polycystic

(C) atrophic

(D) cannot tell

11. Which of the following is usually shown in 3D sonography of infantile polycystic kidneys?

(A) multiple tiny cysts

(B) echogenic kidney

(C) enlarged kidney

(D) both B and C

12. Which of the following is true about the ureters on a second-trimester fetus on 3D sonography?

(A) cannot be seen in their entirety

(B) can be imaged in their long axis

(C) have fluid (urine) in there

(D) none of the above

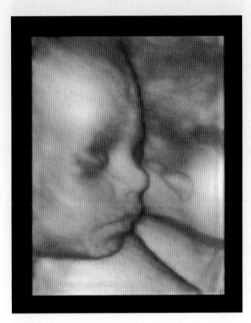

FIGURE 8-41. 3D sonogram of the fetal face.

13. In Fig. 8-41 what is the most common abnormal facial finding?

(A) bilateral cleft lip

(B) bilateral cleft palate

(C) both A and B

(D) neither A nor B

14. Short-axis images through the fetal hard palate may show which of the following characteristics?

(A) teeth buds

(B) cleft palate

(C) cleft lip

(D) all of the above

15. **Which of the following is usually true concerning cleft lip?**

    (A) an isolated anomaly

    (B) life threatening

    (C) associated with brain anomaly

    (D) surgically treatable *in utero*

16. **Which of the following can be said about transparency mode?**

    (A) may help delineation of the extent of the osseous abnormality

    (B) cannot be done since only surface rendition was done

    (C) reverses background colors

    (D) requires additional sweeps

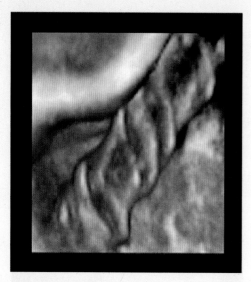

FIGURE 8–42. 3D sonogram of an umbilical cord.

17. **What does the 3D sonogram in Fig. 8–42 show?**

    (A) two umbilical arteries and one umbilical vein

    (B) abnormally loose coiling

    (C) abnormally tight coiling

    (D) none of the above

18. **Which of the following conditions is associated with a single umbilical artery?**

    (A) genitourinary abnormalities

    (B) central nervous system abnormalities

    (C) gastrointestinal abnormalities

    (D) all of the above

19. **Which of the following is true regarding the tightness or "pitch" of umbilical cord coiling?**

    (A) related to rotation of the fetus *in utero*

    (B) varies according to gestational age of the fetus

    (C) predictive of whether or not the fetus has "tumbled" *in utero*

    (D) is not predictive of anything

20. **3D of the umbilical cord is helpful in the diagnosis of which of the following?**

    (A) umbilical cord "knots"

    (B) umbilical cord entanglement in twins

    (C) determines the number of vessels within the cord

    (D) all of the above

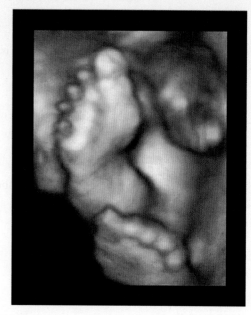

FIGURE 8-43. 3D sonogram of the feet of a near-term fetus.

21. **In Fig. 8-43 what does the image in this sonogram show?**

    (A) abnormal number of toes

    (B) typical "sandal" gap anomaly of the Down's fetus

    (C) both A and B

    (D) normal feet and toes

22. **Which of the following can be associated with club feet?**

    (A) meningomyelocele

    (B) many types of karyotypic anomalies

    (C) normal fetus

    (D) all of the above

23. Rockerbottom feet can be associated with which of the following conditions?

    (A) meningomyelocele

    (B) many types of karyotypic anomalies

    (C) normal fetus

    (D) all of the above

24. The relationship of the long bones of the leg to the foot is

    (A) best shown on 3D

    (B) best shown on 2D

    (C) is difficult to show when there is polyhydramnios

    (D) none of the above

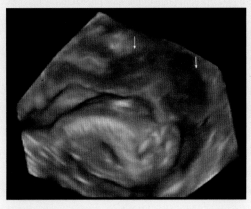

FIGURE 8–44. 3D placental sonogram.

25. What are the arrows pointing to in Fig. 8–44?

    (A) a large retroplacental hematoma

    (B) a 3D scanning artifact

    (C) a large marginal sinus hemorrhage

    (D) none of the above

26. This condition may be associated with which of the following?

    (A) severe maternal compromise

    (B) severe fetal compromise

    (C) both A and B

    (D) none of the above

27. Retroplacental hemorrhage is typically seen associated with which of the following conditions?

    (A) maternal hypertension (eclampsia)

    (B) trauma to abdomen

    (C) both A and B

    (D) amniocentesis

28. In patients with retroplacental hemorrhage, it is important to determine which parameters?

    (A) extent of retroplacental hemorrhage (relative to basal plate surface area)

    (B) the area of hemorrhage

    (C) both A and B

    (D) none of the above

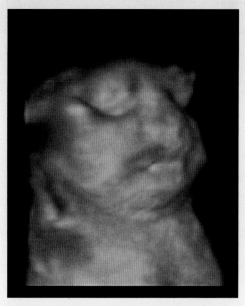

FIGURE 8–45. 3D sonogram of a second-trimester fetus.

29. What is the diagnosis of the fetus shown in Fig. 8–45?

    (A) hydrocephalus

    (B) 3D artifact

    (C) bilateral cleft palate

    (D) none of the above

30. Anencephaly is *not* closely associated with which one of the following findings?

    (A) meningomyelocele

    (B) agenesis of corpus callosum

    (C) decreased maternal serum alpha fetoprotein

    (D) maternal diabetes

31. Anencephaly is thought to be the result of which of the following?

    (A) failure of the anterior neuropore to close properly

    (B) failure of the posterior neuropore to close properly

    (C) maternal trauma

    (D) maternal hypertension

32. **Anencephaly is an example of which of the following?**

    (A) neural tube defect

    (B) normal embryonic stage

    (C) an inherited disorder

    (D) all of the above

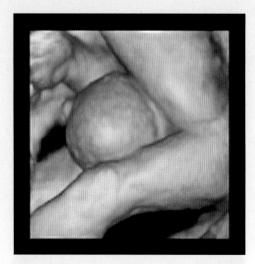

FIGURE 8–46. 3D sonogram of a fetus at 29-weeks' gestation.

33. **What is the diagnosis for the fetus shown in Fig. 8–46?**

    (A) omphalocele

    (B) scrotal mass

    (C) gastroschisis

    (D) none of the above

34. **Omphalocele may be associated with which of the following?**

    (A) karyotypic anomalies

    (B) ectopic heart (cordis)

    (C) diaphragmatic hernia

    (D) all of the above

35. **Gastroschisis is characterized by which of the following?**

    (A) eccentric herniation of the umbilical cord

    (B) higher probability of karyotypic anomaly than omphalocele

    (C) bowel covered by membrane

    (D) none of the above

36. **Omphaloceles may:**

    (A) contain liver and bowel

    (B) be transient and regress

    (C) may be both A and B

    (D) are neither A nor B

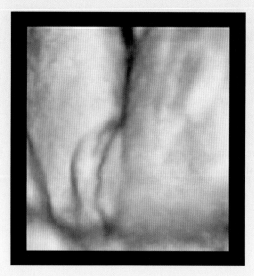

FIGURE 8–47. 3D sonogram of the fetal perineum.

37. **What is the sex of the fetus shown in Fig. 8–47?**

    (A) male

    (B) female

    (C) ambiguous

    (D) cannot be determined

38. **Which of the following is true regarding sonographic evaluation of fetal gender?**

    (A) helpful if karyotypic anomaly is suspected

    (B) endorsed by the AIUM as an indication for routine 3D sonography

    (C) usually misleading

    (D) none of the above

39. **Hypospadias may be associated with which of the following?**

    (A) hydronephrosis

    (B) renal anomalies

    (C) both A and B

    (D) none of the above

40. **Which type of 3D processing best depicts external genitalia?**

    (A) surface rendering

    (B) transparency mode

    (C) tomographic made

    (D) none of the above

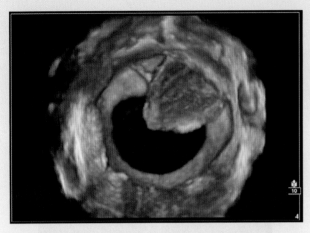

FIGURE 8–48. Multiplanar image and 3D surface volume of an ovary.

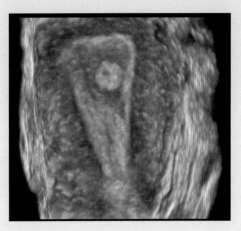

FIGURE 8–49. 3D uterine sonogram obtained in the coronal plane.

41. What is the most likely diagnosis of the finding in Fig. 8–48?

 (A) hemorrhagic cyst

 (B) ovarian tumor

 (C) neither A nor B

 (D) mature follicle

42. The low-level echoes within the mass probably represent which of the following?

 (A) hemorrhage

 (B) mucin

 (C) sebum

 (D) cannot be determined

43. Which of the following does the wall contain?

 (A) papillary excrescence

 (B) dermal sinus

 (C) blood clot

 (D) none of the above

44. What is the most common type of tumor that contains a papillary excrescence?

 (A) borderline serous cystadenoma

 (B) dermoid cyst

 (C) follicular cyst

 (D) hemorrhagic cyst

45. What is the most likely diagnosis of the finding in Fig. 8–49?

 (A) polyp

 (B) pedunculated submucosal fibroid

 (C) uterine septum

 (D) none of the above

46. Polyps may be associated with which of the following?

 (A) infertility

 (B) pain and bleeding

 (C) carcinoma

 (D) all of the above

47. Which of the following is the most appropriate treatment of a polyp?

 (A) wire-loop resection

 (B) dilation and curettage

 (C) don't ask me; I'm just a sonographer

 (D) hysteroscopic removal with polyp forceps

48. What is the best way to distinguish fibroids from polyps?

 (A) They are more echogenic than polyps

 (B) polyps may contain tiny cystic spaces

 (C) blood supply

 (D) none of the above

49. What abnormality is seen in Fig. 8–50?

    (A) endometrial polyp

    (B) submucosal fibroid

    (C) adhesion

    (D) cannot be determined

50. What is the relative chance that a polyp is cancerous?

    (A) low

    (B) high

    (C) cannot be determined based on 3D

    (D) none of the above

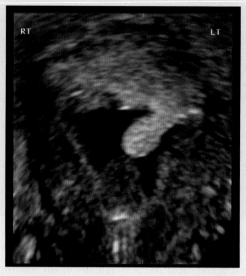

FIGURE 8–50. 3D sonogram obtained during sonohysterography.

Answers and Explanations

At the end of each explained answer, there is a number combination in parentheses. The first number identifies the reference source; the second number or set of numbers indicates the page or pages on which the relevant information can be found.

1. **(A)** This is a surface-rendered image. *(1:90)*

2. **(D)** None of the above. This is a normal 12-week fetus whose abdominal wall is intact after physiologic herniation of bowel that was completed one week earlier. *(1:90)*

3. **(D)** None of the above. See explanation in answer 2. *(1:90)*

4. **(C)** None of the above. See explanation in answer 2. *(1:90)*

5. **(A)** This is a surface-rendered image taken in the midsagittal plane. *(2:687)*

6. **(A)** This is the corpus callosum, which forms from posterior to anterior. *(2:687)*

7. **(D)** None of the above. See explanation in answer 6. *(2:687)*

8. **(C)** Cannot tell the position of the fetus. *(2:687)*

9. **(C)** This is a coronal image of normal kidneys. *(2:687)*

10. **(A)** Normal. See explanation in answer 9. *(2:687)*

11. **(D)** The kidneys are enlarged and echogenic due to multiple dilated renal tubules. *(2:687)*

12. **(A)** Cannot be seen in their entirety. It is difficult to delineate the entire ureter on 3D. *(2:267)*

13. **(D)** This fetus is normal. *(1:113)*

14. **(D)** The cleft lip is best shown on 3D. *(1:113)*

15. A cleft lip is usually an isolated anomaly but can be associated with a sporadic karyotypic abnormality. *(1:113)*

16. **(A)** Transparency mode is used to delineate bony abnormalities. *(1:90)*

17. **(A)** This 3D sonogram of the umbilical cord shows two umbilical arteries and one umbilical vein. *(1:99)*

18. **(D)** All can be associated with a single umbilical artery. *(1:99)*

19. **(A)** The tightness of the coil of the umbilical cord is related to fetal movement *in utero*. *(1:99)*

20. **(D)** 3D is helpful in all of these. *(1:99)*

21. **(D)** These are normal feet and toes. *(1:98)*

22. **(D)** All of these are associated with a club foot. *(1:116)*

23. **(D)** See answer to question 22. *(1:116)*

24. **(A)** 3D is helpful in showing the relationship of the long bones of the leg to the foot. *(1:116)*

25. **(C)** There is a large marginal sinus hemorrhage. *(1:138)*

26. **(B)** This can severely compromise fetal well-being. *(1:138)*

27. **(C)** Both conditions may result in retroplacental hemorrhage. *(1:138)*

28. **(C)** Both are important parameters. *(1:138)*

29. **(D)** This fetus has anencephaly; none of the choices is correct. *(1:111)*

30. **(C)** The alpha-fetoprotein level is decreased. *(1:111)*

31. **(A)** Anencephaly is thought to be a true result of failed closure of the anterior neuropore. *(1:111)*

32. **(A)** Anencephaly is an example of a neural tube defect. Meningomyelocele is another. *(1:111)*

33. **(A)** This is an omphalocele. *(1:115)*

34. **(D)** Omphaloceles may be associated with all of the conditions listed. *(1:115)*

35. **(A)** Gastroschisis involves eccentric herniation of the umbilical cord from a weakening in the right side of the cord insertion. It is usually an isolated defect. *(1:115)*

36. **(A)** Omphaloceles may involve liver and bowel. *(1:115)*

37. **(B)** This shows labia major on a female fetus. *(1:100)*

38. **(A)** It may be helpful to diagnose a specific karyotypic abnormality. *(1:100)*

39. **(C)** Hypospadias involves abnormal penile opening of the urethra and can be associated with renal anomalies and hydronephrosis. *(1:115)*

40. **(A)** Surface rendering best shows external genitalia. *(1:115)*

41. **(B)** This is an ovarian mass with a papillary excrescence. *(1:45)*

42. **(A)** Low-level echoes are arising from hemorrhage. *(1:45)*

43. **(A)** The wall has a large papillary excrescence. *(1:45)*

44. **(A)** Papillary excrescences are frequently seen in borderline serous ovarian cystadenoma *(1:45)*

45. **(A)** This shows a polyp. *(1:61)*

46. **(D)** All of these may be associated with a polyp. *(1:61)*

47. **(D)** They can be removed hysteroscopically with polyp forceps. If there is a pedunculated submucosal fibroid, wire-loop resection is typically performed. *(1:61)*

48. **(B)** Polyps typically contain tiny cystic spaces representing glandular elements. *(1:61)*

49. **(A)** This is an endometrial polyp. *(1:61)*

50. **(A)** Low. Only 3% of polyps are cancerous. *(1:61)*

9

Fetal Echocardiography

Teresa M. Bieker

Study Guide

INTRODUCTION

Congenital heart disease is a leading cause of infant mortality, with a reported incidence of approximately 1 in 100 live births.[1] However, these numbers are based on live-born infants and, therefore, probably underestimate the true incidence in the fetus.[2] Early fetal loss and stillbirths are often the result of complex cardiac defects or chromosomal defects, which have an associated heart defect. For this reason, the incidence of congenital heart disease in the fetus has been reported to be as much as five times that found in live-born children[1] (Table 9–1).

In utero diagnosis of congenital heart disease allows a variety of treatment options to be considered, including delivery at an appropriate facility, termination, and in some cases, *in utero* therapy.[3] Conversely, a normal fetal echocardiogram in the setting of an increased risk factor provides reassurance for both the patient and the physician.

INSTRUMENTATION AND TECHNIQUE

The American Institute of Ultrasound in Medicine (AIUM) Technical Bulletin on the performance of a basic fetal cardiac ultrasound recommends that a four-chamber view and both the right and the left ventricular outflow tracts be obtained on all obstetrical ultrasound exams.[4] Evaluation of a four-chamber view alone may substantially decrease the detection rate of some major cardiac malformations.

When risk factors increase the likelihood of congenital heart disease, a formal and more detailed fetal echocardiogram should be performed.

Various reports advocate evaluation of the fetal heart at different gestational ages[5]; however, the AIUM Technical Bulletin recommends that fetal echocardiographic exams be performed between 18 and 22 weeks of gestation.[4] During this period, optimum image quality and, therefore, diagnostic accuracy are achieved. It should be borne in mind that even at 18 weeks of gestation, the fetal heart is a very small structure. Before this age, many cardiac structures may be too small to evaluate accurately.[6] Recent advances in ultrasound have led to first-trimester screening of the fetal heart. Cardiac position, as well as a four-chamber view and outflow tracts, can be evaluated by a transabdominal or endovaginal approach. Obtaining these views, however, is dependent on fetal size and position.[7] In addition, cardiac lesions such as coarctation of the aorta and hypoplastic left heart syndrome may be progressive lesions.[8,9] Therefore, scanning the fetus too early in gestation may result in a false-negative diagnosis.

Later in gestation, the echocardiographic exam may be hindered by increased attenuation from the fetal skull, ribs, spine, and limbs, as well as decreased amniotic fluid as pregnancy progresses.[6]

Equipment

Fetal echocardiography requires the use of high-resolution ultrasound equipment.[10] Preferred transducer frequencies usually range from 5 to 7 MHz, depending on gestational age, maternal body habitus, and the amount of amniotic fluid present. Equipment utilized for fetal echocardiography should have M-mode and pulsed Doppler capabilities to provide physiologic assessment, as well as color Doppler capabilities to assess spatial and directional information. All of these modalities are vital to performing a complete and accurate examination.

Indications

A family history of congenital heart disease is the most common indication to perform a fetal echocardiogram. Recurrence risk for fetuses varies depending on the type of lesion and their relationship to the affected relative.

493

TABLE 9–1 • Frequency of Congenital Heart Lesions Among Affected Abortuses and Stillborn Infants	
Defect	**Frequency (%)**
Ventricular septal defect	35.7
Coarctation of the aorta	8.9
Atrial septal defect	8.2
Atrioventricular septal defect	6.7
Tetralogy of Fallot	6.2
Single ventricle	4.8
Truncus arteriosus	4.8
Hypoplastic left heart	4.6
Complete transposition of the great arteries	4.3
Double outlet right ventricle	2.4
Hypoplastic right heart	1.7
Single atrium	1.2
Pulmonic stenosis	0.7
Aortic stenosis	0.5
Miscellaneous	10.6

Modified from Hoffman JIE. Incidence of congenital heart disease: II. Prenatal incidence. *Pediatr Cardiol.* 1995; 16:155–165.

TABLE 9–2 • Recurrence Risk in Siblings for any Congenital Heart Defect		
	Suggested Risk (%)	
Defect	**If One Sibling Affected**	**If Two Siblings Affected**
Aortic stenosis	2	6
Atrial septal defect	2.5	8
Atrioventricular canal	3	10
Coarctation of the aorta	2	6
Ebstein anomaly	1	3
Endocardial fibroelastosis	4	12
Hypoplastic left heart	2	6
Pulmonary atresia	1	3
Pulmonary stenosis	2	6
Tetralogy of Fallot	2.5	8
Transposition	1.5	5
Tricuspid atresia	1	3
Truncus arteriosus	1	3
Ventricular septal defect	3	10

Adapted from Nora JJ, Fraser FC, Bear J, et al. *Medical Genetics: Principles and Practice.* 4th ed. Philadelphia: Lea & Febiger; 1994:371.

The risk of congenital heart disease for a fetus with an affected sibling is approximately 2–4%.[11,12] If two or more siblings are affected, this risk increases to approximately 10% (Table 9–2). When the mother of the fetus has a congenital heart abnormality, the recurrence risk is also approximately 10–12%.[12] An affected father carries a lower risk (Table 9–3).[11,12]

Exposure to known cardiac teratogens also increases the risk of having a fetus with a cardiac defect.[13] The list of substances considered teratogenic is extensive.[14] Specific occurrence risk varies with length and type of exposure, as well as the specific substance involved.

Chromosomal abnormalities have been reported to occur in 13% of live-born infants with a congenital heart defect.[15,16] The incidence of abnormal karyotype in the fetus with a congenital heart abnormality is approximately 35%.[2,17] Fetuses with an increased nuchal translucency during a first-trimester ultrasound also have an increased risk for congenital heart defects.[18]

The specific type and occurrence risk of a congenital heart defect vary depending on the chromosomal abnormality. Trisomy 21 is associated with a 40–50% occurrence of congenital heart disease,[15] whereas in trisomy 13 and trisomy 18, the association is almost 100%.[19] As with teratogenic agents, the list of abnormal karyotypes and syndromes associated with cardiac defects is extensive.[14]

Several maternal conditions may also carry an inherent risk to the fetus. Congenital heart disease is increased fivefold among infants of diabetic mothers,[17] whereas phenylketonuria has a reported risk of 12–16%.[20]

Complete heart block in the fetus is associated with maternal collagen vascular disease (systemic lupus erythematosus).

TABLE 9-3 • Suggested Offspring Recurrence Risk for Congenital Heart Defects Given One Affected Parent

	Suggested Risk (%)	
Defect	Father Affected	Mother Affected
Aortic stenosis	3	13–18
Atrial septal defect	1.5	4–4.5
Atrioventricular canal	1	14
Coarctation of the aorta	2	4
Pulmonary stenosis	2	4–6.5
Tetralogy of Fallot	1.5	2.5
Ventricular septal defect	2	6–10

Adapted from Nora JJ, Fraser FC, Bear J, et al. *Medical Genetics: Principles and Practice.* 4th ed. Philadelphia: Lea & Febiger; 1994:371.

TABLE 9-4 • Incidence of Associated Congenital Heart Defects Occurring with Extracardiac Malformations in Infants

System or Lesion	Frequency of CHD (%)
Central nervous system	
Hydrocephalus	4.5–14.8
Dandy–Walker malformation	2.5–4.3
Agenesis of the corpus callosum	14.9
Meckel–Gruber syndrome	13.8
Gastrointestinal	
Tracheoesophageal fistula	14.7–39.2
Duodenal atresia	17.1
Jejunal atresia	5.2
Anorectal anomalies	22
Imperforate anus	11.7
Ventral wall	
Omphalocele	19.5–32
Gastroschisis	0–7.7
Diaphragmatic hernia	9.6–22.9
Genitourinary	
Renal agenesis (bilateral)	42.8
Renal agenesis (unilateral)	16.9
Horseshoe kidney	38.8
Renal dysplasia	5.4
Ureteral obstruction	2.1

Modified from Copel JA, Pilu G, Kleinman CS. Congenital heart disease and extracardiac anomalies: associations and indications for fetal echocardiography. *Am J Obstet Gynecol.* 1986; 154:1121–1132.

In these patients, circulating antinuclear antibodies of the SSA or SSB types damage the developing conduction tissue.[21]

Maternal infections such as human parvovirus and cytomegalovirus also have a reported association with cardiac defects in the fetus.[22]

Another indication for performing a fetal echocardiogram is the presence of extracardiac anomalies in a fetus.[23] The overall incidence of extracardiac malformations in children identified as having a congenital heart abnormality ranges from 25% to 45% (Table 9-4).[23] Cardiac abnormalities such as atrioventricular septal defects are associated with extracardiac defects in more than 50% of cases, while atrial septal defects, ventricular septal defects, tetralogy of Fallot, and cardiac malpositions are associated with extracardiac malformations in about 30% of cases.[23]

A suspected structural or rhythm abnormality seen in the fetal heart on a routine obstetrical examination should also warrant a formal fetal echocardiogram to rule out an underlying structural abnormality or, in some cases, to implement *in utero* therapy.

Nonimmune hydrops fetalis is also an indication for fetal echocardiography. In some cases, it may reflect structural heart disease, while in others, it is the result of a dysrhythmia.[21] Finally, massive polyhydramnios is a recognized indication for fetal echocardiography.[21] An increase in amniotic fluid may be the result of congestive heart failure, but it is more likely related to associated defects in the fetus, such as those that cause difficulty in swallowing or compression of the esophagus. Although there are several predisposing indications to perform a fetal echocardiogram, up to 90% of congenital heart disease occurs in unselected "normal" obstetric patients.[1] Therefore, routine obstetric scanning should identify the majority of fetuses with cardiac lesions that will need a formal fetal echocardiogram.

Position

A fetal echocardiographic exam should always begin by determining fetal position. Unlike a pediatric or adult patient, the fetus cannot be placed in a standard position, nor can the heart be evaluated consistently from routine angles. Although the fetus may move throughout the exam, establishing basic position will allow the examiner to identify various cardiac structures more quickly.[6] Once fetal position is determined, the location and orientation of the heart should be established. In a cross-sectional transverse view of the fetal chest, the correct orientation for the fetal heart is with the apex pointing to the left and the bulk of the heart occupying the left chest. The normal angle of the fetal heart, relative to midline is 45 ± 20°.[24] The left atrium should be located closest to the fetal spine and the right ventricle nearest to the anterior chest wall. This normal orientation is termed *levocardia*.

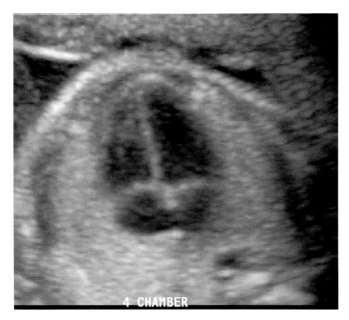

FIGURE 9–1. Apical four-chamber view showing the interventricular and interatrial septae parallel to the ultrasound beam.

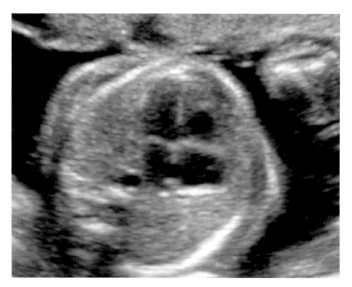

FIGURE 9–2. Apical four-chamber view showing a "pseudo" interventricular septal defect, caused by the septum being parallel to the sound beam.

The normal fetal heart should occupy approximately one-third of the fetal thorax.[25] Fetal cardiac size can be calculated by measuring the diameter or the circumference of the heart and comparing it to the diameter or circumference of the fetal chest, respectively. When calculating this ratio, both measurements must be obtained from the same image.

Scanning Technique

The first view to obtain when beginning a fetal echocardiographic examination is the four-chamber view.[14] There are two different four-chamber views. The apical four-chamber view and the subcostal four-chamber view. The apical four-chamber view is obtained in a transverse view of the fetal chest, with the transducer imaging the fetal heart from either the anterior or the posterior aspect.

In the apical four-chamber view, all four cardiac chambers can be visualized (Fig. 9–1). In addition, color or pulsed Doppler interrogation of the mitral and tricuspid valves can be performed. Doppler should be performed on the atrial side of the valves to assess for valvular insufficiency, whereas Doppler distal to the valves should be done to evaluate for stenosis or atresia. The two superior pulmonary veins should also be identified entering the left atrium from this projection. The two inferior pulmonary veins are usually not visualized on a fetal echocardiogram.

The apical four-chamber view is not optimal for evaluating the interventricular septum (IVS). In this view, the angle of incidence of the sound beam is parallel to the interventricular septum and may result in an artifactual dropout of echoes at the level of the membranous portion, simulating a "pseudo" septal defect (Fig. 9–2).[26]

By sliding the transducer cephalad from an apical four-chamber view, the aorta and pulmonary artery should be visualized side by side (Fig. 9–3). This confirms that both are present and normally of equal size.

The subcostal four-chamber view is obtained by imaging the fetal chest in a transverse projection from the anterior chest wall and angling the transducer slightly cephalad (Fig. 9–4). This view also allows identification and comparison of both atria and ventricles. It is ideal for obtaining M-mode measurements of the ventricles and interventricular septum by placing an M-mode cursor perpendicular to the septum at the level of the atrioventricular valves (Fig. 9–5).

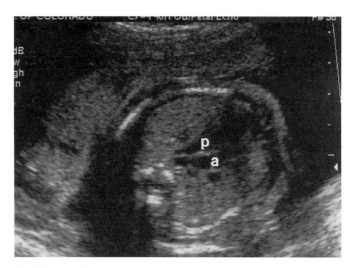

FIGURE 9–3. Three vessel view. The aorta (a) and pulmonary artery (p) can be seen as two parallel structures by angling the transducer cephalad from the apical four-chamber view. The superior vena cava is seen in cross section. This view allows you to confirm that both great vessels are present and are of similar size.

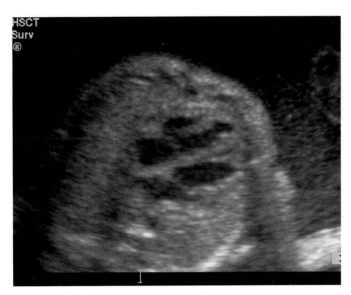

FIGURE 9–4. Subcostal four-chamber view with the interventricular and interatrial septae perpendicular to the sound beam.

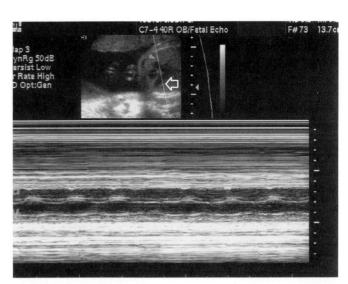

FIGURE 9–6. M-mode tracing through the right atrial (a, arrowhead) and left ventricular (v, open arrow) wall simultaneously to assess the response of each in the setting of a dysrhythmia.

Atrial measurements can be obtained by moving the M-mode cursor through both atria. The subcostal four-chamber view is also preferable for evaluating a fetal dysrhythmia by placing the M-mode cursor through an atrial wall and a ventricular wall simultaneously (Fig. 9–6). This allows visualization of the timing of dysrhythmic events and may aid in making a definitive diagnosis.

Either pulsed Doppler or color Doppler can be used to evaluate the foramen ovale in the subcostal projection. Documentation of flow from the right atrium to the left atrium by either modality rules out restriction of the foraminal flap (Fig. 9–7). It is also valuable in assessing altered flow direction secondary to a structural defect. A spectral Doppler tracing will display normal foraminal flow as being twice the fetal heart rate.

The interventricular septum (IVS) is best evaluated in the subcostal four-chamber view since the ultrasound beam is perpendicular to the intraventricular septum. Color Doppler is the best means of achieving this because it allows a large area to be evaluated simultaneously (Fig. 9–8). Pulsed Doppler may not detect flow across a septal defect if the sample volume is not precisely located.

Larger ventricular septal defects may be detected with gray scale imaging alone; however, many remain undetected by any means. Even when a ventricular septal defect is present, the pressures in the fetal heart are such that no flow may be appreciated across the interventricular septum.

Obtaining a subcostal four-chamber view is critical in performing a complete fetal echocardiogram. By angling the transducer

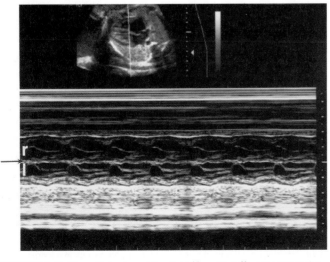

FIGURE 9–5. M-mode tracing of the right (r) and left (l) ventricles at the level of the atrioventricular valves. Arrow = interventricular septum (IVS).

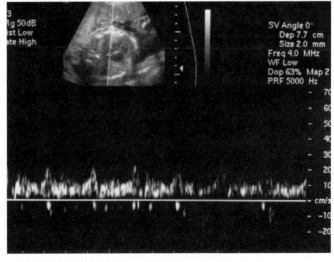

FIGURE 9–7. Pulsed Doppler tracing of the foramen ovale documenting flow from the right atrium into the left atrium.

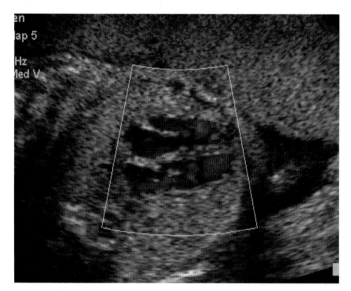

FIGURE 9-8. Color Doppler image showing no flow crossing the intact interventricular septum.

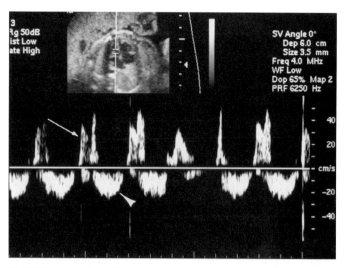

FIGURE 9-10. Pulsed Doppler tracing showing the mitral valve inflow (arrow) simultaneously with the aortic valve (arrowhead) outflow.

systematically toward the fetal right shoulder from this view, most of the remaining fetal heart views are obtained.

A slight angulation from the subcostal four-chamber view toward the fetal right shoulder will result in visualization of a long-axis view of the proximal aorta. In this view, continuity of the anterior wall of the aorta with the interventricular septum and the posterior wall with the anterior leaflet of the mitral valve can by determined (Fig. 9–9). The aortic valve can be interrogated with pulsed Doppler in this view, both proximally looking for aortic insufficiency, and distally to detect stenosis or atresia.

The long-axis view of the aorta also provides another means of evaluating a dysrhythmia. By utilizing a wide sample gate and placing the pulsed Doppler cursor between the mitral and aortic valves, both left ventricular inflow and outflow can be evaluated simultaneously (Fig. 9–10). The inflow through the mitral valve will reflect rhythm disturbances occurring in the atria; whereas, the left ventricular outflow through the aorta reflects the ventricular response. Being able to visualize both events simultaneously may help in differentiating the type of dysrhythmia present.

The right ventricular outflow tract is visualized next by rotating the transducer further in the direction of the fetal right shoulder. In the normal fetus, this view demonstrates the pulmonary artery coursing cephalad, leftward, and posteriorly from the right ventricle (Fig. 9–11). The course of the pulmonary artery should cross

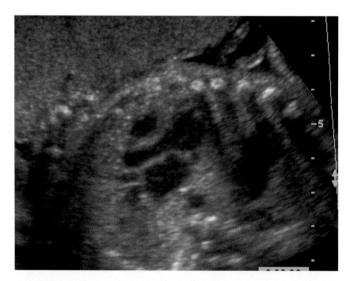

FIGURE 9-9. Long-axis view of the aorta arising from the left ventricle. Continuity can be appreciated between the anterior wall of the aorta and the interventricular septum, and the posterior wall of the aorta with the anterior leaflet of the mitral valve.

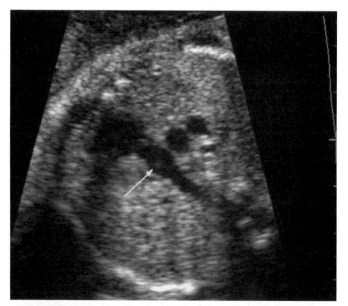

FIGURE 9-11. Continuous angulation of the transducer toward the fetal right shoulder from the long-axis view of the aorta, results in a long-axis view of the pulmonary artery (arrow) arising from the right ventricle. This is the three-vessel view.

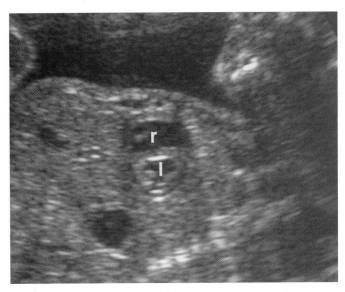

FIGURE 9-12. Sagittal view of the fetus, showing a short-axis view of the right (r) and left (l) ventricles.

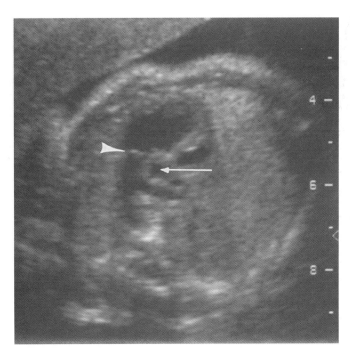

FIGURE 9-13. Angulation toward the fetus's left shoulder from the short-axis view of the ventricles (Fig. 9–12), results in a short-axis view of the great vessels. The pulmonary artery (arrowhead) can be seen normally draping over the aorta (arrow).

the aorta in the normal fetus. In other words, by angling the transducer from the long-axis view of the aorta to the long-axis view of the pulmonary, the great vessels should "criss-cross" directions if they are correctly oriented. Color or pulsed Doppler are again used in this projection to evaluate the valve proximally for pulmonic insufficiency and distally for pulmonic stenosis or atresia.

A further rightward rotation of the transducer will result in a sagittal view of the fetal thorax and thus a short-axis view through the ventricles (Fig. 9–12). The echogenic moderator band should be apparent near the apex to help in identifying the right ventricle.

The short-axis view of the ventricles is useful for obtaining measurements of the ventricular free walls and interventricular septum, as well as chamber size. Color Doppler should be used in this view to again evaluate the interventricular septum for defects. With the color Doppler activated, the ventricles should be scanned from the apex to the level of the atrioventricular valves. If color is seen crossing the septum, pulsed Doppler can be used to confirm a septal defect.

From the short-axis view of the ventricles, a short-axis view of the great vessels can be obtained by angling the transducer slightly toward the fetal left shoulder (Fig. 9–13). In this view, the aorta appears as a circular structure with the pulmonary artery draping over it. The aortic, pulmonic, and tricuspid valves are usually well visualized in this projection. The main pulmonary artery can often be seen bifurcating into the ductus arteriosus and the right pulmonary artery. This view provides a reasonable angle from which the pulmonary and tricuspid valves can be interrogated with pulsed Doppler for insufficiency or stenosis or atresia. The great vessels can also be evaluated for size discrepancy in the short-axis view.

Simultaneous M-mode through the aorta, and left atrium is another useful method for evaluating fetal dysrhythmias

(Fig. 9–14). The atrial contraction will be depicted in atrial wall movement, while the ventricular response is reflected in the motion of the aortic valve.

In the normal heart, the short-axis view of the great vessels confirms the perpendicular relationship of the aorta to the pulmonary artery, thereby excluding such defects as complete or *d*-transposition of the great arteries or truncus arteriosus.

The aortic arch view is obtained from a sagittal plane of the fetal torso, with the transducer angled from the left shoulder to

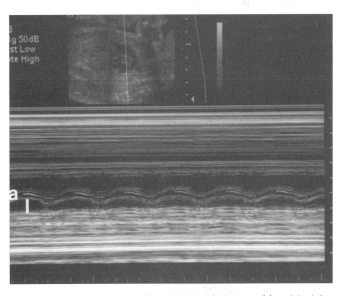

FIGURE 9-14. Simultaneous M-mode through the aorta (a) and the left atrium (l) is a useful means of assessing a dysrhythmia.

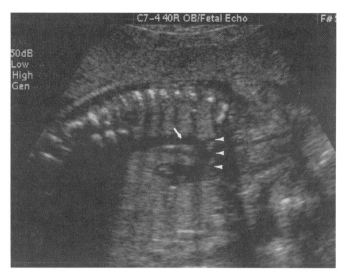

FIGURE 9–15. Sagittal view of the aortic arch (arrow) with the three brachiocephalic vessels (arrowheads) arising from it.

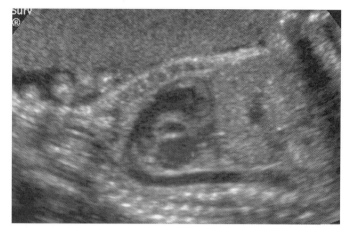

FIGURE 9–16. Sagittal view of the ductal arch with a flatter appearance than the aortic arch.

the right hemithorax. The aortic arch can be differentiated from the flatter, broader, more caudally located ductal arch by identifying the three brachiocephalic vessels arising from its superior aspect (Fig. 9–15). The aortic arch has been described as having a rounded "candy cane" appearance.[25]

Pulsed Doppler should be used to evaluate the arch from the aortic valve to the descending aorta, looking for areas of increased or decreased velocities. Of particular importance is the section of the arch between the origin of the left subclavian artery and the insertion of the ductus arteriosus, as this is where most *in utero* coarctations occur. It should be borne in mind, however, that diagnosis of coarctation of the aorta is extremely difficult, and a coarctation may be present even in the setting of a normal appearing aortic arch, with normal velocities. When evaluating the aortic arch, it is also important to remember to confirm a left-sided location of the descending aorta.

The ductal arch view is obtained by returning to a more anteroposterior axis of the thorax. It is often helpful to image the short-axis view of the great vessels and then angle the transducer slightly until the pulmonary artery/ductus arteriosus confluence connects with the descending aorta (Fig. 9–16). The ductal arch has a flatter appearance than the aortic arch. It is often referred to as having a "hockey stick" appearance.[25] The ductal arch is composed the pulmonary artery, ductus arteriosus, and the descending aorta.

The final view that should be obtained is the right atrial inflow view, allowing visualization of the inferior and superior vena cavae. This is achieved by sliding the transducer rightward from the aortic arch while remaining in a sagittal plane of the fetus (Fig. 9–17).

Pulsed Doppler

Pulsed Doppler substantially enhances the ability to detect cardiac malformations *in utero*. It is an effective means of quanti-

tating flow velocity in the cardiac vessels and across the heart valves, as well as determining flow direction. It is also a useful adjunct in differentiating dysrhythmias.[21] In a standard fetal echocardiogram, pulsed Doppler should be used to evaluate all four cardiac valves, both proximal and distal to the valve. Pulsed Doppler interrogation of the foramen ovale should be done to document the presence of flow into the left atrium. The ductus arteriosus and aortic arch should also be interrogated to document the presence and normality of flow. In addition, pulsed Doppler of the pulmonary veins can be used to confirm their presence and course into the left atrium.

Technical factors to consider include attempting to place the Doppler cursor in the area of interest at an angle as close to 0° as possible by using transducer angulation and the angle correction capabilities of the equipment used. The sample gate should be set small enough so that interference from wall noise and transmitted flow from adjoining vessels or valves can be minimized. Wall filter should be set to eliminate unnecessary noise without losing essential low flow information, and velocity scale should be set to record maximum velocities accurately.

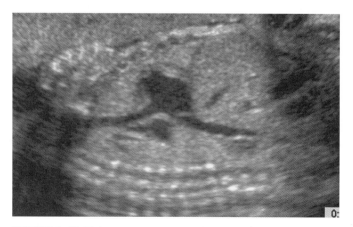

FIGURE 9–17. Right atrial inflow view showing the inferior vena cava and the superior vena cava entering the right atrium.

Color Doppler

Color Doppler also plays an essential role in fetal echocardiography by providing a more efficient and expedient means of assessing normal and abnormal flow patterns in the fetal heart. Color Doppler supplies information on the presence or absence of flow, flow direction, and flow patterns. By superimposing color over the gray-scale image, morphologic and hemodynamic information can be assessed simultaneously.

Color Doppler allows visualization of flow in entire structures, such as the aortic arch, thus making it much more time efficient than pulsed Doppler. This efficiency is also prudent when imaging a fetus because color Doppler imaging produces lower peak intensities than pulsed Doppler.

Color Doppler can simplify the investigation of valvular stenosis or insufficiency, again, by sampling a large area and identifying areas of turbulence or flow reversal. In some cases, color may aid in visualizing such cardiac structures as the outflow tracts, which may be difficult to see with gray-scale imaging alone. Also, it may occasionally lead to detection of an abnormality not obvious on the gray-scale image, such as valvular stenosis, small ventricular septal defects, and flow reversal within the aortic and ductal arches.

Equipment used for fetal echocardiography should have specific fetal cardiac capabilities utilizing higher pulse repetition frequencies, which allow color imaging at a frame rate fast enough to evaluate the rapid fetal heart rate. Using a narrow color field or reducing the image depth, when possible, may be necessary to maintain an adequate frame rate.

It is important to remember that color Doppler will only provide mean velocity information; therefore, pulsed Doppler is a necessary adjunct to color Doppler to provide quantitative information regarding peak velocities.

Power Doppler

Power Doppler, in general, may hold several advantages over color Doppler such as increased sensitivity, lack of aliasing, and direction independence. In the fetal heart, however, flow direction and maximum velocities are essential in making an accurate diagnosis. Therefore, power Doppler is typically not useful except for establishing the presence of blood flow.

M-Mode

Although M-mode echocardiography is not routinely necessary in fetal echocardiographic examinations, it is essential to differentiate some dysrhythmias.[27] By placing the M-mode cursor through both an atrial and ventricular wall or structure simultaneously, the response of both structures can be visualized, aiding in identifying the type of dysrhythmia. M-mode can also be used to acquire measurements of chamber size and wall thickness; however, it is not absolutely necessary because these measurements can also be obtained from two-dimensional (2D) images.

M-mode is also helpful in evaluating contractility in heart abnormalities, which may affect wall motion, such as cardiomyopathies, and is a quick and accurate method of measuring fetal heart rate.

3D and 4D Ultrasound

The advances in three-dimensional (3D) and four-dimensional (4D) ultrasound have recently been applied to evaluate the fetal heart.

Two-dimensional imaging of the fetal heart remains the gold standard; however, there are advantages to 3D volume imaging. By obtaining a volume set of the fetal heart, a third scan plane is obtained. This may be advantageous when a fetus is in a difficult position.[28,29]

Several 3D/4D techniques have been applied to scan the fetal heart. The most common include spatiotemporal image correlation and multiplanar reconstruction.

Spatiotemporal image correlation (STIC): The transducer performs a sweep and a volume set is acquired. The images are then correlated with the fetal heart rate and a complete cardiac cycle is produced.[28,29]

Multiplanar reconstruction: A volume set is obtained and all three image planes are displayed on the screen. The sonographer or physician can then manipulate each plane as needed to obtain a surface rendering in a fourth image.[28,29]

ANATOMY AND PHYSIOLOGY

Several important structural and physiologic differences exist between the fetal and adult cardiovascular systems.[14] Unlike the adult, fetal oxygen and carbon dioxide exchange takes place in the placenta. For oxygenated blood to reach the systemic circulation and deoxygenated blood to return to the placenta for oxygenation, the fetal cardiovascular system contains several shunts not present in the adult.

In utero, oxygenated blood travels from the placenta to the fetus via the umbilical vein. After entering the fetus, the majority of this blood travels through the ductus venosus, bypassing the liver, and entering the inferior vena cava. The remainder of this oxygenated blood enters the liver and mixes with the portal circulation.

After entering the inferior vena cava, this oxygenated blood mixes with deoxygenated blood returning from the lower extremities of the fetus. It then enters the right atrium. As it enters the right atrium, the majority of blood is shunted across the foramen ovale into the left atrium. A smaller amount of blood mixes with the desaturated blood returning from the fetal head and upper extremities. This blood travels into the right atrium and into the pulmonary artery. Resistance to blood flow is high *in utero*; therefore, the majority of the blood that enters the pulmonary artery passes directly into the descending aorta via the ductus arteriosus.

The blood that was shunted through the foramen ovale into the left atrium mixes with a small amount of desaturated blood returned from the lungs by way of the pulmonary veins. This blood then enters the left ventricle and then the aorta. As this blood travels through the aortic arch, a majority passes through the head and neck vessels to supply the fetal head and upper extremities. The remainder continues down the descending aorta, mixes with blood from the ductus arteriosus, and flows out of the fetus by way of the umbilical arteries to the placenta.

The three shunts present *in utero*, the ductus venosus, the foramen ovale, and the ductus arteriosus, all normally close after birth. The ductus arteriosus closes almost immediately after birth. This results in increased pressure within the left atrium which combined with decreased pressure in the right atrium causes the foramen ovale to close. Complete fusion of the foramen ovale is usually complete by 1 year of age. The umbilical arteries also close immediately after birth. This leads to closure of the ductus venosus.

CONGENITAL CARDIAC ABNORMALITIES

Ventricular Septal Defect

The pooled reported frequency of congenital heart lesions among affected abortuses and stillborn infants shows that ventricular septal defect (VSD) is the most common type of heart defect found (Table 9–1).[14]

In children, VSDs account for 20–57% of cases of congenital heart defects.[2] Unfortunately, it is also one the most commonly missed defects *in utero*. The sonographic diagnosis of a VSD is based on identifying an interruption in the ventricular septum. This area of dropout may be bordered by a hyperechoic specular reflector, representing the blunted edge of the intact portion of the septum (Fig. 9–18A). The subcostal four-chamber view is often the most useful view in detecting a VSD.

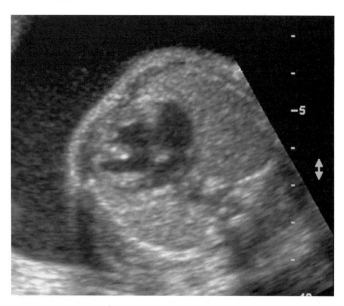

FIGURE 9–18A. Subcostal, four-chamber view showing an anechoic area in the membranous portion of the interventricular septum representing a ventricular septal defect.

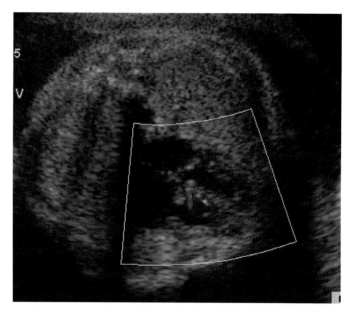

FIGURE 9–18B. Subcostal, four-chamber view of a small membranous ventricular septal defect shown by color Doppler.

VSDs are classified into membranous and muscular defects. Membranous VSDs occur at the base of heart, near the valves. Membranous VSDs are the most common type and usually occur in isolation. Muscular VSDs are located in the muscular septum, at the apex of the heart. Muscular VSDs are divided into four types: inlet, outlet, trabecular, and apical defects. They are typically multiple and are characterized by their location.[14]

VSDs vary in size and may be singular or multiple. Obviously, smaller defects are more difficult to recognize *in utero*. In addition, spontaneous closure of a VSD may occur during later gestation. Therefore, a defect that was present earlier in pregnancy may not be present when reevaluated.

Pulsed and color Doppler are useful in making the diagnosis of a VSD. In fact, some small defects that are virtually unseen by 2D alone may be visualized with the utilization of color (Fig. 9–18B). However, it should be borne in mind that because of the near equal pressures of the right and left ventricles *in utero*, flow across a small VSD may not be appreciated by either color or pulsed Doppler.

Atrial Septal Defect

Atrial septal defects (ASDs) account for approximately 6.7% of congenital heart disease in live-born infants.[30] Overall, ASDs are twice as common in females as in males. It is difficult to make the diagnosis of ASD *in utero* because of the normal atrial shunt, the foramen ovale, which allows blood flow from the right atrium to the left atrium in the fetus. Most *in utero* ASDs are best visualized in the subcostal four-chamber view (Fig. 9–19).

An ostium secundum ASD would appear as a larger than expected area of dropout in the vicinity of the foramen ovale. An ostium primum ASD would result in the absence of the lower portion of the atrial septum, just above the atrioventricular

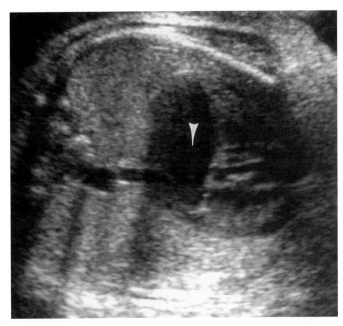

FIGURE 9–19. Subcostal, four-chamber view showing an anechoic area (arrowhead) in the interatrial septum representing an atrial septal defect.

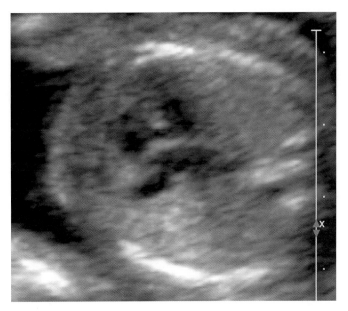

FIGURE 9–20A. Apical four-chamber view in a fetus with an atrioventricular septal defect. A singular atrioventricular valve can be seen closing within a ventricular and atrial septal defect.

valves. As with VSDs, color Doppler may be a useful adjunct in making the diagnosis.

Atrioventricular Septal Defect

Atrioventricular septal defect (AVSD) refers to a constellation of cardiac malformations that include abnormal development of the interatrial septum, the interventricular septum, and the atrioventricular (mitral and tricuspid) valves. It is also referred to as an atrioventricular canal defect or endocardial cushion defect. Approximately 30% of AVSDs in the fetus are associated with polysplenia.[3] Of these, most are accompanied by complete heart block. Chromosomal abnormalities, especially Down syndrome, are associated in up to 78% of cases.[3] When an AVSD is present without complete heart block, it is more likely to be associated with abnormal chromosomes.

A complete AVSD can usually be appreciated from either a subcostal or an apical four-chamber view (Fig. 9–20A). The endocardial cushion is absent, creating a wide opening within the center of the heart (Fig. 9–20B). The continuity between the interatrial and interventricular septa and the atrioventricular valves is lost. Instead of identifying separate mitral and tricuspid valves, one single multileaflet valve is seen.

A partial form of AVSD occurs less frequently. With this, two atrioventricular valves are present; however, their leaflet formation is always abnormal. This may be difficult to appreciate by ultrasound, with the presence of an atrial and a ventricular septal defect being the only clue that an abnormality is present. In a partial AVSD, the apical four-chamber view is useful in demonstrating the abnormal insertion level of the atrioventricular valves. In the normal heart, the tricuspid valve has a more apical insertion than the mitral valve. When a partial

AVSD is present, the two atrioventricular valves appear to insert at the same level.[5]

Additional echocardiographic views of the heart such as a short-axis view and long-axis views of the aorta and pulmonary artery, may be useful in defining the extent of the AVSD, as well as identifying associated cardiac malformations.

Hypoplastic Left Heart Syndrome

Hypoplastic left heart syndrome (HLHS) refers to a group of structural abnormalities affecting the left side of the heart. Its hallmark is a small left ventricle, which can be accompanied by

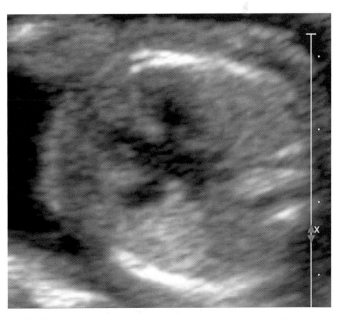

FIGURE 9–20B. Apical four-chamber view in the same fetus. The valve is open showing the large endocardial cushion defect.

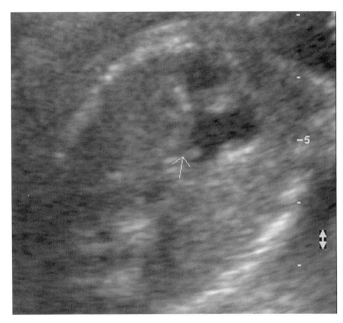

FIGURE 9–21. Apical four-chamber view in a fetus with hypoplastic left heart syndrome. The left heart (arrow) is nearly obliterated, whereas the right ventricle and right atrium are enlarged.

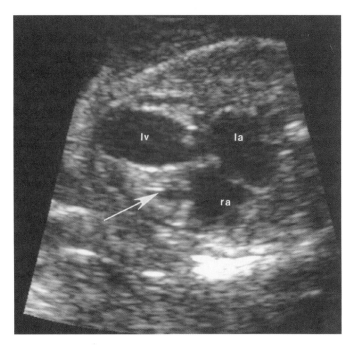

FIGURE 9–22. Subcostal, four-chamber view in a fetus with hypoplastic right heart syndrome. The right ventricle (arrow) is nearly obliterated, whereas the right atrium (ra), left atrium (la) and left ventricle (lv) are enlarged.

aortic atresia, a hypoplastic ascending aorta, an atretic or hypoplastic mitral valve, and a small left atrium (Fig. 9–21).[4] HLHS results from decreased blood flow into or out of the left ventricle. This lack of blood flow results in the underdevelopment of the left ventricle.[6] Sonographically, a very small left ventricle is usually seen. This is apparent in either a four-chamber view or a short-axis view of the ventricles.

When a small left ventricle is identified, accompanying abnormalities of the mitral and aortic valves must be determined. With valve atresia or hypoplasia, the valve orifice will appear smaller than normal for gestational age. Color and pulsed Doppler will demonstrate a lack of blood flow through the valve. The aorta itself will also appear small or atretic. In some cases, the walls of the aorta will appear more hyperechoic than expected. Blood flow through the ascending aorta may be absent or reversed. Reversal of flow represents blood flowing through the ductus arteriosus and then retrograde through the ascending aorta.

HLHS has a very poor prognosis, carrying a 25% mortality rate within the first week of life. All untreated infants die within the first 6 weeks. Treatment of this lesion usually involves surgical repair via a two-stage Norwood procedure or heart transplantation.[10]

Hypoplastic Right Heart

Hypoplastic right heart is the result of either pulmonary atresia with intact ventricular septum or tricuspid atresia.[14] As with HLHS, it occurs when normal blood flow into or out of the ventricle is compromised. Sonographic findings include a small right ventricle accompanied by a small or atretic and pulmonary artery and valve. Either an apical or a subcostal four-chamber

view is most useful in assessing this abnormality (Fig. 9–22). Color and pulsed Doppler will confirm the absence of blood flow across the pulmonary valve.

In tricuspid atresia, flow will be absent or substantially decreased across the tricuspid valve (Fig. 9–23). The pulmonic valve is usually stenotic, so an increased velocity may be appreciated distal to the valve. If severe stenosis is present, no flow may be detectable, making differentiation from pulmonary atresia difficult. Color Doppler is essential for evaluating the interventricular septum for defects. As stated previously, this should be done in a subcostal four-chamber view.

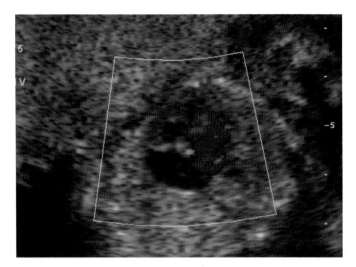

FIGURE 9–23. Apical, four-chamber view showing tricuspid atresia. There is no flow across the echogenic, nonmobile tricuspid valve.

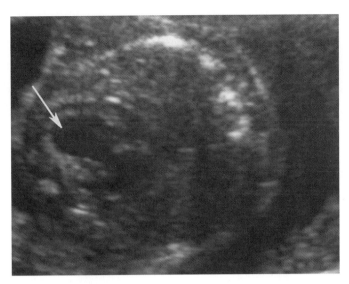

FIGURE 9–24. Subcostal, four-chamber view showing the single ventricle (arrow) present in a univentricular heart.

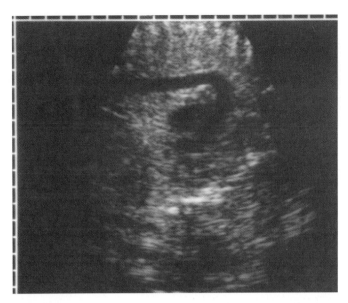

FIGURE 9–25. Sagittal view of the aortic arch showing a normal appearing arch in the setting of a coarctation of the aorta.

Both tricuspid atresia and pulmonary atresia with intact ventricular septum are associated with a large left atrium and a dilated, often hypertrophied, left ventricle. The aortic root may be dilated with either entity. This left-sided enlargement is a result of the vast quantity of blood being forced across the foramen ovale because it is unable to enter the right ventricle.[10] Retrograde blood flow within the ductus arteriosus is also possible because of the increased flow through the aorta and the accompanying decreased or absent flow through the pulmonary artery.

Univentricular Heart

Univentricular heart is defined as the presence of two atrioventricular valves or a common atrioventricular valve emptying into a single ventricle. From either four-chamber view, only three chambers are present, two atria and one large ventricle (Fig. 9–24).

If two atrioventricular valves are identified, but one appears atretic, the most likely diagnosis is tricuspid or mitral atresia, which is usually considered a defect separate from a univentricular heart. The aorta and pulmonary artery are almost always transposed in the setting of a univentricular heart. Pulmonary atresia or stenosis is also common. Univentricular heart has been associated with asplenia or polysplenia in 13% of cases.[11]

Coarctation of the Aorta

When the diagnosis of coarctation of the aorta is made *in utero* or in early infancy, it is easily correctable, but if left undetected, the effects can be devastating. Coarctation is a narrowing of the aortic lumen, which results in an obstruction to blood flow. In 98% of cases, this narrowing occurs between the origin of the left subclavian artery and the ductus arteriosus.[12] The severity of a coarctation can range from a slight narrowing of the distal end of the arch to severe hypoplasia of the entire arch.

Intuitively, the *in utero* diagnosis of a coarctation seems straightforward. It is, however, extremely difficult. Subtle changes associated with coarctation, such as a narrowing of the aortic arch, may not be appreciated, even when the arch is well visualized (Fig. 9–25). This may be caused by the physiological shunts present in the fetal heart, allowing for the severity of the narrowing not to present until after birth.

These shunts may also explain why Doppler velocities may not be affected in the presence of a coarctation. Interestingly, one of the most reliable signs of a coarctation *in utero* to be reported is a right ventricular dimension greater than that expected for a gestational age (Fig. 9–26). Pulmonary artery size may also be increased.[13]

This finding may be subtle; therefore, measurements of the ventricles and great vessels should always be performed in the fetus at risk for coarctation such as those with Turner syndrome (XO) or a prior family history of left heart anomalies. It is also important to remember that coarctation of the aorta is often a progressive lesion, with the distal arch becoming more hypoplastic as pregnancy advances. Reversal of blood flow through the foramen ovale is often, but not always, present with a coarctation.

Aortic and Pulmonic Stenosis

Congenital aortic stenosis is an obstruction of the left ventricular outflow tract. Aortic stenosis is classified into three types: valvular, subvalvular, and supravalvular stenosis. Sixty to 70% of patients with aortic stenosis have valvular stenosis. On ultrasound, aortic stenosis may appear as a thickened or immobile valve. Flow distal to the aortic valve is increased in velocity. With severe stenosis, no flow or reversed flow may be seen.[14]

Congenital pulmonic stenosis is an obstruction or narrowing of the right ventricular outflow tract. Pulmonary stenosis is

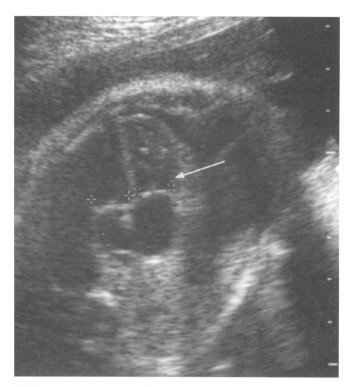

FIGURE 9–26. Apical four-chamber view in a fetus with coarctation of the aorta. The only clue in this case was a right ventricle (arrow) that was slightly larger than expected for gestational age.

classified as obstructive or valvular. A thickened valve or muscular ring may be seen by ultrasound. By pulsed Doppler, there is increased velocity distal to the valve. Pulmonic stenosis can been found in the recipient twin of twin-to-twin transfusion syndrome.[14,31]

Ebstein Anomaly

Ebstein anomaly is defined as the inferior displacement of the tricuspid valve leaflets from their normal location. Ebstein anomaly is an uncommon cardiac lesion, with a reported incidence of 1 in 20,000 live births.[15] It has often been associated with maternal lithium use; however, more recent data have shown this association to be substantially less than previously reported.[16]

The sonographic diagnosis of Ebstein anomaly is usually straightforward. Apical displacement of the tricuspid valve leaflets is readily apparent from either four-chamber view (Fig. 9–27). This results in "atrialization" of the right ventricle, which, along with the tricuspid insufficiency that is almost always present, causes an often massively enlarged right atrium. This is turn, causes the axis of the heart to be severely levocardic, giving the heart a very horizontal position within the fetal chest. Pulmonary atresia or stenosis, as well as dysrhythmias are not uncommon with Ebstein anomaly. Ebstein anomaly frequently causes *in utero* cardiac dysfunction, resulting in cardiomegaly and hydrops fetalis.

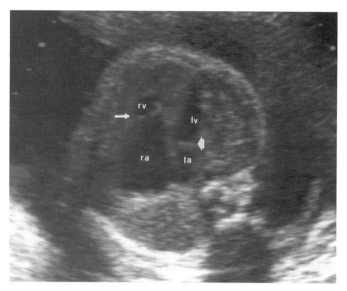

FIGURE 9–27. Apical four-chamber view in a fetus with Ebstein anomaly. The tricuspid valve (arrow) is displaced apically, causing atrialization of the right atrium (ra) and a small right ventricle (rv). la = left atrium, lv = left ventricle.

Tetralogy of Fallot

Tetralogy of Fallot consists of four classic structural defects: a ventricular septal defect, aortic override of the VSD, pulmonary stenosis, and right ventricular hypertrophy.[14] Because of the normal shunts present in the fetus, the right ventricular hypertrophy may not occur *in utero*. To diagnose this malformation *in utero*, an aortic root overriding the interventricular septum must be identified (Fig. 9–28). It is often not possible

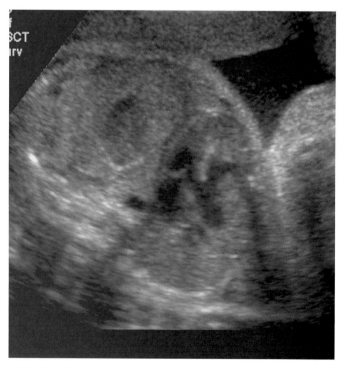

FIGURE 9–28. Apical view of the heart in a fetus with tetralogy of Fallot showing the aorta overriding a ventricular septal defect.

to make this diagnosis solely from a four-chamber view, either apical or subcostal. The VSD may be seen on the four-chamber view; however, color Doppler should be used to confirm that the defect is real and not artifactual. A slight angulation of the transducer toward the fetus' right shoulder from a subcostal four-chamber view, or cephalad from an apical four-chamber view should allow the overriding aorta to be appreciated. Dilatation of the aortic root is usually present in later gestation.[17]

Once an overriding aorta has been observed, the diagnosis of tetralogy of Fallot relies on the evaluation of the right ventricular outflow tract. This is usually best accomplished in either a long-axis view of the pulmonary artery or a short-axis view of the great vessels. The pulmonary artery will appear small, often so much so that it cannot be identified. Pulsed Doppler interrogation of the pulmonic valve may show a greatly increased velocity, indicative of stenosis, or absence of flow in the setting of severe stenosis or atresia. Retrograde flow through the ductus arteriosus may also be present. Making an accurate diagnosis of tetralogy of Fallot relies on identifying the pulmonary artery. If a pulmonary artery cannot be visualized, the differential diagnosis would include pulmonary atresia with a VSD. If there is no main pulmonary artery arising from the right ventricle but smaller pulmonary artery branches are seen arising from the overriding aorta, the diagnosis is truncus arteriosus.

When the diagnosis of tetralogy of Fallot is established, the laterality of the aortic arch should be determined because approximately 25% of cases are associated with a right-sided aortic arch.[19]

Truncus Arteriosus

Truncus arteriosus is rare. It is an embryological failure that results in a single great vessel arising from the heart.[14] The systemic, pulmonary, and coronary circulations are all supplied by this single great vessel. Sonographically, truncus arteriosus appears very similar to tetralogy of Fallot. A VSD is present, and the singular great vessel overrides the defect, similar to the aorta in tetralogy of Fallot (Fig. 9–29). The difference is that the pulmonary artery arises from this great vessel, not the right ventricle. Depending on the type of truncal defect present, the number and position of the pulmonary arteries on the great vessel will vary.[32]

The *in utero* diagnosis of truncus arteriosus may be challenging. The definitive diagnosis can be made only if the origin of the pulmonary artery can be identified arising from the large, single great vessel. Because of the inherent technical factors associated with fetal echocardiography, this may be difficult.

As with tetralogy of Fallot, identification of the overriding great vessel is usually accomplished with slight angulation from either the apical or the subcostal four-chamber view. Several views, including long- and short-axis views of the right outflow tract, must be obtained to confirm the absence of a pulmonary artery. Evaluation of the aortic arch is also important. A right-sided arch has been reported in 15–30% of cases.

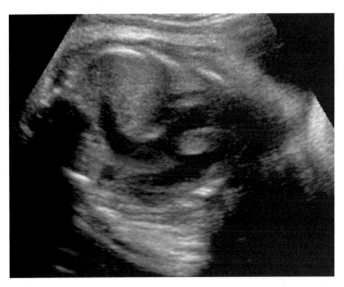

FIGURE 9–29. Subcostal view of the heart in a fetus with truncus arteriosus showing a single truncal vessel overriding a ventricular septal defect.

Interruption of the aortic arch has also been associated with truncus arteriosus.[32]

Complete Transposition of the Great Arteries

Eighty percent of fetuses with transposition of the great arteries have complete or *d*-transposition.[20] In this setting, the connections between the atria and ventricles are normal, meaning that the right atrium connects through the tricuspid valve to the right ventricle, and the left atrium connects through the mitral valve to the left ventricle. However, the aorta arises from the right ventricle, and the pulmonary artery arises from the left ventricle. This results in two parallel circulations that will only allow mixing of venous and arterial blood through the ductus arteriosus, interatrial, or interventricular connections.

The four-chamber views are often normal in the presence of complete transposition. The diagnosis is made by identifying the aorta arising from the right ventricle and connecting to the aortic arch and descending aorta, and identifying the pulmonary artery arising from the left ventricle and then branching into the left and right pulmonary arteries. From a long-axis view of the great vessels, the aorta and pulmonary artery will appear to run in a parallel fashion (Fig. 9–30). The short-axis view, at the level of the great vessels, is also useful in making this diagnosis. In this view, both the pulmonary artery and aorta appear as circular structures adjacent to each other, instead of their normal relationship of the pulmonary artery draping over the aorta. A ventricular septal defect is present in 20% of cases, so color Doppler should be used to assess the interventricular septum thoroughly.[21]

Congenitally Corrected Transposition of the Great Arteries

Congenitally corrected or *l*-transposition of the great arteries comprises the remaining 20% of transposition cases.[20] In corrected transposition, the great vessels arise from the correct sides;

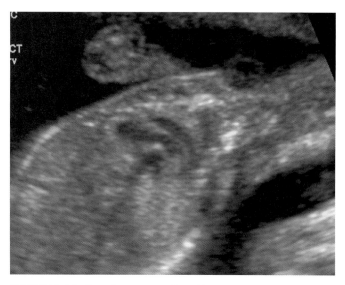

FIGURE 9–30. Complete transposition of the great arteries. The aorta and pulmonary arteries are running parallel.

however, the left and right ventricles and the left and right atrio-ventricular valves are transposed. In other words, the right atrium is connected to the left ventricle, and the left atrium is connected to the right ventricle. The aorta then arises from the left-sided right ventricle, and the pulmonary artery arises from the right-sided left ventricle. Blood circulation in this abnormality is in series, as it is in the normal heart; therefore, surgical correction is not required unless associated cardiac anomalies are present.

Sonographic identification of this abnormality can be subtle. Correct identification of the cardiac chambers is crucial in making this diagnosis. In the normal heart, the tricuspid valve insertion is slightly more apical than the mitral valve (Fig. 9–31). The right ventricle also has a prominent moderator band near the apex that is usually seen on fetal echocardiography. If these findings appear to be left sided, the diagnosis of corrected trans-

position should be considered. As with complete transposition, the great vessels exit the heart in a more parallel relationship than seen in the normal heart. This may be appreciated on a short-axis view of the great vessels but is far more subtle than in complete transposition. It is not uncommon to miss the diagnosis of corrected transposition *in utero*, particularly when no other cardiac defects are present.

VSDs have been reported in about 50% of patients with corrected transposition. Pulmonic stenosis and abnormalities of the mitral and tricuspid valves are also common.[20]

Double Outlet Right Ventricle

Double outlet right ventricle (DORV) is a condition in which more than 50% of both the aortic root and the main pulmonary artery arise from the right ventricle. A ventricular septal defect is almost always present.[22]

This, again, is one of many cardiac defects easily missed when only a four-chamber view is obtained. The long-axis views of the aorta and pulmonary artery are most useful in identifying both great vessels as arising from the right ventricle (Fig. 9–32). In DORV, the most common relationship of the great vessels is side by side, with the aorta right and lateral to the pulmonary artery. When this occurs, the normal perpendicular course of the great vessels is lost. As with transposition of the great arteries, they will appear parallel to each other. Differentiating DORV from transposition relies on identifying both great vessels as arising from the right ventricle. This can be challenging *in utero*. As with all congenital cardiac abnormalities, the surgical intervention depends heavily on the presence or absence of other cardiac anomalies. Therefore, a thorough interrogation of the fetal heart must be undertaken.

Double outlet left ventricle, in which both the aortic root and the main pulmonary artery arise from the left ventricle, has also been reported, but it is exceedingly rare.[23]

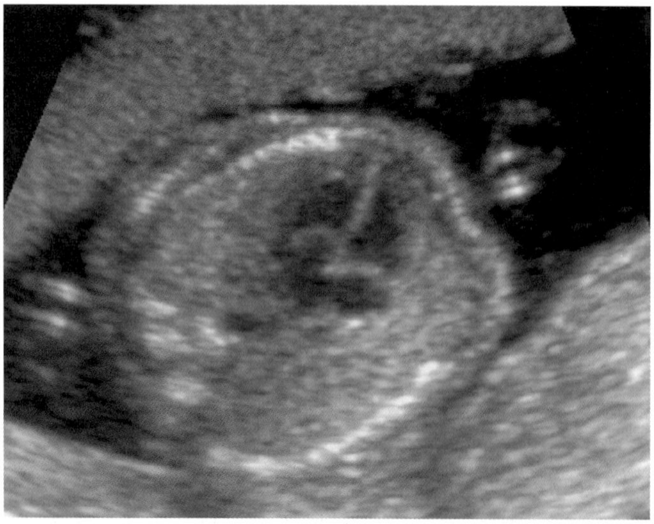

FIGURE 9–31. Corrected transposition of the great arteries. Note how the tricuspid valve is slightly superior to the mitral valve. In the normal heart, the tricuspid valve is more apical.

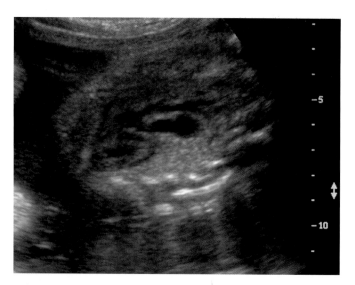

FIGURE 9–32. Double outlet right ventricle in a fetus. The aorta and the pulmonary artery are both arising from the right ventricle.

Total Anomalous Pulmonary Venous Connection

Total anomalous pulmonary venous connection (TAPVC) is an anomaly in which all of the pulmonary veins drain either directly into the right atrium or into channels that terminate in the right atrium.[24] In the normal heart, venous return is to the left atrium. TAPVC is rare and, as with many other congenital cardiac anomalies, is a difficult diagnosis to make in the fetus.

The diagnosis relies on the inability to identify any pulmonary veins entering the left atrium and the identification of all four pulmonary veins entering the right atrium or abnormally converging and entering the superior vena cava, inferior vena cava, portal vein, or ductus venosus.

If any pulmonary veins are seen entering the left atrium, or if all pulmonary veins are not seen entering an ectopic structure, the diagnosis of TAPVC is excluded. Partial anomalous pulmonary venous connection may be present in this setting, but cannot be definitively ascertained *in utero*.

The pulmonary veins are best identified in either a subcostal or an apical four-chamber view. Usually only the two superior veins are identified *in utero* (Fig. 9–33), adding to the difficulty of making this diagnosis. Enlargement of the right ventricle and pulmonary artery may be secondary signs of TAPVC.[24]

When enlargement of these structures is present and the normal pulmonary veins cannot be identified as they drain into the left atrium, the possibility of TAPVC should be entertained. Using color Doppler to identify an abnormal convergence of veins posterior to the right atrium may also be useful.

Cardiac Axis and Position

As stated previously, determining cardiac axis and position is one of the first steps in performing a fetal echocardiogram.

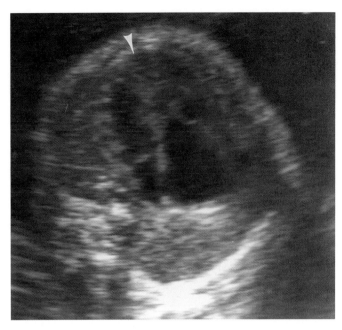

FIGURE 9–34. Severe levocardia in a fetus with Ebstein anomaly. The apex of the heart (arrowhead) is angled too far to the left chest.

Abnormal cardiac axis or position may be an important clue that a structural defect is present.[14]

Normal cardiac axis is termed levocardia, meaning the apex of the heart points to the left side of the fetal chest. Even if a heart is levocardic, if its axis is > 45 ± 20° to the left, an abnormality may be present. Cardiac anomalies that result in severe levocardia are usually those that cause an enlarged right atrium, such as Ebstein anomaly (Fig. 9–34). It is thought that this enlargement causes the heart to shift and lie more horizontally. Mesocardia occurs when the apex of the heart points midline. Mesocardia is uncommon but has been associated with transposition of the great vessels[14] (Fig. 9–35).

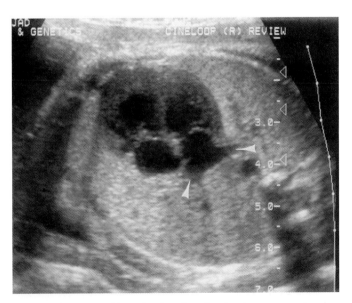

FIGURE 9–33. Apical four-chamber view showing the two normal superior pulmonary veins appropriately entering the left atrium.

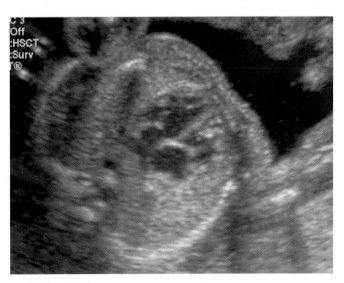

FIGURE 9–35. Four-chamber view showing mesocardia, with the apex of the heart pointing midline.

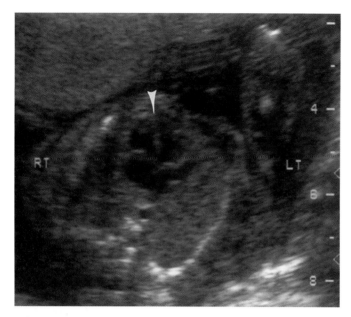

FIGURE 9–36. Dextrocardia of the fetal heart. The apex of the heart (arrowhead) is pointing incorrectly to the right chest.

The terms dextrocardia or dextroversion refer to the apex of the heart pointing abnormally to the right (Fig. 9–36). Isolated dextrocardia is associated with a structural cardiac abnormality in 95% of cases.[14] Dextrocardia associated with abdominal situs abnormalities carries a lower risk. Dextroposition is present when the apex of the heart points normally to the left side of the fetal chest, but the heart itself is positioned in the right chest (Fig. 9–37).

When dextroposition is present, two possibilities should be considered. Either the heart is being displaced to the right by a left-sided thoracic defect such as a diaphragmatic hernia or a cystic adenomatoid malformation, or the heart is filling a potential space in the right thorax. This may be indicative of an absent or hypoplastic right lung.

Whenever a fetal echocardiogram is performed, special attention should be paid to identifying cardiac axis and position. Any deviation from normal may be indicative of an underlying intra- or extracardiac defect.

Dysrhythmias

The normal fetal heart rate is regular and between 100 and 180 beats per minute (bpm). A dysrhythmia is present if the fetal heart rate is noted to be abnormally fast, slow, or irregular. Dysrhythmias are detected in approximately 1% of fetuses.[30]

Most dysrhythmias are benign; however, in a small number of cases, they may be life threatening. M-mode is the most useful method of assessing the type of dysrhythmia present. As stated previously, the M-mode cursor should be placed simultaneously through a structure in the fetal heart that represents an atrial beat (atria wall or atrioventricular valve) and the ventricular response (ventricle wall or semilunar valve).

Premature atrial contractions (PACs) are the most common dysrhythmia encountered in the fetus (Fig. 9–38).[14] They have been associated with a redundant foraminal flap, as well as maternal use of caffeine, cigarettes, or alcohol.[33] Rarely, PACs may evolve into a sustained tachycardia; however, most resolve around the time of delivery and seldom present a problem in the newborn. Tachycardias are the second most common dysrhythmia seen in the fetal population. Tachycardias are classified as:

- Supraventricular tachycardia (SVT)—heart rate of 180–280 bpm, with atrioventricular concordance (Fig. 9–39)
- Atrial flutter—atrial heart rate of 280–400 bpm, with variable ventricular response (Fig. 9–40)

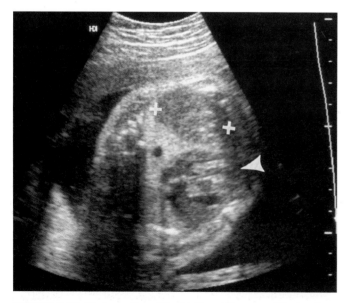

FIGURE 9–37. Dextroposition of the fetal heart. The apex of the heart (arrowhead) is pointing correctly to the left chest; however, the entire heart is being displaced into the right chest by the mass in the left chest (calipers).

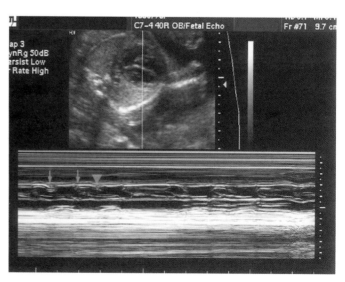

FIGURE 9–38. M-mode tracing of premature atrial contractions in a fetus. Normally spaced atrial beats (arrows) can be seen followed by a premature beat (arrowhead).

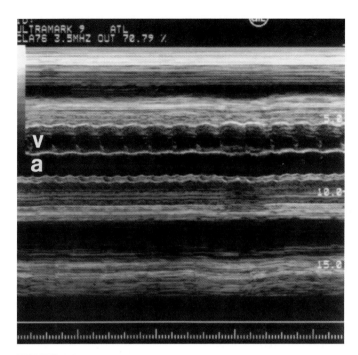

FIGURE 9–39. M-mode tracing of supraventricular tachycardia in a fetus. Both the ventricular (v) and atrial (a) rates were 240 beats per minute.

- Atrial fibrillation—atrial heart rate of >400 bpm, with variable ventricular response

Sustained SVT can result in fetal hydrops or death and represents a fetal medical emergency.[34] SVT is associated with structural heart disease in 5–10% of cases.[35]

The treatment of SVT *in utero* is difficult. Immediate medical therapy should be implemented if there are signs of fetal compromise. Digoxin has been the initial drug of choice when treating fetal SVT; however, several other medications are available and may be used in place of or in combination with digoxin.

Bradycardia may also be encountered in the fetus. Transient bradycardia is often encountered during the course of an ultrasound examination secondary to pressure from the transducer. The bradycardia is resolved when the transducer is removed. This entity should not be confused with pathologic bradycardias that result in a sustained slow heart rate.

Ninety-six percent of fetuses with sustained bradycardia will have second- or third-degree heart block.[14] Second-degree heart block is commonly referred to as a 2:1 or 3:1, etc., heart block, referring to the fact that the ventricular rate will be a submultiple of the atrial rate. In other words, two atrial contractions will occur for every one ventricular contraction, or three atrial contractions will occur for every one ventricular contraction (Fig. 9–41).

Third-degree, or complete, heart block is present when there is complete dissociation between the atrial and ventricular rates, with the atrial rate being faster. Approximately 50% of fetuses with complete heart block have significant structural heart disease, specifically, atrioventricular septal defects, corrected transposition of the great arteries, cardiac tumors, or a cardiomyopathy.[14] Complete heart block associated with an atrioventricular septal defect is highly suggestive of polysplenia syndrome.[36] In fetuses with complete heart block without structural defects, there is a high association with maternal connective tissue diseases such as lupus.[37]

Second- and third-degree heart block are difficult to treat *in utero*. Increasing fetal heart rate through the maternal administration of sympathomimetic agents and placement of an *in utero* pacemaker have been attempted, but with dismal results.[38] Administration of maternal steroids has also been reported.[39]

The prognosis for fetuses with complete heart block and structural heart disease is poor. In fetuses without structural heart disease, outcome is dependent on the atrial and ventricular rate and the presence of fetal hydrops.

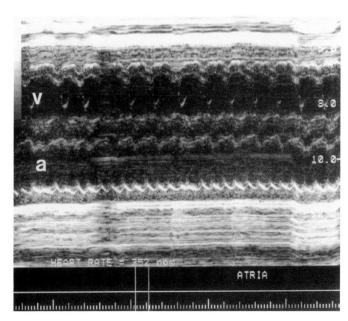

FIGURE 9–40. M-mode tracing of a fetal heart with atrial flutter. The atrial (a) rate was 352 beats per minute, while the ventricular (v) rate was 180 beats per minute.

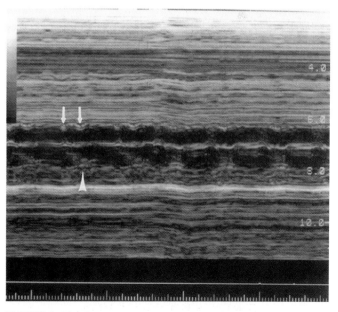

FIGURE 9–41. M-mode tracing of a fetal heart with a 2:1 heart block. The atrial rate is 120 beats per minute, whereas the ventricular rate is 60 beats per minute.

References

1. Hoffman JIE. Incidence of congenital heart disease: II. Prenatal incidence. *Pediatr Cardiol.* 1995; 16:155-165.

2. Allan LD, Crawford DC, Anderson RH, et al. Spectrum of congenital heart disease detected echocardiographically in prenatal life. *Br Heart J.* 1985; 54:523-526.

3. Allan LD. Fetal cardiology. *Ultrasound Obstet Gynecol.* 1994; 4: 441-444.

4. AIUM Technical Bulletin: performance of the fetal cardiac ultrasound examination. American Institute of Ultrasound in Medicine. *J Ultrasound Med.* 1998; 17:601-607.

5. Dolkart LA, Reimers FT. Transvaginal fetal echocardiography in early pregnancy: normative data. *Am J Obstet Gynecol.* 1991; 165:688-691.

6. DeVore GR, Medearis AL, Bear MB. Fetal echocardiography: factors that influence imaging of the fetal heart during the second trimester of pregnancy. *J Ultrasound Med.* 1993; 12:659-663.

7. McAuliffe FM, Trines J, Nield LE, et al. Early fetal echocardiography—a reliable prenatal diagnosis tool. *Am J Obstet Gynecol.* 2005; 193:1253-1259.

8. Allan LD. Diagnosis of fetal cardiac abnormality. *Br J Hosp Med.* 1988; 40:290-293.

9. Fliedner R, Kreiselmaier P, Schwarze A, et al. Development of hypoplastic left heart syndrome after diagnosis of aortic stenosis in the first trimester by early echocardiography. *Ultrasound Obstet Gynecol.* 2006; 28:106-109.

10. Fyfe DA, Kline CH. Fetal echocardiographic diagnosis of congenital heart disease. *Pediatr Clin North Am.* 1990; 37:45-67.

11. Nora JJ, Fraser FC. Cardiovascular disease. In: *Medical Genetics: Principles and Practice.* 3rd ed. Philadelphia: Lea & Febiger; 1989:321-337.

12. Nora JJ, Nora AH. Maternal transmission of congenital heart diseases: new recurrence risk figures and the question of cytoplasmic inheritance and vulnerability to teratogens. *Am J Cardiol.* 1987; 59:459-463.

13. Reed KL. Introduction to fetal echocardiography. *Ob Gyn Clin N Am.* 1991; 18:811-822.

14. Drose JA. *Fetal Echocardiography.* Philadelphia: WB Saunders; 1998:1-300.

15. Berg KA, Boughman JA, Astemboroski JA, et al. Implications for prenatal cytogenetic analysis from Baltimore–Washington study of liveborn infants with confirmed congenital heart defects (CHD). *Am J Hum Genet.* 1986; 39:A50.

16. Berg KA, Clark EB, Astemboroski JA, et al. Prenatal detection of cardiovascular malformations by echocardiography: an indication for cytogenetic evaluation. *Am J Obstet Gynecol.* 1988; 159:477-481.

17. Stewart PA, Wladimiroff JW, Reuss A, et al. Fetal echocardiography: a review of six years' experience. *Fetal Ther.* 1987; 2:222-231.

18. Makrydimas G, Sotiriadis A, Huggon IC, et al. Nuchal translucency and fetal cardiac defects: a pooled analysis of major fetal echocardiography centers. *Am J Obstet Gynecol.* 2005; 192:89-95.

19. Nicolaides K, Shawwa L, Brizot M, et al. Ultrasonographically detectable markers of fetal chromosomal defects. *Ultrasound Obstet Gynecol.* 1993; 3:56-59.

20. Levy HL, Waisbren SE. Effects of untreated maternal phenylketonuria and hyperphenylalaninemia on the fetus. *N Engl J Med.* 1983; 309:1269-1274.

21. Nyberg DA, Emerson DS. Cardiac malformations. In: Nyberg DA, Mahony BS, Pretorius DH, eds. *Diagnostic Ultrasound of Fetal Anomalies: Text and Atlas.* Chicago: Yearbook Medical Publishers, Inc.; 1990:300-341.

22. Drose JA, Dennis MA, Thickman D. Infection in utero: ultrasound findings in 19 cases. *Radiology.* 1991; 178:369-374.

23. Coper JA, Pilu G, Kleinman CS. Congenital heart disease and extracardiac anomalies: associations and indications for fetal echocardiography. *Am J Obstet Gynecol.* 1986; 154:1121-1132.

24. Comstock CH. Normal fetal heart axis and position. *Obstet Gynecol.* 1987; 70:255-257.

25. DeVore GR. The prenatal diagnosis of congenital heart disease—a practical approach for the fetal sonographer. *J Clin Ultrasound.* 1985; 13:229-245.

26. Brown DL, DiSalvo DN, Frates MC, et al. Sonography of the fetal heart: normal variants and pitfalls. *AJR.* 1993; 160:1251-1255.

27. Allan LD, Joseph MC, Boyd EG, et al. M-mode echocardiography in the developing human fetus. *Br Heart J.* 1982; 47:573-583.

28. Yagel S, Cohen SM, Shapiro I, et al. 3D and 4D ultrasound in fetal cardiac scanning: a new look at the fetal heart. *Ultrasound Obstet Gynecol.* 2007; 29:81-95.

29. Tutschek B, Sahn DJ. Three-dimensional echocardiography for studies of the fetal heart: present status and future perspectives. *Cardiol Clin.* 2007 May; 25(2):341-355.

30. Southhall DP, Richard J, Hardwick RA, et al. Prospective study of fetal heart rate and rhythm patterns. *Arch Dis Child.* 1980; 55:506-511.

31. Nizard J, Bonnet D, Fermont L, et al. Acquired right heart outflow tract anomaly without systemic hypertension in recipient twins in twin-twin transfusion syndrome. *Ultrasound Obstet Gynecol.* 2001 Dec; 18(6):669-672.

32. Rowland TW, Hubbel JP, Nadas AS. Congenital heart disease in infants of diabetic mothers. *J Pediatr.* 1973; 83:815-820.

33. Steward PA, Wladimiroff JW. Fetal atrial arrhythmias associated with redundancy/aneurysm of the foramen ovale. *J Clin Ultrasound.* 1988; 16:643-650.

34. Allan LD. Cardiac ultrasound of the fetus. *Arch Dis Child.* 1984; 59:603-605.

35. Beall MH, Paul RH. Artifacts, blocks, and arrhythmias confusing nonclassical heart rate tracings. *Clin Obstet Gynecol.* 1986; 29: 83-85.

36. Machado MV, Crawford DC, Anderson RH, et al. Atrioventricular septal defect in prenatal life. *Br Heart J.* 1988; 59:352-355.

37. McCue CM, Mantakas ME, Tingelstad JB, et al. Congenital heart block in newborns of mothers with connective tissue disease. *Circulation.* 1977; 56:82-85.

38. Carpenter RJ, Strasburger JF, Farson A, et al. Fetal ventricular pacing for hydrops secondary to complete atrioventricular block. *J Am Coll Cardiol.* 1986; 8:1434-1440.

39. Kaaja R, Julkunen HA, Ammala P, et al. Congenital heart block: successful prophylactic treatment with intravenous gamma globulin and corticosteroid therapy. *Am J Obstet Gynecol.* 1991; 165:1333-1335.

Questions

GENERAL INSTRUCTIONS: For each question, select the best answer. Select only one answer for each question, unless otherwise specified.

1. Which of the following should be the first step when performing a fetal echocardiogram?

    (A) fetal heart rate

    (B) fetal position

    (C) gestational age

    (D) amount of amniotic fluid present

2. What is the most important view when performing a fetal echocardiogram?

    (A) aortic arch

    (B) subcostal four-chamber view

    (C) long-axis view of the aorta

    (D) ductal arch

3. Pulsed Doppler can be used to interrogate all valves proximally for which of the following?

    (A) stenosis

    (B) atresia

    (C) contractility

    (D) insufficiency

4. In addition to a four-chamber view, all routine obstetrical ultrasound exams should include which views?

    (A) aorta and pulmonary artery

    (B) mitral and tricuspid valves

    (C) anterior and posterior pulmonary veins

    (D) aortic and ductal arches

5. To assess for a fetal dysrhythmia, the M-mode cursor should be placed simultaneously through which structures?

    (A) mitral and tricuspid valves

    (B) right and left ventricles

    (C) atrial and ventricular wall

    (D) foraminal flap

6. The normal direction of blood flow through the foramen ovale is from which direction?

    (A) right atrium to left atrium

    (B) left atrium to right atrium

    (C) right ventricle to left ventricle

    (D) left ventricle to right atrium

7. All are indications for performing a fetal echocardiogram, *except*

    (A) mother with lupus

    (B) mother with diabetes

    (C) mother with cytomegalovirus

    (D) mother with influenza

8. Which chromosomal abnormality carries the highest risk of an associated congenital heart defect?

    (A) trisomy 21

    (B) trisomy 18

    (C) Turner syndrome

    (D) DiGeorge syndrome

9. Equipment used for fetal echocardiography should be equipped with all of the following modalities, *except*.

    (A) pulsed Doppler

    (B) color Doppler

    (C) power Doppler

    (D) M-mode

10. Congenital cardiac abnormalities occur in approximately how many live births?

    (A) 1/400

    (B) 1/300

    (C) 1/200

    (D) 1/100

11. What is the most common type of congenital heart disease found in abortuses and stillbirths?

    (A) atrial septal defect

    (B) ventricular septal defect

    (C) atrioventricular septal defect

    (D) coarctation of the aorta

12. What is the most appropriate view to interrogate the interventricular septum?

   (A) apical four chamber

   (B) subcostal four chamber

   (C) short axis of the great vessels

   (D) three vessel view

13. A fetal echocardiogram should be performed at approximately how many weeks of gestation?

   (A) 10–12 weeks

   (B) 15–16 weeks

   (C) 18–22 weeks

   (D) 24–28 weeks

14. The apex of the normal heart points in which direction?

   (A) toward the left

   (B) toward the right

   (C) superior

   (D) posterior

15. Compared to midline, what is the angle of the normal fetal heart?

   (A) 20°

   (B) 45°

   (C) 70°

   (D) 90°

16. Which term describes the normal position of the heart?

   (A) levocardia

   (B) dextrocardia

   (C) mesocardia

   (D) dextroposition

17. The normal fetal heart occupies

   (A) 1/4 of the chest

   (B) 2/3 of the chest

   (C) 1/3 of the chest

   (D) 1/2 of the chest

18. The apical four-chamber view is obtained when the septae of the heart are positioned in which direction?

   (A) toward the fetus's right

   (B) parallel to the ultrasound beam

   (C) toward the fetus's left

   (D) perpendicular to the ultrasound beam

19. The apical four-chamber view is *not* the ideal view to visualize which of the following?

   (A) all four chambers

   (B) the mitral and tricuspid valves

   (C) chamber size

   (D) the interventricular septum

20. The sonographer has obtained a subcostal four-chamber view and then angles toward the fetus's right shoulder. What view will be visualized first?

   (A) cross-section view of the ventricles

   (B) short-axis view of the aorta with the pulmonary artery crossing over

   (C) right ventricular outflow tract

   (D) long-axis view of the aorta

21. What is the correct orientation of the great vessels?

   (A) run parallel to each other

   (B) crisscross

   (C) join to form one vessel

   (D) originate from the right ventricle

22. The moderator band can be identified in which cardiac chamber?

   (A) left ventricle

   (B) left atrium

   (C) right ventricle

   (D) right atrium

23. Which view is *least* accurate to identify interventricular septal defects?

   (A) subcostal four-chamber view

   (B) long axis of the proximal aorta

   (C) short-axis view of the ventricles

   (D) short-axis view of the great vessels

24. While demonstrating a short-axis view of the great vessels, the main pulmonary artery is often seen bifurcating into which structures?

   (A) ductus arteriosus and the right pulmonary artery

   (B) right and left pulmonary arteries

   (C) ductus arteriosus and the left pulmonary artery

   (D) ductus arteriosus and the aorta

25. Which does *not* describe the appearance of the aortic arch?

    (A) Brachiocephalic vessels are visualized.

    (B) It has an appearance of a candy cane.

    (C) It is superior to the ductal arch.

    (D) It has an appearance of a hockey stick.

26. Which abnormality can be identified in the portion of the aortic arch just distal to where the ductus arteriosus inserts?

    (A) aortic valve insufficiency

    (B) aortic coarctation

    (C) aortic stenosis

    (D) pulmonary valve insufficiency

27. The ductal arch is composed of all of the following *except*.

    (A) the descending aorta

    (B) the pulmonary artery

    (C) the ascending aorta

    (D) the ductus arteriosus

28. Which relative with history of heart defect puts the fetus at the greatest risk?

    (A) one sibling

    (B) the father

    (C) the mother

    (D) the paternal grandmother

29. Which is *not* an indication for a fetal echocardiography exam?

    (A) nonimmune hydrops

    (B) maternal diabetes

    (C) suspicion of abnormal chromosomes

    (D) suboptimal heart views on a 12-week ultrasound

30. Which is *not* an advantage of using color Doppler during a fetal echocardiography exam?

    (A) identifying areas of turbulence

    (B) indicating direction of flow

    (C) indicating peak velocity

    (D) identifying small ventricular septal defects

31. In which situation is M-mode *not* helpful?

    (A) measuring chamber size

    (B) measuring wall thickness

    (C) documenting dysrhythmias

    (D) documenting direction of flow

32. In the fetus, much of the blood bypasses the liver by traveling through which structure?

    (A) foramen ovale

    (B) ductus venosus

    (C) ductus arteriosus

    (D) ligamentum venosum

33. Pulsed Doppler of the pulmonary veins is useful in determining flow in which direction?

    (A) into the left atrium

    (B) out of the left atrium

    (C) into the right atrium

    (D) out of the right atrium

34. What is the best Doppler angle when performing pulsed Doppler on the fetal heart?

    (A) 90°

    (B) 60°

    (C) 30°

    (D) 0°

35. The sample gate for the pulsed Doppler cursor is set

    (A) small so that many vessels can be interrogated at once

    (B) large so that many vessels can be interrogated at once

    (C) large to ensure the vessel of interest is obtained

    (D) small to avoid interference while obtaining the vessel of interest

36. Oxygenated blood flows from the placenta to the fetus by way of which structure?

    (A) umbilical vein

    (B) umbilical artery

    (C) ductus venosum

    (D) ductus arteriosus

37. Which describes the blood that enters the right atrium in the fetus?

    (A) deoxygenated blood

    (B) oxygenated blood

    (C) oxygenated and deoxygenated blood

    (D) maternal blood

38. Which is *not* a shunt present in the fetus?

    (A) ductus venosum

    (B) foramen ovale

    (C) ductus arteriosus

    (D) umbilical vein

39. **Which modality is least useful in diagnosing a ventricular septal defect?**

    (A) 2D imaging

    (B) color Doppler

    (C) pulsed Doppler

    (D) M-mode

40. **An atrioventricular septal defect includes abnormal development of all of the following *except*.**

    (A) aortic arch

    (B) interatrial septum

    (C) interventricular septum

    (D) atrioventricular valves

41. **In hypoplastic left heart syndrome, what is a cause of the left ventricle becoming hypoplastic?**

    (A) decreased blood flow into or out of the left ventricle

    (B) increased blood flow into or out of the left ventricle

    (C) decreased blood flow due to a closed foramen ovale

    (D) a large ventricular septal defect

42. **In a fetus with hypoplastic left heart syndrome, abnormalities may be seen in which valves?**

    (A) aortic and pulmonary

    (B) mitral and tricuspid

    (C) tricuspid and pulmonary

    (D) mitral and aortic

43. **With hypoplastic left heart syndrome, blood flow through the ascending aorta is usually**

    (A) absent or reversed

    (B) high velocity

    (C) normal

    (D) low velocity

44. **Atrioventricular septal defects are commonly associated with which condition?**

    (A) lupus

    (B) oligohydramnios

    (C) polysplenia

    (D) polyhydramnios

45. **Which chromosomal abnormality is most commonly associated with an atrioventricular septal defect?**

    (A) trisomy 13

    (B) trisomy 18

    (C) trisomy 21

    (D) Turner syndrome

46. **Which heart anomaly has the best prognosis?**

    (A) Ebstein anomaly

    (B) isolated ventricular septal defect

    (C) truncus arteriosus

    (D) undetected coarctation of the aorta

47. **Which heart anomaly usually has the poorest prognosis?**

    (A) hypoplastic left heart syndrome

    (B) hypoplastic right heart syndrome

    (C) mild aortic stenosis

    (D) isolated atrial septal defect

48. **Which structure could be small with hypoplastic right heart syndrome?**

    (A) aortic valve

    (B) pulmonary valve

    (C) aorta

    (D) pulmonary veins

49. **What effect is demonstrated with pulse Doppler, when a valve is stenotic**

    (A) decreased velocity proximal to the valve

    (B) decreased velocity distal to the valve

    (C) increased velocity proximal to the valve

    (D) increased velocity distal to the valve

50. **Which is *not* visualized with hypoplastic right heart syndrome?**

    (A) antegrade flow through the foramen ovale

    (B) large left-sided heart

    (C) increased flow through the pulmonary artery

    (D) dilated aortic root

51. **Which condition is almost always present with a univentricular heart?**

    (A) transposition of the great vessels

    (B) coarctation of the aorta

    (C) hypoplastic left heart syndrome

    (D) Ebstein anomaly

52. **Which is *not* associated with a univentricular heart?**

    (A) two normal atrioventricular valves

    (B) pulmonary stenosis

    (C) asplenia

    (D) polysplenia

53. **Which describes coarctation of the aorta?**

    (A) absence of the aorta

    (B) an aneurysm of the aorta

    (C) narrowing of the aortic lumen

    (D) enlargement of the aortic lumen

54. **The majority of coarctations of the aorta occur between which structures?**

    (A) thoracic and abdominal aorta

    (B) aortic valve and the ductus arteriosus

    (C) right subclavian artery and the ductus arteriosus

    (D) left subclavian artery and the ductus arteriosus

55. **Which is *not* a sign of coarctation of the aorta?**

    (A) enlarged right ventricle

    (B) enlarged left ventricle

    (C) increased velocities in the aorta

    (D) narrowing of the aorta

56. **Coarctation of the aorta is most common in which genetic condition?**

    (A) Turner syndrome

    (B) Edwards syndrome

    (C) trisomy 13

    (D) trisomy 21

57. **Which describes Ebstein anomaly?**

    (A) inferior displacement of the mitral valve

    (B) superior displacement of the mitral valve

    (C) inferior displacement of the tricuspid valve

    (D) superior displacement of the tricuspid valve

58. **Ebstein anomaly has been associated with maternal use of which substance?**

    (A) lithium

    (B) alcohol

    (C) codeine

    (D) tobacco

59. **Which defect is *not* seen in a newborn with tetralogy of Fallot?**

    (A) ventricular septal defect

    (B) overriding aorta

    (C) pulmonary stenosis

    (D) aortic stenosis

60. **Which tetralogy of Fallot defect may *not* be present *in utero*?**

    (A) large ventricular septal defect

    (B) atrial septal defect

    (C) right ventricular hypertrophy

    (D) overriding aorta

61. **Which defect is present with truncus arteriosus?**

    (A) coarctation of the aorta

    (B) hypoplastic right heart

    (C) atrial septal defect

    (D) ventricular septal defect

62. **What is an accurate description of truncus arteriosus?**

    (A) a single vessel arising from the heart; the pulmonary arteries arise from this great vessel

    (B) a single vessel arising from the heart; the aorta arises from this great vessel

    (C) two vessels arise from the heart; running parallel

    (D) two vessels arise from the heart and crisscross

63. **A right-sided aortic arch is not seen in which condition?**

    (A) truncus arteriosus

    (B) congenitally corrected transposition of the great vessels

    (C) tetralogy of Fallot

    (D) situs inversus above the diaphragm

64. **Truncus arteriosus can be mistaken for which other anomaly?**

    (A) transposition of the great vessels

    (B) tetralogy of Fallot

    (C) Ebstein anomaly

    (D) univentricular heart

65. **Which view *cannot* be obtained with complete transposition of the great vessels?**

    (A) apical four chamber

    (B) subcostal four chamber

    (C) short-axis view of the great vessels

    (D) aortic arch

66. **With complete transposition of the great vessels**

    (A) the atria, ventricles, and valves are in the appropriate location; the aorta arises from the right ventricle, the pulmonary artery from the left ventricle

    (B) the atria, ventricles, and valves are in the appropriate location; the aorta arises from the left ventricle, the pulmonary artery from the right ventricle

    (C) the atria, ventricles, and valves are transposed; the aorta arises from the right ventricle, the pulmonary artery from the left ventricle

    (D) the atria, ventricles, and valves are transposed; the aorta arises from the left ventricle, the pulmonary artery from the right ventricle

67. **To identify congenitally corrected transposition of the great vessels, the moderator band can be seen in the**

    (A) right-sided left ventricle

    (B) left-sided left ventricle

    (C) right-sided right ventricle

    (D) left-sided right ventricle

68. **With congenitally corrected transposition of the great vessels**

    (A) the atria, ventricles, and valves are in the appropriate location; the aorta arises from the left ventricle, the pulmonary artery from the right ventricle

    (B) the atria, ventricles, and valves are in the appropriate location; the aorta arises from the right ventricle, the pulmonary artery from the left ventricle

    (C) the right atrium and left ventricle are connected, the left atrium and right ventricle are connected; the aorta arises from the right-sided left ventricle; the pulmonary artery from the left-sided right ventricle

    (D) the right atrium and left ventricle are connected, the left atrium and right ventricle are connected; the aorta arises from the left-sided right ventricle; the pulmonary artery from the right-sided left ventricle

69. **What is the best view to identify double outlet right ventricle?**

    (A) long-axis views of the aorta and pulmonary artery

    (B) apical four-chamber view

    (C) subcostal four-chamber view

    (D) long-axis view of the pulmonary artery

70. **With double outlet right ventricle, the great vessels run**

    (A) right to left

    (B) left to right

    (C) parallel

    (D) perpendicular

71. **When total anomalous pulmonary venous connection occurs, the pulmonary veins drain into which structure?**

    (A) right ventricle

    (B) left ventricle

    (C) right atrium

    (D) left atrium

72. **Which anomaly is most likely to be identified *in utero* if only a four-chamber heart view is obtained?**

    (A) double outlet right ventricle

    (B) tetralogy of Fallot

    (C) transposition of the great vessels

    (D) hypoplastic left heart syndrome

73. **In severe levocardia, the heart is pointed toward the**

    (A) left at a 45° angle

    (B) left at an angle greater than 65°

    (C) right at a 45° angle

    (D) right at an angle greater than 65°

74. **Which term is used when the apex of the heart is pointed toward the right side?**

    (A) levocardia

    (B) levoposition

    (C) dextrocardia

    (D) dextroposition

75. **The heart can be displaced to the right side of the chest due to all of the following *except*.**

    (A) tricuspid insufficiency

    (B) diaphragmatic hernia

    (C) cystic adenomatoid malformation

    (D) hypoplastic right lung

76. **What is the most common type of dysrhythmia?**

    (A) supraventricular tachycardia

    (B) tachycardia

    (C) atrial flutter

    (D) premature atrial contractions

77. **If supraventricular tachycardia is sustained, it can lead to which anomaly?**

    (A) hypoplastic right heart

    (B) hypoplastic left heart

    (C) oligohydramnios

    (D) hydrops

78. **Pressure from the transducer may cause which transient dysrhythmia?**

    (A) premature atrial contractions

    (B) atrial flutter

    (C) bradycardia

    (D) tachycardia

79. **Which of the following describes a second-degree heart block of 3:1?**

    (A) two atrial contractions for every one ventricular contraction

    (B) three atrial contractions for every one ventricular contraction

    (C) two ventricular contractions for every one atrial contraction

    (D) three ventricular contractions for every one atrial contraction

80. **Which is *not* associated with complete heart block?**

    (A) chordae tendineae

    (B) atrial septal defect

    (C) cardiac tumors

    (D) polysplenia

Answers and Explanations

At the end of each explained answer, there is a number combination in parentheses. The first number identifies the reference source; the second number or set of numbers indicates the page or pages on which the relevant information can be found.

1. **(B)** A fetal echocardiogram should always begin by determining fetal position. Once fetal position is determined, situs (position of the heart and stomach) and cardiac structures can be accurately identified. (*Study Guide: 469*)

2. **(B)** In the subcostal four-chamber view, all four chambers can be identified along with the interventricular and interatrial septae. Subcostal four-chamber is the best view to evaluate for ASDs and VSDs, because the septae are perpendicular to the transducer. The long-axis views are important in determining appropriate position of the outflow tracts. (*Study Guide: 470*)

3. **(D)** When valves are insufficient, complete closure of the valve does not occur. Blood, therefore, flows back and can be detected with pulsed Doppler proximal to the valve. (*Study Guide: 474*)

4. **(A)** A four-chamber heart view does *not* exclude all anomalies. To increase the chance of identifying abnormalities, outflow tracts must be obtained. Long-axis views of the aorta and pulmonary artery should be seen "criss-crossing." (*Study Guide: 467*)

5. **(C)** Dysrhythmias involve both the atria and ventricle. An atrial beat and a ventricular response can be evaluated if the M-mode cursor is placed through both the atria and ventricle. (*Study Guide: 469*)

6. **(A)** Blood flows from the right atrium into the left atrium. The foraminal flap opens into the left atrium. (*Study Guide: 474*)

7. **(D)** Complete heart block is associated with mothers who have lupus. Diabetic mothers are more likely to have babies with congenital heart disease, VSD's double-outlet right ventricle, cardiomyopathies, and truncus arteriosus. Cytomegalovirus is associated with dilated cardiomyopathy. (*Study Guide: 467*)

8. **(B)** Trisomies 13 and 18 are associated with heart defects almost 100% of the time. Trisomy 21 has a 40–50% defect rate. (*Study Guide: 468*)

9. **(C)** Pulsed and color Doppler and M-mode are essential tools for a fetal echocardiogram. Even though power Doppler can have higher sensitivity, it has increased flash artifact and cannot determine direction of flow. (*Study Guide: 467*)

10. **(D)** Congenital heart defects occur in 1/100 live births. (*Study Guide: 467*)

11. **(B)** Ventricular septal defects are the most common heart defect, occurring in approximately 20–57% of heart defect cases. (*Study Guide: 475*)

12. **(B)** In the subcostal four-chamber view, the septa are perpendicular to the transducer; therefore, it is more likely a defect will be identified. In the apical four-chamber view, the chambers are identified, but the septae is parallel to the transducer. In this position, a pseudodefect is often seen. (*Study Guide: 470*)

13. **(C)** A fetal echocardiogram should be performed between 18 and 22 weeks. Before this time, the heart is too small to visualize accurately. After 22 weeks, artifact from bony structures and decreased fluid volume makes evaluation difficult. (*Study Guide: 467*)

14. **(A)** The apex of the heart points toward the left. This is termed levocardia. Dextrocardia is when the apex points toward the right. (*Study Guide: 469*)

15. **(B)** The heart sits in the chest at an angle approximately 45°. The angle, however, can vary 20° in either direction. (i.e., 25°–65°). (*Study Guide: 469*)

16. **(A)** Levocardia is the normal orientation of the fetal heart. Dextrocardia occurs when the heart is in the right chest and the apex points toward the right. When the heart is situated in the midline and the apex points midline, this is termed mesocardia. Dextroposition is when the heart is in the right chest but the apex points toward the left. (*Study Guide: 469*)

17. **(C)** The normal fetal heart occupies one-third of the fetal chest. (*Study Guide: 469*)

18. **(B)** The apical four-chamber view is obtained with a transverse view of the chest. The heart (apex) is directed toward or away from the transducer. In other words, the interventricular and interatrial septa run parallel to the beam of the transducer. (*Study Guide: 469*)

19. **(D)** An apical four-chamber view of the heart allows visualization of all four chambers, the size of the chambers, and the mitral and tricuspid valves. The ventricular septum is not well visualized because the septum is parallel to the transducer. (*Study Guide: 469*)

20. **(D)** Once a subcostal four-chamber view is obtained, the transducer can be rotated toward the fetus's right shoulder. The first view seen will be a long-axis view of the aorta (left ventricular outflow tract). If rotation continues, the long axis of the pulmonary artery will be visualized (right

ventricular outflow tract). A short-axis view of the ventricles will be seen next. The short-axis view of the aorta with the pulmonary artery crossing over completes the rotation. (*Study Guide: 470*)

21. **(B)** The great vessels should be documented criss-crossing. If the great vessels run parallel, this could indicate transposition of the great vessels. Truncus arteriosus is when one vessel arises from the ventricle. When both vessels arise from the right ventricle, this is termed double outlet right ventricle. (*Study Guide: 471*)

22. **(C)** The moderator band is located in the right ventricle. This can be helpful in determining situs, especially with congenitally corrected transposition of the great arteries. (*Study Guide: 480*)

23. **(D)** The subcostal four-chamber view, long-axis view of the aorta, and the short-axis view of the ventricles are all useful in determining pathology of the ventricular septum. The short-axis view of the great vessels does not demonstrate the ventricular septum. It is, however, beneficial in determining correct orientation of the great vessels. (*Study Guide: 470*)

24. **(A)** In the fetus, the main pulmonary artery bifurcates into the ductus arteriosus and the right pulmonary artery. (*Study Guide: 472*)

25. **(D)** The aortic arch does not have the appearance of a hockey stick. The ductal arch is flat and broader, much like a hockey stick. (*Study Guide: 473*)

26. **(B)** The majority of coarctations occur just distal to where the ductus arteriosus inserts into the aorta. Aortic valve insufficiency is obtained proximal to the aortic valve. Aortic stenosis occurs at the level of the aortic valve. Pulmonary valve insufficiency would be identified in the right ventricle, proximal to the pulmonary valve. (*Study Guide: 477*)

27. **(C)** The ductal arch has a hockey stick appearance. The pulmonary artery, ductus arteriosus, and the descending aorta comprise the ductal arch. (*Study Guide: 473*)

28. **(C)** The most common indication for a fetal echocardiogram is family history. The risk for a reoccurring heart defect is highest when the mother has a defect (10–12%). The percentages are lower with other family members. (*Study Guide: 467*)

29. **(D)** Suboptimal heart views on a 12-week ultrasound are not an indication for a fetal echocardiogram. At 12 weeks, the fetal heart is small and structures are difficult to visualize. If the heart is suboptimal on an 18- to 20-week ultrasound, a fetal echocardiogram should be performed. (*Study Guide: 467*)

30. **(C)** Peak velocities can only be obtained with pulsed Doppler. Color Doppler, however, can help in determining areas of increased velocity or turbulence. (*Study Guide: 474*)

31. **(D)** M-mode is not useful in determining direction of flow. Color or pulsed Doppler can be used to determine direction. (*Study Guide: 474*)

32. **(B)** In the fetus, oxygenated blood travels from the umbilical veins through the ductus venosus, bypassing the liver. This blood then enters the inferior vena cava. The blood that enters the liver mixes with the portal system. Once the fetus is born, the ductus venosus closes and becomes the ligamentum venosum of the liver. (*Study Guide: 474*)

33. **(A)** The pulmonary veins enter the left atrium. Pulsed Doppler is helpful in determining appropriate direction and location of the pulmonary veins. (*Study Guide: 474*)

34. **(D)** The Doppler angle should be as close to zero as possible. With a 90° angle, a Doppler signal cannot be obtained. (*Study Guide: 474*)

35. **(D)** The Doppler gate should be small to avoid interference of other structures and vessels. (*Study Guide: 474*)

36. **(A)** Blood flows from the placenta to the fetus by way of the umbilical vein. The umbilical arteries return blood back to the placenta. The ductus venosum is a shunt that allows blood to bypass the liver. The ductus arteriosus shunts blood from the pulmonary artery to the descending aorta. (*Study Guide: 474*)

37. **(C)** Oxygenated blood flows from the placenta through the umbilical vein. Most of this blood bypasses the liver via the ductus venosum and enters the inferior vena cava (IVC). Deoxygenated blood from the lower extremities travels up the IVC and mixes with the oxygenated blood. This oxygenated and deoxygenated blood then enters the right atrium. (*Study Guide: 475*)

38. **(D)** The umbilical vein is not considered a shunt. It carries blood from the placenta to the fetus. The ductus venosus allows blood to bypass the liver. It closes shortly after birth and becomes the ligamentum venosum in the liver. The foramen ovale shunts blood from the right atrium to the left atrium. The ductus arteriosus is a shunt between the pulmonary artery and the descending aorta. It also closes shortly after birth and becomes the ligamentum arteriosum. Closure of the ductus arteriosus causes a pressure change in the heart. After birth the pressure is higher in the left side of the heart, causing the foramen ovale to close. (*Study Guide: 475*)

39. **(D)** M-mode is not very useful in identifying a ventricular septal defect in the fetus. It is useful in determining heart rate and rhythm, chamber size, and wall thickness. (*Study Guide: 474*)

40. **(A)** An atrioventricular septal defect is an abnormal development of the interatrial septum, interventricular septum, and the atrioventricular valves (tricuspid and mitral valves). (*Study Guide: 476*)

41. **(A)** With hypoplastic left heart syndrome (HLHS), there is a decrease in the blood flow coming in or out of the ventricle. The decrease in flow results in underdevelopment of the ventricle. (*Study Guide: 476*)

42. **(D)** Because HLHS affects the left heart, the mitral and aortic valves can be abnormal. (*Study Guide: 476*)

43. **(A)** With HLHS, the flow through the ascending aorta may be absent or reversed. This is caused by the blood flowing back through the ductus arteriosus into the ascending aorta. (*Study Guide: 476*)

44. **(C)** Atrioventricular septal defects are associated with polysplenia approximately 30% of the time. (*Study Guide: 476*)

45. **(C)** Approximately 78% of AVSDs are associated with Down syndrome (trisomy 21). (*Study Guide: 476*)

46. **(B)** An isolated ventricular septal defect has the best prognosis. With Ebstein anomaly, the displacement of the tricuspid valve can lead to an enlarged right atrium, pulmonary atresia or stenosis, and cardiomegaly. Truncus arteriosus has a poor prognosis when left untreated. When treated, there is still mixing of oxygenated and deoxygenated blood. If a coarctation of the aorta is untreated it can be fatal. (*Study Guide: 475*)

47. **(A)** Hypoplastic left heart syndrome has the poorest prognosis. If left untreated, it is uniformly fatal. The poor prognosis is because of the small left heart, hypoplastic mitral valve, and ascending aorta. Hypoplastic right heart syndrome, however, has a better prognosis with a survival rate of approximately 25%. A *mild* aortic stenosis and an isolated atrial septal defect are treatable and have a good prognosis. (*Study Guide: 476*)

48. **(B)** With hypoplastic right heart syndrome, the pulmonary artery and valve can be small or atretic. The aorta and pulmonary veins are not affected by hypoplastic right heart syndrome since they are left-sided structures. (*Study Guide: 477*)

49. **(D)** When a valve is stenotic, the velocity will be increased distal to the valve. The sample gate can be placed proximal to the valve to determine valvular regurgitation. (*Study Guide: 474*)

50. **(C)** With the decrease of size and flow through the right side of the heart, there is decreased flow through the pulmonary artery. (*Study Guide: 477*)

51. **(A)** A univentricular heart has two atria and one ventricle. Often, when a univentricular heart is present, there is transposition of the great vessels coming off this one ventricle. (*Study Guide: 477*)

52. **(A)** With a univentricular heart, two atrioventricular valves may be seen. One, however, is usually atretic, indicating tricuspid or mitral atresia. This atresia is not related to the univentricular heart but is considered a separate pathology. Pulmonary stenosis, asplenia, and polysplenia are all associated with a univentricular heart. (*Study Guide: 477*)

53. **(C)** Coarctation is a narrowing of the aorta. Coarctation is often difficult to diagnosis *in utero*. (*Study Guide: 477*)

54. **(D)** Approximately 98% of coarctations occur between the left subclavian artery and the ductus arteriosus. (*Study Guide: 477*)

55. **(B)** Coarctation of the aorta is often difficult to visualize *in utero*. A narrowing of the aorta or increased velocities in the aorta can help to confirm the diagnosis. A large right ventricle may be a secondary sign of a coarctation. (*Study Guide: 477*)

56. **(A)** Coarctation of the aorta is most commonly seen with Turner syndrome. (*Study Guide: 477*)

57. **(C)** Ebstein anomaly is a right-sided heart anomaly. The tricuspid valve is displaced inferiorly. (*Study Guide: 478*)

58. **(A)** Maternal use of lithium has been associated with Ebstein anomaly. (*Study Guide: 478*)

59. **(D)** The four criteria for tetralogy of Fallot are a ventricular septal defect, overriding aorta, pulmonary stenosis, and right ventricular hypertrophy. (*Study Guide: 478*)

60. **(C)** Right ventricular hypertrophy may not be seen *in utero* because of the presence of fetal shunts. An atrial septal defect is not a defect associated with tetralogy of Fallot. (*Study Guide: 478*)

61. **(D)** Ventricular septal defects are present with truncus arteriosus. The single vessel overrides this defect. (*Study Guide: 479*)

62. **(A)** With truncus arteriosus, a single vessel arises from the heart. The pulmonary arteries then branch off this single vessel. (*Study Guide: 479*)

63. **(B)** Congenitally corrected transposition of the great vessels occurs when ventricles are switched. The aorta arises from the left-sided right ventricle and follows the normal course toward the left side. With truncus arteriosus, a right-sided aortic arch is seen in approximately 15–30% of cases. Tetralogy of Fallot has a right side aortic arch in 25% of cases. With situs inversus of the chest, all anatomy above the diaphragm would be transposed. (*Study Guide: 478–480*)

64. **(B)** Truncus arteriosus and tetralogy of Fallot appear similar sonographically. Both pathologies have a single vessel overriding a ventricular septal defect. Truncus arteriosus, however, occurs when the pulmonary arteries arise from this single vessel; where with tetralogy of Fallot, the pulmonary artery arises from the right ventricle. A univentricular heart's vessels are often transposed. (*Study Guide: 478, 479*)

65. **(C)** With complete transposition of the great vessels, the great arteries arise from the heart in a parallel fashion; therefore, a normal short-axis view of the great vessels cannot be obtained. A normal four-chamber heart can be identified. This stresses the point of why outflow tracts should always be obtained. (*Study Guide: 479*)

66. **(A)** With complete transposition of the great vessels, the atria, ventricles, and valves are in the appropriate location. The aorta arises from the right ventricle, and the pulmonary artery arises from the left ventricle. This differs from congenitally corrected transposition of the great vessels. With congenitally corrected transposition, the right atrium

and left ventricle are connected, and the left atrium and right ventricle are connected. The aorta arises from the left-sided right ventricle, and the pulmonary artery arises from the right-sided left ventricle. Identification of the moderator band in the right ventricle is helpful in the diagnosis of congenitally corrected transposition of the great vessels. (*Study Guide: 479*)

67. **(D)** The moderator band will always be located in the right ventricle. In congenitally corrected transposition of the great vessels, the right ventricle is located on the left side of the chest. (*Study Guide: 480*)

68. **(D)** With congenitally corrected transposition, the right atrium and left ventricle are connected, and the left atrium and right ventricle are connected. The aorta arises from the left-sided right ventricle, and the pulmonary artery arises from the right-sided left ventricle. Identification of the moderator band in the right ventricle is helpful in the diagnosis of congenitally corrected transposition of the great vessels. With complete transposition of the great vessels, the atria, ventricles and valves are in the appropriate location. The aorta arises from the right ventricle, and the pulmonary artery arises from the left ventricle. (*Study Guide: 480*)

69. **(A)** When the long-axis views of the aorta and pulmonary artery are obtained, both great arteries would be visualized arising from the right ventricle. Four-chamber views of the heart will not demonstrate double outlet right ventricle. (*Study Guide: 480*)

70. **(C)** Double outlet right ventricle occurs when both great arteries arise from the right ventricle running parallel. (*Study Guide: 480*)

71. **(C)** The pulmonary veins normally drain into the left atrium. When total anomalous pulmonary venous connection is present, all four pulmonary veins will drain into the right atrium, or other venous structures. (*Study Guide: 480*)

72. **(D)** Of the choices listed, hypoplastic left heart syndrome would be the most likely diagnosed *in utero* when only a four-chamber heart view is visualized. All of the other pathologies listed can be diagnosed with careful interrogation of the outflow tracts. (*Study Guide: 476*)

73. **(B)** Severe levocardia is defined as the heart's apex pointing toward the left at an angle greater than the normal 45° ± 20°. Severe levocardia is commonly seen with Ebstein anomaly, or other cardiac lesions that cause right-sided enlargement. (*Study Guide: 481*)

74. **(C)** Dextrocardia is when the heart is in the right chest, and the apex of the heart is pointed toward the right. Levocardia is the normal position of the heart. Severe levocardia is defined as the heart's apex pointing toward the left at an angle greater than the normal 45° ± 20°. Dextroposition is when the heart's apex points toward the left, but the heart is in the right chest. (*Study Guide: 481*)

75. **(A)** A diaphragmatic hernia and cystic adenomatoid malformation can push the heart into the right chest. Hypoplastic right lung causes a potential space on the right side that the heart can move into. Tricuspid insufficiency will not cause abnormal cardiac axis or position. (*Study Guide: 481*)

76. **(D)** The most common dysrhythmia is premature atrial contractions (PACs). PACs can be caused by maternal use of caffeine, cigarettes or alcohol, or by a redundant foraminal flap. The majority of PACs resolve by delivery. (*Study Guide: 482*)

77. **(D)** Supraventricular tachycardia occurs when the fetal heart rate is 180–280 bpm, and there is also atrial–ventricular concordance. If SVT remains throughout pregnancy, fetal hydrops or death can occur. (*Study Guide: 482*)

78. **(C)** Transducer pressure can lead to bradycardia. When pressure is released, normal rate returns. (*Study Guide: 482*)

79. **(B)** A second-degree heart block of 3:1 occurs when there are three atrial contractions for every one ventricular contraction. (*Study Guide: 482*)

80. **(A)** Atrial septal defects, cardiac tumors, and polysplenia are all associated with complete heart block. Chordae tendineae are cord-like tendons that connect the papillary muscles to the tricuspid valve. (*Study Guide: 482*)

10

Breast Sonography

Lawrence E. Mason

Study Guide

INTRODUCTION

For many years, breast sonography has been an important tool in the management of breast disorders. In recent years, its role in the workup of breast disorders has become more defined as technical advances has improved in spatial and temporal resolution. It is now required by the American College of Radiology that a breast imaging facility offer breast sonography to be considered for accreditation. Without the potentially harmful effects of ionizing radiation, the role of sonography in breast imaging will continue to evolve as technical advances occur.

EPIDEMIOLOGY OF BREAST CANCER[1]

It is our primary role as sonographers and physicians to provide our best efforts to educate patients on the detection of breast disorders, namely breast cancer. Except for skin cancer, breast cancer is the most common cancer among women. The chance of developing invasive breast cancer at sometime in a woman's life is about 1 in 8 (13% of women).[1] At this time, there are more than 2 million breast cancer survivors in the United States. Women living in North America have the highest rate of breast cancer in the world.

INDICATIONS FOR BREAST SONOGRAPHY

Breast sonography is used as an adjunct to mammography and physical examination. The most common indications to perform an ultrasound exam are the presence of a palpable mass or discovery of an abnormality on mammography. Ultrasound is useful to determine if a mass is cystic or solid, which helps determine management. Ultrasound guidance for aspirations and biopsies is also an indication. Also, ultrasound is the first imaging study in the evaluation of breast mass in pregnant or lactating women, under the age of 30 and in women following mastectomy with a complaint on the side of the mastectomy.

Indications for breast ultrasound include:

- Identification and characterization of palpable abnormalities
- Identification and characterization of clinical and mammographic findings
- Guidance for procedures
- Follow up a finding from a breast MRI or other examination of the breast

EXAMINER QUALIFICATIONS

All examiners performing breast ultrasound examinations, including those assisting physicians with ultrasound guided breast biopsy procedures, are encouraged to meet minimum criteria (Table 10–1).[2]

When breast sonography is performed by an experienced examiner, patients with breast related complaints can be appropriately triaged for clinical follow up, biopsy or referred for surgery as necessary. However, the detection of breast cancer and breast disorders is a daunting task for the inexperienced breast sonographer and the responsibility for the detection of breast disorders does not rest exclusively on the shoulders of the sonographer. The sonographer's primary function is to document limited anatomic regions of the breast with knowledge of normal anatomy. In fulfilling this role, the sonographer should be able to bring to the attention of the physician areas of interest that require further evaluation. In the majority of cases, a breast sonogram will require correlation of the sonographic findings with the clinical and mammographic findings prior to the patient leaving the department. This will often necessitate

TABLE 10–1 • Criteria for Breast Ultrasound Examinations	
Qualifications	**Sonographer or Mammography Technologist: Breast Ultrasound**
Initial	ARDMS certification and current registration, or ARRT post-primary certification and current registration in breast sonography, or ARRT certification and current registration (or unrestricted state license) and MQSA qualified AND Five Continuing education units (CEUs)/ Continuing medical education (CMEs) specific to breast ultrasound
Continuing experience	Regular performance of breast sonographic exams

an interaction between the physician and the patient which may include additional imaging.

If the examiner thinks that the sonographic findings do not agree with the indication for the examination (i.e., the exam was performed for a 3 cm mass on a mammogram, but only a 1 cm simple cyst is seen on ultrasound), the patient may be instructed to wait until the physician can verify the concordance of the findings. Alternatively, the patient should be instructed to return at a later time with the understanding that the examination is incomplete.

The physician is not required to be present during breast ultrasound examinations performed by American Registry for Diagnostic Medical Sonography (ARDMS) sonographers or American Registry of Radiologic Technologists (ARRT) with certification in breast sonography. However, a physician must be in the department during breast ultrasound examinations performed by ARRT technologists without advanced registry in breast sonography. In all situations, the physician is ultimately responsible to see that the appropriate images are obtained.[2]

EQUIPMENT REQUIREMENTS

Equipment used for practice of breast ultrasound should have the following features[3]:

1. High-resolution, real-time, linear array transducer
2. Center frequency of at least 7 MHz
3. Adjustable focal zone(s)

Linear array, broad bandwidth transducers with a minimum center frequency of 7 MHz are required for breast sonography. However, a center frequency of 10 MHz or greater is preferred. Transducers in the range of 7 to 15 MHz are utilized for breast imaging and the higher frequencies help demonstrate ductal anatomy. Broad bandwidth provides for high resolution superficial scanning with beam penetration to depth settings of 4 cm or greater. At 7.5 MHz, a linear array transducer suitable

for breast imaging should have penetration to a depth of at least 4 cm. Higher frequency transducers (>10 MHz) are focused at a depth of 3 cm or less, optimizing resolution of superficial masses. Whereas higher frequencies are more suitable to resolve smaller and superficial structures, the drawback is the frequency-dependent attenuation of deeper breast tissue, which restricts the ability of the beam to adequately display deeper breast structures and lesion detail.

Even with high resolution transducers, use of an acoustic standoff pad often improves the resolution of superficial, near-field lesions. Copious usage of gel may be more suitable than standoff pads for the evaluation of superficial lesions, particularly those in locations where skin folds preclude an even surface contour. Harmonic and compound imaging techniques may also be useful in addressing artifacts in breast sonography. Spatial resolution of the sonographic images and edge shadowing (i.e., shadowing from adjacent echogenic interfaces) may be improved through the use of spatial compounding, while harmonic imaging may reduce the echoes seen within a lesion to improve the accuracy of diagnosis (i.e., a fluid-filled cystic mass will appear more anechoic with harmonic imaging).

The ability to adjust the focal zone is important for accurate display of breast lesions. If the focal zone is not properly set in the mid portion of the lesion, artifactual echoes may occur within cysts. This can occur despite optimization of other settings.

TECHNIQUE

Patient Positioning

Generally, the patient is placed in the supine position with the hand on the ipsilateral side of the breast to be examined placed behind the head. The patient is then rolled into a contralateral posterior oblique position. This helps reduce breast thickness and bring posterior lesions closer to the skin surface, thus reducing the limitations of a high frequency transducer. This positioning technique is most effective for lesions in the lateral tissue but is also useful for those in the medial tissue. For evaluation of the medial breast tissue, placing the patient's ipsilateral arm by the side often optimizes the examination. Rolling the patient into a posterior oblique position ipsilateral to the side to be examined may also be helpful for examination of the medial tissue and this may be a more comfortable position for a prolonged examination.

Sonographic Evaluation of Palpable Lesions

Patients are often referred for sonographic evaluation of areas of palpable concern. These areas may be noticeable to the patient, but often these areas are noticeable only to the referring clinician who has requested the examination. This scenario poses an issue to the sonographer as the sonographer may not be able to elicit any true concerns from the patient. For this reason, it is recommended that sonographers attempt to receive graphic or written documentation of where the area of interest is with respect to the nipple/areolar complex (i.e., distance from the nipple) and according to the clock face designation of the breast.

In addition, it may be necessary for the interpreting physician to verify by physical examination that the area to be evaluated is the area of clinical interest. This may necessitate a physical examination by a physician prior to the patient leaving the department. Correlation of imaging findings with clinical findings is paramount to ensure that an abnormality is not overlooked.

The technique of the examination of a palpable lesion is not significantly different than that of a nonpalpable lesion. For lesions that can be reliably palpated, the examiner should attempt to fix the lesion between two fingers. This will aid in decreasing the mobility of a lesion and improve diagnostic accuracy. This technique is especially useful for lesions that are superficial, mobile or subjectively small (i.e., <1 cm). For lesions within the skin, use of a standoff pad or a generous amount of gel may be necessary. At the least, the focal zone should be brought as close to the surface as possible, the depth should be minimized and the image appropriately magnified.

Also, examination of the area of palpable interest is often facilitated if the area is localized by physical examination with the patient in the position which allows the lesion to be most easily palpated. The patient may then be repositioned as necessary. In the evaluation of an area of palpable interest, the examination may be performed with the patient in a variety of recumbent, upright and standing positions to assure the examiner that the area of interest is in fact being appropriately evaluated.

IDENTIFICATION, LABELING AND DOCUMENTATION OF THE EXAM

Each examination is required to note the following on each image[3]:

- Patient's first and last names (required)
- Identification number and/or date of birth (required)
- Examination date (required)
- Facility name and location
- Designation of right or left breast
- Location of the lesion or area of interest using diagrammatic, clock face or other consistent notation, including distance from the nipple
- Scan plane/transducer orientation-radial/antiradial; longitudinal/transverse (required)
- Initials (or ID) of the sonographer performing the breast ultrasound exam and/or the physician performing the biopsy

Documentation of a mass/lesion requires the following:

- Each lesion should be noted in two orthogonal planes, both with and without calipers
- The maximal dimension of the mass should be measured as should the mass in three planes
- The focal zone should be set to the depth of the lesion

All abnormalities should be documented in two orthogonal planes. For the breast, imaging and description of lesions in the radial and anti-radial plane correlates with the ductal anatomy of the breast as both have an axis radiating from the nipple in a spoke-like fashion. Using radial and antiradial imaging with notation of clock face position and distance from the nipple allows a finding to be accurately localized. The clock face position can be used to identify the location of a lesion in the breast. It is important to remember that the clock face is superimposed, without reorientation, on both breasts in the same manner, thus the lateral right breast and medial left breast correspond to the 9 o'clock position.

The distance of the lesion from the nipple in centimeters is also required for proper documentation. To estimate the distance from the nipple, the length of the transducer footprint should be known and an estimate of the distance from the nipple can be assessed by knowledge of the transducer position (i.e., 1.5 transducer lengths from the nipple equals 9 cm from the nipple if the transducer is 6 cm in length).

Also, at least two sets of images of a lesion should be obtained: one with and one without measurements (calipers obscure the marginal detail). When documenting a negative examination of an area of palpable concern, an image should be taken at the exact location of the palpable area, and clearly labeled to indicate that the image corresponds to the palpable area. If the ultrasound examination is being performed for a targeted lesion or palpable abnormality, the corresponding quadrant of the breast should be examined. If a breast survey exam of the entire breast is performed, images should be acquired from all four quadrants. Images labeled 12, 3, 6, and 9 o'clock or upper outer, upper inner, lower inner or lower outer quadrant are appropriate.

Documentation of Ultrasound Guided Biopsies

Biopsies performed with the assistance of ultrasound may be performed with or without a device which employs a forceful thrust through breast tissue into or through the area of interest. The mechanism by which the biopsy device produces a forceful thrust is referred to as 'firing.' Often, biopsy devices that do not feature a firing mechanism have the ability to suction tissue into a portion of the needle. After suctioning tissue into the needle, a cutting device is activated thus producing a tissue sample. These instruments are referred to as 'vacuum-assisted' biopsy devices. The necessary image documentation differs slightly depending upon which type of device is used to perform a biopsy (Table 10–2).[4]

TABLE 10–2 • Required Clinical Images: Core Needle Biopsy (Non-vacuum & Vacuum)	
Non-Vacuum Device	**Vacuum Device**
Pre-biopsy images of mass in two orthogonal views	Pre-biopsy images of mass in 2 orthogonal views
Pre-fire image of needle adjacent to the lesion in the long axis	Sonogram showing the needle adjacent to or within the mass in the long axis
Post-fire image of needle in lesion in the long axis	

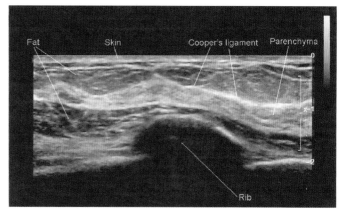

FIGURE 10–1. Cooper's ligaments extend from the parenchyma to the skin. Note the superficial rim of echogenicity at the rib and deeper shadow associated with calcification.

CORRELATING THE FINDINGS

The size and location of all lesions should be closely correlated with the abnormalities found on physical exam and other imaging modalities, namely mammography. Often, sonographic findings may be noted that were not previously identified on other imaging modalities. It is important to note these findings while continuing a search for an abnormality that would correlate with the reason for which the examination was requested. If this was an imaging finding, consultation with the radiologist/interpreting physician is necessary prior to the patient leaving the department. This will help reduce interpretation error and reduce delays in the diagnosis of breast diseases, namely cancer. Usually, size and location are the two lesion characteristics which aid the most in establishing confidence that what is seen sonographically correlates with what is seen on other modalities.

BREAST ANATOMY

The breast is a glandular organ composed primarily of fat, fibrous and glandular tissue with the capacity to alter its composition as a response to various factors. Hormonal stimuli effect the premenopausal changes and the age-related replacement of the glandular elements with fatty tissue. These changes contribute to the variable sonographic appearance of breast tissue at different stages of development. The fibroglandular composition of the breast is the primary variable that determines the attenuation characteristics of the breast tissue.

The breast parenchymal structure consists of 15–20 lobes that converge at the nipple in a radial arrangement, similar to the spokes of a wheel. One major duct, with an approximate 2 mm diameter, drains each lobe. Typically, 5–10 major collecting ducts open at the nipple.

The arterial supply is derived from numerous perforating arterial branches including the internal thoracic (internal mammary), lateral thoracic, and 3rd–5th intercostals arteries. The most medial of these is the internal thoracic (internal mammary) artery.

Sonographic Anatomy of the Breast

Skin. Skin is seen as two thin echogenic lines bordering a central hypoechoic region (Figs. 10–1 and 10–2). Normal thickness is <2 mm, however, in the lower breast at the junction of the inferior skin of the breast and the chest wall (inframammary fold) and in the region of the nipple (periareolar) up to 3 mm thickness is allowed.

Cooper's Ligaments. Cooper's ligaments are seen as thin, discrete echogenic lines radiating through the breast parenchyma extending toward the skin (Figs. 10–1 and 10–2). These ligaments help attach the parenchyma to the overlying skin and are best seen in the subcutaneous region where surrounding hypoechoic fat helps better visualize their appearance. They are often difficult to visualize within the hyperechoic parenchyma.

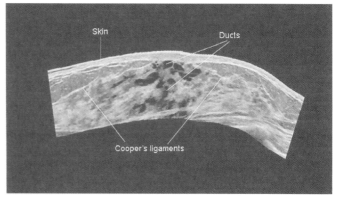

FIGURE 10–2. Prominent ducts are normally seen in the retroareolar region.

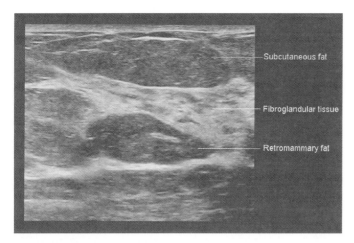

FIGURE 10-3. The typical appearance of fat (subcutaneous and retromammary) and parenchyma.

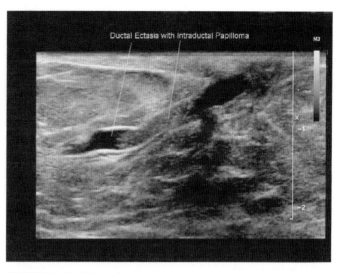

FIGURE 10-5. Dilated ducts may be seen with a detectable abnormality.

Breast Parenchyma (Fibroglandular Tissue). The breast parenchyma appears as areas of increased echogenicity located between the subcutaneous fat and retromammary fat (Figs. 10–2 and 10–3). The majority of the parenchyma is in the area deep to the nipple and in the lateral breast. Fibroglandular tissue usually occupies the majority of the volume of the breast in younger women and decreases with age. Hormone replacement therapy in postmenopausal women contributes to the persistence of fibroglandular tissue within the breast.

Duct. Ducts are seen as tubular, anechoic structures visible most prominently in the region beneath the nipple where they typically measure 2–3 mm in greatest diameter (Fig. 10–2). Ductal ectasia exists when ducts are >3 mm in diameter (Fig. 10–4). Ducts increase in diameter as a normal phenomenon during pregnancy and lactation. Evaluation for the presence of an intraductal mass is indicated if there is ductal ectasia in other settings (Fig. 10–5).

Fat. Fat is seen primarily in the subcutaneous and retromammary (between parenchyma and chest wall) regions (Figs. 10–2 and 10–3). The gain setting of the ultrasound unit should be set so that fat is hypoechoic with a medium to light gray appearance. The amount of fat within the breast decreases during pregnancy and lactation.

Ribs. The ribs appear as hypoechoic structures with a superficial curvilinear echogenic line on the side closest to the chest muscles and breast (Fig. 10–1). Marked posterior acoustic shadowing is present deep to the rib. Often, a central echogenic focus may be seen within the hypoechoic rib. The ribs are positioned immediately deep to the chest wall muscles.

Chest Wall Muscles. The chest wall muscles are located deep to the breast tissue and superficial to the ribs. Morphologically, they are plate-like and demonstrate a striated appearance with a dominant hypoechoic echotexture and internal echogenic lines (Fig. 10–6). The chest wall musculature is composed

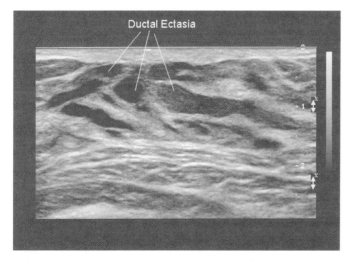

FIGURE 10-4. Dilated ducts may be seen without a detectable abnormality.

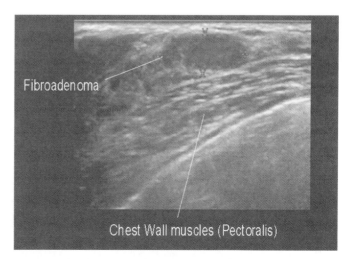

FIGURE 10-6. Typical appearance of the pectoralis muscle. Note the oval, parallel, circumscribed mass. This proved to be a benign fibroadenoma.

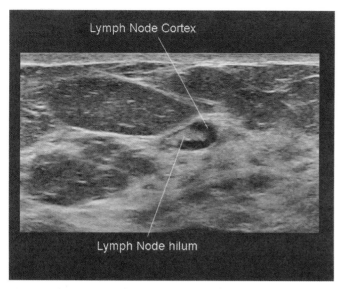

FIGURE 10–7. The typical appearance of an intramammary lymph node on gray-scale imaging is see in this image. Note the bean-shape of the lymph node with an echogenic hilum and hypoechoic periphery.

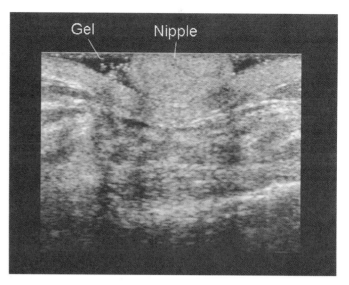

FIGURE 10–9. Imaging the nipple often requires the use of a standoff pad or copious amounts of gel.

primarily of the pectoralis muscles which extend horizontally from a midline location toward the axillae.

Lymph Nodes. Lymph nodes (Fig. 10–7) are oval, bean-shaped structures with a hypoechoic periphery (cortex) and a central echogenic region (hilum). These structures are normal when seen in the breast, particularly in the upper outer quadrant and axilla. Mass-like thickening of the peripheral cortex, gross change in shape (i.e., becomes globular) and absence of the echogenic hilum are abnormal findings. Assessment with color Doppler often yields detectable flow at the hilum where vessels enter and exit the lymph node (Fig. 10–8).

Nipple. The nipple often produces posterior acoustic shadowing distal to underlying tissue in normal circumstances. Proper

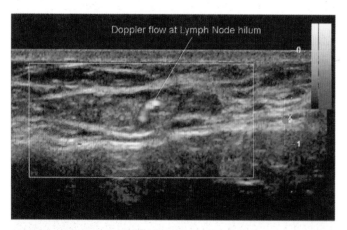

FIGURE 10–8. The typical appearance of an intramammary lymph node on Doppler imaging is see in this image. Note the kidney-bean shape with an echogenic hilum and hypoechoic periphery. Color Doppler sonography often depicts a vessel coursing into the hilum.

examination requires a standoff pad or abundant gel for effective visualization (Fig. 10–9).

LESION CHARACTERISTICS

Appropriate description of a lesion's characteristics is paramount for the communication of an examination's findings. Each characteristic should be assessed individually. Keeping characteristics separate under different descriptor categories helps get an overall impression of the lesion in question. Alternatively, the presence of a suspicious descriptor should prompt a more thorough evaluation to ensure that no other suspicious characteristics exist. An accurate portrayal of the lesion in question is needed to determine the most appropriate management and it is not infrequent that a single suspicious characteristic prompts intervention which can lead to the diagnosis of a malignancy. Characteristics suggestive of a malignant and benign processes (Tables 10–3 and 10–4) as well as those typically describing a simple cyst (Table 10–5) can be found in the included tables.

Shape[5]

Lesion shape may be classified as round or oval (Table 10–5). Round masses have a spherical or globular shape (Fig. 10–10). Oval masses have an elliptical shape and may have two or three gentle undulations (Fig. 10–11). All other masses are characterized as irregular.

Orientation[5]

Parallel orientation (Fig. 10–13) describes a mass which has its longest dimension parallel to the skin i.e., wider than tall. Nonparallel orientation describes a mass whose long axis is not

TABLE 10-3 • Descriptors Suggestive of Malignancy

Category	Descriptor
Shape	Irregular
Orientation	Not parallel (taller than wide)
Margins	Not circumscribed
Lesion boundary	Echogenic halo
Posterior acoustic features	Shadowing
Surrounding tissue	Cooper's ligament changes Architectural distortion Edema Skin thickening Skin retraction

TABLE 10-4 • Descriptors Suggestive of Benignancy

Category	Descriptor
Shape	Round Oval
Orientation	Parallel (wider than tall)
Margins	Circumscribed
Posterior acoustic features	None/enhancement
Surrounding tissue	N/A

TABLE 10-5 • Descriptors of A Simple Cyst

Category	Descriptor
Shape	Round Oval
Margins	Circumscribed
Echogenicity	Anechoic
Lesion boundary	Abrupt interface
Posterior acoustic features	Enhancement
Surrounding tissue	N/A

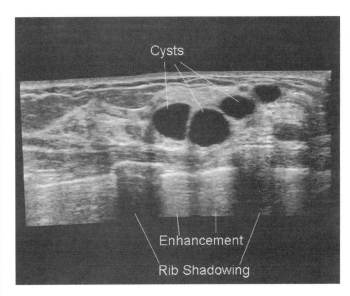

FIGURE 10-10. Round circumscribed, anechoic masses with posterior acoustic enhancement are seen in this image. These masses represent cysts.

parallel to the skin, i.e., taller than wide; this includes round lesions.

Margins[5]

A mass described as circumscribed is one whose margins are well defined and sharp with an abrupt transition between the mass and the adjacent tissue. The margins of a non-circumscribed mass can be described as indistinct (no clear demarcation with surrounding tissue), angular (sharp corners with adjacent tissue), microlobulated (scalloped appearance) or spiculated (sharp lines projecting from the mass) (Fig. 10–12).

Lesion Boundary[5]

The presence of an echogenic transition zone interposed between the mass and the adjacent tissue is referred to as an

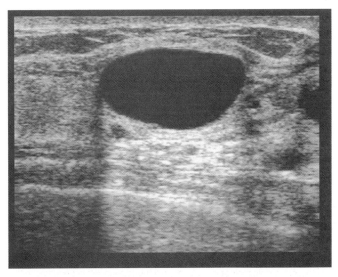

FIGURE 10-11. Oval circumscribed, anechoic mass with enhanced through transmission and distal acoustic enhancement.

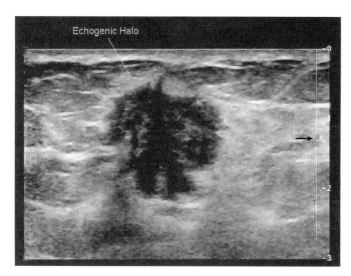

FIGURE 10–12. An irregular, complex mass with spiculated and angular margins and an echogenic halo is depicted. Note the focal zone (black arrow at the right of the image) positioned at the center of the mass. This was an invasive cancer.

'echogenic halo' (Fig. 10–12). Its absence suggests the presence of an abrupt interface (Figs. 10–11 and 10–13).

Echogenicity[5]

Anechoic defines a mass without any internal echoes (Fig. 10–11). Hyperechoic describes a mass whose interior has elements with increased echogenicity relative to fat or similar echogenicity to that of fibroglandular tissue (Fig. 10–14). Isoechoic describes a mass with echogenicity the same as fat, while hypoechoic describes a mass with low level internal echoes present that are less than the echogenicity of fat (Fig. 10–13). Complex describes a mass with both anechoic and hypo-/iso-/hyperechoic components (Fig. 10–12).

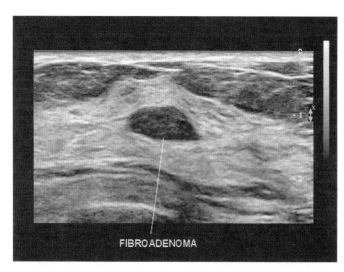

FIGURE 10–13. Note the oval, circumscribed, parallel, hypoechoic mass depicted in this image. No surrounding tissue abnormality is seen. This was a benign fibroadenoma.

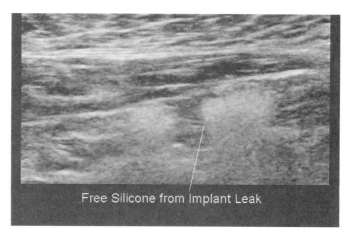

FIGURE 10–14. Free silicone can be seen in axillary or intramammary lymph nodes or in breast tissue. There is poor visualization of structures beneath the silicone-filled lymph nodes.

Posterior Acoustic Features[5]

If there is increased echogenicity of the tissue deep to the mass, this is termed posterior acoustic enhancement (Figs. 10–10 and 10–11). A reduction in echogenicity of the tissue deep to the mass (not including the tissue deep to the edges of the mass) is termed posterior acoustic shadowing. Some lesions do not demonstrate posterior acoustic features and others demonstrate a combination of such features.

Surrounding Tissue[5]

Dilatation of the ducts (ductal ectasia, Fig. 10–4) or changes in the branching pattern can be seen with certain processes. Also, Cooper's ligament changes can manifest as an increase in thickness or disruption, particularly in the presence of an inflammatory process. As the breast retains fluid, edema may manifest as branching hypoechoic lines throughout an enlarged breast (Fig. 10–15). Disruption of normal anatomic planes

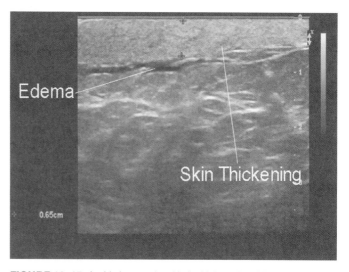

FIGURE 10–15. In this image, the skin is thickened and fluid is seen beneath the skin surface.

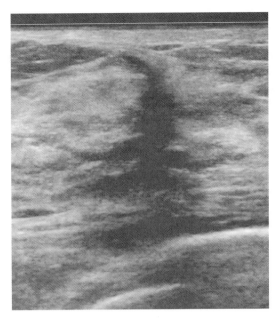

FIGURE 10–16. Post surgical breast scar. Distortion of the tissue with an irregular hypoechoic appearance in this image due to a surgical scar.

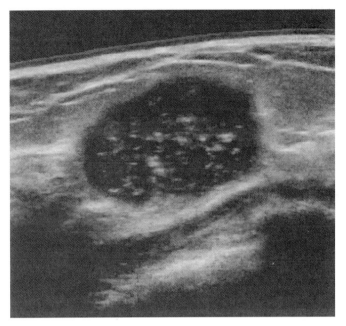

FIGURE 10–18. Complicated breast cyst. Multiple hyperechoic foci are seen in this largely anechoic mass representative of a complicated cyst.

is termed architectural distortion (Fig. 10–16) and is commonly seen in malignancy and in postsurgical cases. Skin thickening (Fig. 10–15), whether focal or diffuse, is also noteworthy as is evidence of skin retraction in which the skin surface may have an irregular, pulled-in appearance.

Calcifications[5]

Calcifications (Fig. 10–17) are often difficult to visualize and characterize with ultrasound. They appear as echogenic foci whose

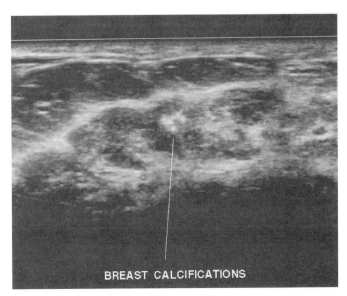

FIGURE 10–17. Discrete echogenic foci seen in this image represent calcifications.

ability to produce posterior acoustic shadowing is primarily dependant upon size. Calcifications which measure >0.5 mm in diameter are termed macrocalcifications and those which measure <0.5 mm in diameter are termed microcalcifications. If calcifications are visualized, it is important to note whether they are seen in association with a mass.

Unique Instances[5]

Clustered microcysts often have an appearance of a cluster of tiny anechoic foci of diameter >2–3 mm with thin (<0.5 mm thickness) intervening septations and no solid contents. Complicated cysts (Fig. 10–18) are most commonly characterized as masses with homogeneous, low-level internal echoes which may have fluid-fluid levels that shift with changes in the patient's position. Masses in or on the skin include sebaceous or epidermal inclusion cysts; these are often seen as entities at least partially contiguous with the dermis. The echogenic lines of the skin may separate to include a portion of the mass, thus confirming the location of the mass within the skin. Foreign bodies such as surgical clips, biopsy markers, implants (Fig. 10–19) or extruded implant material such as silicone should be described. Surgical clips and biopsy markers appear as discrete echogenic foci with variable posterior acoustic shadowing primarily dependent on size. Extruded silicone has a typical 'dirty shadowing' or 'snowstorm' appearance and can be seen in regional lymph nodes (Fig. 10–14).

Doppler[5]

Detecting vascularity within a lesion can help determine whether are solid components. However, the absence of Doppler flow

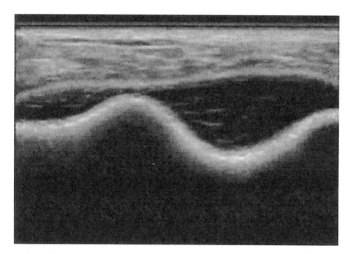

FIGURE 10–19. The capsule of an intact breast implant with overlying extracapsular fluid is depicted in this image. Fluid may be seen adjacent to normal, intact implants and does not signify the presence of a rupture.

does not exclude the presence of a solid portion. Reactive tissue changes from a nearby process may manifest as diffusely increased vascularity and demonstrate an increased Doppler signal.

BREAST MASSES

Cysts

Cysts are the most common breast masses, particularly in premenopausal women. The classic description of a simple cyst is that of a round, circumscribed, anechoic mass with posterior acoustic enhancement and no adjacent architectural distortion. Due to their fluid-filled nature, cysts lack internal vascularity on Doppler evaluation and can usually be deformed with gentle pressure. When any of these characteristics are not present, the diagnosis of a cyst should be in question. As experience grows, it may be seen that cysts assume a variety of shapes and have a range of echogenicity. These atypical characteristics may be suspicious depending upon the circumstance and may prompt an aspiration under sonographic guidance. If the cyst collapses completely following aspiration, this is diagnostic of a breast cyst. However if there is incomplete collapse of the cyst or a solid portion is seen in or adjacent to the cyst, biopsy of the solid portion is indicated. Recurrent, symptomatic cysts may be surgically excised. Hemorrhagic cysts often contain echogenic fluid or debris which may appear solid, thus prompting intervention when detected.

Fibroadenomas

Fibroadenomas are the most common solid breast masses. The classic description of a fibroadenoma is that of an oval, circumscribed, hypoechoic mass with its long axis oriented parallel to the breast tissue. A macrolobulated (i.e., a few large lobulations) contour may be seen. The peak age for detection is ages 20 to 30 years, but they can be seen well into the eighth and ninth decades of life. Solid masses often have overlapping features, thus making the exclusion of a different entity, particularly breast carcinoma, difficult. Biopsy is often needed to obtain a diagnosis. Certain characteristics of a solid mass such as recurrence following removal, postmenopausal enlargement and >2 cm of growth in a year are atypical findings which raise the suspicion for the presence of a mass other than a benign fibroadenoma.

Carcinoma

The sonographic detection of breast cancer is of utmost importance and not without pitfalls. A full description of the appearance of breast carcinoma would be beyond the scope of this text. Additionally, breast masses can appear different with variations in tissue density and echogenicity. Masses associated with an ill-defined border, an echogenic halo, margins that are sharp and angular, spiculation, posterior acoustic shadowing or adjacent architectural distortion are suspicious for malignancy. Also, any solid mass seen within a duct is suspicious and should be further evaluated. Subtle changes in the architecture of the breast (i.e., thickening of the adjacent Cooper's ligaments) are often the best clues that an aggressive, malignant process is ongoing, but detection of such findings often requires an experienced examiner with a discriminating eye.

SUMMARY

Breast sonography is a useful tool in the workup of breast disorders. As operator experience increases, the ability of the sonographer to differentiate subtle abnormalities of the breast will develop. With an understanding of technique and breast anatomy, adherence to the examination requirements and knowledge of the necessary language for appropriate characterization of the findings, a solid foundation for a developing breast sonographer is set.

References

1. American Cancer Society. Overview: Breast Cancer. 2006. Available: http://www.cancer.org/docroot/CRI/CRI_2_1xasp?dt=5(09/26/2006).

2. American College of Radiolog. Breast Ultrasound Accreditation Program requirements. 2007. Available: http://www.acr.org/accreditation/breast/breast_ultrasound_regs.aspx).

3. American College of Radiology. *ACR Practice Guidelines for the Performance of a Breast Ultrasound Examination* (Revised 2002). Reston, VA: Guidelines and Standards Committee; 1994.

4. American College of Radiology *ACR Practice Guideline for Performance of Ultrasound-Guided Percutaneous Breast Interventional Procedure* (Amended 2006). Reston, VA:1996.

5. American college of Radiology. ACR BI-RAD®—US Lexicon Classification Form Reston, VA:2006.

Questions

GENERAL INSTRUCTIONS: For each question, select the best answer. Select only one answer for each question unless otherwise instructed.

1. Which of the following is *not* an indication for breast ultrasound?

    (A) guidance for a breast biopsy

    (B) a patient had a breast sonogram last year and prefers it over a mammogram

    (C) an abnormality is palpated by the patient's physician

    (D) an abnormality is palpated by the patient

2. Which of the following statements is true regarding focal zone setting in breast sonography?

    (A) the focal zone should be set above the level of the lesion being imaged

    (B) the focal zone should be set at the level of the lesion being imaged

    (C) there should only be one focal zone used for maximum image optimization

    (D) the focal zone placement is not critical in sonographic breast imaging

3. What breast lesion is an acoustic standoff pad most helpful?

    (A) deep within the breast tissue

    (B) axillary in location

    (C) superficially positioned within the breast

    (D) mobile upon palpation

4. Each breast lesion should be measured in which of the following scan planes?

    (A) radial, antiradial

    (B) radial, transverse

    (C) sagittal, transverse

    (D) longitudinal, antiradial

5. A sonographic exam demonstrating a 2 cm anechoic, circumscribed mass at the 4 o'clock position in the left breast is compared to the patient's mammogram which suggested a 2 cm spiculated mass at the 9 o'clock position. Which of the following should the sonographer do?

    (A) tell the patient she has a cyst and there is nothing to worry about

    (B) tell the patient that the mammogram was a false positive and she should be followed up with sonography for future evaluation of the mass

    (C) take images of all abnormalities and tell the patient she may leave and return next year for her follow-up mammogram

    (D) discuss the differences in location and characteristics of the masses seen on the mammogram and sonogram with the interpreting physician.

6. Which of the following best describes the thickness of normal skin overlying the breast?

    (A) 2–3 cm

    (B) 1–2 cm

    (C) 5–10 mm

    (D) 2–3 mm

7. While preparing to perform a sonographic exam on a patient who was referred for evaluation of a palpable abnormality, the patient states she cannot feel the area reliably while lying down. Which of the following should the sonographer do?

    (A) ask the patient to try and find the lesion lying down because this is the best position for the sonographic exam

    (B) ask the patient to find it sitting up because it is usually the easiest position

    (C) ask the patient to find the lesion in whatever position necessary and attempt to image it from this position

    (D) examine the entire breast without attempting to localize the palpable abnormality

8. Which of the following sonographic features suggests malignancy?

    (A) round

    (B) posterior acoustic enhancement

    (C) spiculated

    (D) circumscribed

9. What minimum center frequency in MHz is required for transducers used in breast sonography

    (A) 6

    (B) 7

    (C) 8

    (D) 9

    (E) 10

10. In order for a breast mass to be characterized as anechoic it must:

    (A) not contain any internal echoes

    (B) demonstrate reverberation artifacts at the near-field edge

    (C) produce refraction artifacts on the lateral borders

    (D) demonstrate reduced echogenicity deep to the mass

11. What is the approximate chance of a woman developing invasive breast cancer in her lifetime?

    (A) 1 in 8

    (B) 1 in 15

    (C) 1 in 40

    (D) 1 in 100

12. Positioning to reduce the breast thickness of the upper outer quadrant can be achieved by placing the patient in which of the following positions?

    (A) place the ipsilateral hand behind the head and roll the patient into an ipsilateral posterior oblique position

    (B) place the contralateral hand behind the head and roll the patient into an ipsilateral posterior oblique position

    (C) place the ipsilateral hand behind the head and roll the patient into a contralateral posterior oblique position

    (D) place the contralateral hand behind the head and roll the patient into a contralateral oblique position

13. Which of the following information is not required documentation for diagnostic sonograms?

    (A) laterality (right or left breast)

    (B) clock face notation

    (C) distance from the nipple

    (D) scan plane orientation

    (E) patient's last name only

14. Using the length of the transducer's footprint may provide a means to determine what sonographic feature of breast abnormalities?

    (A) depth of the lesion

    (B) distance of the lesion from the nipple

    (C) the transverse diameter of the lesion

    (D) the depth at which to place the focal zone for best optimization

15. The utilization of the radial/antiradial scan planes provides the best demonstration of what breast anatomy?

    (A) the lobes of the glandular tissue

    (B) Cooper's ligaments

    (C) the ductal anatomy of the breast

    (D) the terminal ductal lobular units

16. Which two characteristics are most helpful to establish concordance between a lesion seen on ultrasound and mammography?

    (A) margins and density

    (B) echogenicity and distance from the nipple

    (C) margins and echogenicity

    (D) size and location

17. The mass in Fig. 10–20 can best be described as:

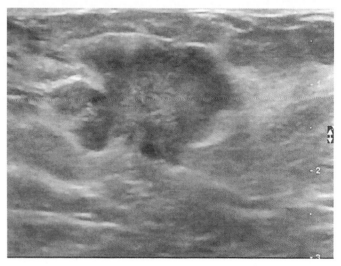

FIGURE 10–20.

    (A) irregular

    (B) circumscribed

    (C) macrolobulated

    (D) spiculated

18. The mass in Fig. 10–21 is best described as:

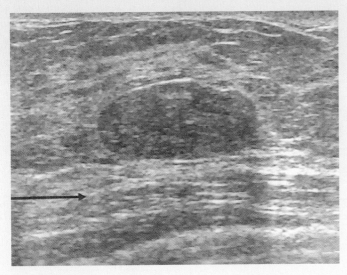

FIGURE 10–21.

(A) round

(B) circumscribed

(C) posteriorly enhancing

(D) spiculated

19. In Fig. 10–21, what structure is the arrow pointing to?

(A) Cooper's ligaments

(B) pectoralis muscle

(C) fibroglandular tissue

(D) skin

20. This image in Fig. 10–22 demonstrates:

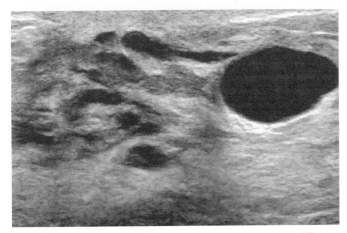

FIGURE 10–22.

(A) dilated ductal anatomy

(B) a simple cyst with breast implant rupture

(C) multiple, irregular cysts

(D) a single cyst with dilated ductal anatomy

21. What abnormal finding is not demonstrated in Fig. 10–23?

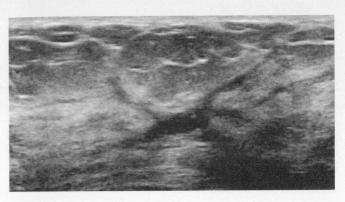

FIGURE 10–23.

(A) architectural distortion

(B) posterior acoustic attenuation

(C) angular margins

(D) calcifications

22. An asymptomatic patient receives a breast sonogram as additional workup. The exam reveals a mass with multiple internal punctuate echogenic foci. What do these foci most likely represent?

(A) calcifications

(B) gas

(C) artifact

(D) fat

23. Sonography is the recommended initial imaging modality for the evaluation of an area of palpable interest in patients younger than what age?

(A) 30

(B) 40

(C) 50

(D) 60

24. Which of the following terms is not an appropriate descriptor of breast lesion shape?

(A) oblong

(B) round

(C) oval

(D) irregular

25. If sonographic scanning in the upper outer quadrant of the breast demonstrates findings suspicious for a tubular structure, which of the following techniques should be used to further evaluate it?

    (A) imaging in an orthogonal plane
    (B) use of Doppler
    (C) adjusting the gray scale
    (D) adjusting the focal zone

26. What type transducer should be used for breast sonography?

    (A) curved
    (B) linear
    (C) vector
    (D) curvilinear

27. Echogenicity of a mass is assessed relative to which of the following structures?

    (A) Cooper's ligaments
    (B) skin
    (C) fat
    (D) muscle

28. The appearance of hazy, echogenic material with posterior acoustic shadowing seen in an augmented breast should raise the suspicion for which of the following?

    (A) malignancy
    (B) scar
    (C) fibrocystic disease
    (D) implant rupture

29. An image from a sonogram performed on a patient referred for evaluation of a palpable abnormality reveals an oval, circumscribed hypoechoic mass-like area with mixed internal echogenicity seen deep to the pectoralis muscle. What does these findings most-likely represent?

    (A) fibroadenoma
    (B) cyst
    (C) invasive malignancy
    (D) lymph node
    (E) rib

30. Which of the following statements is true regarding a biopsy performed with a vacuum-assisted device?

    (A) pre-fire and post-fire images should be obtained.
    (B) pre-fire images only should be obtained.
    (C) post-fire images only should be obtained.
    (D) images demonstrating the needle in or adjacent to the mass should be obtained.

31. Which of the following statements is true regarding a breast cyst post-aspiration?

    (A) there is no need to acquire a post-aspiration image.
    (B) a post-aspiration image should only be obtained if a small amount of fluid remains.
    (C) a post-aspiration image should only be obtained if there is question if a solid component is present.
    (D) a post-aspiration image should be obtained routinely.

32. During imaging of an area of concern, there is evidence of interruption of the Cooper's ligaments. An irregular hypoechoic region with angular margins and posterior acoustic shadowing is seen, but no mass is visualized. Which of the following is the most appropriate descriptor for this appearance?

    (A) spiculation
    (B) architectural distortion
    (C) dirty shadowing
    (D) normal parenchyma

33. The finding discussed in question 32 is most likely to be seen in which of the following scenarios?

    (A) benign lesions
    (B) post-surgical change
    (C) young, asymptomatic patients
    (D) pregnant patients with a palpable mass

Answers and Explanations

1. **(B)** Breast sonography is an adjunct to mammography in the detection of breast disorders. It is not an examination that is used in place of mammography, but rather in addition and is not used alone as a screening tool. A, C and D are all indications for breast sonography. (*Study Guide*)

2. **(B)** Placement of the focal zone at the level of the lesion or region of interest optimizes visualization of the lesion characteristics. (*Study Guide*)

3. **(C)** The use of an standoff pad improves visualization of superficial lesions within the near field, which is sometimes referred to as the sonographic 'blind spot'. (*Study Guide*)

4. **(A)** Radial and antiradial are the preferred scan planes for imaging the breast anatomy primarily based on the ductal anatomy of the breast as it converges toward the nipple. The annotation of the clock face orientation for imaging denotes transducer placement for radial/antiradial scan planes. (*Study Guide*)

5. **(D)** All sonographic findings should be discussed with the interpreting physician. (*Study Guide*)

6. **(D)** Skin thickness is normally no more than 2–3 mm. (*Study Guide*)

7. **(C)** Localizing a palpable lesion is paramount to the performance of an adequate exam. It is also important to stabilize the lesion so that it may be adequately examined. This is often best achieved by scanning the patient in the position in which the lesion is best felt. (*Study Guide*)

8. **(C)** Spiculated borders of a breast mass are considered abnormal and concerning for malignancy. (*Study Guide*)

9. **(B)** A minimum center frequency of 7 MHz is required for breast sonography, although higher frequencies should be employed when possible. Superficial lesions or smaller breast mass would not require as much penetration and a higher frequency would be appropriate. (*Study Guide*)

10. **(A)** The term anechoic indicates 'without echoes' and therefore, for a lesion to be deemed such, it should not produce any echoes within. Cysts may produce reverberation artifacts in the near-field edge, but this is not a requirement to be deemed anechoic. (*Study Guide*)

11. **(A)** The chance of developing breast cancer in a woman's life is approximately 1 in 8. (*Study Guide*)

12. **(C)** This position permits placement of the breast tissue on a level surface and reduces breast thickness in the upper outer quadrant. (*Study Guide*)

13. **(E)** All images are considered part of a patient's medical record and should document the patient's full name. (*Study Guide*)

14. **(B)** The distance of a lesion from the nipple should be documented with as much accuracy as possible. By knowing the length of the transducer's footprint that distance can be assessed by placing the edge of the transducer at the nipple and evaluating the relationship of the lesion's position to the transducer edge in terms of a ratio of the transducer length. (*Study Guide*)

15. **(C)** The ductal anatomy of the breast converges toward the nipple. The implementation of the radial and antiradial scan planes provides longitudinal and transverse orientation with respect to breast anatomy. (*Study Guide*)

16. **(D)** In order to compare sonographic findings with mammography, it is important to verify that location and the lesion size are consistent in order to prevent errors of discordance. (*Study Guide*)

17. **(A)** The lesion is not circumscribed. Macrolobulation is typically benign descriptor that is best reserved for an oval benign-appearing mass such as a suspected fibroadenoma. A spiculated appearance is typically seen with more hypoechoic masses, posterior acoustic shadowing and architectural distortion, similar to that seen with postsurgical scarring. (*Study Guide*)

18. **(B)** The lesion is oval and circumscribed, typical for a fibroadenoma. (*Study Guide*)

19. **(B)** The pectoralis muscle is demonstrated posterior to the breast tissue and is recognized by internal echogenic striations. (*Study Guide*)

20. **(D)** This image demonstrates a well-circumscribed anechoic lesion with posterior enhancement suggesting a breast cyst. In close proximity to the cyst, there are tubular hypoechoic structures suggesting dilated ducts are present. (*Study Guide*)

21. **(D)** There are no calcifications suggested in this image, although there is distortion of the normal breast tissue with angular margins and some posterior acoustic shadowing/attenuation. (*Study Guide*)

22. **(A)** Artifactual internal echogenicity and fat are rarely punctuate in appearance. Additionally, gas would be unlikely in an asymptomatic patient. (*Study Guide*)

23. **(A)** Younger patients typically have dense glandular breast tissue, which prevents mammography from clearly identifying abnormalities even if palpable. The use of sonography

can not only evaluate the area of interest, but also correlate any findings with palpation while reducing the patient's exposure to ionizing radiation. *(Study Guide)*

24. **(A)** Oblong is not an accepted descriptor of lesion shape. *(Study Guide)*

25. **(B)** Imaging in the orthogonal plane is necessary for any evaluation in breast sonography, normal or abnormal. The use of Doppler will help determine if this finding is a vessel or a duct. *(Study Guide)*

26. **(B)** Linear array transducers provide the best resolution and are particularly useful in superficial structures, such as the breast, when a wide field of view is not essential. *(Study Guide)*

27. **(C)** Fat is hypoechoic relative to the mammary/glandular tissue. The gray scale and gain settings should be set to demonstrate fat as the medium level echo and compare all other tissue/findings to its echogenicity. *(Study Guide)*

28. **(D)** Free silicone has the appearance of 'dirty shadowing', which is described in this question. *(Study Guide)*

29. **(E)** The ribs and chest wall are the only structures which are typically identified deep to the pectoralis muscle. Lymph nodes in this region are not commonly identified by ultrasound. *(Study Guide)*

30. **(D)** Vacuum-assisted devices do not 'fire' when obtaining the specimen. *(Study Guide)*

31. **(D)** This protocol is important to determine and document the completeness of the aspiration. *(Study Guide)*

32. **(B)** Spiculation is used to describe the margins of a mass when the tissue surrounding the mass is altered and has angular characteristics. Architectural distortion is best used when a mass is not appreciated, but the tissue is similarly altered. *(Study Guide)*

33. **(B)** Architectural distortion is usually seen post-surgically or in association with a malignancy. *(Study Guide)*

11

Abdominal Vascular Sonography

Marsha M. Neumyer

Study Guide

INTRODUCTION

Over the past two decades, there has been an explosive advancement in ultrasound transducer technology that has contributed to improved tissue penetration and image resolution. These developments have allowed exploration of the abdominal vasculature with ease and accuracy. Real-time two-dimensional imaging, complemented with spectral, color, and power Doppler, provides excellent depiction of anatomy, tissue texture and density, acoustic characteristics associated with pathology, blood flow patterns, and alterations in flow direction. All of these features have value in differentiating normal tissue from lesions associated with vascular disorders, and in classification of the hemodynamic patterns detected in the circulatory system of the abdomen.

This chapter addresses the arterial and venous vascular systems in the abdomen separately. The discussion of each system covers, individually, the anatomy of the vessels within that system, common vascular disorders, sonographic and spectral Doppler characteristics, and current usage of correlating imaging modalities. Hopefully, this arrangement will allow the student to relate disease processes to functional structure and anatomy and to the signature Doppler spectral waveforms and flow patterns associated with alterations in vascular resistance that occur normally and in response to disease.

ABDOMINAL AORTA

Anatomy

The abdominal aorta begins at the aortic hiatus of the diaphragm as a continuation of the thoracic aorta, coursing in the left paramedian scan plane in approximately 70% of the population. It parallels the inferior vena cava (IVC), which lies to its right.[1,2] It can be differentiated from the IVC by its rigid

contour, pulsatility, and thicker, echogenic walls. At the level of the fourth lumbar vertebra, it bifurcates into the right and left common iliac arteries. The right iliac artery lies superior to the left iliac vein, a situation that serves as a precursor to left iliac vein thrombosis in many patients. In normal adults, the diameter of the aorta averages 2 cm proximally tapering to about 1.5 cm at the level of the bifurcation. The common iliac arteries have an average diameter of 1 cm.[3] The diameter of the abdominal aorta varies somewhat with age, gender, race, and body habitus and may be ectatic or smaller than normal throughout its length. Because the diameter of a vessel impacts velocity parameters, it is important to consider vessel size in diagnostic vascular examinations.

In most patients, the abdominal aorta can be imaged in the longitudinal plane throughout its length. Proximally, the aorta can be visualized just inferior to the diaphragm. The celiac and superior mesenteric arteries arise proximally from the anterior wall of the aorta, while the renal arteries originate from the lateral or posterolateral wall in its midsegment. The small inferior mesenteric artery originates from the anterolateral aspect of the mid-to-distal aorta (Fig. 11–1). Aortic diameter measurements are best determined from cross-sectional images, which allow documentation of both anteroposterior and transverse dimensions.

Sonographic and Spectral Doppler Characteristics

A sonographic image of the aorta will demonstrate walls with linear reflectivity. In a normal vessel, the lumen is anechoic and the walls are smooth (Fig. 11–2). Because the proximal aorta gives rise to branches that supply blood to the low-resistance vascular beds of the liver, spleen, and kidneys, the Doppler spectral waveform from this segment of the vessel may feature forward flow throughout the cardiac cycle. Below the renal arteries, blood flow from the aorta is supplying the high-resistance vascular beds fed by the lumbar and lower extremity

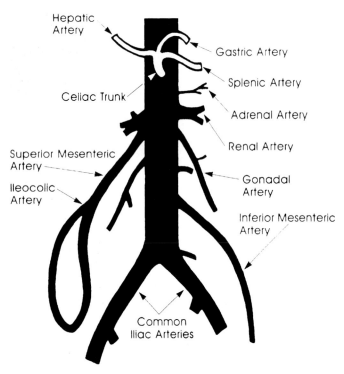

FIGURE 11–1. Diagram of abdominal aorta and aortic branches.

arteries and the spectral pattern will normally be triphasic (Fig. 11–3). This pattern, which characterizes peripheral arterial flow, exhibits rapid systolic upstroke, a sharp systolic peak, rapid systolic deceleration to a reversed flow component, and forward diastolic flow. If there is a loss of vessel elasticity or compliance proximal to the Doppler sample site, or if there is increased peripheral resistance distally, the forward diastolic flow component may be absent. Peak systolic velocity in the abdominal aorta normally ranges from 70 to 140 cm/s dependent on age, gender, body habitus, and cardiac output.[4]

Aortic Disease

Stenosis and Occlusion.
Narrowing of the lumen of the aorta may be caused by atherosclerotic disease, webs, or extrinsic

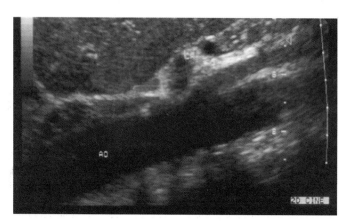

FIGURE 11–2. Real-time image of the abdominal aorta.

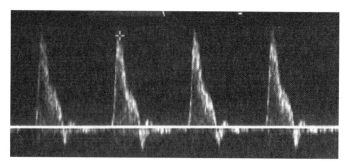

FIGURE 11–3. Doppler spectral waveform from the normal infrarenal abdominal aorta.

compression. Two-dimensional real-time imaging will detail atherosclerotic disease as either acoustically homogeneous plaque along the wall of the aorta consistent with fatty or fibro-fatty lesions or as brightly echogenic deposits that may demonstrate acoustic shadowing. These features are characteristic of complex, calcified plaque. Narrowing of the lumen due to stenosis or compression can be visualized with color-flow or power Doppler imaging. Flow-limiting stenosis causes an increase in peak systolic and end-diastolic velocities and loss of the reversed flow component of the normal triphasic Doppler spectral waveform. Disordered or turbulent flow results in spectral broadening throughout systole (Fig. 11–4). A comparison of pre-stenotic and stenotic velocities will demonstrate at least a twofold increase in peak systolic velocity when the diameter of the aorta is narrowed by more than 50% and at least a fourfold increase when the luminal diameter is compromised by more than 75%.[5] Classic post-stenotic turbulence and decreased velocity are noted in association with both lesions.

Aortic occlusion is characterized by longitudinal, rather than cross-sectional, pulsation, intraluminal echoes, and absence of flow documented by optimized spectral, color, or power Doppler. The spectral waveform immediately proximal to the occlusion exhibits a high-resistance pattern with low or no diastolic flow and a "thump of the stump" appearance. If the aorta is reconstituted distal to the occlusion, the signal in the patent segment of the aorta will be monophasic with delayed systolic upstroke, a blunt systolic peak, and delayed runoff (Fig. 11–5).

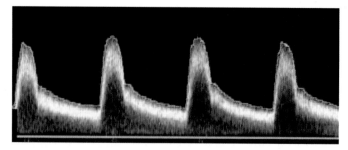

FIGURE 11–4. Doppler spectral waveform from flow-reducing abdominal aortic stenosis. Note spectral broadening throughout systole.

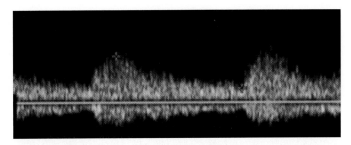

FIGURE 11–5. Doppler spectral waveform distal to aortic occlusion.

Aneurysm. An aneurysm is defined as an abnormal focal dilation of a vessel. All three layers of the arterial wall (intima, media, and adventitia) remain intact with a true aneurysm. In contrast, a false, or pseudoaneurysm, is described as a tear involving two or all three layers of the arterial wall allowing blood to escape into the surrounding tissues. True aneurysms are most often associated with atherosclerosis, smoking, diabetes, hypertension, hyperlipidemia, pregnancy, trauma, or infection.[3] Pseudoaneurysms characteristically result from trauma or surgery but may be mycotic in origin.

The abdominal aorta is considered aneurysmal when its diameter exceeds 3 cm or is one and one-half times larger than the more proximal segment.[3] Visceral and peripheral arterial aneurysms are frequently associated with abdominal aortic aneurysmal disease.

Most aneurysms develop in the infrarenal segment of the aorta, superior to the aortic bifurcation, although they may be found in the juxtarenal or suprarenal segments or involve the iliac arteries.

Abdominal aortic aneurysms (AAAs) are most common in elderly (older than 65 years) male smokers. Aneurysmal dilation is quite often discovered incidentally during routine physical examinations. Patients may be asymptomatic or present with a pulsatile abdominal mass; back or abdominal pain that radiates down the leg; a "throbbing" sensation in the abdomen (abdominal bruit); shortness of breath; or numbness in the extremities.[6]

Aortic aneurysms are at risk for rupture when their diameter exceeds 6 cm.[3] Rupture is considered a surgical emergency; there is a 50% mortality rate in current surgical practice. Patients usually experience acute abdominal or back pain that becomes worse when they assume an upright position.[6] A cyanotic-appearing discoloration may be apparent in the groin region.

Classification of True Aneurysms. Aneurysms are classified according to their anatomical configuration. *Fusiform* aneurysms are most often spindle-shaped, with stretching of the aortic walls occurring concentrically. This anatomic configuration accounts for approximately 90% of aortic aneurysms. *Saccular* aneurysms are characterized by an outpouching from the anterior aortic wall (Fig. 11–6). The aorta is considered to be

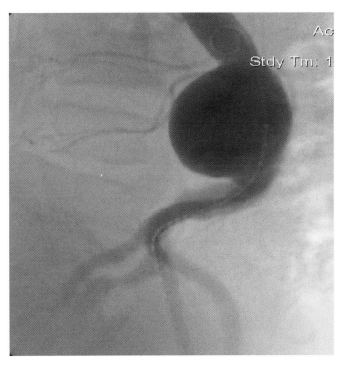

FIGURE 11–6. Arteriogram demonstrating a saccular aortic aneurysm.

ectatic when it is diffusely dilated along its length with diameter measurements averaging 3–6 cm.[3,6]

Other complications that may result in dilation of the aorta include mycotic infections and intimal tears. Mycotic aneurysms can result from any infection but are commonly associated with *Staphylococcus, Escherichia coli,* or *Salmonella* and have been found with cases of pancreatitis.[6] The majority of mycotic aneurysms are saccular and are most often located in the suprarenal segment of the aorta.

If the walls of an aneurysm are calcified, or if the aneurysm displaces surrounding organs or structures, it may be identified on plain film but that is not the modality of choice for initial screening. If leakage or rupture of an aneurysm is suspected, this can best be demonstrated with computed tomography (CT) or magnetic resonance imaging (MRI). CT scanning is most commonly chosen prior to surgical repair to facilitate choice and sizing of graft material, as well as location and patency of aortic branch vessels.

Sonographic and Doppler Characteristics of AAAs. Sonography is the procedure of choice for identification of abdominal aneurysmal disease and for monitoring for aneurysm enlargement. B-mode imaging will define the area(s) of aortic dilation and allow classification of the aneurysm (Fig. 11–7). Maximal anteroposterior and transverse diameters should be documented with care taken to measure along the axis of the aorta and not the axis of the spine.[3] Thrombus and atherosclerotic debris within the aneurysmal sac should be documented and notes taken of the presence of aortic dissection or free fluid within the abdomen, which could indicate rupture.

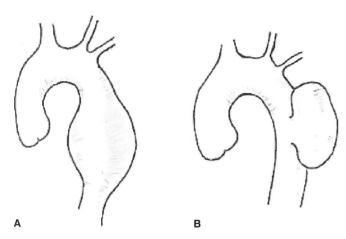

FIGURE 11–7. Diagrams illustrating (**A**) fusiform and (**B**) saccular aortic aneurysms.

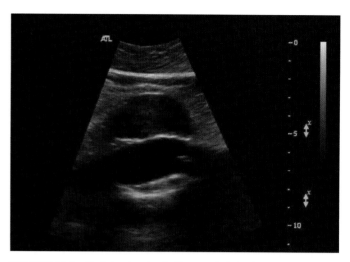

FIGURE 11–9. Real-time longitudinal image of abdominal aorta illustrating echogenic walls of an aortic endograft and the residual aneurysm sac.

Color-flow imaging facilitates recognition of the swirling bidirectional flow pattern common to true aneurysms (Fig. 11–8). Spectral Doppler demonstrates disordered bidirectional flow with peak systolic velocity slightly reduced when compared to the proximal adjacent normal segment of the aorta.

Surgical and Endovascular Repair of Aortic Aneurysms. Historically, the majority of AAAs have been repaired surgically with resection or grafts. In recent years, endovascular repair with percutaneous insertion of aortic stent grafts has been successfully used in selective patients. The grafts may be modular or bifurcated and are inserted through the femoral artery into the aorta over a catheter, excluding the aneurysm.[3,7] Attachment of the graft to the wall of the aorta is achieved with balloon dilation. The graft is anchored to the arterial wall, proximally and distally, by metallic barbs. The residual aneurysm sac remains, surrounding the aortic stent graft. Occasionally, blood may re-enter the aneurysm sac via leaks (endoleaks) at the attachment sites, through aortic branch vessels such as the inferior mesenteric or lumbar arteries, or through the graft wall. If the leak is severe, it may place the aneurysm at risk for rupture.

Sonographic and Doppler Characteristics of Aortic Stent Grafts. High-resolution real-time imaging demonstrates the residual aortic aneurysm sac (Fig. 11–9). The sac will contain acoustically homogeneous material; sonolucent areas or hypoechoic regions may appear within the sac if endoleaks are present. The brightly echogenic walls of the aortic stent graft are easily identified in the majority of patients (see Figure 11–9). If a bifurcated graft has been used, the limbs of the graft are apparent within the aneurysm sac and may have been crossed to stabilize the graft. Color-flow imaging will facilitate confirmation of patency of the body and limbs of the graft and, when optimized for slow flow, can be used to identify flow within the residual aneurysm sac. Power Doppler is a valued tool for confirmation of endoleaks. Spectral Doppler is used to demonstrate the flow patterns within the stent graft, direction and source of flow associated with endoleaks, and the difference in spectral pattern recorded in endoleaks compared to the flow pattern in the stent graft.

Dissection. Aortic dissection occurs when there is a tear in the intima or between the intima and media allowing the layers to separate from the arterial wall.[3,7] Blood is then able to course between the separated layers and the remaining arterial wall, creating a true lumen and a false lumen. This condition has a high rate of mortality; however, 50% of treated patients have a 10-year survival rate.[6] Dissection may occur secondarily to trauma, aortic catheterization, or surgical procedures but is commonly associated with Marfan syndrome, hypertension, aortic coarctation, bicuspid aortic valve, atherosclerosis, pregnancy, cystic medial necrosis, and arteritis.

The DeBakey classification is commonly used to describe the extent and severity of the aortic compromise[3] (Fig. 11–10).

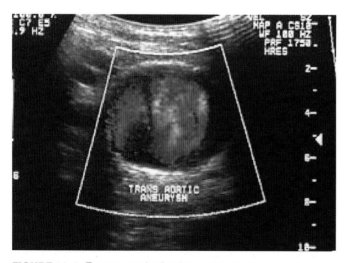

FIGURE 11–8. Transverse color-flow image of abdominal aorta illustrating bidirectional (yin-yang) flow pattern.

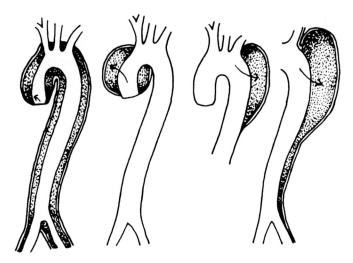

FIGURE 11-10. DeBakey classification of aortic dissection.

- Type I dissection involves the ascending aorta, aortic arch, and descending aorta
- Type II dissection involves only the ascending aorta
- Type III dissection involves the descending thoracic aorta and may extend into the abdominal aorta

Sonographic and Doppler Characteristics. The real-time image will detail the echogenic intima separated from the aortic wall (Fig. 11–11). Color-flow imaging facilitates identification of the true and false lumens. Flow direction may reverse in the false lumen if there is only one tear; however, there may be multiple points of entry and exit and flow patterns may be complex. Doppler spectral waveforms should demonstrate antegrade flow in the true lumen with evidence of spectral broadening. Turbulent flow and elevated velocity are not commonly seen in the true lumen unless the lumen is significantly narrowed. The spectral waveforms in the false lumen may demonstrate increased resistance with low or absent diastolic flow if an outflow channel is not present. Because the false lumen often

thromboses, it is important to determine, to the extent possible, whether the aortic branch vessels originate from the true or the false lumen.

Confirmation of aortic dissection is most often achieved with standard contrast arteriography or dynamic contrast or helical CT imaging.

SPLANCHNIC ARTERIES (CELIAC AND MESENTERIC ARTERIES)

Celiac, Common, Hepatic, Splenic, Left Gastric

Anatomy. The celiac artery is the first major branch of the abdominal aorta. It arises from the anterior aortic wall approximately 2 cm below the diaphragm at about the level of the twelfth thoracic vertebra and the first lumbar vertebra. The celiac artery (a.k.a. celiac axis, celiac trunk) is most often 2–3 cm in length. Approximately 1–2 cm from its origin, it divides into the common hepatic, splenic, and left gastric arteries. The splenic artery supplies blood to the spleen, pancreas, left half of the greater omentum, greater curvature of the stomach, and part of the fundus of the stomach. The common hepatic artery supplies the liver, gallbladder, stomach, pancreas, duodenum, and greater omentum.[1,2]

Sonographic and Doppler Characteristics. The celiac artery can be located as it arises from the anterior wall on a longitudinal image of the proximal aorta. It is best demonstrated, however, in the transverse scan plane of the aorta, as it is quite often tortuous. At its bifurcation into the common hepatic and splenic arteries, it assumes a "seagull" appearance, as these branches arise almost perpendicular to the celiac trunk (Fig. 11–12).

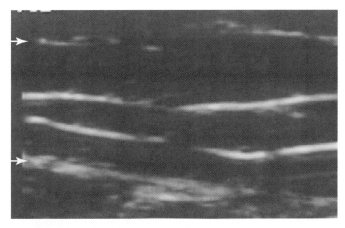

FIGURE 11-11. Real-time image of aortic dissection. Echogenic intima noted to be separated from arterial wall (arrows).

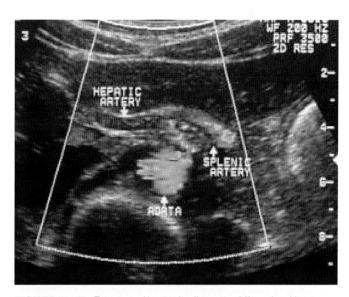

FIGURE 11-12. Transverse image of celiac artery bifurcation. Note "seagull" appearance created by position of the common hepatic and splenic arteries.

The splenic artery, the largest branch of the celiac, is most often tortuous. It courses along the posterosuperior margin of the pancreas and terminates within the hilum of the spleen.[1,2] It is most easily imaged along its course in the transverse plane beneath the body of the pancreas. The distal segment of the artery can be interrogated in the splenic hilum using a left lateral scan plane with a splenic window.

From its origin at the celiac bifurcation, the common hepatic artery courses along the superior border of the pancreatic head.[1,2] It gives rise to the gastroduodenal artery between the duodenum and the anterior surface of the head of the pancreas. It then courses superiorly and gives rise to the right gastric artery before entering the porta hepatis where it becomes the proper hepatic artery. The proper hepatic artery branches into the right and left hepatic arteries within the liver. These branches then divide into the segmental and subsegmental hepatic artery branches that course parallel to the bile ducts and portal vein branches.[1,2] The hepatic artery can be imaged from its origin to its termination within the liver. Its course and flow patterns are best delineated with color-flow imaging. The intrahepatic branches are most easily interrogated using a coronal oblique image plane.

The left gastric artery is occasionally seen longitudinally for approximately 1–2 cm but is not commonly visualized sonographically due to its small diameter and anatomic course.[6] The artery courses along the lesser curvature of the stomach, sending branches to the anterior and posterior segments of the stomach and esophagus.[1,2]

The celiac artery and its branches supply the low-resistance vascular beds of the liver and spleen. For this reason, these vessels will normally demonstrate a low-resistance waveform pattern characterized by constant forward diastolic flow (Fig. 11–13). The peak systolic velocity is <200 cm/s with an end-diastolic velocity <55 cm/s. Flow is laminar in the absence of significant disease. Postprandially, there is little to no increase in systolic or diastolic velocities, as the liver and spleen do not alter their vascular resistance in response to digestion.[5]

Superior and Inferior Mesenteric Arteries

Anatomy. The superior mesenteric artery (SMA) arises from the anterior wall of the aorta approximately 1–3 cm inferior to the celiac artery origin at about the level of the first lumbar vertebra.[1,2] In a small percentage of patients, the celiac artery and SMA may share a common trunk or the right hepatic artery may originate from the proximal segment of the SMA, also known as a replaced hepatic artery. Just beyond its origin, the SMA arcs anteriorly and then courses inferiorly to parallel the anterior aortic wall to the level of the ileocecal valve.[1,2] From the transverse scan plane of the aorta, it can be seen that the SMA lies anterior to the left renal vein and duodenum and posterior to the pancreas. Unlike the celiac, the SMA has multiple branches that supply the pancreas, duodenum, jejunum, ileum, cecum, and the ascending and transverse colon. However, because of their small size, these vessels are not typically visualized sonographically.

The inferior mesenteric artery (IMA) originates from the left anterolateral wall of the aorta. It provides important collateral pathways when there is occlusive disease in the celiac or SMA circulation. The IMA is normally smaller in diameter than the SMA and can most often be identified from the transverse scan plane using surface anatomy as a landmark. Color-flow imaging facilitates identification of the artery's origin approximately two finger widths above the level of the umbilicus. The IMA supplies the left third of the transverse colon, the descending colon, sigmoid colon, and most of the rectum.[1,2]

Sonographic and Doppler Characteristics. The SMA can be visualized along its length from a longitudinal image plane. It will appear as a tubular structure that courses parallel to the anterior aortic wall originating just distal to the origin of the celiac artery (Fig. 11–14). It courses posterior to the splenic vein and pancreas and left of the superior mesenteric vein. From a transverse image plane, it is located superior to the left renal vein and appears disc-like with a dense echogenic ring caused by a fatty collar. From this image plane, it is noted that a portion of the body of the pancreas drapes over the SMA.

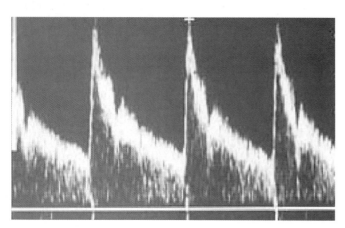

FIGURE 11–13. Classic low-resistance Doppler spectral waveform of the celiac artery.

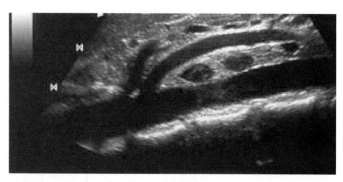

FIGURE 11–14. Real-time image of abdominal aorta demonstrating origins of the celiac and superior mesenteric arteries. Also note the adjacent lymphadenopathy.

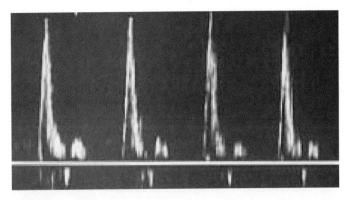

FIGURE 11-15. High-resistance spectral waveform pattern from a normal fasting superior mesenteric artery.

Because the SMA supplies the muscular tissues of the duodenum, jejunum, and colon, it will exhibit a high resistance flow pattern characterized by low diastolic flow in its fasting state (Fig. 11-15). Following ingestion of a meal, vascular resistance decreases to meet the metabolic demands for additional blood flow that are associated with digestion (Fig. 11-16). To meet this demand, systolic and diastolic velocities normally increase at least twofold. Doppler spectral waveforms from the IMA mimic those of the SMA in both the fasting and postprandial states.

Splanchnic Arterial Disease

Stenosis and Occlusion. Flow-limiting disease involving the celiac artery and its branches or the SMA and IMA is most often caused by atherosclerosis and is commonly located at the vessel origins or at points of bifurcation. While the prevalence of mesenteric occlusive disease is low, women are affected more often than men, and in general, mesenteric disease is a problem of the elderly. Under normal circumstances, the visceral arteries receive 25–30% of the cardiac output and, in the fasting condition, contain one-third of the total blood volume.[6,7] When the flow demand in the gastrointestinal circulation cannot be met due to arterial stenosis or occlusion

(usually in at least two of the three major splanchnic vessels), patients complain of postprandial abdominal angina, i.e., pain associated with ingestion of a meal. As a result of pain associated with eating, they develop a "fear of food" syndrome and subsequent gastrointestinal impairment and significant weight loss. Even though the progression of atherosclerotic disease may be slow and insidious, the vascular compromise can lead to bowel infarction. Occasionally, patients suffer acute occlusion of the mesenteric arteries and will present with severe abdominal pain. This should be considered a surgical emergency as delayed revascularization may result in gastrointestinal catastrophe.

Flow impairment may also be caused by compression of the splanchnic arteries. During normal respiration, the celiac artery may be intermittently compressed by the median arcuate ligament of the diaphragm. The ligament slides off the celiac artery allowing it to return to normal diameter when the patient takes a deep breath. The proximal superior mesenteric artery may be compressed in the mesentery or the duodenum may be "trapped" between the SMA and the aorta. This leads to SMA compression syndrome, which is characterized by an epigastric bruit, colicky abdominal pain, and occasionally malabsorption.

The visceral arterial circulation is richly collateralized with a network of vessels that connect the celiac and its branches with the branches of the superior and inferior mesenteric arteries.[2] When the celiac artery is critically stenosed or occluded, the pancreaticoduodenal arcade, a complex of small arteries surrounding the pancreas and duodenum, provides a collateral pathway. Collateral flow through branches of the inferior mesenteric artery via the arc of Riolan or the marginal artery of Drummond, or the pancreaticoduodenal arcade may be apparent when there is occlusion of the superior mesenteric artery.

Sonographic and Doppler Characteristics. Although disease may be found in any segment of the visceral arteries, atherosclerotic disease occurs most often at the vessel origins as an extension of plaque found on the aortic wall. B-mode imaging will detail the location and extent of plaque. The severity of luminal compromise may be estimated visually using color or power Doppler to define residual lumen. If stenosis is severe, a color bruit that is characterized by a mosaic color pattern and perivascular color artifact may be apparent.

Flow-limiting stenosis (>60–70% diameter reduction) of the celiac artery will demonstrate peak systolic velocities in excess of 220 cm/s and end-diastolic velocities >55 cm/s.[3,5,7] A post-stenotic signal must be confirmed to differentiate elevated velocities due to focal stenosis from those associated with collateral compensatory flow. Median arcuate ligament compression of the celiac artery will result in high-velocity signals during normal respiration with return to normal velocity ranges when the patient takes a deep breath.

Peak systolic velocity in the SMA will be >275 cm/s with an end-diastolic velocity exceeding 45 cm/s when the diameter

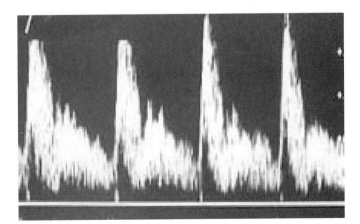

FIGURE 11-16. Low-resistance spectral waveform pattern from a postprandial superior mesenteric artery. Note the increase in diastolic flow.

of the SMA is reduced more than 70%.[3,5,7] As with the celiac artery, a post-stenotic signal must be confirmed to ensure identification of focal flow-limiting disease.

Arterial occlusion should be confirmed using spectral, color, or power Doppler optimized to show low-velocity flow.

Standard contrast arteriography with selective lateral views of the aorta provides confirmation of stenosis or occlusion of the visceral arteries and defines the presence and extent of collateral circulation prior to revascularization. In recent years, CT scanning has demonstrated a valuable role in localization of disease and display of relational anatomy.[8]

RENAL ARTERIES

Anatomy

The renal arteries arise from the lateral, posterolateral, or anterolateral wall of the abdominal aorta at the level of the second or third lumbar vertebrae.[1,2] Most often they are single, but in approximately 35% of the population, there may be multiple renal arteries on each side.[5,6] This anomaly occurs more often on the left than on the right. The right renal artery is longer than the left and courses superiorly in its proximal segment and then courses posterior to the IVC to enter the hilum of the right kidney. The left renal artery courses through the flank posterior to the left renal vein to enter the hilum of the left kidney. The main renal artery gives rise to branches that supply blood to the adrenal gland and the ureter and then divides into anterior and posterior branches within the renal hilum. These in turn subdivide into the segmental arteries within the renal sinus and then give rise to the interlobar arteries that parallel the renal pyramids. The interlobar arteries divide into the arcuate arteries that curve around the bases of the pyramids. The arcuate arteries further subdivide into the small lobular arteries that supply the renal cortex.[1,2,5]

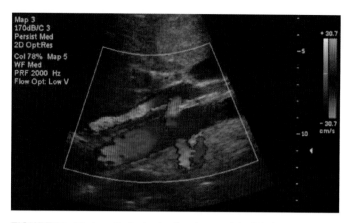

FIGURE 11–18. Longitudinal color-flow image of the inferior vena cava and abdominal aorta demonstrating origins of renal arteries from the coronal plane.

Sonographic and Doppler Characteristics

The proximal-to-mid segments of the renal arteries can most often be visualized from the transverse scan plane of the aorta at the level of the left renal vein (Fig. 11–17). Alternatively, the proximal segments of the arteries can be seen arising laterally from the aorta by scanning in a coronal plane through the liver so that the IVC and aorta are superimposed on each other (Fig. 11–18). The origin of the right renal artery can frequently be visualized on longitudinal images of the IVC as a small disc-shaped structure lying posterior to the IVC (Fig. 11–19). The distal-to- mid segments of the renal arteries are best seen with transverse imaging of the kidney using a subcostal or intercostal approach.[5,7] Quite often this approach will provide excellent images of the length of the renal artery from the hilum to its origin at the lateral wall of the aorta (Fig. 11–20). In an adult, kidney length is normally 11–13 cm and the width is 5–7 cm (Fig. 11–21). The anteroposterior thickness averages 2–3 cm, with the left organ being slightly larger than the right.[6]

The normal renal arterial waveform exhibits the classic features associated with flow to low-resistance end-organs; it

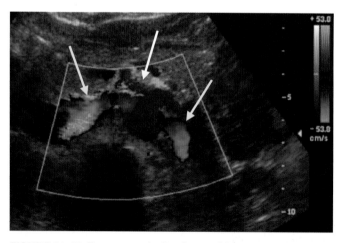

FIGURE 11–17. Transverse color-flow image of the proximal to mid segments of the renal arteries (yellow arrows) at the level of the left renal vein (white arrow).

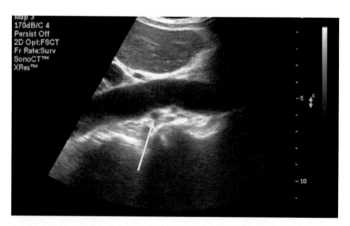

FIGURE 11–19. Real-time longitudinal image of the inferior vena cava. Note the disc-like appearance of the right renal artery posteriorly (yellow arrow).

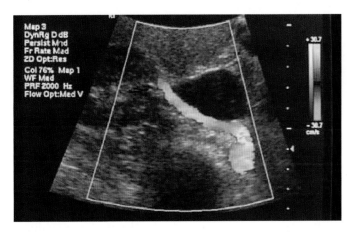

FIGURE 11–20. Color-flow image of the right renal artery as it courses from the hilum of the kidney to the aortic wall.

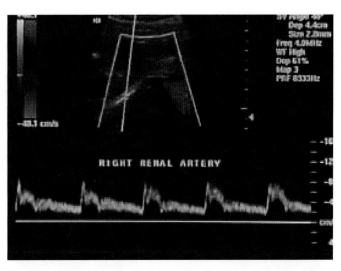

FIGURE 11–22. Color-flow image and Doppler spectral waveforms from a normal renal artery. Note the classic low-resistance waveform pattern.

is characterized by constant forward flow throughout diastole (Fig. 11–22). The peak systolic and end-diastolic velocities decrease proportionately from the main renal artery to the segmental arteries within the renal sinus to the arcuate arteries within the cortex of the kidney. Peak systolic velocity within the main renal artery is normally <120 cm/s with end-diastolic velocities averaging 30–50% of the peak systolic velocity.[5,7] A resistive index may be calculated to demonstrate evidence of impedance to arterial inflow. A normal resistive index in an adult is <0.70, while the indices are notably higher in premature infants and children younger than 4 years (0.70–1.0).[6]

Renal Arterial Disease

Stenosis and Occlusion. Atherosclerotic renal artery stenosis is the most common curable cause of renovascular hypertension. Atherosclerotic plaque occurs most frequently at the renal artery ostium (origin) or within the proximal third of the renal artery. Ostial disease represents extension of plaque from the aortic wall. Medial fibromuscular dysplasia of the renal

artery or its segmental branches is the second most common cause of renovascular hypertension.[7] This is a nonatherosclerotic disease entity that causes concentric regions of narrowing and dilation in the mid-to-distal segment of the renal artery (Fig. 11–23). In addition to atherosclerosis and fibromuscular dysplasia, causes of renal artery dysfunction include arteritis, aneurysm, congenital renal artery stenosis, congenital fibrous bands, neoplasms, vascular malformations, emboli, thrombus, trauma, fistulas, pheochromocytoma, neurofibromatosis, middle aortic syndrome, aortic coarctation, irradiation, and perirenal hematoma. Although patients with renal artery stenosis or occlusion may be asymptomatic, the majority present with systolic hypertension (>140 mm Hg), a flank bruit, congestive heart failure, or renal failure, or they are outside the normal age range for hypertension.

Medical renal disease (intrinsic parenchymal disease) should be included in the differential diagnosis for patients

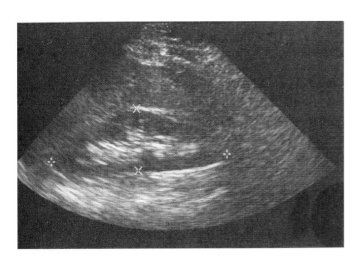

FIGURE 11–21. Gray-scale image of a kidney illustrating measurement of length and thickness.

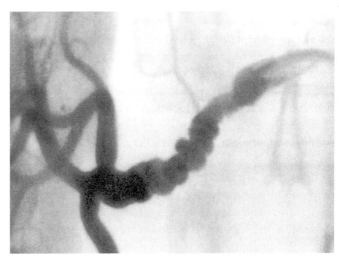

FIGURE 11–23. Arteriogram illustrating the concentric narrowing and dilation associated with renal arterial medial fibromuscular dysplasia.

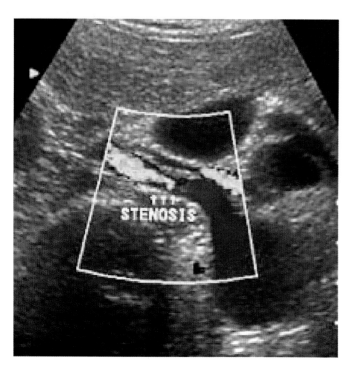

FIGURE 11–24. Color-flow image of the right renal artery demonstrating a region of disordered flow associated with stenosis.

with hypertension. Parenchymal vascular disorders will cause elevated renovascular resistance. This may occur secondary to renal artery stenosis or be the primary etiology for elevated blood pressure.

Sonographic and Doppler Characteristics. B-mode imaging may reveal narrowed segments along the course of the renal artery, but confirmation of stenosis will be facilitated with color or power Doppler imaging (Fig. 11–24). In regions of flow-limiting disease, color Doppler will exhibit disordered flow patterns; a perivascular color artifact may be present if the stenosis is severe enough to cause a bruit. If the renal artery is occluded, no flow should be evident using spectral, color, or power Doppler optimized for slow flow. Low-amplitude, dampened spectral waveforms with tardus parvus ("late to rise") characteristics will be found within the renal parenchyma as a result of collateral flow. As renal artery stenosis progresses, renal length decreases. There is commonly a difference in renal length >3 cm side-to-side. Pole-to-pole length of the kidney will most often be <8 cm if the renal artery is occluded.[5,7]

Flow-limiting renal artery stenosis causes elevation in the peak systolic velocity. This velocity can be compared to the aortic velocity as a ratio of the angle corrected aortic peak systolic velocity recorded at the level of the celiac artery and the highest angle-corrected velocity in the main renal artery. When the renal-aortic velocity ratio (RAR) exceeds 3.5, there is evidence of flow-limiting renal artery stenosis (>60% diameter reduction). Care must be taken to ensure that the aortic peak systolic velocity is >40 cm/s but <100 cm/s, as use of the RAR

when velocity is outside these values will result in overestimation or underestimation of the severity of renal artery stenosis.[7] If the RAR cannot be used to confirm flow-limiting disease due to suspect aortic velocities, attention should be given to the peak systolic velocity in the renal artery and presence or absence of a classic post-stenotic signal. Recognition of hemodynamically significant stenosis is dependent on a renal artery peak systolic velocity >180 cm/s and a post-stenotic signal. Stenosis that is < hemodynamically significant (<60% diameter reducing) can be recognized when the renal artery peak systolic velocity is more than 180 cm/s, but no post-stenotic signal is present.[7]

Renal artery stenosis may also be identified using indirect methods that assess the distal renal artery and its segmental branches. While this technique has not been well validated, it has value in patients in whom the length of the renal artery cannot be adequately interrogated due to excessive abdominal gas, body habitus, post-interventional, or traumatic causes. Using a 0° angle of insonation and a slow sweep speed, Doppler spectral waveforms are recorded from the distal renal artery and the segmental branches within the renal sinus. An acceleration time (time from onset of systole to the early systolic peak, which is seen on the systolic upstroke prior to peak systole) >100 ms indicates >60% diameter reducing renal artery stenosis. An acceleration index may also be used to identify flow-limiting renal artery disease. The index is defined as the change in distance between the onset of systolic flow and the peak systolic velocity divided by the acceleration time. An index <291 cm/s^2 is consistent with significant renal artery stenosis.[7,9]

Many types of medical renal diseases are accompanied by elevation of vascular resistance apparent in the intersegmental and arcuate arteries within the renal parenchyma. Normally, the end-diastolic velocity is at least 30–50% of the peak systolic velocity. As vascular resistance increases, diastolic flow decreases and a ratio of systolic to end-diastolic velocities within the intrarenal vessels will be >0.20.[5,7]

Hydronephrosis is characterized by abnormal dilation of the renal calyces and renal pelvis caused by obstruction of the urinary tract. Sonographically, the renal sinus exhibits a hypoechoic or cystic area that may be variable dependent on the severity of the obstructive process (Fig. 11–25). The resistive index is commonly elevated with values >0.70 in patients with obstructive hydronephrosis but may also be increased in patients with intrinsic renal parenchymal disease, perinephric or subcapsular hematoma, hypotension, and decreased heart rate.[4]

Although standard contrast arteriography remains the gold standard for confirmation of renal artery stenosis and occlusion, other imaging modalities may be used for confirmation of the sonographic examination or clinical findings. These include CT or MRI scanning, radionuclide renography, and intravenous pyelography.

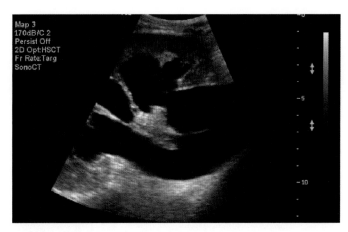

FIGURE 11–25. Real-time image of a kidney with hydronephrosis. Note the cystic appearance of the renal sinus.

INFERIOR VENA CAVA

Anatomy

The common iliac veins come together to form the IVC at approximately the level of the umbilicus or the fourth lumbar vertebra. The distal IVC ascends superiorly toward the diaphragm coursing to the right of the aorta and the spine. Although it will parallel the aorta along most of its course, it curves anteriorly in its proximal segment to enter the right atrium of the heart. The IVC receives blood from the hepatic, renal, right gonadal, right suprarenal, inferior phrenic, and lumbar veins[1,2] (Fig. 11–26). Normally, the IVC diameter is <2.5 cm, with slight increase in diameter above the entry level of the renal veins because of the increased volume of blood

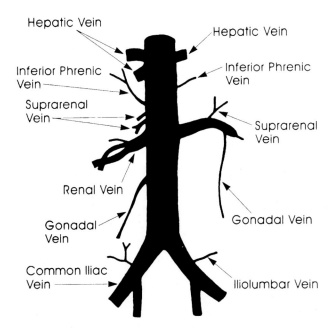

FIGURE 11–26. Diagram of the inferior vena cava illustrating its major branches.

that is returned from the kidneys.[6] Diameter of the IVC is dependent on the patient's body habitus, the stage of respiration, and right atrial pressure. Anatomic anomalies may be noted including duplication (0.2–3.0% of the population) or absence of the IVC (<0.2%) or transposition to the left side (0.2–0.5%).[1,2]

Sonographic and Spectral Doppler Characteristics

The IVC normally appears as an anechoic, tubular structure, the diameter of which varies with changes in respiration. Deep inspiration causes increased abdominal pressure and impedes venous return from the abdomen. This results in dilation of the IVC. Dilation can also occur in the presence of congestive heart failure, tricuspid regurgitation, or any condition that results in increased right atrial pressure.

Spectral Doppler demonstrates pulsatility in the proximal segment of the IVC because of the reflected right atrial pressure. Velocities are variable but remain low. The Doppler spectral waveform in the distal IVC demonstrates phasicity, similar to that seen in the lower extremity veins (Fig. 11–27). Color-flow imaging reveals directional variations associated with respirophasicity in the distal segment of the vein and reflected right atrial pulsations proximally.

Inferior Vena Caval Disease

Thrombosis is the most common vascular problem affecting the IVC and most often results from migration of thromboembolic material from the lower extremities or pelvic veins. IVC thrombosis is likely to occur with any condition that promotes stasis of blood flow in the abdominal veins, trauma to the vein wall, or hypercoagulability (Virchow's triad). Conditions that are associated with these features include dehydration, generalized sepsis, shock, retroperitoneal infection, pelvic inflammatory disease, caval filters or catheters, and extremity or abdominal surgery. Tumor thrombus may also be noted in association with carcinomas of the kidney, adrenal gland, pancreas, or liver. Other malignancies may involve the IVC including ovarian and uterine neoplasms, lymphatic metastases from the prostate, pheochromocytomas, and Wilms' tumor.

While IVC thrombosis may be asymptomatic, the majority of patients will present with lower extremity edema and discomfort or symptoms characteristic of malignant conditions.

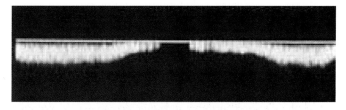

FIGURE 11–27. Doppler spectral waveforms from the infrarenal inferior vena cava. The respirophasicity is similar to that seen in the lower extremity veins.

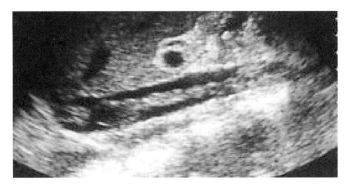

FIGURE 11–28. Real-time longitudinal image of the inferior vena cava demonstrating acute, free-floating thrombus.

Sonographic and Doppler Characteristics. Thrombosis of the IVC causes dilation at the site of outflow obstruction. Acute thrombus will appear hypoechoic and a free-floating thrombus tail may be seen in the very acute phase (Fig. 11–28). The IVC will be noncompressible or partially compressible with transducer pressure applied directly over the vein in the transverse imaging plane. As the thrombus ages, it will initially increase in echogenicity but then progresses through a variety of characteristics ranging from acoustic heterogeneity with anechoic regions to homogeneity. The acoustic features return to heterogeneity and the vein walls contract as the thrombus becomes chronic.

Doppler spectral waveforms demonstrate continuous, nonphasic flow patterns with partial obstruction of the caval lumen. No flow will be demonstrated by optimized spectral, color, or power Doppler when the lumen is totally obstructed. Low-amplitude, continuous waveforms may be recorded distal to the site of thrombosis if recanalization or collateralization of the thrombosed segment has occurred.

Correlative imaging is achieved with venocavography, MRI, or CT scanning.

HEPATIC AND PORTAL VEINS

Anatomy of the Hepatic Veins

The hepatic veins drain into the IVC and are the largest tributaries to the IVC. There are three major hepatic veins: the right, middle, and left. These large veins serve as boundary markers between the hepatic lobes and have multiple smaller branches throughout the liver parenchyma. The left and middle hepatic veins frequently share a common trunk at the IVC confluence, while the right hepatic vein remains independent. Occasionally, an accessory (inferior) right hepatic vein may be noted; one or more of the hepatic veins may be absent. The middle hepatic vein courses within the main interlobar fissure thus, dividing the liver into right and left lobes. The right lobe of the liver is divided into posterior and anterior segments by the right hepatic vein. The left hepatic vein divides the left lobe of the liver into medial and lateral segments.[1,2,5]

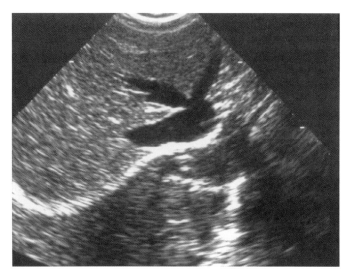

FIGURE 11–29. Real-time image of two hepatic veins at the hepatocaval confluence. The image illustrates the "Playboy bunny" sign.

Sonographic and Spectral Doppler Characteristics. The hepatic veins are best imaged from a subcostal approach, angling the transducer cephalad under the xiphoid process or from a right intercostal plane of view. Most often all three branches can be visualized. When only two branches are imaged from the subcostal approach, the veins mimic the head and ears of a rabbit. This is referred to as the "Playboy bunny sign" (Fig. 11–29). B-mode images normally reveal anechoic tubular structures that lack echogenic walls. While the diameter of the hepatic vein branches may appear small within the parenchyma of the liver, their diameters increase as they course toward the IVC.[6]

The Doppler spectral waveform from normal hepatic veins is pulsatile with two forward-flow cycles corresponding to the two phases of atrial filling. This is followed by a brief period of reversed flow (Fig. 11–30). This "W-shaped" waveform is dependent on variations in central venous pressure. The waveform is also influenced by respiration and compliance of the liver parenchyma. Flow direction in the hepatic veins is normally hepatofugal (away from the liver).

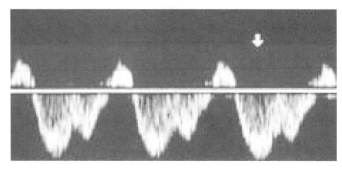

FIGURE 11–30. Classic Doppler spectral waveform pattern from normal hepatic veins.

Anatomy of the Portal Vein

The portal vein is formed by the confluence of the splenic and superior mesenteric veins and carries nutrient-rich blood from the gastrointestinal tract, gallbladder, pancreas, and spleen to the liver where it is processed and filtered. The portal vein is responsible for carrying approximately 75–80% of the blood to the liver, while the hepatic artery supplies the remaining 20%.

Beyond the confluence of the splenic and superior mesenteric veins, the main portal vein courses to the right and cephalad to enter the porta hepatis where it bifurcates into right and left branches. The confluence of the splenic and portal veins is posterior to the neck of the pancreas. The inferior mesenteric vein drains into the splenic vein immediately to the left of this confluence. The coronary (left gastric) vein most often enters the splenic vein superiorly near the superior mesenteric/portal venous confluence and courses in a cranio-caudad plane.[10] The main portal vein lies anterior to the IVC, cephalad to the head of the pancreas, and caudal to the caudate lobe. It enters the liver along with the hepatic artery and common bile duct.[1,2,6,10] This portal triad travels as a unit throughout the liver parenchyma bound together by a collagenous membrane (Glisson's capsule).[6]

Within the porta hepatis, the main portal vein divides into the right and left portal vein branches. The right portal vein divides into anterior and posterior branches; the left divides into medial and lateral branches.[1,2]

Sonographic and Spectral Doppler Characteristics.

The portal vein can be followed sonographically from a transverse plane at the level of the splenic confluence and the porta hepatis. The course of the vein, its branches, and flow direction can be defined by using a right intercostal approach with the transducer angled toward the porta hepatis (Fig. 11–31). It should be noted that in contrast to the hepatic vein walls, the walls of the main portal vein and its branches are echogenic.

This feature is attributed to the acoustic properties of collagen fibers found in the intimal and medial layers of the vein. While hepatic veins are boundary formers and course longitudinally toward the IVC, portal veins branch horizontally and are oriented as branches from the porta hepatis. The diameters of the left and right portal veins are greater at their origin in the region of the porta hepatis; minimal changes in diameter are noted during respiration. The diameter of the main portal vein is normally <13 mm in the segment just anterior to the IVC. An increase in diameter occurs during expiration, while inspiration results in decreased diameter. These changes are regulated by the volume of blood entering the visceral arterial system and the volume outflow through the systemic venous channels.

Doppler spectral waveforms from the portal veins normally demonstrate hepatopetal flow (toward the liver) with minimal phasicity and mean velocity ranging from 20 to 30 cm/s in the supine, fasting patient (Fig. 11–32). Mean velocity decreases slightly with inspiration and increases with expiration. Pulsatility of the portal veins may be apparent in patients with tricuspid insufficiency or congestive heart failure.

Hepatoportal Disease

Budd–Chiari Syndrome.

Obstruction of the outflow veins, or Budd–Chiari syndrome, results from high-grade stenosis or occlusion of some or all of the hepatic veins. Its occurrence is uncommon and is most often caused by membranous obstruction of the suprahepatic or infrahepatic portion of the IVC, but it may be related to tumor invasion or thrombosis. Budd–Chiari syndrome also occurs secondary to pregnancy, use of oral contraceptives, trauma, hypercoagulable states, polycythemia vera, radiation therapy, Behçet's syndrome, or hepatic abscesses. The hepatic veins may recanalize or they may become fibrotic. Parenchymal fibrosis, hemorrhage, and vascular congestion are associated with chronic hepatic veno-occlusive disease. While many patients may remain asymptomatic, the majority will present with right-upper-quadrant discomfort or pain, abdominal

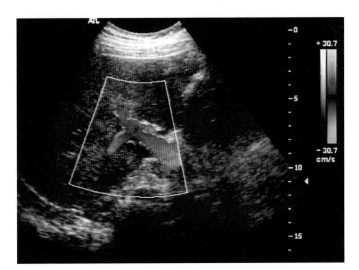

FIGURE 11–31. Color-flow image of the main portal vein from a right intercostal approach.

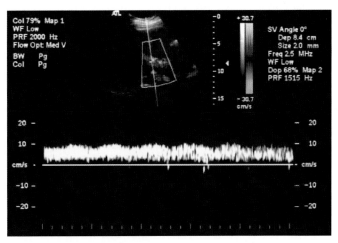

FIGURE 11–32. Color-flow image and Doppler spectral waveforms demonstrating normal hepatopetal flow direction and minimal phasicity.

distention secondary to ascites, hepatomegaly, and superficial collateral veins. Budd–Chiari syndrome can be confirmed with CT or MRI scanning. Both modalities can demonstrate narrowing or absence of the hepatic veins. Venography may be used to confirm partial or complete obstruction of the IVC and the presence and extent of collateralization.

Portal Vein Thrombosis.

Portal vein thrombosis is most commonly associated with biliary atresia, cirrhosis, tumor, trauma, hypercoagulable states, portal hypertension, and inflammatory conditions such as pancreatitis or inflammation of the bowel. Other conditions may lead to thrombosis including dehydration and blood disorders. Interventional procedures such as endoscopic esophageal sclerotherapy or percutaneous injection of ethanol for ablation of hepatocellular carcinoma may occasionally result in portal vein thrombosis. Periportal collaterals may form in the porta hepatis (cavernous transformation) or venous recanalization may be apparent following thrombosis of the extrahepatic portal vein. While cavernous transformation occurs in adults secondary to cirrhosis, pancreatitis, or malignancy, it is not commonly seen in patients with liver disease but, surprisingly, is frequently encountered in patients with healthier livers.[10] It has been noted in neonates in association with omphalitis, systemic infection, abdominal inflammation, or dehydration or as a result of exchange transfusion or umbilical vein catheterization.

Portal venography is most often used to confirm the sonographic findings and to determine portal venous pressure. CT with contrast enhancement and MRI are also used to demonstrate portal vein thrombosis and cavernous transformation.

Portal Hypertension.

Normally, blood pressure within the liver is low (5–10 mm Hg) and commonly only slightly higher than that in the IVC. Portal hypertension causes the blood pressure in the liver to exceed 30 mm Hg as a result of obstruction to venous outflow.[5] In Western countries, cirrhosis is the usual cause of portal hypertension followed by hepatic vein thrombosis and portal venous occlusion. As resistance to normal portal venous flow increases, pressure within the liver increases and alternative routes for blood flow spontaneously develop. Flow in the main portal vein most often becomes hepatofugal in direction and normal portal tributaries enlarge to serve as collateral pathways.

Portal hypertension is classified into three categories: prehepatic, intrahepatic and posthepatic. Prehepatic (presinusoidal) portal hypertension is caused by thrombosis or obstruction of the main portal vein before it enters the liver. Intrahepatic (sinusoidal) portal hypertension is the most common and is due to impedance to portal venous flow within the liver. Posthepatic (post-sinusoidal) portal hypertension occurs secondary to obstruction of the outflow veins or suprahepatic IVC.

Historically, standard contrast angiography has been used for confirmation of portal hypertension, determination of portal venous pressure, and demonstration of portosystemic collater-

als. Angiography is also used to direct placement of coils or foam for embolization of varices and catheters for transjugular intrahepatic portosystemic shunts (TIPSs).

Sonographic and Doppler Characteristics of Hepatoportal Disease.

Budd–Chiari syndrome causes the liver to enlarge and may result in development of ascites. Splenomegaly is usually present and the caudate lobe may be enlarged as a result of increased outflow through the caudate veins. Sonographically, the liver parenchyma appears heterogeneous with increased echogenicity. While intraluminal echoes consistent with thrombus may be apparent in the acute stages, most commonly the hepatic veins are difficult to visualize because of reduced or absent flow. Spectral, color and/ or power Doppler optimized for very low flow should be used to demonstrate the presence of collateral pathways and to confirm patency or occlusion of the hepatic veins. Continuous, low-velocity Doppler spectral waveforms are commonly apparent proximal to stenotic segments while markedly elevated velocities are found at the site of stenosis. This pattern will be altered if the IVC is obstructed; low-velocity signals will be noted even in stenotic segments of the hepatic veins.

If the portal vein is acutely thrombosed, it will be dilated with acoustically homogeneous echoes within the lumen (Fig. 11–33). The thrombotic process may be segmental with sparing of one or more of the main tributaries.[5] Chronic thrombosis may cause the portal vein and its branches to be difficult to visualize because of a decrease in vein diameter and the presence of increased intraluminal echogenicity resulting from fibrosis.

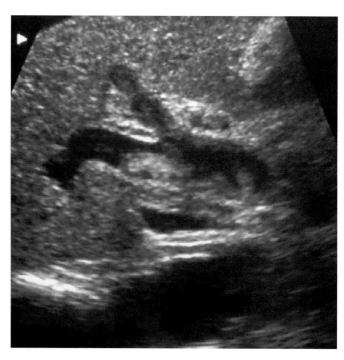

FIGURE 11–33. Real-time image demonstrating acute thrombus within the lumen of the portal vein.

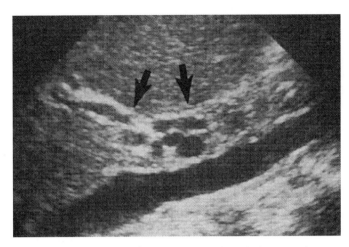

FIGURE 11–34. Real-time image of the porta hepatis demonstrating small, serpiginous venous collaterals. This finding is consistent with cavernous transformation of the portal vein.

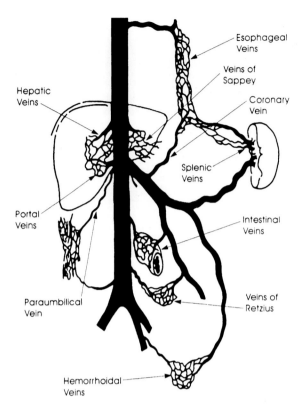

FIGURE 11–35. Diagram illustrating portosystemic collateral pathways.

Total obstruction of the portal vein can be demonstrated with color or power Doppler to show the absence of flow. Thrombosis can then be confirmed with optimized spectral Doppler. Color or power Doppler will demonstrate flow around the thrombus when the vein is partially obstructed. Spectral Doppler waveforms will be nonphasic, consistent with the absence of respiratory variation as a result of increased venous pressure. If cavernous transformation has replaced the main portal vein, multiple small tubular structures will be noted in the porta hepatis (Fig. 11–34). They will appear anechoic but will demonstrate low-velocity, minimally phasic spectral waveforms characteristic of portal venous flow. When flow in the portal vein is compromised, the hepatic artery assumes responsibility for supplying the majority of oxygenated blood to the liver. As a result of flow demand, the hepatic artery may enlarge, vascular resistance in the hepatic artery decreases, and velocity may increase.

Tumor infiltration of the portal vein occurs most often in patients with hepatocellular carcinoma or liver metastases. Color Doppler will define multiple small vessels throughout the tumor-filled portal vein. While cavernous transformation of the portal vein will demonstrate venous signals in the small channels, tumor blood flow is characterized by low-resistance arterial waveforms.

Portal hypertension can be characterized by its sonographic findings. The portal vein is commonly enlarged, decompression of the liver results in changes in normal blood flow patterns and direction of flow, and collateral pathways and varices (enlarged veins) develop (Fig. 11–35). Hepatic cirrhosis results in loss of respirophasicity in the portal vein and its branches. As portal venous pressure increases, the Doppler spectral waveform may become bidirectional, demonstrating both hepatopetal and hepatofugal flow. Continuous hepatofugal portal venous flow is consistent with portal hypertension and velocity commonly is <12 cm/s (Fig. 11–36). Portal vein diameter at the level of

the IVC is frequently greater than 13 mm and respiratory variation in vein diameter disappears.[10] Periportal fibrosis causes increased echogenicity of the portal venous walls and the vein may become comma-shaped. The coronary vein diameter usually increases to exceed 5 mm. Additionally, the diameter of the splenic and superior mesenteric veins may increase to more than 10 mm, but most often, there is <20% increase in diameter of these veins from quiet respiration to deep inspiration. Varices may be noted in the splenic hilum and the region of the gallbladder.

There are other sonographic findings that characterize portal hypertension. Commonly there is fatty infiltration of the liver and portosystemic collaterals are apparent within the liver parenchyma and the splenic hilum (splenorenal and splenocaval), as well as a recanalized paraumbilical vein. Identification of the collateral pathways is facilitated with color

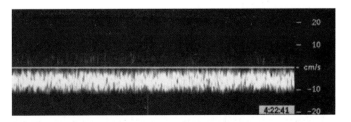

FIGURE 11–36. Doppler spectral waveform demonstrating continuous, low-velocity hepatofugal flow in the portal vein. This finding is suggestive of portal hypertension.

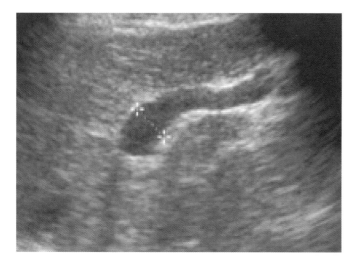

FIGURE 11-37. Gray-scale image of the paraumbilical vein in the long axis within the falciform ligament.

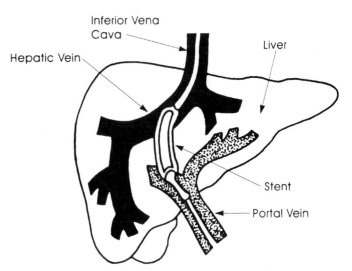

FIGURE 11-38. Diagram illustrating a transjugular intrahepatic portosystemic shunt (TIPS).

flow imaging which will define their presence and confirm flow direction. Splenomegaly may be present (>13 cm), while liver size decreases to <10 cm anteroposteriorly, less than 15 cm in length, and <20 cm in width.[6] Dilated, tortuous superficial veins may be obvious surrounding the umbilicus (caput medusa). These arise from a recanalized paraumbilical vein, which can be imaged in a longitudinal or transverse scan plane in the region of the falciform ligament (Fig. 11-37).[10] The umbilical vein will appear as a "bull's eye" when imaged in the transverse plane.

TRANSJUGULAR INTRAHEPATIC PORTOSYSTEMIC SHUNTS

The current nonsurgical procedure of choice for reduction of venous pressure, variceal bleeding, and ascites is diversion of blood from the portal vein to the systemic venous circulation by way of an intrahepatic shunt. The shunt is created by catheter entry through the right internal jugular vein. The catheter is then advanced to the superior vena cava (SVC) and the hepatic (usually right or middle) vein. The catheter traverses the liver parenchyma and enters the main portal vein. A metallic stent is placed over the catheter and balloon dilated to create a shunt between the portal venous system and the hepatic vein (Fig. 11-38).

Sonographic and Doppler Characteristics of TIPS

Prior to placement of the TIPS, sonography has shown value in confirming patency and flow direction in the portal vein and its branches, demonstration of a recanalized paraumbilical vein or other portosystemic collaterals, varices, and location and extent of ascites. Attention is given to assessment of the internal jugular vein to ensure its patency.

Following placement of the TIPS, the shunt is evaluated to obtain baseline information on shunt velocity, direction of flow in the main portal vein and its intrahepatic branches, and the hepatic veins. Flow velocities in the main portal vein usually exceed 80 cm/s, with a waveform pattern mimicking the pulsatile flow common to the hepatic veins (Fig. 11-39). Because most of the intrahepatic flow will be toward the shunt (low resistance), hepatofugal flow direction is expected in the portal vein branches. Flow in the hepatic veins should remain hepatofugal. A change in normal flow direction in the intrahepatic venous channels signifies shunt dysfunction and stenosis or occlusion of the shunt should be determined.[9]

High-resolution B-mode imaging is used to define location of the shunt within the hepatic and portal veins; the shunt should extend well into both vessels. Sonographically, the shunt will appear as an echogenic tubular structure extending along a curved path from the portal vein to the hepatic vein (Fig. 11-40). Most often, it measures 8-10 mm in diameter.

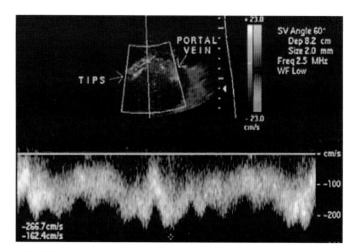

FIGURE 11-39. Color-flow image and Doppler spectral waveforms demonstrating normal flow in a TIPS.

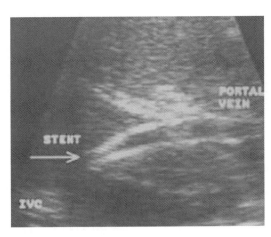

FIGURE 11–40. Real-time image of a TIPS within the parenchyma of the liver. Note the echogenic walls of the shunt.

Recognition of TIPS Dysfunction

Because TIPSs are susceptible to malfunction over time, it is important to maintain a surveillance program to monitor blood flow within the shunt and the intrahepatic vessels. Follow-up evaluations are usually performed at quarterly intervals as long as the shunt remains patent. Shunt dysfunction is most often caused by stenosis of the shunt or hepatic vein or shunt thrombosis. Acute thrombus is acoustically homogeneous and may cause partial or total compromise of the shunt lumen. The presence and extent of the thrombus may be defined with color Doppler imaging, while total obstruction of the shunt must be confirmed with optimized spectral Doppler. The direction of flow in the main portal vein may revert to hepatofugal with decreased velocities and varices may recur.

Intimal hyperplasia is the primary factor in shunt stenosis and is caused by a buildup of collagenous material between the shunt and its endothelial surface. While it commonly occurs in the early post-shunt period, it may develop any time within the first year. Acoustically, it is homogeneous and will be noted to compromise the lumen of the shunt. The extent of compromise can be defined with color-flow imaging and the severity of stenosis determined by velocity spectral waveform parameters.

While problems may be encountered in the portal vein, body of the shunt, or the hepatic outflow vein, most often the obstruction is on the hepatic end of the conduit. B-mode imaging will confirm a reduction in the internal diameter of the shunt when compared to the baseline measurement. Magnified views will facilitate comparative measurements. Color-flow imaging will define narrow segments, regions of disordered flow, and changes in flow direction in the portal and hepatic veins. Additional signs of shunt dysfunction include recurrence of varices and portosystemic collaterals and new onset of ascites.

Changes in velocity and flow direction when compared to the baseline evaluation are key to identification of shunt dysfunction. Depending on the severity of stenosis, velocities may either increase or decrease compared to the previous examination. TIPS velocities are typically higher than those of native

vessels, but an interval increase or decrease in velocity exceeding 50 cm/s has been shown to be consistent with stenosis, while actual velocities <60 cm/s are diagnostic of flow limitation that is clinically significant.[3,9]

RENAL VEINS

Anatomy of the Renal Veins

The renal veins return blood from the kidneys to the IVC. The intrarenal subcapsular veins converge to form the stellate veins. These veins drain into the interlobular veins, which empty into the interlobar veins. The interlobar veins form the main renal vein. The right renal vein courses superiorly to the right renal artery to the lateral wall of the IVC and is the shorter of the two renal veins. The left renal vein courses from the hilum of the left kidney to cross the aorta anteriorly and the pancreas inferiorly before entering the IVC. As it crosses the aorta, it is visualized posterior to the SMA.[1,2] The vein may be compressed in the mesentery between the aorta and SMA, resulting in the "nutcracker sign." Multiple venous branches are common.

Sonographic and Doppler Characteristics

Sonographically, the renal veins appear as anechoic tubular structures extending from the renal hila to the posterolateral walls of the IVC (Fig. 11–41). The renal veins are routinely evaluated with optimized spectral and color Doppler to determine patency and flow direction. The Doppler spectral waveform pattern demonstrates low-velocity respirophasicity with flow away from the renal hilum.

Renal Venous Disorders

Renal Vein Thrombosis. Renal vein thrombosis most commonly occurs secondary to trauma or tumor. Trauma frequently causes extrinsic compression of the vein or endothelial damage, which leads to flow obstruction and thrombosis. Renal tumors

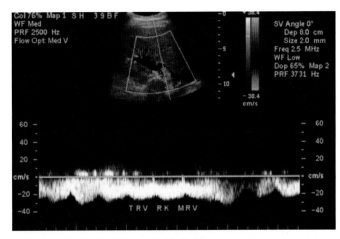

FIGURE 11–41. Color-flow image and Doppler spectral waveforms from a normal renal vein.

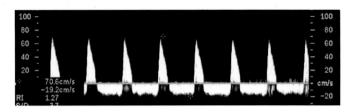

FIGURE 11–42. Doppler spectral waveforms from a renal artery with outflow to a thrombosed renal vein.

often advance to the renal vein. In the neonate, thrombosis may result from infection, dehydration, hypotension, or maternal diabetes. Primary renal disorders including membranous glomerulonephritis and nephrotic syndrome are frequently the etiology for this condition in adults. Systemic causes must also be considered including lupus erythematosus, amyloidosis, diabetes mellitus, and sickle cell anemia.

Renal vein thrombosis is encountered more often in the left renal vein and children are affected more often than adults. Patients may present initially with proteinuria, microscopic hematuria, and epigastric discomfort or pain. Adults may present acutely with dehydration, vascular congestion, or hypercoagulopathies. Clinical symptoms may also include pulmonary embolism.

Sonographic and Doppler Characteristics of Renal Venous Disorders. Acute renal vein thrombosis causes the kidney to increase in size while cortical echogenicity decreases. The renal sinus becomes hypoechogenic, the pyramids are prominent with poor definition and the corticomedullary junction is indistinct. Thrombosis causes the renal vein to dilate. Acute thrombus will appear acoustically homogeneous; chronicity leads to increased echogenicity. Color and power Doppler imaging may facilitate differentiation of partial from total venous obstruction by outlining the filling defect. Continuous, nonphasic flow is associated with partial thrombosis, while the absence of flow due to total obstruction can be confirmed with optimized spectral, color and power Doppler. When the renal vein is thrombosed, the Doppler spectral waveform from the renal artery characteristically demonstrates increased resistance as having a rapid systolic upstroke, rapid deceleration, and reversed, blunted diastolic flow (Fig. 11–42).

LIVER, RENAL, AND PANCREAS TRANSPLANTS

Liver Transplantation

Liver transplantation is the treatment of choice for end-stage liver disease. With current surgical techniques and immunosuppressive therapy, the expected survival rate at 1 year exceeds 85%.[9] Sonography plays a major role in the preopera-

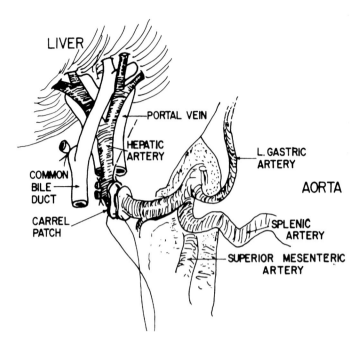

FIGURE 11–43. Diagram illustrating liver transplant procedure.

tive and postoperative evaluation. Children with biliary atresia may have an associated polysplenia syndrome with intestinal malrotation, bilateral symmetry of the major bronchi, and abnormal location of the portal vein to a position anterior to the duodenum. Additionally, the IVC may be interrupted. Hepatic artery anatomic variants and the presence and flow patterns associated with portacaval or mesocaval shunts must be defined. It is critical that these conditions are identified prior to transplantation.

The donor liver may be cadaveric (orthotopic) in origin or the patient may retain his or her own liver and a portion of a donor liver is transplanted (heterotopic). The vascular anatomy and anastomotic sites will differ with each type of procedure. If an orthotopic cadaveric transplant (OLTX) is used, the recipient's liver and gallbladder are removed and a cadaveric donor liver is transplanted (Fig. 11–43). The arterial and venous anastomoses include the extrahepatic portal vein, hepatic artery, and suprahepatic and infrahepatic IVC. Biliary drainage is achieved with a Roux-en-Y cholecystojejunostomy or choledochostomy with a T-tube. With heterotopic transplantation, the vascular anastomoses are to the suprahepatic IVC, hepatic artery, and portal vein. Biliary drainage is temporary through a choledochojejunostomy.[7]

Sonographic and Doppler Characteristics of Liver Transplants. Sonography is generally performed pretransplantation and post-transplantation. Preoperatively, the abdomen is assessed for fluid collections and masses, hepatomegaly, splenomegaly, patency of the hepatic artery, and its branches, portal vein and its branches, superior mesenteric vein, splenic artery and vein, and the IVC. Particular attention is given to the measurements of the liver and spleen and to detection of malignancy. The post-transplant evaluations are directed to confirmation of vessel patency and flow patterns at the anastomotic sites. Flow velocities may be slightly elevated in the early post-transplant period due to vascular accommodation, extrinsic compression due to tissue edema, and slight diameter mismatch. Even so, there is normally no evidence of remarkable velocity increase in any vessel or post-stenotic turbulence associated with flow-limiting compromise of vessel lumen. Color-flow imaging may facilitate identification of the hepatic artery and hepatic veins and confirmation of appropriate flow direction in all vessels.

Recognition of Liver Transplant Complications

Organ Rejection. Rejection of the liver transplant is a primary cause of organ dysfunction. Clinically, patients experience fever, malaise, anorexia, and hepatomegaly. Sonography is neither sensitive nor specific for the identification of hepatic transplant rejection but has value in excluding stenosis or thrombosis of the hepatic artery, portal vein, or IVC, as well as biliary complications. Laboratory tests are valuable in refining the suspected diagnosis and include elevated serum bilirubin, alkaline phosphatase, and serum transaminase. Confirmation of rejection is achieved most commonly with needle biopsy.

Hepatic Artery Thrombosis. Thrombosis of the hepatic artery post-transplant is considered a critical complication as it jeopardizes transplant viability and the possibility of re-transplantation. While it may be difficult to demonstrate intraluminal thrombus with real-time imaging, optimized spectral, color, or power Doppler will confirm absence of flow. Standard contrast angiography has historically been chosen to validate the sonographic findings.

Hepatic Artery Stenosis. Kinking, coiling, or curling of the extrahepatic segment of the hepatic artery may occur as a result of excessive length of the anastomosed vessel. Flow-reducing stenosis can occur in any of the segmental branches of the artery within the liver parenchyma. Color-flow imaging will define regions of disordered flow and occasional evidence of perivascular color artifact characteristic of an arterial bruit associated with chaotic flow patterns. Hepatic arterial Doppler spectral waveforms exhibit peak systolic velocities in excess of 180 cm/s, with evidence of post-stenotic turbulence and a systolic acceleration time >0.8 seconds (Fig. 11–44). Distal to the site of narrowing, the Doppler waveform is usually dampened with low velocity forward diastolic flow (resistive index <0.5).[4,7]

Portal Vein Thrombosis. Post-transplant thrombosis of the portal vein is associated with early transplant failure and a high mortality rate. High-resolution B-mode imaging will demonstrate dilation of the portal vein and acoustically homogeneous intraluminal echoes. The thrombus may be partially or totally

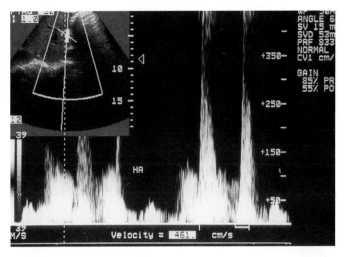

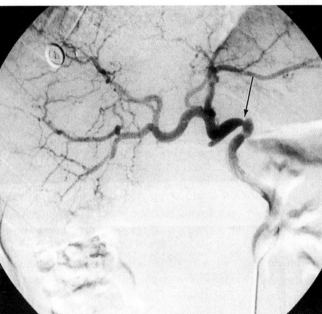

FIGURE 11–44. Arteriogram with associated Doppler spectral waveforms from a liver transplant hepatic artery stenosis.

obstructive. Color or power Doppler imaging may be used effectively to highlight flow around a thrombus that is partially occluding a vein lumen or confirm absence of flow when total obstruction is suspected. Thrombosis may extend beyond the main portal vein and include the right and left branches and their tributaries. Attention should be given to identification of periportal collaterals and patency of the hepatic artery that may continue to provide flow to the liver.

Portal Vein Stenosis. Stenosis of the portal vein is an uncommon complication following liver transplantation. When present, it is most often found in the region of the portal vein anastomosis as an irregularity of the vein wall or a band-like stricture. Aneurysmal dilation and portal hypertension may be associated with chronic stenosis.

Inferior Vena Cava Thrombosis and Stenosis. Flow may be compromised in the IVC post-transplant as a result of an anastomotic stricture or extrinsic compression from tissue edema, hematomas, or fluid collections adjacent to the IVC anastomoses. Real-time imaging will demonstrate acoustically homogeneous or heterogeneous intraluminal echoes dependent on the age of the thrombus. Partial versus total obstruction can be determined with color or power Doppler and confirmed with optimized spectral Doppler interrogation. Luminal compromise may cause elevation of IVC velocities in the region of narrowing with dampening of the distal signal.

Biliary Complications. Obstruction and leaks are the most common biliary complications post-transplantation. Obstruction is considered to be present if the common bile duct diameter exceeds 6 mm. This complication is most often caused by strictures associated with surgical technical errors, infection, chronic rejection, or ischemia. Additional causes may be related to dysfunction of T-tubes or stents, redundancy of the common bile duct, biliary stones, and mucoceles of the remnant of the cystic duct. Bile leaks are identified sonographically as anechoic fluid collections in the biliary system. Bilomas may be present in the gallbladder fossa and porta hepatis. These will appear cyst-like with internal echoes and demonstrate acoustic enhancement. Most often, they are irregularly shaped.

Pseudoaneurysms. Pseudoaneurysms occur when at least two of the three layers of the arterial wall have been punctured, allowing blood to escape into the surrounding tissue. Pseudoaneurysms (false aneurysms) may occur when there is leakage of blood through an anastomotic site or from an artery that has mistakenly been punctured during the transplant procedure or post-transplantation biopsy. This is an uncommon complication and is most often associated with graft needle biopsy or infection. Recognition of pseudoaneurysms is facilitated with color-flow imaging and differentiation of pseudoaneurysm from true aneurysmal dilation is dependent on documentation of a to-and-fro Doppler spectral waveform in the tract that connects the false aneurysm to the punctured artery (Fig. 11–45).

Correlative imaging modalities for confirmation of liver transplant dysfunction are chosen based on the clinical presentation. Standard contrast arteriography is used to demonstrate patency of the primary arteries and veins and for assessment of organ perfusion. Radionuclide scintigraphy has shown value for evaluation of liver perfusion, hepatocyte function, and assessment of bile excretion. While bilomas and abscesses may be identified sonographically, hepatobiliary scintigraphy is used to confirm these lesions. CT imaging has value for confirmation of biliary necrosis; however, cholangiography is the procedure of choice for confirmation of biliary system compromise.

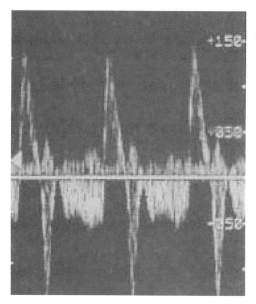

FIGURE 11–45. Characteristic "to-and-fro" Doppler spectral waveform pattern recorded in the neck of a pseudoaneurysm.

Renal Transplantation

Renal transplantation was first introduced in the 1950s and has become the procedure of choice for patients with end-stage renal disease. Survival rates are excellent in the current surgical era as a result of improved surgical procedures and advances in immunosuppression. Multiple causes of post-transplantation renal failure still exist, however, and many of these can be identified sonographically. Real-time imaging, coupled with spectral, color, and power Doppler, has shown value as a tool for preoperative assessment and post-transplantation surveillance of tissue and flow characteristics that are consistent with renal transplant dysfunction.

If a living related donor kidney is used, sonography plays an important preoperative role in ensuring that the arterial and venous circulations are normal and that the recipient aorta and external iliac arteries are free of atherosclerotic debris. Following transplantation, sonographic surveillance is employed to identify increased renovascular resistance associated with acute rejection, acute tubular necrosis (ATN), transplant renal artery stenosis/occlusion, and arteriovenous communication.

In adult patients, the transplanted kidney is most often placed superficially in the right lower abdomen. The donor renal artery is anastomosed to the right external or internal iliac artery while the transplant renal vein is anastomosed to the external iliac vein. Drainage from the ureter into the bladder is achieved via ureteroneocystostomy (Fig. 11–46).

Sonographic and Doppler Characteristics of Renal Transplants.
Since the 1980s, real-time imaging has been used to identify acute renal transplant rejection. The more popular characteristics include increased renal volume, enlargement of

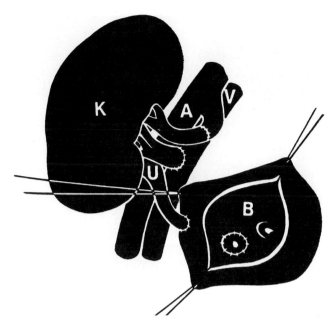

FIGURE 11–46. Diagram illustrating the surgical anastomoses used for renal transplantation. K is kidney; A is arterial; V is vernous; U is ureter; B is bladder.

the renal pyramids, decrease in the amount of renal sinus fat, increased cortical echogenicity, decreased echogenicity of the renal parenchyma, indistinct corticomedullary boundaries, and thickening of the renal pelvis. These criteria are neither sensitive nor specific for renal allograft rejection when correlated histologically.

Greater emphasis has been placed on assessment of the flow patterns within the transplant renal artery and vein and the parenchymal vessels because these patterns alter with increased vascular resistance. Many investigators have shown that elevation of the resistive index is associated with acute transplant rejection, acute tubular necrosis, renal vein thrombosis, obstruction, and extrinsic compression of the renal artery or transplant. Others have concentrated on changes in the Doppler spectral waveform patterns that occur with increased vascular resistance. Sequential monitoring of blood flow patterns has provided recognition of Doppler spectral patterns associated with acute transplant rejection, acute tubular necrosis, transplant renal artery stenosis/occlusion, renal vein thrombosis, and arteriovenous fistulas.[4,9]

Sonographically, the normal renal transplant will appear as an elliptical organ lying in close proximity to the psoas muscle in the lower right iliac fossa. The ureter may be difficult to image unless it is enlarged due to obstruction. The region surrounding the transplant should be surveyed for fluid collections and care should be taken to identify hydronephrosis or inappropriate echogenicity of the renal tissues. Color-flow imaging will facilitate identification of the anastomoses of the transplant renal artery and vein to the external iliac artery and vein and confirmation of flow throughout all segments of the renal medulla and cortex (Fig. 11–47). Arteriovenous fistulas

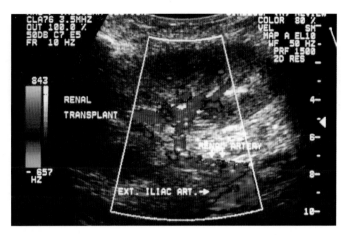

FIGURE 11–47. Color-flow image illustrating the iliac arterial and venous anastomoses and flow within the parenchyma of a renal transplant.

and stenosis associated with kinking or intrinsic narrowing of an artery will present on the color-flow image as regions of disordered flow and mosaic coloration. Tissue infarction is best confirmed with optimized power and spectral Doppler to show absence of flow.

Doppler spectral waveforms from the normal external iliac artery demonstrate phasicity with forward flow in the segment of the artery proximal to the anastomosis of the transplant renal artery. The relatively low resistant flow pattern is caused by the flow demand of the transplanted organ. In the segment of the external iliac artery distal to the renal artery anastomosis, the Doppler spectral waveform will be triphasic, characteristic of the high resistance peripheral arterial system of the lower extremities (Fig. 11–48). The external iliac vein normally demonstrates respirophasicity consistent with venous flow patterns in the extremities.[3,9]

Slight flow disturbance may be apparent at the renal artery anastomosis due to slight deviation of the flow stream. High-velocity, turbulent flow patterns are not normally seen. The Doppler spectral waveform demonstrates a low-resistance pattern with constant forward flow throughout diastole. This pattern is propagated throughout the transplant renal artery and the

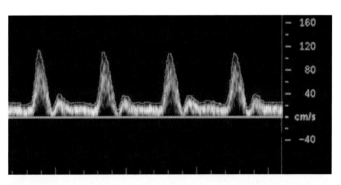

FIGURE 11–48. Doppler spectral waveforms demonstrating the flow pattern in the external iliac artery in the region of the transplant renal artery anastomosis.

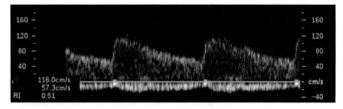

FIGURE 11-49. Normal low-resistance Doppler spectral waveforms from a renal transplant.

vessels within the medulla and cortex of the organ (Fig. 11–49). The peak systolic and end-diastolic velocities decrease proportionately from the main renal artery to the arcuate vessels within the cortex. Although venous respirophasicity may decrease, continuous nonphasic flow is not normal.[3,9]

Recognition of Renal Transplant Complications

Acute Renal Transplant Rejection. Real-time imaging details an enlarged organ with a slightly irregular renal outline, indistinct corticomedullary boundaries, decreased echogenicity of the pyramids, decreased echogenicity of the renal sinus, increased cortical echogenicity, and irregular fluid-filled areas within the renal cortex.

Acute vascular rejection is characterized by proliferative endovasculitis, which causes the arterial intima to thicken. Blood flow is impeded by the arterial narrowing and vascular resistance increases (resistive index >0.8). The increase in resistance is characterized by a decrease in diastolic flow. This is evident in the Doppler spectral waveform pattern throughout the kidney (Fig. 11–50). As the severity of the rejection episode continues to advance, the diastolic flow component of the waveform may deteriorate from low to zero to a reversed flow phase. In the most critical cases of rejection, diastolic flow may be altogether absent. Platelet-fibrin aggregates may form to the extent that the intersegmental and arcuate arteries of the transplant thrombose; this results in organ failure.[9]

Acute Tubular Necrosis. ATN may be difficult to identify with real-time imaging, as the tissues appear normal. Mild ATN is

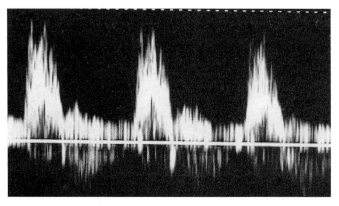

FIGURE 11-50. High-resistance Doppler spectral waveform pattern associated with acute renal transplant rejection.

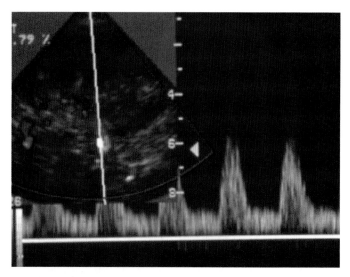

FIGURE 11-51. Doppler spectral waveform pattern associated with moderate acute tubular necrosis. Note the rapid systolic deceleration and increased pulsatility compared to the normal spectral pattern.

characterized by peritubular necrosis and medullary arterial-venous shunting. As the necrotic process becomes more severe, tubular and interstitial edemas are apparent and impedance to arterial inflow to the transplanted organ increases. Resistive indices will increase, but this quantitative method of assessment only signifies increased renovascular resistance and does not define its etiology. We have shown a continuum of Doppler spectral patterns associated with mild, moderate, and severe ATN.[5,9]

Mild ATN produces a spectral pattern that appears normal except for rapid deceleration from the systolic peak to an increased diastolic forward-flow component. This is thought to be the result of the arterial-venous medullary shunting. Moderate ATN is associated with a spectral waveform that demonstrates rapid systolic deceleration and increased pulsatility (Fig. 11–51). As the severity of the necrotic process increases, vascular resistance increases and diastolic flow decreases further. The Doppler spectral pattern for severe ATN demonstrates a reduction in the amount of diastolic flow, amplitude of the signal, and descent of the diastolic flow component. The waveform may be indistinguishable from the pattern associated with severe acute rejection.[5,9]

Transplant Renal Artery Stenosis and Occlusion. Transplant renal artery stenosis has been shown to occur in as many as 12% of cases. This is most often the result of one of two complications. The first is due to sharp angulation of the transplant renal artery at the anastomosis to the external iliac artery. The kinking may result in flow reduction in the renal artery. The second type may result from anastomotic stricture as a consequence of technical error or from progression of atherosclerotic disease in the iliac artery. The second type may also be related to arterial injury during harvesting, chronic rejection, or post-transplant intimal hyperplasia. Clinically, patients present with new onset hypertension, elevated serum creatinine levels, and

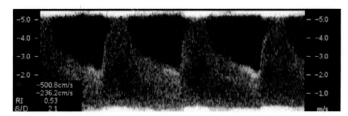

FIGURE 11–52. Flow-reducing transplant renal artery stenosis is characterized by high-velocity, turbulent signals and a renal-iliac artery ratio >3.0.

perhaps a bruit in the region of the transplant renal artery anastomoses.

If anastomotic kinking is present, real-time imaging will define sharp angulation at the anastomotic site; color or power Doppler can be used to confirm narrowing of the arterial lumen. Spectral Doppler waveforms from the external iliac and transplant renal artery reveal high-velocity, turbulent flow and a renal-iliac artery ratio of more than 3.0[5] (Fig. 11–52).

Severe vascular rejection may lead to thrombosis of the transplant renal artery or the vessels within the sinus and cortex of the kidney. Infarction may be complete or segmental. Immediate surgical or lytic intervention is required to salvage the organ. High resolution B-mode imaging details a hyperechoic organ or regions of ischemic tissue. Occlusion of the transplant renal arteries is suggested when there is no evidence of flow using optimized spectral, color, or power Doppler.

Thrombosis of the transplant renal vein is most often caused by surgical technical complications or from extrinsic compression of the vein postoperatively by hematoma, seroma, or tissue edema. Sonographically, the vein appears dilated with acoustically homogeneous intraluminal echoes. Spectral, color, or power Doppler will confirm the absence of flow in the transplant renal vein and throughout the renal parenchymal venous tree. The Doppler spectral waveform from the renal arteries is characterized by a sharp systolic upstroke followed by rapid deceleration to a reversed and blunted diastolic flow component as previously described.

Arteriovenous Fistulas. Acute renal transplant rejection has historically been confirmed with cortical needle biopsy. These procedures may result in development of arteriovenous communications within the parenchyma of the organ. These arteriovenous (AV) fistulas rarely severely compromise blood flow to the kidney and are usually self-limiting. Color-flow imaging can be used to define the presence, size, and effect on the arterial and venous circulation. Doppler spectral waveforms detail the pressure-flow gradient in the fistula as evidenced by high-velocity, turbulent flow in the feeding arteries and pulsatile, arterialized flow patterns in the draining veins.

Pseudoaneurysms. Percutaneous biopsy or anastomotic leakage may result in formation of pseudoaneurysm at the site of arterial puncture or breakthrough. The majority of pseudoaneurysms

are small and self-limiting; the patient remains asymptomatic. Some, however, may be quite large and can compromise flow to the transplanted kidney or rupture. As described earlier, blood escapes from the artery into the surrounding tissue and is connected to the artery by a neck or pedicle. High-pressure flow enters the false aneurysm through the neck during systole and returns to the artery during the low-pressure diastolic phase of the cardiac cycle. This results in the classic "to-and-fro" Doppler spectral waveform that is diagnostic for flow patterns associated with pseudoaneurysms (see Fig. 11–45).

Consistent with liver transplantation, correlative imaging modalities chosen for confirmation of renal transplant dysfunction are based on the clinical presentation. MRI or radionuclide imaging is chosen to evaluate perfusion and functional status of the transplanted kidney. Standard contrast arteriography has historically been used for vascular evaluation, while CT imaging has shown value for both pre-transplantation and post-transplantation assessment.

Pancreas Transplantation

Most often, pancreatic transplantation is performed in patients with end-stage renal disease secondary to type I diabetes and to reverse the complications related to progression of disease. The pancreas is transplanted in conjunction with a renal transplant or may be transplanted alone in diabetic patients who do not have renal failure.

The first segmental pancreas transplantation was performed in 1966 and survival rates have increased in the present era as a result of improved surgical techniques and immunosuppressive regimens. Graft failure is often the consequence of acute rejection, vascular thrombosis, pancreatitis, fluid collections, infection, pseudocysts, and anastomotic leaks. The most serious complications occur in the early post-transplantation period and are commonly related to thrombosis of the splenic vein.

The pancreatic transplant is placed superficially in the pelvic area in a manner similar to that used in renal transplantation. When both organs are transplanted together, the pancreas is placed on the patient's right side and the kidney on the left side (Fig. 11–53). The celiac artery and SMA are harvested from the donor aorta on a Carrel patch and anastomosed to the recipient's external iliac artery. The tail of the pancreas is perfused by the splenic artery, which is left intact during transplantation. The donor portal vein is anastomosed to the external iliac vein; the splenic vein drains the tail of the pancreas transplant. A section of the donor's duodenum is attached to the recipient bladder to achieve exocrine drainage.[9]

Clinical features of acute pancreas transplant rejection include elevated serum amylase, glucose, and lipase levels.

Recognition of Pancreas Transplant Complications

Acute Rejection. In contrast to its use as a valuable aid to detection of acute rejection in renal transplants, sonography has

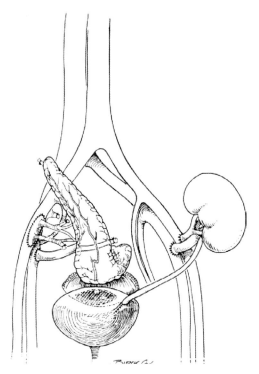

FIGURE 11–53. Diagram illustrating the surgical procedure used for transplantation of a kidney and pancreas. *(Reprinted, with permission, from Neumyer MM: Ultrasonographic Assessment of Renal and Pancreatic Transplants. The Journal of Vascular Technology, 19 (5-6); 321–329, 1995.)*

demonstrated little value in identification of rejection in pancreas transplants. Real-time imaging may demonstrate acoustic inhomogeneity, poor margination of the organ, dilated pancreatic duct, and relative changes in attenuation.

Thrombosis. Thrombosis is most often seen in the early postoperative period but may occur later as a consequence of rejection of the transplanted organ or infection. Venous thrombosis is most serious when it affects the splenic vein and can threaten organ viability.[9] When multiple venous segments are involved, arterial inflow is compromised and organ survival is jeopardized. Color-flow imaging is used to confirm patency of the arterial and venous anastomoses and perfusion of the transplanted organ. Most importantly, it has been the procedure of choice for confirming patency of the splenic vein throughout its tortuous course along the posterior aspect of the organ.[8]

Pancreatitis. Pancreatitis may occur as an inflammatory response to reperfusion of the organ at the time of transplantation. In most cases, this is a mild episode but, if severe, can compromise organ viability. Sonographically, in the acute phase, the pancreas is slightly enlarged with a hypoechoic, fluffy-looking texture as a result of tissue edema. Fibrosis and calcifications may be noted if the condition is long-standing.[6]

Questions

GENERAL INSTRUCTIONS: For each question, select the best answer. Select only one answer for each question unless otherwise specified.

1. Which of the following sonographic features is *not* used to diagnose renal artery occlusion?

    (A) absence of a visible main renal artery

    (B) low-amplitude, low-velocity signals in the kidney

    (C) kidney size >9 cm

    (D) no flow detected by optimized spectral, color, or power Doppler

2. Which of the following terms describes an aorta that is diffusely dilated?

    (A) saccular

    (B) fusiform

    (C) spindle-shaped

    (D) ectatic

3. What is the first major branch of the abdominal aorta?

    (A) lumbar artery

    (B) renal artery

    (C) celiac artery

    (D) superior mesenteric artery

4. Which of the following terms is used to describe concentric, spindle-shaped dilation of the abdominal aorta?

    (A) ectatic

    (B) fusiform

    (C) saccular

    (D) dissecting

5. The branches of which of the following arteries form a "seagull" appearance on a sonographic image?

    (A) inferior mesenteric artery

    (B) renal artery

    (C) superior mesenteric artery

    (D) celiac artery

6. What are the branches of the celiac artery?

    (A) proper hepatic, superior mesenteric, and left gastric arteries

    (B) splenic, left gastric and common hepatic arteries

    (C) right gastric, splenic, and inferior mesenteric arteries

    (D) left gastric, superior mesenteric, and splenic arteries

7. Abdominal pain that increases in severity with an upright position is symptomatic of which of the following conditions?

    (A) aortic dissection

    (B) pancreatitis

    (C) ruptured aortic aneurysm

    (D) acute mesenteric ischemia

8. Where are abdominal aortic aneurysms most often located?

    (A) in the juxtarenal aorta

    (B) in the suprarenal aorta

    (C) in the infrarenal aorta

    (D) at the aortic bifurcation

9. The splanchnic circulation does *not* include which of the following arteries?

    (A) renal, superior, and inferior mesenteric arteries

    (B) gastric, celiac, and superior mesenteric arteries

    (C) celiac, superior, and inferior mesenteric arteries

    (D) superior mesenteric, celiac, and gastroduodenal arteries

10. A 50–74% diameter-reducing stenosis of the abdominal aorta is characterized by which of the following findings?

    (A) a 20% increase in peak systolic velocity compared to the proximal normal arterial segment

    (B) a twofold increase in peak systolic velocity compared to the proximal normal arterial segment

    (C) a fourfold increase in peak systolic velocity compared to the proximal normal arterial segment

    (D) a 50% increase in peak systolic velocity compared to the proximal normal arterial segment

11. **When an aortic stent graft is used to repair an abdominal aortic aneurysm, which of the following statements about the aneurysm is true?**

    (A) It is allowed to remain.

    (B) It is resected.

    (C) It is wrapped around the aortic graft.

    (D) It is ligated and bypassed.

12. **Which of the following findings is *not* usually associated with aortic dissection?**

    (A) pregnancy

    (B) Marfan's syndrome

    (C) hypertension

    (D) advanced age

13. **Real-time images demonstrating the echogenic intima separated from the aortic wall are suggestive of which of the following diagnoses?**

    (A) abdominal aortic aneurysm

    (B) arterial dissection

    (C) false aneurysm

    (D) mycotic aneurysm

14. **The common hepatic artery gives rise to which of the following arteries?**

    (A) gastroduodenal artery and right gastric artery

    (B) coronary artery and celiac artery

    (C) proper hepatic artery and left gastric artery

    (D) gastroduodenal artery and right hepatic artery

15. **The splenic artery does *not* supply blood to which of the following structures?**

    (A) spleen

    (B) gallbladder

    (C) pancreas

    (D) stomach

16. **Which of the following arteries is the largest branch of the celiac artery?**

    (A) gastroduodenal artery

    (B) left gastric artery

    (C) hepatic artery

    (D) splenic artery

17. **The left gastric artery is most often visualized in real-time**

    (A) longitudinally

    (B) arising from the superior mesenteric artery

    (C) inferior to the celiac artery

    (D) along the greater curvature of the stomach

18. **The Doppler spectral waveform from the normal celiac artery is characterized by all of the following *except*.**

    (A) constant forward diastolic flow

    (B) peak systolic velocity <200 cm/sec

    (C) end-diastolic velocity >75 cm/sec

    (D) rapid systolic upstroke

19. **The accompanying Doppler spectral waveform is from a fasting superior mesenteric artery. This waveform is characteristic of**

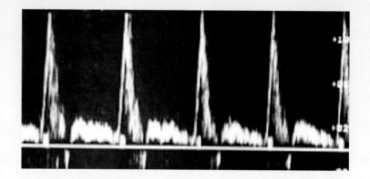

    (A) a normal superior mesenteric artery (SMA)

    (B) more than 70% diameter-reducing SMA stenosis

    (C) a post-stenotic signal

    (D) SMA stenosis that is not hemodynamically significant

20. **Anatomically, the SMA courses**

    (A) anterior to the left renal vein

    (B) posterior to the duodenum

    (C) perpendicular to the aorta

    (D) anterior to the pancreas

21. **Which of the following is *not* a classic symptom associated with chronic mesenteric ischemia?**

    (A) post-prandial pain

    (B) "fear of food" syndrome

    (C) weight loss

    (D) acute, severe abdominal ischemia

22. The Doppler spectral waveform associated with flow-reducing SMA stenosis is *not* characterized which one of the following findings?

    (A) turbulence

    (B) an SMA-aortic ratio >3.5

    (C) peak systolic velocity >275 cm/sec

    (D) end-diastolic velocity >45 cm/sec

23. A high-velocity celiac artery Doppler signal that normalizes with deep inspiration is suggestive of which of the following diagnoses?

    (A) flow-reducing celiac artery stenosis

    (B) portal hypertension

    (C) median arcuate ligament compression

    (D) mesenteric ischemia

24. A collateral pathway to compensate for occlusion of the celiac and/or superior mesenteric artery does *not* include which of the following?

    (A) the arc of Riolan

    (B) the pancreaticoduodenal arcade

    (C) the marginal artery of Drummond

    (D) the inferior epigastric artery

25. Which of the following imaging procedures is historically used for confirmation of visceral artery stenosis or occlusion and demonstration of the extent of collateralization?

    (A) standard contrast arteriography with selective lateral views

    (B) computed tomography

    (C) magnetic resonance imaging

    (D) contrast-enhanced sonography

26. The left renal vein courses

    (A) posterior to the inferior vena cava (IVC)

    (B) posterior to the aorta

    (C) between the aorta and the SMA

    (D) parallel to the superior mesenteric vein

27. The arcuate arteries of the kidney

    (A) subdivide into the intersegmental arteries

    (B) curve around the bases of the pyramids

    (C) lie within the renal hilum

    (D) demonstrate a high-resistance Doppler spectral waveform

28. Renal artery flow-reducing stenosis is indicated if which of the following findings is seen?

    (A) The renal-aortic ratio is <3.0 and the peak systolic velocity is >180 cm/sec.

    (B) The peak systolic renal artery velocity is <180 cm/sec and a post-stenotic signal is found.

    (C) The end-diastolic renal artery velocity is >20 cm/sec and the acceleration time is >1.0.

    (D) The renal-aortic ratio is >3.5 and a post-stenotic signal is found.

29. The renal-aortic velocity ratio can be used to diagnose renal artery stenosis if the aortic velocity is

    (A) <30 cm/sec

    (B) between 40 cm/sec and 100 cm/sec

    (C) >120 cm/sec

    (D) between 30 cm/sec and 80 cm/sec

30. As renal vascular resistance increases, what happens to diastolic flow initially?

    (A) decreases

    (B) reverses

    (C) becomes quasi-steady

    (D) increases

31. The renal resistive index (RI) would *not* usually be increased in patients with which of the following conditions?

    (A) intrinsic renal parenchymal disease

    (B) perinephric or subcapsular hematoma

    (C) decreased heart rate

    (D) mild acute tubular necrosis

32. A Doppler spectral waveform demonstrating high resistance features would normally be found in which of the following arteries?

    (A) hepatic artery

    (B) inferior mesenteric artery

    (C) renal artery

    (D) splenic artery

33. What is the second most common cause of renovascular hypertension?

    (A) ostial atherosclerotic plaque

    (B) anastomotic stenosis

    (C) fibromuscular dysplasia

    (D) renal artery aneurysm

34. Tardus parvus Doppler spectral waveforms within the renal parenchyma indicate which of the following findings?

    (A) renal artery stenosis or occlusion

    (B) medical renal disease

    (C) hydronephrosis

    (D) pyelonephritis

35. Renal artery occlusion is *not* indicated by

    (A) a kidney pole-to-pole length <8 cm

    (B) low-amplitude, low-velocity cortical signals

    (C) a difference in kidney length <2 cm

    (D) absence of color Doppler in imaged renal artery

36. An end-diastolic to systolic velocity ratio of <0.20 from a renal intersegmental artery indicates which of the following diagnoses?

    (A) medical renal disease

    (B) renal artery stenosis

    (C) renal artery occlusion

    (D) fibromuscular dysplasia

37. The common iliac veins come together to form the inferior vena cava at the level of the

    (A) second lumbar vertebra

    (B) fourth lumbar vertebra

    (C) ileocecal valve

    (D) inguinal ligament

38. What is the most common vascular problem affecting the inferior vena cava?

    (A) tumor extension

    (B) thrombosis

    (C) extrinsic compression

    (D) transposition

39. Carcinomas of the kidney, adrenal gland, and liver frequently involve which of the following vessels?

    (A) abdominal aorta

    (B) hepatic veins

    (C) renal arteries

    (D) inferior vena cava

40. Which of the following is *not* likely to cause inferior vena cava thrombosis?

    (A) stasis

    (B) sepsis

    (C) abdominal surgery

    (D) pregnancy

41. In a normal adult, the renal artery resistive index should not be greater than

    (A) 0.03

    (B) 0.35

    (C) 0.70

    (D) 1.05

42. If the inferior vena cava is partially obstructed, the Doppler spectral waveforms will be

    (A) phasic

    (B) pulsatile

    (C) continuous

    (D) absent

43. Which of the following would *not* be used for confirmation of inferior vena cava thrombosis?

    (A) venocavography

    (B) contrast angiography

    (C) magnetic resonance imaging

    (D) computed tomographic scan

44. The liver is divided into right and left lobes by which of the following veins?

    (A) right hepatic vein

    (B) middle hepatic vein

    (C) portal vein

    (D) left hepatic vein

45. The "Playboy bunny" sign refers to the

    (A) hepatic artery

    (B) portal veins

    (C) common bile duct

    (D) hepatic veins

46. Which vessel receives drainage from the hepatic veins?

    (A) inferior vena cava

    (B) portal vein

    (C) splenic vein

    (D) superior mesenteric vein

47. The Doppler spectral waveform from the hepatic veins is normally

    (A) non-phasic
    (B) pulsatile
    (C) quasi-steady
    (D) continuous

48. Which of the following vessels supplies the majority of oxygenated blood to the liver?

    (A) aorta
    (B) hepatic artery
    (C) superior mesenteric artery
    (D) portal vein

49. The portal vein is formed by the confluence of which of the following veins?

    (A) hepatic and splenic veins
    (B) superior mesenteric and splenic veins
    (C) hepatic and superior mesenteric veins
    (D) inferior and superior mesenteric veins

50. Where does the main portal vein lie?

    (A) inferior to the superior mesenteric vein
    (B) inferior to the head of the pancreas
    (C) cephalad to the caudate lobe
    (D) anterior to the inferior vena cava

51. Which three vessels form the portal triad?

    (A) portal vein, superior mesenteric vein, splenic vein
    (B) portal vein, common bile duct, hepatic artery
    (C) portal vein, hepatic artery, superior mesenteric artery
    (D) portal vein, common bile duct, middle hepatic vein

52. Which of the following is true regarding hepatic veins?

    (A) are boundary formers and course horizontally toward the inferior vena cava
    (B) are not boundary formers and are oriented toward the porta hepatis
    (C) are not boundary formers and course longitudinally toward the porta hepatis
    (D) are boundary formers and course longitudinally toward the inferior vena cava

53. Doppler spectral waveforms from the portal veins do *not* normally demonstrate which of the following?

    (A) pulsatility
    (B) minimal phasicity
    (C) hepatopetal flow
    (D) velocity ranging from 20–30 cm/sec

54. Which of the following terms is used to describe obstruction of the hepatic veins?

    (A) fibromuscular dysplasia
    (B) cavernous transformation
    (C) Budd–Chiari syndrome
    (D) hemangioma

55. Which of the following statements describes hepatic veins?

    (A) They can be compressed with a Valsalva maneuver.
    (B) They have thick, echogenic walls.
    (C) They course horizontally within the liver parenchyma.
    (D) They divide the liver into segments.

56. In the Western countries, portal hypertension is most often caused by which of the following?

    (A) hepatitis
    (B) sclerosing cholangitis
    (C) cirrhosis
    (D) hepatocellular carcinoma

57. Cavernous transformation is found in association with

    (A) hepatic vein thrombosis
    (B) portal vein thrombosis
    (C) superior mesenteric vein thrombosis
    (D) inferior vena cava thrombosis

58. What is the normal blood pressure within the liver?

    (A) 5–10 mm Hg
    (B) 20–30 mm Hg
    (C) 0–5 mm Hg
    (D) more than 30 mm Hg

59. What is the most common type of portal hypertension?

    (A) suprahepatic
    (B) extrahepatic
    (C) intrahepatic
    (D) posthepatic

60. Which of the following signs is *not* consistent with portal hypertension?

    (A) portal vein diameter >13 mm
    (B) portal vein velocity <12 cm/sec
    (C) respiratory variation in portal vein signals
    (D) hepatofugal portal venous flow

61. Which of the following causes mycotic aneurysms?

    (A) Marfan's syndrome

    (B) trauma

    (C) penetrating injuries

    (D) infection

62. The paraumbilical vein is a branch of which of the following veins?

    (A) coronary vein

    (B) left gastric vein

    (C) left portal vein

    (D) middle hepatic vein

63. Which of the following veins assumes a "bull's eye" appearance in the transverse image plane in the region of the falciform ligament and after exiting the liver may form the caput medusa in the region of the umbilicus in patients with portal hypertension?

    (A) paraumbilical vein

    (B) coronary vein

    (C) left hepatic vein

    (D) right gastric vein

64. A TIPS is placed in the liver to shunt blood from which of the following veins?

    (A) right hepatic artery to left hepatic vein

    (B) left portal vein to right hepatic artery

    (C) main portal vein to right hepatic vein

    (D) right portal vein to left hepatic vein

65. The color-flow image and Doppler spectral waveforms below are suggestive of which of the following findings?

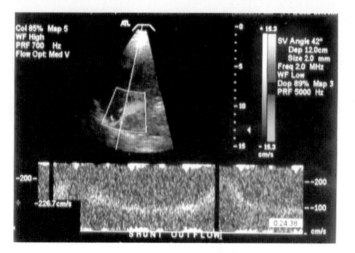

    (A) TIPS stenosis

    (B) obstruction in the hepatic outflow vein

    (C) inferior vena cava thrombosis

    (D) portal vein thrombosis

66. Following placement of a functioning TIPS, flow in the hepatic veins should be

    (A) hepatopetal

    (B) phasic

    (C) hepatofugal

    (D) continuous

67. The B-Mode image below demonstrates

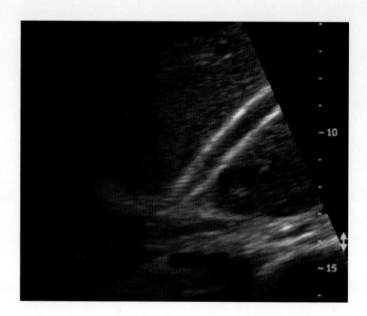

    (A) a TIPS within the liver

    (B) hepatocellular carcinoma

    (C) hemangioma

    (D) stenosis of the right hepatic vein

68. Following placement of a TIPS, velocity within the shunt is 180 cm/sec, flow in the portal vein is 110 cm/sec, flow in the main portal vein is hepatopetal, flow in the left portal and hepatic veins is hepatofugal. What are these findings most consistent with?

    (A) occlusion of the TIPS

    (B) TIPS stenosis

    (C) normally functioning TIPS

    (D) hepatic outflow obstruction

69. Following placement of a TIPS, velocity within the shunt is 55 cm/sec, flow in the portal vein is 58 cm/sec, flow in the main portal vein is hepatopetal, flow in the left portal and hepatic veins is hepatopetal. What are these findings most consistent with?

   (A) occlusion of the TIPS
   (B) TIPS stenosis
   (C) normally functioning TIPS
   (D) hepatic outflow obstruction

70. The Doppler spectral waveform pattern that suggests renal vein thrombosis is characterized by which of the following findings?

   (A) rapid systolic upstroke, rapid deceleration, and low diastolic flow
   (B) delayed systolic upstroke, rapid deceleration, and high diastolic flow
   (C) rapid systolic upstroke, rapid deceleration, and reversed, blunted diastolic flow
   (D) delayed systolic upstroke, rapid deceleration, and high, blunted diastolic flow

71. Which of the following symptoms is *not* associated with renal vein thrombosis?

   (A) hematuria
   (B) pulmonary embolism
   (C) epigastric pain
   (D) fever

72. The Doppler spectral waveforms shown below illustrate

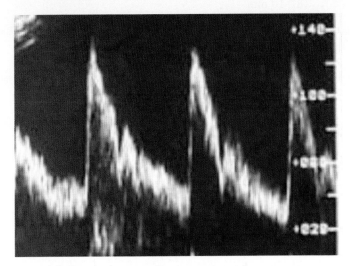

   (A) flow-reducing celiac artery stenosis
   (B) flow-reducing renal artery stenosis
   (C) normal flow in the celiac artery
   (D) normal flow in the renal artery

73. The Doppler spectral waveforms shown below are diagnostic of

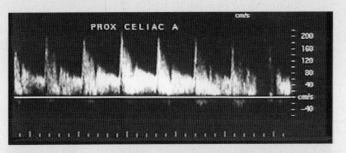

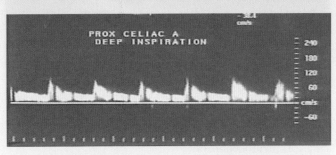

   (A) atherosclerotic stenosis of the celiac artery
   (B) median arcuate ligament compression of the celiac artery
   (C) postprandial celiac artery flow
   (D) collateral compensatory flow in the celiac artery

74. If the urethra is obstructed, which of the following is true?

   (A) Hydronephrosis will not occur.
   (B) Hydronephrosis will be unilateral.
   (C) Hydronephrosis will be bilateral.
   (D) Renal calculi are the cause.

75. Acute renal vein thrombosis is suggested if which of the following is true?

   (A) The renal sinus become hyperechogenic.
   (B) The corticomedullary junction is indistinct.
   (C) The Doppler spectral waveform demonstrates pulsatility.
   (D) The kidney is smaller than normal.

76. The kidney exhibits a hypoechoic, cystic-appearing area within the echogenic renal sinus. What is this finding most consistent with?

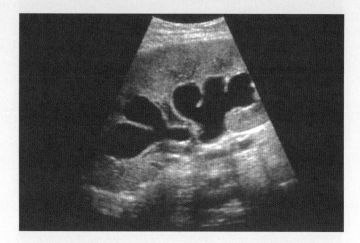

(A) renal calculus

(B) hydronephrosis

(C) renal infarction

(D) renal artery occlusion

77. With obstructive hydronephrosis, the resistive index is

(A) less than 0.50

(B) more than 1.2

(C) more than 3.5

(D) more than 0.70

78. Which of the following terms is used to describe a cadaveric liver transplant?

(A) orthotopic

(B) heterogeneous

(C) heterotopic

(D) homogeneous

79. The arterial and venous anastomoses for a cadaveric liver transplant include the

(A) extrahepatic portal vein, hepatic artery, right hepatic vein, suprahepatic and infrahepatic IVC

(B) the left portal vein, hepatic artery, right hepatic vein, and IVC

(C) extrahepatic portal vein, hepatic artery, suprahepatic and infrahepatic IVC

(D) right portal vein, splenic vein, suprahepatic and infrahepatic IVC

80. Which of the following is *not* a valued tool for confirmation of liver transplant rejection?

(A) sonography

(B) standard contrast arteriography

(C) radionuclide scintigraphy

(D) computed tomography

81. Which of the following is considered a critical complication following liver transplantation?

(A) hepatic artery stenosis

(B) hepatic vein thrombosis

(C) IVC stenosis

(D) hepatic artery thrombosis

82. Post-liver transplantation, the hepatic artery Doppler spectral waveforms demonstrate a peak systolic velocity >180 cm/sec, systolic acceleration time >0.8 sec, and RI <0.5. What are these findings most consistent with?

(A) normal hepatic artery

(B) hepatic artery stenosis

(C) hepatic artery thrombosis

(D) portal vein obstruction

83. Pseudoaneurysms are associated with

(A) an intimal tear

(B) low-resistance Doppler spectral waveforms

(C) to- and fro- flow patterns

(D) a post-stenotic signal

84. The diameter of the portal vein is measured as it crosses anterior to the IVC in a patient lying supine. The diameter should not exceed

(A) 5 mm

(B) 10 mm

(C) 13 mm

(D) 15 mm

85. The gastroduodenal artery is a branch of which of the following arteries?

(A) celiac artery

(B) hepatic artery

(C) splenic artery

(D) gastric artery

86. Which of the following is not a significant cause of renal transplant failure?

(A) acute rejection

(B) acute tubular necrosis

(C) renal artery stenosis

(D) fibromuscular dysplasia

87. In adults, the transplant renal artery is most often anastomosed to which of the following arteries?

    (A) aorta

    (B) common iliac artery

    (C) external iliac artery

    (D) hepatic artery

88. Real-time imaging characteristics of renal transplant rejection include

    (A) decreased renal volume, decreased cortical echogenicity, thickening of the renal pelvis

    (B) decreased renal volume, increased cortical echogenicity, thickening of the renal pelvis

    (C) decreased renal sinus fat, increased cortical echogenicity, thickening of the renal pelvis

    (D) increased renal volume, increased cortical echogenicity, thickening of the renal pelvis

89. The Doppler spectral waveform pattern associated with acute renal transplant rejection demonstrates

    (A) rapid systolic upstroke, rapid deceleration, low or absent diastolic flow

    (B) rapid systolic upstroke, delayed deceleration, forward diastolic flow

    (C) delayed systolic upstroke, rapid deceleration, low or absent diastolic flow

    (D) delayed systolic upstroke, delayed deceleration, forward diastolic flow

90. Moderate ATN is associated with a Doppler spectral pattern demonstrating

    (A) rapid systolic upstroke, rapid deceleration, absent diastolic flow

    (B) rapid systolic upstroke, rapid deceleration, increased pulsatility

    (C) delayed systolic upstroke, delayed deceleration, low or absent diastolic flow

    (D) delayed systolic upstroke, delayed deceleration, acceleration index >3.78

91. Flow-reducing transplant renal artery stenosis is suggested by

    (A) a renal-aortic velocity ratio >3.5

    (B) a peak systolic renal artery velocity >180 cm/sec

    (C) a renal-iliac velocity ratio >3.0

    (D) an end-diastolic to peak systolic velocity ratio >0.2

92. Which of the following does *not* apply to the right renal artery?

    (A) courses posterior to the IVC

    (B) arises from the aortic wall at the level of the first or second lumbar vertebrae

    (C) demonstrates a spectral waveform with constant forward diastolic flow

    (D) gives rise to branches that supply the adrenal, pancreas and ureter

93. Doppler spectral waveforms from a renal transplant arteriovenous fistula are characterized by

    (A) low velocity, low-amplitude arterial signals and pulsatile venous flow

    (B) high-velocity, turbulent arterial signals and low amplitude, continuous venous flow

    (C) high-velocity, turbulent arterial signals and pulsatile venous flow

    (D) low-velocity, low-amplitude arterial signals and continuous venous flow

94. What is the most serious complication of pancreas transplantation?

    (A) superior mesenteric artery stenosis

    (B) hepatic artery thrombosis

    (C) splenic vein thrombosis

    (D) celiac artery stenosis

95. Normally, portal venous flow is

    (A) pulsatile

    (B) hepatopetal

    (C) hepatofugal

    (D) bidirectional

96. Severe portal hypertension may be accompanied by all of the following *except*

    (A) a patent paraumbilical vein

    (B) a patent coronary vein

    (C) increased portal venous flow volume

    (D) a caput medusa

97. TIPSs are used to

    (A) treat recurrent gastrointestinal bleeding and refractory ascites

    (B) treat hepatocellular carcinoma

    (C) shunt blood from the splenic vein to the renal vein

    (D) shunt blood from the jugular vein to the IVC

98. **Renal artery occlusion is suggested by all of the following EXCEPT**

    (A) absence of flow in the renal artery using optimized power Doppler imaging

    (B) low-amplitude, low-velocity Doppler spectral waveforms throughout the renal parenchyma

    (C) a side-to-side difference in renal length of 1.5 cm

    (D) a kidney length <8 cm

99. **The renal artery acceleration index is defined as**

    (A) the time interval from the onset of systole to the early systolic peak

    (B) the time interval from the onset of systole to peak systole divided by Doppler frequency

    (C) the change in distance between the onset of systolic flow and the early systolic peak

    (D) the change in distance between the onset of systolic flow and the peak systolic velocity divided by the acceleration time

100. **The term "flow-reducing stenosis" signifies arterial narrowing of**

    (A) 20–30%

    (B) 30–40%

    (C) 50–60%

    (D) 100%

101. **The postprandial Doppler spectral waveform from the normal SMA will exhibit**

    (A) rapid systolic upstroke, rapid deceleration, reversed diastolic flow

    (B) rapid systolic upstroke, rapid deceleration, forward diastolic flow

    (C) rapid systolic upstroke, delayed deceleration, low diastolic flow

    (D) rapid systolic upstroke, blunt systolic peak, delayed run-off

102. **The best image of the celiac, common hepatic, and splenic arteries is obtained from the**

    (A) transverse plane at the level of the left renal vein

    (B) sagittal plane to the right of midline

    (C) transverse plane at the level of the SMA

    (D) sagittal plane at the level of the SMV

103. **A perivascular color artifact is noted in the region of a transplant renal artery anastomosis. What is this most likely associated with?**

    (A) a bruit

    (B) an arteriovenous fistula

    (C) transplant renal artery occlusion

    (D) a pseudoaneurysm

104. **A "to- and-fro" Doppler spectral waveform is associated with**

    (A) saccular aneurysm

    (B) dissecting aneurysm

    (C) pseudoaneurysm

    (D) fusiform aneurysm

105. **Acute occlusion of a renal artery would likely result in**

    (A) low-amplitude, low-velocity Doppler waveforms throughout the kidney

    (B) increased flow in the contralateral renal artery

    (C) Doppler waveforms with absent diastolic flow in the cortical vessels

    (D) no evidence of collateral flow

106. **An abdominal aortic aneurysm >6 cm in anteroposterior diameter should be**

    (A) followed with sonograms at 6-month intervals

    (B) followed with CT scan at yearly intervals

    (C) treated emergently to prevent risk of rupture

    (D) treated with ultrasound probe compression

107. **What is the second most common cause of renovascular hypertension?**

    (A) fibromuscular dysplasia

    (B) atherosclerotic renal artery stenosis

    (C) renal artery occlusion

    (D) chronic renal failure

108. **The longitudinal image of the aorta seen below illustrates**

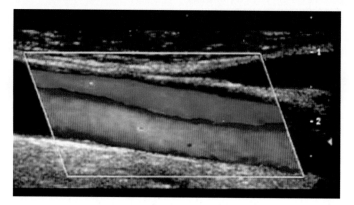

    (A) saccular aneurysm

    (B) fusiform aneurysm

    (C) mycotic aneurysm

    (D) aortic dissection

109. The transverse image of the aorta seen below illustrates

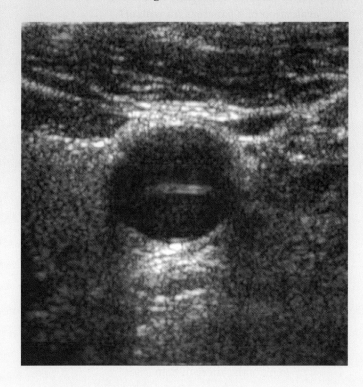

(A) saccular aneurysm
(B) fusiform aneurysm
(C) mycotic aneurysm
(D) aortic dissection

110. Which artery is *not* routinely evaluated during a mesenteric duplex study?

(A) superior mesenteric
(B) splenic
(C) left gastric
(D) celiac

111. In the figure below, the Doppler spectral waveform from the SMA indicates

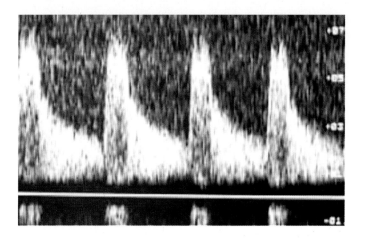

(A) collateralization
(B) fasting state
(C) postprandial state
(D) flow-limiting stenosis

112. A rapid decrease in velocity and turbulent flow distal to arterial stenosis is the result of

(A) a pressure-flow gradient
(B) narrowing of the diameter of the vessel
(C) an increase in kinetic energy at the distal end of the stenosis
(D) tandem lesions

113. What is the best image plane to use for visualization of the left renal vein?

(A) transverse
(B) coronal
(C) oblique
(D) longitudinal

114. The color-flow image seen below illustrates

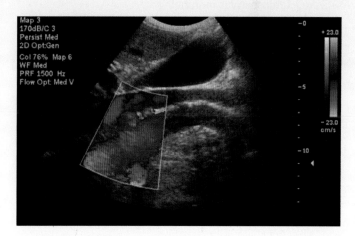

(A) normal renal artery
(B) multiple renal arteries
(C) renal artery occlusion
(D) retroaortic left renal vein

115. The transducer is placed in the right intercostal space directed toward the porta hepatis. The color bar indicates flow toward the transducer is red and flow away is blue. Using this scan plane and color setting, flow in the normal portal vein will be

    (A) blue

    (B) red

    (C) bidirectional

    (D) absent

116. Power Doppler imaging demonstrates all of the following *except*

    (A) power spectrum

    (B) perfusion

    (C) intensity

    (D) direction

117 Distal to an 80% stenosis in the proximal renal artery, the Doppler spectral waveform will exhibit

    (A) rapid systolic upstroke

    (B) early systolic peak

    (C) tardus parvus morphology

    (D) absence of diastolic flow

118. Heterotopic partial transplantation is

    (A) frequently used with pancreas transplantation

    (B) frequently used for patients with renal failure

    (C) the most common type of liver transplantation

    (D) used with cadaveric livers

119. The abdominal aorta is considered aneurysmal if its diameter exceeds

    (A) 1 cm

    (B) 2 cm

    (C) 3 cm

    (D) 1 times the diameter of the proximal normal segment

120. Which vessel is *not* interrogated during routine evaluation of a renal transplant?

    (A) external iliac artery

    (B) external iliac vein

    (C) intersegmental artery

    (D) inferior vena cava

121. Which vessel is not routinely interrogated during evaluation of a pancreas transplant?

    (A) hepatic artery

    (B) splenic vein

    (C) superior mesenteric artery

    (D) portal vein

122. Clinically, patients with portal hypertension may have

    (A) bleeding from gastroesophageal varices

    (B) ascites

    (C) hepatomegaly

    (D) all of the above

123. Increased velocity due to stenosis can be differentiated from collateral compensatory flow by noting that the

    (A) post-stenotic signal is present with a flow-reducing stenosis but not with collateral flow

    (B) high velocity will be seen throughout the visualized length of the artery in both cases

    (C) A but not B

    (D) both A and B

124. Which of the following is a complication associated with aortic stent grafts that may require lifelong follow-up?

    (A) risk of kinking

    (B) crossed limbs

    (C) endoleaks

    (D) stenosis

125. Which of the following is *not* associated with aortic endoleaks?

    (A) flow within the residual aneurysm sac

    (B) increased risk for rupture

    (C) graft and endoleaks waveforms differ

    (D) turbulent chaotic flow pattern

126. The right renal artery can be imaged from

    (A) transverse approach at the level of the left renal vein

    (B) longitudinal image of the IVC from a right paramedian scan plane

    (C) transverse view of the kidney through an intercostal approach

    (D) all of the above

127. **The left portal vein divides into**

    (A) the paraumbilical and coronary veins

    (B) medial and lateral branches

    (C) left gastric and coronary veins

    (D) anterior and posterior branches

128. **The coronary vein enters which of the following veins near the confluence of the superior mesenteric and portal veins?**

    (A) inferior mesenteric

    (B) renal

    (C) portal

    (D) left gastric

129. **The Doppler spectral waveform from the normal portal vein is**

    (A) pulsatile

    (B) minimally phasic

    (C) continuous and non-phasic

    (D) high resistant

130. **In patients with portal hypertension, it is common to find spontaneous venous shunting between the**

    (A) IVC and hepatic artery

    (B) coronary vein and the paraumbilical vein

    (C) splenic vein and renal vein

    (D) superior mesenteric vein and portal vein

131. **Velocity parameters diagnostic of flow-reducing SMA stenosis are**

    (A) peak systolic velocity <250 cm/sec; end-diastolic velocity <45 cm/sec

    (B) peak systolic velocity >275 cm/sec; end-diastolic velocity >55 cm/sec

    (C) peak systolic velocity <250 cm/sec; end-diastolic velocity <45 cm/sec and a post-stenotic signal

    (D) peak systolic velocity >275 cm/sec; end-diastolic velocity >45 cm/sec and a post-stenotic signal

132. **The caput medusa associated with portal hypertension is identified**

    (A) in the region of the portal confluence

    (B) as periportal collaterals in the porta hepatis

    (C) as superficial collaterals surrounding the umbilicus

    (D) as varices in the splenic hilum

133. **Which of the following arteries is *not* part of the renal arterial system?**

    (A) segmental arteries

    (B) arcuate arteries

    (C) cruciate arteries

    (D) interlobar arteries

134. **The adult kidney is normally**

    (A) 8–10 cm in length, 2–4 cm in width, and 4–5 cm in anteroposterior thickness

    (B) 10–14 cm in length, 3–5 cm in width, and 2–3 cm in anteroposterior thickness

    (C) 12–15 cm in length, 2–4 cm in width, and 4–5 cm in anteroposterior thickness

    (D) 11–13 cm in length, 5–7 cm in width, and 2–3 cm in anteroposterior thickness

135. **The peak systolic velocity in the adult aorta is normally**

    (A) 30–70 cm/sec

    (B) 40–100 cm/sec

    (C) 70–140 cm/sec

    (D) 140–160 cm/sec

136. **Elevated resistive index in a renal transplant can be associated with**

    (A) acute rejection

    (B) acute tubular necrosis

    (C) increased transducer pressure over the transplant

    (D) all of the above

137. **The Doppler spectral waveform from the suprarenal aorta may be**

    (A) triphasic

    (B) biphasic

    (C) A but not B

    (D) both A and B

138. **The Doppler spectral waveform pattern for severe acute tubular necrosis is indistinguishable from the pattern associated with severe acute rejection. Both patterns demonstrate**

    (A) rapid systolic upstroke, rapid deceleration, constant forward diastolic flow

    (B) rapid systolic upstroke, rapid deceleration, low diastolic flow

    (C) delayed systolic upstroke, rapid deceleration, constant forward diastolic flow

    (D) delayed systolic upstroke, delayed deceleration, low diastolic flow

139. Which type of aneurysm forms an "outpouching" from the aortic wall?

    (A) mycotic aneurysm

    (B) pseudoaneurysm

    (C) saccular aneurysm

    (D) fusiform aneurysm

140. An epigastric bruit that is present during normal respiration but disappears with deep inspiration is most likely due to

    (A) median arcuate ligament compression of the celiac artery

    (B) atherosclerotic aortic stenosis

    (C) superior mesenteric artery Nutcracker syndrome

    (D) renal artery stenosis

141. The renal-aortic velocity ratio should *not* be used when the aortic peak systolic velocity is

    (A) 50–60 cm/sec

    (B) 90 cm/sec

    (C) less than 30 cm/sec

    (D) 100 cm/sec

142. The inferior mesenteric vein drains into the splenic vein

    (A) to the left of the confluence of the portal and splenic veins

    (B) to the right of the confluence of the portal and splenic veins

    (C) inferior to the confluence of the portal and splenic veins

    (D) superior to the confluence of the portal and splenic veins

143. Which vessel is not usually visualized sonographically?

    (A) inferior mesenteric artery

    (B) cystic vein

    (C) paraumbilical vein

    (D) inferior right hepatic vein

144. Pulsatility of the portal venous Doppler waveform indicates

    (A) right heart failure

    (B) tricuspid regurgitation

    (C) portal hypertension

    (D) all of the above

145. When measured in the cranio-caudad plane, the spleen is considered to be enlarged when its length exceeds

    (A) 8 cm

    (B) 10 cm

    (C) 13 cm

    (D) 15 cm

146. In patients with portal hypertension, the most common portosystemic collateral is the

    (A) paraumbilical vein

    (B) coronary vein

    (C) splenic vein

    (D) cystic vein

147. The coronary vein is considered to be enlarged when its diameter exceeds

    (A) 2 mm

    (B) 4 mm

    (C) 6 mm

    (D) 8 mm

148. The normal flow direction in the coronary vein is

    (A) toward the splenic and portal vein

    (B) away from the splenic and portal vein

    (C) hepatofugal

    (D) toward the inferior vena cava

149. The portal vein travels throughout the liver with the

    (A) middle hepatic vein and left hepatic artery

    (B) hepatic vein and common bile duct

    (C) paraumbilical vein and hepatic artery

    (D) hepatic artery and common bile duct

150. To obtain the correct dimensions of an abdominal aortic aneurysm it is important to scan

    (A) following the axis of the spine

    (B) following the axis of the aorta

    (C) following the axis of the IVC

    (D) all of the above

Answers and Explanations

At the end of each explained answer, there is a number combination in parentheses. The first number identifies the reference source; the second number or set of numbers indicates the page or pages on which the relevant information can be found.

1. **(C)** Renal size decreases as the compromise to blood flow increases. The kidney size is generally <9 cm when the renal artery is occluded. (3:624; 7:461)

2. **(D)** A vessel that is diffusely dilated is considered "ectatic." Saccular, fusiform, and spindle-shaped are terms used to describe the shape of aneurysms. (3:529; 4:253, 254)

3. **(C)** The first major branch of the abdominal aorta is the celiac artery, which originates from the anterior wall of the aorta just inferior to the diaphragm. One to two centimeters distal to the origin of the celiac artery, the superior mesenteric artery arises from the anterior aortic wall. These vessels may share a common trunk. (3:571)

4. **(B)** A concentric, spindle-shaped dilation of the abdominal aorta is termed "fusiform" and is used to describe aneurysms. A saccular aneurysm is created by an outpouching from the aortic wall. Dissecting is a term used to describe a tear in the intimal lining of an artery allowing blood to course between the intima and the media. Ectasia refers to a vessel that is diffusely dilated. (4:253–255).

5. **(D)** The branches of the celiac artery (common hepatic and splenic) form a "seagull" appearance in the transverse imaging plane. They arise almost perpendicular to the celiac trunk at its bifurcation. (2; 6:72)

6. **(B)** The three branches of the celiac artery are the common hepatic, splenic, and left gastric. (4:233)

7. **(C)** Patients with a ruptured aortic aneurysm usually present with abdominal or back pain that worsens in the upright or erect position. (6:82)

8. **(C)** Aortic aneurysms are most often located below the renal arteries and in the common iliac arteries. (3:532)

9. **(A)** The splanchnic circulation supplies blood flow to the gastrointestinal system and is composed of the celiac artery, the superior and inferior mesenteric arteries, and their branches. The renal arteries are part of the urogenital system. (3:571, 572)

10. **(B)** A doubling of velocity across segments of a vessel of similar diameter is consistent with >50% reduction in diameter; a fourfold increase in velocity signifies a narrowing >75%. (5:259, 260)

11. **(A)** The aortic stent graft (endograft) is inserted percutaneously over a catheter advanced into the aorta from the femoral artery. The endograft excludes the aneurysm which remains. With surgical repair, the aneurysm is most often treated with graft replacement of the aorta. (7:482–485)

12. **(C)** Hypertension is not a common cause of aortic dissection although it results in increased pressure on the arterial wall. Because the medial layer of the arterial wall weakens with age, this is the most predisposing condition for aortic dissection. (3:531)

13. **(B)** Arterial dissection is characterized by a tear in the intima of the arterial wall. This allows blood to course between the intima and media, creating a true and false lumen. The intimal flap can be seen on real-time images as an echogenic, pulsating structure within the lumen of the artery. (3:531)

14. **(A)** The common hepatic artery divides into the gastroduodenal artery in the hepatoduodenal ligament and the right gastric artery at the liver hilum. (2; 4:240)

15. **(B)** Gallbladder. The splenic artery supplies blood to the spleen, pancreas, left half of the greater omentum, greater curvature of the stomach, and part of the fundus of the stomach. The common hepatic artery supplies the gallbladder. (4:240; 6:72)

16. **(D)** The splenic artery is the largest branch of the celiac artery. (6:72)

17. **(A)** Approximately 1–2 cm of the left gastric artery may be seen longitudinally. This artery is not routinely examined during evaluation of the mesenteric arterial circulation. (6:73)

18. **(C)** The normal celiac artery Doppler spectral waveform exhibits the characteristics of blood flow to low resistance end organs. It has rapid systolic upstroke, rapid deceleration, and constant forward diastolic flow. The peak systolic velocity is normally <200 cm/sec and the end-diastolic velocity is <55 cm/sec. (3:576; 4:483)

19. **(A)** The waveform demonstrates low diastolic flow and the absence of turbulence. These are features of a normal vessel supplying blood to a high resistance end organ. Flow-reducing superior mesenteric artery (SMA) stenosis would cause the peak systolic and end-diastolic velocities to increase to >275 cm/sec and 45 cm/sec, respectively. A post-stenotic signal would be evident immediately distal to the stenosis as a consequence of the pressure-flow gradient that develops with significant vessel narrowing. (3:573, 577)

20. **(A)** The SMA originates from the anterior wall of the aorta 1–2 cm below the celiac artery and behind the pancreas. It courses anterior to the left renal vein and parallels the aorta as it moves caudally. *(4:243; 7:467)*

21. **(D)** Acute, severe abdominal ischemia is associated with sudden occlusion of one or more of the mesenteric arteries. Chronic mesenteric ischemia has an insidious onset as a consequence of progression of atherosclerotic disease. Clinically, patients present with a triad of symptoms: postprandial pain, "fear of food" syndrome, and weight loss. *(3:572–574; 7:466)*

22. **(B)** The diagnostic criteria for flow-reducing SMA stenosis are peak systolic velocity >275 cm/sec, end-diastolic velocity >45 cm/sec, and a classic turbulent post-stenotic signal. *(3:576; 5:483; 7:471)*

23. **(C)** The median arcuate ligament of the diaphragm can compress the celiac artery origin during respiration. Compression occurs during normal respiration but is relieved with deep inspiration and breath holding because of relaxation of the diaphragmatic crus. While portal hypertension may cause increased hepatic artery velocity, this would not vary with respiration and is uncommonly transmitted to the celiac artery. Flow-reducing celiac artery stenosis, and mesenteric ischemia due to significant disease in one or more mesenteric arteries, would cause velocity elevation in the celiac artery. The velocities would not vary with respiratory maneuvers. *(7:470)*

24. **(D)** The inferior epigastric artery is a collateral pathway for occlusive disease involving the aorto-iliac system. Occlusion of the proximal mesenteric arteries is compensated through collaterals that commonly arise from the inferior mesenteric artery and its branches or through the pancreaticoduodenal arcade. *(3:270; 7:468)*

25. **(A)** Standard contrast arteriography with selective lateral views has historically been used to confirm the sonographic findings and to define collateral pathways prior to revascularization. In recent years, CT scans have been used to localize disease and display relational anatomy. *(8:239, 240)*

26. **(C)** The left renal vein courses from the hilum of the left kidney, crosses the aorta anteriorly between the aorta and SMA, and moves inferior to the pancreas before entering the IVC. *(4:288; 6:77)*

27. **(B)** Arcuate arteries arise from the interlobar arteries. They curve around the base of the pyramids where they give rise to the lobular arteries that supply the cortex of the kidney. Their flow pattern is normally low resistance like that of the main renal artery and its larger branches. *(4:245; 5:676)*

28. **(D)** Flow-reducing renal artery stenosis is indicated if the renal-aortic ratio is >3.5, the peak systolic renal artery velocity is >180 cm/sec, and there is a post-stenotic signal. *(5:664; 7:460, 461)*

29. **(B)** If the renal-aortic velocity ratio is used to determine severity of renal artery stenosis, care must be taken to assure that the aortic velocity is between 40 and 100 cm/sec. Use of velocities outside those values in the calculation can result in over or under-estimation of the severity of disease. Example: renal artery velocity = 150 cm/sec and the aortic velocity = 30 cm/sec. The renal-aortic ratio = 5.0, suggesting significant renal artery stenosis. Similarly, if the renal artery velocity = 320 cm/sec and the aortic velocity = 120 cm/sec, the renal-aortic ratio will be 3.0 and flow-limiting renal artery stenosis would not be indicated. *(7:460).*

30. **(A)** This inverse relationship is caused by the impedance to arterial inflow that results from intrinsic disease. Such conditions are generally associated with endovasculitis and interstitial edema. In cases of marked renovascular resistance, the diastolic flow component of the Doppler spectral waveform may approach zero or reverse. *(5:664)*

31. **(D)** The Doppler spectral waveform associated with mild acute tubular necrosis may be indistinguishable from the signal recorded in a normal kidney. Most often, there is increased diastolic flow as a result of arterial-venous shunting. This is evident in a normal resistive index (RI). As AT progresses in severity, renovascular resistance increases and the RI is elevated. *(4:247; 5:680)*

32. **(B)** The fasting, normal inferior mesenteric artery demonstrates a high resistance waveform pattern typical of arteries feeding resting, muscular tissues (fasting SMA, peripheral arteries). The features of such waveforms are rapid systolic upstroke, rapid deceleration, and low diastolic flow. There may be a brief period of early diastolic flow reversal. The hepatic, renal and splenic arteries supply high flow demand organs and their waveform is characterized by constant forward diastolic flow. *(3:577, 578; 5:696)*

33. **(C)** The most common curable cause of renal-related hypertension is atherosclerotic renal artery stenosis. The second most common cause is due to medial fibromuscular dysplasia. This is a non-atherosclerotic disease entity that commonly affects the mid-to-distal segment of the renal artery in young, hypertensive women. *(7:458)*

34. **(A)** The term "tardus parvus" refers to the delayed systolic upstroke and run-off evident in the dampened Doppler spectral waveforms recorded distal to flow-limiting stenosis or arterial occlusion. Medical renal disease, hydronephrosis and pyelonephritis cause increased renovascular resistance. The resultant waveform would demonstrate low diastolic flow. *(3:620)*

35. **(C)** When kidney size differs by more than 3.0 cm, occlusion of the renal artery on the side with the smaller kidney should be suspected. A small kidney with absent Doppler signals in the renal artery and dampened signals within the renal parenchyma from collateral vessels is consistent with renal artery occlusion. *(7:457)*

36. **(A)** A diastolic to systolic velocity ratio <0.20 is consistent with renal parenchymal disease (medical renal disease). Renal artery stenosis, occlusion, and fibromuscular dysplasia do not result in elevated vascular resistance in the kidney unless there is associated medical renal disease. (7:462)

37. **(B)** The right and left common iliac veins come together to form the IVC at the level of the fourth or fifth lumbar vertebrae. (4:200)

38. **(B)** The pathologic condition that most often affects the inferior vena cava is thrombosis. Primary tumors of the IVC are uncommon but tumor extension or compression of the IVC may occur. (3:545)

39. **(D)** Carcinomas of the kidney, adrenal gland, and liver often extend into the inferior vena cava via paracaval lymph nodes. (3:545)

40. **(D)** Pregnancy can result in extrinsic compression of the inferior vena cava but prolonged, severe stasis is uncommon and caval thrombosis is an infrequent complication of pregnancy. Stasis due to prolonged inactivity, including surgery, can lead to venous thrombosis. Conditions that lead to dehydration, such as sepsis, promote development of thrombosis. (6:186)

41. **(C)** A resistive index less than 0.70 is considered normal for an adult. (5:677).

42. **(C)** Continuous, non-phasic Doppler spectral waveforms will be recorded when the lumen of the inferior vena cava is partially compromised. (3:546, 547)

43. **(B)** Contrast arteriography would not be a procedure of choice for confirmation of inferior vena caval thrombosis. Arteriography will enhance definition of the lumen of arteries, but it is limited in its ability to define filling defect or absence of flow in the outflow circulation. (3:283)

44. **(B)** The right hepatic vein divides the right lobe of the liver into anterior and posterior segments. The middle hepatic vein divides the liver into right and left lobes. The left hepatic vein separates the medial and lateral segments of the left lobe of the liver. The portal vein enters the liver through the porta hepatis. (3:520)

45. **(D)** The "Playboy bunny" sign refers to the real-time image of at least two of the three major hepatic veins obtained with oblique, cephalic angulation of the transducer from a right paramedian approach under the xiphoid process. (6:76)

46. **(A)** The three major hepatic veins drain into the inferior vena cava. The portal vein is formed by the confluence of the splenic and superior mesenteric veins and carries oxygenated blood into the liver. (3:520; 7:438)

47. **(B)** The spectral waveform from the normal hepatic veins demonstrates somewhat chaotic, pulsatile flow. There are two cycles of forward flow toward the heart as a result of reflections of right atrial and ventricular diastole. These

are followed by a third cycle which is brief and reversed, accompanying atrial systole. (3:523)

48. **(D)** The portal vein carries more than 50% of the oxygen required by the liver. While its responsibility for blood supply to the liver may increase when the portal venous flow is compromised, the hepatic artery most often supplies only 30% of the blood flow. The aorta and SMA do not provide flow directly to the liver. (10:319)

49. **(B)** The portal vein is formed by the confluence of the superior mesenteric and splenic veins. (2; 3:518)

50. **(D)** The portal vein lies anterior to the IVC, cephalad to the head of the pancreas, and caudal to the caudate lobe. (2; 7:438)

51. **(B)** The portal triad is composed of the portal vein, the hepatic artery, and the common bile duct. (7:439; 10:317)

52. **(D)** Hepatic veins are boundary formers which divide the segments of the liver. They course longitudinally toward the inferior vena cava, increasing in diameter as they approach the hepato-caval confluence. Portal veins course horizontally toward their origin at the porta hepatis. (2; 3:520)

53. **(A)** Portal venous flow exhibits low velocity, minimally phasic variation as a result of respiration-related changes in thoracic pressure. Flow direction is normally hepatopetal (toward the liver). Pulsatility is common to the hepatic venous circulation. (3:520)

54. **(C)** Occlusion of one or more of the hepatic veins is termed Budd–Chiari syndrome. Cavernous transformation may follow portal vein thrombosis and appears as periportal collaterals in the porta hepatis. Hemangioma is a benign tumor of the liver. Fibromuscular dysplasia is a non-atherosclerotic disease entity that causes concentric narrowing and dilation of arteries. This condition is observed in renal and carotid arteries. (3:602; 4:294)

55. **(D)** Hepatic veins divide the liver into segments, coursing longitudinally toward the vena cava. For this reason, they are considered "boundary formers." Unlike the portal veins which have echogenic walls due to the collagen within their boundaries, the hepatic vein walls lack echogenicity. The veins usually are not compressed during a Valsalva maneuver, which increases abdominal pressure. (7:441)

56. **(C)** In Western nations, portal hypertension is most often caused by cirrhosis. Cirrhosis may be caused by hepatitis, but is not the direct cause of portal hypertension. Hepatocellular carcinoma and sclerosing cholangitis may be found in association with portal hypertension but are not the primary causes of this condition. (3:588)

57. **(B)** Portal vein thrombosis may be followed by development of serpiginous periportal collaterals within the hepatic hilum. This is referred to as cavernous transformation. (7:441)

58. (A) Normal blood pressure within the liver is 5–10 mm Hg. Portal hypertension is present when the pressure gradient from the portal vein to the hepatic veins or IVC exceeds 10 mm Hg. *(3:585; 10:319)*

59. (C) The most common type of portal hypertension is intrahepatic due to sinusoidal obstruction resulting from cirrhosis. *(3:585)*

60. (C) Portal hypertension causes the portal vein velocity to decrease due to increased resistance to flow and the flow pattern becomes continuous as respiratory variation disappears as a result of increased hepatic pressure. The portal vein enlarges to >13 mm in diameter and with severe disease, the flow direction in the portal vein reverses to decompress the liver. *(3:588; 10:320)*

61. (D) Mycotic aneurysms are arterial dilations that are infected. Marfan syndrome is associated with stretching and weakening of the aortic wall which may lead to development of an aneurysm. Injuries that cause penetration of the arterial wall may result in pseudoaneurysms. *(6:82)*

62. (C) Left portal vein. The paraumbilical (umbilical) vein is a branch of the left portal vein. It serves as a collateral pathway for decompression of the liver in patients with portal hypertension. It carries blood away from the liver, exiting in the ligamentum teres and forming a network of veins surrounding the umbilicus (caput medusa). *(3:591; 4:295)*

63. (A) The paraumbilical (umbilical) vein is a branch of the left portal vein. It serves as a collateral pathway for decompression of the liver in patients with portal hypertension. The coronary vein (left gastric vein) is another important collateral pathway in patients with portal hypertension. *(3:591)*

64. (C) Most often flow is shunted from the main portal vein to the right hepatic vein to empty into the systemic venous circulation (IVC). This is an effective, nonsurgical method used to decompress the liver in patients with portal hypertension. *(7:442)*

65. (A) The color-flow image and peak systolic velocity (>250 cm/sec) suggest stenosis of the TIPS. Velocities are normally in the range of 65–220 cm/sec with flow directed toward the shunt. *(7:442; 9:290)*

66. (C) Flow direction should remain normal, or hepatofugal, following placement of a TIPS. Hepatopetal flow would suggest that the shunt is not functional and flow will be diverted in the hepatic and portal vein to allow the liver to decompress. Flow is normally pulsatile in the hepatic veins. Continuous, non-phasic signals suggest obstruction to venous outflow. *(9:291)*

67. (A) The echogenic walls of the TIPS are apparent within the liver parenchyma. Hepatic venous stenosis is best demonstrated with color flow imaging. A hemangioma

is a benign liver tumor. Hepatocellular carcinoma would not have echogenic boundaries. *(9:290)*

68. (C) Peak systolic velocity in a normally functioning TIPS ranges from 65 to 220 cm/sec. Flow is shunted toward the TIPS. Therefore, flow direction in the portal vein will be hepatopetal. Flow direction in the hepatic veins should remain hepatofugal. *(9:291)*

69. (B) These findings suggest TIPS stenosis. Normally, velocity in the main portal vein exceeds 100 cm/sec. Flow direction is hepatopetal. In this case, the shunt velocity has deteriorated to <60 cm/sec. This is consistent with compromised shunt flow. The direction of flow in the hepatic veins is hepatopetal, suggesting collateral flow to compensate for shunt dysfunction. *(9:291)*

70. (C) Renal arterial inflow may remain normal even though the renal vein is thrombosed. Given this, the Doppler spectral waveform demonstrates rapid systolic upstroke, rapid deceleration, but because outflow through the venous system is compromised, the diastolic flow is reversed and blunted. This is consistent with impedance to outflow through the renal vein. *(7:454)*

71. (B) Patients with renal vein thrombosis may initially have proteinuria, epigastric pain, fever, and hematuria. Renal vein thrombosis is seen more frequently in children than adults. *(6:212)*

72. (C) The Doppler spectral waveform demonstrates peak systolic velocity <200 cm/sec, end-diastolic velocity <55 cm/sec, and the absence of a post-stenotic signal. These findings are consistent with normal flow in the celiac artery. *(3:579, 580)*

73. (B) Note should be taken of the decrease in peak systolic velocity associated with deep inspiration. These findings are suggestive of median arcuate ligament compression of the origin of the celiac artery. The celiac artery velocity does not alter significantly in the postprandial state because the liver and spleen do not participate immediately in meeting the metabolic needs associated with digestion. Fixed stenosis and collateral compensatory flow are not affected by changes in respiration. *(3:581, 582)*

74. (C) If the urethra is obstructed, hydronephrosis will be bilateral because the urethra is the conduit for both ureters. Renal calculi are generally not chronically obstructive at ureteral level. *(6:186).*

75. (B) In cases of acute renal vein thrombosis, the kidney enlarges and becomes hypoechogenic. The pyramids are prominent but the corticomedullary junction is indistinct. With partial obstruction of the renal vein, the Doppler spectral waveform demonstrates absence of respirophasicity. Unlike the findings with renal artery occlusion, the renal size is most often unaffected. *(3:624, 625)*

76. **(B)** In hydronephrosis, the kidney exhibits a cystic area within the echogenic renal sinus. This acoustic difference may be mild, moderate, or severe, dependent on the severity and length of the obstruction. Renal infarction produces wedge-shaped flow defects at the level of the renal hilum that may extend to the level of the renal cortex. Renal artery occlusion is evidenced by an absence of flow in the main real artery. Collateral flow may be documented within the renal parenchyma. Renal calculi are most often echogenic with sharp, marginated acoustic shadowing. (6:186)

77. **(D)** With obstructive hydronephrosis, the resistive index is most often >0.70. (4:86)

78. **(A)** A cadaveric liver transplant is termed orthotopic. The recipient's liver and gallbladder are excised and the cadaveric liver is transplanted. When heterotopic transplantation is used, the recipient's liver remains in place and a portion of the donor liver is transplanted. The terms "heterogeneous" and "homogeneous" refer to acoustic properties of atherosclerotic plaque or other tissue. (5:721)

79. **(C)** Because the recipient's liver is removed, an orthotopic liver transplant requires at least three anastomoses: the extrahepatic portal vein, hepatic artery, and the suprahepatic IVC. A fourth anastomosis at the infrahepatic IVC may be necessary. (5:721)

80. **(A)** Sonography may define many of the vascular problems associated with liver transplant dysfunction, but it lacks sensitivity for diagnosis of liver transplant rejection. (7:443–445)

81. **(D)** The hepatic artery provides blood flow to the liver transplant. Thrombosis of the hepatic artery places the organ in jeopardy of failure. Hepatic artery and IVC stenoses can be compensated through collateral pathways. Thrombosis of a hepatic vein has little consequence while portal vein thrombosis may threaten the survival of the transplanted organ and recipient. (7:443)

82. **(B)** The elevation in peak systolic velocity, accompanied by delayed systolic upstroke as evidenced by the systolic acceleration time >0.8 and a low resistive index, is consistent with flow-limiting hepatic artery stenosis. There would be no evidence of flow if the hepatic artery were thrombosed. Portal vein obstruction would not cause delayed acceleration in the hepatic artery. (4:242)

83. **(C)** The "to- and-fro" spectral Doppler flow pattern in the neck of a pseudoaneurysm is diagnostic. The pattern is the result of high-pressure arterial flow entering the neck during systole and exiting to the lower pressure of the parent artery during diastole. This produces a rapid systolic upstroke and reverse diastolic flow ("to-fro") pattern. Although spectral broadening is apparent due to rapid changes in direction, a post-stenotic signal is not present. Low resistance Doppler waveforms are associated with high flow demand organs and arteriovenous communications. An intimal tear may lead to arterial dissection. (3:393)

84. **(C)** The diameter of the portal vein, measured just above the IVC with the patient in quiet respiration, is normally <13 mm. With deep inspiration, the diameter may increase to 15–16 mm. (10:321)

85. **(B)** The common hepatic artery divides into the gastroduodenal artery and the proper hepatic artery at the level of the hepatoduodenal ligament. (4:240)

86. **(D)** Renal medial fibromuscular dysplasia affects the mid-to-distal segments of the native renal artery, but is not associated with renal transplant dysfunction. (5:684–694; 9:322)

87. **(C)** The external iliac artery is most often chosen as the anastomotic vessel for the transplant renal artery. The transplant renal artery may be anastomosed to the aorta in children. (5:685; 9:324)

88. **(D)** Renal transplant rejection is suggested sonographically by an increase in renal volume, increased cortical echogenicity, an indistinct corticomedullary boundary, and thickening of the renal pelvis. (4:268)

89. **(A)** The Doppler spectral waveform pattern associated with acute renal transplant rejection is characterized by rapid systolic upstroke, rapid deceleration, and low or absent diastolic flow. Acute rejection is associated with endovasculitis and accumulation of interstitial fluid. These factors cause elevation of renovascular resistance. This impedes arterial inflow to the kidney and diastolic flow, consequently, decreases. (5:685–688)

90. **(B)** Moderate ATN is associated with slight increase in renovascular resistance. The Doppler spectral waveform is characterized by rapid systolic upstroke, rapid deceleration, and increased pulsatility as a result of increased resistance to arterial inflow. (5:688, 689)

91. **(C)** Transplant renal artery stenosis is suggested by a renal artery to iliac artery velocity ratio >3.0. Answers (A) and (B) are related to flow-limiting stenosis in a native renal artery. A diastolic to systolic velocity ratio is used to confirm medical renal disease. (5:691)

92. **(D)** The right renal artery has branches that supply blood to the adrenal and ureter, but not the pancreas. All other statements are true regarding this artery. (5:662; 7:452–456)

93. **(C)** Because of the transmission of high-pressure arterial flow into the low-pressure venous circulation, renal transplant arteriovenous fistulae demonstrate high-velocity turbulent arterial signals and pulsatile venous flow. (3:631)

94. **(C)** Splenic vein thrombosis is the most serious complication of pancreas transplantation as it threatens organ survival. While arterial inflow is maintained via multiple channels, drainage of the organ is principally through the splenic venous circulation. (9:327–329)

95. **(B)** Portal venous flow is normally toward the liver, or hepatopetal in direction. (10:319)

96. **(C)** Portal venous flow volume decreases with portal hypertension. Flow is diverted to the systemic circulation via collaterals such as the coronary vein and paraumbilical vein. Superficial venous collaterals are often apparent surrounding the umbilicus (caput medusa). (10:322)

97. **(A)** TIPSs are used to treat recurrent gastrointestinal bleeding and refractory ascites due to portal hypertension. The shunt is intrahepatic and carries blood from the portal vein to a hepatic vein for drainage into the systemic venous circulation (IVC). (9:289–291; 10:324)

98. **(C)** As renal artery stenosis progresses to occlusion, kidney size decreases due to restricted blood flow. A difference in kidney size >3.0 cm should raise suspicion of compromised blood flow on the side with the smaller organ. Kidney length is most often <8 cm. Unless the occlusion was acute, low-amplitude, low-velocity collateral flow signals will be found throughout the renal parenchyma. (7:457)

99. **(D)** The renal acceleration index is defined as the change in distance between the onset of systolic flow and the peak systolic velocity divided by the acceleration time. It is used to predict significant proximal renal artery stenosis. (9:314)

100. **(C)** A decrease in pressure and flow occurs in most vessels in the arterial system when the diameter of the artery is narrowed by 50–60%. This approximates a 75–80% area reduction. (3:10)

101. **(B)** Post-prandially, vascular resistance decreases in the tissues fed by the SMA. The Doppler spectral waveform reflects the change by altering its normally high resistance flow pattern to a low resistance pattern. This is characterized by rapid systolic upstroke, rapid deceleration, and forward diastolic flow. (5:700–702)

102. **(C)** The "seagull sign" formed by the celiac artery and its primary branches, the common hepatic and splenic arteries, can best be seen from a transverse image plane at the level of the SMA. The transducer should be angled slightly cephalad as the celiac artery arises from the anterior aortic wall approximately 1–2 cm proximal to the SMA. (3:513; 7:468, 469)

103. **(A)** Color artifact in the tissues surrounding arteries is most often due to turbulence associated with rapid disturbed flow. The chaotic flow causes vibration of the arterial wall and surrounding tissues and the movement is color encoded. This feature is used to identify the presence of bruits associated with significant flow disturbance, which can occur with sharp angulation of a vessel or flow-limiting stenosis. Although an arteriovenous fistula is possible, it is more likely that kinking or stenosis at the anastomotic site is responsible for the disturbed flow. Pseudoaneurysms are diagnosed by the "to- and-fro" flow pattern found in the neck that connects the pseudoaneurysm to the parent artery. (4:450)

104. **(C)** The "to- and-fro" Doppler spectral waveform is diagnostic of a pseudoaneurysm. It is caused by the change in pressure and flow direction within the neck of the false aneurysm as blood moves into the aneurysm in systole and returns through the neck to the native artery in diastole. (3:392)

105. **(D)** Acute occlusion of the renal artery would most likely result in the absence of collateral flow within the organ. Collateral vessels develop in patients who have flow-limiting disease and are evident as low-velocity, low-amplitude waveforms throughout the kidney. Absent diastolic flow indicates elevated renovascular resistance and medical renal disease. (7:457)

106. **(C)** There is a reported rupture rate of 10% per year for abdominal aortic aneurysms measuring >6 cm in diameter. For this reason, large aneurysms should be treated emergently to prevent risk of rupture. (3:532)

107. **(A)** The second most common cause of renovascular hypertension is fibromuscular dysplasia. This non-atherosclerotic disease entity most commonly affects the mid-to-distal segment of the renal artery and is found predominantly in younger women. (7:458)

108. **(D)** The color flow image illustrates an aortic dissection which is seen as "true" and "false" channels within the aortic lumen. The channels are separated by an Intimal flap. A saccular aneurysm appears as an "outpouching" from the aortic wall. Fusiform aneurysms are spindle-shaped as a result of concentric dilation of the artery. Mycotic aneurysms are infected aneurysms whose shapes are variable.

109. **(D)** The transverse image illustrates an echogenic flap of intima within the lumen of the aorta. This flap, created by a tear in the intima, allows blood to flow between the intima and media in true and false channels. (3:531)

110. **(C)** The left gastric artery is not routinely evaluated during a mesenteric duplex study. The artery is difficult to image unless it has enlarged as a result of increased flow volume when there is occlusive disease in the hepatic, splenic, or celiac arteries. (3:513, 514)

111. **(D)** The Doppler spectral waveform from the SMA represents flow-reducing SMA stenosis (peak systolic velocity >275 cm/sec, end-diastolic velocity >45 cm/sec, and a post-stenotic signal). This waveform demonstrates significantly elevated systolic velocity and pan-systolic spectral broadening consistent with turbulent flow. The end-diastolic velocity is well above 45 cm/sec. A post-stenotic signal is not shown. Velocities at the values illustrated in this study would not be consistent with those seen as a result of collateralization or eating. A fasting SMA waveform is characterized by low diastolic flow. (7:471)

112. **(A)** A rapid decrease in velocity and turbulent flow patterns distal to arterial stenosis are characteristic of a post-stenotic signal. This flow pattern is caused by a decrease in pressure and flow that occurs when the diameter of an artery is significantly reduced. Kinetic energy is decreased at the distal end of a stenosis. When tandem lesions are present, the entrance and exit effect on energy as blood moves through the lesions results in major energy loss distally. (5:160–168)

113. **(A)** The left renal vein can best be seen from a transverse image plane just inferior to the SMA. It will be noted to cross the aorta anteriorly in most patients. In a small percentage of patients, the left renal vein is retro-aortic or bifid with one limb crossing the aorta anteriorly and the other inferiorly. *(7:454)*

114. **(B)** The color-flow image illustrates two renal arteries on the right side. Multiple renal arteries occur in approximately 20% of the population and, for reasons that are not well understood, are more common on the left side. *(7:456)*

115. **(B)** In the normal portal vein, flow is hepatopetal in direction (toward the liver). Using the scan plane and transducer orientation described, the sound beam is pointed toward the direction of flow. The color bar indicates flow toward the transducer is red. *(10:318, 319)*

116. **(D)** Power Doppler is based on the intensity of the returned Doppler signal and the difference between that intensity and the signal returned from surrounding tissue. As such, it is not as angle-dependent as color Doppler because that modality relies on color-encodement of shifted frequencies. Power Doppler excels at demonstrating low-velocity flow, tissue perfusion, and vessel wall-to-lumen interfaces. Flow is highlighted by summing forward and reverse velocities relevant to the sound beam to produce a power spectrum. The shortcoming of power Doppler is that it cannot illustrate flow direction. *(3:78)*

117. **(C)** Distal to an 80% stenosis, the Doppler spectral waveform will assume a tardus parvus morphology. This is characterized by delayed systolic upstroke and delayed run-off. The early systolic peak is not apparent. Absence of diastolic flow is consistent with elevated renovascular resistance, which does not always accompany renal artery stenosis. *(3:622)*

118. **(C)** Heterotopic partial transplantation is the most common type of liver transplantation. Patients retain their liver and receive a portion of a liver from a donor. Orthotopic transplantation is used for cadaveric liver transplants. *(5:721–724)*

119. **(C)** The abdominal aorta is considered if its diameter exceeds 3 cm or is 1.5 times larger than the proximal normal segment. *(3:554)*

120. **(D)** The IVC is not routinely interrogated during examination of a renal transplant. The vessels of interest are the inflow artery and vein (external iliacs), the transplant renal artery and vein, and the vessels within the renal parenchyma. *(9:322, 323)*

121. **(A)** The hepatic artery is not routinely interrogated during evaluation of a pancreas transplant. The celiac and superior mesenteric arteries are anastomosed to the recipient iliac and should be routinely evaluated to ensure arterial perfusion of the pancreas transplant. The venous drainage is through the portal venous system. Patency of the splenic vein must be confirmed, because thrombosis of this vessel has an impact on organ survival. *(5:728)*

122. **(D)** Dependent on the severity of portal venous compromise, patients may present with variceal bleeding, ascites, hepatomegaly, splenomegaly, and extensive collateral circulation. *(10:321)*

123. **(C)** The classic flow profile associated with significant arterial stenosis is characterized by increased velocity at the site of stenosis, post-stenotic turbulence, followed by return to laminar flow. Collateral compensatory flow will exhibit elevated velocity throughout the visualized length of the collateral vessel. There is no evidence of a pressure-flow gradient, and therefore, a post-stenotic signal is not present. *(5:165–167)*

124. **(C)** A complication of aortic stent grafts (endografts) that is not encountered with surgical repair of abdominal aortic aneurysms is risk of blood re-entering the residual aneurysm sac. Blood within the sac is termed an "endoleak." Endoleaks have been associated with all of the devices on the market and have appeared as long as 4–5 years after aneurysm repair. For this reason, it is likely that aortic stent grafts will require lifelong follow-up with sonography and/or other imaging modalities that have adequate sensitivity for endoleak detection. *(7:482)*

125. **(D)** Turbulent, chaotic flow patterns are not associated with endoleaks. Dependent on the source and classification of the endoleaks, flow patterns usually demonstrate high resistance with low diastolic flow or a to- and-fro flow pattern associated with changes in pressure gradients between the residual aneurysm sac and the feeding artery. The Doppler spectral waveform from the endoleak will differ in morphology from the spectral waveform recorded in the body or limb of the aortic stent graft. *(3:556, 557)*

126. **(D)** The right renal artery can be imaged satisfactorily in most patients from a transverse plane at the level of the left renal vein or from a right intercostal approach through a transverse image of the kidney. Additionally, it should be recognized that the right renal artery courses posterior to the IVC. The artery can be seen in cross-section from a longitudinal image of the IVC. This image plane is used for percutaneous placement of IVC filters under ultrasound guidance. *(3:614, 615)*

127. **(B)**

128. **(D)**

129. **(B)**

130. **(C)** When blood pressure is elevated in the liver, the organ will attempt to decompress through spontaneous shunting, which directs flow away from the liver into the systemic venous circulation. A common pathway is from the splenic vein to the left renal vein, which empties into the IVC. *(7:437)*

131. **(D)** Current diagnostic criteria for identification of flow-reducing SMA stenosis are: Peak systolic velocity >275 cm/sec, end-diastolic velocity >45 cm/sec, and a post-stenotic signal. *(7:467–469)*

132. **(C)** The caput medusa associated with portal hypertension is associated with superficial collateral veins surrounding the umbilicus. The veins originate within the liver from a recanalized umbilical vein, a branch of the left portal vein. *(10:321, 322)*

133. **(C)** The cruciate arteries are part of the peripheral arterial system. The segmental, interlobar and arcuate arteries are found within the renal parenchyma. *(5:676)*

134. **(D)** The adult kidney is normally 11–13 cm in length, 5–7 cm in width, and 2–3 cm in anteroposterior thickness. The size of the kidney decreases with progression of renal artery stenosis. *(6:170)*

135. **(C)** The peak systolic velocity in the adult aorta is normally between 70 and 140 cm/sec. The velocity decreases with age. *(4:240)*

136. **(D)** Elevated resistive index (RI) is consistent with impedance to arterial inflow to the kidney. This can be caused by the endovasculitis and interstitial fluid accumulations associated with acute rejection or the peritubular necrosis that is a signature of ATN. It should also be noted that pressure applied with the transducer to the tissues over the renal transplant is transmitted into the organ and increases resistance to arterial inflow. This is translated to elevated RI. *(5:685)*

137. **(D)** Blood flow in the suprarenal aorta is entering arterial branches that supply the low resistance vascular beds of the liver, spleen, and kidneys. The only high-resistance organ supply in a fasted patient is that of the superior mesenteric artery. Because the majority of flow is to high-demand end organs, the spectral pattern in the suprarenal abdominal aorta may be biphasic. Waveform morphology is in large part dependent on the compliance of the aorta and its branch arteries and the level of flow demand expressed by the fasting liver, spleen, and gastrointestinal circulation. Because of this, high-resistance triphasic waveforms, which are generally seen in the infrarenal aorta, may also be evident in the suprarenal segment. *(3:575, 576)*

138. **(B)** As the necrotic process associated with acute tubular necrosis progresses from moderate to severe, resistance to arterial inflow to the kidney increases. This is reflected in the Doppler spectral waveform which demonstrates rapid systolic upstroke and rapid deceleration because the obstructive process is distal to the renal artery. The amount, amplitude, and descent of the diastolic flow component are reduced and diastolic flow will be low or absent, dependent on the severity of disease. *(9:324)*

139. **(C)** A saccular aneurysm forms an outpouching from the aortic wall. While pseudoaneurysms may appear as outpouchings, they are distinguished from true saccular aneurysms by a puncture of one or more of the layers of the arterial wall, allowing blood to escape into the surrounding tissues. A fusiform aneurysm is characterized by concentric dilation of the artery. *(3:532)*

140. **(A)** The celiac artery arises from the anterior aortic wall. During normal respiration, the median arcuate ligament of the diaphragm can slide over the proximal celiac artery. This extrinsic compression causes narrowing of the arterial lumen and velocity increases. With deep inspiration, the ligament slides off the artery and normal blood flow is restored. *(7:470)*

141. **(C)** To prevent overestimation or underestimation of severity of renal artery stenosis, the renal-aortic ratio should only be used when the aortic velocity is between 40 cm/sec and 100 cm/sec. *(7:460)*

142. **(A)** The inferior mesenteric vein drains into the splenic vein to the left of the confluence of the portal and splenic veins. *(10:317)*

143. **(B)** The cystic vein, a branch of the portal vein, drains into the gallbladder. It is usually not visualized sonographically. When drainage of the vein is compromised in patients with portal hypertension, varices can develop in the gallbladder wall. Search for these varices during sonographic evaluation may support the diagnosis of portal hypertension. *(10:318)*

144. **(D)** Pulsatility of the Doppler spectral waveform recorded in the portal vein is abnormal and most often suggests right heart failure, tricuspid regurgitation, a fistula between the hepatic vein and portal vein, or portal hypertension. The portal venous flow pattern is normally minimally phasic with respiratory variation. *(10:318)*

145. **(C)** Splenomegaly is diagnosed when the length of the spleen exceeds 13 cm. The measurement should be made from a cranio-caudad image plane to ensure accuracy. *(10:320)*

146. **(B)** The coronary vein is the most common collateral pathway in patients with portal hypertension and is found in >80% of patients. The paraumbilical (umbilical) vein is also an important pathway for decompression of the liver. *(10:321)*

147. **(C)** The coronary vein is considered to be enlarged when its diameter exceeds 6 mm. *(10:321)*

148. **(A)** When pressure increases in the liver, the flow direction in the coronary vein may reverse. Normal flow direction is toward the splenic and portal veins. *(10:321)*

149. **(D)** The portal vein courses throughout the liver with the hepatic artery and common bile duct. Together, they form the portal triad. The three structures are covered by Glisson's capsule, which is acoustically echogenic, accounting for the brightness of the walls of the triad. *(6:94, 95)*

150. **(B)** Because the aorta may be tortuous, the correct dimensions of abdominal aortic aneurysms can be obtained by following the axis of the aorta rather than the axis of the spine. *(3:533)*

12

Cerebrovascular Sonography

George L. Berdejo, Joshua Cruz, Fernando Amador, and Evan C. Lipsitz

Study Guide

ANATOMY

Aorta

The systemic circulation begins with the left side of the heart.[1–4] The aortic arch is the first segment of the aorta, which is the longest artery in the body. The aorta is divided into four main segments:

1. Ascending aorta or aortic trunk
2. Aortic arch
3. Descending or more commonly known as the thoracic aorta
4. Abdominal aorta

The great vessels include the aortic arch and its three major branches that include the following:

1. Innominate artery or brachiocephalic trunk
2. Left common carotid artery (CCA)
3. Left subclavian artery

CEREBROVASCULAR CIRCULATION

Anterior Circulation

The anatomy of the cerebrovascular circulation consists of both intracranial and extracranial vessels (Fig. 12–1). The extracranial cerebrovascular arteries can be further divided into the carotid artery circulation, which supplies blood to the anterior part of the brain, and the vertebrobasilar circulation, which supplies blood to the posterior part of the brain. The anterior and posterior portions of the brain are connected by the circle of Willis.

Except for the origin of the common carotid arteries, the right and left carotid artery circulation are identical. The right carotid artery circulation begins at the level of the right clavicle where the brachiocephalic trunk divides and becomes the right common carotid artery (CCA) and right subclavian artery. The left CCA and the left subclavian artery both originate directly from the aortic arch. Bilaterally, the CCA courses anteriorly to the superior level of the thyroid gland. Here, the CCA bifurcates into the internal carotid artery (ICA) and the external carotid artery (ECA).

The primary role of the ICA is to perfuse the ophthalmic artery, anterior portion of the brain, and the circle of Willis. The origin of the ICA is slightly dilated; hence, the term the carotid bulb or carotid sinus. The bulb may encompass the most distal segment of the CCA. This is an important anatomical site, as it is here where carotid artery disease is most likely to develop. The ICA continues to course anterolaterally until it enters the skull through the carotid canal. There are no branches of the ICA outside of the skull. Intracranial branches of the internal carotid include the anterior choroidal, posterior communicating, and ophthalmic arteries. The ophthalmic artery, which perfuses the eye, originates at the carotid siphon. The carotid siphon appears as an "S"-shaped curve. The termination of the ICA forms the lateral aspects of the circle of Willis (Fig. 12–2), and this is where the origins of the middle and anterior cerebral arteries are located.

The external carotid artery courses superiorly and anteriorly and yields several branches, which primarily feed the thyroid, tongue, tonsils, and ears (Table 12–1). The ECA does not perfuse the brain and is, even when disease is present, not considered a source of transient ischemic attack or cerebrovascular accident.

The ECA can become an important source of collateral blood flow in the presence of severe ipsilateral internal carotid artery disease.[5,6] In rare cases; ECA stenosis can result in symptoms in patients with ipsilateral ICA occlusion and, therefore, should be carefully evaluated in those patients.

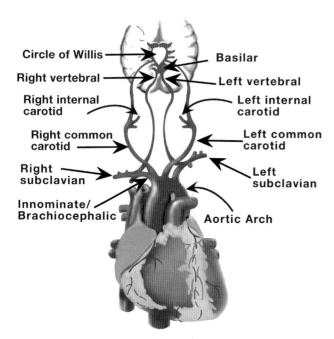

FIGURE 12–1. Diagram showing the relationship and anatomic locations of the intracranial and extracranial carotid vessels.

Posterior Circulation

The posterior circulation of the brain, also known as the vertebrobasilar system, includes the vertebral arteries that originate from the proximal subclavian arteries.[7–9] Both the right and left vertebral arteries course on either side of the vertebral column and through openings in each of the transverse processes of the cervical vertebrae. As the vertebral arteries enter the base of the skull, they join to form the basilar artery. The basilar artery then terminates at the circle of Willis where the right and left posterior cerebral arteries originate.

Intracranial Circulation

The circle of Willis is a very small network of vessels that is about the size of a quarter and may serve as a collateral pathway in the

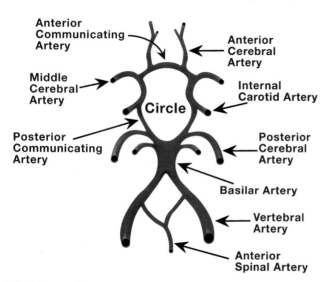

FIGURE 12–2. The circle of Willis.

TABLE 12–1 • External Carotid Artery Branches

1. Superior thyoid
2. Ascending pharyngeal
3. Occipital
4. Facial
5. Maxillary
6. Posterior auricular
7. Lingual
8. Superficial temporal

presence of significant disease. The circle of Willis is formed by the (1) termination of the right and left ICAs, (2) right and left anterior cerebral arteries (ACA-A1), (3) anterior communicating artery (ACom), (4) right and left posterior communicating arteries (PCom), and (5) posterior cerebral arteries (PCAs). The middle cerebral artery (MCA) originates off the circle of Willis at the termination of the ICA and is not considered to be a part of the circle of Willis (Fig. 12–2).

Collateral Pathways

Collateral pathways are abundant in the cerebrovasculature.[5,6] Other pathways include connections between the supraorbital and frontal arteries (branches of the ophthalmic artery), and the superficial temporal artery, a branch of the ECA. The occipital branch of the ECA communicates with the atlantic branch of the vertebral arteries.

In addition to collateral pathways, there is also a compensation factor to consider. Since the intracranial circulation is perfused by four main vessels, the bilateral flow of the ICA and vertebral arteries may increase in any of these vessels to compensate for the presence of hemodynamically significant disease in the others. Therefore, an understanding of all circulatory factors in the carotid system must be taken into consideration for a complete diagnostic picture.

PHYSIOLOGY AND HEMODYNAMICS

Peripheral resistance of a vascular bed is one factor that determines the amount of blood flow to a region of the body. The resistance is primarily controlled by the vasoconstriction and vasodilatation of the arterioles within that vascular bed. Vasodilatation decreases the peripheral resistance allowing blood to move in that direction. Vasoconstriction increases the resistance and blood tends to move in the direction of lower resistance. The resistance within a given system is reflected in the diastolic component of the Doppler spectral waveform.

The brain is a very low resistance vascular bed that allows for continuous blood supply throughout the cardiac cycle, so we should expect there to be continuous forward flow throughout diastole in all vessels that directly provide blood to the brain

(Fig. 12–3).[10] These include the ICA and vertebral arteries, which in general will yield very similar Doppler spectral waveforms. The ECA, however, perfuses the areas of the face and smaller structures of the head and generally will yield very little flow in diastole. Accordingly, there is a distinct difference in the Doppler waveforms that represent these vessels. It is extremely important for the examiner to recognize this difference so as to allow proper identification of the bifurcation vessels. Since the CCA is common to the ICA and ECA, it yields characteristics belonging to both vessels (Fig. 12–4).

MECHANISMS OF DISEASE

Risk Factors for Stroke

Some stroke risk factors are hereditary, while others are a function of natural processes. Still others result from a person's lifestyle. Non-modifiable risk factors include age, heredity and

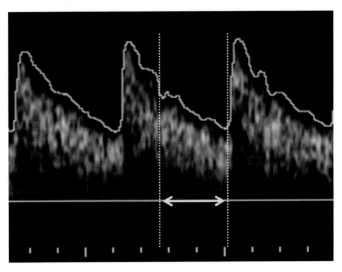

FIGURE 12–3. Spectral waveform from the internal carotid artery. The diastolic flow component of the cardiac cycle is outlined by the dotted yellow lines. Note that there is continuous forward flow (flow above the baseline) throughout the cardiac cycle.

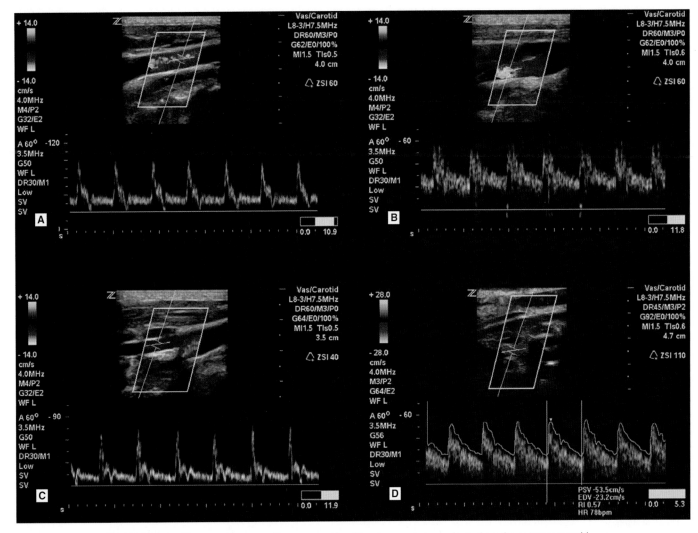

FIGURE 12–4. Ultrasound images with corresponding Doppler spectral waveforms from the common carotid (**A**), internal carotid (**B**), external carotid (**C**), and vertebral (**D**) arteries.

race, gender, and prior stroke, transient ischemic attack (TIA), or heart attack.[11]

Advancing age is a risk factor for stroke. The chance of having a stroke approximately doubles for each decade of life after age 55 years. While stroke is common among the elderly, many people younger than 65 years also suffer strokes.

Heredity (family history) and race plays an important role. It is well known that stroke risk is greater if a parent, grandparent, sister, or brother has had a stroke. African Americans have a much higher risk of death from a stroke than Caucasians. This is partly because African Americans have higher risks of high blood pressure, diabetes, and obesity.

Stroke is more common in men than in women. In most age-groups, more men than women will have a stroke in a given year. However, more than one-half of total stroke deaths occur in women. At all ages, more women than men die of stroke. Use of birth control pills and pregnancy pose special stroke risks for women.

The risk of stroke for someone who has already had one is many times that of a person who has not. Episodes of TIA are "warning signs" that produce stroke-like symptoms but no permanent damage. This is discussed further in the text. TIAs are strong predictors of stroke and a person who has had one or more TIAs is almost ten times more likely to have a stroke than someone of the same age and sex who has not. Recognizing and treating TIAs can reduce the risk of a major stroke.

The modifiable risk factors for stroke include hypertension, diabetes, cigarette smoking, hyperlipidemia, carotid artery stenosis, atrial fibrillation, excessive alcohol consumption, and physical inactivity (Table 12–2).[12]

The most important controllable risk factor is hypertension, which increases the risk of stroke twofold to fourfold.[13] This higher risk is seen in both systolic and diastolic hypertension, as well as in isolated systolic hypertension in the elderly. Blood pressure control significantly reduces the risk

of stroke; it has been shown to prevent 30 strokes for every 1,000 patients treated. Many people believe the effective treatment of high blood pressure is a key reason for the accelerated decline in the death rates for stroke. According to the current recommendation of the Stroke Council of the American Heart Association (AHA), blood pressure should be maintained at <140/90 mm Hg.[11]

Diabetes mellitus is an independent risk factor for stroke. Diabetes increases stroke risk 1.8- to 6-fold. Many people with diabetes also have high blood pressure and blood cholesterol and are overweight. This increases their risk even more. While diabetes is treatable, the presence of the disease still increases the risk of stroke.

In recent years, studies have shown cigarette smoking to be an important risk factor for stroke. Approximately 27% of men and 22% of women in the United States smoke cigarettes. Smokers have a relative risk of stroke in the range of 1.8, and the estimated population attributable risk of stroke due to smoking is 18%. The nicotine and carbon monoxide in cigarette smoke damage the cardiovascular system in many ways. The use of oral contraceptives combined with cigarette smoking greatly increases stroke risk. Fortunately, this increased risk disappears within 5 years of smoking cessation.[11,12]

Hyperlipidemia is a risk factor for a stroke. Lipid disorders have been shown to increase the risk of stroke by 1.8- to 2.6-fold. Most of the information regarding the effect of lowering cholesterol on stroke risk comes from secondary analyses of trials on the prevention of coronary disease, but it is prudent to use these guidelines when evaluating patients for stroke risk. Tighter control of hyperlipidemia is indicated for patients who have a history of stroke or cardiovascular disease.[12]

Carotid or other artery disease results in an increased risk for stroke, as the carotid arteries supply blood to the brain. A carotid artery narrowed by fatty deposits from atherosclerosis may become blocked by a blood clot. Carotid artery disease is also called carotid artery stenosis. Peripheral artery disease can result in the narrowing of blood vessels carrying blood to leg and arm muscles. People with peripheral artery disease have a higher risk of carotid artery disease, which raises their risk of stroke.

Atrial fibrillation is a heart rhythm disorder that raises the risk for stroke. The heart's upper chambers do not beat effectively, which can let the blood pool and clot. If a clot breaks off, enters the bloodstream, and lodges in an artery leading to or in the brain, a stroke can result. People with coronary artery disease or heart failure have a higher risk of stroke than those with hearts that work normally. Dilated cardiomyopathy (an enlarged heart), heart valve disease, and some types of congenital heart defects also raise the risk of stroke.

Sickle cell disease is a genetic disorder that mainly affects African American and Hispanic children. "Sickled" red blood cells are less able to carry oxygen to the body's tissues and organs. These cells also tend to stick to blood vessel walls, which can block arteries to the brain and cause a stroke. Stroke

---

TABLE 12–2 • Risk Factors: Modifiable and Non-Modifiable

- Advanced age
- Atrial fibrillation
- Carotid artery stenosis
- Cigarette smoking
- Diabetes
- Excessive alcohol consumption
- Family history of stroke
- Heart disorders
- History of transient ischemic attacks
- Hypercholesterolemia
- Hyperlipidemia
- Hypertension
- Obesity
- Physical inactivity
- Use of oral contraceptives

is the second leading killer of people younger than 20 years who suffer from sickle cell anemia.[14]

Physical inactivity and obesity can increase the risk of high blood pressure, high blood cholesterol, diabetes, heart disease, and stroke.

Atherosclerosis

Atherosclerosis is a chronic systemic disease that affects the arterial system and occurs within the arterial wall, typically within or beneath the intima. There are various characteristics of the disease, among them location. Atherosclerosis is commonly seen at origins and bifurcations of vessels. Since flow divides and changes its laminar characteristics, a shearing force is created at the flow divider, which over time is responsible for the wear of the intima.[15] For this reason the carotid bifurcation is a prime location for carotid artery disease. It is a chronic inflammatory response in the walls of arteries, in large part due to the accumulation of macrophage white blood cells and promoted by low-density (especially small particle) lipoproteins (plasma proteins that carry cholesterol and triglycerides) without adequate removal of fats and cholesterol from the macrophages by functional high-density lipoproteins (HDLs). It is commonly referred to as a "hardening" of the arteries.

Plaque formation may begin as simple layers of lipids called fatty streaks that are deposited in the wall. Over time, plaques on the walls may progress to a more fibrous component that includes the accumulation of lipids, collagen, and fibrin that is soft and gelatinous in texture appearing as a hypoechoic structure along the arterial wall. Over time, the plaque may proliferate further into the lumen causing narrowing, also known as stenosis. The walls may harden secondary to a more calcium and collagen component. Unstable plaques or plaques that have areas that are weak, compared to more firm or well-integrated plaque within the wall, potentially can be a source of embolic debris.[15]

Atherosclerosis is caused by the formation of multiple plaques within the arteries.[15,16] The atheromatous plaque is divided into three distinct components:

1. The atheroma, which is the nodular accumulation of a soft, flaky, yellowish material at the center of large plaques, composed of macrophages nearest the lumen of the artery
2. Underlying areas of cholesterol crystals
3. Calcification at the outer base of older/more advanced lesions.

Atherosclerosis typically begins in early adolescence and is usually found in most major arteries, yet is asymptomatic and not detected by most diagnostic methods during life. Autopsies of healthy young men that died during the Korean and Vietnam Wars showed evidence of the disease.[17,18] It most commonly becomes seriously symptomatic when interfering with the coronary circulation supplying the heart or cerebral circulation supplying the brain and is considered the most important underlying cause of strokes, heart attacks, various heart diseases including congestive heart failure, and most cardiovascular diseases, in gen-

eral. Atheroma in arm or, more often, leg arteries, which results in decreased blood flow, is called peripheral artery occlusive disease.

According to U.S. data for the year 2004, for about 65% of men and 47% of women, the first symptom of atherosclerotic cardiovascular disease is heart attack or sudden cardiac death (death within one hour of onset of the symptom). Most artery flow-disrupting events occur at locations with less than 50% residual lumen.

Embolus

An embolus can be a solid, liquid, or a gas that travels through the bloodstream. Embolic strokes are usually caused by a blood clot that forms elsewhere in the body or plaque debris and travels through the bloodstream to the brain. Embolic strokes often result from heart disease or heart surgery and occur rapidly and without any warning signs. About 15–50% of embolic strokes occur in people with atrial fibrillation; the rest are attributable to a variety of causes, including (1) left ventricular dysfunction secondary to acute myocardial infarction or severe congestive heart failure, (2) paradoxical emboli secondary to a patent foramen ovale, and (3) atheroemboli. These latter vessel-to-vessel emboli often arise from atherosclerotic lesions in the aortic arch, carotid arteries, and vertebral arteries. In paradoxical embolism, a deep vein thrombosis embolizes through an atrial or ventricular septal defect in the heart then into the brain.[19] This phenomenon may manifests itself as symptoms of TIA or even cerebrovascular accident (CVA), more commonly known as a stroke. By identifying these lesions with duplex ultrasound, the risks associated with significant atherosclerotic disease can be prevented with appropriate treatment.

Subclavian Steal Syndrome

Subclavian steal syndrome refers to the reversal of flow in the ipsilateral vertebral artery to supply the distal subclavian artery in the presence of a proximal subclavian or innominate artery obstruction (Fig. 12–5). This phenomenon demonstrates the hemodynamic effects of severe stenosis and the compensatory nature of the circulatory system. Patients with this condition experience vertebrobasilar symptoms in response to exercise of the ipsilateral arm. It is more common on the left since the left subclavian is an isolated artery and does not communicate with the carotid artery. Therefore, the anatomy of the innominate artery is protective. Arm ischemia is rare in these patients, although a significant difference in blood pressure often exists between the two arms. A decreased radial artery pulse, combined with symptoms of vertebrobasilar insufficiency exacerbated by arm exercise, is pathognomonic. The diagnosis is confirmed angiographically by late films demonstrating filling of the distal subclavian by retrograde vertebral blood flow or by duplex ultrasound detection of reversed flow in the vertebral artery.[20] A vertebral artery Doppler signal can also yield an alternating (toward and away) flow pattern (Fig. 12–6). This alternating pattern can transition to complete flow reversal with exercise of the ipsilateral upper extremity or after reactive hyperemia testing and

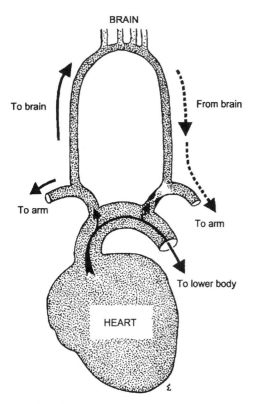

FIGURE 12–5. This diagram depicts the anatomy and physiology of a subclavian steal. Flow in the right vertebral artery is antegrade (toward the brain) to the basilar. Flow then reverses in the contralateral vertebral to perfuse the left subclavian artery in the presence of a hemodynamically significant stenosis in the left subclavian artery proximal to the left vertebral artery origin.

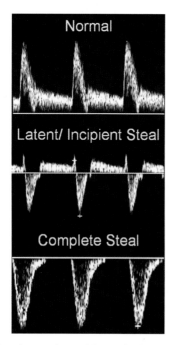

FIGURE 12–6. Doppler waveforms of the vertebral artery in various degrees of subclavian artery stenosis. Top is a normal waveform. Middle is an alternating flow waveform, and bottom demonstrates complete reversal of flow.

can be demonstrated by observation of the vertebral artery Doppler signal after exercise or release of a blood pressure cuff that has been inflated to a suprasystolic blood pressure for approximately 3 minutes. A standard transcranial Doppler evaluation with particular attention to the blood flow direction and the velocities in the vertebral arteries and the basilar artery can also be useful. Blood flow is normally away from the transducer (suboccipital approach) in the vertebrobasilar system. If flow is toward the transducer at rest or with provocative maneuvers, there is evidence of a steal.[21]

Dissection

Dissection is a nonatherosclerotic condition that is usually the result of trauma that causes a sudden tear in the intimal lining of the vessel. The intima then separates from the media and adventitia (Fig. 12–7). This separation creates a "false" lumen wherein blood may pulsate. The dissection may extend proximally or distally and may remain asymptomatic or may thrombose and cause neurological symptoms when it is flow limiting.

Aneurysm

An aneurysm is defined as a permanent focal dilation of an arterial segment greater than 50% of the diameter of the normal adjacent vessel. Aneurysms of the extracranial carotid artery are rare (Fig. 12–8); several decades ago, such aneurysms were often attributed to syphilitic arteritis and peritonsillar abscess. Currently, the most common causes are trauma, cystic medial necrosis, fibromuscular dysplasia, and atherosclerosis.[22] Neurologic manifestations are varied and include (1) cranial nerve involvement, which may produce dysarthria (hypoglossal nerve), hoarseness (vagus nerve), dysphagia (glossopharyngeal nerve), or tinnitus and facial tics (facial nerve); (2) compression of the cervical sympathetic chain and Horner's syndrome; and (3) ischemic syncopal attacks, resulting from embolism or interference with blood flow. Commonly, patients with an extracranial carotid aneurysm present to their physician with a cervical or parapharyngeal mass. Sometimes, an unsuspecting physician will perform a needle biopsy, which is followed by significant bleeding, hematoma formation,

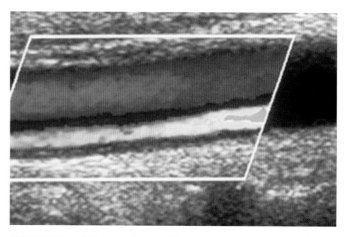

FIGURE 12–7. This is an ultrasound image of a common carotid artery dissection with two patent flow lumens.

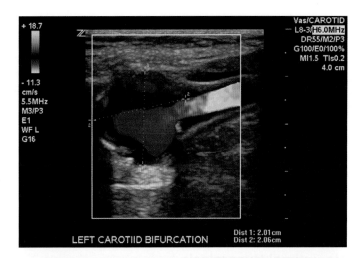

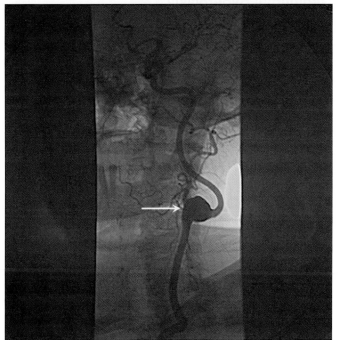

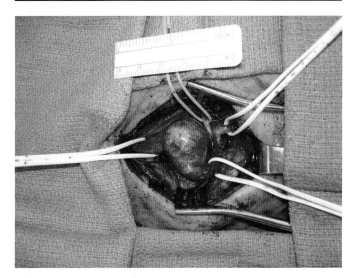

FIGURE 12-8. Patient with an internal carotid artery aneurysm. The top figure is a sagittal ultrasound image of an internal carotid artery aneurysm. The middle image is the confirmatory arteriogram, and the bottom image shows the intraoperative finding.

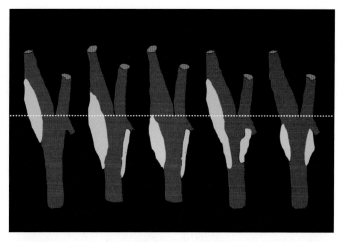

FIGURE 12-9. This cartoon illustrates the variable location of the carotid "bulb" outlined in aqua blue. Note that although the level of the bifurcation (dotted white line) is unchanged, the bulb may encompass any or all parts of the bifurcation, internal or external carotid arteries. Therefore, the level at which the common carotid artery divides into the internal and external carotid arteries should be referred to as the carotid bifurcation and not the carotid "bulb."

or stroke.[23] An aneurysm of the carotid artery must not be misdiagnosed as a large carotid bulb. Note that the carotid bulb presents in various sizes and locations (Fig. 12–9). In addition, a comparison to the contralateral side is helpful.

Carotid Body Tumors

Haller introduced glomus tumors of the head and neck into the medical record in 1762 when he described a mass at the carotid bifurcation that had a glomus body-like structure. In 1950, Mulligan renamed this type of neoplasm a chemodectoma to reflect its origins from chemoreceptor cells. In 1974, Glenner and Grimley renamed the tumor paraganglioma on the basis of its anatomic and physiologic characteristics. They also created a classification method based on the location, innervation, and microscopic appearance of the tumors.

Carotid body tumors, also called chemodectomas, are vascular tumors that arise from the paraganglionic cells in the outer layer of the carotid artery at the bifurcation level (Fig. 12–10).

This disease, which may be hereditary, is more common in South America than in North America. Tumors can become sizable before causing symptoms, such as a painless, pulsating mass in the upper neck, and eventually can cause difficulty in swallowing. Ten percent of these tumors occur on both sides of the carotid artery. Although these can be noted on duplex ultrasonography,[24,25] they are definitively diagnosed using computed tomography (CT) or magnetic resonance imaging (MRI) scans, and sometimes angiography.[26] These tumors are generally benign; only about 5–10% are malignant. Treatment includes surgery and occasionally radiation therapy.[27]

Fibromuscular Dysplasia

Fibromuscular Dysplasia (FMD) is a non-atherosclerotic disease that usually affects the media of the arterial wall due to

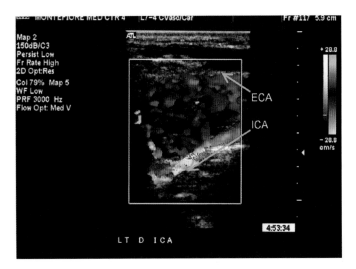

FIGURE 12–10. Color-flow duplex image of a carotid body tumor. Note the typical splaying of the bifurcation vessels secondary to the location of the tumor between the ICA and ECA, which are indicated by the green arrows. Hypervascularity is evident by the color Doppler.

abnormal cellular development that causes stenosis of the renal arteries, carotid arteries, and less commonly, other arteries of the abdomen and extremities. This disease can cause hypertension, strokes, and arterial aneurysm and dissection.

FMD is often diagnosed incidentally in the absence of any signs or symptoms during an imaging study. Angiography with contrast will show a characteristic "string of beads" morphology in a vessel affected by FMD (Fig. 12–11). This pattern is caused by multiple arterial dilations separated by concentric stenosis.

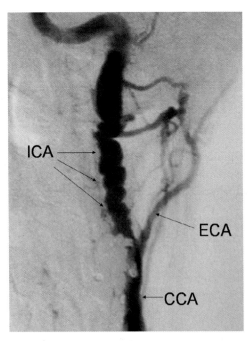

FIGURE 12–11. Angiographic presentation of fibromuscular dysplasia. Notice the classic "string of beads" appearance in the distal segment of the extracranial internal carotid artery (ICA). (ECA: external carotid artery; CCA: common carotid artery.)

FMD tends to occur in females between 14 and 50 years of age. However, it has been found in children younger than 14 years, both male and female. Up to 75% of all patients with FMD will have disease in the renal arteries.[28] The second most common artery affected is the carotid artery. More than one artery may have evidence of FMD in 28% of people with this disease.[29] All relevant arteries should be checked if found.

In the carotid system, it predominantly occurs in the mid segment of the ICA, it is bilateral in approximately 65% of the cases, and it is usually found in females. Color Doppler imaging may reveal a turbulent flow pattern adjacent to the arterial wall, with absence of atherosclerotic plaque in the proximal and distal segments of the ICA.[21,24,25]

Neointimal Hyperplasia

Neointimal hyperplasia accounts for most re-stenoses occurring within the first 2 years following vascular intervention. Development of the a neointimal hyperplastic lesion involves the migration of smooth muscle cells from the media to the neointima, their proliferation, and their matrix secretion and deposition. Thus, mechanisms of smooth muscle cell migration are key to the formation of neointima, early re-stenosis, vessel occlusion, and ultimate failure of vascular interventions. This is often a factor in patients who experience re-stenosis after carotid endarterectomy.[30]

SIGNS AND SYMPTOMS

Physical Examination

Physical examination of the extracranial carotid circulation includes palpation of common carotid, internal carotid artery, and temporal artery pulses. Acquisition of the bilateral brachial artery blood pressures can be performed routinely or per a prescribed algorithm and can be useful in the evaluation of patients with suspected vertebrobasilar symptoms as mentioned earlier. Auscultation of the carotid arteries is also part of the physical examination. Patients with evidence of cerebrovascular disease may in fact be asymptomatic. An asymptomatic stenosis is defined as any pre-occlusive lesion in the CCA, carotid bifurcation artery, or ICA in a patient with no ipsilateral monocular or cerebral hemispheric symptoms.

Cervical or carotid bruit is often the only indication for screening in patients with suspected hemodynamically significant carotid artery disease. Information about the incidence of carotid bruit in asymptomatic patients is available from the Framingham study. This study found that 3.5% of men and women had carotid bruits at 44–54 years of age. This increased to 7.0% at 65–79 years.[31]

Auscultation is performed by placing a stethoscope over the carotid artery. The patient is asked to take a deep breath and hold while the examiner listens for bruits (Fig. 12–12). A bruit is the result of vibration in the tissue that is transmitted to the surface of the skin. Bruits in the neck can be the result of the

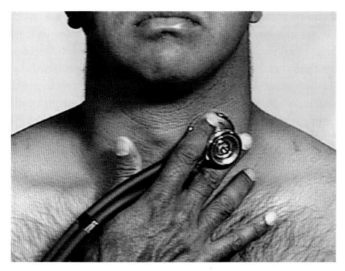

FIGURE 12–12. A stethoscope is placed over the cervical carotid artery and the examiner listens while the patient takes a deep breath.

turbulent blood flow that is seen distal to a hemodynamically significant stenosis. They can also be heard in patients with loops, coils, kinks, and tortuosity of the ICA, or they can be cardiac in origin. Not all patients with these findings however will present with a carotid bruit. Other causes may include external compression from thoracic outlet syndrome, arteriovenous malformations, and tumor.[32,33]

Auscultation for carotid artery bruit during routine examination has a low specificity that requires the support of ultrasound investigation. Due to the relatively low prevalence of carotid artery disease in the community; a national screening

program is not cost-effective. However, patients in whom a bruit is heard should have further investigations in order to prevent the sequelae of carotid artery disease.[34,35]

Acute neurological deficits are differentiated as TIAs or strokes, based on whether the deficit resolves within or persists longer than 24 hours. A TIA is any neurological dysfunction that lasts for less than 24 hours and completely resolves. Transient symptoms however are often a precursor to more serious complications. The neurological dysfunction may be described by the patient as some variation of a motor or sensory deficit (Table 12–3). TIAs typically last for just a few minutes or even seconds and result from deprivation of blood supply to a focal area in the anterior circulation of the brain. This may be caused by emboli or severe stenosis in the carotid circulation, either intracranial or extracranial. Patients may suffer from repeated symptoms that are similar in nature but worsen or occur with increased frequency. These are referred to as crescendo TIA and is important to identify, as this may be a sign of impending stroke.

Other temporary symptoms involve the vertebrobasilar system (posterior circulation). Symptoms include vertigo, syncope, ataxia, drop attacks, and any other symptom that is bilateral in nature. Although these types of symptoms are indications for cerebrovascular evaluation, they typically will not be caused by carotid disease, as there are many other differential diagnoses.[36]

CVA, commonly referred to as stroke, is defined as any motor or sensory deficit that lasts longer than 24 hours and does not completely resolve. Seventy-five percent of patients with stroke have experienced a previous TIA. CVA is essentially a result of necrosis or death of brain tissue. Major CVA can be debilitating, resulting in permanent paralysis and potentially death. In addition, it is quite

TABLE 12–3 • Common Signs and Symptoms of Cerebrovascular Disease (Transient Ischemic Attacks and Strokes)	
Signs or Symptoms	Definition
Amaurosis fugax	Transient blindness, either partial or complete often "shade coming down over one eye"; caused by embolism to the ophthalmic artery or one of its branches
Hemiparesis/hemiplegia	Unilateral paralysis either partial or complete
Hemianopia	Blindness in one-half of the field of vision; can be bilateral or unilateral and may be from middle cerebral artery occlusion
Dysarthria	Difficulty with speech secondary to impaired muscles used for speech
Dysphasia	Difficulty with the coordination of speech or failure to arrange words in context
Dysphagia	Difficulty with swallowing
Ataxia	Unsteady gait
Diplopia	Double vision
Vertigo	Loss of equilibrium sometimes described as the room spinning

possible for patients to have had a stroke and never have suffered any symptoms. Most of these are found incidentally on a CT scan of the head that is usually performed for some other reason.

TESTING FOR CEREBROVASCULAR DISEASE

Duplex Ultrasound Technique[37,38]

The examination is explained and a history (risk factors, symptoms) is obtained from the patient. Arm pressures are recorded bilaterally (<20 mm Hg difference is within normal limits) and the presence of cervical bruits if present is documented.

Suggested instrument setups for carotid duplex imaging are as follows: (1) use a high-frequency (5–10 MHz) linear array transducer, (2) image orientation: head to the left of the monitor, (3) color assignment: although color is based on the direction of blood flow (toward or away) in relation to the transducer, red is usually assigned to arteries and blue to venous blood flow, (4) the color scale (pulse repetition frequency [PRF]) should be adjusted throughout the examination to evaluate the changing velocity patterns, (5) the wall filter is set low, (6) the color *box* width affects frame rates (number of image frames per second), so the color display should be kept as small as possible, and (7) the color gain should be adjusted throughout the examination as the signal strength changes.

Duplex evaluation is primarily done in the long axis since the assessment of the carotid system requires Doppler insonation throughout the CCA, ICA, and origin of the ECA. The vertebral arteries also are included, especially in the presence of vertebrobasilar symptoms. The examination is performed with the patient in the supine position (Fig. 12–13). Anything that restricts access to the entirety of the extracranial carotid system from the base of

the neck to the angle of the mandible is removed (Fig. 12–14). Pillows may be used to support the neck; however, the patient's head should be positioned such that the chin is pointed up and the head slightly turned away from the side being examined.

The examination begins with a transverse sweep of the carotid system examining the vessels of interest from the origin of the common carotid artery to its bifurcation where the origins of the internal and external carotid artery are identified. This allows for a preview of all the vessels and surrounding structures (Fig. 12–15). Any abnormalities including extracarotid pathology and thyroid masses are noted. The sonographic appearance and size of these structures are included in a final report. Location of plaque, plaque characteristics, and location of the bifurcation are assessed as well.

Sagittal to the long axis of the vessel, follow the course of the CCA from its origin (or as proximal as can be obtained) to the bifurcation. The origin of the right CCA almost always can be imaged since its origin is from the innominate artery (Fig. 12–16). In contrast, because access is limited secondary to depth and adjacent bony and muscular structures, the left CCA may be very difficult to visualize. Imaging with a sector transducer is an alternative and should be used when a significant stenosis is suspected at the origin of the left CCA. Using color-flow Doppler imaging as a guide, interrogate the length of the CCA with pulsed Doppler, noting peak systolic and end diastolic velocities. The CCA bifurcation is a common place for atherosclerotic plaque and is also the site of what is commonly referred to as the carotid bulb, although the location of the bulb itself may be variable (see Fig. 12–9). This area should be assessed from multiple views. At this point the ICA and ECA are followed individually, and it is important to distinguish the ICA from the ECA. Although the spectral waveform pattern is the primary determinant, other parameters are useful (Table 12–4).

Follow the course of the ICA from its origin at the CCA bifurcation as far distal as possible. Using color-flow Doppler as

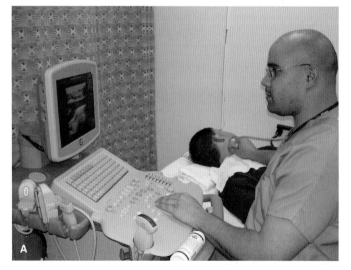
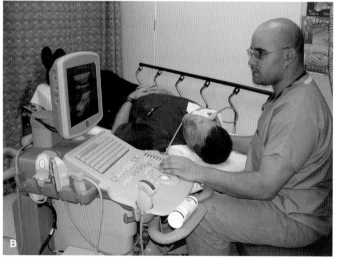

FIGURE 12–13. The examination is performed in the supine position while the examiner is either (**A**) at the head of the patient or (**B**) standing or sitting beside the patient.

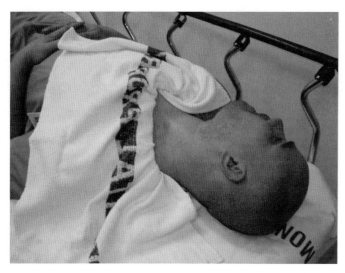

FIGURE 12–14. All restrictive garments such as turtleneck shirts and jewelry are removed to allow easy access to the neck, and the patient's head is turned slightly away from the side that is examined.

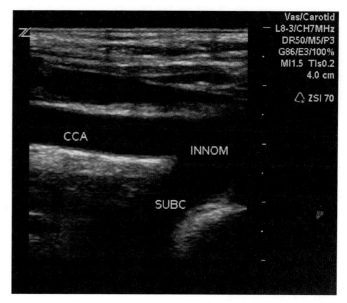

FIGURE 12–16. Ultrasound image of the right common carotid artery off the innominate.

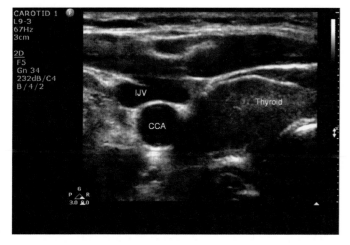

FIGURE 12–15. Transverse ultrasound image of the common carotid artery and surrounding structures.

a guide, interrogate the length of the vessel with pulsed Doppler and measure the peak systolic and end-diastolic velocities. Imaging from a posterolateral or lateral approach usually provides the best image. Where significant plaque is visualized, multiple views and Doppler assessment are imperative to ensure the data obtained is accurate and reproducible. Typically atherosclerotic disease occurs within the first few centimeters of the ICA, and elevated velocities at this segment in the presence of disease will be categorized based primarily on the spectral Doppler velocities. The distal ICA may be difficult to image secondary to depth and tortuosity. The clinical implication of tortuosity has yet to be proven as a significant finding; however, it should be noted that normal flow disturbances occur and elevated velocities may be recorded as a result of rapid changes in Doppler angles between the insonation beam and the acute changes in geometry of the blood vessel (Fig. 12–17).[39] Consideration is, therefore, recommended before interpreting high velocities as indicative of hemodynamically significant disease.

TABLE 12–4 • Differentiating the ICA from the ECA*

Characteristics	ICA	ECA
Extracranial branches	None	Yes (eight in number)
Doppler waveform	ICA yields a low-resistance waveform with continuous forward flow throughout the cardiac cycle and will always have more diastolic flow than the ECA in normal conditions	ECA yields a high-resistance waveform with less diastolic flow than internal; sometimes a reversed flow component in early diastole
Size and location at bifurcation	Larger and located posterior and lateral to the ECA	

*Tapping on the superficial temporal artery causes oscillations in the ECA waveform (although this is thought to be a very weak parameter). As oscillation is sometimes noted in both the ICA and the ECA.

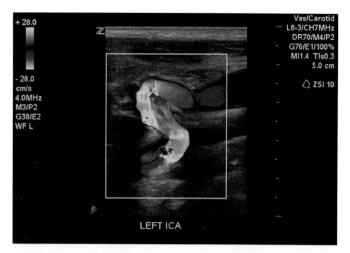

FIGURE 12–17. Color duplex image of a tortuous internal carotid artery (ICA). Notice the changes in the color-flow pattern that indicate rapid changes in the Doppler angle and not necessarily elevated velocities associated with stenosis.

FIGURE 12–19. Long-axis view of the vertebral artery. Note that the bony structures indicated by the green arrows result in acoustic shadowing.

Look for other visual evidence of disease on the B-mode image and for the presence of post-stenotic turbulence.

A Doppler waveform is obtained at the origin of the ECA. This is done to document patency and to help distinguish this vessel from the ICA (Fig. 12–18).

The vertebral artery lies deeper than the CCA and can be located by angling the transducer slightly laterally from a longitudinal view of the mid/proximal CCA. To reliably identify the vertebral artery, it should be followed distally, and periodic shadowing should be visualized from the transverse processes of the vertebrae (Fig. 12–19). The vertebral artery is accompanied by the vertebral vein and proper identification of the artery is made by evaluation of the Doppler signal. Once the vertebral artery has been correctly identified, it should be followed as far

proximally as possible. The use of color Doppler will greatly assist in locating the vertebral artery and its origin, as well as in evaluating the direction of blood flow.

Doppler interrogation of the carotid system is performed in the longitudinal plane using a 60° angle between the ultrasound beam and the vessel walls, as well as the angle cursor parallel to the vessel wall (placement of the Doppler sample volume parallel to the color jet has not undergone extensive validation criteria). Using a constant Doppler angle permits comparison of repeated studies in the same individual. Insonation angles >60° should never be used for data acquisition and analysis, as significant measurement error is introduced in even small changes in the Doppler angle of insonation when it is >60°. The Doppler sample volume is moved slowly through the artery searching for the highest velocity. The color Doppler display will help guide the proper placement of the sample volume and is useful in locating sites of disease as evidenced by the presence of aliasing of the color-flow image.

Doppler signals are recorded from the proximal, mid, and distal CCA; the origin of the ECA; the proximal, mid, and distal ICA; the origin of the vertebral artery; and the subclavian artery bilaterally. In a normal vessel, the Doppler sample volume placement should be at the center of the lumen. The pulsed Doppler sample volume placement width is set at 1–2 mm to detect discrete changes in blood flow and minimize artifactual spectral broadening. When a stenosis is identified, a thorough interrogation of the stenotic area is performed. In the presence of disease, color-flow Doppler imaging should be used as a guide to aid in the optimal placement of the pulsed Doppler sample volume where the highest velocity may be obtained. Be sure to profile the lesion by moving the sample volume back and forth through the lesion to elicit the highest velocity within the stenosis. A Doppler waveform is obtained at the site of stenosis, where highest velocity is suspected

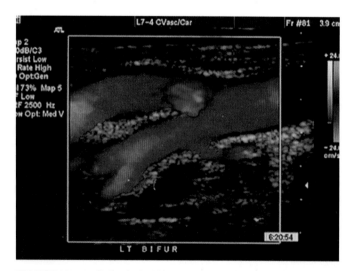

FIGURE 12–18. Color duplex illustrating branches of the external carotid artery. This is helpful for identification of the internal carotid artery versus the external carotid artery.

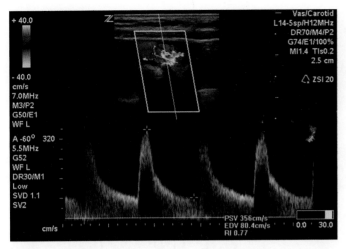

FIGURE 12–20. Internal carotid artery stenosis evident by the significant elevation of the velocity.

(Figs. 12–20 and 12–21), and a second Doppler waveform obtained distal to the lesion for documentation of post-stenotic turbulence that almost always accompanies a hemodynamically significant stenosis. It is important to evaluate all Doppler signals bilaterally to correctly perform a carotid duplex imaging examination.

The location of any plaque, as well as its surface characteristics (smooth versus irregular) and echogenicity (homogeneous, heterogeneous, or calcified), visualized during the examination should be described (Fig. 12–22).

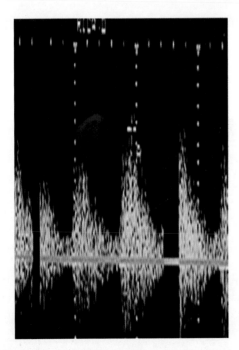

FIGURE 12–21. Spectral Doppler waveform that demonstrates post-stenotic turbulence as evident by flow above and below the baseline; spectral broadening; and irregular picket-fence configuration of the envelope of the spectral waveform throughout the cardiac cycle.

Interpretation and Diagnostic Criteria

The accurate interpretation of a carotid duplex imaging examination depends on the quality and the completeness of the evaluation. Often the patient's body habitus will affect the quality of the image and the sonographer's ability to search the entire carotid system with Doppler. The sonographer must know when and be prepared to switch transducers when necessary to complete the carotid examination and have a complete understanding of the equipment controls to optimize the duplex imaging system. In addition to the peak systolic velocity, end-diastolic velocity, direction of blood flow, and the shape of the Doppler spectral waveform should be compared at the same level bilaterally. Abnormal waveform shape (increased or decreased pulsatility) may be an indicator of more proximal (innominate, subclavian) or distal (intracranial) disease (Fig. 12–23).

To determine the degree of stenosis present, a complete Doppler evaluation of the artery is necessary. There should be an elevated velocity through the narrowed segment and post-stenotic disturbances distal to the stenosis. The highest velocity obtained from a stenosis is used to classify the degree of narrowing. Doppler signals obtained distal to the area of post-stenotic flow disturbance may be normal or diminished, and the upstroke of the distal Doppler spectral waveform may be slowed.

University of Washington criteria were traditionally used to categorize disease from the origin of the internal carotid artery (Table 12–5). However, because the carotid endarterectomy trials [North American Symptomatic Carotid Endarterectomy Trial (NASCET),[40] Asymptomatic Carotid Atherosclerosis Study (ACAS),[41] European Carotid Surgery Trial (ECST)[42]] used specific thresholds for surgical treatment, ultrasound criteria for ICA stenosis more than 70% and more than 60% were needed to classify patients. Investigators have found that an ICA/CCA peak systolic velocity (PSV) ratio is useful in grading ICA stenosis more than 70%[43] and more than 60%, respectively[44] (Table 12–6). The ratios are calculated using the highest PSV from the origin of the ICA divided by the highest PSV from the CCA (approximately 2–3 cm proximal to the bifurcation).

In the presence of a contralateral ICA occlusion, the velocity from the ipsilateral ICA may be elevated. This may lead to overestimating the extent of ipsilateral ICA disease.[45,46] To avoid overestimation of the ICA stenosis, new velocity criteria have been suggested. A PSV of more than 140 cm/s is used for a stenosis >50% diameter reduction and an end-diastolic velocity of >155 cm/s for a stenosis greater than 80% diameter reduction of the lumen.[46]

Anatomic features, such as a high carotid bifurcation (<1.5 cm from the angle of the mandible), excessive distal extent of plaque (>2.0 cm above the carotid bifurcation), or a small distal ICA diameter (≤0.5 cm), or a redundant or kinked ICA can complicate carotid endarterectomy. In the past, arteriography was the only preoperative study capable of imaging these

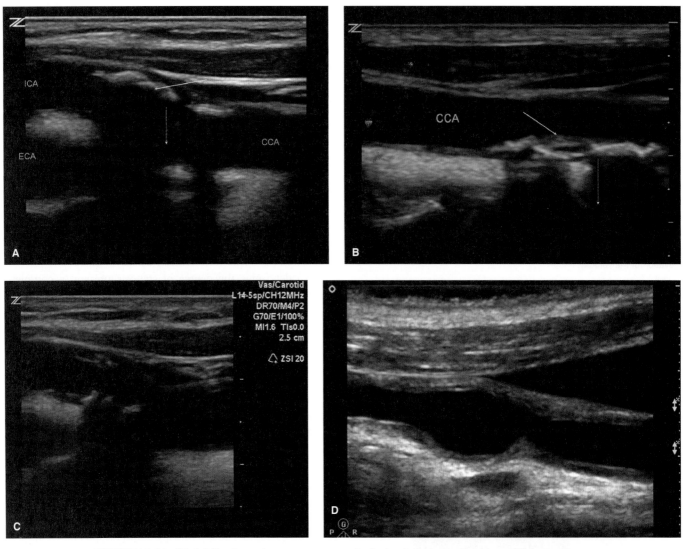

FIGURE 12–22. (**A**) Calcific plaque that creates an acoustic shadow indicated by the arrows. (**B**) A smooth plaque that is heterogeneous in texture with a calcific component that causes an acoustic shadow indicated by the dotted arrow. (**C**) A plaque with an irregular border and heterogeneous in texture. (**D**) A smooth and predominantly homogeneous plaque. (CCA: common carotid artery; ECA: external carotid artery; ICA: internal carotid artery.)

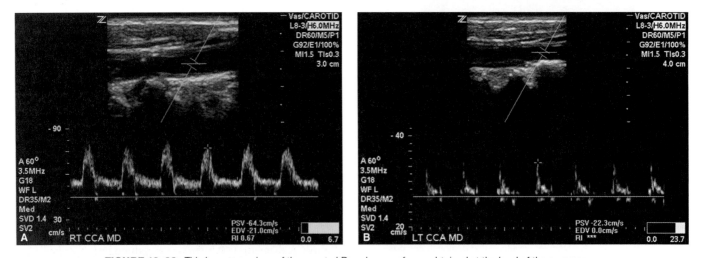

FIGURE 12–23. This is a comparison of the spectral Doppler waveforms obtained at the level of the common carotid artery (CCA) bilaterally in a patient with a left internal carotid artery (ICA) occlusion. (**A**) Normal spectral Doppler waveform of the right CCA. (**B**) On the contralateral side, a high-resistance spectral Doppler waveform with no diastolic flow suggestive of the distal ICA occlusion on the ipsilateral side.

TABLE 12–5 • Strandness Criteria for Grading ICA Stenosis

Diameter Reduction	Peak Systolic Velocity	End-Diastolic Velocity
<50%	<125 cm/s	
50–79%	≥125 cm/s	
80–99%		>140 cm/s
Occlusion	no signal	no signal

features. Accordingly, in the presence of ICA stenosis, other important information to include in the evaluation and interpretation of a carotid duplex imaging examination is (1) the location of the bifurcation relevant to the angle of the mandible (or some other external landmark), (2) the distal extent of the plaque beyond the ICA origin, (3) patency and diameter of the distal ICA, (4) the presence of tortuosity or kinking of the vessels, and (5) plaque characteristics (e.g., smooth versus irregular surface, calcification). This information is particularly relevant in patients undergoing carotid endarterectomy based on the duplex scan findings alone.[47]

Diagnosis of ICA Occlusion

Atherosclerosis is by far the most common cause of occlusion of the extracranial carotid arteries; however, fibromuscular dysplasia and dissection are additional causes. Most occlusions occur in the ICA.[48] ICA occlusion is not amenable to surgical intervention and a false-positive diagnosis will preclude the potential for treatment in this patient population. It is, therefore, important for patient management to differentiate between high-grade stenosis versus occlusion of the ICA. Differentiation of these two clinical entities was a major concern in ultrasound in the era before color-flow Doppler. However, with the advent of and technological advances in the 2D image and in color and power Doppler imaging, ICA occlusion can now very accurately be distinguished from high-grade stenosis.[48–50]

In the presence of a suspected ICA occlusion, the artery should be evaluated with spectral Doppler, color Doppler, and power Doppler to rule out the presence of trickle flow. Secondary ultrasound characteristics of an ICA occlusion include echogenic material filling the lumen, lack of arterial pulsations, reversed color blood flow near the origin of the occlusion, and the loss of diastolic blood flow in the ipsilateral CCA (Figs. 12–23A and B and 12–24).

To reach this level of accuracy, it is important to employ several technical strategies[51]: (1) The ultrasound instrument must be adjusted to allow for the detection of very low flow velocities. The operator must take care to ensure the appropriate pulse repetition frequency (PRF); this is referred to as the scale on some instruments. The wall filter must be adjusted so it does not exclude low-frequency signals. (2) The operator must make sure to obtain the best possible image of the vessel in question and inspect the lumen for any evidence (2D or Doppler) of active blood flow. This may require multiple angle views and approaches so that both the 2D and Doppler analysis have been optimized. (3) The operator must interrogate all visualized segments of the ICA with spectral Doppler. If flow is detected, be careful to ensure the correct flow direction so as to not mistake an adjacent vein for a patent ICA. (4) The operator must use both the sagittal and transverse planes to evaluate the suspected occlusion for any potential flow channels. (5) If possible, the operator should image the very distal ICA. In the presence of a suspected occlusion, the presence of antegrade flow distally is likely to mean that a patent lumen proximally has been overlooked.

CCA occlusion/stenosis occurs much less often than ICA occlusion and it can be accompanied by stroke or other neurologic events or it can be asymptomatic. Often these patients present after radiation therapy to the neck region and atherosclerosis is a less likely cause.

Pitfalls in the diagnosis of ICA occlusion include calcific plaques (Fig. 12–25). These will cause acoustic shadowing that limits or prevents visualization of the vessel of interest. Other pitfalls include high bifurcations and deep vessels that can limit the investigation and a pulsatile jugular vein that can be mistaken for a patent ICA.

TABLE 12–6 • NASCET and ACAS Criteria for Grading ICA Stenosis

Diameter Reduction	ICA/CCA PSV Ratio
70–99%	>4[40]
60–99%	>3.2[41]

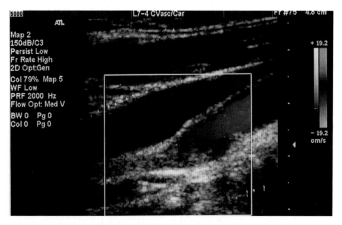

FIGURE 12–24. Color duplex image of a carotid artery occlusion.

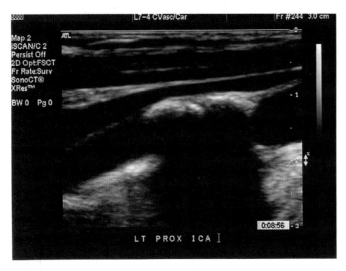

FIGURE 12-25. Color duplex image of a calcific plaque that in many cases limits and sometimes prohibits adequate visualization of the carotid bifurcation. These plaques must be imaged from multiple approaches to achieve an adequate evaluation.

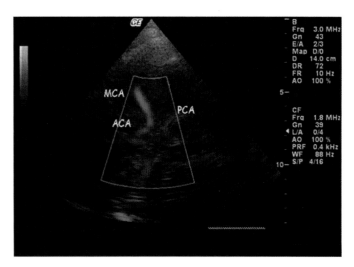

FIGURE 12-26. Power Doppler image of a portion of the circle of Willis.

Transcranial Doppler and Imaging

Routine transcranial Doppler (TCD) ultrasound examination of the intracranial arteries was demonstrated to be possible in 1982.[52] TCD, and more recently, transcranial color Doppler and power imaging, gives detailed information about the flow velocity in brain arteries and veins (Fig. 12–26). This hemodynamic information is routinely used in the diagnosis of cerebrovascular disease. Used to help in the diagnosis of emboli, stenosis, vasospasm from a subarachnoid hemorrhage (bleeding from a ruptured aneurysm), and other problems, this relatively quick and inexpensive test is growing in popularity in the United States.[53,54] It is often used in conjunction with other tests such as MRI, magnetic resonance angiography, carotid duplex ultrasound, and CT scans.

One fact to keep in mind when utilizing TCD is that the value obtained for a particular artery is the velocity of blood flowing through the vessel, and unless the diameter of that vessel is established by some other means, it is not possible to determine the actual blood flow. Thus, TCD is primarily a technique for measuring relative changes in flow. The utility of the technique is now well established for a number of different disease processes.[54-64]

Two methods of recording may be used for this procedure. The first uses the B-mode image in combination with the Doppler information. Once the desired blood vessel is found, blood flow velocities may be measured with a pulsed Doppler, which records velocities over time. This is referred to as transcranial Doppler imaging (TCDI) and is performed using the duplex scanner. The second method of recording uses only the Doppler probe function, relying instead on the training and experience of the clinician in finding the correct vessels. This is referred to subsequently as TCD.

The operator must be aware that the Doppler spectral waveforms obtained during a TCDI examination are based on hemo-dynamics, and that the waveforms obtained do not provide anatomic information. TCDI is an advancement of intracranial ultrasound techniques since it combines the hemodynamic information with anatomic landmarks, enabling the accurate identification of the intracranial arteries. Increases in intracranial arterial velocity may be due to but not limited to increased volume flow without a lumen diameter change, a decrease in lumen diameter (stenosis) without a change in volume flow, or by a combination of an increase in volume flow and a decrease in lumen diameter.

The accurate interpretation of a patient's TCDI examination may be difficult without knowledge of the location and the extent of atherosclerotic disease present in the extracranial vasculature.

The TCD technique was introduced as a method to detect cerebral arterial vasospasm following subarachnoid hemorrhage. During the past 20 years, the list of clinical applications for transcranial Doppler has grown (Table 12–7) and the addition of new areas of research will permit better understanding of intracranial cerebrovascular hemodynamics.

Examination Protocols and Techniques

Transcranial Doppler Imaging (TCDI).[65-67] The quality of the intracranial image depends on proper adjustment of many instrument controls. Increasing the power setting and the color gain to the appropriate level during a TCDI study are probably the most important instrument control adjustments. Adjusting the focal zone in the range of 6–8 cm will improve the image and color resolution. Maintaining a small image sector width and color box width will keep the highest possible frame rates. Checking for the appropriate color PRF, sensitivity, and persistence settings are also very important to obtain good quality color Doppler intracranial images.

The color display is important because it assists in the proper placement of the Doppler sample volume. The interpretation of the TCDI examination is made from the Doppler spectral waveform information. Therefore, Doppler signals are

TABLE 12-7 • Transcranial Doppler Applications

1. Diagnosis of intracranial vascular disease
2. Monitoring vasospasm in subarachnoid hemorrhage
3. Screening of children with sickle cell disease
4. Assessment of intracranial collateral pathways
5. Evaluation of the hemodynamic effects of extracranial occlusive disease on intracranial blood flow
6. Intraoperative monitoring
7. Detection of cerebral emboli
8. Monitoring evolution of cerebral circulatory arrest
9. Documentation of subclavian steal
10. Evaluation of the vertebrobasilar system
11. Detection of feeders of arteriovenous malformations
12. Monitoring anticoagulation regimens or thrombolytic therapy
13. Monitoring during neuroradiologic interventions
14. Testing of functional reserve
15. Monitoring after head trauma

obtained from various depths along the artery's path (Table 12–8). The color Doppler display helps guide the operator, as the Doppler sample volume is "swept" through the intracranial arteries to obtain the Doppler spectral waveforms. At each depth setting, it is important to adjust the position of the sample volume on the color display and angle the transducer to optimize the Doppler signal.

Conventional color orientation for TCDI examinations is set for shades of red indicating blood flow toward the transducer and shades of blue indicating blood flow away from the transducer. By keeping this color assignment constant, intracranial blood flow direction in the arteries can be readily recognized. The appearance of intracranial arterial blood flow is dependent on many instrument controls that can affect its presentation. Therefore, estimations of arterial size are not accurate from the color Doppler display.

The Doppler evaluation of the intracranial arteries is performed with a low-frequency (2–3 MHz) phased-array imaging transducer. A large sample volume is used to obtain a good signal-to-noise ratio. With TCDI, a smaller gate (i.e., 5–10 mm) can be placed on a specific arterial segment that is readily identified from a color-flow image. Intracranial arterial velocities acquired with TCDI are acquired assuming a zero-degree angle.

Additionally, with the use of TCDI, many investigators are reporting results using peak systolic and end-diastolic velocities instead of the traditionally accepted mean velocities (time average peak velocities). Each institution will have to decide which velocity value to report and adjust the diagnostic criteria accordingly.

Transcranial Doppler (TCD) is a "blind" technique that encompasses many of the concepts described above but employs a Doppler probe, only without the image component to analyze the intracranial vasculature.[66,67] Using various windows (Fig. 12–27) and depths, mean velocities are acquired and a diagnosis can be rendered (see Table 12–8).

Miscellaneous Tests

Large observational studies and atherosclerosis regression trials of lipid-modifying pharmacotherapy have established that intima-media thickness (IMT) of the carotid and femoral arteries, as measured noninvasively by B-mode ultrasound, is a valid surrogate marker for the progression of atherosclerotic disease.[68] IMT is a measurement that can be obtained at the level of the carotid bifurcation (Fig. 12–28). Although automated software is required to ensure accurate and reproducible data to assess a patient's risks for such events, we can comment on the integrity of the vessel wall and look for variations of wall thickness along its length. Measuring the IMT is simply a screening tool and is mentioned here as an attempt to increase awareness of it and its utilization.[69]

TABLE 12-8 • Mean Velocities Using Various Doppler US Approachs

Window	Artery	Depth (mm)	Mean Velocity (cm/s)
Transtemporal	Middle cerebral	30–67	62 ± 12
	Anterior cerebral	60–80	50 ± 11
	Terminal internal carotid	60–67	39 ± 9
	Posterior cerebral	55–80	39 ± 10
	Posterior communicating		
	Anterior communicating		
Transorbital	Ophthalmic	40–60	21 ± 5
	Internal carotid (siphon)	60–80	47 ± 10
Suboccipital	Vertebral	40–85	38 ± 10
	Basilar	>80	41 ± 10
Submandibular	Distal internal carotid	35–70	37 ± 9

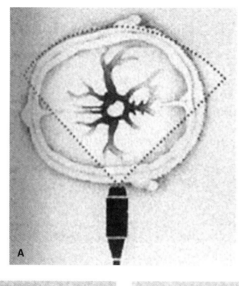

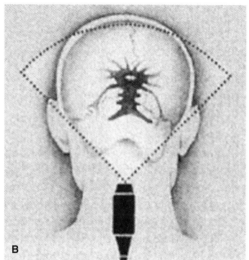

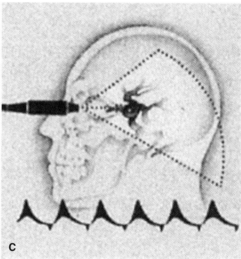

FIGURE 12–27. Transcranial Doppler is accomplished using the following approaches: (**A**) transtemporal, (**B**) suboccipital, (**C**) transorbital.

Other tests used in the diagnosis and management of patients with known or suspected cerebrovascular diseases include contrast arteriography, magnetic resonance angiography (MRA) and computed tomography (CTA).

Arteriography is the gold standard for the preoperative assessment of patients considered for carotid interventions, although the reported complications of stroke and death range between 0.2% and 0.7%. Noninvasive modalities such as MRA, combined duplex ultrasound and TCD, and duplex ultrasound alone are attractive because they avoid the contrast and catheter-related complications associated with arteriography. In many institutions, duplex ultrasound has emerged as the sole preoperative imaging study prior to carotid and other arterial and venous interventions.[46,70]

Arteriography is a catheter-based technique that may include assessment of the aortic arch as well as selected injections of individual subclavian and carotid arteries with anteroposterior,

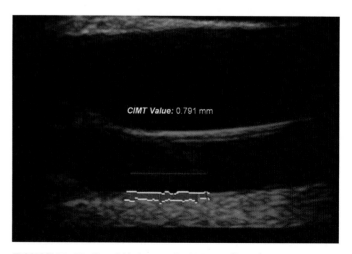

FIGURE 12–28. Carotid intima-media thickness (CIMT) measurement using proprietary software (Prowin).

lateral, and oblique views to evaluate the intracranial and extra-cranial vessels (Fig. 12–29).[20,71]

CT of the head is useful in identifying silent infarcts, determining the timing of surgery, evaluating the risk of surgery, and ruling out other causes of disease or symptoms. CT provides radiographic images of the body from many angles. A computer combines the pictures into two- and three-dimensional images. This test can also be performed with the administration of contrast dye to highlight the cerebrovasculature.[19]

MRA is increasingly being used as a noninvasive method for analyzing the carotid bifurcation. Many studies comparing duplex, MRA, and angiography have now been performed. While initial reports on MRA suggest it to be accurate for identifying carotid occlusion, MRA appears less reliable than duplex for categorizing stenosis in areas of moderate to severe narrowing where flow is turbulent, and it tends to overestimate disease. MRA remains an adjunct to duplex or angiography.[72–75]

Treatment

The management options for patients with carotid artery stenosis include the following on their own or in combination: (1) conservative management (risk factor modification), (2) carotid endarterectomy (CEA), or (3) balloon angioplasty and stenting (CAS).[13]

The standard surgical procedure is CEA, while the newer minimally invasive endovascular intervention is called carotid artery angioplasty with stenting. Common indications for these procedures include transient ischemic attacks (TIAs) or cerebrovascular accidents (CVAs, strokes), although CEA can also be performed in asymptomatic patients with carotid stenosis. CAS is typically reserved for more high risk patients.[13]

CEA is the removal of plaque on the inside of an artery. The internal, common, and external carotid arteries are clamped, the lumen of the ICA is opened, and the atheromatous plaque substance removed. The artery is closed, hemostasis achieved, and the overlying layers closed. Many surgeons use a temporary shunt to provide blood supply to the brain during the procedure. The procedure may be performed under general or local anesthesia. The latter allows for direct monitoring of neurological status by intraoperative verbal contact and testing of grip strength. With general anesthesia, indirect methods of assessing cerebral perfusion must be used, such as electroencephalography (EEG), TCD analysis, and carotid artery stump pressure monitoring. At present, there is no good evidence to show any major difference in outcome between local and general anesthesia.

Angioplasty and stenting of the carotid artery is undergoing investigation as alternatives to CEA (Fig. 12–30). CAS is a less invasive procedure that can be performed via a percutaneous approach or through a small incision for intra-arterial access. A catheter is advanced into the carotid artery to the area of stenosis. This catheter has a balloon at its tip, which may vary in size. When the balloon is advanced over the lesion, the balloon is inflated. Inflation of the balloon compresses the plaque in the artery and makes a larger opening inside the artery to restore the lumen for improved blood flow. A stent (a tiny, expandable metal coil) is often deployed at the site to help keep the artery from narrowing or closing again (recoil).

Because of the potential for emboli to the brain that may cause stroke, embolic prevention devices (EPDs) should be used during CAS. One type of EPD has a filter-like basket attached to a catheter that is positioned in the artery in order to "catch" any clots or small debris that might break loose from the plaque during the procedure. This technique may help reduce the incidence of stroke during CAS.[76]

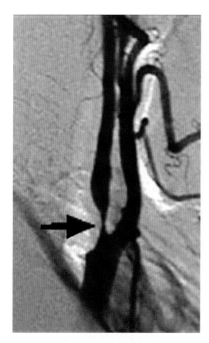

FIGURE 12–29. Angiographic diagnosis of an internal carotid artery stenosis.

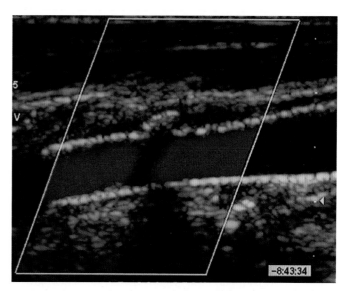

FIGURE 12–30. Ultrasound image of a carotid stent. Notice the plaque that has been pushed against the wall as a result of balloon angioplasty.

Intraoperative Carotid Duplex Imaging

The assessment of the CEA site by duplex imaging for technical adequacy has been shown to be an effective method to improve the results of the operation. Intraoperative duplex imaging identifies disturbed blood flow and anatomic abnormalities such as residual plaque, thrombus, and platelet aggregation. The detection of peak systolic velocities >150 cm/s with the presence of an anatomic defect warrants correction because of its potential to progress. Investigators have reported that the use of intraoperative carotid duplex imaging has had a favorable impact on the stroke rate and incidence of restenosis of the carotid artery; however, it is recommended that each institution should establish its own diagnostic criteria whether for use in the operating room or for diagnosis of atherosclerotic lesions.[77–79]

References

1. Stephens RB, Stillwell DL. *Arteries and Veins of the Human Brain.* Springfield, IL: Charles C Thomas; 1969.

2. McVay CB. *Anson and McVay Surgical Anatomy.* 6th ed. Philadelphia: WB Saunders; 1984.

3. Clemente CD (ed). *Gray's Anatomy of the Human Body.* 30th American ed. Philadelphia: Lea and Febiger; 1985.

4. Meyer JS (ed). *Modern Concepts of Cerebrovascular Disease.* New York: Spectrum Books; 1975.

5. Fields WS, Breutman ME, Weibel J. *Collateral Circulation to the Brain.* Baltimore: Williams & Wilkins; 1965.

6. Strandness DE Jr. *Collateral Circulation in Clinical Surgery.* Philadelphia: WB Saunders; 1969.

7. Bendick PJ, Glover JL. Vertebrobasilar insufficiency: Evaluation by quantitative duplex flow measurements. *J Vasc Surg.* 1987; 5:594-600.

8. Bendick PJ, Glover JL. Hemodynamic evaluation of vertebral arteries by duplex ultrasound. *Surg Clin North Am.* 1990; 70:235-244.

9. Bendick PJ. Duplex examination. In: Berguer R, Caplna LR, eds. *Vertebrobasilar Arterial Disease,* pp. 93-103. St. Louis: Quality Medical Publishers; 1992.

10. Strandness DE Jr. Extracranial artery disease. In: Strandness DE Jr, ed. *Duplex Scanning in Vascular Disorders,* 2nd ed, pp. 113-157. New York: Raven Press; 1993.

11. Hallett JW, Brewster DC, Darling RC. *Handbook of Patient Care in Vascular Surgery.* 3rd ed. Boston: Little, Brown & Co; 1995.

12. Goldstein LB, Adams R, Becker K, et al. Primary prevention of ischemic stroke: a statement for healthcare professionals from the Stroke Council of the American Heart Association. *Circulation.* 2001; 103:163-182.

13. Fazel P, Johnson K. Current role of medical treatment and invasive management in carotid atherosclerotic disease. *Proc (Bayl Univ Med Cent)* 2008; 21(2):133-138.

14. National Institute of Neurological Disorders and Stroke (NINDS) (1999). Stroke: Hope Through Research.

15. Maton A, Hopkins J, McLaughlin CW, et al. *Human Biology and Health.* Englewood Cliffs, NJ: Prentice Hall; 1993.

16. Patterson RF. Basic science in vascular disease. *J Vasc Technol.* 2002; 26(1).

17. Tuzcu EM, Kapadia SR, Tutar E, et al. High prevalence of coronary atherosclerosis in asymptomatic teenagers and young adults: evidence from intravascular ultrasound. *Circulation.* 2001; 103(22):2705-2710.

18. Fishbein MC, Schoenfield LJ. Heart Attack Photo Illustration Essay. Available at: MedicineNet.com.

19. Feigin VL. Stroke epidemiology in the developing world. *Lancet.* 2005; 365(9478):2160-2161.

20. Panetta TF. Cerebrovascular disease. In: Sales CM, Goldsmith J, Veith FJ, eds. *Handbook of Vascular Surgery.* St. Louis, MO: Quality Medical Publishing; 1994.

21. Katz ML. Extracranial/intracranial cerebrovascular evaluation. In: Hagen-Ansert SL, ed. *Textbook of Diagnostic Ultrasonography.* 5th ed. St. Louis, MO: Mosby; 2001.

22. Smullens SW. Surgically treatable lesions of the extracranial circulation, including the vertebral artery. *Radiol Clin North Am.* 1986; 23:453-460.

23. Ito M, Nitta T, Sato K, Ishii S. Cervical carotid aneurysm presenting as transient ischemic and recurrent laryngeal nerve palsy. *Surg Neurol.* 1986; 25:346-350.

24. Gritzmann N, Herold C, Haller J, et al. Duplex sonography of tumors of the carotid body. *Cardiovasc Intervent Radiol.* 1987; 10(5):280-284.

25. Jansen JC, Baatenburg de Jong RJ, Schipper J, et al. Color Doppler imaging of paragangliomas in the neck. *J Clin Ultrasound.* 1997 Nov-Dec; 25(9):481-485.

26. Alkadhi H, Schuknecht B, Stoeckli SJ, Valavanis A. Evaluation of topography and vascularization of cervical paragangliomas by magnetic resonance imaging and color duplex sonography. *Neuroradiology.* 2002 Jan; 44(1):83-90.

27. Antonitsis P, Saratzis N, Velissaris I, et al. Management of cervical paragangliomas: review of a 15-year experience. *Langenbecks Arch Surg.* 2006 Aug; 391(4):396-402. Epub 2006 May 6.

28. Fenves AZ, Ram CV. Fibromuscular dysplasia of the renal arteries. *Curr Hypertens Rep.* 1999 Dec; 1(6):546-549.

29. Lüscher TF, Keller HM, Imhof HG, et al. Fibromuscular hyperplasia: extension of the disease and therapeutic outcome. Results of the University Hospital Zurich Cooperative Study on Fibromuscular Hyperplasia. *Nephron.* 1986; 44 Suppl 1:109-114.

30. Samson RH, Yungst Z, Showalter DP. Homocysteine, a risk factor for carotid atherosclerosis, is not a risk factor for early recurrent carotid stenosis following carotid endarterectomy. *Vasc Endovascular Surg.* 2004 Jul-Aug; 38(4):345-348

31. Gillett M, Davis WA, Jackson D, et al; Prospective evaluation of carotid bruit as a predictor of first stroke in type 2 diabetes: the Fremantle Diabetes Study. *Stroke.* 2003 Sep; 34(9):2145-2151. Epub 2003 Aug 7.

32. Murie JA, Sheldon CD, Quin RO. Carotid artery bruit: association with internal carotid stenosis and intraluminal turbulence. *Br J Surg.* 1984 Jan;71(1):50-52.

33. LaBan MM, Meerschaert JR, Johnstone K. Carotid bruits: their significance in the cervical radicular syndrome. *Arch Phys Med Rehabil.* 1977 Nov; 58(11):491-494.

34. Magyar MT, Nam EM, Csiba L, et al. Carotid artery auscultation—anachronism or useful screening procedure? *Neurol Res.* 2002 Oct; 24(7):705-708.

35. Hill AB. Should patients be screened for asymptomatic carotid artery stenosis? *Can J Surg.* 1998 Jun; 41(3):208-213.

36. Soteriades ES, Evans JC, Larson MG, et al. Incidence and prognosis of syncope. *N Engl J Med.* 2002 Sep 19; 347(12):878-885.

37. Labropoulos N, Erzurum V, Sheehan MK, Baker W. Cerebral vascular color flow scanning technique and applications. In: Mansour MA, Labropoulos N, eds. *Vascular Diagnosis.* Chapter 9. Philadelphia, PA: Elsevier Saunders; 2005.

38. SVU Vascular Technology Professional Performance Guideline. Extracranial Cerebrovascular Duplex Ultrasound Evaluation. Available at: http://www.svunet.org.

39. Hoskins SH, Scissons RP. Hemodynamically significant carotid disease in duplex ultrasound patients with carotid artery tortuosity. *J Vasc Technol.* 2007; 31(1):11-15.

40. North American Symptomatic Carotid Endarterectomy Trial Collaborators: Beneficial effect of carotid endarterectomy in symptomatic patients with high grade carotid stenosis. *N Engl J Med.* 1991; 325:445-453.

41. Executive Committee Asymptomatic Carotid Atherosclerosis Study. Endarterectomy for asymptomatic carotid artery stenosis. *JAMA.* 1995; 273:1421.

42. Randomized trial of endarterectomy for recently symptomatic carotid stenosis: final results of the MRC European Carotid Surgery Trial (ECST). *Lancet.* 1998; 351:1379-1387.

43. Moneta GH, Edwards JM, Chitwood RW, et al. Correlation of North America Symptomatic Carotid Endarterectomy Trial (NASCET) angiographic definition of 70-99% internal carotid artery stenosis with duplex scanning. *J Vasc Surg.* 1995; 17:152-159.

44. Moneta GH, Edwards JM, Papanicolaou G, et al. Screening for asymptomatic carotid internal carotid artery stenosis: duplex criteria for discriminating 60-99% stenosis. *J Vasc Surg.* 1995; 21:989-994.

45. Fujitani RM, Mills JL, Wang LM, Taylor SM. The effect of unilateral internal carotid artery occlusion upon contralateral duplex study: criteria for accurate interpretation. *J Vasc Surg.* 1992; 16:459-468.

46. Spadone DP, Barkmeier LD, Hodgson KJ, et al. Contralateral internal carotid artery stenosis or occlusion: pitfall of correct ipsilateral classification—a study performed with color-flow imaging. *J Vasc Surg.* 1990; 11:642-649.

47. Wain RA, Lyon RT, Veith FJ, et al. Accuracy of duplex ultrasound in evaluating carotid artery anatomy before endarterectomy. *J Vasc Surg.* 1998 Feb; 27(2):235-242; discussion 242-244.

48. Chang YJ, Lin SK, Ryu SJ, et al. Common carotid artery occlusion: evaluation with duplex sonography. *Am L Neuroradiol.* 1995; 16:1099-1105.

49. Mattos MA, Hodgson K, Ramsey DE, et al. Identifying total carotid occlusion with colour flow duplex scanning. *Eur J Vasc Surg.* 1992; 6:204-210.

50. Lee DH, Gao FQ, Rankin RN, et al. Duplex and color Doppler flow sonography of occlusion and near occlusion of the carotid artery. *Am J Neuroradiol.* 1996; 17:1267-1274.

51. Zwiebel WJ, Pellerito JS. Carotid occlusion, unusual carotid pathology and tricky carotid cases. In: Zwiebel WJ, Pellerito JS, eds. *Introduction to Vascular Ultrasonography.* Chapter 10. Philadelphia, PA: Elsevier Saunders; 2005.

52. Aaslid R, Markwalder TM, Nornes H. Noninvasive transcranial Doppler ultrasound recording of flow velocity in basal cerebral arteries. *J Neurosurg.* 1982 Dec; 57(6):769-774.

53. Sloan MA, Alexandrov AV, Tegeler CH, et al. Therapeutics and Technology Assessment Subcommittee of the American Academy of Neurology. Assessment: transcranial Doppler ultrasonography: report of the Therapeutics and Technology Assessment Subcommittee of the American Academy of Neurology. *Neurology.* 2004 May 11; 62(9):1468-1481.

54. Newell D, Aaslid R. *Transcranial Doppler.* New York: Raven Press; 1992.

55. Babikian VL, Feldmann E, Wechsler LR, et al. Transcranial Doppler ultrasonography: year 2000 update. *J Neuroimaging.* 2000 Apr;10(2):101-115.

56. Adams RJ, McKie VC, Hsu L, et al. Prevention of a first stroke by transfusions in children with sickle cell anemia and abnormal results on transcranial Doppler ultrasonography. *N Engl J Med.* 1998; 339:5-11.

57. Alexandrov AV, Bladin CF, Norris JW. Intracranial blood flow velocities in acute ischemic stroke. *Stroke.* 1994; 25:1378-1383.

58. Alexandrov AV, Demchuck AM, Wein TH, Grotta JC. The accuracy and yield of transcranial Doppler in acute cerebral ischemia. *Stroke.* 1999; 30:238.

59. Wilterdink JL, Feldmann E, Furie KL, et al. Transcranial Doppler ultrasound battery reliably identifies severe internal carotid artery stenosis. *Stroke.* 1997; 28:133-136.

60. Razumovsky AY, Gillard JH, Bryan RN, Hanley DF, Oppenheimer SM. TCD, MRA and MRI in acute cerebral ischemia. *Acta Neurol Scand.* 1999; 99:65-76.

61. Di Tullio M, Sacco RL, Venketasubramanian N, et al. Comparison of diagnostic techniques for the detection of patent foramen ovale in stroke patients. *Stroke.* 1993; 24:1020-1024.

62. Petty GW, Mohr JP, Pedley TA, et al. The role of transcranial Doppler in confirming brain death: sensitivity, specificity, and suggestions for performance and interpretation. *Neurology.* 1990; 40:300-303.

63. Ducrocq X, Hassler W, Moritake K, et al. Consensus opinion on diagnosis of cerebral circulatory arrest using Doppler-sonography: Task Force Group on cerebral death of the Neurosonology Research Group of the World Federation of Neurology. *J Neurol Sci.* 1998; 159:145-150.

64. Ringelstein EB. CO_2-reactivity: dependence from collateral circulation and significance in symptomatic and asymptomatic patients. In: Caplan LR, Shifrin EG, Nicolaides, Moore WS, eds. *Cerebrovascular Ischemia: Investigation and Management,* pp. 149-154. London: Med-Orion; 1996.

65. Spencer MP. Transcranial Doppler monitoring and causes of stroke from carotid endarterectomy. *Stroke.* 1997; 28:685-691.

66. Katz ML, Alexandrov AV. *A Practical Guide to Transcranial Doppler Examinations.* Littleton, CO: Summer Publishing Company; 2003.

67. Katz ML. Intracranial cerebrovascular evaluation. In: *Textbook of Diagnostic Ultrasonography.* St. Louis, MO: Mosby; 2001.

68. Bots ML, Hoes AW, Koudstaal PJ, et al. Common carotid intima-media thickness and risk of stroke and myocardial infarction: the Rotterdam Study. *Circulation.* 1997; 96:1432-1437.

69. Bortel L. What does intima-media thickness tell us? *J Hypertens.* 2005; 23:37-39.

70. Hingorani A, Ascher E, Marks N. Preprocedural imaging: new options to reduce need for contrast angiography. *Semin Vasc Surg.* 2007 Mar; 20(1):15-28.

71. Redmond PL, Kilcoyne RF, Rose JS, et al. Principles of angiography. In: Rutherford RB, ed. *Vascular Surgery*. 3rd ed, pp. 143-157. Philadelphia: WB Saunders; 1989.

72. Khaw KT. Does carotid duplex imaging render angiography redundant before carotid endarterectomy. *Br J Radiol*. 1997; 70:235-238.

73. Alvarez-Linera J, Benito-León J, Escribano J, et al. Prospective evaluation of carotid artery stenosis: elliptic centric contrast-enhanced MR angiography and spiral CT angiography compared with digital subtraction angiography. *AJNR Am J Neuroradiol*. 2003 May; 24(5):1012-1019.

74. Hirai T, Korogi Y, Ono K, et al. Prospective evaluation of suspected stenoocclusive disease of the intracranial artery: combined MR angiography and CT angiography compared with digital subtraction angiography. *AJNR Am J Neuroradiol*. 2002 Jan; 23(1):93-101.

75. Saloner D. Preoperative evaluation of carotid artery stenosis: comparison of contrast-enhanced MR angiography and duplex ultrasonography with digital subtraction angiography. *AJNR Am J Neuroradiol*. 2003 Jun-Jul; 24(6):1034-1035.

76. Yadav JS, Wholey MH, Kuntz RE, et al. Protected carotid-artery stenting versus endarterectomy in high-risk patients. *N Engl J Med*. 2004; 351:1493-1501.

77. Bandyk DF, Mills JL, Gahtan V, Esses GE. Intraoperative duplex scanning of arterial reconstructions: Fate of repaired and unrepaired defects. *J Vasc Surg*. 1994; 20:426-433.

78. Baker WH, Koustas AG, Burke K, et al. Intraoperative duplex scanning and late carotid artery stenosis. *J Vasc Surg*. 1994; 19:829-833.

79. Kuntz KM, Polak JF, Whittemore AD, et al. Duplex ultrasound criteria for the identification of carotid stenosis should be laboratory specific. *Stroke*. 1997; 28:597-602.

Questions

GENERAL INSTRUCTIONS: For each question, select the best answer. Select only one answer for each question unless otherwise specified.

1. **What is the annual rank of stroke in the United States as a cause of death?**

    (A) 1st with 800,000 deaths

    (B) 2nd with 600,500 deaths

    (C) 3rd with 500,000 deaths

    (D) none of the above

2. **The emphasis of stroke as a national issue is based on which of the following?**

    (A) defining the stroke as ischemic or hemorrhagic

    (B) preventing long-term disability

    (C) deciding which treatment is to be used

    (D) early diagnosis and treatment to prevent long-term disability

3. **Which of the following imaging modalities is the newest technique for early determination of a stroke as hemorrhagic or ischemic?**

    (A) ultrasound of the carotid arteries

    (B) computerized axial tomography (CT)

    (C) magnetic resonance imaging (MRI) diffusion imaging

    (D) digital subtraction arteriography (DSA)

4. **Which of the following best defines stroke?**

    (A) a sudden increase of blood flow to the brain causing syncope

    (B) a sudden increase in blood flow to the brain causing eye damage

    (C) any motor sensory deficit lasting greater than 24 hours

    (D) any motor sensory deficit lasting less than 24 hours

Match the following terms with the correct definition.

5. Transient ischemic attack (TIA) _____

6. Stroke in evolution (SIE) _____

7. Reversible ischemic neurologic deficit (RIND) _____

8. Completed stroke _____

9. Acute brain death _____

    (A) neurologic symptoms that last longer than 24 hours, but completely resolve

    (B) this is caused by either lack of blood supply or effect of blood outside of normal vessels

    (C) ischemic neurologic symptoms that last less than 24 hours and completely resolve

    (D) stable neurologic deficit that had sudden onset and persists longer than 3 weeks

    (E) ischemic neurologic symptoms that actively worsen during a period of observation

10. **Which of the following is currently the major cause of vascular disease?**

    (A) hypertension

    (B) intracerebral hemorrhage

    (C) smoking more than one pack of cigarettes per day

    (D) atherosclerosis

11. **Internal carotid artery symptoms include all of the following *except*?**

    (A) paralysis on the contralateral side

    (B) decreased level of consciousness

    (C) amaurosis fugax

    (D) ataxia

12. **Which of the following is a neurologic symptom related to atherosclerotic disease in the posterior circulation (vertebrobasilar disease)?**

    (A) amaurosis fugax

    (B) contralateral extremity weakness

    (C) orthostatic hypotension

    (D) vertigo

13. Continuous wave (CW) Doppler or pulse wave (PW) Doppler is not used in which of the following?

    (A) periorbital Doppler

    (B) extracranial arteries

    (C) ocular pneumoplethysmography

    (D) transcranial Doppler

14. Ocular pneumoplethysmography (OPG) can be used to detect which of the following?

    (A) hemodynamically significant lesions (greater than 60%)

    (B) for the assessment of collateral circulation

    (C) both A and B

    (D) none of the above

15. Color Doppler units provide which of the following information?

    (A) real-time imaging

    (B) Doppler waveform analysis

    (C) color depiction of the flow characteristics

    (D) all of the above

    (E) both B and C

16. The optimal transducer for high-resolution gray-scale image is obtained by which frequency transducer?

    (A) 2.5 MHz linear array

    (B) 5 MHz curved array

    (C) 5 MHz linear array

    (D) 7.5 MHz linear array

17. Doppler information in the extracranial arterial system is best achieved using which of the following angles?

    (A) 60–70° angle to the artery

    (B) 0° angle to the artery

    (C) 45–60° angle to the artery

    (D) 20–35° angle to the artery

18. Which of the following is the most utilized of the Doppler criteria for estimation of percentage diameter stenosis?

    (A) end diastolic velocity

    (B) peak diastolic velocity divided by end diastolic velocity

    (C) peak systolic velocity

    (D) none of the above

19. What is mandatory when using velocity to represent the Doppler shift?

    (A) angle correction

    (B) high-frequency linear array transducer

    (C) electronic steering of transducer

    (D) both B and C

20. Which of the following is one of the artifacts with pulsed Doppler in a hemodynamically significant stenosis?

    (A) spectral broadening

    (B) turbulence

    (C) aliasing

    (D) both A and B

21. Aliasing occurs when high frequencies exceed the Nyquist limit and may be corrected by which of the following?

    (A) increasing the transducer frequency and increasing the sample volume

    (B) positioning the sample volume deeper by transducer manipulation

    (C) change in probe position, decreasing the depth, increasing the PRF, increasing the Doppler angle or lowering the frequency

    (E) none of the above

22. Which of the following are two advantages of power Doppler?

    (A) extremely sensitive to high flow state of intracranial arteries

    (B) more sensitive frequency shift information

    (C) beneficial in defining occlusive vessels

    (D) is not dependent on beam angle and free from aliasing artifact

    (E) both A and B

    (F) both C and D

Match the following three layers of an artery wall with the correct definition.

23. Media _____   (A) elastic inner layer

24. Adventitia _____   (B) layer of muscle and elastic tissue

25. Intima _____   (C) outer loose filmy layer

26. Which of the following terms best describes variable plaque morphology?

    (A) soft (homogeneous low-level gray echoes)

    (B) dense (highly echogenic)

    (C) calcified (increased echogenicity with acoustic shadowing)

    (D) ulcerated (irregular margins or craters)

    (E) heterogeneous

27. The cerebrovascular vessels arise from which of the following?

    (A) vertebral artery

    (B) costocervical trunk

    (C) internal thoracic

    (D) aortic arch

28. Branches of the subclavian artery include

    (A) vertebral

    (B) internal thoracic

    (C) thyrocervical and costocervical trunk

    (D) dorsal scapular

    (E) all of the above

Match the following to Fig. 12–31.

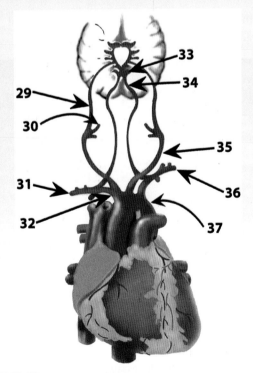

FIGURE 12–31.

29. _____

30. _____

31. _____

32. _____

33. _____

34. _____

35. _____

36. _____

37. _____

    (A) basilar artery

    (B) right external carotid artery

    (C) left subclavian artery

    (D) right common carotid artery

    (E) left vertebral artery

    (F) right subclavian artery

    (G) left common carotid artery

    (H) aortic arch

    (I) brachiocephalic trunk

    (J) right internal carotid artery

38. Which of the following is the most important branch of the carotid system?

    (A) internal carotid artery

    (B) vertebral artery

    (C) common carotid artery

    (D) external carotid artery

Match the following extracranial arteries with the correct spectral analysis description.

39. internal carotid artery _____

40. external carotid artery _____

41. common carotid artery _____

42. carotid bulb _____

    (A) exhibits a complicated turbulent flow pattern

    (B) demonstrates a rapid increase in velocity during systole with a clear window and a continuous antegrade flow during diastole

    (C) combination of the pattern of internal and external carotid arteries

    (D) demonstrates a brisk systolic upstroke, sharp peak, abrupt downstroke

Match the following extracranial waveforms with the proper normal waveform.

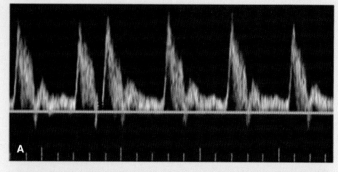

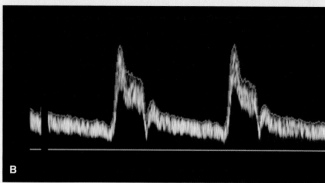

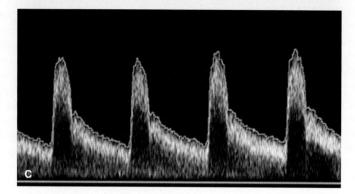

43. external carotid artery _____

44. internal carotid artery _____

45. common carotid artery _____

46. Which of the following radiographic modalities is the method of choice for opacifying the entire cerebral arterial system?

   (A) carotid duplex examination with transcranial Doppler

   (B) computerized axial tomography with contrast

   (C) magnetic resonance imaging with contrast

   (D) digital subtraction angiography

Place the transverse scans of the extracranial carotid arteries in the proper order according to examination protocol.

47. _____   (A) origin of the vertebral artery

48. _____   (B) carotid bifurcation with internal and external carotid arteries

49. _____   (C) common carotid artery

50. _____   (D) carotid bulb

51. _____   (E) brachiocephalic artery and bifurcation of the subclavian and carotid arteries

Place the following longitudinal scans of the extracranial carotid arteries in the proper order according to examination protocol.

52. _____   (A) vertebral artery from origin and as far distal as possible

53. _____   (B) carotid bifurcation (carotid bulb and proximal portion of internal and external carotid arteries)

54. _____   (C) external carotid artery as far distal as possible

55. _____   (D) common carotid artery (from clavicle to mandible)

56. _____   (E) internal carotid artery as far distal as possible

Match the following gray-scale image to the normal extracranial carotid arteries.

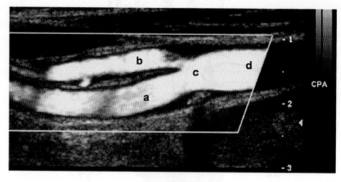

57. _____ external carotid artery.   A

58. _____ internal carotid artery   B

59. _____ common carotid artery.   C

60. _____ carotid bulb   D

61. Which of the following terms is used to describe normal flow in the normal carotid artery?

   (A) laminar

   (B) turbulent

   (C) helical

   (D) parabolic

62. **Which of the following is the first major branch of the internal carotid artery with clinical significance?**

(A) middle cerebral artery

(B) anterior cerebral artery

(C) ophthalmic artery

(D) posterior communicating artery

63. **The internal carotid artery supplies blood to which of the following structures?**

(A) cerebral hemispheres of the brain only

(B) cerebral hemispheres of the brain, eyes and accessory organs, forehead, and part of the nose

(C) posterior portion of the brain and face

(D) none of the above

64. **The external carotid artery supplies blood to which of the following structures?**

(A) cerebellum

(B) scalp, face, and most of the neck

(C) face, eyes, and temporal portion of the brain

(D) all of the above

65. **Which of the following maneuvers will identify that the Doppler signal is coming from the external carotid artery?**

(A) swallowing

(B) compression of the mandibular artery

(C) temporal tapping

(D) none of the above

66. **Which common carotid artery arises directly from the aortic arch?**

(A) the right common carotid artery

(B) the left common carotid artery

(C) the right subclavian artery

(D) the left innominate artery

67. **Nonatheromatous causes of turbulent flow in the carotid arteries may include which of the following?**

(A) sudden increase in the diameter of the vessel

(B) kinking of the internal carotid artery

(C) tortuosity of the internal carotid artery

(D) all of the above

(E) none of the above

68. **An increased resistivity index in the common carotid artery may indicate which of the following?**

(A) stenotic disease proximal to the sample site

(B) stenotic disease distal to the sample site

(C) disease at the sample site

(D) sample volume site placed too close to the arterial wall

69. **Which of the following are factors affecting the Doppler shift frequency?**

(A) Doppler angle

(B) transducer

(C) velocity of the red blood cells

(D) both B and C

(E) A, B, and C

70. **What is the most common site for atherosclerotic plaque formation?**

(A) distal internal carotid artery

(B) distal common carotid artery

(C) carotid bifurcation

(D) vertebral artery origin

71. **Which branch of the internal carotid artery is in the cervical section of the neck?**

(A) ophthalmic

(B) cavernous

(C) posterior communicating

(D) none of the above

72. **The gradual decrease in blood flow due to narrowing does *not* produce symptoms until it reaches the point of "critical stenosis." Which of the following diameter reductions constitute a critical stenosis?**

(A) 20% diameter reduction

(B) 30–45% diameter reduction

(C) 70% diameter reduction ("critical" is a >70% diameter reduction; but hemodynamically significant is >50%?)

(D) 25–30% diameter reduction ("critical" is a <70% diameter reduction; but hemodynamically significant is <50%?)

Identify the following plaque morphology with the
appropriate image.

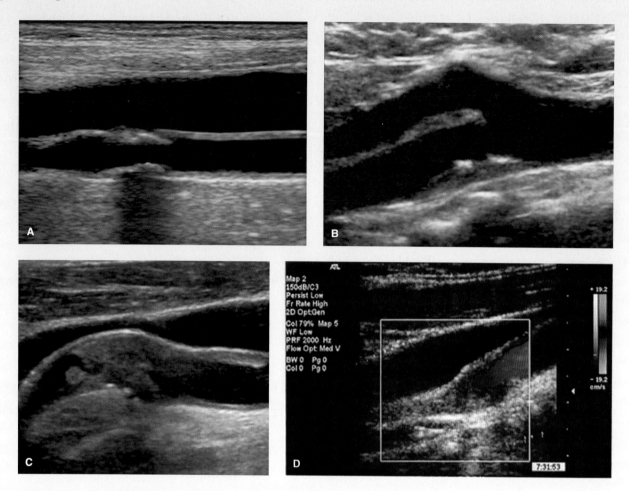

73. soft _____

74. dense _____

75. calcified _____

76. ulcerated _____

77. intraplaque hemorrhage _____

Match the following with the appropriate image:

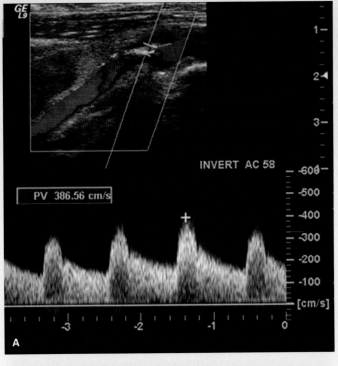

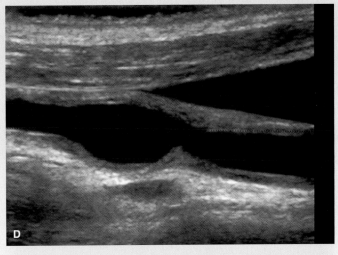

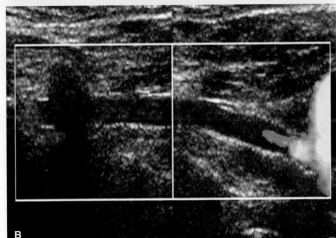

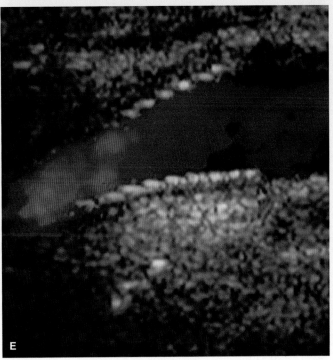

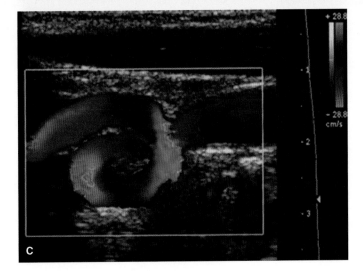

78. critical stenosis _____

79. occlusion of ICA _____

80. reversal of flow in bulb proximal to ICA occlusion _____

81. moderate stenosis by diameter reduction _____

82. mild stenosis by diameter reduction _____

83. **Distal to a critical stenosis, the spectral analysis depicts which of the following characteristics?**

    (A) peak systole velocities decrease

    (B) end diastole velocities decrease

    (C) turbulent flow is present in the spectral analysis

    (D) all of the above

84. **Which of the following best describes carotid body tumors?**

    (A) rare neoplasms

    (B) composed of paraganglionic tissue

    (C) occur only at the carotid bifurcation

    (D) both A and B

    (E) all of the above

85. **Which of the following variations of the extracranial carotid artery is associated with the symptom of ischemia?**

    (A) coiling of the internal carotid artery

    (B) kinking of the internal carotid artery

    (C) tortuosity of the internal carotid artery

    (D) all of the above

86. **According to the North American Symptomatic Carotid Endarterectomy Trial (NASCET), which one of the following is the most common treatment to risk reduction for stroke?**

    (A) identifying and operating on appropriately severe common carotid bifurcation lesions.

    (B) treating all patients with aspirin therapy and perform carotid Doppler exam once a year

    (C) once the stenosis reaches a moderate level, perform the endarterectomy before symptoms occur

    (D) none of the above

Match the following vessels to Fig. 12–32.

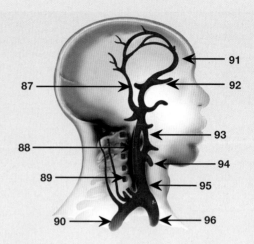

FIGURE 12–32.

87. _____

88. _____

89. _____

90. _____

91. _____

92. _____

93. _____

94. _____

95. _____

96. _____

(A) superficial temporal artery

(B) supraorbital artery

(C) subclavian artery

(D) internal carotid artery

(E) ophthalmic artery

(F) common carotid artery

(G) external carotid artery

(H) superior thyroid artery

(I) brachiocephalic trunk

(J) vertebral artery

97. **Which of the following is *not* a branch of the subclavian?**

    (A) vertebral

    (B) internal thoracic

    (C) thyrocervical trunk

    (D) costocervical trunk

    (E) hypophyseal

98. **The extracranial posterior circulation is composed of which of the following?**

    (A) paired vertebral arteries in the back of the neck

    (B) basilar artery

    (C) brachiocephalic

    (D) both B and C

99. **Subclavian steal syndrome causes which of the following symptoms?**

(A) ataxia

(B) limb paralysis

(C) vertigo

(D) syncope

(E) all of the above

(F) both C and D

100. **Which of the following is the hallmark sign of the subclavian steal syndrome?**

(A) difference of blood pressure (10–20 mm Hg) between the two arms

(B) decreased peripheral pulse in the affected upper extremity

(C) difference of blood pressure (20–30 mm Hg) between the two arms

(D) all of the above

(E) both A and B

(F) both B and C

101. **Which of the following are Doppler waveform characteristics of the subclavian steal syndrome?**

(A) deceleration, reversed, or alternating flow in the contralateral vertebral artery

(B) decreased velocities/frequencies at the site of subclavian stenosis

(C) diminished waveform distal to the stenosis or occlusion

(D) all of the above

(E) both A and C

102. **Which of the following will be depicted in the normal vertebral artery spectral analysis?**

(A) high-resistant flow similar to external carotid artery

(B) monophasic flow

(C) low-resistance waveform pattern similar to the internal carotid artery

(D) none of the above

103. **Normally the vertebrobasilar system provides what percentages of blood flow to intracranial system?**

(A) 40%

(B) 10–20%

(C) 20–30%

(D) none of the above

104. **In which view can the vertebral artery be visualized?**

(A) medial to the jugular

(B) transverse just lateral to the common carotid artery

(C) longitudinal plane at the level of the common carotid with the transducer angled laterally until the vertebral is seen passing through the transverse processes

(D) both A and C

(E) both B and C

105. **When is subclavian steal syndrome asymptomatic?**

(A) when exercising contralateral side

(B) when exercising ipsilateral side

(C) at rest

(D) none of the above

Match the following arteries in Fig. 12–33.

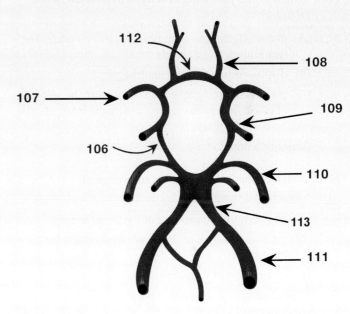

FIGURE 12–33.

106. _____

107. _____

108. _____

109. _____

110. _____

111. _____

112. _____

113. _____

(A) anterior cerebral artery

(B) posterior communicating artery

(C) anterior communicating artery

(D) middle cerebral artery

(E) basilar artery

(F) internal carotid artery

(G) vertebral artery

(H) posterior cerebral artery

114. **Which of the following transducer is required for performing a transcranial Doppler examination?**

    (A) high-frequency continuous-wave transducer

    (B) high-frequency linear array

    (C) low-frequency (2 MHz) transducer

    (D) appropriate computerized software for calculations

    (E) both C and D

115. **Which of the following does the suboccipital window examine?**

    (A) vertebral arteries

    (B) posterior communicating arteries

    (C) basilar artery

    (D) both A and C

    (E) both A and B

116. **Which of the following best describes transcranial Doppler?**

    (A) invasive technique that measures and visualizes the major intracranial vessels

    (B) displays intracerebral hemorrhages

    (C) noninvasive technique used to measure the velocity of blood flow in the major intracranial brain vessels by using Doppler

    (D) both B and C

117. **Which of the following is an advantage of transcranial imaging?**

    (A) observation of narrowing of the vessel lumen

    (B) visual assessment of the transcranial vessels for localization

    (C) observation of vessel tortuosity

    (D) calculation of the vessel lumen

    (E) all of the above

    (F) both B and D

118. **Which of the following arteries is the largest branch of the cerebral internal carotid artery?**

    (A) ophthalmic artery

    (B) middle cerebral artery

    (C) anterior cerebral artery

    (D) all of the above

119. **The middle cerebral artery supplies blood to which of the following lobes?**

    (A) occipital lobe

    (B) frontal lobe

    (C) temporal lobe

    (D) parietal lobe

    (E) A, B, and C

    (F) B, C, and D

120. **The middle cerebral artery is divided into which of the following segments?**

    (A) M1

    (B) M2

    (C) M3

    (D) A-1

    (E) A, B, and C

121. **The posterior communicating artery anastomoses with which of the following arteries?**

    (A) anterior cerebral artery

    (B) posterior cerebral artery

    (C) posterior cerebral artery and middle cerebral artery

    (D) both A and C

122. **The ophthalmic artery forms extensive anastomoses with which of the following arteries?**

    (A) anterior communicating artery

    (B) anterior cerebral artery

    (C) middle cerebral artery

    (D) external carotid artery

123. **The anterior cerebral artery and its branches supply blood to which of the following structures?**

    (A) frontal and parietal lobes

    (B) corpus callosum

    (C) septum pellucidum

    (D) basil ganglia

    (E) anterior limb of the internal capsule

    (F) all of the above

    (G) A, B, and C

124. **The vertebral arteries unite to form which of the following arteries?**

    (A) posterior communicating artery

    (B) posterior cerebral artery

    (C) basilar artery

    (D) both A and C

125. **The various parts of the brainstem are supplied by which of the following arteries?**

    (A) middle cerebral artery

    (B) posterior communicating artery

    (C) basilar artery

    (D) all of the above

126. The basilar artery does not give rise to which one of the following arteries?

    (A) anterior inferior cerebellar artery

    (B) posterior communicating artery

    (C) superior cerebellar artery

    (D) posterior cerebral arteries

127. Which of the following are the anastomotic arteries that are formed by the major cerebral arteries?

    (A) middle cerebral and anterior communicating artery

    (B) vertebral and basilar arteries

    (C) anterior cerebral and anterior communicating arteries

    (D) circle of Willis

    (E) both A and C

Match the following collateral pathway systems that supply blood by existing anastomoses in the brain.

128. right-to-left anastomoses provide redistribution of blood flow between the sides of the body and occur via _____

129. carotid-to-vertebral anastomoses via _____

130. subclavian-to-carotid and subclavian-to-vertebral anastomoses _____

131. ICA-to-ECA ipsilateral anastomoses _____

132. optical anastomoses can provide collateral flow between _____

(A) involve the deep cervical artery, spinal branches of the vertebral arteries, and the ascending cervical artery

(B) superorbital and supratrochlear arteries

(C) anterior communicating and basilar arteries

(D) posterior communicating arteries

(E) anterior cerebral artery, middle cerebral artery, and posterior communicating artery

133. Pulsatility index represents the degree of

    (A) pliability of the artery

    (B) stenosis of the artery

    (C) peripheral resistance

    (D) all of the above

134. A pulsatility index of >1.2 may indicate which of the following findings?

    (A) increased intracranial pressure

    (B) vasospasm

    (C) hypercapnia

    (D) aortic insufficiency

    (E) all of the above

135. Transtemporal window allows insonation of the

    (A) middle cerebral artery (M1–M2 segments)

    (B) anterior cerebral artery

    (C) posterior cerebral artery and C1 segment of the carotid siphon

    (D) distal ICA

    (E) A, B, and C

136. Suboccipital window allows insonation of which of the following?

    (A) carotid siphon (C2, C3, and C4)

    (B) vertebral arteries

    (C) basilar artery

    (D) B and C

    (E) A, B, and C

137. Submandibular window allows insonation of which of the following?

    (A) ophthalmic artery

    (B) carotid siphon

    (C) retromandibular ICA (distal)

    (D) both A and B

138. Transorbital window allows insonation of which of the following?

    (A) ophthalmic artery

    (B) carotid siphon (C2, C3, and C4)

    (C) anterior communicating artery

    (D) both A and B

    (E) all of the above

Match the following acoustic windows with the proper name.

139. transorbital window _____

140. transtemporal window _____

141. transoccipital window _____

142. Each transcranial Doppler examination includes all of the following *except*

(A) color Doppler imaging

(B) spectral waveform analysis with notation of depth, speed, and direction of flow

(C) mean velocity

(D) measurements of all arteries in the circle of Willis

Match the direction of flow for the following vessels.

143. carotid siphon _____

144. ICA bifurcation _____

145. M1 segment of MCA _____

146. vertebral artery _____

147. basilar artery _____

148. ACA _____

149. PCA, P1 segment _____

150. PCA, P2 segment _____

151. ophthalmic artery _____

(A) flow is bidirectional

(B) away from the probe

(C) toward the probe

(D) can flow in any direction

152. **Which of the following will occur with the occlusion or a critical stenosis of the ipsilateral extracranial carotid artery?**

(A) Middle cerebral artery velocity is decreased or absent.

(B) Middle cerebral artery end diastole is increased.

(C) Ophthalmic artery will decrease in flow or may have reverse flow.

(D) Both A and C

(E) Both A and B

153. **Subclavian steal syndrome can be detected in which of the following intracranial vessels?**

(A) cervical vertebrals

(B) intracranial vertebral arteries

(C) basilar artery

(D) all of the above

(E) both B and C

154. **Intracranial vessel stenosis will exhibit which of the following characteristics?**

(A) focal increase in the mean blood flow velocity distal to the stenosis

(B) focal increase in the mean blood flow velocity at the site of the vessel stenosis

(C) color-flow Doppler will show multiple color patterns

(D) all of the above

(E) both A and C

(F) both B and C

155. **Which of the following intracranial vessels is the most common to occlude and is seen with acute stroke?**

(A) basilar artery

(B) anterior cerebral artery

(C) ophthalmic artery

(D) middle cerebral artery

156. **Transcranial color Doppler can be used to examine which of the following conditions?**

(A) brain death

(B) vasospasms

(C) arteriovenous malformations

(D) embolus

(E) all of the above

Answers and Explanations

At the end of each explained answer, there is a number combination in parentheses. The first number identifies the reference source; the second number or set of numbers indicates the page or pages on which the relevant information can be found.

1. **(C)** Stroke is ranked in the United States as the third leading cause of death annually. *(1:561)*

2. **(D)** The emphasis of stroke as a national issue is on early diagnosis and treatment to prevent long-term disability. *(2:491)*

3. **(C)** The newest technique for early determination of a stroke, a hemorrhagic or transient ischemic attack is magnetic resonance imaging diffusion imaging. *(2:491)*

4. **(C)** Any sensory or motor deficit lasting more than 24 hours. *(2:491)*

5. **(C)** Transient ischemic attack is an acute neurologic symptom that lasts less than 24 hours and completely resolves. *(3:107, 108)*

6. **(E)** Stroke in evolution is ischemic symptoms that actively worsen during a period of observation. *(3:107, 108)*

7. **(A)** Reversible ischemic neurologic deficit is a neurologic symptom that lasts longer than 24 hours and completely resolves. *(3:107, 108)*

8. **(D)** Completed stroke is a stable neurologic deficit that had sudden onset and persists longer than 3 weeks. *(3:107, 108)*

9. **(B)** Acute brain death is caused by either lack of blood supply or effect of blood outside of normal vessels. *(3:119, 243)*

10. **(D)** Atherosclerosis is the major cause of vascular disease. *(3:254)*

11. **(D)** Ataxia, also called dystaxia, is a symptom of vertebrobasilar insufficiency, not internal carotid artery symptoms. *(5:173)*

12. **(D)** Vertigo is a neurologic symptom of vertebrobasilar disease. *(5:1227)*

13. **(C)** Ocular pneumoplethysmography is used with pressure cups over the ocular globe. *(Study Guide)*

14. **(C)** Ocular pneumoplethysmography is used to detect hemodynamically significant lesions (>60%) and in the assessment of collateral flow. *(Study Guide)*

15. **(D)** All of the above. Color Doppler units provide real-time imaging, Doppler waveform analysis, and color depiction of the flow characteristics. *(Study Guide)*

16. **(D)** A 7.5 MHz linear array is the optimal transducer for high-resolution gray-scale imaging of the carotid arteries. *(Study Guide)*

17. **(C)** 45–60° angle to the artery gives the best Doppler information. *(Study Guide)*

18. **(C)** Peak systolic velocity is the most utilized of the Doppler criteria for estimation of percentage diameter reduction. *(Study Guide)*

19. **(A)** Angle correction is mandatory when using velocity to represent Doppler shift. *(3:43)*

20. **(C)** Aliasing is an artifact that occurs with pulsed Doppler in a hemodynamically significant stenosis. *(3:48)*

21. **(C)** Change in probe position, decreasing the depth, increasing the pulse repetition frequency, increasing the Doppler angle, or lowering the frequency can correct aliasing. *(3:43, 44)*

22. **(F)** Both C and D. Two advantages of power Doppler are: it is beneficial in defining occlusive vessels and it is not dependent on beam angle and free from aliasing artifact. *(3:45)*

23. **(B)** The arterial layer of muscle and elastic tissue is the media. *(Study Guide)*

24. **(C)** The outer loose filmy layer of the artery wall is the adventitia. *(Study Guide)*

25. **(A)** The elastic inner layer of the artery wall is the intima. *(Study Guide)*

26. **(E)** Variable plaque morphology is described as heterogeneous (inhomogeneous) which sonographically appears as a non-uniform echo texture *(3:162–164)*

27. **(D)** The aortic arch is the vessel from which the cerebrovascular vessels arise. *(3:134)*

28. **(E)** All of the above. The vertebral, internal thoracic, thyrocervical, costocervical, and dorsal scapular all arise from the subclavian artery. *(3:134)*

29. **(J)** Right internal carotid artery. *(Study Guide)*

30. **(B)** Right external carotid artery. *(Study Guide)*

31. **(F)** Right subclavian artery. *(Study Guide)*

32. **(I)** Brachiocephalic trunk. *(Study Guide)*

33. **(A)** Basilar artery. *(Study Guide)*

34. **(E)** Left vertebral artery. (*Study Guide*)

35. **(G)** Left common carotid artery. (*Study Guide*)

36. **(C)** Left subclavian artery. (*Study Guide*)

37. **(H)** Aortic arch. (*Study Guide*)

38. **(C)** The common carotid artery is the main branch of the carotid system. (*3:133–135*)

39. **(B)** The internal carotid artery demonstrates a rapid increase in velocity during systole with a clear window and continuous antegrade flow during diastole. (*3:133–135*)

40. **(D)** The external carotid artery has a brisk systolic upstroke, sharp peak, and abrupt downstroke because it supplies a high-resistance system. (*3:133–135*)

41. **(C)** The common carotid artery combines the pattern of the internal and the external carotid artery. (*3:133–135*)

42. **(A)** The Carotid "bulb" exhibits a complicated turbulent flow pattern. (*Study Guide*)

43. **(B)** External carotid artery. (*3:134*)

44. **(C)** Common carotid artery. (*3:134*)

45. **(A)** Internal carotid artery. (*3:134*)

46. **(D)** Digital subtraction angiography is the radiographic modality that is the method of choice for opacifying the entire cerebral arterial system. (*Study Guide*)

The following are the transverse scans of the extracranial carotid arteries in the proper order according to the examination protocol:

47. **(E)** Brachiocephalic artery and bifurcation of the subclavian and carotid arteries (*3:134*)

48. **(C)** Common carotid artery. (*3:134*)

49. **(D)** Carotid bulb. (*3:134*)

50. **(B)** Carotid bifurcation with internal and external arteries. (*3:134*)

51. **(A)** Origin of the vertebral artery. (*3:134*)

The following longitudinal scan of the extracranial arteries in the proper order according to examination protocol:

52. **(D)** Common carotid artery from clavicle to mandible. (*3:133–136*)

53. **(B)** Carotid bifurcation (carotid bulb and proximal portion of internal and external carotid arteries. (*3:133–136*)

54. **(E)** Internal carotid artery as far distal as possible. (*3:133–136*)

55. **(C)** External carotid artery as far distal as possible. (*3:133–136*)

56. **(A)** Vertebral artery from origin as far distal as possible. (*3:133–136*)

57. **(A)** External carotid artery. (*3:133–136*)

58. **(B)** Internal carotid artery. (*3:133–136*)

59. **(C)** Common carotid artery (*3:133–136*)

60. **(D)** Carotid bulb. (*3:133–136*)

61. **(A)** Laminar flow is the normal flow pattern in the carotid artery. (*3:133–136*)

62. **(C)** Ophthalmic artery is the first major branch of the internal carotid artery with clinical significance. (*3:133–136*)

63. **(B)** Cerebral hemispheres of the brain, eyes and accessory organs, forehead, and part of the nose are supplied by blood from the internal carotid artery. (*3:133–136*)

64. **(B)** Scalp, face, and most of the neck are supplied blood from the external carotid artery. (*3:134*)

65. **(C)** Temporal tapping is the maneuver to identify that the Doppler signal is coming from the external carotid artery. (*3:143, 144*)

66. **(B)** The left common carotid artery. (*3:134*)

67. **(D)** All have the above. Turbulent flow does not necessarily have to be caused by atheromatous plaque. Sudden increase in the diameter of the blood vessel can cause turbulence. This can be seen in the carotid bulb region where the boundary layer separates from the arterial wall with an inherent reversal of flow. Tortuous arteries also can cause turbulence as blood flow is forced to change direction. Carotid kinks can cause turbulence as the arterial lumen is narrowed. (*3:6*)

68. **(B)** An increased resistivity index in the common carotid artery can indicate stenotic or occlusive disease distal to the sample site. Total occlusion of the internal carotid artery can cause a decrease in diastolic flow in the common carotid artery because of increased resistance to flow. (*3:174*)

69. **(E)** Doppler shift frequencies are affected by Doppler angle, transducer frequency, and the velocity of the red blood cells. (*3:43*)

70. **(C)** Carotid bifurcation is the most common site for atherosclerotic plaque formation. (*3:134*)

71. **(D)** None of the above. The internal carotid artery does not have a branch in the cervical section. (*3:134*)

72. **(C)** 50% diameter reduction ("critical" is a >70% diameter reduction; but hemodynamically significant is >50%?) (*3:172*)

Identification of the plaque morphology:

73. **(E)** Soft. *(3:157)*

74. **(C)** Dense. *(3:157)*

75. **(A)** Calcified. *(3:157)*

76. **(B)** Ulcerated. *(3:157)*

77. **(D)** Intraplaque hemorrhage. *(3:157)*

78. **(B)** Critical stenosis. *(3:157)*

79. **(D)** Occlusion of the internal carotid artery. *(3:157)*

80. **(E)** Reversal of flow in bulb proximal to internal carotid artery occlusion. *(3:180)*

81. **(C)** Moderate stenosis by diameter reduction. *(3:180)*

82. **(A)** Mild stenosis by diameter reduction. *(3:180)*

83. **(D)** All of the above. Distal to a critical stenosis, the spectral analysis depicts peak systole velocities decrease, end-diastole velocities decrease, and turbulent flow is seen in the spectral analysis. *(3:174)*

84. **(D)** Carotid body tumors are composed of paraganglionic tissue and are rare neoplasms. *(3:139)*

85. **(B)** Kinking of the internal carotid artery is associated with the symptom of ischemia. *(3:139)*

86. **(A)** Identifying and operating on appropriately severe common carotid bifurcation lesions is the most common treatment to risk reduction for stroke according to NASCET. *(3:135)*

87. **(A)** The superficial temporal artery. *(3:136)*

88. **(D)** The internal carotid artery. *(3:136)*

89. **(J)** The vertebral artery. *(3:136)*

90. **(C)** The subclavian artery. *(3:136)*

91. **(B)** The supraorbital artery. *(3:136)*

92. **(E)** The ophthalmic artery. *(3:136)*

93. **(G)** The external carotid artery. *(3:136)*

94. **(H)** The superior thyroid artery. *(3:136)*

95. **(F)** The common carotid artery. *(3:136)*

96. **(I)** The brachiocephalic trunk. *(3:136)*

97. **(E)** The hypophyseal is not a branch of the subclavian. *(3:136)*

98. **(A)** The extracranial posterior circulation is composed of paired vertebral arteries in the back of the neck. *(3:136)*

99. **(E)** The subclavian steal syndrome causes ataxia, limb paralysis, vertigo, and syncope as symptoms. *(3:12, 113)*

100. **(E)** The hallmark sign of the subclavian steal syndrome is the difference of blood pressure (10–20 mm Hg) between the two arms and decreased peripheral pulse in the affected upper extremity. *(3:12, 113)*

101. **(E)** The Doppler waveform characteristics of the subclavian steal syndrome include deceleration, reversed, or alternating flow in the contralateral vertebral artery and diminished waveform distal to the stenosis or occlusion. *(3:12, 113)*

102. **(C)** The normal vertebral artery spectral analysis will depict low-resistance waveform pattern similar to the internal carotid artery. *(3:148, 149)*

103. **(B)** Normally the vertebrobasilar system provides a 10–20% percentage of blood flow to the intracranial system. *(3:148-149)*

104. **(C)** The vertebral artery can be visualized by the longitudinal plane at the level of the common carotid with the transducer angled laterally until the vertebral is seen passing through the transverse processes. *(3:148, 149)*

105. **(C)** The subclavian steal syndrome is asymptomatic at rest. *(3:12, 113)*

106. **(B)** The posterior communicating artery. *(3:136)*

107. **(D)** The middle cerebral artery. *(3:136)*

108. **(A)** The anterior cerebral artery. *(3:136)*

109. **(F)** The internal carotid artery. *(3:136)*

110. **(H)** The posterior cerebral artery. *(3:136)*

111. **(G)** The vertebral artery. *(3:136)*

112. **(C)** The anterior communicating artery. *(3:136)*

113. **(E)** The basilar artery. *(3:136)*

114. **(E)** The transcranial Doppler examination requires low frequency (2 MHz) and the appropriate software for spectral analysis calculations and computations. *(3:148, 149)*

115. **(D)** The suboccipital window examines vertebral arteries and basilar artery. *(3:134–137)*

116. **(C)** The transcranial Doppler is described as a noninvasive technique to measure the velocity of blood flow in the major intracranial brain vessels by using pulsed-waved Doppler. *(3:246)*

117. **(E)** Transcranial imaging has the advantage of observation of the narrowing of the vessel lumen, visual assessment of the transcranial vessels for localization, observation of vessel tortuosity, and calculation of the vessel lumen. *(3:239–241)*

118. **(B)** The middle cerebral artery is the largest branch of the cerebral internal carotid artery. *(3:133, 134)*

119. **(F)** The middle cerebral artery supplies blood to the frontal lobe, the temporal lobe, and the parietal lobe. *(3:136)*

120. **(E)** The middle cerebral artery is divided into M1, M2, and M3 segments. *(3:136)*

121. **(B)** The posterior communicating artery anastomoses with the posterior cerebral artery. *(3:136)*

122. **(D)** The ophthalmic artery forms extensive anastomoses with the external carotid artery. *(3:136)*

123. **(F)** All of the above. The anterior cerebral artery and its branches supply the frontal and parietal lobes, the corpus callosum, the septum pellucidum, the basil ganglia, and the anterior limb of the internal capsule. *(3:136)*

124. **(C)** The vertebral arteries unite with the basilar artery. *(3:136–138)*

125. **(C)** The basilar artery supplies the various parts of the brainstem. *(3:136–138)*

126. **(B)** The basilar artery does not give rise to the posterior communicating artery. *(3:136–138)*

127. **(D)** The anastomotic arteries that are formed by the major cerebral arteries is the circle of Willis. *(3:136–138)*

128. **(C)** Right-to-left anastomoses provide redistribution of blood flow between the sides of the body and occur via anterior communicating and basilar arteries. *(3:138)*

129. **(D)** Carotid-to-vertebral anastomoses via posterior communicating arteries. *(3:136)*

130. **(A)** Subclavian-to-carotid and subclavian-to-vertebral anastomoses involve the deep cervical artery, spinal branches of the vertebral arteries, and the ascending cervical artery. *(3:136)*

131. **(B)** ICA-to-ECA ipsilateral anastomoses superorbital and supratrochlear arteries. *(3:180)*

132. **(E)** Optical anastomoses can provide collateral flow between anterior cerebral artery, middle cerebral artery, and posterior communicating artery. *(4:1228)*

133. **(C)** Pulsatility index represents the degree of peripheral resistance. *(3:236)*

134. **(E)** A pulsatility index of >1.2 may indicate an increased intracranial pressure, vasospasm, hypercapnia, and aortic insufficiency. *(3:236)*

135. **(E)** Transtemporal window allows insonation of the middle cerebral artery (M1-M2 segments), anterior cerebral artery, and posterior cerebral artery and C1 segment of the carotid siphon. *(3:122, 123)*

136. **(D)** Suboccipital window allows insonation of vertebral arteries and basilar artery. *(3:151, 152)*

137. **(C)** Submandibular window allows insonation of the retromandibular internal carotid artery (distal). *(3:151, 152)*

138. **(D)** Transorbital window allows insonation of ophthalmic artery and carotid siphon (C2, C3, and C4). *(Study Guide)*

139. **(C)** Mean velocity. *(3:151, 152)*

140. **(A)** Color doppler imaging. *(3:151, 152)*

141. **(B)** Spectral waveform analysis with notation of depth, speed, and direction. *(3:151, 152)*

142. **(D)** Measurements of all arteries in the circle of Willis. *(3:151)*

143. **(D)** The carotid siphon can flow in any direction. *(Study Guide)*

144. **(A)** Internal carotid artery bifurcation flow is bidirectional. *(Study Guide)*

145. **(C)** M1 segment of MCA flow is toward the probe. *(Study Guide)*

146. **(B)** Vertebral artery flow is away from the probe. *(3:143–145)*

147. **(B)** Basilar artery flow is away from the probe. *(3:143–145)*

148. **(B)** Anterior cerebral artery (ACA) flow is away from the probe. *(3:143–145)*

149. **(C)** Posterior cerebral artery (PCA), P1 segment flows toward the probe. *(3:143–145)*

150. **(B)** PCA, P2 segment flow is away from the probe. *(3:143–145)*

151. **(C)** Ophthalmic artery flow is toward the probe. *(3:143–145)*

152. **(D)** With the occlusion or a critical stenosis of the ipsilateral extracranial carotid artery, the middle cerebral artery velocity is decreased or absent, and ophthalmic artery will decrease in flow or may have reverse flow. *(3:143–145)*

153. **(E)** Subclavian steal syndrome can be detected in intracranial vessels of the intracranial vertebral arteries and basilar artery. *(3:12, 113)*

154. **(F)** Intracranial vessel stenosis will exhibit characteristics of focal increase in the mean blood flow velocity at the site of the stenosis and color-flow Doppler will show multiple color patterns. *(4:1533)*

155. **(D)** The middle cerebral artery is the most common intracranial vessel to occlude and is seen with acute stroke. *(4:1522)*

156. **(E)** All of the above. Transcranial color Doppler can be used to examine conditions of brain death, vasospasms, arteriovenous malformations, and embolus. *(3:119–243)*

References

1. AbuRahma FA, Bergam JJ. *Noninvasive Vascular Diagnosis: A Practical Guide to Therapy.* 2nd ed. New York : Springer-Verlag; 2006.

2. Hof PR, Mobbs CV. *Handbook of Neurobiology of Aging.* Philadelphia, PA: Elsevier Health Sciences; 2009.

3. Zwiebel WJ, Pellerito JS. *Introduction to Vascular Ultrasonography.* 5th ed. Philadelphia, PA: Elsevier Saunders; 2005.

4. Brunicardi CF. *Schwartz's Principles of Surgery.* 9th ed. New York: McGraw Hill; 2010.

5. *Dorland's Illustrated Medical Dictionary.* 31st ed. Philadelphia, PA: Elsevier Health Sciences; 2010.

13

Sonography of the Peripheral Veins

George L. Berdejo, Joshua Cruz, and Evan C. Lipsitz

Study Guide

ANATOMY OF BLOOD VESSELS[1–8]

Blood vessels act as the conduits through which blood is pumped by the heart. The vessels fall naturally into three general categories:

1. Arteries are vessels that convey blood **away from the heart** and toward the tissues. According to size and structure, large, medium, and small arteries (arterioles) are recognized. A transition vessel between arteries and capillaries is formed by the meta-arteriole. Because of the content of smooth muscle in their walls, medium and smaller arteries play an important role in the regulation of blood pressure and blood flow.

2. The capillaries permeate the body organs and tissues and act as the vehicles for exchange of materials between blood and cells.

3. Veins convey blood from the tissues and **toward the heart**. They act as volume conduits rather than pressure vessels.

Capillaries

Capillaries are composed of an endothelial tube supported by a few reticular fibers. They measure about 7–9 microns in diameter and are the most numerous of the body's blood vessels. There are quite literally miles of capillaries in the body, and they present a very large surface area to the flow of blood. Because of their extreme thinness, capillaries serve as the vessels through which exchange of materials between cells and blood occurs. The large surface area of the capillaries ensures a slow flow of blood through vessels, permitting time for exchanges to occur.

Venules, or small veins, drain the capillary beds. These vessels typically have two layers of tissue in their walls: endothelium and a surrounding layer of collagenous connective tissue. Medium-sized veins acquire a thin media containing scattered smooth muscle cells and a prominent adventitia. Large veins are almost always adventitia. Veins have little pressure to withstand and are easily collapsed. Veins of the arms, legs, and viscera are provided with valves to ensure blood flow toward the heart. Medium and large vessels of both types possess a system of blood vessels that nourish the tissue in their walls. These constitute the vasa vasorum: literally blood vessels to blood vessels.

Vessel Walls

The vessels of the arterial and venous systems are basically tubes. The largest of these tubes have walls composed of three layers, or coats. The walls of the next largest consist of two of these coats. The walls of the smallest vessel consist of only one coat that is so thin that it is composed of a single layer of cells. The layers are given the same names in both the arterial and the venous system, but their size, strength, and composition are somewhat different.

The outermost layer of the vessel wall is called the tunica adventitia. *Tunica* is the Latin word for coat; *adventitia* is Latin for extraneous or coming from abroad. Although *tunica adventitia* is the form most commonly used to describe the outside layer, some anatomy books use the term *tunica externa*.

We are accustomed to thinking of blood vessels as conduits that carry blood to or away from other structures. However, blood vessels are composed of living tissue, so they also require nourishment. The adventitia of both veins and arteries is nourished by minute vessels called vasa vasorum.

The middle of the vessel wall consists of a layer called the tunica media. The name of this layer is easy to remember. It comes from the same Latin root as the word *medium*, which

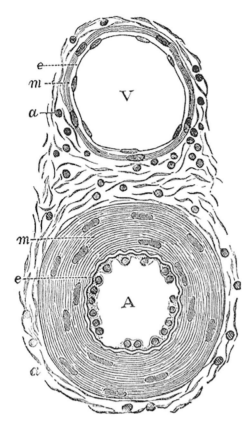

FIGURE 13–1. Cross sectional image of a vein and artery. Note the differences in the 3 layers of the vessel walls.

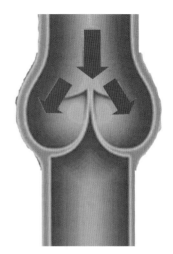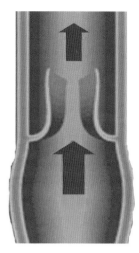

FIGURE 13–2. Vein valve closed (left). Vein valve open (right).

means in the middle. The innermost layer of a blood vessel is called the tunica intima, coming from the Latin word for *within*.

Although the three layers of the venous walls have the same names as those of the arteries, there are some differences in structure. In a vein, the adventitia is considerably thinner and much less strong. The tunica media of veins is also much thinner and weaker than the arterial media, and it contains far less elastic tissue. This makes sense, as arteries must withstand the pulsations of the heart, while veins are usually non-pulsatile and need less elasticity (Fig. 13–1).

The venous and the arterial tunica intima consists of a single-celled endothelium. However, the major difference between the venous and the arterial tunica intima is the presence of vein valves.

The most significant feature of venous structure is the presence of bicuspid valves (Fig. 13–2). These valves are oriented to permit blood to flow in a cephalad direction only. When functioning properly, they do not allow retrograde flow down the leg. Valves in the perforating veins direct blood from the superficial to the deep system only. Just cephalad to and surrounding the valve cusps, the vein is dilated to form a small sinus. This aids the function of the valve by facilitating their closure. Without the dilated area, the valves when open would be closed approximated to the venous wall. Because blood flow at the base of the

valve cusp is relatively stagnant, venous thrombi tend to form in the valve sinuses. Valves are much more numerous in the veins below the knee than in the more proximal veins. The vena cava and the common iliac veins have no valves. Only about one-fourth of the external iliac veins contain a valve and about three-fourths of the femoral veins have a valve. One to four valves are present in the superficial femoral vein, one to three in the popliteal, about seven in the peroneal, and nine in the anterior and posterior tibial veins. A valve is constantly present in the profunda femoris vein just before it joins the femoral vein to form the common femoral vein. Within the terminal 2–3 cm of the great saphenous vein, there are one or two valves. The remainder of this vein contains 10–20 valves, most of which are below the knee. The small saphenous vein has 6–12 valves.

VENOUS ANATOMY

The veins are the back half of the closed loop circulatory system. Blood flows through the veins toward the heart and that is how we will trace the course of each system of the venous circulation, starting with the periphery and working back toward the heart. As veins join with other veins, they get bigger.

In discussing the venous portion of the peripheral systemic circulation, we will deal with three different groups or systems: the deep veins, the superficial veins, and the perforating or communicating veins (Fig. 13–3).

Deep Veins

The deep veins are so called because of where they are in relation to skin and muscle. All veins lie under the skin, but some veins are more deeply situated than others. The deep veins are those that lie under both skin and fascia. The major deep veins are analogs of the corresponding arteries.

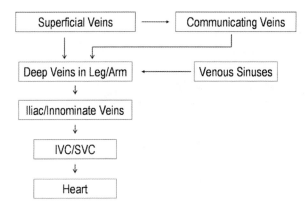

FIGURE 13-3. Venous flow pattern in the lower extremity.

In the extremities, deep veins are surrounded by muscle, a fact that is important to the flow of venous blood. Deep veins of the body lie next to the major arteries and almost always share their names. There are four exceptions to the arterial/deep venous similarity and three of them occur more or less as a group in the upper half of the body. There are two exceptions in name and two in number. The two name exceptions are the internal jugular vein/common carotid artery equivalent and the vena cava/aorta equivalent. Number exceptions are one innominate artery versus two innominate veins and one infrapopliteal artery on each side versus two or more infrapopliteal veins (Fig. 13–4).

Anatomy of the Upper Extremity. Blood returning from the digital or finger veins empties into a venous network in the hand called the palmar arch. Just as in the arterial system, there is both a deep and a superficial arch in the hand and these unite to form the beginning of the radial and ulnar veins of the forearm.

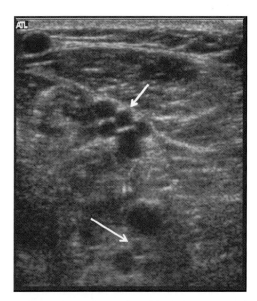

FIGURE 13-4. Transverse sonogram of the tibial veins. White arrows pointing to arteries with adjacent deep veins.

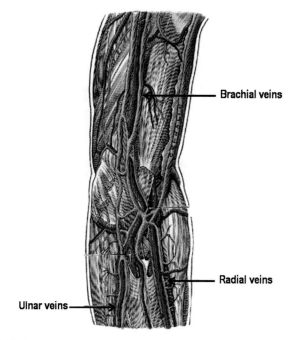

FIGURE 13-5. Deep venous anatomy of the upper and lower arm.

The radial (thumb side) and ulnar (pinky side) veins move proximally in the forearm next to the arteries and they generally join in the area just below the antecubital fossa to form the brachial vein (Fig. 13–5). The brachial vein has no superficial component, and therefore, some anatomists consider it to be the first of the true deep veins of the upper extremity. It courses up the arm beside the brachial artery gradually increasing in size as it goes along.

Where the brachial vein enters the axilla or armpit, it takes on the name of its new location and becomes the axillary vein (Fig. 13–6). As it emerges from the axilla and crosses the outer border of the first rib, it is called the subclavian vein. The subclavian vein courses underneath the clavicle to the base of the neck where the first of the artery/deep venous exceptions is encountered.

In the arterial circulation, there is a vessel on each side of the neck called the common carotid artery. In the deep venous circulation, there is no carotid vein to correspond with that artery. Instead, the right and left internal jugular veins run alongside the carotid arteries. On the right side, the right subclavian vein joins the right internal jugular vein to form the right innominate vein. On the left side where there is no equivalent innominate artery however, the left subclavian and left internal jugular veins form the left innominate vein. The right and left innominate veins anastomose to form the third of the arterial deep venous exceptions, the superior vena cava (Fig. 13–7).

The two venae cavae are the venous equivalent of the aorta. Just as all blood supplied by the arterial system comes from the heart by way of the aorta, all blood drained by the venous system returns to the heart by way of the vena cava. The superior vena cava, which is formed by the anastomosis of the two

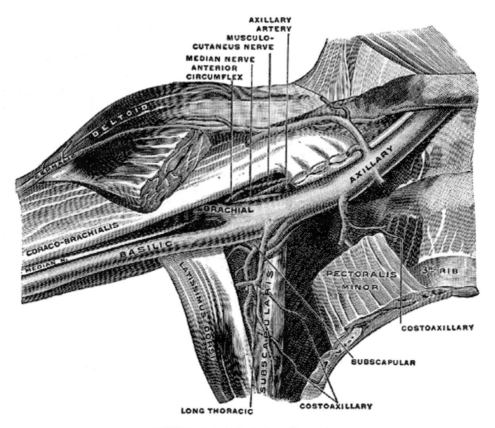

FIGURE 13-6. Veins in the axillary region.

innominate veins, is the larger of the two. The inferior vena cava, which drains the abdomen, will be discussed later. The superior vena cava is so named because it receives the venous return from the upper portion of the body (head, neck, thorax, and upper extremities) and is situated above or superior to the heart. The plural form, venae cavae, is generally used in speaking of the superior and inferior venae cavae together.

Anatomy of the Lower Extremity. To find the last arterial/ deep venous exception, it is necessary to go to the distal lower extremity in the calf. In the foot, a deep and superficial arch structures receive venous drainage from the toes. At the ankle, we find the first of the exclusively deep veins. Just as in the arterial circulation, the leg contains anterior tibial, posterior tibial, and peroneal veins, but the arterial system has only one of each. The venous system has several of each; two, occasionally three, and sometimes four anterior tibial, posterior tibial, and peroneal veins may be found in the leg in normal individuals. This multiplicity of named deep veins in the leg contributes to the difficulty of assessing small deep venous thromboses in this area. These veins move proximally along the leg next to the arteries whose names they share. Large spindle-shaped veins called soleal sinusoids collect the venous drainage from the soleus muscle and terminate in the posterior and peroneal veins. The veins draining the gastrocnemius muscle are tributaries of the popliteal vein. These large muscular sinusoids are important physiologically because they act as the principal bellows of

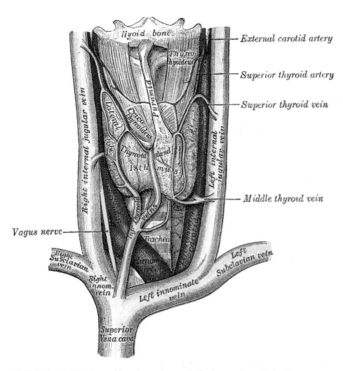

FIGURE 13-7. Internal jugular veins, subclavian and central veins.

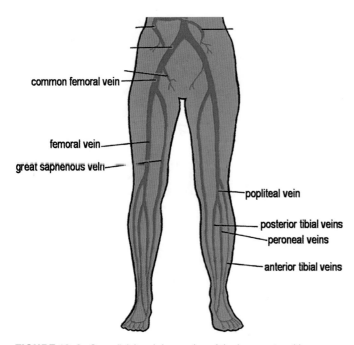

FIGURE 13-8. Superficial and deep veins of the lower extremities.

the muscle pump and pathologically because they are a favored site for the formation of thrombus (Fig. 13–8).

The joining of the leg veins is similar to the division of the infrapopliteal arteries. The popliteal artery first divides to form the anterior tibial artery and then the tibial peroneal trunk, which then divides to become the posterior tibial and peroneal arteries. In the venous system, the posterior tibial and peroneal veins come together first and are then joined by the anterior tibial veins. All these veins join to form the popliteal vein (Fig. 13–8).

The popliteal vein leaves the fossa and enters the thigh as the femoral vein. The femoral vein is a deep vein. It runs through the adductor canal along the medial side of the superficial femoral artery. As the femoral vein moves proximally, it joins the profunda or deep femoral vein and enters the region of the groin. There, it becomes the common femoral vein. The femoral vein in the thigh and the common femoral vein are always situated medial to the superficial femoral and common femoral arteries (Fig. 13–8).

Moving proximally to the level of the inguinal ligament, the common femoral vein becomes the external iliac vein. It then joins with the internal iliac or hypogastric vein to become the common iliac vein. Finally, at the level of the umbilicus, the right and left common iliac veins anastomose to form the beginning of the inferior vena cava (Fig. 13–9).

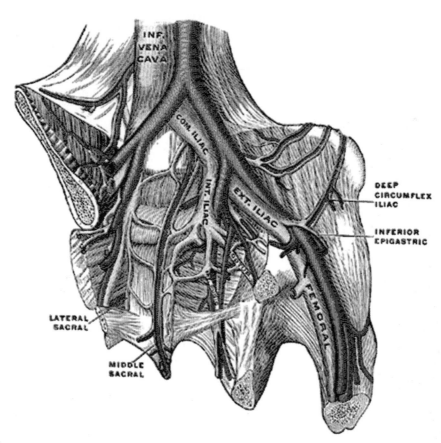

FIGURE 13-9. Demonstrating the anatomy of the venous system in the pelvis and lower abdomen.

The inferior vena cava and the abdominal aorta are paired vessels, both of which arise from paired vessels at their distal margins; however, there is only so much room in which the six major vessels can exist. The right common iliac artery actually lies atop the left common iliac vein so that the inferior vena cava and the aorta can lie side-by-side (Fig. 13–9). This position sometimes causes compression of the left common iliac vein (May Thurner syndrome) and may occasionally be a factor in certain noninvasive tests of the lower extremity.

The inferior vena cava moves proximally through the abdomen gathering returned blood from different visceral and pelvic veins. As it reaches the level of the heart, it joins with the superior vena cava to empty all the returning venous blood into the right atrium where it begins the circulatory cycle all over again.

Superficial Veins

The superficial veins are those that are located under the skin, but above the fascia. These veins can sometimes be seen beneath the skin, especially if they become distended as varicose veins.

Upper Extremities. In the hand, as already mentioned, there are superficial as well as deep venous structures called palmar arches. In the forearm, the superficial veins form a complex network spreading out over the circumference of the limb. In the arm, these four arm veins join to form two larger superficial veins.

The superficial veins running along the lateral aspect of the arm are called the cephalic veins, while those in the medial aspect are called the basilic veins. The pattern of distribution for the superficial veins of the upper extremity is different for each person and can differ from one side to the other in the same individual. The main trunk of the cephalic vein empties into the subclavian vein and the main trunk of the basilic veins empty into the deep venous system via the axillary; however, both these terminations can be variable (Fig. 13–10).

Lower Extremities. The lower extremity also has two sets of superficial veins. Starting posterior to the lateral malleolus and running along the posterior aspect of the leg are the veins that form the small saphenous network. The posterior lateral and posterior branches of the small saphenous vein join, then move deep into the interior of the leg by perforating the fascia at the upper third of the calf. The small saphenous network empties into the popliteal vein usually at the middle portion of the popliteal fossa; however, this can vary and sometimes occurs well above the knee (Fig. 13–11).

Beginning again at the dorsum of the foot, but this time anterior to the medial malleolus is the great saphenous vein. This superficial vein is an extremely important one, especially in surgery where it is used as material for bypass grafts (lower extremity or coronary). Its branches or tributaries extend over the anterior medial and lateral aspects of the limb, but the course of its main trunk is reasonably well defined. After its origin in the foot, the great saphenous vein passes superiorly along the medial aspect of the leg. In the area of the knee, it swings

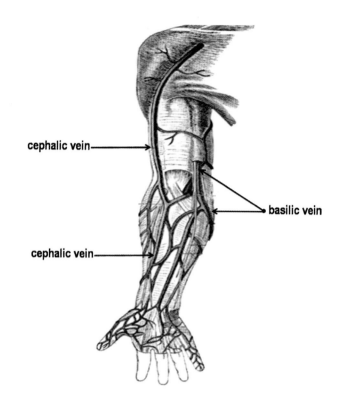

FIGURE 13–10. Demonstrating superficial veins of the arm and forearm.

toward the back of the limb. The great saphenous network connects with the deep venous system a few centimeters below the inguinal ligament. Like the small saphenous network, it must penetrate the fascia to reach the deep veins (Fig. 13–11). The greater saphenous vein is the longest vein in the body.

Draining into the saphenous veins are numerous tributaries, which lie more superficially in the subcutaneous tissue. One of these veins, the posterior arch vein, deserves special mention because it represents the superficial connection of the three ankle perforating veins, which are of major importance in the genesis of venous stasis ulceration. The posterior arch vein begins behind the medial malleolus and passes up the medial aspect of the calf to enter the great saphenous vein at the knee level. The confluence of the cephalad end of the great saphenous vein with the deep venous system is called the saphenofemoral junction. This junction is very important, as a thrombus in the greater saphenous vein may propagate into the deep venous system by means of the saphenofemoral junction.

In addition to their depths, the deep and superficial veins differ in another way, especially in the lower limbs. The walls of the saphenous veins are somewhat stronger than those of the deep veins in the leg. This makes sense when you consider their relative position. The deep veins are buried within the muscle masses of the lower limbs under the fascial layer and they are supported by these structures. The superficial veins have only a thin covering of skin for protection and support. However, the strength of the saphenous veins is limited; they cannot carry large amounts of blood at any one time.

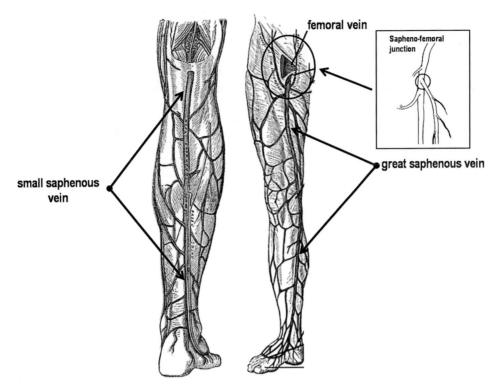

FIGURE 13–11. Small saphenous vein and tributaries. Great saphenous vein and branches. *(Reprinted with permission from Gray H. In: Goss CM, ed. Anatomy of the Human Body. Philadelphia: Lea & Febiger; 1973: 717,718.)*

Perforating Veins

Connecting the deep and superficial systems is a series of perforating or communicating veins. These perforating veins allow blood in the superficial veins to remain at manageable levels. These veins penetrate the fascia, hence, the name perforating. In the thigh, there is a constant perforating vein known as the Hunterian perforator that connects the femoral vein to the greater saphenous vein. More numerous and more important are the perforating veins in the calf.

When functioning properly, valves in the perforating or communicating veins direct the flow from the superficial veins toward the deep system only (Fig. 13–12).

NORMAL VENOUS HEMODYNAMICS[9,10]

In order to understand the changes that occur with disease, a general understanding of normal venous hemodynamics needs to be achieved. The pressure within any blood vessel is a result of, in part, the dynamic pressure produced by the contraction of the left ventricle. Unlike the arterial system, this component in the venous system is relatively low, around 15–20 mm Hg in the venules and 0–6 mm Hg in the right atrium. In any position other than horizontal, hydrostatic pressure plays a major role in determining the pressure within the veins. Hydrostatic pressure is due to the weight of the column of blood within the vessel.

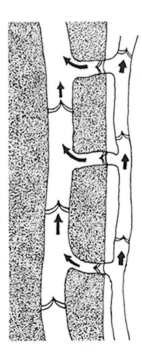

FIGURE 13–12. Venous flow pattern. Superficial to deep veins via the perforators.

Hydrostatic pressure is equal to the density of the blood multiplied by the acceleration due to gravity multiplied by the height of the column of blood. In the human body, the level of the right atrium is used as the reference point by which to measure hydrostatic pressure. When supine, the arteries and veins are all approximately the same height as the heart. Therefore, the hydrostatic pressure is negligible and the pressure will approximate the dynamic pressure. The pressure within the veins at the level of the ankle is about 15 mm Hg. When standing, an individual who is approximately 6 feet tall will add a hydrostatic pressure of 102 mm Hg at the ankle level (Fig. 13–13).

Because veins are collapsible tubes, their shape is determined by transmural pressure. Transmural pressure is equal to the difference between the pressure within the vein and the tissue pressure. At low transmural pressures (when a person is supine), a vein will assume a dumbbell shape. As the pressure within a vein increases, the vein will become elliptical. At high transmural pressures (while standing), the vein will become circular. As venous transmural pressure is increased from 0 to 15 mm Hg, the volume of the vein may increase by more than 250%. A small increase in pressure is required to change an elliptical vein into a high volume circular vein; however, a significant increase in pressure is required to stretch the venous wall once the vein has assumed a circular configuration.[8–10]

VENOUS PRESSURE AND FLOW

The first characteristic we associate with arterial flow is pulsatility; however, the direct influence of the pulsating heart on the venous system is minimal. Most veins do not yield pulsatile flow, but there are two full and one partial exceptions to that rule. Because of the proximity to the heart, the internal jugular vein and subclavian vein are normally pulsatile. The axillary vein may or may not be pulsatile depending on the individual. Pulsatility in the axillary vein is not considered abnormal but rather an individual variation. Non-pulsatility is normal in all but the great veins. The characteristic of flow typical of veins is called phasicity.

The term phasicity in reference to the venous system refers to the ebb and flow that occurs in normal veins in response to respiration. All deep veins normally exhibit phasicity, even those that are somewhat pulsatile. Respiration has this ebb-and-flow influence because unlike the strong-walled arteries, veins are collapsible.

The two phases of respiration are inspiration (breathing in) and expiration (breathing out). The way in which the blood moves in phase with respiration differs according to the part of the body affected and the position in which the body is placed.

When a body is standing upright, breathing produces pressure gradients that influence the movement of venous blood. As the lungs fill with air during inspiration, the thoracic cavity expands. When the thorax expands, the diaphragm drops, and consequently the abdominal cavity becomes smaller. The veins located within the chest and abdomen are affected by these changes in pressure. As the thoracic cavity gets larger, pressure within it decreases and pressure within the right atrium and the thoracic portion of the vena cava is also reduced. At the same time, the abdominal cavity is getting smaller, raising the pressure within the abdomen and the abdominal veins.

Fluids move from areas of high pressure to areas of low pressure. During inspiration, the result is collapse of the inferior vena cava and decreased or no flow from the lower extremities. With expiration, the process reverses itself; the intra-abdominal pressure decreases and the intrathoracic pressure increases, resulting in increasing venous blood flow to the heart from the lower extremities and in general decreased flow from the upper extremities.[8,9]

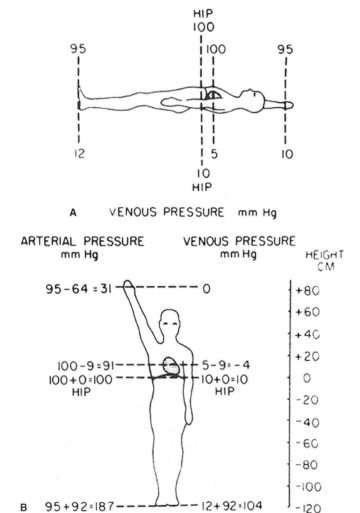

FIGURE 13–13. Graph showing changes in venous pressure caused by changes in body position. *(Reprinted with permission from Strandness DE. Sumner DS.* Hemodynamics for Surgeons. *New York: Grune & Stratton; 1975: 123.)*

Venous Return from the Upper Extremities

Respiration affects venous return from the upper extremities, but to a lesser extent than it affects the lower body. Again, phasicity in the upper extremity veins also can vary according to circumstances. In the brachial vein for instance, inspiration may produce either a reduced or an increased sound. If the lowered or negative intrathoracic pressure causes more blood to move from the brachial vein to the subclavian vein, flow from the brachial vein will increase. Sometimes, however, expansion of the lungs on inspiration will physically compress the subclavian vein. When this happens, less venous blood will move from the chest into the arms and the sound on the brachial vein will diminish. From a clinical standpoint, this is important in that phasic changes should be detectable in all deep veins in relation to breathing.

Venous Return from the Lower Extremities

In the presence of a deep venous thrombosis, venous pressure is increased due to an increase in venous resistance. The change in venous resistance will depend on the location of the obstructed venous segment, the length of the obstruction, and the number of veins involved. Oscillations in the venous flow from the leg may be reduced or absent and flow may become continuous.

Edema is a consistent sign of increased venous pressure. The Starling equilibrium equation describes the movement of fluid across the capillary. Forces that act to move fluid out of the capillary are the intracapillary pressure and the interstitial osmotic pressure. Forces that favor the reabsorption of fluid from the interstitium are the interstitial pressure and the capillary osmotic pressure. Normally, the forces are balanced so that there is little overall fluid loss out of the vascular space into the interstitial space. While standing, the increased capillary pressure is no longer balanced by the reabsorptive forces and fluid loss from the vascular system occurs. Edema formation is limited by the action of the muscle of the calf muscle pump. Contraction of the calf muscles acts to empty the veins and decrease venous pressure. In the presence of venous thrombosis, venous pressure is increased. This increased venous pressure will be transmitted back through the vascular system to the capillary level resulting in increased capillary pressure which will lead to edema formation. Use of compression stockings will decrease interstitial pressure, which will favor increased fluid reabsorption. This decreases edema formation. Elevating the legs will reduce the intracapillary pressure by reducing the hydrostatic pressure, which will also limit edema formation.[8]

VENOUS DYNAMICS WITH EXERCISE

The calf muscle pump aids in the return of blood from the legs against the force of gravity. The muscles act as the power source. The intramuscular sinusoids (especially the gastrocnemius and soleus) and the deep and superficial veins all play a part in this mechanism. The valves are necessary to ensure efficient action of the muscle pump. Closure of the valves in the deep veins decreases the length of the column of blood, which aids in reducing venous pressure. At rest, blood pools in the leg and it is only propelled passively by the dynamic pressure gradient created by the contraction of the left ventricle. Contraction of the calf muscles can generate pressures >200 mm Hg. This compresses the veins forcing blood upward in both the deep and superficial veins. The valves are closed in the perforating veins and in the veins in the distal calf to prevent reflux of blood. Upon relaxation, since these veins in the calf are empty, blood is drawn into this area from the superficial veins via perforators. More distal veins also help fill the calf veins upon relaxation.[8,10]

VENOUS RESISTANCE

When distended, the cross-sectional area of the vein is about three to four times that of the corresponding arteries. It is not surprising then that the extrapulmonary veins contain about two-thirds of the blood in the body. Nevertheless, it is somewhat surprising that despite their large diameter, veins offer about the same resistance to flow as arteries. This is explained by the collapsible nature of the vein walls. Veins are seldom completely full. In the partially empty state, they assume a flattened or elliptical cross-section, which offers a great deal more resistance to blood flow than a circular cross-section. The ability to go from an elliptical to a circular cross-section is distinctly advantageous. It permits the veins to accommodate a great increase in blood flow without an increase in the pressure gradient from the periphery to the heart. In other words, as the rate of flow increases, the vein becomes more circular, lessening resistance.

DEEP VEIN THROMBOSIS: MECHANISMS OF DISEASE AND PATHOLOGY

Etiology, Pathology, and Pathophysiology of Deep Vein Thrombosis[11]

Venous obstruction is almost always the result of venous thrombosis. Less frequently, extrinsic compression may lead to total obstruction, such as on the subclavian vein, sometimes due to a thoracic outlet issue, although this is rare. This is sometimes referred to as effort thrombosis or Paget–Schroetter syndrome[12,13] (Fig. 13–14). Compression can also occur in the area of the left common iliac vein (May Thurner syndrome[14,15]). Deep vein thrombosis in the lower limbs is a relatively common condition and is particularly important because of the risk of pulmonary embolism. In the past, it was thought that deep venous thrombosis inevitably caused chronic edema, hyperpigmentation, and other changes of chronic venous insufficiency. Now, it is well known that approximately one-third of thrombi will lyse quickly. In vein segments that experience total lysis within 3–5 days, valvular function is often maintained.[16] Because of the risk for pulmonary embolization, urgent diagnosis is made

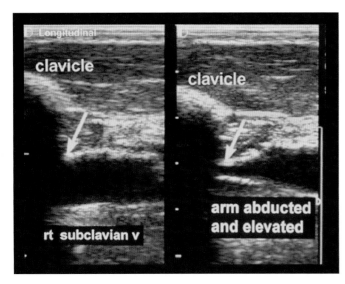

FIGURE 13–14. Sonograms demonstrating normal subclavian vein on the left image and compression with abduction of upper extremity on right image.

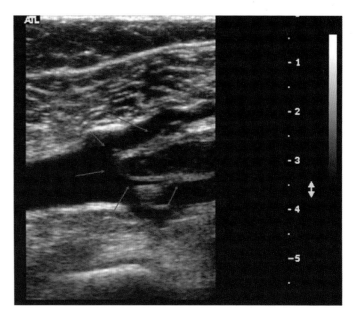

FIGURE 13–15. Sonogram with red arrows demonstrating thrombus within the lumen of a vein.

by imaging techniques and treatment is by immediate anticoagulation. Acute anticoagulation is achieved with heparin and chronic anticoagulation with warfarin. Thrombolytic therapy may be used in special clinical situations.[17–23]

Deep vein thrombi can vary from a few millimeters in length to long tubular masses that fill the main veins. They can form in veins >1 or 2 mm in diameter and generally in large or medium sized vessels. Thrombi begin as microscopic nidi, and then grow by an additive process and become visible. Small thrombi are commonly found in valve pockets throughout various deep veins of the leg and thigh and in saccules of soleal veins. It is from these that the long tubular structures grow. Initially, there is propagation in the direction of the venous stream by deposition of successive layers of thrombus coagulum from the blood, the primary microscopic nidus thus becomes visible. Additional further layers, both longitudinally and circumferentially, increase the length and diameter of the thrombus. Such thrombi at first are attached to the vein only at their points of origin and float almost freely in the blood system (Fig. 13–15). If further propagation occurs, venous obstruction may result and this often leads to retrograde thrombosis back to the next patent vessel.[24,25]

Pathophysiology of Calf Vein Thrombosis. Despite observations that most thrombi begin in the calf and that proximal thrombi are often an extension of calf vein thrombosis, limited data suggest that there are pathophysiological differences between proximal and isolated calf vein thrombosis. Patients with isolated calf vein thrombosis have fewer risk factors and a lower incidence of malignancy. Among 499 patients with an acute deep vein thrombosis, those with calf vein thrombosis had a median of one risk factor in comparison to two risk factors in those with proximal thrombosis.[16] Consistent with these observations, patients with isolated vein thrombosis appear to

be less hypercoagulable. Such data suggest the isolated calf vein thrombi are not simply early thrombi that have yet to propagate but rather reflect a more limited prothrombotic state.

Incidence of Deep Vein Thrombosis[26,27]

Clinically recognized acute deep vein thrombosis has been estimated to have an incidence of up to 250,000–300,000 new cases per year in the United States. A number of studies have focused specifically on the epidemiology of venous thromboembolism (VTE). In these studies, involving predominantly Caucasian populations, the incidence of first-time symptomatic VTE directly standardized for age and sex to the U.S. population ranged from 71 to 117 cases per 100,000 population.[27–32]

Based on potential differences in the incidence of acute and chronic complications, these episodes are commonly defined as involving the proximal lower extremity veins, extending from the popliteal to the iliac vein confluence or isolated to the calf veins. Isolated calf vein thrombosis may involve the peroneal, posterior tibial or anterior tibial veins, the gastrocnemius veins, or the soleal veins. Although lower extremity deep vein thrombosis is thought to usually originate in the calf veins, most *symptomatic* thromboses involve the proximal veins. The incidence of isolated calf vein thrombosis has varied among series but has rarely been insignificant. As many as one-third of thrombi detected by duplex ultrasonography are isolated to the calf veins.[16]

Risk Factors

Patient's with one or more elements of Virchow's triad (Table 13–1) are susceptible to thrombosis.[33–35] Most cases arise during the course of another illness and a connection with

TABLE 13–1 • Virchow's Triad

Virchow's triad can be summarized as follows:

- Venous stasis
  - More time for clotting
  - Small clots not washed away
  - Increased blood viscosity
- Vessel wall damage
  - Accidental trauma
  - Surgical trauma
- Blood coagulability increase
  - Increase in tissue factor
  - Presence of activated factors
  - Decrease in coagulation inhibitors (antithrombin III [ATIII])

confinement to bed and advancing age has been known for a long time. Post-trauma, orthopedic, gynecologic, obstetric, and surgical patients are at risk, but many medical patients such as those with heart attacks, congestive heart failure, acute strokes, and paraplegia are as well. Additionally, deep vein thrombosis occurs as a primary state in healthy ambulatory men and women without apparent cause, and it is now recognized as a hazard in patients taking therapeutic estrogen and in women taking oral contraceptives. Other recognized predisposing factors are obesity and previous thrombosis (Table 13–2).

Isolated iliac vein thrombosis is thought to be rare. However, it is well known that pregnancy and pelvic abnormality such as cancer, trauma, and recent surgery can also predispose to iliac vein thrombosis.[36] The true incidence of isolated pelvic deep vein thrombosis in these patients, however, is not known, as duplex diagnosis of iliac thrombosis is often difficult and its accuracy, compared to the diagnosis of lower extremity deep vein thrombosis, is yet to be established.

While axillary-subclavian venous thrombosis represents a small fraction of all cases of deep vein thrombosis, in fact it is an important clinical entity. In the past, it was thought to be benign and self-limiting, and conservative measures were advocated. More recently, it has been recognized that considerable morbidity may occur and aggressive management is dominant in today's practice.[37] Similarly, in the past, spontaneous axillary-subclavian venous thrombosis, referred to as effort thrombosis, was associated with a variety of physical activities. Now because of central lines and pacemaker wires, a more frequent cause is traumatic and iatrogenic. In fact, this element of axillary-subclavian venous thrombosis is so common that it is felt that between one-third and two-thirds of patients with subclavian lines or catheters develop deep vein thrombosis. Some patients with upper extremity venous thrombosis will have abnormal clotting factors (Fig. 13–16).

TABLE 13–2 • Risk Factors for Venous Thromboembolism

	Risk Factors for Venous Thromboembolism			
Stasis/Endothelial Injury	Thrombotic Disorders	Medical Conditions	Drugs	Other
Indwelling vein devices	Activated Protein C resistance	Malignancy (solid tumor and myeloproliferative disorders)	Oral contraceptive use	Advancing age
Surgery (especially pelvic or orthopedic)	Factor V Leiden	Pregnancy	Hormone replacement therapy	
Major trauma, fractures	Prothrombin gene mutation G20210A	Myocardial infarction	Chemotherapy (including tamoxifen)	
Prolonged travel	Hyperhomocysteinemia	Congestive heart failure		
Paralysis (including anesthesia >30 minutes	Anticardiolipin antibodies	Stroke		
Varicose veins	Lupus anticoagulant	Obesity		
History of DVT	Elevated factor VIII level	Inflammatory bowel disease		
Prolonged bed rest	Protein C deficiency Protein S deficiency Dysfibrogenemia Dysplasminogenemia	Nephrotic syndrome History of DVT Heparin induced thrombocytopenia Paroxysmal nocturnal hemoglobinuria		

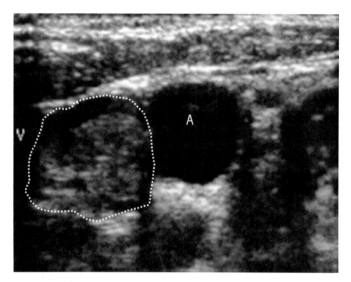

FIGURE 13–16. Transverse sonogram of deep vein thrombosis in the upper extremity.

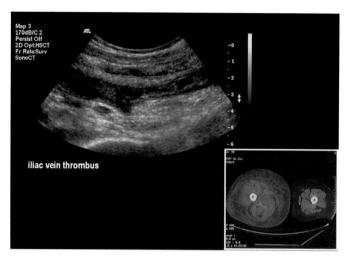

FIGURE 13–17. Sonogram of an iliac vein thrombus. In lower right edge of the image is a corresponding CT scan with increased size of the right leg in this patient with phlegmasia.

Symptoms and Physical Findings

Difficulty in diagnosing deep vein thrombosis is based on the presence of nonspecific symptoms in many patients. The clinical presentation of deep vein thrombosis can be totally asymptomatic or may progress to flagrant phlegmasia cerulea dolens and venous gangrene. The clinical diagnosis based on a physical examination is known to be notoriously inaccurate. Homans' sign (calf pain with passive dorsiflexion of the foot) is also a poor predictor for the presence of deep vein thrombosis. This has led to the investigation and use of pretest probability algorithms. Wells et al. suggested an algorithm based on the determination of pre-test probability and compression ultrasound screening.[38] When thrombi develop in the deep venous system of the lower extremity, the findings may include acute inflammation, pain, and/or swelling, or it may be an entirely bland pathologic process. While the thrombus can produce a venous occlusion, such blockage may be partial or so well compensated that the distal limb swelling does not occur. Therefore, definitive diagnosis remains elusive except by imaging techniques.

The findings of deep vein thrombosis will vary with the location of the thrombus as well as whether it occurs in isolated fashion or in multiple venous segments. It is the proximal iliofemoral veins that present the greatest risk for fatal pulmonary embolism and often produce the most dramatic manifestations (Fig. 13–17). There can be massive swelling, pain, and tenderness of the lower extremity. Phlegmasia cerulean dolens is a severe form of iliofemoral thrombus that causes significant obstruction to venous outflow. This is characterized by cyanosis, which rarely progresses to gangrene. Phlegmasia alba dolens is another form characterized by arterial spasm and a pale cool leg with diminished pulses. Thrombi in the distal or calf veins present the least risk for pulmonary embolus.[39]

Superficial Thrombophlebitis. The terminology describing this entity is appropriate because it truly describes an inflammatory process. It is commonly believed that thrombosis of the deep and superficial venous system represents the same process. However, there does not appear to be any evidence to support that theory.

Contributing Factors. The most common cause of superficial thrombophlebitis is intravenous infusions that inflict a chemical injury on the vein wall that leads to inflammation and then inevitably thrombosis of the involved vein or veins. In the lower limbs, superficial thrombophlebitis most commonly occurs in varicose veins. This commonly follows a traumatic event that may or may not be severe. The development of migratory superficial phlebitis may be the first sign of an underlying malignancy (Trousseau's sign) [40] and has also been associated with Buerger's disease (thromboangiitis obliterans).[41]

Risk Factors and Clinical Manifestations. Varicose veins in the lower extremity and intravenous therapy in the upper extremity predispose a patient to phlebitis. The clinical presentation of superficial thrombophlebitis consists of severe pain, redness, inflammation, swelling, and pyrexia (fever). This is evident simply on physical examination of the involved area, and because the process leads to the development of thrombosis, a palpable cord is often seen.

Differential Diagnosis. The most common entities that can be confused with superficial thrombophlebitis are lymphangitis and cellulitis. In most case, the differential diagnosis is not too difficult, particularly if the examiner realizes that cellulitis and lymphangitis do not typically lead to thrombosis of the superficial veins.

Diagnostic Approach. Phlebitis in a superficial vein is readily diagnosed clinically. Physical diagnosis of superficial thrombophlebitis can be made by detecting an erythematous streaking in the distribution of the superficial veins. Tenderness is present and the extent of thrombus is identified by a palpable cord. Because superficial thrombophlebitis leads to thrombosis of the involved veins, continuous-wave Doppler is the ideal method for establishing the diagnosis. The finding of a patent vein in the area of inflammation rules out phlebitis. Although the diagnosis can be made by physical examination, accurate estimation of the proximal extent of the disease process or deep venous involvement is based on objective testing in the vascular laboratory. If there is any concern over the extent of the thrombosis, particularly whether it involves the deep venous system, it is important to use duplex scanning to depict both the thrombus and its proximal extent.

Clinical Implications. Although the initial diagnosis can be made clinically, it is now known that approximately 20% of patients with superficial vein thrombosis will have an associated occult deep vein thrombosis. Further, in approximately one-third of those who present with only superficial phlebitis initially, the thrombus will eventually extend into the deep venous system via the saphenofemoral junction or perforating vein. Phlebitis of the long saphenous vein above the knee is particularly susceptible to progression to deep vein thrombosis. Therefore, it is prudent to perform a duplex examination for deep vein thrombosis and in selective cases, a follow-up examination in patients with suspected or proven ascending superficial phlebitis.

Evaluation of the lower extremity venous system for deep vein thrombosis has revealed thrombosis of the great saphenous vein in approximately 1% of limbs. Thus, examination of the saphenofemoral junction should be part of the examination of the lower extremity venous system when deep vein thrombosis is suspected.

Upper Extremity Findings. Symptomatic patients with axillary-subclavian venous thrombosis often present with a swollen forearm, upper arm, and shoulder. A visible pattern of venous distention may be present across the anterior aspect of the shoulder and chest wall. There may be venous distention of the antecubital veins as well as those in the hand. If a tender palpable cord is present in the neck and/or axilla, this is due to a superficial thrombophlebitis accompanying the deep vein thrombosis. A bluish or cyanotic discoloration is commonly present in the hand and fingers and an aching pain in the forearm, exacerbated by exercise is also a common complaint.

PULMONARY EMBOLISM

Pulmonary embolism (PE) is a common medical condition that can contribute substantially to individual patient morbidity and mortality as well as global healthcare costs. There are an estimated 600,000 cases of PE each year in the United States, with an in-hospital case-fatality rate attributable to PE of approximately 2%.[42,43] These statistics clearly underestimate the extent of the problem, as this does not include patients with deep vein thrombosis, many more patients with PE die *with* PE (even if not *from* PE), and the mortality with these conditions continues to increase after hospital discharge. In fact, mortality rates from 3 months to 3 years after hospital discharge frequently range from 15% to 30%.[43–45] For patients with hemodynamic compromise, the mortality with PE is substantially higher, in the range of 20% to 30%, while still in the hospital.[42] Mortality rates are higher in men than women and in African-American individuals compared with Caucasian individuals, yet mortality rates overall are declining temporally.[46–49]

Ninety percent of PEs arise from deep vein thrombosis of the lower extremities and pelvis; the rest originate from the upper extremities, heart, or pulmonary arteries. While in most patients with established PE, diagnosis of deep vein thrombosis may be confirmed by noninvasive testing or venography, and only about 30% will present with clinical manifestations of venous thrombosis. In the appropriate clinical setting, suspicion usually is aroused by the sudden onset of chest pain, dyspnea, and hemoptysis and by low P_{O_2}.[50–53] Findings, however, have almost no predictive value. Tachycardia, tachypnea, and low P_{CO_2} are perhaps more indicative of pulmonary embolism.[54,55]

TREATMENT

The treatment of acute deep vein thrombosis is directed at preventing its primary complications, recurrent venous thromboembolism, and the post-thrombotic syndrome. Without appropriate treatment, 20–50% of patients with proximal thrombosis will sustain a pulmonary embolism. The data with respect to calf vein thrombosis is less sound, although the incidence of pulmonary embolism is thought to be significantly less than for proximal deep vein thrombosis.[50–53]

The embolic potential of isolated calf vein thrombosis continues to be debated; however, approximately 20% of such thrombi will propagate to a more proximal level at which point the risk for pulmonary embolus is increased. Although the incidence of post-thrombotic sequelae may be less than after proximal thrombosis, between one-fourth and one-half of patients will have mild to moderate symptoms 1–3 years later. Isolated calf vein thrombosis should, therefore, not be regarded as trivial and cannot be ignored.

Current consensus recommendations in patients without contraindications include antithrombotic treatment, including unfractionated heparin, warfarin, low-molecular-weight heparin, and thrombolytic agents presently to treat venous thromboembolic disease. However, improved anticoagulants are being developed. Gradient elastic stockings, filters, stents, and thrombectomies can also be used in the therapeutic armamentarium, when appropriate. Thrombolytic therapy is suggested for patients with massive iliofemoral deep vein thrombosis at risk of limb gangrene. Venous thrombectomy is suggested in related patients with massive iliofemoral deep vein thrombosis at risk of gangrene. These modalities are often employed in patients with massive, severely symptomatic phlegmasia cerulea or alba dolens. Placement of an inferior vena cava filter is suggested for patients with a contraindication for, or complication of, anticoagulant therapy as well as recurrent or progression of deep vein thrombosis despite adequate anticoagulation. Serial noninvasive follow-up to exclude proximal propagation is a reasonable alternative in patients with contraindications to anticoagulation.[17]

Lower Extremity Venous Duplex Ultrasound

Full diagnostic capabilities for the ultrasound evaluation and diagnosis of deep vein thrombosis include Doppler spectral analysis, color-flow Doppler imaging transducer compression, and high resolution B-mode imaging. Normal ultrasound findings include unidirectional flow, compressibility of the vein, and a lumen free of internal echoes. In order to demonstrate the compressibility of a normal vein, minimal external compression is needed with the transducer in the transverse position (Fig. 13–18). Unidirectional flow is best demonstrated with color-flow Doppler imaging. Doppler spectral analysis is beneficial in evaluating venous flow, which normally changes during the respiratory cycle as described above.

For the average person, a 5 MHz linear transducer is the scan head of choice. Often, transducers are changed during an examination depending on the depth of the vessel and the patient's body habitus. For larger patients, a lower frequency transducer of 2.5 MHz or 3.75 MHz can be used with the trade-off of slightly reduced resolution.

Examination Protocol. The following protocol has been described in detail in the Society for Vascular Ultrasound's Vascular Technology Professional Performance Guideline.[56] The routine protocol calls for careful examination of the common femoral vein, great saphenous vein, deep femoral vein origin, femoral vein in the thigh, popliteal vein, and the calf veins including the posterior tibial and peroneal veins.

The examination is performed with the patient in the supine position and the examination table in slight reverse Trendelenburg with the leg externally rotated (Fig. 13–19). This is the position of choice for viewing the common femoral vein, femoral vein in the thigh, deep femoral vein, great saphenous vein, popliteal vein, and the anterior and distal posterior tibial veins. The patient may be turned prone or lateral to view the popliteal vein, peroneal and proximal posterior tibial veins, and small saphenous and soleal veins.

When indicated, and if possible, the iliac veins are also evaluated. The anterior tibial veins are not routinely evaluated, as in the absence of symptoms in their distribution, their

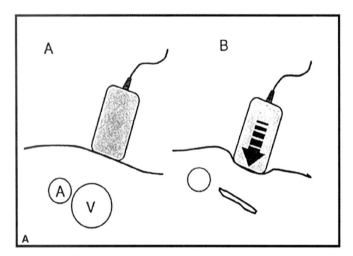

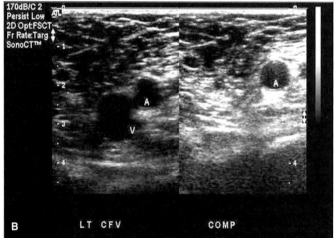

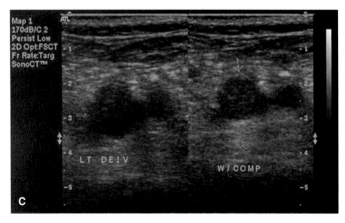

FIGURE 13–18. (**A**) schematic illustrating external compression with the transducer in the transverse position, (*a*) non-compression (*b*) compression. (**B**) Sonogram demonstrating the effect of non-compression and compression a normal vein. (**C**) Sonogram demonstrating the effect of compression on a vein with thrombus.

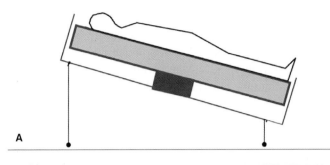

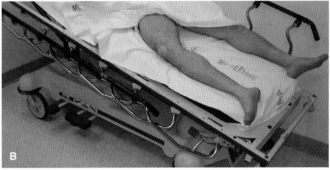

FIGURE 13–19. (**A**) Examination table in reverse Trendelenburg position. (**B**) Patient lying down in a reverse Trendelenburg position.

involvement in the thrombotic process is rare. The sonographer should carefully study all vessels using a combination of long- and short-axis images. Special care must be taken not to miss duplicated vessels. This is especially true of the femoral vein in the thigh and the popliteal vein below the knee (Fig. 13–20). Several reports have demonstrated that multiple femoral veins were present in 177 (46%) of 381 venograms, a much higher rate than the generally accepted frequency of duplication of 20–25%.[57,58]

Images with and without compression and using the color flow to detect directional flow are all useful. Doppler spec-

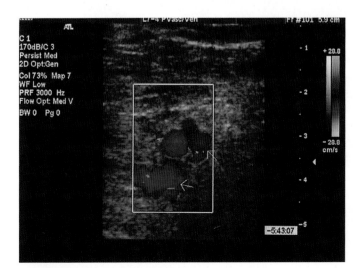

FIGURE 13–20. Duplex image of a duplicated popliteal vein.

tral analysis helps in assessing phasicity and augmentation responses and is particularly helpful as a secondary means of evaluating the patency of the iliac veins. Although the great saphenous vein is not included in the deep venous system, its origin is often visualized because of the risk of saphenous thrombophlebitis extending into the deep system.[56–59]

DIFFERENTIAL DIAGNOSES[60–71]

In this patient population, the vascular laboratory is accustomed to primarily evaluate for the presence of deep vein thrombosis. Incidental findings of other abnormalities have been reported; however, a search for these entities is neither routine nor standard protocol. A systematic search for alternative causes of the patient's signs or symptoms and official reporting of these findings is beneficial to the patient and may avoid additional testing or prolonged hospitalization.

Some of the differential diagnoses that may be present in a patient with suspected deep vein thrombosis include cellulitis, true or false aneurysms, arterial venous fistulas and feeder sources for hematomas. In addition, the surrounding tissues may contain masses such as cysts and hematomas and enlarged lymph nodes may also be present.

Incidental Pathology

Cellulitis is rarely associated with DVT.[60] In these cases, the vascular laboratory may be asked to exclude deep vein thrombosis or evaluate for the presence of abscess formation. Soft tissue thickening and edema are a common finding in these patients. Abscess typically presents as a discrete fluid collection with variable echogenicity. There may be neovascularity of the wall.[61]

In the case of conspicuous swelling of the extremity, lymphedema can be suspected when markedly enlarged lymph nodes are visualized in the groin with normal venous hemodynamics. The inguinal nodes lie in the groin near the femoral vessels and appear enclosed in a dense fibrous capsule (Fig. 13–21). Lymphadenopathy is an enlargement of lymph nodes, which can be the result of an inflammatory or a neoplastic process. Swelling and localized tenderness can occur secondary to lymphatic obstruction or extrinsic venous compression. It may be possible to distinguish a benign enlarged lymph node from a malignant lymph node by shape and vascular patterns. A benign node generally will maintain an ovoid shape with bright echoes reflecting the hilum and surrounding hypoechogenic regions for the remainder of the node. Vascularity is seen entering in the hilar region. With malignancy, the node may become more spherical with loss of the echogenic hilum and more irregular vascularity.

A bursa is a sac of fluid. Dilated bursae communicating with the knee form cysts in the area of the popliteal fossa. These popliteal cysts commonly cause pain, swelling, and tenderness. Popliteal cysts are avascular, which may be helpful in the

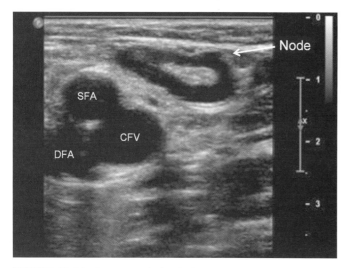

FIGURE 13–21. Sonogram of a inguinal node near the femoral vessels.

diagnosis of a structure in this region. They are found in patients with osteoarthritis, rheumatoid arthritis, and injury to the knee. Dilated bursae that lie between the gastrocnemius muscle and the semi-membranous tendons, posterior and medial to the

knee joint are known as Baker's cysts. Baker's cysts have an oval and often septated appearance that is mostly hypoechoic in character and are typically located posteromedial to the popliteal vessel in the popliteal space. Ruptured cysts can dissect downward into the muscular fascial planes of the calf muscles producing irregular borders and pointed inferior end and may yield the appearance of a thrombosed vessel. Therefore, care should be taken to demonstrate that it is distinct from the vein and artery (Fig. 13–22).

Following trauma to an extremity, extravascular blood may accumulate. The resulting hematoma may appear quite similar to a Baker's cyst yet can become more echogenic with time. Characteristically, they appear as heterogeneous areas within a muscle or between muscle planes, although their appearance can be quite variable (Fig. 13–23). Differentiation between a hematoma and abscess is not possible based on ultrasound alone and usually requires aspiration for a definitive diagnosis.

Peripheral masses that develop acutely are usually accompanied by a history of previous trauma or surgical intervention. The incidence of pseudoaneurysm complication is 0.5–1.0% and the most common site is the common femoral artery. This mass is easily recognized by persistent circular swirling of blood between the site of rupture and the arterial lumen.

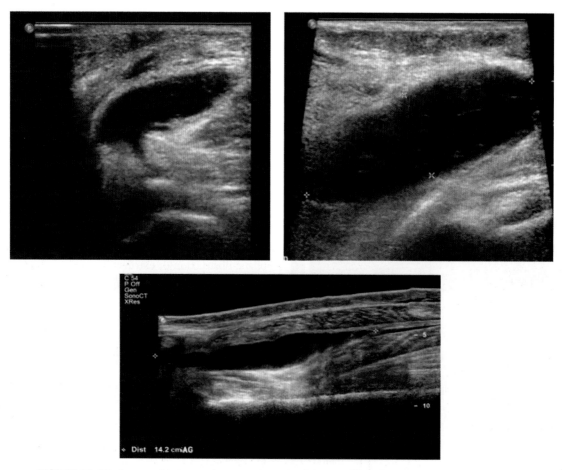

FIGURE 13–22. Sonographic images demonstrating various shapes of Baker's cyst.

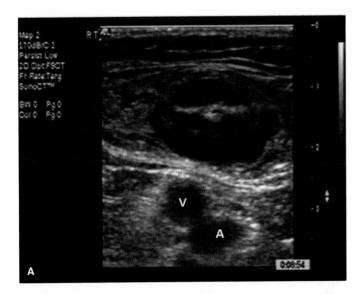

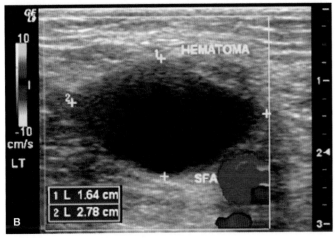

FIGURE 13–23. (**A** & **B**) Sonographic variations of hematomas.

False aneurysms are at risk for expanding, can cause localized compression of adjacent structures, and may rupture. True venous aneurysms are rare and obvious from their overtly large size. Arteriovenous fistulas (AVFs) are also common following catheter insertion and can be identified by high-velocity turbulent signals within the vein, high-velocity, low-resistance flow within the communicating neck, and an easily visible color Doppler bruit. Congenital AVFs are rarely seen and are usually diagnosed early in life. These entities are discussed in detailed in Chapter 14.

On rare occasions extravascular sources such as tumors can cause extrinsic compression and swelling. These masses are difficult to differentiate clinically from deep venous thrombosis. Sonographically, hypervascularization and enhanced color fill within these structures are suggestive of this problem and warrant further investigation. This phenomenon is often noted at the iliac vein level and should be suspected in patients with abnormally continuous venous flow within the common femoral vein when there is no evidence of deep vein thrombosis noted in the legs. These findings should prompt examination of the iliac veins to exclude a compression syndrome versus a thrombotic process or a combination of the two (Fig. 13–24).

DIFFERENTIATION OF ACUTE VERSUS CHRONIC DEEP VEIN THROMBOSIS

Duplex ultrasound is the most common method utilized today for the diagnosis of acute deep vein thrombosis.[72] Three diagnostic criteria have been utilized to document the presence of *acute* deep vein thrombosis (Fig. 13–25).

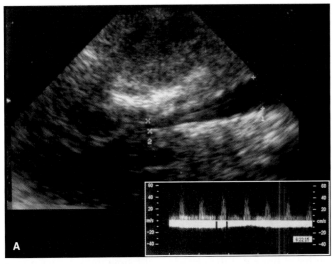

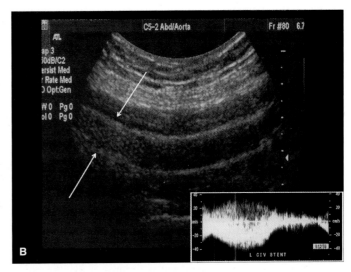

FIGURE 13–24. (**A**) Extrinsic compression of the iliac vein. Spectral Doppler on lower right of image demonstrate a continuous flow. (**B**) White arrows pointing to a stent repair in a iliac vein. Bottom right image demonstrate normal phasic flow pattern.

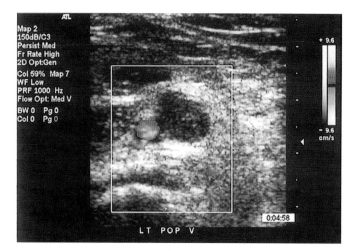

FIGURE 13–25. Color Duplex image demonstrating acute deep vein thrombosis.

1. Intraluminal echoes are seen.
2. The vein is incompressible. The vein will sometimes be significantly distended (often the diameter of the vein will be up to twice that of the accompanying artery). Increased vein size is a very specific sign of an acute process; however, not all patients with acute deep vein thrombosis will present with this finding.
3. There is no Doppler (color or spectral) evidence of active blood flow.

In most laboratories, the result of the duplex scan is the basis for clinical decisions regarding the need for anticoagulant therapy in patients suspected of deep vein thrombosis.

The ability of duplex imaging to differentiate between acute and chronic disease is critical to its use in patients with symptoms of recurrent deep venous obstruction. In the lower extremity, the diameter of the vein appears to be an important factor. Van Gemmeren et al.[73] compared duplex scan results to either histologic criteria or patient history and symptoms. A significant correlation was found between the age of thrombosis and the venous diameter. When thrombosis was less than 10 days old, the venous diameter was at least twice that of the diameter of the accompanying artery. Two other criteria, echogenicity and margin of the vein wall, were not reliable indicators.

To increase the utility of duplex imaging in patients with recurrent disease, a baseline follow-up study should be obtained in all patients with deep venous obstruction. Gaitini et al. recommended a follow-up study 6–12 months following an acute episode.[74] An alternative approach is to obtain a baseline study at the time anticoagulant therapy is discontinued. If the patient presents with recurrent symptoms, it may be possible to interpret the results of the duplex examination without comparison to a baseline study.[75]

UPPER EXTREMITY VENOUS DUPLEX ULTRASOUND

After explaining the procedure to the patient, obtain a pertinent history and perform a physical examination of the extremities. Remove clothing so that access is not limited to the arm and neck on either side. If an indwelling catheter is in place, remove the bandages or dressings and cover the area with a sterile skin cover. The examination should be performed in a routine systematic fashion commencing at the internal jugular vein down to the innominate veins through the chest and into the arm and forearm if indicated. The asymptomatic side is always evaluated first. Comparison to the side contralateral to the involved symptomatic extremity at the same level with the patient in a similar position (supine or close to supine is best) is critical. Because the innominate, subclavian, and axillary veins are deep and protected by overlying anatomic structures and are in close proximity to the clavicle, compression ultrasound is not possible. Color and Doppler spectral flow patterns can used to assess patency of these veins. Compression techniques can be reserved to assess the more peripheral, easily compressed deep and superficial veins in the arm.

Hemodynamics

Spontaneous flow should be present in the innominate, subclavian, and internal jugular veins. In addition, the flow signals are pulsatile due to their proximity to the right atrium. Venous flow does not reduce as dramatically during expiration in the upper extremity (particularly medial to the clavicle) and phasicity normally seen in lower extremity veins may not be appreciated. Augmentation from compression maneuvers is reduced when compared to the lower extremity veins due to the smaller venous volume of the upper extremities.

Protocol[57,76–79]

Begin the scan with the patient in the supine position and the arm at the patient's side. Using a 5 or 7 MHz linear-array transducer, the internal jugular vein is identified in the mid-neck in the transverse plane. This vessel should be examined from the level of the mandible to its confluence with the subclavian vein while compressing the vessel intermittently to assess it for the presence of intraluminal thrombus. Anatomic structures may prevent compressibility of the very proximal internal jugular vein. Spectral waveforms are obtained in the long axis carefully noting the direction and pattern of the venous flow as the internal and external jugular veins serve as major collateral pathways to shunt flow to the contralateral side in the presence of innominate vein occlusion. Venous flow is frequently pulsatile due to the proximity of this vein to the heart.

Using color Doppler, scan in a medial direction along the cephalad border of the clavicle and follow the subclavian vein into the innominate vein. This part of the scan is performed using a small footprint transducer with a 5 MHz imaging

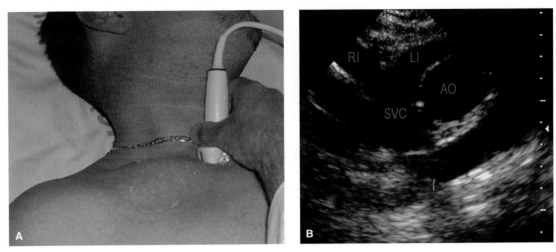

FIGURE 13–26. (A) Transducer position at the suprasternal notch. **(B)** Sonogram of the superior vena cava (SVC) using the suprasternal notch approach.

frequency. The right innominate vein is oriented vertically and the left assumes a more horizontal plane. Color flow should outline the flow channel even when the vessel walls are poorly seen. In some patients, the innominate vein may be followed to the superior vena cava, although most often only a small section of this vein may be visualized (Fig. 13–26).

The subclavian vein is then located inferior to the clavicle and followed to the outer border of the first rib where it becomes the axillary vein (Fig. 13–27). Compression maneuvers can be attempted; however, most often color and spectral Doppler will need to be used as these vessels may be resistant to compression despite the absence of clot. If the subclavian or axillary vein are not clearly seen, abduct the arm 90° from the torso and bend the arm in a pledge position to free the vessels from compression from surrounding structures. In the transverse and then longitudinal view, observe the vessel looking for

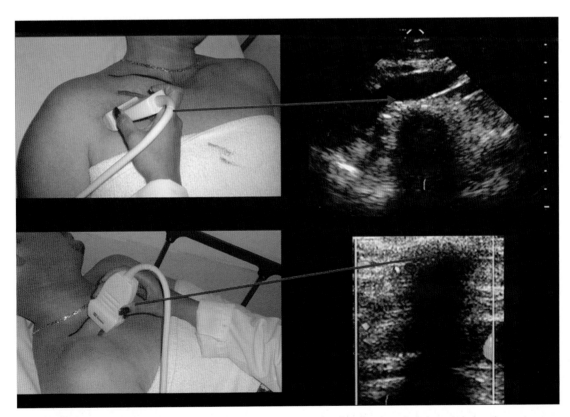

FIGURE 13–27. Demonstrate transverse and sagittal approach to imaging the subclavian vein below the clavicle (left) with corresponding sonograms (right).

the presence of internal echoes that may represent thrombus. Wall motion should also be observed as often as the vein walls will coapt in response to breathing.

The axillary vein can be followed through the deltopectoral groove into the arm where it becomes the brachial vein. The brachial veins are adjacent to the brachial artery and may be difficult to see because of their small size. They are best imaged in the transverse plane and should be compressed in a manner similar to that of the lower extremity veins to their termination at the elbow.

The cephalic vein is imaged at its confluence with the axillary vein. This vessel is best imaged using a high-frequency (7 to 10 MHz) transducer and is evaluated for patency using the compression technique. It is often very small and too superficial to image unless it is thrombosed. An occlusive tourniquet can be placed proximally on the upper arm to dilate this vein and make it easier to see. If signs or symptoms of cephalic vein thrombosis are present, the symptomatic segments of the vein should be imaged. The basilic and the brachial veins are continuous with the axillary vein in the upper arm, allowing these vessels to be seen in the same scan plane. The basilic vein is more posterior and is closer to the skin; however, once it has penetrated the fascia, it will be as deep as the brachial veins.

The forearm veins may be evaluated if the patient is symptomatic in this region. These veins are small and often difficult and tedious to visualize and evaluate. They are best identified by using the color-flow scan to find the adjacent artery and then using augmentation techniques to confirm the presence of flow.

Photoplethysmography techniques assess reflux and differentiate between superficial and deep vein incompetency. These techniques provide indirect information about location and extent of venous insufficiency. These methods are less time consuming than the color-flow Doppler for screening the bilateral lower extremities and can be of great value when there are a large number of patients. Photoplethysmography (PPG) involves the use of a photoelectric cell placed above the medial malleolus. This photocell actually has an infrared light emitting diode and a photodetector that is attached to an amplifier and a strip chart recorder in the direct current (DC) mode. The patient is placed in a sitting position with the legs hanging in a dependent, non-weight-bearing position. Either the patient dorsiflexes the foot to contract the calf muscles or the calf is squeezed to empty the veins. The leg is allowed to relax and the refilling time of the veins is recorded. The normal venous refilling time is 20 seconds or greater. Less than 20 seconds indicates venous incompetency[80] (Fig. 13–28). Venous incompetency can be confined to the superficial veins or involve the deep veins. It is important to discriminate which systems are involved since the superficial veins can be surgically corrected but the deep veins cannot be surgically corrected. If the initial examination is positive for incompetency the test is repeated with a tourniquet placed above the knee to occlude the superficial veins. If the test with the tourniquet is positive it indicates the deep system is also incompetent.

Air plethysmography (APG)[81,82] is a technique that allows the measurement of limb volume changes with different maneuvers. The device consists of a cuff that is placed around the leg, a calibrated pressure transducer, and an analog chart recorder that provides a visual display. Parameters derived from performing various APG measurements with positional changes include the venous filling index, which quantitates venous reflux, the ejection fraction, which correlates with calf muscle pump function, and the residual volume fraction, which correlates with ambulatory calf venous pressure. Venous occlusion techniques allow the measurement of arterial flow into the limb and the venous outflow fraction, which can be used to evaluate venous obstruction. Differentiation of pathology in the deep venous system from that in the superficial venous system is possible. APG has been validated in the evaluation of venous insufficiency in the legs and has a place in the evaluation of symptomatic patients suspected of having deep venous thrombosis. The ability of the device to quantitate absolute arterial flow to the lower extremity makes it useful in evaluating operative results and following disease progression.

Venography (phlebography)[83,84] is defined as radiography of the veins after injection of contrast medium. It is now used infrequently because ultrasound studies are a less invasive way to get the needed diagnostic information. There are two types of venography *ascending* and *descending* depending on the injection site. Ascending venography will be injected into a peripheral vein and the contrast material carried centripetal by the venous flow. Descending venography will be injected into a proximal vein in the leg and the contrast media carried distally by induced retrograde venous flow.

The normal venogram of the lower extremity demonstrates the deep and superficial system, as well as the external and common iliac veins. In some instances, special maneuvers (compression or muscular contraction) may be required to delineate the venous structures fully. The veins are quite variable among different individuals but are usually shown as deep venous trunks that are well defined and easily recognized. The valves are best seen after muscular contraction. The perforators will be defined between the deep venous trunks and the superficial veins.

CHRONIC VENOUS DISEASE

Venous insufficiency can be conveniently divided into primary venous insufficiency (varicose veins, telangiectasias) and chronic venous insufficiency (skin changes, secondary venous dysfunction).[85] About 10–30% of the US population has some variant of venous disease.[86] The American Venous Forum has developed the CEAP classification to help define the different degrees of venous insufficiency by different categories: C (clinical state), E (etiology), A (anatomy), P (pathophysiology).

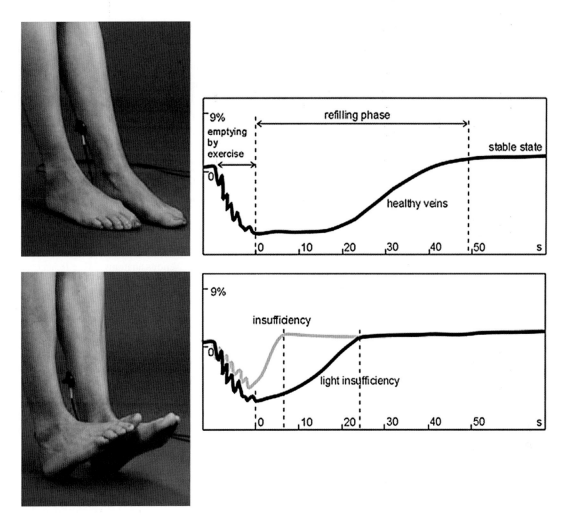

FIGURE 13–28. Images of photoplethysmography (PPG). Left upper photo demonstrate the feet in a resting position and the lower left photo demonstrate the feet in a dorsiflexion position in order to empty the calf. On the top upper right is a normal response to calf exercise. On the bottom right is an abnormal response to venous valvular incompetency.

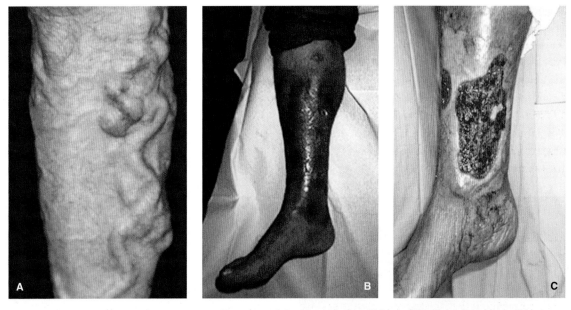

FIGURE 13–29. Images of various manifestations of chronic venous insufficiency. (**A**) large varicose veins. (**B**) Hyperpigmentation. (**C**) Venous ulcerations.

The major components of pathophysiology in venous insufficiency are obstruction and vascular incompetence. These components may lead to venous hypertension, which is presently thought to be responsible for significant signs and symptoms in this disease class.

Signs and Symptoms. Varicose veins are dilated veins within subcutaneous tissue, which can be divided into primary (normal deep system) and secondary (abnormal deep symptoms). Symptoms that may be associated with varicose veins include heaviness, itching, tiredness, burning, and cramps. Chronic venous insufficiency may be manifested by varicose veins alone or by hyperpigmentation, edema, ulceration, and lipodermatosclerosis (Fig. 13–29).[85]

History and physical examination as above can identify the diagnosis of venous insufficiency but in general cannot identify the presence, location, or extent of vascular incompetency or obstruction. Duplex scanning has become the single most important noninvasive adjunctive tool in answering these questions and, thus, provides the appropriate medical or surgical approach in this clinical setting.

The exam may be completed in two parts.[87,88] First, a supine protocol can be utilized to identify patency versus venous obstruction. In the second part of the exam, the proximal great saphenous can be evaluated with Valsalva in reversed Trendelenburg position, but the remainder of the exam should be completed in the standing position with the weight on the leg that is not being examined. In general, reflux >0.5 seconds, is consistent with the venous insufficiency, and this may further be classified into mild, moderate and severe, according to reflux duration (Fig. 13–30).[89]

Management of venous insufficiency can be noninvasive or invasive, depending on the underlying condition of the patient. Noninvasive options include leg elevation, compression, and topical treatment. Invasive approaches include sclerotherapy, skin grafting, stripping of superficial veins, open subfascial perforator surgery, subfascial endoscopic perforator surgery (SEPS), and deep vein reconstruction.[90] A relatively new development in the treatment of saphenous vein reflux is minimally invasive catheter directed endovenous obliteration.[91]

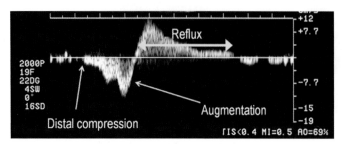

FIGURE 13–30. Doppler image demonstrating venous reflux.

References

1. Pieri A, Massimo G, Santinim M. Ultrasonographic anatomy of upper extremity veins. *J Vasc Technol.* 2002; 26(3):173-180.

2. Ricci S, Georgiev M. Ultrasound anatomy of the superficial veins of the lower limb. *J Vasc Technol.* 2002; 26(3):183-199.

3. Pieri A, Gatti M, Santini M, Marcelli F, Carnemolla A. Ultrasonographic anatomy of the deep veins of the lower extremity. *J Vasc Technol.* 2002; 26(3):201-211.

4. Hollinshead WH. *Textbook of Anatomy.* 3rd ed. New York: Harper and Row; 1974; 75.

5. Kadir S. *Diagnostic Angiography.* Philadelphia: WB Saunders; 1986; 541.

6. DeWeese JA, Rogoff SM, Tobin CE. *Radiographic Anatomy of Major Veins of the Lower Limb.* Rochester, NY: Eastman Kodak; 1965.

7. Blackburn DR. Venous anatomy. *J Vasc Technol.* 1988; 12:78-82.

8. Oliver MA. Anatomy and physiology. In: Talbot SR, Oliver MA, eds. *Techniques of Venous Imaging.* Pasadena, CA: AppletonDavies; 1992; 11-20.

9. Hemodynamics of the normal arterial and venous system. In: *Duplex Scanning in Vascular Disorders.* 3rd ed. Philadelphia, PA: Lippincott, Williams & Wilkins; 2002; 32-60.

10. Strandness DE Jr, Sumner DS. *Hemodynamics for Surgeons.* New York: Grune & Stratton; 1975; 120-160.

11. Deep venous thrombosis and the post thrombotic syndrome. In: *Duplex Scanning in Vascular Disorders.* 3rd ed. Philadelphia, PA: Lippincott, Williams & Wilkins; 2002; 169-190.

12. Urschel HC Jr, Razzuck MA. Paget-Schroetter syndrome: what is the best management? *Ann Thorac Surg.* 2000; 69:1663-1668.

13. Vijaysadan V, Zimmerman AM, Pajaro RE. Paget-Schroetter syndrome in the young and Active. *J Am Board Fam Med.* 2005; 18(4):314-319.

14. May R, Thurner J. The cause of the predominantly sinistral occurrence of thrombosis of the pelvic veins. *Angiology.* 1957; 8(5):419-427.

15. Fazel R, Froehlich JB, Williams DM, Saint S, Nallamothu BK. Clinical problem-solving. A sinister development—a 35-year-old woman presented to the emergency department with a 2-day history of progressive swelling and pain in her left leg, without antecedent trauma. *N Engl J Med.* 2007; 357(1):53-59.

16. Meissner M, Caps M, Bergelin RO, et al. Early outcome after isolated calf vein thrombosis. *J Vasc Surg.* 1997; 26:749

17. Oliver MA. Medical management of acute deep vein thrombosis. *J Vasc Technol.* 2002; 26:227-229.

18. Buller et al. Seventh ACCP Conference on antithrombotic and thrombolytic therapy. *Chest.* 2004; 126:4015-4285.

19. Weitz JW. Orally active direct thrombin inhibitors. *Semin Vasc Med.* 2003; 3:131-137.

20. Ridker PM, Goldhaber SZ, Danielson E, et al. Long-term, low intensity warfarin therapy for the prevention of recurrent venous thromboembolism. *N Engl J Med.* 2003; 349:631-639.

21. Kearon C, Ginsberg GS, Kovacs MJ, et al. Comparison of low-intensity warfarin therapy with conventional intensity warfarin therapy for long term prevention of recurrent venous thromboembolism. *N Engl J Med.* 2003; 349:631-639.

22. Weitz JI. New anticoagulants for treatment of venous thromboembolism. *Circulation.* 2004; 110[suppl I]:I-19-I26.

23. Thromboembolic Risk Factors (THRIFT) Consensus Group. Risk of and prophylaxis for venous thromboembolism in hospital patients. *BJM.* 1991; 305:567-574.

24. Kim SH, Bartholomew JR. Venous thromboembolism. Disease management project. Cleveland, OH: Cleveland Clinic; 2010.

25. Turpie AGG, Chin BSP, Lip GYH. Clinical review. ABC of antithrombotic therapy. Venous thromboembolism: pathophysiology, clinical features, and prevention. *BMJ* 2002; 325:887-890.

26. White RH. The Epidemiology of venous thromboembolism. *Circulation.* 2003; 107:I-4.

27. Anderson FA Jr, Wheeler HB, Goldberg RJ, et al. A population-based perspective of the hospital incidence and case-fatality rates of deep vein thrombosis and pulmonary embolism. The Worcester DVT Study. *Arch Intern Med.* 1991; 151:933-938.

28. Silverstein MD, Heit JA, Mohr DN, et al. Trends in the incidence of deep vein thrombosis and pulmonary embolism: a 25-year population-based study. *Arch Intern Med.* 1998; 158:585-593.

29. Bounameaux H, Hicklin L, Desmarais S. Seasonal variation in deep vein thrombosis. *BMJ.* 1996; 312:284-285.

30. Coon WW. Epidemiology of venous thromboembolism. *Ann Surg.* 1977; 186:149-164.

31. Gillum RF. Pulmonary embolism and thrombophlebitis in the United States, 1970–1985. *Am Heart J.* 1987; 114:1262-1264.

32. Kierkegaard A. Incidence and diagnosis of deep vein thrombosis associated with pregnancy. *Acta Obstet Gynecol Scand.* 1983; 62:239-243.

33. Dickson BC. Venous thrombosis: on the history of Virchow's triad. *UTMJ.* 2004; 81:166-171.

34. Owen CA. *A History of Blood Coagulation.* Rochester: Mayo Foundation for Medical Education and Research; 2001; 169-180.

35. Rosendaal F. Venous thrombosis: a multicausal disease. *Lancet.* 1999; 353(9159):1167-1173.

36. Meissner M, Caps M, Bergelin R, Manzo R, Strandness DE Jr. Early outcome after isolated calf vein thrombosis. *J Vasc Surg.* 1997; 26(5):749-756.

37. Hingorani A, Ascher E, Lorenson E, DePippo P, Salles-Cunha S, Scheinman M, Yorkovich W, Hanson J. Upper extremity deep venous thrombosis and its impact on morbidity and mortality rates in a hospital-based population. *J Vasc Surg.* 1997 Nov; 26(5):853-860.

38. Wells PS, Anderson DR, Bormanis J, et al. Value of assessment of pretest probability of deep-vein thrombosis in clinical management. *Lancet.* 1997; 350:1795-1798.

39. Patel AV. Diseases of the venous and lymphatic systems. In: Sales CM, Goldsmith J, Veith FJ, eds. *Handbook of Vascular Surgery.* St. Louis, MO: Quality Medical Publishing, Inc; 1994.

40. Del Conde I, Bharwani LD, Dietzen DJ, Pendurthi U, Thiagarajan P, López JA. Microvesicle-associated tissue factor and Trousseau's syndrome. *J Thromb Haemost.* 2007; 5:70-74.

41. Olin JW. Thromboangiitis obliterans (Buerger's disease). *N Engl J Med.* 2000; 343:864-849.

42. Saeger W, Genzkow M. Venous thromboses and pulmonary embolisms in post-mortem series: probable causes by correlations of clinical data and basic diseases. *Pathol Res Pract.* 1994; 190:394-399.

43. Kniffin WD Jr, Baron JA, Barrett J, et al. The epidemiology of diagnosed pulmonary embolism and deep venous thrombosis in the elderly. *Arch Intern Med.* 1994; 154:861-866.

44. Cushman M, Tsai A, Heckbert SR, et al. Incidence rates, case fatality, and recurrence rates of deep vein thrombosis and pulmonary embolus: the Longitudinal Investigation of Thromboembolism Etiology (LITE). *Thromb Haemost.* 2001; 86(suppl 1):OC2349.

45. Hansson PO, Welin L, Tibblin G, et al. Deep vein thrombosis and pulmonary embolism in the general population. "The Study of Men Born in 1913." *Arch Intern Med.* 1997; 157:1665-1670.

46. Nordstrom M, Lindblad B, Bergqvist D, et al. A prospective study of the incidence of deep-vein thrombosis within a defined urban population. *J Intern Med.* 1992; 232:155-160.

47. White RH, Zhou H, Kim J, et al. A population-based study of the effectiveness of inferior vena cava filter use among patients with venous thromboembolism. *Arch Intern Med.* 2000; 160:2033-2041.

48. White RH, Zhou H, Romano PS. Incidence of idiopathic deep venous thrombosis and secondary thromboembolism among ethnic groups in California. *Ann Intern Med.* 1998; 128:737-740.

49. Murin S, Romano PS, White RH. Comparison of outcomes after hospitalization for deep venous thrombosis or pulmonary embolism. *Thromb Haemost.* 2002; 88:407-414.

50. Fedullo PF, Tapson VF. Clinical practice. The evaluation of suspected pulmonary embolism. *N Engl J Med.* 2003; 349:1247-1256.

51. Carson JL, Kelley MA, Duff A, et al. The clinical course of pulmonary embolism. *N Engl J Med.* 1992; 326:1240-1245.

52. Goldhaber SZ. Pulmonary embolism. *N Engl J Med.* 1998; 339:93-104.

53. Horlander KT, Mannino DM, Leeper KV. Pulmonary embolism mortality in the United States, 1979–1998: an analysis using multiple-cause mortality data. *Arch Intern Med.* 2003; 163:1711-1717.

54. Turkstra F, Kuijer PMM, van Beek EJR, Brandjes DPM, ten Cate JW, Büller HR. Diagnostic utility of ultrasonography of leg veins in patients suspected of having pulmonary embolism. *Ann Intern Med.* 1997; 12:775-781.

55. Wells PS, Anderson DR, Rodger M, et al. Derivation of a simple clinical model to categorize patients probability of pulmonary embolism: increasing the models utility with the SimpliRED d-dimer. *Thromb Haemost.* 2000; 83:416-420.

56. Vascular Technology Professional Performance Guidelines. Lower Extremity Venous Duplex Evaluation. Available: http://www.svtnet.org.

57. Nix L, Troillet R. The use of color in venous duplex examination. *J Vasc Technol.* 1991; 15:123-128.

58. Zwiebel W. Technique for extremity venous ultrasound examination. In: *Introduction to Vascular Ultrasonography.* 5th ed. Philadelphia: Elsevier Saunders; 2005.

59. Labropoulos N, Tassiopoulos AK. Vascular diagnosis of venous thrombosis. In: *Vascular Diagnosis.* 1st ed. Philadelphia: Elsevier Inc; 2005.

60. Glover JL, Bendick PJ. Appropriate indications for venous duplex ultrasonographic examinations. *Surgery.* 1996 Oct; 120(4):725-730.

61. Polak JP. *Peripheral Vascular Sonography.* 2nd ed. Philadelphia: Lippincott, Williams & Wilkins; 2004; 204-209.

62. Gocke J. Lower extremity venous ultrasonography. In: Mohler ER, Gerard-Herman M, Jaff MR, eds. *Essentials of Vascular Laboratory Diagnosis.* Danvers, MA: Blackwell Futura; 2005; 199.

63. Zweibel WT. Nonvascular pathology encountered during venous sonography. In: Zweibel WT, Pellerito JS, eds. *Introduction of Vascular Technology*. Philadelphia, PA: Elsevier Saunders; 2005; 501-512.

64. Daigle RJ. *Techniques in Noninvasive Vascular Diagnosis*. Littleton, CO: Summer Publishing; 2002; 89-91.

65. Bluth EI. Leg swelling with pain or edema. In: Bluth EI et al, eds. *Ultrasonography in Vascular Diseases*. New York, NY: Thieme; 2001.

66. Labropoulos N, Tassiopoulos AK. Vascular diagnosis of venous thrombosis. In: Mansour MA, Labropoulos N, eds. *Vascular Diagnosis*. Ch. 41. Elsevier Saunders; 2005; 435-437.

67. Hodge M et al. Incidental finding during venous duplex examination: solitary fibrous tumor or arteriovenous malform in the left lower extremity. *J Vasc Ultrasound*. 2007; 31(1):41-44.

68. Mansour MA. Vascular diagnosis of abdominal and peripheral aneurysms. In: Mansour MA, Labropoulos N, eds. *Vascular Diagnosis*. Ch. 35. Elsevier Saunders; 2005.

69. Kim-Gavino CS, Vade A, Lim-Dunham J. Unusual appearance of a popliteal venous aneurysm in a 16 year old patient. *J Ultrasound Med*. 2006; 25:1615-1618.

70. Arger PH, Lyoob SD, eds. *The Complete Guide to Vascular Ultrasound*. Philadelphia, PA: Lippincott, Williams & Wilkins; 2004; 26.

71. Shaw M et al. Case study: cystic adventitial disease of the popliteal artery. *J Vasc Ultrasound*. 2007; 31(1):45-48.

72. Gaitini D. Current approaches and controversial issues in the diagnosis of deep vein thrombosis via duplex Doppler ultrasound. *J Clin Ultrasound*. 2006 Jul-Aug; 34(6):289-297.

73. van Gemmeren D, Fobbe F, Ruhnke-Trautmann M, Hartmann CA, Gotzen R, Wolf KJ, Distler A, Schulte KL. Diagnosis of deep leg vein thrombosis with color-coded duplex sonography and sonographic determination of the duration of the thrombosis. *Z Kardiol*. 1991 Aug; 80(8):523-528.

74. Gaitini D, Kaftori JK, Pery M, Markel A. Late changes in veins after deep venous thrombosis: ultrasonographic findings. *Rofo*. 1990 Jul; 153(1):68-72.

75. Cavezzi A, Labropoulos N, Partsch H, Ricci S, Caggiati A, Myers K, Nicolaides A, Smith PC; UIP. Duplex ultrasound investigation of the veins in chronic venous disease of the lower limbs—UIP consensus document. Part II. Anatomy. *Vasa*. 2007 Feb; 36(1):62-71.

76. Nack T, Needleman L. Comparison of duplex sonography and contrast venography for evaluation of upper extremity venous disease. *J Vasc Technol*. 1992; 16(2):69-73.

77. Falk RL, Smith DF. Thrombosis of upper extremity thoracic inlet veins: diagnosis with duplex Doppler sonography. *Am J Roentgenol*. 1987; 149:677-682.

78. Froehlich JB, Zide RS, Persson AV. Diagnosis of upper extremity deep vein thrombosis using a color Doppler imaging system. *J Vasc Technol*. 1991; 15(5):251-253.

79. Knudson GJ et al. Color Doppler sonographic imaging in the assessment of upper extremity deep vein thrombosis. *Am J Roentgenol*. 1990; 154:399-403.

80. Gerlock AJ, Giyanani VL, Krebs CA. *Applications of Noninvasive Vascular Techniques*. Philadelphia: WB Saunders; 1988.

81. Asbeutah AM, Riha AZ, Cameron JD, McGrath BP. Quantitative assessment of chronic venous insufficiency using duplex ultrasound and air plethysmography. *J Vasc Ultrasound*. 2006; 30(1):23-30.

82. Katz MR, Comerota AJ, Kerr R. Air plethysmography (APG®): a new technique to evaluate patients with chronic venous insufficiency. Dept of Surgery, Temple University Hospital, Philadelphia, PA. *J Vasc Technol*. 1991; 15(1):23-17.

83. Kim D, Orron DE, Porter DH. Venographic anatomy, technique and interpretation. In: Kim D, Orron DE, eds. *Peripheral Vascular Imaging and Intervention*. St. Louis: Mosby-Year Book; 1996; 269-349.

84. Abrams HI. *Angiography*. 2nd ed. Vol. II. Boston: Little Brown; 1971; 1251-1271.

85. Bergan JJ et al. Chronic venous insufficiency. In: Merli GJ, Weitz HH, Carasasi AC, eds. *Peripheral Vascular Disorders*. Philadelphia, PA: Saunders; 2004; 123-129.

86. Arcelus TI, Caprini TA. Nonoperative treatment of chronic venous insufficiency. *J Vasc Technol*. 2002; 26:231-238.

87. Manzo R. Duplex evaluation of chronic disease. In: Strandness DE, ed. *Duplex Scanning in Vascular Diseases*. Philadelphia, PA: Lippincott; 2002.

88. Neumyer MM. Ultrasound diagnosis of venous insufficiency. In: Zwiebel WT, Pellerito JS, eds. *Introduction of Vascular Technology*. Ch. 26. Philadelphia, PA: Elsevier Saunders; 2005.

89. Thrush A, Hartshorne T. *Peripheral Vascular Ultrasound*. London: Churchill Livingstone; 1999.

90. Belcaro G, Nicolaides AN, Veller M. *Venous Disorders*. London: Saunders; 1995.

91. Kabnick LS. New horizons in the treatment of saphenous vein reflux. *J Vasc Technol*. 2002; 239-246.

Questions

GENERAL INSTRUCTIONS: For each question, select the best answer. Select only one answer for each question, unless otherwise indicated.

1. All deep veins of the lower leg have at least how many valves

    (A) 10

    (B) 7

    (C) 5

    (D) 2

2. What is the longest vein in the body?

    (A) cephalic vein

    (B) femoral vein

    (C) great saphenous vein

    (D) inferior vena cava (IVC)

3. The popliteal vein passes through what structure to become the femoral vein?

    (A) profunda hiatus

    (B) adductor canal

    (C) Scarpa's triangle

    (D) flexor hallucis longus

4. Which of the following veins is *not* part of the superficial venous system?

    (A) great saphenous vein

    (B) femoral vein

    (C) short saphenous vein

    (D) basilic vein

5. Which of the following is *not* typically exhibited by normal veins of the lower extremity above the knee?

    (A) spontaneous flow

    (B) phasic flow

    (C) pulsatile flow

    (D) compressibility

6. What percentage of blood in the body can be found within the venous system?

    (A) 60–65%

    (B) 50–65%

    (C) 70–75%

    (D) 75–80%

7. All of the following are true of veins *except*?

    (A) Veins have thicker walls than arteries.

    (B) Veins are distensible.

    (C) Veins are collapsible.

    (D) Veins can be divided into deep and superficial systems.

8. Which of the following complications is the primary clinical concern in deep vein thrombosis (DVT)?

    (A) claudication

    (B) pulmonary embolism (PE)

    (C) valve competency

    (D) loss of extremity

9. Duplex scanning of the deep venous system of the lower extremities is usually performed with the patient in which of the following positions?

    (A) supine position with the leg straight

    (B) supine position with the leg externally rotated

    (C) supine position with the leg internally rotated

    (D) prone position with the leg internally rotated

10. The outermost layer of the vein wall is called the tunica

    (A) media

    (B) intima

    (C) adventitia

    (D) endothelium

11. A spontaneous venous signal may not be heard in which one of the following vessels?

    (A) external iliac vein

    (B) posterior tibial vein

    (C) deep femoral vein

    (D) common femoral vein

12. Which of the following terms best describes a normal venous signal in the lower extremity?

    (A) continuous

    (B) phasic

    (C) pulsatile

    (D) oscillating

13. Extensive iliofemoral thrombosis producing a tight leg edema, severe pain, and cyanotic mottled skin is commonly referred to as?

    (A) Raynaud's phenomenon

    (B) claudication

    (C) Byrum trace syndrome

    (D) phlegmasia cerulea dolens

14. Deep vein thrombosis often destroys the venous valves sometimes resulting in post-phlebitic syndrome, which can lead to all of the following *except*

    (A) thin vessel walls

    (B) chronic induration

    (C) stasis dermatitis

    (D) ulcers

15. During inspiration, as the intra-abdominal pressure increases

    (A) blood flows smoothly throughout the body, at the moment of exhalation the valves close, and then quickly reopen again

    (B) blood flow from the lower extremities decreases while increasing the flow from the upper part of the body

    (C) blood flow from the lower extremities increases while decreasing the flow from the upper part of the body

    (D) but there is no significant effect on the venous flow patterns

16. Which of the following *cannot* be used to evaluate chronic venous insufficiency?

    (A) photoplethysmography

    (B) air plethysmography

    (C) duplex ultrasound

    (D) CT scan

17. Which of the following is *not* a component of "Virchow's triad"?

    (A) injury to the vessel wall

    (B) hypercoagulability

    (C) immobility of extremity

    (D) stasis

18. Which vessels' distal landmark is the area between the medial malleolus and the Achilles tendon near the skin surface?

    (A) anterior tibial veins

    (B) posterior tibial veins

    (C) short saphenous vein

    (D) great saphenous vein

19. Which layer of the vein wall are the venous valves attached to?

    (A) tunica adventitia

    (B) tunica intima

    (C) tunica media

    (D) tunica lateral

20. A Greenfield filter, is normally placed in the

    (A) right internal jugular

    (B) inferior vena cava

    (C) superior vena cava

    (D) external iliac of thrombosed leg

21. The subclavian vein gives off what branch just before becoming the axillary vein?

    (A) costocoracoid vein

    (B) basilic vein

    (C) cubital vein

    (D) cephalic vein

22. The gastrocnemius plexus drains the blood from the gastrocnemius muscle and empties into which of the following vessels?

    (A) posterior tibial vein

    (B) anterior tibial veins

    (C) popliteal vein

    (D) peroneal vein

23. The dynamic venous pressure normally measures about 15–20 mm Hg in the venules. What does it normally measure in the right atrium?

    (A) 15–20 mm Hg

    (B) 100 mm Hg

    (C) 0 mm Hg

    (D) 50 mm Hg

24. Which of the following is *least* likely to compromise blood flow on the basis of compression?

    (A) Baker's cyst

    (B) lymph nodes

    (C) varicose veins

    (D) hematomas

25. Which of the following is *not* a normal characteristic of veins?

    (A) phasicity

    (B) spontaneity

    (C) compressibility

    (D) augmentation

    (E) continuous signal without respiratory movements

26. There are no valves present in which of the following veins?

    (A) innominate veins

    (B) axillary vein

    (C) external jugular vein

    (D) internal jugular vein

27. The superficial veins of the lower extremities can be demonstrated sonographically within 1–2 cm of the skin surface; where do they lie?

    (A) within the subcutaneous fat

    (B) within the connective tissue sheath

    (C) just below the subcutaneous fat

    (D) just above the deep fascia

28. The Brescia–Cimino fistula is created surgically between which of the following vessels?

    (A) distal ulnar artery and basilic vein

    (B) cephalic vein and the radial artery

    (C) proximal radial artery and transpose basilic vein

    (D) brachial artery and cephalic vein

29. Deep vein thrombosis of the upper extremity is becoming more frequent because of which of the following?

    (A) Increased number of patients having radiation therapy and complications

    (B) Increased incidence of trauma patients with complications

    (C) Increased incidence of thoracic outlet syndrome

    (D) Increased use of central venous catheters

30. Which of the following describes the normal route of venous flow in the lower extremity?

    (A) superficial veins to perforator veins to the deep veins

    (B) deep veins to the perforator veins to the superficial veins

    (C) deep veins to superficial veins to perforator veins

    (D) superficial veins to the deep veins to perforator veins

31. Which of the following veins is a continuation of the dorsalis pedis and lies between the tibia and fibula on top of the interosseous membrane?

    (A) popliteal vein

    (B) anterior tibial vein

    (C) short saphenous vein

    (D) peroneal vein

32. Which one of the following is most likely to lead to hemodialysis access failure?

    (A) a large outflow vein

    (B) perigraft collection

    (C) outflow vein stenosis

    (D) the "steal syndrome"

33. What is sclerotherapy?

    (A) surgical removal of the superficial veins

    (B) use of support stockings and appropriate exercise

    (C) injection of superficial veins with agent to induce thrombosis

    (D) injection of deep and superficial veins with agent to induce thrombosis

34. Which of the following is *not* a cause of chronic venous insufficiency?

    (A) varicose veins

    (B) surgery

    (C) post-thrombotic syndrome

    (D) chronic recurrent thrombosis

35. Which one of the following is *not* used to augment veins?

    (A) distal compression of the vein

    (B) coughing

    (C) Valsalva maneuver

    (D) compression of the vein with the transducer probe

36. Venography shows a clot in the venous system as

    (A) an echogenic mass within the vein

    (B) a filling defect within the vein

    (C) a heterogeneous mass within the vein

    (D) a dilated vein with a spongy appearing mass in the lumen

37. Acute thrombus is soft and may be compressed to a certain extent. Chronic thrombus

    (A) is not compressible to any extent
    (B) may be easily compressed to a certain extent
    (C) will easily compress completely
    (D) with some difficulty (pressure) will compress completely

38. Chronic venous insufficiency may be characterized by all of the following *except*

    (A) absence of leg pain
    (B) varicose veins
    (C) chronic swelling of the leg
    (D) cutaneous hyperpigmentation

39. Which of the following is *not* believed to be a contributing factor to primary varicose veins?

    (A) abnormal wall weakness
    (B) increased distending force
    (C) large arteriovenous fistulas
    (D) multiple arteriovenous fistulas

40. Ascending venography cannot be used for which of the following?

    (A) to assess the function of the proximal valves in the lower extremity
    (B) to determine the location of incompetent perforator
    (C) to localize recanalized channels indicating previous thrombophlebitis
    (D) to determine the absence or presence of varicosities

41. Which of the following terms describes varicose veins with competent deep vein valves and incompetent superficial veins?

    (A) secondary varicose veins
    (B) primary varicose veins
    (C) first varicose veins
    (D) thigh varicose veins

42. Which vein(s) arise(s) from and drain the plantar venous arch and superficial venous net of the foot?

    (A) anterior tibial veins
    (B) posterior tibial veins
    (C) great saphenous vein
    (D) short saphenous vein

43. Which vein receives both the superficial and deep venous systems of the upper extremity?

    (A) innominate vein
    (B) cephalic vein
    (C) brachial vein
    (D) subclavian vein

44. The axillary veins consist of 5% smooth muscle, whereas veins in the feet consist of

    (A) 60–80% smooth muscle
    (B) 35–50% smooth muscle
    (C) 25–45% smooth muscle
    (D) 75–85% smooth muscle

45. Each toe has two dorsal digital and two plantar veins that unite to form the dorsal metatarsal veins that join to form which of the following?

    (A) dorsal metatarsal venous arch
    (B) superficial dorsal venous arch
    (C) deep dorsal venous arch
    (D) plantar–dorsal venous arch

46. The communicating veins or "perforators" are located throughout the leg; in most legs, there are

    (A) more than 50 of these veins
    (B) more than 1000 of these veins
    (C) more than 100 of these veins
    (D) more than 500 of these veins

47. The only point in the body (in any position except upright) where the arteriovenous pressure gradient remains the constant (83 mm Hg) is the hydrostatic indifferent point (HIP), which is located

    (A) at the external jugular
    (B) at the hip
    (C) at the aorta bifurcation
    (D) just below the diaphragm

48. After thrombus fills the vein and adheres to the wall of the vessel, it will then contract, and recanalization will begin. How long does this generally take?

    (A) about 10 days after formation
    (B) about 3 days after formation
    (C) about 5 days after formation
    (D) about 12 days after formation

49. Which of the following is *not* among the most significant risk factor for deep vein thrombosis?

    (A) obesity
    (B) the use of oral contraception
    (C) diabetes
    (D) smoking
    (E) pregnancy

50. Deep vein thrombus can originate anywhere in the venous system, but studies have shown the single most common site to be which of the following?

    (A) soleal sinusoids
    (B) posterior tibial vein
    (C) iliofemoral veins
    (D) saphenous–femoral junction

51. The veins in the sole of the foot form the planter cutaneous arch, which drains into the medial and lateral marginal veins, which in turn empty into

    (A) great and short saphenous veins
    (B) anterior and posterior tibial veins
    (C) anterior tibial vein and short saphenous vein
    (D) great saphenous vein

52. What type of venography offers the ability of assessing valvular functions?

    (A) posterior venography
    (B) descending venograph
    (C) ascending venograph
    (D) visceral venograph

53. Which one of the organs listed below does *not* empty blood through the portal vein?

    (A) spleen
    (B) gallbladder
    (C) renal
    (D) pancreas

54. In what anatomic region is/are the venous valves found?

    (A) tunica intima
    (B) tunica media
    (C) tunica adventitia
    (D) both A and C

55. The right ovarian vein drains directly into the inferior vena cava. The left ovarian vein drains into which of the following veins?

    (A) the right ovarian vein
    (B) the left internal iliac vein

    (C) the inferior vena cava
    (D) the left renal vein

56. A functioning valve is competent if

    (A) it simultaneously opens and closes
    (B) it allows both forward and reverse venous flow
    (C) it will not allow reversal of venous blood flow
    (D) it stays open continuously allowing continuous venous flow

Questions 57 through 64: Match the structures in Fig. 13–31 with the terms in Column B.

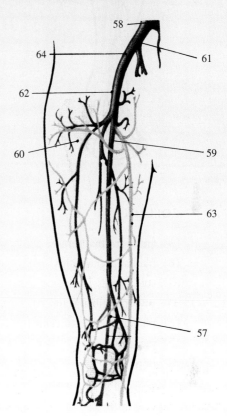

FIGURE 13–31.

COLUMN A   COLUMN B

57. _____   (A) popliteal vein

58. _____   (B) great saphenous vein

             (C) femoral vein

59. _____   (D) distal inferior vena cava

60. _____   (E) internal iliac vein

             (F) deep femoral vein (profunda)

61. _____   (G) external iliac vein

62. _____   (H) common femoral vein

63. _____

64. _____

Questions 65 through 72: Match the structures in Fig. 13–32 with the terms in Column B.

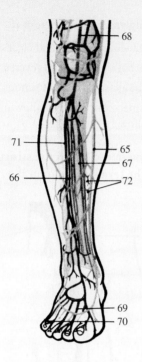

FIGURE 13–32.

COLUMN A	COLUMN B
65. _____	(A) anterior tibial veins
	(B) plantar digital veins
66. _____	(C) soleal veins
67. _____	(D) posterior tibial veins
	(E) plantar metatarsal veins
68. _____	(F) peroneal veins
69. _____	(G) popliteal vein
	(H) great saphenous vein
70. _____	
71. _____	
72. _____	

Questions 73 through 76: Match the letters on the sonogram with the structures in column A

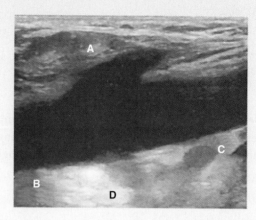

FIGURE 13–33.

COLUMN A

73. posterior enhancement _____

74. common femoral vein _____

75. great saphenous vein _____

76. femoral vein _____

77. **Which of the following is shown in the compression image in Fig. 13–34?**

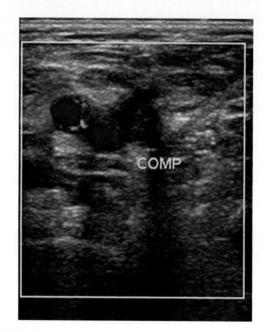

FIGURE 13–34.

(A) normal response to compression maneuver

(B) thrombosed common femoral vein

(C) vascularized lymph node

(D) groin pseudoaneurysm

78. Fig. 13–35 represents which of the following?

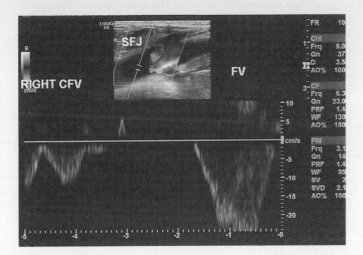

FIGURE 13–35.

(A) normal phasic flow

(B) refluxing saphenous vein

(C) normal response to distal compression

(D) pulsatile venous flow

79. Fig. 13–36 represents which of the following?

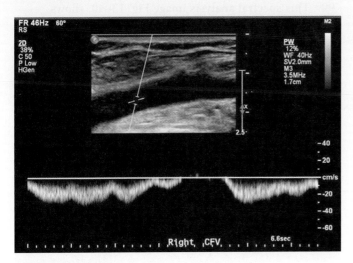

FIGURE 13–36.

(A) normal phasic flow

(B) incompetent valves

(C) normal response to distal compression

(D) pulsatile venous flow

80. Posterior to the neck of the pancreas, what two veins join to form the portal vein?

(A) splenic vein and hepatic vein

(B) hepatic vein and superior mesenteric vein

(C) hepatic vein and celiac vein

(D) splenic vein and superior mesenteric vein

Questions 81 through 94: Match the letter in Column B with the appropriate veins as seen in Fig. 13–37.

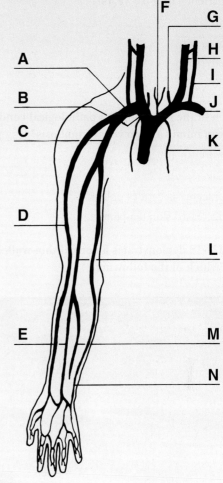

FIGURE 13–37.

COLUMN A

81. Ulna _____

82. Left subclavian _____

83. Vertebral _____

84. Cephalic _____

85. External jugular _____

86. Axillary _____

87. Basilic _____

88. Radial _____

89. Internal jugular _____

90. Brachiocephalic _____

91. Brachial _____

92. Inferior thyroid _____

93. Right subclavian _____

94. Internal thoracic _____

COLUMN B

(A)

(B)

(C)

(D)

(E)

(F)

(G)

(H)

(I)

(J)

(K)

(L)

(M)

(N)

95. What percentage of patients with deep vein thrombosis will be likely to develop venous insufficiency in 5–10 years?

    (A) 50%
    (B) 60%
    (C) 70%
    (D) 80%

96. Which of the following is a pathological condition that can mimic a deep vein thrombosis?

    (A) aortic aneurysm
    (B) Baker's cyst
    (C) phlegmasia cerulea dolens
    (D) decreased skin temperature

97. Fig. 13–38 demonstrates a normal thin-walled vein with which of the following?

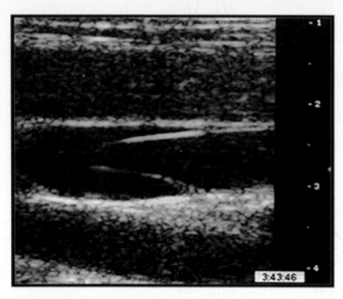

FIGURE 13–38.

    (A) a closed valve
    (B) a opened valve
    (C) the early stages of a thrombosis
    (D) an artifact

98. This compression image in Fig. 13–39 at the mid-thigh represents which of the following?

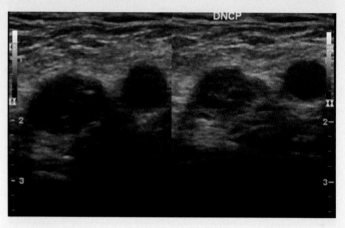

FIGURE 13–39.

    (A) An artifact within the lumen
    (B) incompressibility of a vein segment
    (C) compressibility of a vein segment
    (D) Rupture of vein segment due to transducer compression

99. This spectral analysis image Fig. 13–40 shows venous flow with

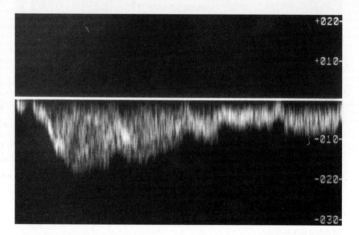

FIGURE 13–40.

    (A) normal respiratory movements
    (B) augmentation
    (C) collateral flow pattern
    (D) vein pulsatility

100. Fig. 13–41 is a gray-scale image of the common femoral vein (C) at the saphenous–femoral junctions. What is the arrow pointing to?

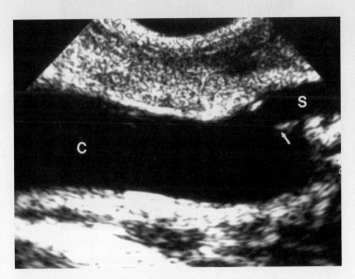

FIGURE 13–41.

(A) plaque at the saphenous–femoral junction

(B) an artifact

(C) open valves at the saphenous–femoral junction

(D) early stages of thrombosis at the saphenous–femoral junction

101. The spectral analysis of the portal vein in Fig. 13–42 shows normal respiratory movements and

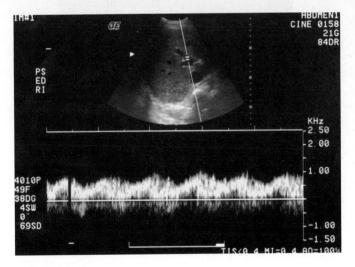

FIGURE 13–42.

(A) blood flow away from the liver

(B) flow that is bidirectional

(C) pulsatility

(D) blood flow toward the liver

102. The image in Fig. 13–43 is of the common femoral vein with a Doppler waveform demonstrating

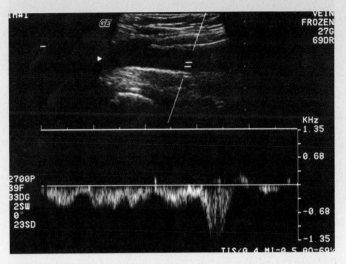

FIGURE 13–43.

(A) normal distal augmentation

(B) augmentation demonstrating venous insufficiency

(C) normal phasic waveform

(D) augmentation demonstrating proximal thrombus

103. The spectral analysis of the middle hepatic vein in Fig. 13–44 shows the characteristics of

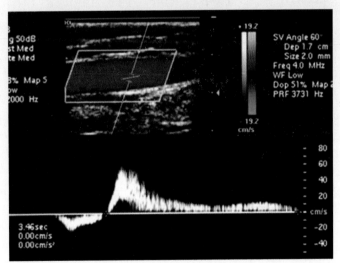

FIGURE 13–44.

(A) augmentation demonstrating reflux

(B) pulsatile Doppler waveform

(C) normal phasic waveform

(D) continuous Doppler waveform

104. **What is shown in the image in Fig. 13–45?**

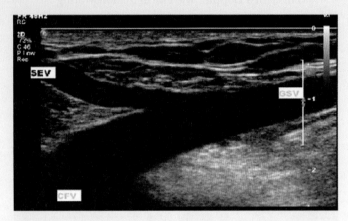

FIGURE 13–45.

    (A) popliteal trifurcation

    (B) confluence of the deep femoral and femoral veins

    (C) sapheno-popliteal junction

    (D) sapheno-femoral junction

105. **What is shown in the image in Fig. 13–46?**

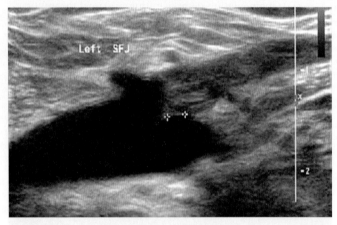

FIGURE 13–46.

    (A) normal sapheno-femoral junction

    (B) occlusion of the great saphenous vein

    (C) chronic occlusion of the saphenous vein

    (D) static valve at the sapheno-femoral junction

106. **After an episode of deep vein thrombosis, the venous valves are destroyed and become incompetent. This is termed**

    (A) thrombophlebitis

    (B) Raynaud's phenomenon

    (C) post-phlebitic syndrome

    (D) phlegmasia cerulea dolens

107. **Fig. 13–47 represents**

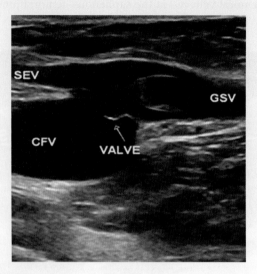

FIGURE 13–47.

    (A) reflux in the femoral vein

    (B) thrombus in the common femoral vein

    (C) thrombus in the proximal great saphenous vein

    (D) normal great saphenous vein

108. **Fig. 13–48 represents**

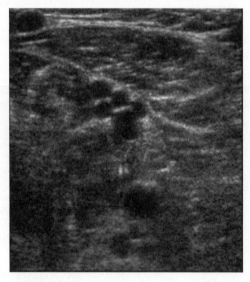

FIGURE 13–48.

    (A) a large Baker's cyst

    (B) a ruptured gastrocnemius muscle

    (C) multiple veins in the calf (posterior tibial and peroneal veins)

    (D) soleal vein thrombosis

109. Identify the findings in Fig. 13–49.

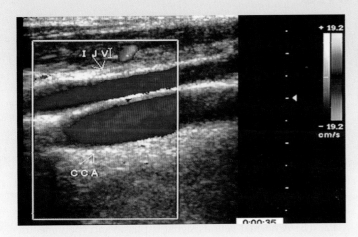

FIGURE 13–49.

   (A) normal flow dynamics of the neck vessels

   (B) partially occluded external jugular vein

   (C) partially occluded internal jugular vein

   (D) retrograde internal jugular vein flow

110. Identify the findings in Fig. 13–50.

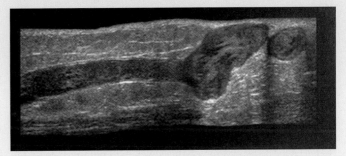

FIGURE 13–50.

   (A) normal appearance of the short saphenous vein in the foot

   (B) occluded, varicose superficial vein

   (C) partially occluded deep vein in the leg

   (D) an occluded popliteal vein behind the knee

Answers and Explanations

At the end of each explained answer, there is a number combination in parentheses. The first number identifies the reference source; the second number or set of numbers indicates the page or pages on which the relevant information can be found.

1. **(A)** All deep veins of the lower leg contain at least ten valves. As many as 10–15 may be present in each vein. They are usually paired and communicate with the superficial system. (*Study Guide*)

2. **(C)** The longest vein in the body is the great saphenous vein located in lower extremities. The largest vein in the body is the inferior vena cava (IVC) located in the abdomen. (*Study Guide*)

3. **(B)** The popliteal vein extends upward through the adductor (Hunter's) canal to become the femoral vein. The flexor hallucis longus are tendons in close proximity to the interosseous membrane in the distal third of the lower leg. The femoral vein ascends into Scarpa's triangle, then crosses behind the artery to assume a more medial position. (*Study Guide*)

4. **(B)** The femoral vein located in the lower extremities, is part of the deep venous system. The great and short saphenous veins are also in the lower extremities. The basilic vein is found in the upper extremity. (*Study Guide*)

5. **(C)** Normally the veins are not pulsatile. Exceptions include cardiac disease, extreme bradycardia and overtransfusion, which can cause pulsatility. Variations in the diameter of veins are caused by respiration, rather than the cardiac cycle. (*Study Guide*)

6. **(D)** Seventy-five to 80% of the blood volume is contained within the venous system. The ability of the veins to adjust shape and size makes it ideally suited for the storage of blood. (*Study Guide*)

7. **(A)** Veins have thinner walls with very little muscle, resulting in their being both distensible and collapsible. They can also be divided into deep and superficial systems, unlike arteries. (*Study Guide*)

8. **(B)** The primary clinical concern in DVT is the complication of pulmonary embolism. Claudication is an arterial disease. Valvular incompetence frequently results from a DVT. (*Study Guide*)

9. **(B)** Duplex scanning of the deep vein system of the lower extremities is usually performed with the patient supine and the leg externally rotated. It is important that the leg also be relaxed for ease of blood flow. The popliteal vein can be visualized with the patient in a prone position. (*Study Guide*)

10. **(C)** The tunica adventitia, the outer layer, is the strongest part of the vein wall. It is composed of collagen fibers. Tunica media is the middle layer. Tunica intima is the inner layer that contains the venous valves. (*Study Guide*)

11. **(B)** A spontaneous venous signal may not be heard at the posterior tibial vein at the ankle. In this location, the blood flow rate may be below the sensitivity of the Doppler velocity detectors. Most Doppler velocity detectors cannot detect movement below 6 cm/s. (*Study Guide*)

12. **(B)** A normal venous signal is phasic and spontaneous. A continuous venous signal indicates either internal obstruction of flow or external compression of the vein proximal to the position of the transducer. (*Study Guide*)

13. **(D)** Phlegmasia cerulea dolens produces a clinical pattern of tight leg edema, severe pain, and cyanotic mottled skin when extensive iliofemoral thrombosis occurs. Raynaud's syndrome is a functional vasospastic disorder affecting the small arteries and arterioles of the extremities. (*Study Guide*)

14. **(A)** In patients who have had previous episodes of deep vein thrombosis the vessel walls are thickened not thinned. Post-phlebitic syndrome often leads to chronic induration, stasis dermatitis, and ulcers in later years. Symptoms of this condition appear between 18 months and 10 years after the thrombotic event. (*Study Guide*)

15. **(B)** Respiration causes the diaphragm to descend. This increases intra-abdominal pressure, decreasing blood flow from the lower extremities while increasing the flow from the upper part of the body. (*Study Guide*)

16. **(D)** CT scan cannot evaluate chronic venous insufficiency. Photoplethysmography, Doppler, ultrasound, descending contrast venography, ascending contrast venography, and ambulatory venous pressure can evaluate chronic venous insufficiency. (*Study Guide*)

17. **(C)** Immobility of extremity is not one of the categories of "Virchow's triad." Rudolf Virchow was the German pathologist who introduced the theory between 1845 and 1856. There are many risk factors that may increase a patient's chances of developing thrombosis, but all factors should fit into one of the three categories. (*Study Guide*)

18. **(B)** The posterior tibial veins' distal landmark is the area between the medial malleolus and the Achilles tendon. After identifying the vessels, they can be followed up the medial surface of the calf. The veins are paired, one vein on either side of the posterior tibial artery. (*Study Guide*)

19. **(B)** The tunica intima (inner layer) is the thin layer of endothelial cells that contains the venous valves. The

valves consist of two leaflets that maintain the blood flow in one direction, toward the heart. (*Study Guide*)

20. **(B)** The filter is placed in the inferior vena cava (via the jugular or femoral approach) to prevent the upward extension of clot to the lung. The Greenfield filter consists of a small cone-shaped filter that is placed usually below the levels of the renal veins in the IVC. (*Study Guide*)

21. **(D)** As soon as the subclavian vein branch of the cephalic vein, its name change to the axillary vein. This happens at the outer border of the first rib. Usually, only one valve is found in the axillary vein. (*Study Guide*)

22. **(C)** The gastrocnemius plexus empties into the popliteal vein. The soleus plexus veins empty into the posterior tibial vein. (*Study Guide*)

23. **(C)** The right atrium pressure is normally 0 mm Hg and is termed central venous pressure. When it measures 0 mm Hg, the blood flows from the systemic veins into the right atrium. (*Study Guide*)

24. **(C)** Varicose veins cannot compromise the flow of a vessel by external compression. Baker's cyst, tumors, or hematomas often produce external compression that can compromise the flow. (*Study Guide*)

25. **(E)** Vein characteristics include phasicity, spontaneity, compressibility, and augmentation. They do not have a continuous signal without respiratory motion; this is characteristic of collateral venous flow. (*Study Guide*)

26. **(A)** There are no valves in the innominate veins. Valves are present in the external and internal jugular veins, axillary veins, and the subclavian vein. (*Study Guide*)

27. **(A)** The superficial veins of the lower extremities lie within 1–2 cm of the skin surface within the subcutaneous fat. The system consists of dorsal venous arch, marginal veins, and lesser and greater saphenous veins. (*Study Guide*)

28. **(B)** The Brescia–Cimino fistula is created surgically between the cephalic vein and the radial artery at the wrist. It has a 3-year patency rate of 80–90%, and is the most durable dialysis access. It requires 3 to 6 weeks to mature. (*Study Guide*)

29. **(D)** Deep vein thrombosis is occurring more frequently due to the increased use of central venous catheters. (*Study Guide*)

30. **(A)** The veins of the lower extremity flow from the superficial veins through the perforators(communicating veins) to the deep veins. Valves maintain the flow in one direction. Flow in the opposite directions is abnormal. (*Study Guide*)

31. **(B)** The anterior tibial vein is a continuation of the dorsalis pedis and lies between the tibial and fibula, located in the anterior compartment just on top of the interosseous membrane. In the upper part of the calf, they join the popliteal vein. (*Study Guide*)

32. **(C)** Outflow vein stenosis. (*Study Guide*)

33. **(C)** Sclerotherapy is the injection of a sclerosing agent into the superficial veins to damage the endothelium and cause thrombosis which organizes and closes the veins. (*Study Guide*)

34. **(B)** Surgery. Some of the causes of chronic venous insufficiency are varicose veins, chronic recurrent thrombosis, and post-thrombotic syndrome. Venous stasis, the result of the failure of the venous pump mechanism, reflects chronic venous insufficiency. (*Study Guide*)

35. **(D)** Compression of the vein with the transducer probe is a maneuver used to confirm patency and rule out the presence of clot. It is not the maneuver used for augmentation. Distal compression, Valsalva, or cough maneuvers are the methods for augmenting the veins. (*Study Guide*)

36. **(B)** Venous thrombus or clot obstructs the draining vein and creates a filling defect on the venogram. (*Study Guide*)

37. **(A)** Chronic thrombus is not compressible to any extent. (*Study Guide*)

38. **(A)** Absence of leg pain. Venous stasis is characterized by chronic swelling of the leg, malleolar ulceration, cutaneous hyperpigmentation, varicose veins, and leg pain. Venous stasis leads to chronic venous insufficiency. (*Study Guide*)

39. **(C)** Small not large arteriovenous fistulas have been suggested as a possible contributing factor to primary varicose veins. Other factors are abnormal wall weakness, increased distending force, and multiple arteriovenous fistulas. Primary varicose veins are associated with venous valvular incompetency. (*Study Guide*)

40. **(A)** Ascending venography cannot assess the function of the proximal valves in the lower extremity. Only descending venography can offer that capability. Ascending venograph can offer the location of incompetent perforators; localize recanalized channels indicating previous thrombophlebitis and the absence or presence of varicosities. (*Study Guide*)

41. **(B)** Varicose veins with competent deep vein valves and incompetent superficial veins are termed primary varicose veins. Veins with both incompetent superficial and deep vein valves are termed secondary varicose veins. (*Study Guide*)

42. **(B)** The posterior tibial veins arise from and drain the plantar venous arch and superficial venous net of the foot. They also receive the peroneal veins farther up the calf. (*Study Guide*)

43. **(D)** The subclavian vein receives both the superficial and deep venous system of the upper extremity. An occlusion of this vein blocks both these major systems. Acute pain,

swelling, and edema of the entire upper extremity can occur. (*Study Guide*)

44. **(A)** The feet contain 60–80% smooth muscle. Veins consist largely of smooth muscle and have relatively little elastin. (*Study Guide*)

45. **(B)** The dorsal digital and plantar veins unite to form the dorsal metatarsal veins that join to form the superficial dorsal venous arch. The plantar cutaneous arch eventually drains into the greater and lesser saphenous veins. (*Study Guide*)

46. **(C)** Normally, there are more than 100 communicating veins located throughout most limbs. They are mainly <2 mm in diameter and are usually described in groups. (*Study Guide*)

47. **(D)** The hydrostatic indifferent point (HIP) is just below the diaphragm. It is the only point that remains constant. (*Study Guide*)

48. **(C)** Generally about 5 days after the thrombus fills the vein, it will start to contract. The next step is recanalization. Valves within the thrombus are usually destroyed. (*Study Guide*)

49. **(C)** The significant causes for DVT are multiple: Surgery, oral contraceptive pills, smoking, prolonged bed rest, pregnancy and obesity. Diabetes is not among the most significant risk factor for DVT. (*Study Guide*)

50. **(A)** The soleal sinusoids are the most common site to develop a DVT according to recent studies. DVTs can originate any place with the venous system. (*Study Guide*)

51. **(A)** The plantar cutaneous arch empties into the great and short saphenous veins. The superficial dorsal venous arch also ends up at the great and short saphenous veins. (*Study Guide*)

52. **(B)** The descending venography offers the ability of assessing valvular functions. It directly visualizes the venous valves. (*Study Guide*)

53. **(C)** The renal system does not go through the portal vein. The spleen, stomach, pancreas, gallbladder, and intestines do send their blood to the liver by way of the portal vein. (*Study Guide*)

54. **(A)** The inherent semilunar venous valves are found in the tunica intima; the innermost lining of the vein. (*Study Guide*)

55. **(D)** The left ovarian vein drains into the left renal vein. The right empties directly into the inferior vena cava. (*Study Guide*)

56. **(C)** Valves are competent if they do not allow reversal of flow. The valves ensure flow in the forward direction toward the heart. (*Study Guide*)

57. **(A)** Popliteal vein (*Study Guide*)

58. **(B)** Great saphenous vein (*Study Guide*)

59. **(C)** Femoral vein (*Study Guide*)

60. **(F)** Profunda (deep) femoral vein (*Study Guide*)

61. **(E)** Internal iliac vein (*Study Guide*)

62. **(H)** Common femoral vein (*Study Guide*)

63. **(D)** Distal inferior vena cava (*Study Guide*)

64. **(G)** External iliac vein (*Study Guide*)

65. **(H)** Great saphenous vein (*Study Guide*)

66. **(F)** Peroneal veins (*Study Guide*)

67. **(D)** Plantar digital veins (*Study Guide*)

68. **(G)** Popliteal vein (*Study Guide*)

69. **(E)** Plantar metatarsal veins (*Study Guide*)

70. **(B)** Posterior tibial veins (*Study Guide*)

71. **(A)** Anterior tibial veins (*Study Guide*)

72. **(C)** Soleal vein (*Study Guide*)

73. **(D)** Posterior enhancement (*Study Guide*)

74. **(B)** common femoral vein (*Study Guide*)

75. **(A)** Great saphenous vein (*Study Guide*)

76. **(C)** Femoral vein (*Study Guide*)

77. **(B)** Thrombosed common femoral vein (*Study Guide*)

78. **(C)** Normal response to distal compression (*Study Guide*)

79. **(A)** Normal phasic flow (*Study Guide*)

80. **(D)** The splenic vein and the superior mesenteric vein join posterior to the neck of the pancreas to form the portal vein. The main portal vein courses toward the right, superiorly, and anteriorly. (*Study Guide*)

81. **(M)** Ulna vein (*Study Guide*)

82. **(J)** Left subclavian vein (*Study Guide*)

83. **(G)** Vertebral vein (*Study Guide*)

84. **(D)** Cephalic vein (*Study Guide*)

85. **(H)** External jugular vein (*Study Guide*)

86. **(C)** Axillary vein (*Study Guide*)

87. **(N)** Basilic vein (*Study Guide*)

88. **(E)** Radial vein (*Study Guide*)

89. **(H)** Internal jugular vein (*Study Guide*)

90. **(B)** Brachiocephalic vein (*Study Guide*)

91. **(L)** Brachial vein (*Study Guide*)

92. **(F)** Inferior thyroid vein (*Study Guide*)

93. **(A)** Right subclavian vein (*Study Guide*)

94. **(K)** Internal thoracic vein (*Study Guide*)

95. **(D)** About 80% of patients with deep vein thrombosis will be likely to develop venous insufficiency in the next 5–10 years. The incidence of serious venous problems is increasing in the United States according to recent studies. (*Study Guide*)

96. **(B)** Baker's cyst is a pathological condition that can mimic a deep vein thrombosis. It can also be easily demonstrated by ultrasound, along with the patency of the deep veins. (*Study Guide*)

97. **(B)** An opened valve (*Study Guide*)

98. **(B)** Incompressibility of a vein segment (*Study Guide*)

99. **(A)** Normal respiratory movement. It is phasic with respiration and controlled by intra-abdominal pressure. (*Study Guide*)

100. **(C)** Fig. 13–41 is a gray-scale image of the common femoral vein at the saphenous–femoral junction, with an arrow pointing to open valves at the junction. The margins of the valves are positioned in the direction of blood flow, and lie flat against the wall as long as the flow is going toward the heart. The valves close when the flow reverses. (*Study Guide*)

101. **(D)** The spectral analysis of the portal vein in Fig. 13–42 show normal respiratory movements and blood flow toward the liver. This is called hepatopetal flow. (*Study Guide*)

102. **(A)** The image in Fig. 13–43 is of the common femoral vein with a Doppler waveform demonstrating normal augmentation distal to the transducer. Squeezing the distal portion of the extremity forces the flow of the blood to increase at a rapid speed. (*Study Guide*)

103. **(A)** Augmentation demonstrating reflux (*Study Guide*)

104. **(D)** Fig. 13–45 is an image of a sapheno-femoral junction. (*Study Guide*)

105. **(B)** Fig. 13–46 pictures occlusion of the great saphenous vein. (*Study Guide*)

106. **(C)** Deep vein thrombosis results in the post-phlebitic syndrome and venous incompetency. The venous valves are destroyed with deep vein thrombosis leading to venous incompetency. In later years, there will be chronic induration, stasis, dermatitis, and ulceration associated with venous incompetency. (*Study Guide*)

107. **(C)** Fig. 13–47 represents thrombus in the proximal great saphenous vein.

108. **(C)** Fig. 13–48 represents multiple veins in the calf (posterior tibial and peroneal veins)

109. **(D)** Fig. 13–49 shows retrograde internal jugular vein flow.

110. **(B)** Fig. 13–50 shows occluded, varicose superficial vein.

14

Peripheral Arterial Sonography

George L. Berdejo, Fernando Amador, Joshua Cruz, and Evan C. Lipsitz

Study Guide

ANATOMY OF THE ARTERIAL CIRCULATION

The circulatory system is a closed system of tubes that carry oxygenated blood away from the heart to the tissues of the body and then return deoxygenated blood to the heart. The system consists of arteries (large elastic tubes) dividing into medium size muscular arteries and into smaller arteries that branch into arterioles that branch into microscopic vessels termed capillaries. Vasa vasorum are small vessels that nourish the media and the adventitia. The systemic circulation includes all the arteries and arterioles that carry oxygenated blood from the left ventricle to the systemic capillaries plus the veins and venules that carry deoxygenated blood returning to the right atrium after flowing through the organs and tissue. Subdivisions of the systemic circulation are the coronary, cerebral and the hepatic portal circulation.[1]

The composition of large and medium-size arteries include:

- *intima (tunica interna)* The intima is the innermost layer and is a monolayer of flattened endothelial cells and a thin underlying matrix of collagen and elastic fibers.
- *media (tunica media)* The media is a thick middle layer of varying amounts of smooth muscle, collagen, and elastic fibers. It has an outer border of external elastic membrane separating it from the adventitia.
- *adventitia (tunica externa)* The adventitia is the outermost layer of an artery composed of collagen and elastin, which provides the strength of the arterial wall (Fig. 14–1).[2]

The composition of the arteries provides two important functional properties: elasticity and contractility. The ventricles of the heart contract and eject blood from the heart, and the large arteries expand and accommodate the increased blood flow. The ventricles relax, and the elastic recoil of the arteries forces the blood onward. As the sympathetic stimulation is increased, the smooth muscle of the artery contracts and narrows the vessel lumen, which is termed vasoconstriction. Conversely, as the sympathetic stimulation decreases, the smooth muscle relaxes and the vessel dilates; this is termed vasodilatation.[2]

All systemic arteries arise from the heart and branch from the aorta and are termed according to their location. The aorta is divided into the ascending aorta, aortic arch, the descending aorta, thoracic aorta, and the abdominal aorta. The lower abdominal aorta bifurcates into the common iliac arteries to supply the pelvis and lower extremities. The arteries of the pelvis include the following: the common iliac arteries, internal iliac (hypogastric) arteries, and external iliac arteries.[3]

THE AORTA

The systemic circulation begins with the left side of the heart.[4–6] As blood passes through the mitral valve during diastole, the left ventricle expands to allow blood to accumulate. During the systolic contraction of the left ventricle, blood will pass through the aortic valve and into the aortic arch. The aorta is the longest artery in the body. The aorta is divided into four main segments (Fig. 14–2):

1. Ascending aorta or aortic trunk
2. Aortic arch
3. Descending or more commonly known as the thoracic aorta
4. Abdominal aorta

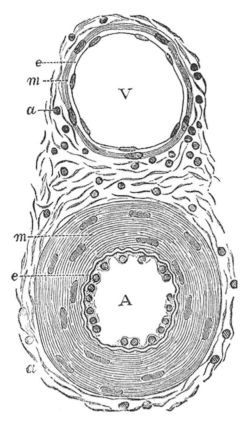

FIGURE 14–1. Transverse section of a small artery (A) and vein (V) of a child. The intima, media and adventitia are represented by the lowercase letters *e*, *m* and *a* respectively. *(Figure from Wikipedia Commons in the public domain.)*

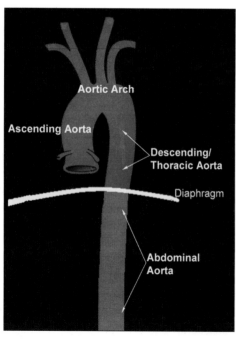

FIGURE 14–2. Cartoon displaying the four segments of the aorta.

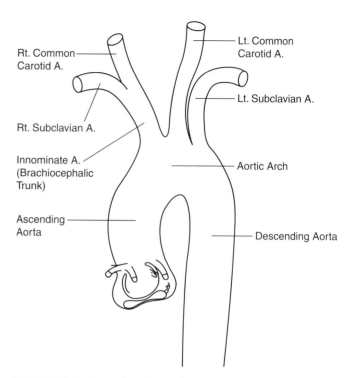

FIGURE 14–3. The aortic arch vessels include the innominate artery, which divides and gives off the right common carotid and right subclavian arteries. The next major vessel is the left common carotid and the last major arch vessel is the left subclavian artery.

The great vessels include the aortic arch and its three major branches that include the following (Fig. 14–3):

1. Innominate artery or brachiocephalic trunk
2. Left common carotid artery (CCA)
3. Left subclavian artery

The abdominal aorta begins at the aortic hiatus of the diaphragm, in front of the lower border of the body of the last thoracic vertebra, and descending in front of the vertebral column, ends on the body of the fourth lumbar vertebra, commonly a little to the left of the middle line by dividing into the two common iliac arteries. It diminishes rapidly in size, in consequence of the many large branches that it gives off. The major branches of the abdominal aorta are the celiac, superior mesenteric, renal, lumbar, and inferior mesenteric arteries.

The celiac artery and the superior and inferior mesenteric arteries are unpaired, while the renals are paired. The celiac artery is a short trunk, about 1.25 cm in length, which arises from the front of the aorta, just below the aortic hiatus of the diaphragm, and passing nearly horizontally forward, divides into three large branches, the left gastric, the common hepatic, and the splenic; it occasionally gives off one of the inferior phrenic arteries. The renals emerge immediately distal to the level of the superior mesenteric artery to perfuse the right and left kidney.

Arterial supply of the pelvis and lower extremities (Figs. 14–4 and 14–5).

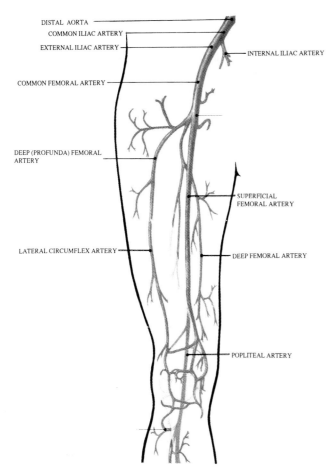

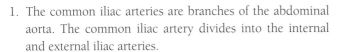

FIGURE 14–4. Anatomy of the arterial circulation from the distal abdominal aorta to the popliteal artery below the knee.

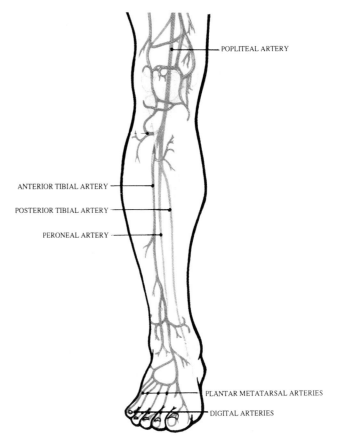

FIGURE 14–5. Anatomy of the major arteries below the knee.

1. The common iliac arteries are branches of the abdominal aorta. The common iliac artery divides into the internal and external iliac arteries.

2. The internal iliac arteries supply the pelvic wall, perineum, pelvic organs, and some areas of the gluteal and thigh.

3. The external iliac arteries. The two main branches are the inferior epigastric artery and deep circumflex iliac artery.

4. The common femoral artery is a continuation of the external iliac artery. It divides into the superficial and deep femoral arteries.

5. The deep femoral artery serves as an important collateral when there is significant disease in the superficial femoral artery.

6. The superficial femoral artery is a continuation of the common femoral artery. It courses the length of the thigh passing through the adductor canal or Hunter's canal at the distal third of the thigh, where it becomes the above the knee popliteal artery.

7. The popliteal artery is a continuation of the superficial femoral artery. The popliteal artery divides into the anterior tibial artery and tibioperoneal trunk. There are multiple branches around the knee area genicular branches, muscular branches, and sural arteries.

8. The anterior tibial artery is a branch of the popliteal artery. It runs along the along the anterior aspect of the tibia. The anterior tibial artery becomes the dorsalis pedis artery at the foot.

9. The tibioperoneal trunk is the second branch of the distal popliteal artery. The tibioperoneal trunk branches into the posterior tibial and peroneal arteries.

10. The posterior tibial artery extends down the medial and posterior region of the lower leg. Distal to the medial malleolus it divides into the medial and lateral plantar arteries and it feeds the sole of the foot.

11. The peroneal artery extends down the lateral and posterior region of the lower leg, along the fibula. The peroneal artery branches into anterior and posterior perforators. The peroneal feeds the lateral lower leg and the calcaneus (heel) area.

12. The plantar arch is comprised of the deep and the lateral plantar artery. The deep plantar artery is a branch of the dorsalis pedis artery. The lateral plantar arch is a branch of the posterior tibial artery. They supply the digits, skin and muscle of the foot.

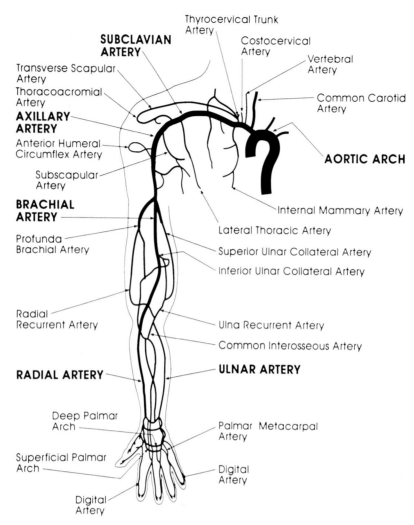

FIGURE 14–6. Arterial anatomy of the upper extremities. Major vessels are in bold print.

Arterial Supply of the Upper Extremities (Fig. 14–6)

The right subclavian artery arises from the brachiocephalic trunk. The left subclavian artery is the third branch of the aortic arch. The subclavian artery extends under the clavicle and gives off five branches:

1. Vertebral artery
2. Internal mammary
3. Dorsal scapular
4. Thyrocervical
5. Costocervical

The axillary artery, a continuation of the subclavian artery, gives off branches that feed muscle of the chest and shoulder.

1. Superior thoracic
2. Thoraco-acromial
3. Lateral thoracic
4. Subscapular
5. Anterior circumflex humeral
6. Posterior circumflex humeral

The brachial artery is a continuation of the axillary artery, which extends to the elbow and bifurcates into the radial and ulnar artery below the antecubital fossa. The ulnar and radial arteries are the main arteries of the forearm.

The radial artery courses along the lateral side of the forearm to the wrist and at the hand it forms the deep palmar arch. The ulnar artery courses along the medial side of the forearm to the wrist and at the hand forms the superficial palmar arch. In the hand the volar and digital arteries supply muscle and skin of the hand and digits.

PHYSIOLOGY AND HEMODYNAMICS

The physiology of circulation is termed hemodynamics. Blood flows as a result of the difference in energy or pressure. The arterial system represents the high energy/pressure, and the

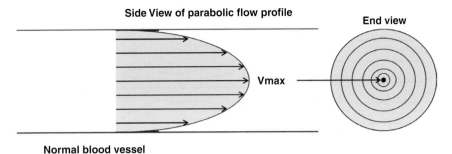

FIGURE 14–7. Laminar flow, sometimes known as streamline flow, occurs when a fluid flows in parallel layers, with no disruption between the layers. Note the fastest moving flow is in the center of the vessel resulting in a parabolic flow profile.

veins represent the low energy/pressure. Energy/pressure levels decrease from the arterial to venous ends because of the lost energy as a result of blood viscosity and its inertia. There are layers and particles inherent in the vessels that create resistance and cause a loss of energy. The energy is restored by the pumping action of the heart to maintain the arterial energy/pressure difference required for the blood flow. Blood flow through the arterial system is termed *laminar flow* and is defined as blood movement in concentric layers with the highest velocity in the center of the vessel creating a parabolic flow profile[7] (Fig. 14–7). There are several laws that govern blood flow and influence the results of the Doppler evaluation of the arterial system.

Poiseuille's Law states that in a cylindric tube model, the mean linear velocity of laminar flow is directly proportional to the energy difference between the ends of the tube and the square of the radius. It is inversely proportional to the length of the tube and viscosity of the fluid. Volume flow is proportional to the fourth power of the vessel radius[7,8] (Fig. 14–8). Small changes in the radius can result in large changes in flow. Laminar flow may be disturbed or turbulent.

The factors affecting the development of turbulence are expressed by the Reynolds number (Fig. 14–9). The development of turbulence depends mainly on the size of the vessel and the velocity of flow. Laminar flow is stable, and the streamline tends to remain intact, whereas turbulent flow has broken discontinuous streamlines that produce eddy currents (circular, backward movements of the fluid) and vortices (radial rotation of the fluid within a body of fluid) (Fig. 14–10). The stability of a fluid can be reasonably predicted by the Reynolds number. Laminar flow tends to be disturbed if the Reynolds number exceeds 2,000.[7,8]

In cases of arterial stenosis specific characteristics are seen. Proximal to the stenosis, blood forms a velocity gradient across the vessel lumen as it moves. The flow velocity increases upon entering the stenosis because of the decreased cross-sectional area. Inside the stenosis, the flow may be increased but remain stable. It maintains its streamlines and organization. Distally where the lumen is restored, there is an unstable flow pattern. At the orifice of the stenosis, there is usually flow separation that produces a stagnant region around the narrowing. In the center of the stenosis, the high-velocity jet flows into the larger opening and creates flow reversals, eddy currents, and vortices. As the flow continues down the vessel, the energy present in the flow turbulence dissipates and stability returns to the flowing blood.

Bernoulli's equation plays a central role in the quantitative applications of Doppler. The equation makes the assumption that the total energy along a streamline is constant. The energy simply changes from one form to another as the conditions of the streamline changes.

Bernoulli's equation states that the moving fluid shifts energy from one form to another, depending on the conditions. The total energy remains constant. If the flow is vertical, the hydrostatic pressure makes contribution.[8,9]

$$Q = \frac{(P_1 - P_2)\, \pi r^4}{8L\eta}$$

Q = Flow
P_1 = Proximal Pressure
P_2 = Distal Pressure
π = Pi, a constant
r = Radius
L = Length
η = Viscosity

FIGURE 14–8. Poiseuille's equation.

$$Re = \frac{v \times r}{\dfrac{n}{p}}$$

Re = Reynolds Number
v = Velocity of Blood (cm/sec)
r = Radius (cm)
n = Viscosity (poises)
p = Density

FIGURE 14–9. The equation for Reynolds number.

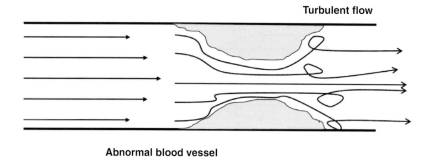

FIGURE 14–10. The hemodynamics of stenosis. Exit effects beyond the stenosis result in swirling and eddying of the blood flow (turbulence).

Bernoulli's Principle

$$P_1 + \rho g h_1 + 1/2pv_1{}^2 = P_2 + \rho g h_2 + 1/2pv_2{}^2 + heat,$$

where P = pressure

        $\rho g h$ = hydrostatic pressure

        $1/2pv^2$ = kinetic energy

The sum of velocity and kinetic energy of a fluid flowing through a tube is constant.

The volume of blood flow through tissue in a given period of time (milliliters per minute) is termed the blood flow. The velocity of blood flow (centimeters per second) is inversely related to the cross-sectional area of the blood vessel such that:

$$V = Q/A,$$

where V is velocity, Q is flow, and A is the area of the vessel. Therefore, the blood flows slowest where the cross-sectional area is greatest. Blood pressure (BP) is the pressure exerted by blood on the wall of a blood vessel. Blood pressure is created by the contraction of the ventricles. In the aorta of a resting young adult, BP rises to approximately 120 mm Hg during systole (contraction) and drops to approximately 80 mm Hg during diastole (relaxation). If the carbon monoxide rises, the blood pressure rises. If the total volume of blood in the system decreases, the BP decreases. As blood flows into small arteries, the resistance increases and the pressure within the arteries begins to fall. The expansion and contraction of arteries after each systole of the left ventricle creates a pressure wave termed the pulse, which is transmitted down the aorta into the peripheral arteries. Normally, the pulse rate is the same as the heart rate. Resting pulse is between 70 and 80 beats per minute. Tachycardia is the term for a rapid resting heart or pulse rate (>100/min) and brachycardia is the term for a slow resting heart or pulse rate (<60/min). If pulses are missed, it is irregular.[9] Blood pressure is usually measured in the left brachial artery using a sphygmomanometer.

MECHANISMS OF DISEASE

Risk Factors.[10,11] There are several risk factors that contribute to the development of atherosclerosis, some of which can be controlled, and some that cannot. Risk factors include:

- Documented atheroma in any artery
- Diabetes

- Dyslipidemia (cholesterol and triglyceride level disturbances)
- Higher fibrinogen blood concentrations
- Homocysteine in the upper half of the normal range, and especially elevated levels
- Aging and male gender (women have more problems after menopause, but hormone replacement therapy worsens rather than improves the risk)
- Tobacco smoking, even just once a day. This is probably the most important risk factor for peripheral vascular disease. Smoking accelerates the atherosclerotic process and causes vasospasm.
- First-degree relatives with heart disease or a stroke at a relatively young age
- High blood pressure
- Obesity (especially central obesity, i.e. fat at waist level, especially intra-abdominal (around the intestines)
- Being physically less active, especially aerobic exercise
- Several internal chemical markers indicating ongoing inflammation may also relate to relative risk

These risk factors, judging from clinical trials, operate synergistically to promote earlier and more severe disease yet still miss many who become disabled from the consequences of atherosclerosis.

Most humans develop atherosclerosis. Usually only "high-risk" patients are advised to change dietary choices, exercise, lose weight, take cholesterol-lowering mediation and lower blood sugar levels.

Atherosclerosis

Atherosclerosis is a chronic systemic disease that affects the arterial system and occurs within the arterial wall, typically within or beneath the intima. There are various characteristics of the disease, among them location. Atherosclerosis is commonly seen at origins and bifurcations of vessels. Since flow divides and changes its laminar characteristics, a shearing force is created at the flow divider and over time, this is responsible for the wear of the intima.[12]

It is a chronic inflammatory response in the walls of arteries, in large part due to the accumulation of macrophage white blood cells and promoted by low-density (especially small particle) lipoproteins (plasma proteins that carry cholesterol and triglycerides) without adequate removal of fats and cholesterol from the macrophages by functional high-density lipoproteins (HDLs). It is commonly referred to as a "hardening" of the arteries.

Plaque formation may begin as simple layers of lipids called fatty streaks that are deposited in the wall. Over time plaque on the walls may progress to a more fibrous component that includes the accumulation of lipids, collagen, and fibrin that is soft and gelatinous in texture appearing as a hypoechoic structure along the arterial wall. Over time the plaque may proliferate further into the lumen causing narrowing, also known as stenosis. The walls may harden secondary to a more calcium and collagen component. Unstable plaques or plaques that have areas that are weak, compared to more firm or well-integrated plaque within the wall, potentially can be a source of embolic debris.[12]

It is caused by the formation of multiple plaques within the arteries.[11,12] The atheromatous plaque is divided into three distinct components:

1. The atheroma, which is the nodular accumulation of a soft, flaky, yellowish material at the center of large plaques, composed of macrophages nearest the lumen of the artery

2. Underlying areas of cholesterol crystals

3. Calcification at the outer base of older/more advanced lesions

Atherosclerosis typically begins in early adolescence and is usually found in most major arteries, yet is asymptomatic and not detected by most diagnostic methods during life. Autopsies of healthy young men that died during the Korean and Vietnam Wars showed evidence of the disease.[13,14] It most commonly becomes seriously symptomatic when interfering with the coronary circulation supplying the heart or cerebral circulation supplying the brain and is considered the most important underlying cause of strokes, heart attacks, various heart diseases including congestive heart failure, and most cardiovascular diseases, in general. Atheroma in arm, or more often, leg arteries, that results in decreased blood flow, is called peripheral artery occlusive disease (PAOD).

According to U.S. data for the year 2004, for about 65% of men and 47% of women, the first symptom of atherosclerotic cardiovascular disease is heart attack or sudden cardiac death (death within one hour of onset of the symptom). Most artery flow disrupting events occur at locations with less than 50% residual lumen.

Embolism is defined as an obstruction in a vessel from a foreign substance (blood clot). Most arterial embolisms are of cardiac origin and often seen in patients with atrial fibrillation, after a myocardial infarction, ventricular aneurysm, bacterial endocarditis, mechanical heart valves, atrial myxoma, and paradoxical emboli. Other sources of embolism are aneurysms or atherosclerotic plaques. Common locations of cardio-emboli

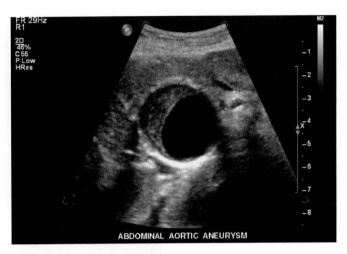

FIGURE 14–11. Transverse ultrasound image of an abdominal aortic aneurysm with laminated thrombus seen on the lateral wall to the left (patient's right).

are the aortic bifurcation, iliacs, femoral bifurcation, and popliteal artery.

Aneurysms are a permanent localized dilation of an artery with an increase in diameter of at least 50% compared to an adjacent segment. The dilation involves all three layers of the artery. Common places to find aneurysms are the infrarenal aorta, femoral, and popliteal arteries. A fusiform aneurysm is a circumferential dilation of an artery. A saccular aneurysm is outer bulge of a discrete part of the artery.

Abdominal aortic aneurysms (AAAs) are primarily found in the infrarenal aorta. If the diameter of the aorta is >3 cm or twice the size of the adjacent segment it can be considered aneurysmal (Fig. 14–11). The risk factors for developing an aortic aneurysm are age (>65 years), gender (male > female), hypertension, family history, smokers, and the presence of chronic obstructive pulmonary disease. The larger the aneurysm, the greater the risk of rupture. AAAs >5 cm in diameter have a 25% rupture rate within 5 years. In addition to rupture, other complications of AAA are occlusion, embolization that may cause blue-toe syndrome, compression of adjacent peri-abdominal structures, infection and aortocaval fistula.[15]

Pseudoaneurysm (false aneurysm) is a contained hematoma that is often the result of injury to the artery, either traumatic or iatrogenic (Fig. 14–12). Arteriovenous fistula is a communication between an artery and an adjacent vein. These are common complications post-cardiac catheterization. The most common place to see a pseudoaneurysm is in the groin. Pseudoaneurysms are simply diagnosed and treated using ultrasound techniques. Historically, duplex-guided manual compression had routinely been used to correct these lesions; however, in recent years, ultrasound-guided thrombin injection has been employed.[16] Depending on the anatomy of the arteriovenous fistula, these may also be treated using duplex-guided manual compression.[17]

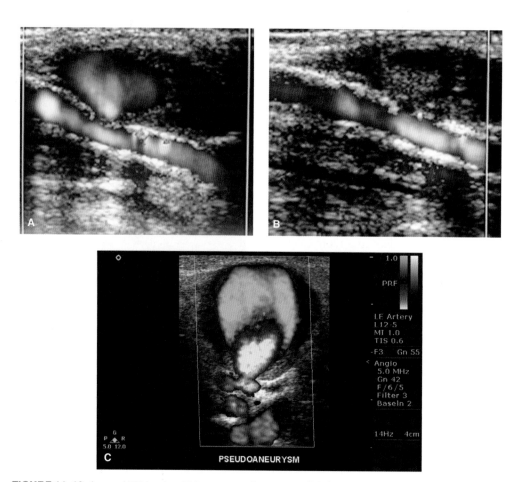

FIGURE 14–12. In panel "**A**" is a brachial artery pseudoaneurysm (PSA). Although there is flow within the sac, thrombus, seen to the right of the image, has started to form within the sac. Panel "**B**" shows a post-compression scan. The PSA sac is now completely filled with thrombus after 10 minutes of duplex-guided manual compression. Panel "**C**" shows a femoral artery PSA with very little thrombus formation.

A mycotic aneurysm is caused by an infectious process that involves the arterial wall. They often occur in multiple sites and are usually seen as a complication of bacterial endocarditis. In children, ultrasound or magnetic resonance imaging may be used to identify and monitor treatment of the aneurysm because of the noninvasive nature and lack of radiation. The mycotic aneurysm exhibits the same ultrasound characteristics as the aneurysm.

Dissection is a non-atherosclerotic condition that is usually a result of trauma that causes a sudden tear in the intimal lining of the vessel (Fig. 14–13). The intima then separates from the media and adventitia. This separation creates a "false" lumen whereby blood may pulsate. Since there is no place for pulsatile flow in the false lumen, it may extend proximally or distally or may thrombose. The risk of thrombosis may cause hemodynamic changes in the true lumen and cause neurological symptoms when the dissection involves the carotid arteries.[15]

Nonatherosclerotic Lesions[18]

Arteritis is a disease that is characterized by inflammation of the blood vessels. This inflammatory response may lead to occlu-

sion or narrowing of arterial lumen. Takayasu's arteritis is a type of vasculitis or arteritis that affects large vessels as well as the aorta and its main branches (brachiocephalic, common carotid and subclavian arteries). It is most common in young Asian

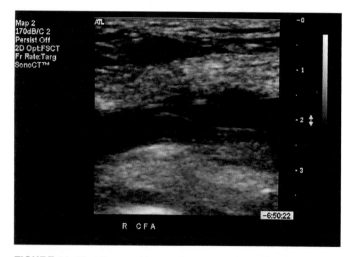

FIGURE 14–13. Ultrasound image of a common femoral artery with dissection (linear echo) that extends proximally (to the left of the image) into the external iliac artery.

women. Cardiovascular symptoms may include hypertension, diminished peripheral pulses and aortic regurgitation.

Behçet's syndrome is a multisystem vasculitis that affects the arteries and veins. It presents with ulcer of the genital and mouth and other skin lesions. Recurrent superficial and deep vein thrombosis is common and may include cerebral venous thrombosis.

Polyarteritis nodosa is a vasculitis that involves the medium and small muscular arteries. It may lead to aneurysmal formation, renal dysfunction, congestive heart failure, and new onset of hypertension.

Kawasaki disease is a vasculitis that may affect large, medium, and small arteries, but it is more frequent in the coronary arteries. It predominately affects boys. It presents with an unexplained fever, rash, erythema of the palms/soles, oral mucous changes (strawberry tongue and fissure lips).

Thromboangiitis obliterans (Buerger's disease) is a segmental inflammatory disease that affects the small and medium-sized arteries and veins and nerve in the upper and lower extremities. It is a highly cellular inflammatory thrombus within the blood vessel, but it spares the vessel walls. It primarily occurs in young male (younger than 40 years) heavy smokers. It begins with ischemia of the distal arteries and veins of the extremities. Patients may present with rest pain, ischemic ulcers, or thrombophlebitis.

Raynaud's phenomenon is characterized by episodic vasospasm on exposure to cold or with emotional stress. The classic presentation is blanching of the digits (white), and the pallor is replaced by cyanosis (blue) due to an ischemic response and finally the digits turn red during hyperemic phase, although these changes may not necessarily occur in series (Fig. 14–14).

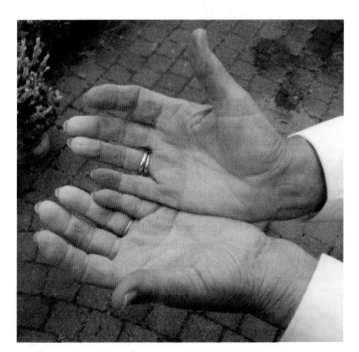

FIGURE 14–14. The hands of a patient with Raynaud's phenomenon. Note the different color changes in this patient demonstrating the various stages of the color change.

Raynaud's phenomenon is classified as primary (not associated with any other disease) and secondary (associated with underlying disease, connective tissue disorder, arterial occlusive disease, trauma, neurologic disorders, drugs, and toxins). The most common site of occurrence is the fingers. Other sites include the toes, nose, and ears. The risk factors associated with the disorder are female sex, family history, and exposure to cold weather. Patients with primary Raynaud's present with symptoms bilaterally (symmetric attacks) involving both hands precipitated by exposure to cold or emotional stress, as well as normal digit pressures. Secondary Raynaud's presents with abnormal digit pressures, is asymmetric in patients with embolization and trauma, and presents with bilateral or symmetric symptoms in patients with systemic disorder.

Thoracic outlet syndrome (TOS) refers to symptoms that are produced by obstruction of the vascular or neurologic bundle serving the arm as it passes from the thoracocervical region to the axilla. The subclavian vessels and the lower trunk of the brachial plexus pass through three triangular channels, which make up the thoracic outlet. Neurogenic is the most common, whereas venous and arterial are most rare. Neck and upper extremity trauma is the most common factor in neurogenic TOS. Other cases are associated with congenital and acquired anatomic variations. Most of the patients are female and present with pain, paresthesias, and weakness typically involving the hand. Compression of the subclavian vein at the thoracic outlet may occur and cause effort thrombosis (Paget–Schroetter syndrome) of the subclavian vein.

Entrapment syndrome is caused by a congenital abnormality between the popliteal artery and the medial head of the gastrocnemius muscle. It is most commonly considered in young athletic male patients who present with calf pain when exercising. The symptoms are usually unilateral.

Cystic adventitial disease most commonly affects the popliteal artery. The cyst arises from the media or subadventitial layer with expansion into the adventitia causing stenosis or occlusion of the vessel. It is most common in young men (approximately 40 years).

HISTORY AND PHYSICAL EXAMINATION[15,18]

The value of a history and physical examination should not be underestimated in establishing a correct diagnosis. This part of the patient evaluation also builds the foundation on which further diagnostic tests and therapeutic interventions may be planned.

In the vast majority of cases, an accurate anatomic diagnosis can be made on the basis of a thorough history with confirmation by a directed physical examination. The availability and wide array of sophisticated diagnostic tests available at the present time may facilitate the tendency for all practitioners to rely on the results of these tests and not on the physical examination. It is important for all practitioners to maintain their history taking and physical examination skills, and it is only through the frequent performance of these tasks that this can be achieved. Although much of the following discussion does not fall under the purview of the sonographer/vascular technologist, the more knowledgeable and skilled one is in patient assessment, the more likely he or she is to obtain meaningful test results. Finally, an accurate history and physical exam serve as a "control" for all vascular diagnostic ultrasound or physiologic tests, which are by nature operator dependent.

History

The first priority in the evaluation of the patient is to adequately assess the patient's chief complaint and history of present illness, i.e., the reason the patient is seeking medical attention and all the events relating to this complaint. When acquiring a patient history, the examiner must pay close attention to patient demographics such as age (atherosclerosis often present after age 40) and sex (some diseases are more common in males than females).

Patients may present with complaints of pain, numbness or weakness, swelling, discoloration, ulceration, or other symptoms. Whatever the chief complaint, all the aspects and characteristics of the presenting complaint should be elucidated. This includes location and radiation, where the symptom is, and whether it radiates to another part of the body. The quality and quantity (severity) of the symptom must be assessed; i.e., is it burning, dull, sharp, aching, etc? The temporal pattern is critical; i.e., when did the symptoms first begin, how long have they been present, are they constant or intermittent, is it experienced frequently or infrequently, and are the symptoms improving, worsening, or remaining static? Mitigating factors that relieve or aggravate the symptom should be evaluated. Finally, symptoms in the abstract are not the critical issue, but rather, the impact on the patient's lifestyle must be evaluated. For example, for some patients, two to three block claudication might be only a minor nuisance, while for others it might be severely disabling.

A complete history also must include the patient's past medical history, past surgical history, medications, and allergies. Specific inquiries relating to risk factors for vascular disease should be made. These include the presence of diabetes, hypertension, elevated cholesterol, cigarette smoking, and markers of atherosclerotic problems such as myocardial infarction, previously documented coronary artery disease, angina, chest pain, transient ischemic attacks, and/or stroke. Any history of deep vein thrombosis or phlebitis should be obtained as well as a history of clotting problems and blood transfusions. The presence of renal dysfunction should be evaluated since many patients may ultimately come to angiography, and since patients who are on dialysis generally having extensive vascular calcification. Surgical history is also of importance with special attention to previous vascular and cardiac procedures. This will obviously have an impact on the availability of vein for use as a conduit, as well as provide the basis for the surgical or interventional

treatment planning. Medications are, of course, of importance, as these may contribute to or mask certain symptoms. A social history including the patient's living arrangements, occupation, and support systems may also be of critical importance, especially if aggressive treatment is warranted to treat the symptoms. A brief family history may be relevant, especially relating to a history of coagulopathy or excessive bleeding.

Signs and Symptoms. Pain is the most common chief complaint regardless of whether the occlusive disease is acute or chronic. Pain may present as either intermittent claudication or pain at rest.

Acute arterial occlusion is a sudden and complete blockage of a main arterial supply to the extremity. The most common etiology of an acute occlusion may be embolic or thrombotic (bypass graft or native artery). Most emboli originate in the heart (atrial fibrillation, recent myocardial infarct). Thrombosis of a diseased artery or a bypass graft is common. Another cause for acute occlusion is vascular trauma. The initial presentation is characterized by the presence of the six Ps (Table 14–1). Patients with embolic events tend to have a history of cardiac disease with no significant underlying peripheral arterial disease. Symptoms are of rapid onset. The patient with an acute thrombosis is likely to have had a previous vascular procedure either endovascular or open. In this group of patients, onset may be more gradual secondary to the development of collaterals from the chronic disease.

Chronic arterial disease often presents as intermittent claudication. This word is derived from the Latin, *claudico*, meaning to limp, and is pain that is brought on by exercise and relieved with rest. It is often described as a cramping sensation or a feeling of tiredness or heaviness. It is reproduced by the same level of exercise and is relieved within 2–5 minutes of rest.

The pathophysiology of claudication is that of muscle ischemia caused by diminished oxygen delivery. An occlusion or stenosis of the arteries supplying a particular muscle group will limit flow; therefore, the increased metabolic demands during exercise cannot be met.[12] Most patients with calf claudication have occlusion of the superficial femoral artery. Bilateral thigh or buttock claudication associated with erectile dysfunction is known as the Leriche syndrome and is consistent with aorto-iliac disease. The impotence is the result of inadequate blood flow through the hypogastric artery.

TABLE 14–1 • Sign and Symptoms of Acute Arterial Disease
1. Pain
2. Poikliothermia (cold extremity)
3. Pallor (pale or white)
4. Pulselessness
5. Paresthesias (numbness, tingling sensation)
6. Paralysis (rigor)

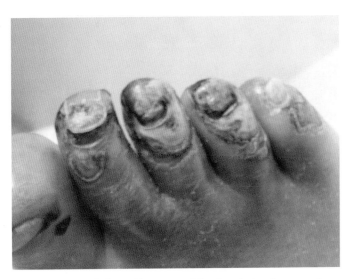

FIGURE 14–15. Patient with severe multilevel occlusive disease and gangrenous toes.

Ischemic rest pain is easily differentiated from claudication. Rest pain is a constant pain described as a severe aching or burning in the foot. The pain usually localizes to the metatarsal heads but may be worse in the location of a gangrenous toe or ischemic ulcer. This pain often intensifies at night and may be relieved by dependency (i.e., hanging the foot over the side of the bed). Rest pain is of far greater consequence than is claudication. Whereas the latter may remain a benign condition, rest pain heralds the onset of gangrene and demands immediate attention.

Tissue loss and gangrene are the most severe forms of ischemia (Fig. 14–15). Patients with tissue loss often present with multilevel occlusive disease. Arterial ischemic ulcers are often localized in the distal toes, heel, or sole and dorsum of the foot. Gangrene usually appears as a focal black or dark blue spot over a toe. If not treated, it may spread to other toes, foot, and in severe cases the entire leg. There are two types of gangrene: (1) wet which is associated with infection and (2) dry which is non-infected. Other causes of leg ulcers are diabetic neuropathy, venous disease, and infection.

Symptoms of spinal stenosis, sciatica, osteoarthritis, or causalgia may be indistinguishable from those of vasculogenic claudication, hence, the term "pseudoclaudication," and may have to be ruled out as differential diagnoses. Diabetic neuropathy may be confused with rest pain; however, the pain associated with diabetic neuropathy is not relieved by changes in position and the patients often lack the associated physical findings seen in patients with peripheral vascular disease.

Physical Examination

The lower extremities should be carefully evaluated. Physical exam should include palpation, auscultation and inspection. This includes a pulse examination as well as a thorough inspection of the extremities themselves. Pulse palpation is probably the most important part of the physical examination.

The absence of a pulse is indicative of a more proximal occlusion (e.g., absence of the common femoral artery pulse indicates aorto-iliac occlusive disease). Femoral, popliteal, dorsalis pedis, and posterior tibial arteries are palpated and graded according to the following scale: 0 is a non-palpable pulse, 1+ is a diminished, but palpable pulse, 2+ is a normal pulse, 3+ is a bounding pulse, and 4+ is an excessively bounding pulse. A Doppler signal may be used to augment the pulse evaluation but is generally of little value since any flow will produce a signal and only in the presence of a completely occluded artery will the signal be completely absent. In order to perform an accurate pulse examination, both the patient and the examiner need to be in a comfortable and relaxed position. Special attention needs to be paid to any muscle fasciculation, which can often be mistaken for a palpable pulse. If the presence of a palpable pulse is uncertain, the pulse may be counted out to a separate examiner who is palpating the radial or femoral pulse or the pulsations on electrocardiogram or other monitor can be observed. In the upper extremity, pulses should be examined at the subclavian artery (above the middle of the clavicle). The axillary artery should be palpated in the groove between the biceps and triceps muscle, the brachial artery pulse can be palpated at the antecubital fossa, and the ulnar and radial arteries should be palpated at the wrist on the medial and lateral aspects, respectively.

Palpation is also helpful in assessing the temperature of the extremity. The examiner should use the back of the same hand to assess the temperature of each extremity being examined to compare any difference between them.

Auscultation with a stethoscope is performed to assess for the presence of a bruit. A bruit indicates the presence of a hemodynamically significant stenosis (note that the absence of a bruit does not exclude the presence of significant arterial occlusive disease). Auscultation should be performed at the abdomen, groin to detect any significant aorto-iliac disease, and at popliteal fossa to detect any popliteal artery disease. Auscultation over the iliac and femoral arteries should be performed to assess bruits, which may be suggestive of stenoses. In the presence of such a stenosis, a combination procedure with stenting of the iliacs and a peripheral bypass may be warranted.

Inspection of the lower extremity may reveal signs of acute or chronic arterial insufficiency. The patient's foot and toes should be carefully examined. Special attention should be noted in between the toes for any broken skin.

In chronic arterial insufficiency, trophic changes such as muscle atrophy, hair loss, thickened toe nails, ulcerations, or gangrene should also be noted.

In acute lower extremity ischemia, patients may present with skin mottling, cyanosis, pallor, or muscle weakness.[19,20]

Inspection of the upper extremity can reveal important information about arterial perfusion. In an acute event, the upper extremity may be pallid with diminished motor and sensory functions. In chronic processes, ulceration, gangrene, and muscle atrophy in the forearm and wrist may be noted.

Upper extremity pulses including the axillary, brachial, radial, and ulnar pulses should be palpated, and if there is any question of upper extremity pathology, differential blood pressures should be checked in the arms. An Allen's test is performed to assess the collateral circulation between the radial and ulnar artery distributions.

The abdomen should be palpated for epigastric or lower quadrant masses. In a thin patient, the aortic pulsation may be prominent and can be mistaken for aneurysmal dilatation. In general, any pulsatile mass in the lower quadrants is an iliac artery aneurysm until proven otherwise. The abdomen may be auscultated for bruits, which are suggestive of renal or visceral artery stenoses, although these may be nonspecific findings.

Further examination of the lower extremity includes close inspection of the leg for swelling or lesions. This includes evaluation of the heels and careful evaluation of the skin between the toes. Chronic venous stasis changes or chronic arterial changes are noted, as is the presence of lymphedema, varicosities, and overall skin quality. Finally, venous filling and capillary refill can be used to roughly assess the adequacy of the circulation in the absence of palpable pulses.

TESTING OF THE UPPER AND LOWER EXTREMITIES

Doppler Evaluation[21,22]

Continuous-wave (CW) Doppler provides information on motion and flow. CW waveform analysis can provide localized information in patients with an incompressible vessel due to wall calcification. A CW transducer has two crystals, one constantly transmitting and the other constantly receiving. It is capable of recording all frequency shifts without aliasing. Range ambiguity (entire length is evaluated, not a specific depth) is a limitation. Flow that is moving toward the probe is represented as a positive Doppler shift or flow above the baseline. Flow that is moving away from the probe is represented as a negative Doppler shift and below the baseline. CW Doppler can be heard audibly, recorded by a chart strip recording, or recorded on film. It is usually a simple analog waveform without the distribution of frequencies that are displayed in the spectral analysis. Zero-crossing detectors display an average of the flow velocity (mean frequency, not peak frequency).

The magnitude of the Doppler shift is proportional to the angle of incidence, the smaller the angle, the higher the Doppler shift (0° will produce the highest Doppler shift) and vice-versa (if the angle is 90°, there is no Doppler shift because the cosine of 90° is 0).

Pulsed-Wave Spectral Analysis

Spectral analysis is the method of choice for displaying the Doppler signals. It is a mathematical computation of the reflected pulse that displays individual frequencies and is computed

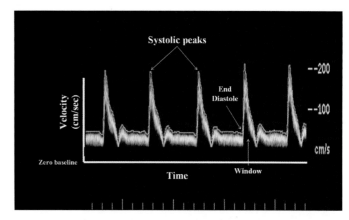

FIGURE 14–16. This image demonstrates the various components of the spectral Doppler waveform.

using the fast Fourier transform (FFT) method. It displays all of the Doppler shift frequencies as a bright echo or a shade of gray. It displays time on the horizontal axis and velocity or frequency shift on the vertical axis. In essence, it is a frequency spectrum of the cardiac cycle. The spectral analysis demonstrates the presence, direction, and characteristics of the blood flow (Fig. 14–16). In the vascular examination, the spectral waveform analysis has the capabilities of showing the degree of stenosis, site of occlusion, type of vessel, flow disturbances and turbulence, peripheral resistance, and relative flow velocity.

Patient Positioning

The optimal position for the vascular evaluation is supine with the extremities at the same level as the heart. The room should be warm (to avoid vasoconstriction). For the lower extremity evaluation, the hip should be externally rotated and the knee slightly bent to allow access to the vessels of interest on the medial aspect of the leg. The leg can be straightened to evaluate the anterior tibial artery as needed. For the upper extremity evaluation, the arms should be at the patient's side and relaxed.

Technique

CW Doppler evaluation of the lower extremities is performed with a 5 to 10 MHz transducer, the frequency to be determined by the depth of the vessel being evaluated. Gel is applied to the area in question. The probe is held at a 45–60° angle to the skin and fine movements are made to elicit the best possible signal.

In the lower extremity, Doppler waveforms are obtained from the following vessels:

- Common femoral artery (CFA)
- Superficial femoral artery (SFA)
- Popliteal artery (PopA)
- Posterior tibial artery (PTA)
- Dorsalis pedis artery (DPA)

If no signals are elicited from the DPA or PTA, waveforms from the peroneal artery can be recorded (Fig. 14–17).

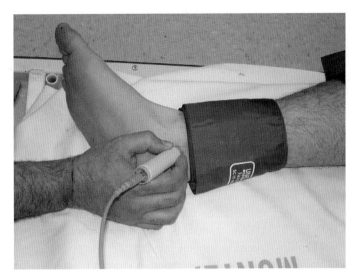 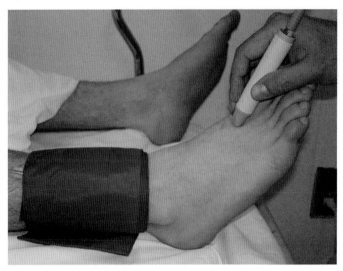

FIGURE 14–17. These images demonstrate the proper technique for examination of the pedal arteries. On the left the anterior tibial artery is being evaluated in the distal leg as it crosses the extensor crease. On the right, the posterior tibial artery is found medial and immediately distal to the medial malleolus. The Doppler probe is held at a 45°–60° angle to the vessel.

In the upper extremity, Doppler waveforms are obtained from the following vessels:

- Subclavian artery
- Axillary artery
- Brachial artery
- Ulnar artery
- Radial artery

Qualitative Interpretation

The Doppler waveform of the arteries in the arms and legs is a graphic representation of the pulsatile blood flow within them. As peripheral arterial occlusive disease progresses, the pulsatility diminishes until it is completely lost.

Normal waveforms are triphasic or biphasic at rest and demonstrate a sharp systolic rise, sharp diastolic drop that goes below the baseline (indicative of good peripheral resistance), and in some cases, a second forward-flow component in diastole (indicative of good arterial compliance).

As arterial disease progresses, the systolic flow begins to decrease and there is a loss of flow reversal (Fig. 14–18).

Quantitative Interpretation

Pulsatility index (PI) can also be used to evaluate peripheral arterial disease. A decrease in the PI may indicate more proximal disease (Fig. 14–19).

$$PI = (peak\ systolic\ velocity - peak\ diastolic\ velocity)/mean\ velocity$$

Normal PI values:

- Common femoral artery >5
- Popliteal artery >8
- Posterior tibial artery >14

PI below these values suggests proximal occlusive disease. PI interpretation at the common femoral artery may be affected in the presence of concomitant superficial femoral artery occlusive disease; therefore, the prediction of proximal disease in this setting may be unreliable.

Acceleration time (AT) in the common femoral artery is used to predict the presence of hemodynamically significant aorto-iliac lesions. AT is calculated by measuring the time from the onset of systole to peak systole.

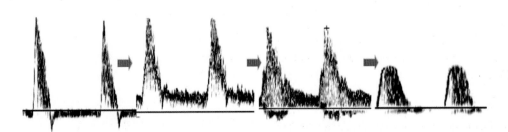

FIGURE 14–18. Spectrum of changes seen in the spectral Doppler waveform with increasing degrees of stenosis (left is normal to right abnormal).

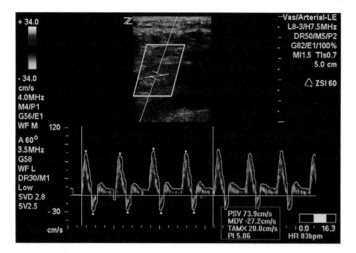

FIGURE 14–19. Calculation of the pulsatility index (PI) using information from four cardiac cycles as marked by the outlined spectra and the yellow calipers. The PI, in the red box, is 5.06 and is within normal limits.

Normal AT in the common femoral artery is <122 ms (Fig. 14–20). AT in the common femoral artery >144 ms suggests an occlusive disease process above that level. As disease progresses, the waveforms dampen and the acceleration time increases.

In experienced hands, Doppler waveform analysis is a simple screening test to evaluate for the presence and approximate location of peripheral arterial disease; however, there are limitations and pitfalls to this technique and they are as follows:

1. It requires skill and experience. This is a very technologist-dependent examination that requires skill and training to learn the proper probe positioning and the location of the vasculature, and that requires familiarity with the audible signs of the various disease processes and their severity.

2. It sometimes cannot differentiate stenosis from occlusion.

3. It is rendered useless if there is not direct contact with the skin over the vessel (inaccessible vessels secondary to bandage, casts, open wounds).

4. In patients with uncompensated congestive heart failure (CHF), all the waveforms may be damped and the location of the disease may not be detectable.

5. In patients with venous hypertension, the venous signals may be pulsatile and can be confused with arterial signals.

Segmental Pressures[22]

Segmental pressures are an indirect noninvasive test that indicates the level and degree of arterial disease and can evaluate disease progression. This test can be performed using a three- (thigh, calf ankle) or a four-cuff method (high thigh, above knee, below knee, and ankle), on the lower extremity (Fig. 14–21). The three-cuff method may not differentiate between iliac/common femoral and superficial femoral lesions. The patient should be in the supine position to eliminate the effect of gravity (hydrostatic pressure) and erroneous blood pressure measurements. The head should be slightly elevated. The patient should rest 15–20 minutes to permit stabilization of the pressures. The hip should be externally rotated and the knee slightly bent to facilitate proper Doppler probe placement. The room should be kept warm to avoid the complications of vasoconstriction. Pressures are obtained while the patient is at rest using a CW Doppler probe in the range of 5–10 MHz. A sphygmomanometer is used to measure pressure with a Doppler probe placed at the posterior tibial or dorsalis pedis artery to record the pressure as each individual cuff is activated. The pressure obtained is the pressure underneath the cuff that has been inflated. The cuff at each site is inflated until the systolic pressure sound disappears. The pressure in the cuff is then slowly released (2–3 mm Hg/sec) until the sound or the Doppler waveform returns. This measurement is recorded. Bilateral brachial pressures are used as the standard and should be within 20 mm Hg of each other. If there is a greater difference in the bilateral brachial measurements, this would indicate upper extremity arterial disease. The highest value of the normal two pressures is used as the standard.[22]

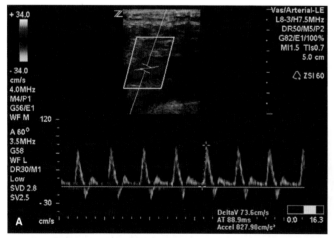
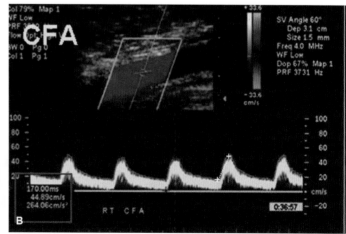

FIGURE 14–20. The acceleration time in (**A**) is 88.9 ms. In (**B**) in a patient with iliac artery occlusion, the acceleration time is 170 ms.

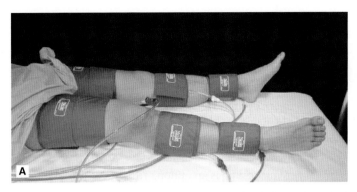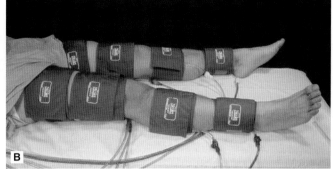

FIGURE 14–21. In "**A**" is a patient being evaluated using a three-cuff technique that employs one 20-cm length cuff on the thigh. In "**B**," the four-cuff method, two 12-cm cuffs are used on the thigh. Both techniques employ 10–12 cm cuffs around the calf and ankle.

In the upper extremity, with a cuff on the upper arm and forearm, the pressures are obtained by first placing the probe at the antecubital fossa to obtain the brachial artery pressure. The probe is placed at the wrist at the medial side to obtain the ulnar artery pressure and on the lateral side to obtain the radial artery pressure. The cuff should be inflated 20–30 mm Hg suprasystolic and deflated slowly (2–3 mm Hg/sec) until the signal comes back and the pressure is recorded. Digit pressures can be obtained by placing a small digital cuff over the base of the finger and then using a photoplethysmography (PPG) sensor to detect the return of flow.

Interpretation

In the upper extremity, the study is normal if there is a pressure gradient of <20 mm Hg between the right and the left brachial pressure or between the upper arm and forearm ipsilaterally. The normal finger-to-brachial index is more than 0.80. A pressure gradient of 20 mm Hg or greater between brachial pressures suggests a more proximal obstruction (innominate, subclavian, axillary, or brachial artery) in the arm with the lower pressure. A pressure gradient of 20 mm Hg or greater between the upper arm and forearm suggests an obstruction in the segment between the cuffs. A gradient of greater than >15–20 mm Hg between the radial and ulnar arteries suggests obstruction in the vessel with the lower pressure. Any finger-to-brachial index of <0.80 suggests the possibility of hemodynamically significant disease on that side.

In the lower extremity, when using a four-cuff technique, the normal upper thigh pressure is 20–30 mm Hg greater than the brachial pressure. This is because the narrow size of the bladder artifactually elevates the thigh pressure. With the four-cuff technique, the thigh pressure should be equal to or a little higher than the brachial artery pressure.

A pressure gradient of 20 mm Hg or less is considered within normal limits. The normal ankle brachial index (ABI) and toe brachial index (TBI) are more than 1.0 and more than 0.70, respectively. The study is abnormal if there is a pressure gradient of 20 mm Hg or greater between adjacent segments ipsilaterally or if there is a horizontal (right versus left) differ-

ence of 20 mm Hg or greater at the same level (Fig. 14–22). In the four-cuff technique, an upper thigh pressure 20 mm Hg lower than the brachial pressure indicates inflow disease (aorto-iliac or common femoral artery).

Limitations and pitfalls associated with this technique are as follows:

- It cannot distinguish stenosis from occlusion.
- It does not provide information regarding specific location for disease but only provides an approximate location.

Segmental Pressure Examination

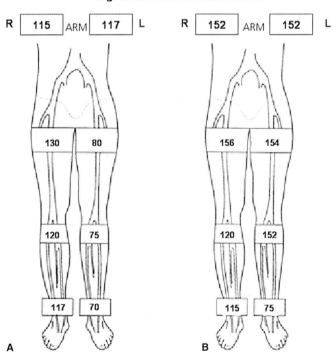

FIGURE 14–22. Segmental blood pressure measurement test. **A**, segmental leg pressures in a normal right extremity (ankle brachial index [ABI]: 117/117 = 1.00) and one with a significant left iliac artery stenosis or occlusion (ABI: 70/117 = 0.60). Horizontal and vertical pressure gradients exist at the thigh. **B**, segmental leg pressures in a patient with a right superficial femoral artery stenosis and a distal left tibial artery occlusion.

- In patients with calcified vessels, pressures may be erroneously elevated due to medial wall calcification (especially true in diabetic and end-stage renal disease patients).

- Patients with surgical incisions may not able to tolerate the pressures.

- Extensive bandages or casts may preclude the ability to wrap the cuffs.

- Improper size of the cuff may result in falsely low or high pressures.

- Inability to elicit a signal distal to the cuff will not allow for the acquisition of a pressure.

Ranges of disease are as follows:

Normal: systolic ankle pressure is equal to or greater than brachial systolic pressure (a ratio of ≥1.0)

Claudication: ABI between 0.5 and 0.9 indicates claudication (often requires exercise testing).

Severe occlusive disease: ABI of <0.5 indicates severe occlusive disease (usually does not require exercise testing).

Pressure gradient of >20 mm Hg between cuff levels indicates a hemodynamically significant lesion.

Bilateral pressure gradients should be approximately equal for comparison.

Exercise testing is an important adjunct to the segmental pressure evaluation, as it can help differentiate patients with true claudication from those with other differential diagnoses (pseudoclaudication). Exercise helps to unmask occlusive disease that is not apparent at rest. It is beneficial in patients with normal or borderline ABIs at rest who present with claudication-type symptoms. By monitoring the ankle systolic pressure pre-exercise and post-exercise, we are able to determine the severity of the arterial occlusive disease process. The magnitude of the immediate pressure drop after exercise and the time for recovery to resting pressure are proportional to the severity of arterial disease.

Technique

After the segmental pressure evaluation identifies the appropriate patient for exercise testing, cuffs are placed at the bilateral ankle and bilateral upper arm. Resting pressures are recorded at the brachial artery, the dorsalis pedis artery (DPA), and the posterior tibial artery (PTA) bilaterally (if symptomatically) or on the symptomatic side only. The highest ankle pressure and the higher of the brachial artery pressures are used to calculate the ABIs. The patient is asked to walk on the treadmill at 2 mph at a 12% incline for 5 minutes or until symptoms force the patient to stop. Immediately after exercise and at 2, 5, and 10 minutes thereafter, the ankle and brachial pressures are recorded until the pressures return to the resting values.

After exercise, pressures should increase slightly or remain equal in comparison to the resting pressures. Any pressure drop is considered abnormal. In patients whose pressures return to resting values within 2–6 minutes, single-level disease is suspected. Pressures that return to resting value after 10 minutes are more likely due to multilevel occlusive disease.

Contraindications to the exercise test are shortness of breath, recent history of myocardial infarction, elevated blood pressure of more than 200 mm Hg systolic and more than 100 mm Hg diastolic, inability or unwillingness to exercise, and patients with symptoms or other findings at rest (ulceration, rest pain).

In patients who are unable to exercise or are disabled, reactive hyperemia testing is an option. The patient is tested in the supine position. After acquisition of the resting pressures, a thigh cuff is inflated to suprasystolic pressure for 3–5 minutes. The thigh cuff is then deflated and an ankle pressure is recorded immediately after cuff deflation.

In normal patients, a drop in ankle pressure of up to 30% may be noticed. Any drop in pressure of up to 50% of the resting ankle pressure may be seen in patients with single-level disease. A more than 50% ankle pressure drop may be noticed in patients with multilevel disease.

Although it may be useful in some patients, the exercise test is preferred. Reactive hyperemia may be limited in patients who cannot tolerate the pressure exerted by the thigh pressure cuff. In addition, although the exam may uncover an occult stenosis, it may not be clear whether the stenosis is in fact the cause of the patient's symptoms, as the pressure drop was not brought on by exercise.

PLETHYSMOGRAPHY[21,22]

Plethysmography provides subjective information about the overall perfusion to the limb. It is not affected by medial calcinosis and is often better tolerated than segmental pressures. It is generally a measurement of volume changes in the extremities for measuring blood flow. It has been used in the past for venous flow studies and venous reflux studies and is now used primarily for arterial studies. Limitations include constant movement (voluntary or involuntary) that may affect the contour of the waveforms, inability to differentiate between stenosis and occlusion, decreasing accuracy in the presence of multilevel disease, excessive bandages, casts, and open wounds, and changes in the pulse waveform contour (may assume an obstructive contour) that can occur in cold rooms.

There are several types of plethysmography. *Air plethysmography* uses airflow to measure volume changes in a limb. It is performed using pneumatic cuffs inflated to a low pressure (~65 mm Hg) that measure the relative changes in pressure in a limb. These instruments provide a good arterial pulse contour waveform.[22] The normal pulse contour has a rapid systolic upstroke, with a prominent dicrotic notch and a down slope that bows toward the baseline in diastole. As disease progresses, changes in the waveform are noted. In mild disease, the rapid systolic upstroke is present and a down slope that bows toward the baseline in diastole is seen; however, the dicrotic notch is

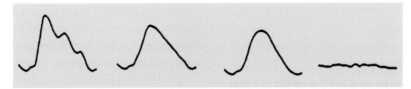

FIGURE 14–23. From left to right are the changes seen in the pulse volume waveforms with increasing levels of disease. Far left is normal. Loss of the dichroitic notch is the first evidence of disease and is seen in the second waveform. The third waveform reveals blunting of the waveform peak on the far right in severe disease there is severe diminution of the pulse volume waveform.

absent. Moderate disease yields a rounded systolic peak, loss of the dicrotic notch, and the down slope bows away from the baseline. In patients with severe disease, there is reduced pulsatility in the waveform with a flattened systolic peak and a delayed rise time (Fig. 14–23).

Photoplethysmography is performed using a small photocell placed on the extremity, which contains an infrared light (light-emitting diode [LED] and a phototransistor) (Fig. 14–24). This photocell identifies subcutaneous flow and produces a pulse contour that can be recorded.[21] This technique is frequently used in vascular examinations to detect blood flow when it becomes difficult with conventional techniques. For example, in diabetics where toe pressure must be obtained, the photocell is placed on the toe to obtain a Doppler signal and take a pressure recording.

It is an extremely useful examination in patients with calcified vessels. Medial calcification does not extend into the digital arteries, making it possible to measure systolic toe pressures. In the upper extremity evaluation of the digit, perfusion helps to differentiate fixed arterial disease from vasospastic disorder (cold exposure or stress related).[21]

DUPLEX IMAGING

The clinical role of duplex scanning in the vascular patient has expanded from its earliest applications as the noninvasive exam of choice for the evaluation of atherosclerotic disease of the carotid artery to evaluation of virtually the entire vascular system.

Patients with lower extremity arterial occlusive disease typically undergo a combination of invasive and noninvasive tests prior to lower extremity revascularization. While the patient's symptoms and the results of these tests are used to decide when surgery is needed, the surgery is usually planned on the basis of diagnostic arteriography alone. Arteriography accurately defines the location of stenotic and occluded arterial segments and is considered the gold standard for selecting the location of a graft's proximal and distal anastomoses. However, arteriography poses the risks of contrast-induced renal dysfunction, puncture site complications. Arteriography also poses a risk for catheter and guidewire-induced vessel wall injury and allergic reactions. In addition, both standard and digital angiographic techniques occasionally fail to visualize patent low-flow distal arterial segments.[23–26]

Duplex ultrasound with color (CDU) can also be used to image the lower extremity and pelvic arteries, is safer and less expensive than arteriography, and is also noninvasive. Many studies have shown the clinical utility of CDU for preoperative assessment prior to carotid endarterectomy and for endovascular treatment of short, focal lesions of the aorto-iliac and femoropopliteal arteries. We and others have used CDU as the sole

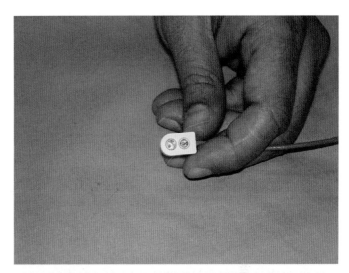

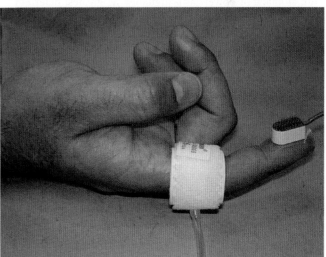

FIGURE 14–24. On the top is the face of the photocell with light-emitting diode and phototransistor. Below is the technique used for acquisition of a digital pressure. The signal from the diode photocell is monitored as the cuff is inflated.

imaging technique to evaluate patients prior to lower extremity revascularization.[27–30]

IMAGING THE AORTIC BIFURCATION AND ILIAC ARTERIES

Abdominal scanning requires technical expertise and a thorough understanding of anatomy, physiology, and hemodynamics. Increasing sophistication and refinement of ultrasound technology have allowed for the accurate examination of the deep abdominal and pelvic vasculature, and color-flow duplex evaluation of the abdominal aorta and iliac arteries is now performed routinely in most vascular laboratories. Color Doppler vascular ultrasound can routinely interrogate and reliably quantify disease in the aorta and iliac arteries.

Indications

The patient referred for evaluation of the aortic bifurcation and iliac arteries may be referred for the purpose of ruling out aneurysm, atherosclerotic occlusive disease, or dissection. Other indications include follow-up of a known abdominal aortic aneurysm, surveillance of lower extremity (LE) revascularization or documentation of disease progression.

Symptoms

The patient can present with one or a combination of the following symptoms: abdominal, flank, or groin pain; a pulsatile abdominal mass; severe disabling buttock or thigh claudication; impotence; manifest signs of lower extremity ischemia; or may be asymptomatic.

Patient Preparation

Recent abdominal surgery, obesity, and respiratory motion are known limitations to abdominal and pelvic scanning. However, stomach or bowel gas is arguably the greatest deterrent to visualization. To avoid or minimize this limitation and obtain optimal images, it is important that patients be adequately prepared for the procedure. This can often be accomplished with an 8-hour fast.

Equipment/Transducer Selection: An ultrasound duplex scanner with high-resolution imaging capability, excellent color Doppler penetration, and low-frequency transducer availability (frequency selection will vary according to body habitus) is essential to the evaluation. The operating frequency and type of transducer used will vary. In general low-frequency (2.0–3.5 MHz) transducers, phased- or curved-array transducers facilitate better color/spectral penetration; however, they sacrifice image quality. High-frequency (>5 MHz) linear arrays produce excellent two-dimensional images; however, the Doppler penetration capability is inferior. Often more than one transducer is necessary to perform a complete and optimal exam.

Patient Positioning/Image Acquisition.[31] Examination of the abdominal aorta begins by placing the patient in the supine position and visualizing the entire length of the abdominal aorta in the short-axis view. The transducer can be placed immediately inferior to the xiphoid process and rotated 90° and slightly left of the midline for long-axis views of the aorta (a depth of field of 10–12 cm should allow visualization in most patients). The left lateral decubitus position is considered the best approach for visualization of the aorta and its branches, as the liver is used to provide an acoustic window into the abdomen. (Note: a variety of positions may be required for full visualization of the aorto-iliac vasculature. These may include supine, lateral decubitus, flank approach, or prone translumbar.)

Examination of the external iliac artery starts with the patient in the supine position. At the inguinal ligament, the common femoral artery and vein are identified in the transverse plane. The external iliac artery can then be followed proximally using the longitudinal axis, as it dives deep into the pelvis to its confluence with the hypogastric artery where they form the common iliac artery. The common iliac artery is followed proximally to its confluence with the contralateral common iliac artery to form the aorta.

The lower extremity vasculature is evaluated from the common femoral through the pedal arteries (Fig. 14–25). The CDU examination results are used as a map or a duplex arteriogram, which is then used by the vascular surgeon to make therapeutic decisions (Fig. 14–26).

Blood flow analysis should be performed using both spectral and color Doppler because they are complementary. Once the color-flow image has been optimized, spectral Doppler is used to obtain detailed information of blood flow. A beam angle of 60° is recommended for interrogation of the blood flow. When used consistently, this helps to reduce intraobserver and interobserver variability. Flow should be sampled at regular intervals 1–2 cm throughout the area of interest and at points of flow disturbance documented by color Doppler. In general, there are three stenosis classifications for the aortic and iliac artery stenosis: <50%, >50%, or occluded. These are based on a combination of the B-mode examination and flow-velocity data. In general, a focal twofold increase in velocity from one segment to another with a change in spectral waveform configuration and poststenotic turbulence suggests the presence of more than 50% stenosis. A greater than twofold increased velocity with no poststenotic turbulence suggests stenosis less than 50%. If there is disagreement between the B-mode finding and the Doppler data, classification should be made based on the spectral Doppler data. Inability to elicit Doppler or visual evidence of active blood flow under optimal two-dimensional and Doppler settings suggests complete occlusion.

These techniques have allowed the performance of limb salvage procedures in selected patients without the need for diagnostic arteriography. Improvements in vascular ultrasound imaging promise to minimize or eliminate the need for arteriography in many high-risk patients.

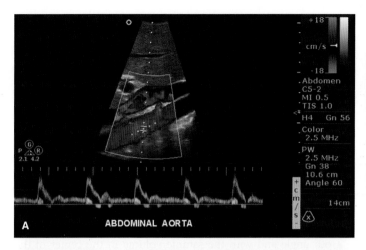

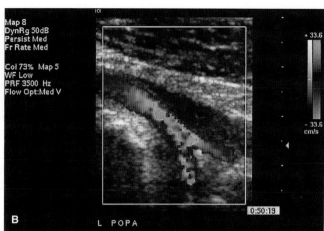

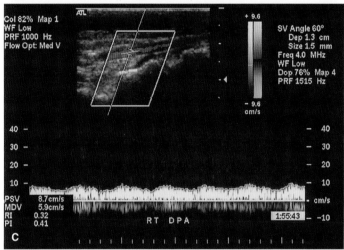

FIGURE 14–25. Ultrasound images from different levels in the arterial tree. **A** is a long-axis image and spectral waveform from the abdominal aorta at the level of the renal arteries. **B** is a color-flow image of the below the knee popliteal artery at the origins of the anterior tibial artery and tibioperoneal trunk. **C** is a low-flow dorsalis pedis artery in a patient with multilevel occlusive disease. The peak velocity is 8 cm/sec.

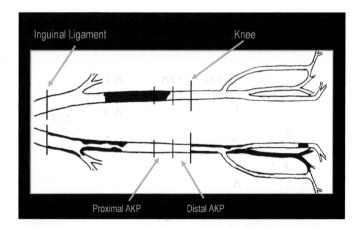

FIGURE 14–26. Diagram that depicts the results of a duplex arterial mapping. On the right, the patient has proximal superficial femoral artery (SFA) disease, with straight line flow through the popliteal artery. Below the knee the patient has an occluded peroneal artery and a short occlusion of the distal posterior tibial artery. The anterior tibial artery is patent and without stenosis throughout its length to the level of the foot. On the left, the patient has an SFA occlusion with reconstitution of the above the knee popliteal artery and three vessel runoff to the foot.

LOWER EXTREMITY DUPLEX IMAGING

The most common application of this technique is for the evaluation of the vein bypass graft. It can also be used to identify the exact anatomical location of arterial occlusive disease and to differentiate stenosis from occlusion, for assessment of dialysis access grafts, to assess and define pulsatile masses including aneurysms and pseudoaneurysms and to identify iatrogenic arteriovenous fistulas.[16,17,29,32]

Bypass Graft Imaging[32]

The goal of vein graft surveillance is to identify lesions that may ultimately lead to vein graft occlusion. The rationale for graft surveillance is the progressive nature of atherosclerosis and the tendency of both vein and prosthetic bypass grafts to develop flow-limiting lesions. Duplex ultrasound in conjunction with some form of indirect testing is the recommended surveillance method following lower extremity bypass grafting. At present, frequent surveillance is recommended in the first postoperative year with the initial scan being performed intraoperatively. Studies have shown that grafts followed in a surveillance program have a higher patency rate than those followed only clinically.

Interpretation criteria for identifying stenotic lesions have traditionally focused on identification of focally elevated peak systolic velocities at a site of a stenosis or abnormally low peak systolic velocities somewhere within the distal portion of the graft. A peak systolic velocity of >45 cm/sec has been popularized as an indicator of impending graft failure; however, disagreement exists that this value represents an appropriate threshold for all vein grafts. Others have advocated the use of flow volume measurements in a predetermined part of the distal graft as a better indicator of impending graft failure, while some have suggested that the significance of change over time, not an absolute velocity or flow value may be a more sensitive indicator. Most interpretation criteria have been developed for the *in situ* saphenous vein bypass graft. The same principles can be applied to the reversed vein graft; however, differences in graft diameter and hemodynamics must be considered. There are no established criteria for evaluation of prosthetic grafts and controversy exists in this area. Liberal use of arteriography during the learning phase is suggested to develop criteria that work best in individual laboratories. In general, any doubling of velocity from a normal site proximal to the stenosis is consistent with a 50% diameter reduction; however, this assumes a constant diameter.

Exam Preparation and General Considerations. Prior to the evaluation, it is helpful to be familiar with the type of graft being examined. The important elements of this information include the sites of the proximal and distal anastomoses, the type of conduit, and the location of the graft in the leg. Superficial grafts such as *in situs* or grafts that are tunneled subcutaneously are best evaluated with high frequency transducers (7.5–10 MHz). Lower frequency (3–5 MHz) transducers are best for grafts tunneled anatomically. For grafts anastomosed to the above knee popliteal or peroneal arteries, it may be necessary to employ a sector or curved array transducer to identify the distal anastomosis and outflow vessel. To avoid the complications of infection, a sterile couplant sheet can be used for imaging in the early postoperative period.

Technical Protocol. The examination starts by identifying the mid portion of the graft in the leg in the transverse orientation. The graft is then followed proximally to its confluence with the inflow vessel where the proximal anastomosis is identified. At this point, the transducer is rotated sagittally and the inflow vessel is assessed. The entire length of the graft through the distal anastomosis and outflow artery is then interrogated using both the gray-scale image and simultaneously Doppler spectral analysis (Fig. 14–27). Doppler waveforms are obtained using a 60° angle and with the sample volume in the center of the vessel and the cursor parallel to the vessel wall. Any angle that varies from the standard should be noted and used on follow-up studies for comparison. The peak systolic and end diastolic velocity is recorded from waveforms obtained at predetermined sites in the graft, anastomotic sites, and inflow and outflow vessels. Data is also recorded at all areas of abnormality as determined by color or spectral Doppler.

Color-Flow Doppler. The use of color Doppler is recommended, as it provides observation of the graft from a large field of view and significantly reduces the time required to evaluate the graft. The color-flow map is used as a guide for the placement of the sample volume and when proper settings are used will easily identify areas of high velocity and turbulent flow. The pulse repetition frequency is lowered until aliasing occurs and then adjusted appropriately to allow good color saturation with the highest velocities seen in the center of the graft. Stenosis is suspected when there is 1) narrowing of the color-flow channel; 2) shift toward the colors representing higher velocities; 3) change in color due to aliasing; 4) prolonged duration of color throughout the cardiac cycle; and 5) color-flow bruit (Fig. 14–28).

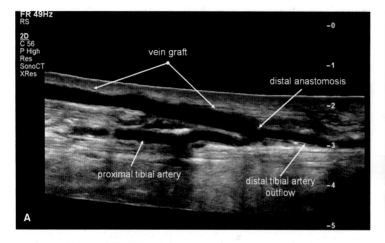
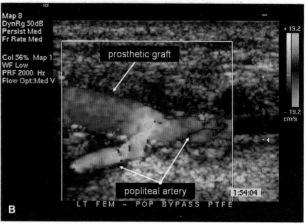

FIGURE 14-27. A is a gray-scale image of the distal anastomosis of a femoral to posterior tibial artery reversed saphenous vein graft. **B** is a color-flow image at the distal anastomosis of a femoro-popliteal polytetraflouroethylene (PTFE) prosthetic graft. There is flow beyond the anastomosis moving both retrograde and prograde in the popliteal artery.

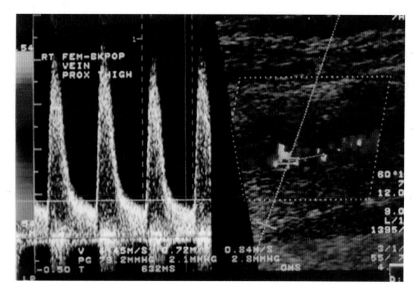

FIGURE 14–28. Color-flow image of a stenotic lesion in a vein graft.

All abnormal color changes are evaluated by spectral Doppler to determine whether an actual velocity increase has occurred keeping in mind that changes in vessel alignment with respect to the scanning lines can cause a color change due to the alteration in Doppler angle. Additionally all sites of flow disturbance are evaluated via the B-mode scan to identify the type of lesion present in the graft conduit. It is imperative to remember that although the B-mode image and color-flow information provide important anatomic information and serve as guides to sample volume placement, the severity of the stenotic lesion is categorized only by Doppler spectral waveform analysis.

Causes of Vein Graft Failure. Graft failure can occur by three mechanisms: occlusion by thrombosis, hemodynamic failure, and structural failure (aneurysmal degeneration). The frequency of graft failure is highest within the first 10–14 days (4–10%) post-implantation, decreases progressively in the first year, and is approximately 2–4% per year thereafter. Technical errors (suture stenosis, intimal flaps, retained thrombus, graft entrapment, torsion) are the most common causes of failure in the early postoperative period (within 30 days). Late failure can be due to myointimal hyperplasia from preexisting vein graft lesions or atherosclerosis that can develop de novo in vein grafts or disease progression in adjacent native arteries but is most typically seen in the distal runoff bed (Fig. 14–29). It is the period between 30 days and 2 years that occlusive lesions develop and for this reason a more aggressive surveillance protocol is employed.

Hemodynamics. Doppler signals will undergo normal changes in the diastolic component of the flow waveform over time. In the early postoperative period, the Doppler waveform may demonstrate continuous forward flow throughout diastole because of a hyperemic response seen after revascularization of a severely ischemic limb. Subsequent visits may reveal a change to the more normal peripheral multiphasic type of waveform with reversal of flow in diastole. This of course is dependent on the status of the outflow tract. The peak systolic velocities will not change significantly.

If significant decreases (20–30 cm/sec) in the peak velocities, as recorded from an index site, are noted, a problem in the graft or adjacent vessels must be suspected. In general, a delayed upstroke (prolonged rise time) infers a problem proximal to the transducer, whereas a decrease in diastolic flow suggests a distal lesion. Staccato waveforms, representing to and from motion of blood, are seen proximal to high-grade lesions or occlusion and are usually followed by immediate thrombosis of the graft. This phenomenon can be distinguished from the normal triphasic waveform by its low amplitude and the very short duration of each flow component.

An effective surveillance program must be applicable to all patients, practical in terms of time, effort, and cost and should

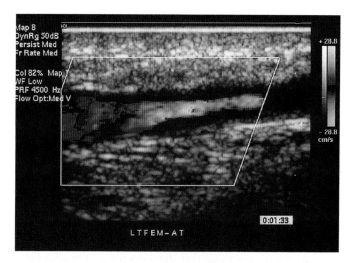

FIGURE 14–29. Color-flow image of a patient with a myointimal hyperplastic lesion at the proximal anastomosis of a vein graft as demonstrated by the echo-lucency on the near and far walls of the graft.

provide a means for detecting, grading severity, and assessing progression of lesions. The ultimate goal is detection of the threatened graft before thrombosis occurs.

Lower Extremity Arterial Mapping for Occlusive Disease

Despite the surgeon's comfort in the easy-to-interpret format of a conventional arteriogram, compelling reasons exist to research the feasibility of alternatives to this "gold standard" test. Arteriography is expensive, uncomfortable for patients, and encumbered with significant potential complications including bleeding, hematoma, or pseudoaneurysm formation, arterial dissection, embolization, and contrast induced nephrotoxicity.[23–26] Duplex ultrasonography, on the other hand, is an inexpensive, noninvasive, well-tolerated modality that is capable of accurately distinguishing between normal, stenotic, and occluded vessels.

The rationale for supposing that duplex arterial mapping (DAM) can serve a similar purpose to conventional preoperative arteriography is based on two genres of studies in which both tests are performed in the same patients. The first type of study evaluates whether DAM can accurately evaluate individual arteries and detect 50% or greater stenoses or occlusions when compared to the de facto gold standard of arteriography.[27,28, 33–38] A signature study representative of this genre was performed by Moneta et al.[39] who compared duplex arterial mapping with arteriography in 150 consecutive patients under consideration for lower extremity revascularization. The authors summarized that for vessels proximal to the crural arteries, duplex technology could adequately visualize 99% of the arteries. The sensitivity for duplex ultrasound in documenting a 50% or greater lesion ranged from 89% in the iliac arteries to a low of 67% within the popliteal artery. Stenoses could be distinguished from occlusions in almost all cases (98%). In the crural vessels, DAM was able to visualize the anterior tibial, posterior tibial, and peroneal arteries 94%, 96%, and 83% of the time, respectively. The sensitivity of duplex ultrasound for documenting continuous patency of these vessels was 90%, 90%, and 82%, respectively. More recent studies employing newer generation duplex scanners have yielded improved results, especially within the infrapopliteal vasculature where it is now possible to not only document continuous patency of a vessel but also distinguish between greater or less than 50% stenoses.[29]

Knowledge of the presence, degree, and location of arterial stenoses does not necessarily mean that all manners of lower extremity revascularizations can be performed based on duplex examinations alone. However, studies including one performed in our own laboratory have sought to answer the question "Can duplex scan arterial mapping replace contrast arteriography as the test of choice before infrainguinal revascularization?"[29]

Our study concluded that the need for a femoropopliteal versus an infrapopliteal bypass could be correctly predicted by DAM in 90% of the patients studied. Our study concluded that the need for a femoropopliteal versus an infrapopliteal bypass could be correctly predicted by DAM in 90% of the patients studied. Moreover, both of the anastomotic sites for the bypass were correctly predicted by means of DAM in 90% of the patients who had femoropopliteal bypasses versus only 24% of the patients who underwent infrapopliteal bypasses. We concluded that DAM could reliably predict which patients required femoropopliteal bypasses versus infrapopliteal bypasses.

In the following section, we describe the technique used in our laboratory to perform DAM. In addition, the clinical utility of this modality when compared to conventional arteriography is explored.

TECHNIQUE FOR DUPLEX ARTERIAL MAPPING

Prior to DAM, patients are advised to perform an overnight fast, wear loose-fitting clothing, and expect the examination to last an average of 45 minutes. At the time of the study, the patient is placed supine on a standard examination table. We utilize ATL HDI 3,000 and 5,000 (Advanced Technology Labs, Bothell, Washington) color duplex scanners and start the examination with a broadband L7-4 MHz linear-array transducer. First, the common femoral artery on the symptomatic side is insonated. A femoral artery acceleration time >133 cm/sec^2 is our criteria to initiate the mapping by scanning the aorto-iliac system. A femoral artery acceleration time <133 cm/sec^2 rules out the presence of significant aorto-iliac occlusive disease,[40] and if the patient is free of symptoms or findings (decreased femoral pulse) suggesting aorto-iliac disease, we begin by mapping the infrainguinal vasculature only.

For infrainguinal mapping, the leg is externally rotated to facilitate investigation of the thigh and medial calf vessels and returned to its neutral position to evaluate the anterior tibial artery. Different transducers (L12-5 broadband linear or CL 10-5 curved array) are used when necessary to image the more distal vasculature. In this fashion, the common, deep, and superficial femoral, above and below knee popliteal, anterior, and posterior tibial, peroneal, and dorsalis pedis arteries are all imaged in continuity.

A combination of B-mode and color-flow imaging is used to locate the vessels within the appropriate anatomic region and facilitate accurate placement of the sample volume. In the presence of aliasing or narrowing of the color-flow channel, a spectral Doppler waveform is obtained and the systolic blood flow velocities are noted proximal to and within the area being interrogated. If the area of interest demonstrates a peak systolic velocity at least twice as great as that within the adjacent proximal segment, a >50% stenosis is documented. This has been adapted from Jager, Phillips, and Martin and is detailed in Table 14–2.[38] In the presence of an elevated peak systolic velocity, but one that is not doubled, a <50% stenosis

TABLE 14-2 • Stratification of % Arterial Stenosis	
% Stenosis	**Velocity Ratio**
Normal	Triphasic waveform with no spectral broadening
1–19%	Normal waveform with slight spectral broadening and peak velocities increased less than 30% more than the adjacent proximal segment
20–49%	Spectral broadening with no window under the systolic peak, peak velocity less than 100% of the proximal adjacent segment
50–99	Peak velocity 100% more than the adjacent proximal segment and reversed flow component is usually absent; monophasic waveform and reduced velocity beyond the stenosis
Occlusion	No flow in the imaged artery, monophasic pre-occlusive thump; velocities markedly diminished and waveforms monophasic beyond the occlusion

is diagnosed. Finally, the absence of any color-flow signal within a vessel confirms the presence of an occlusion. Our technologists also note the presence and degree of calcification within the vasculature and the location of large collateral vessels distal to occlusions.

The significant portions of the examination are recorded on tape for documentation and further surgeon review if desired, and the results are presented on an easy to interpret graphical representation of the lower extremity vasculature.

Patients who are going to undergo surgery without arteriography have the skin site overlying the distal anastomosis marked with a pen after the surgeon has reviewed the study results and chosen the desired outflow vessel.

Several important technical limitations of DAM must be noted. Examinations may be challenging or impossible to perform in patients with an obese body habitus, severe vascular calcification, or open wounds overlying the course of the named vessels. In addition, the proximal portion of the anterior tibial artery may be difficult or impossible to image, as it traverses the interosseous membrane and the terminal branches of the peroneal artery may not be seen secondary to their small size and deep location within the leg. The degree and extent of mural calcification, exclusive of vessel size, may have a significant impact on the pre-bypass decision-making process; however, there is no widely accepted way to measure or grade calcification. There is also no current means to distinguish between the suitability of crural vessels with similar duplex grades of stenoses to harbor the distal anastomosis of a bypass graft. Finally, duplex arterial mapping is a technically demanding study that requires a large amount of experience to perform accurately.

Considerable practice combined with surgeon feedback and during the learning curve, comparison of DAM findings to angiography (when performed) is mandatory.

Computerized Axial Tomography (CT)[41,42]

CT units have an x-ray tube, two scintillation detectors, a line printer, teletyper, and a computer and magnetic disc unit that are used to attain a series of detailed visualizations of the tissues of the body at any depth desired. It is painless and noninvasive and requires no special preparation; however, there is associated radiation. The body is scanned in two planes simultaneously at various angles. The computer calculates tissue absorption, displays a printout of the numerical values, and produces a visualization of the tissues that demonstrates the densities of the various structures. Tumor masses, infarctions, bone displacement, and accumulations of fluid may be detected.

Angiography, Arteriography, and Digital Subtraction Angiography (DSA)

Angiography or arteriography is defined as "the roentengenographic visualization of blood vessels following introduction of contrast material and is used as a diagnostic aid."[23,43] It is a radiology procedure where a rapid sequence of films is obtained after injection of contrast material through a catheter that is introduced percutaneously through the femoral or axillary arteries. The catheter tip is placed into the selective artery or its branches. Early films show the contrast material in the major arteries followed by subsequent filling of the smaller arteries. Angiography has the ability to demonstrate intrinsic vascular abnormalities such as atherosclerotic plaques, strictures, occlusions, and malformations. In the extremities, it can also assess the degree of collateral circulation and the patency of the distal vessels. It has long been considered the "gold standard" for vascular examinations and is usually done before surgery or interventional techniques. In some instances, it also solves such diagnostic dilemmas as vasospastic disorders versus occlusive disease of the hands, Buerger's disease, ergotism, temporal arteritis, and periarteritis nodosa. However, angiography is invasive and has some inherent risks with radiation exposure.

Magnetic Resonance Imaging (MRI)

Magnetic resonance imaging shows proton density in the body and obtains dynamic studies of certain physiologic functions. Basically, it induces transitions between energy states by causing certain atoms to absorb and transfer energy. This is done by directing a radiofrequency pulse at a substance placed within a large magnetic field. The various measures of time required for material to return to a baseline energy state (relaxation time) can be translated by a complex computer algorithm to a visual image. Magnetic resonance images can be obtained in the transverse, coronal, or sagittal planes. It can penetrate bone without significant attenuation with the underlying tissue clearly imaged. There is no associated radiation.[44]

Treatment for Peripheral Vascular Disease

Treatment programs are tailored to each individual and take into account the needs of the patient and family. The treatment will depend on factors such as the severity of the symptoms, the degree of arterial narrowing or blockage, the impact of the disease on the patient's lifestyle/quality of life, and the patient's overall health. Treatment for patients with peripheral vascular disease may include:

- Controlling risk factors through lifestyle changes and medication
- Endovascular therapy or surgery to reopen arteries of the legs or arms

Controlling Risk Factors and Lifestyle Changes

Peripheral vascular disease is a common condition among people who have diabetes and those who smoke. Diabetics must control their blood sugar levels and smokers must quit smoking completely. Other essential lifestyle changes are diet and exercise. Diet changes include reducing the amount of cholesterol-containing (fatty) foods and, for overweight people, reducing calories to decrease weight. Exercise helps in weight loss and in building a stronger circulatory system and improving blood flow. Even though peripheral vascular disease may cause pain during exercise, a program of daily walking for short periods may help the person maintain or regain function. Patients with peripheral vascular disease, particularly those with diabetes, also must carefully monitor their feet for cuts or wounds and avoid tight-fitting shoes.

Medications

Patients with peripheral vascular disease may benefit from medications to reduce the risk of heart attack and stroke. Among the more commonly prescribed drugs are antiplatelet drugs. These medications make the blood platelets less likely to stick together. Aspirin is the most common, least expensive of these drugs, and typically has the fewest potential side effects. Anticoagulants are prescription drugs that prevent blood clots by affecting the proteins in the body's clotting system and require careful monitoring. The drugs include heparin, which is used short term, and warfarin (Coumadin), which is used long term. Cholesterol-lowering drugs decrease the amount of cholesterol, especially low-density lipoprotein (LDL) (the "bad" form of cholesterol). These drugs decrease the primary material that make up deposits that narrow or plug arteries and create atherosclerosis. Examples of these drugs are niacin, statins, fibrates, and bile acid sequestrants. Calcium channel blockers help to dilate arteries and control high blood pressure. Vitamins such as folate, B_6, and B_{12} help to decrease homocystine in the blood. In specific situations, other dietary supplements may be prescribed, such as L-arginine and omega-3 fatty acids.[45]

Endovascular Therapy and Surgery

Angioplasty and stenting is the mechanical widening of a narrowed or totally obstructed blood vessel and has come to include all manners of vascular interventions typically performed in a minimally invasive or percutaneous method. It is often called percutaneous transluminal angioplasty (or PTA). PTA is most commonly performed to treat narrowing in the leg arteries, especially the common iliac, external iliac, superficial femoral, and popliteal arteries, but can also be used to treat narrowing in veins.

This procedure is performed via a puncture of the femoral artery or less commonly the brachial or radial artery. Using various wires, sheaths, and catheters, the interventionalist identifies the narrowed or blocked artery, stretches it open with a balloon, and may or may not place a stent in the area to prevent it from collapsing again. Balloon angioplasty and stenting has generally replaced invasive surgery as the first-line treatment for peripheral vascular disease (Fig. 14–30).[46]

Surgery is the appropriate option for those patients with severe peripheral vascular disease that interferes with daily activities and is not amenable to less invasive forms of intervention. Surgery may include endarterectomy or bypass grafting.

Endarterectomy is a surgical procedure to remove the atheromatous plaque material, or blockage, in the lining of an artery constricted by the buildup of fatty deposits. It is carried out by separating the plaque from the arterial wall. Endarterectomy is performed with or without a patch graft. This procedure is more invasive than angioplasty and can be used when a very short segment of an artery is blocked or severely clogged. The surgeon identifies the location of the blockage and then makes an incision over the area. The clogged artery is opened and the diseased segment removed. The artery is closed, or if this will make it too narrow, a small patch of vein or prosthetic graft material is inserted as a cap to maintain a large enough opening for the flow of blood.

Surgical bypass treats narrowed arteries by directly creating a detour, or bypass, around a section of the artery that is blocked. Leg artery bypass surgery involves taking a vein from the body or an artificial vein to construct a bypass around a blocked main leg artery. The bypass is, in effect, a secondary system to allow blood to flow to the distal extremity. The vein or graft is sutured in place proximal and distal to the obstruction (Fig. 14–31). It requires at least two incisions, one above and one below the blocked artery. Sometimes, especially when veins are used, longer incisions are necessary.

Inflow operations are performed to restore blood flow in the presence of aorto-iliac occlusive disease. Aorto-bifemoral grafts originate from the aorta and take blood to the femoral arteries at the groins. Aorto-bifemoral grafting is the most successful type of inflow operation but is also the most invasive. A prosthetic graft is anastomosed to the aorta. The graft has two limbs that are then tunneled under the abdominal muscles to the groins to be anastomosed to the femoral arteries.

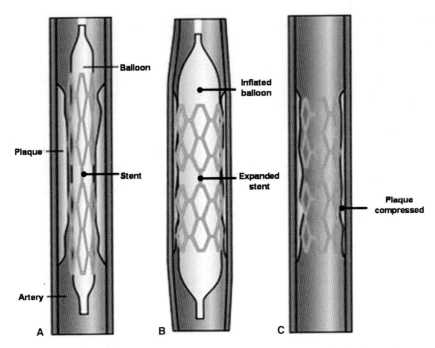

FIGURE 14–30. (**A**) Collapsed balloon and stent are advanced to the level of stenosis within the vessel. (**B**) Balloon is inflated and stent is deployed pushing plaque against wall of artery. (**C**) Plaque is compressed and lumen has been restored.

Axillobifemoral grafts originate from the axillary arteries and take blood to the femoral arteries. This is sometimes the best option in very elderly or very unfit patients as it is a less traumatic alternative to aorto-bifemoral grafting. Femoro-femoral crossover grafts originate from a normal femoral artery in the groin of one leg and take blood to the femoral artery in the groin of the opposite leg.

Outflow operations are performed to restore blood flow to the more distal leg. Femoro-popliteal bypass grafts originate from the femoral artery in the groin and take blood to the popliteal artery either just above or below the knee. Femoro-distal or femoro-crural bypass grafts originate from the femoral artery at the groin or in the thigh and take blood to one of the three calf blood vessels (anterior and posterior tibial arteries and peroneal artery).[47]

Aortic Aneurysms

The definitive treatment for an aortic aneurysm is surgical repair. This typically involves opening the dilated portion of the aorta and inserting a synthetic (Dacron or Gore-Tex) graft. Once the graft is sewn into place, the aneurysmal sac is closed around the artificial tube.

The determination of when surgery should be performed is complex and case-specific. The overriding consideration is

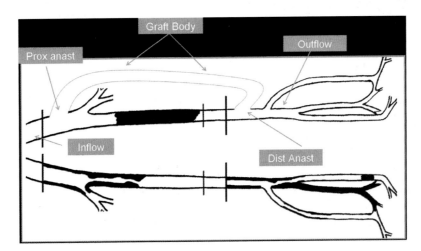

FIGURE 14–31. Bypass graft (dotted orange line) in the left lower extremity. Proximal anastomosis is at the common femoral artery and the distal anastomosis is at the below the knee popliteal artery.

when the risk of rupture exceeds the risk of surgery. The diameter of the aneurysm and its rate of growth and other coexisting medical conditions are all important factors in the determination. A rapidly expanding aneurysm should be operated on as soon as feasible, since it has a greater chance of rupture. Slowly expanding aortic aneurysms may be followed by routine diagnostic testing (CT scan or ultrasound imaging). If the aortic aneurysm grows at a rate of more than 1 cm/yr, surgical treatment is considered.

Current treatment guidelines for abdominal aortic aneurysms suggest elective surgical repair when the diameter of the aneurysm is >5 cm. However, recent data suggests medical management for abdominal aneurysms with a diameter of <5.5 cm.[48]

In recent years, endoluminal treatment of abdominal aortic aneurysms has emerged as a less invasive alternative to open surgical repair. The first endoluminal exclusion of an aneurysm took place in Argentina by Dr. Parodi and his colleagues in 1991. The endovascular treatment of aortic aneurysms involves the placement of an endovascular graft and stent via a percutaneous or open technique (usually through the femoral arteries) into the aneurysmal portion of the aorta. This technique has been reported to have a lower mortality rate compared to open surgical repair and is now being widely used in individuals with comorbid conditions that make them high-risk patients for open surgery. Some centers also report very promising results for the specific method in patients that do not constitute a high surgical risk group.

There have also been many reports concerning the endovascular treatment of ruptured abdominal aortic aneurysms, which are usually treated with an open surgery repair due to the patient's impaired overall condition. Mid-term results have been quite promising.[49] However, according to the latest studies, the procedure does not carry any overall survival benefit.[50]

While the endovascular repair of abdominal aortic aneurysms offers many benefits (Table 14–3), there are several potential complications of this technique. The most significant of these complications are endoleak and graft migration, which have been described for all of the endovascular grafts that have been used to date for endovascular abdominal aortic aneurysm repair.

TABLE 14–4 • Endoleak Types

Type 1a, 1b	Endoleak whose origin is at the proximal (1a) or distal (1b) stent attachment site
Type 2	Endoleak originating from a branch vessel. Possible sources include patent lumbar (posterior to the endovascular graft sonographically), inferior mesenteric (anteriolateral to the endovascular graft sonographically), accessory renal or hypogastric arteries or other patent branches of the abdominal aorta. These are best seen in the transverse orientation.
Type 3	Endoleak that originates at the junctions between components of modular devices or from fabric tears within the graft.
Type 4	Transgraft flow or flow that fills the aneurysm sac due to porosity of the graft.
Endotension	Increase in aneurysm size in the absence of endoleak.

An endoleak is defined as flow outside of the endovascular graft that perfuses and pressurizes the aneurysm sac. This ongoing pressurization of the aneurysm sac carries with it the persistent risk of aneurysm enlargement and rupture. The presence of an endoleak, therefore, negates the primary goal of the endovascular procedure and results in an aneurysm that remains inadequately treated. Several types of endoleaks have been described (Table 14–4). Although other complications of endovascular abdominal aortic aneurysm repair have been described, (Table 14–5) considerable progress in patient selection and surgical technique has reduced the overall rate of these problems. Currently, the optimal method for post-endovascular graft screening and the most reliable method for detecting endoleak and complications are subject to debate. CT is favored in some centers and color Doppler ultrasound in others[51–56] (Fig. 14–32).

TABLE 14–3 • Advantages of Endovascular Graft Exclusion of Abdominal Aortic Aneurysms

- Performed from remote site and avoids laparotomy
- Small incisions (femoral, brachial, or carotid artery cut down for access)
- No prolonged aortic clamping
- Decreased or no intensive care unit stay
- Decreased length of stay (1–2 days for endovascular vs 6–8 days for open repair)
- Decreased time to resumption of normal activity level

TABLE 14–5 • Complications Associated with Endovascular Repair of Abdominal Aortic Aneurysms

Aneurysm growth
Embolization
Fabric tears
Graft infection
Graft migration
Hook fracture
Limb thrombosis
Limb separation
Endoleak*

*Common to all endovascular grafts used to date.

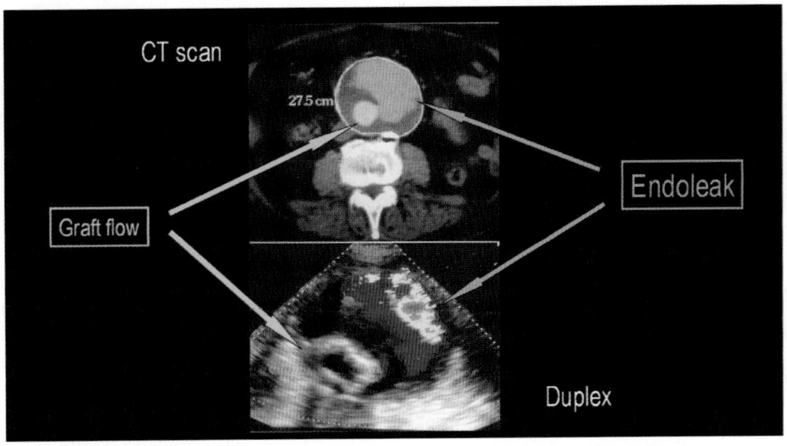

FIGURE 14-32. Top is a CT scan in a patient with an endovascular graft placed to exclude an abdominal aortic aneurysm. Contrast is seen in both the graft as well as the aneurysm sac. Bottom is a color flow image in the same patient that reveals color flow in the graft (blue) and in the aneurysm sac. These findings are diagnostic of endoleak.

The authors wish to acknowledge Anna Sander for her assistance in the preparation of this manuscript.

References

1. Powis RL, Schwartz RA. *Practical Doppler Ultrasound for the Clinician*. Baltimore: Williams & Wilkins; 1991; 52.

2. Hallet JW, Brewster DC, Darling RC. *Handbook of Patient Vascular Surgery*. 3rd ed. Boston: Little, Brown; 1995; 6.

3. Williams PL, Warwick R, Dyson M, et al., eds. *Gray's Anatomy*. 37th ed. New York: Churchill Livingstone; 1989.

4. Stephens RB, Stillwell DL. *Arteries and Veins of the Human Brain*. Springfield, IL: Charles C Thomas; 1969.

5. McVay CB. *Anson and McVay Surgical Anatomy*. 6th ed. Philadelphia: WB Saunders; 1984.

6. Clemente CD, ed. *Gray's Anatomy of the Human Body*. 30th American ed. Philadelphia: Lea and Febiger; 1985.

7. Zwiebel WJ, Pellerito JS. *Introduction to Vascular Ultrasonography*. 5th ed. Philadelphia: WB Saunders; 2005.

8. Hedrick WR, Hykes DL, Strachman DE. *Ultrasound Physics and Instrumentation*. 3rd ed. St. Louis, MO: Mosby; 1995.

9. Tortora GJ, Grabowski SR. *Principles of Anatomy & Physiology*. 7th ed. New York: HarperCollins; 1993.

10. Hackam DG, Anand, SS. Emerging risk factors for atherosclerotic vascular disease. A critical review of the evidence. *JAMA*. 2003; 290:932-940.

11. Patterson RF. Basic science in vascular disease. *J Vasc Technol*. 2002; 26(1).

12. Maton A, Hopkins J, McLaughlin CW, Johnson S, Warner MQ, LaHart D, Wright JD. *Human Biology and Health*. Englewood Cliffs, NJ: Prentice Hall; 1993.

13. Tuzcu EM, Kapadia SR, Tutar E, et al. High prevalence of coronary atherosclerosis in asymptomatic teenagers and young adults: evidence from intravascular ultrasound. *Circulation*. 2001; 103(22):2705-2710.

14. Fishbein MC, Schoenfield LJ. Heart attack photo illustration essay. Available: MedicineNet.com.

15. Sales CM, Goldsmith J, Veith FJ. *Handbook of Vascular Surgery*. St. Louis, MO: Quality Medical Publishing; 1994.

16. Kang SS, Labropoulos N, Mansour MA, Baker WH. Percutaneous ultrasound guided thrombin injection: a new method for treating postcatheterization femoral pseudoaneurysms. *J Vasc Surg*. 1998 Dec; 28(6):1120-1121.

17. Berdejo GL, Wengerter KR, Marin ML, Suggs WD, Veith FJ. Color flow duplex guided manual occlusion of iatrogenic arteriovenous fistulas. *J Vasc Technol*. 1995; 19(2):79-83.

18. Hutt JRB, Davies AH. Nonatherosclerotic vascular disease. In: Davies and Brophy, eds. *Vascular Surgery*. London: Springer; 2006.

19. Hobson RW, Veith FJ, Wilson SE, eds. *Vascular Surgery: Principles and Practice*. Marcel Dekker; October 2003.

20. Hirsch AT, Criqui MH, Treat-Jacobson D, et al. Peripheral arterial disease detection, awareness and treatment in primary care. *JAMA*. 2001 Sep 19; 286(11):1317-1324.

21. Gerlock AJ, Giyanani VL, Krebs CA. *Applications of Noninvasive Vascular Techniques*. Philadelphia: WB Saunders; 1988.

22. Needham T. Physiologic testing of lower extremity arterial disease: segmental pressures, plethysmography and velocity waveforms. In: Mansour AM, Labropoulos N, eds. *Vascular Diagnosis*. Philadelphia, PA: Elsevier Saunders; 2005.

23. Hessel SJ, Adams DF, Abrams HL. Complications of angiography. *Radiology* 1981; 138:273-281.

24. Sigstedt B, Lunderquist A. Complications of Angiographic Examinations. *AJR Am J Roentgenol*. 1978; 130:455-460.

25. Formanek G, Frech RS, Amplatz K. Arterial thrombus formation during clinical percutaneous catheterization. *Circulation*. 1990; 41:833-839.

26. Lang EK. A survey of the complications of percutaneous retrograde arteriography. *Radiology* 1963; 81:257-263.

27. Larch E, Minar E, Ahmadi R, Schnurer G, Schneider B, Stumpflen A, et al. Value of color duplex sonography for evaluation of tibioperoneal arteries in patients with femoropopliteal obstruction: a prospective comparison with antegrade intraarterial digital subtraction angiography. *J Vasc Surg*. 1997; 25:629-636.

28. Karacagil S, Lofberg AM, Granbo A, Lorelius LE, Bergqvist D. Value of duplex scanning in evaluation of crural and foot arteries in limbs with severe lower limb ischaemia—a prospective comparison with angiography. *Eur J Vasc Endovasc Surg.* 1996; 12: 300-303.

29. Wain R, Berdejo GL, Delvalle WN, Lyon RT, Sanchez LA, Suggs WD, et al. Can duplex scan arterial mapping replace contrast arteriography as the test of choice before infrainguinal revascularization. *J Vasc Surg.* 1999; 29:100-109.

30. Ascher E, Mazzariol F, Hingorani Salles-Cunha S, Gade P. The use of duplex arterial mapping as an alternative to conventional arteriography for primary and secondary infrapopliteal bypasses. *M J Surg.* 1999; 178:162-165.

31. Cramer MM. Color flow duplex examination of the abdominal aorta: atherosclerosis, aneurysm, and dissection. *J Vasc Technol.* 1995; 19(5).

32. Cato R, Kupinski AM. Graft assessment by duplex ultrasound scanning. *J Vasc Technol.* 1994; 18(5):307-310.

33. Cossman DV, Ellison JE, Wagner WH, Carroll RM, Treiman RL, Foran RF, et al. Comparison of contrast arteriography to arterial mapping with color-flow duplex imaging in the lower extremities. *J Vasc Surg.* 1989; 10:522-529.

34. Polak JF, Karmel MI, Mannick JA, O'Leary DH, Donaldson MC, Whittemore AD. Determination of the extent of lower-extremity peripheral arterial disease with color assisted duplex sonography: comparison with angiography. *AJR Am J Roentgenol.* 1990; 155:1085-1089.

35. Hatsukami TS, Primozich JF, Zierler E, Harley JD, Strandness DE. Color doppler imaging of infrainguinal arterial occlusive disease. *J Vasc Surg.* 1992; 16:527-533.

36. Pemberton M, London NJM. Colour flow duplex imaging of occlusive arterial disease of the lower limb. *Br J Surg.* 1997; 84:912-919.

37. Sensier Y, Fishwick G, Owen R, Pemberton M, Bell PRF, London NJM. A comparison between colour duplex ultrasonography and arteriography for imaging infrapopliteal arterial lesions. *Eur J Endovasc Surg.* 1998; 15:44-50.

38. Jager KA, Phillips DJ, Martin RL. Noninvasive mapping of lower limb arterial lesions. *Ultrasound Med Biol.* 1985; 11:515-521.

39. Moneta GL, Yeager RA, Antonovic R, Hall LD, Caster JD, Cummings CA, et al. Accuracy of lower extremity arterial duplex mapping. *J Vasc Surg.* 1992; 15:275-284.

40. Kupper CA, Dewhirst N, Burnham SJ. Doppler spectral waveforms for recording peripheral arterial signals: the preferred method. *J Vasc Technol.* 1989; 13:69-73.

41. Hoff FL, Mueller K, Pearce W. Computed tomography in vascular disease. In: Ascer E, ed. *Haimovici's Vascular Surgery.* 5th ed. Malden, MA: Blackwell Publishing; 2004.

42. Prokop M, Schaefer-Prokop C. *Spiral and Multislice Computed Tomography of the Body.* Thieme Publishers; 2002.

43. Neiman HL, Lyons J. Fundamentals of angiography. In: Ascer E, ed. *Haimovici's Vascular Surgery.* 5th ed. Malden, MA: Blackwell Publishing; 2004.

44. Karmacharya JJ, Velazquez OC, Baum RA, Carpenter JP. Magnetic resonance angiography. In: Ascer E, ed. *Haimovici's Vascular Surgery.* 5th ed. Malden, MA: Blackwell Publishing; 2004.

45. Stoyioglou A, Jaff MR. Medical treatment of peripheral arterial disease: a comprehensive review. *J Vasc Interv Radiol.* 2004; 15(11):1197-1207.

46. Lumsden AB, Lin P, eds. *Endovascular Therapy for Peripheral Vascular Disease.* Blackwell Publishing; 2006.

47. Ascer E, ed. *Haimovici's Vascular Surgery.* 5th ed. Malden, MA: Blackwell Publishing; 2004.

48. Mortality results for randomised controlled trial of early elective surgery or ultrasonographic surveillance for small abdominal aortic aneurysms. The UK Small Aneurysm Trial Participants. *Lancet.* 1998 Nov 21; 352(9141):1649-1655.

49. Veith FJ, Gargiulo NJ. Endovascular aortic repair should be the gold standard for ruptured AAAs, and all vascular surgeons should be prepared to perform them. *Perspect Vasc Surg Endovasc Ther.* 2007 Sep; 19(3):275-282.

50. Rutherford RB. Randomized EVAR trials and advent of level I evidence: a paradigm shift in management of large abdominal aortic aneurysms? *Semin Vasc Surg.* 2006 Jun; 19(2):69-74.

51. Berdejo GL, Lyon RT, Ohki T, Sanchez LA, Wain RA, Del Valle WN, Marin ML, Veith FJ. Color duplex ultrasound evaluation of transluminally placed endovascular grafts for aneurysm repair. *J Vasc Technol.* 1998; 22(4):201-207.

52. Sato DT, Goff CD, Gregory RT, et al. Endoleak after aortic stent graft repair: Diagnosis by color duplex ultrasound vs. CT scan. *J Vasc Surg.* 1998; 28(4):657-663.

53. Lyon RT, Berdejo GL, Veith FJ. Ultrasound imaging techniques for evaluation of endovascular stented grafts. In: Parodi JC, Veith FJ, Marin ML, eds. *Endovascular Grafting Techniques.* Media, PA: Williams & Wilkins; 1999.

54. Wolf YG, Johnson BL, Hill BB, Rubin GD, Fogarty TJ, Zarins CK. Duplex ultrasonography vs. CT angiography for postoperative evaluation of endovascular abdominal aortic aneurysms repair. *J Vasc Surg.* 2000 Dec; 32(6):1142-1148.

55. Zanetti S, DeRango P, et al. Role of duplex scan in endoleak detection after endoluminal aortic repair. *Eur J Vasc Endovasc Surg.* 2000; 19:531-535.

56. Berdejo GL, Lipsitz EC. Ultrasound assessment following endovascular aortic aneurysm repair. In: Zwiebel and Pellerito, eds. *Introduction to Vascular Ultrasonography.* Philadelphia, PA: Elsevier Saunders; 2005.

Questions

GENERAL INSTRUCTIONS: For each question, select the best answer. Select only one answer for each question, unless otherwise instructed.

1. **What determines the Doppler shift frequency?**

   (A) flow toward the transducer

   (B) flow away from the transducer

   (C) difference between the reflected and transmitted frequencies

   (D) the velocity of the moving particles toward the transducer

2. **The Doppler effect creates**

   (A) change in frequency or Doppler shift when the reflector moves relative to the transducer

   (B) increase in frequency as the reflector moves away from the transducer

   (C) maximum frequency shift at 90°

   (D) requires angle correction for frequency measurements

3. **Continuous-wave Doppler has how many crystals in the transducer?**

   (A) one

   (B) two

   (C) three

   (D) four

4. **If flow is toward the transducer, what will the frequency shift be?**

   (A) lower

   (B) same

   (C) variable

   (D) higher

5. **If the transmitted frequency is raised, what is the Doppler shift?**

   (A) increases

   (B) decreases

   (C) remains the same

   (D) will not be detected

6. **Maximum Doppler shift frequency occurs at which of the following angles?**

   (A) 90°

   (B) 180°

   (C) 0°

   (D) 75°

7. **What instrumentation is used for measurement of volume changes in the extremities to demonstrate blood flow?**

   (A) continuous-wave Doppler

   (B) color-flow Doppler

   (C) plethysmography

   (D) pulse volume recording

8. **All of the following are true of spectral analysis except**

   (A) mathematical display of the frequency components in the Doppler signal

   (B) computer using the fast Fourier transform method

   (C) demonstrates the presence, direction, and characteristics of blood flow

   (D) does not provide measurements of the blood flow

9. **Name the components of the spectral analysis labeled in Fig. 14–33.**

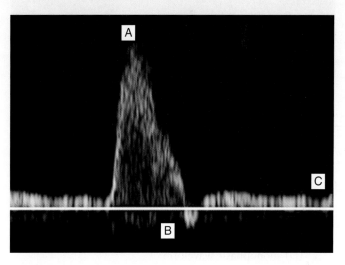

FIGURE 14–33. Spectral analysis waveform.

   (A) _____

   (B) _____

   (C) _____

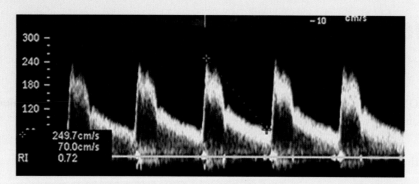

FIGURE 14–35. Spectral analysis waveform.

10. What does the spectral broadening seen on the spectral analysis mean?

(A) normal arterial waveform

(B) increased bandwidth caused by disturbed flow

(C) decreased bandwidth caused by disturbed flow

(D) increased bandwidth caused by laminar flow

11. Which of the following statements about aliasing is *false*?

(A) velocities exceed the Nyquist limit

(B) wraparound of the waveform

(C) higher velocities appear on the negative side of the baseline

(D) not controlled by the pulse repetition rate

12. Which of the following is demonstrated in Fig. 14–34?

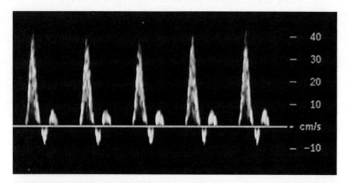

FIGURE 14–34. Spectral analysis waveform.

(A) spectral broadening

(B) aliasing

(C) turbulence

(D) monophasic waveform

(E) triphasic waveform

13. Which of the following is demonstrated in Fig. 14–35?

(A) spectral broadening

(B) aliasing

(C) monophasic waveform

(D) triphasic waveform

14. Which of the following is demonstrated in Fig. 14–36?

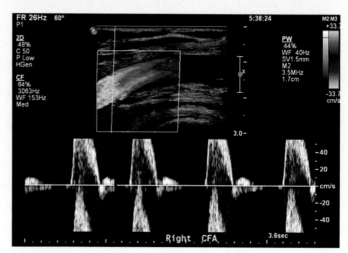

FIGURE 14–36. Spectral analysis waveform.

(A) dampened waveform

(B) aliasing of the waveform

(C) monophasic waveform

(D) triphasic waveform

15. Which of the following is demonstrated in Fig. 14–37?

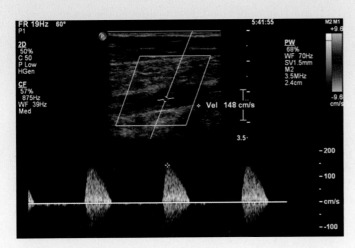

FIGURE 14–37. Spectral analysis waveform.

(A) laminar flow

(B) aliasing

(C) monophasic waveform

(D) biphasic waveform

(E) triphasic waveform

16 Which of the following is demonstrated in Fig. 14–38?

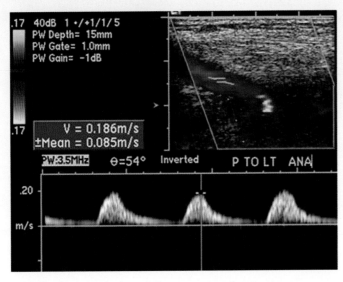

FIGURE 14–38. Spectral analysis waveform.

(A) spectral broadening

(B) aliasing

(C) triphasic waveform

(D) monophasic waveform

17. Which of the following is shown in Fig. 14–39?

$$FS = \frac{2\ v\ Fo}{c+}\ \cos\theta$$

FIGURE 14–39. Physics equation.

(A) Doppler equation

(B) Poiseuille's law

(C) Reynolds number

(D) Bernoulli's equation

18. A radiology procedure where a balloon catheter is placed in a vessel and dilated to eliminate stenotic lesions is called

(A) digital subtraction angiography

(B) magnetic resonance imaging

(C) positron emission tomography

(D) percutaneous transluminal angioplasty

19. What interventional procedure using a vascular catheter for introduction of a substance or device is used to control bleeding or stop the blood flow?

(A) transjugular intrahepatic portosystemic shunt

(B) embolization

(C) percutaneous angioplasty

(D) thrombolytic therapy

20. Which of the following terms describes the physiology of circulation?

(A) fluid dynamics

(B) circulatory system

(C) hemodynamics

(D) coronary circulation

21. Blood movement in concentric layers with the highest velocity in the center of the vessel that creates a parabolic flow profile is

(A) laminar flow

(B) disorganized flow

(C) boundary layer separation

(D) turbulent flow

22. **What type of plethysmography identifies subcutaneous blood flow?**

    (A) air

    (B) strain gauge

    (C) impedance

    (D) photoplethysmography

23. **In the poststenotic flow zone, there may be frank swirling movements, which are called**

    (A) collateral flow

    (B) vortices

    (C) reversed flow

    (D) laminar flow

24. **Which of the following statements about the Reynolds number is *false*?**

    (A) defines the point where flow changes from laminar to disturbed

    (B) is less than 2,000 in the normal arterial circulation

    (C) is not included in the basic principles of fluid dynamics

    (D) predicts the stability of a fluid

25. **Laminar flow tends to be disturbed if the Reynolds number exceeds what value?**

    (A) 500

    (B) 700

    (C) 1,000

    (D) 1,500

    (E) 2,000

26. **Which term describes a turbulence in the blood flow distal to a narrowing of the vessel?**

    (A) poststenotic turbulence

    (B) velocity jet

    (C) laminar flow

    (D) dampened flow

27. **How is the velocity of blood flow related to the cross-sectional area of the blood vessel?**

    (A) inversely

    (B) directly related

    (C) not related

    (D) variable

28. **Blood pressure is**

    (A) volume of blood flowing through the vessel

    (B) average pressure throughout the cardiac cycle

    (C) pulse pressure in circulatory system

    (D) pressure exerted by blood on the wall of a blood vessel

29. **In a resting young adult, what is normal blood pressure?**

    (A) 100 mm Hg during systole and 50 mm Hg during diastole

    (B) 120 mm Hg during systole and 40 mm Hg during diastole

    (C) 150 mm Hg during systole and 70 mm Hg during diastole

    (D) 120 mm Hg during systole and 70 mm Hg during diastole

30. **The expansion and contraction of arteries after each systole of the left ventricle creates a pressure wave termed**

    (A) cycle

    (B) waveform

    (C) pulse

    (D) mean

31. **The resting pulse is**

    (A) between 50 and 100 pulses per minute

    (B) over 100 pulses per minute

    (C) under 50 beats per minute

    (D) between 25 and 75 pulses per minute

32. **Predisposing factors for arterial disease do *not* include**

    (A) smoking

    (B) aging

    (C) diabetes

    (D) family history of arterial disease

    (E) hypertension

    (F) bradycardia

33. **What is the most common symptom of lower extremity arterial disease?**

    (A) ulceration

    (B) absence of pulses

    (C) claudication

    (D) cyanosis

34. Which of the following is *not* one of the classic five Ps for acute arterial ischemia?

(A) pain

(B) pallor

(C) pressure

(D) paresthesias

(E) paralysis

(F) pulselessness

35. The ankle brachial index is used in which examination?

(A) strain gauge plethysmography

(B) peripheral angiography

(C) peripheral venous evaluation

(D) segmental pressure arterial examination

36. If a patient falls into a claudication category on the segmental pressure examination, what additional testing is done?

(A) color flow Doppler

(B) peripheral angiography

(C) exercise with a treadmill or hyperemia testing

(D) impedance plethysmography

37. In performing the segmental arterial pressure examination, where is the pressure recording obtained?

(A) site where the cuff is inflated and deflated

(B) at the posterior tibial artery

(C) site below where the cuff is inflated and deflated

(D) site above where the cuff is inflated and deflated

38. In segmental arterial studies, the cuff at each site is inflated until the systolic pressure, sound, or Doppler waveform does what?

(A) appears

(B) disappears

(C) remains constant

(D) none of the above

39. What is used as the standard pressure for segmental arterial studies?

(A) posterior tibial artery systolic pressure

(B) common femoral artery systolic pressure

(C) brachial artery systolic pressure

(D) anterior tibial artery systolic pressure

40. What should the bilateral brachial pressures be?

(A) 5 mm Hg

(B) 10 mm Hg

(C) 25 mm Hg

(D) 50 mm Hg

41. What does an ankle brachial index of 0.6–0.9 indicate?

(A) normal value

(B) claudication

(C) severe occlusive disease

(D) occlusion

42. What does an ankle brachial index of 0.5 or less indicate?

(A) normal value

(B) claudication

(C) severe occlusive disease

(D) occlusion

43. In peripheral arterial disease and the vessels of the lower extremity are calcified with falsely elevated values on the segmental pressure recordings, what is required?

(A) color-flow Doppler

(B) strain gauge plethysmography

(C) brachial pressures

(D) toe pressures

44. What is the normal toe pressure?

(A) equal to the brachial pressure

(B) equal to the ankle index pressure

(C) 60% of the brachial pressure

(D) 75% of the brachial pressure

45. What effect does normal exercise have on blood flow?

(A) increases

(B) decreases

(C) remains unchanged

(D) creates a high variable

46. Composition of the arteries does *not* include

(A) intima

(B) media

(C) adventitia

(D) internal capsule

47. As sympathetic stimulation is increased, the smooth muscle of the artery contracts and narrows the vessel lumen. This is called

(A) vasodilatation

(B) vascular narrowing

(C) vasoconstriction

(D) vasospasm

48. Which artery is present only on right side of the upper extremity?

(A) brachiocephalic

(B) subclavian

(C) thyrocervical

(D) costocervical

49. Which arterial vessel is a direct continuation of the subclavian?

(A) vertebral

(B) common carotid

(C) axillary

(D) brachiocephalic

50. What are the terminal branches of the brachial artery?

(A) axillary and subclavian

(B) palmar and digital

(C) radial and ulna

(D) radial and palmar

51. Which arterial vessel is a continuation of the external iliac and supplies the psoas major muscle, inferior epigastric, and deep circumflex?

(A) common femoral

(B) superficial femoral

(C) profunda femoral

(D) popliteal

52. Which vessel lies posterior to the medial aspect of the ankle?

(A) anterior tibial

(B) peroneal

(C) posterior tibial

(D) dorsalis pedis

53. Ischemia is secondary to

(A) excessive blood flow

(B) normal blood flow

(C) loss of blood flow

(D) none of the above

54. An embolism is

(A) sudden blocking of artery by clot or foreign material

(B) atherosclerotic plaque formation

(C) trauma to an artery with resulting occlusion

(D) dissection of an artery caused by trauma

55. What type of pain is present during exertion and disappears upon cessation of activity?

(A) rest pain

(B) claudication pain

(C) trauma pain

(D) normal exercise

56. Which of the following causes the majority of arterial diseases?

(A) genetic origin

(B) atherosclerosis

(C) cardiac disease

(D) diabetes

57. Blood flow and pressures are not significantly diminished until at least what percentage of the cross-sectional area of the vessel is obliterated?

(A) 25%

(B) 50%

(C) 75%

(D) 95%

58. Other factors that influence a critical stenosis are

(A) length of the stenosis

(B) blood viscosity

(C) peripheral resistance

(D) both A and C

(E) all of the above

59. What is the most common site of atherosclerotic occlusion in the lower extremity?

(A) common femoral artery bifurcation into superficial and deep femoral artery

(B) profunda (deep) femoral artery

(C) distal superficial femoral artery in the adductor canal

(D) popliteal artery

60. Which artery in the lower extremity passes through the interosseous membrane and courses along the anterolateral aspect of the leg?

(A) posterior tibial

(B) anterior tibial

(C) peroneal

(D) dorsalis pedis

61. Which of the following terms describes a stenosis or occlusion of the subclavian artery proximal to the vertebral artery?

    (A) subclavian steal syndrome
    (B) thoracic outlet syndrome
    (C) vertebral-basilar occlusive disease
    (D) vertebral artery stenosis

62. Subclavian steal is characterized by which of the following findings?

    (A) turbulent erratic waveforms throughout the vertebrals
    (B) a monophasic waveform of the subclavian artery
    (C) a high-grade stenosis with increased velocities
    (D) reversal of blood flow within the vertebral artery

63. What is the hallmark clinical sign of subclavian artery stenosis?

    (A) pain in the upper extremity
    (B) numbness in the upper extremity
    (C) difference in blood pressure of <10 mm Hg
    (D) absence of upper extremity pulses

64. Intrinsic compression of the vessels by the clavicle, first rib, and the scalene muscles is characteristic of which of the following syndromes?

    (A) subclavian steal syndrome
    (B) thoracic outlet syndrome
    (C) subclavian aneurysms
    (D) Raynaud's disease

65. Positioning maneuvers (military, hyperabduction, and Adson) are used during diagnostic testing for which of the following syndromes?

    (A) Raynaud's disease
    (B) subclavian steal syndrome
    (C) thoracic outlet syndrome
    (E) Raynaud's phenomenon

66. Which of the following is a functional vasospastic disorder that affects the small arteries of the extremities?

    (A) Raynaud's disease or syndrome
    (B) Raynaud's phenomenon
    (C) thoracic outlet syndrome
    (D) subclavian steal syndrome

67. Which of the following is an obstructive arterial disease that has an underlying systemic or vascular abnormality?

    (A) Raynaud's disease
    (B) Raynaud's phenomenon

    (C) thoracic outlet syndrome
    (D) subclavian steal syndrome

68. Which of the following does not have a true arterial wall and usually result from trauma or previous surgical reconstruction?

    (A) aneurysm
    (B) dissection
    (C) pseudoaneurysm
    (D) arteriovenous malformation

69. Which type of aneurysm is associated with an infectious process?

    (A) pseudoaneurysm
    (B) mycotic
    (C) dissecting
    (D) fusiform

70. Which type of aneurysm has two lumens?

    (A) pseudoaneurysm
    (B) mycotic
    (C) dissecting
    (D) saccular

71. In the evaluation of arterial reconstruction and grafts, what provides quantification of the flow of the entire extremity?

    (A) color-flow Doppler
    (B) spectral waveform analysis
    (C) ankle brachial index
    (D) duplex scanning

72. What does a decrease in peak systolic flow velocity of <45 cm/sec in the arterial graft indicate?

    (A) patency of the graft
    (B) stenosis of the graft
    (C) occlusion of the graft
    (D) increased potential for graft failure

73. Which of the following terms describes a communication between the artery and the vein?

    (A) pseudoaneurysm
    (B) aneurysm
    (C) arteriovenous fistula
    (D) dissection

74. The resistive index is used to quantify

(A) arterial flow

(B) peripheral resistance

(C) turbulence

(D) volume of flow

75. Tachycardia means

(A) rapid heart rate

(B) slow heart rate

(C) normal heart rate

(D) irregular heart rate

76. Which of the following is *not* a noninvasive testing procedure?

(A) Doppler

(B) plethysmography

(C) segmental pressures

(D) angiography

77. The ankle brachial index is

(A) brachial systolic pressure divided by the ankle systolic pressure

(B) the ankle systolic pressure divided by the brachial systolic pressure

(C) brachial diastolic pressure divided by the ankle diastolic pressure

(D) ankle diastolic pressure divided by the brachial diastolic pressure

78. What is required before the performance of the vascular noninvasive examination?

(A) evaluation of blood pressure

(B) process screening

(C) patient history

(D) billing procedures

79. In performance of the segmental pressure examination of the lower extremities, how many cuffs are preferred?

(A) 2

(B) 3

(C) 4

(D) 5

80. What chemical substance are in contrast agents used to increase reflectivity and improve the ultrasound image?

(A) iodine

(B) saline

(C) barium sulfate (BaSO4)

(D) air microbubbles

81. What are the two major pathways of the cardiovascular system?

(A) arterial and venous

(B) systemic and pulmonary circulation

(C) cerebrovascular and systemic circulation

(D) cerebrovascular, systemic, and pulmonary circulation

82. Which layer of the artery is the muscle layer?

(A) intima

(B) media

(C) adventitia

(D) tunica externa

83. What is the first branch of the subclavian?

(A) thyrocervical

(B) internal mammary

(C) costocervical trunk

(D) vertebral

Questions 84 and 85: Match the structures in Fig. 14–40 with the terms in Column B.

MEDIAL   LATERAL

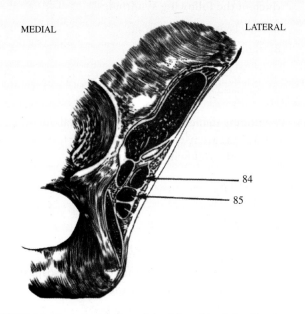

FIGURE 14–40. Lateral surface of the right pelvic girdle. *(Reprinted with permission from Gray H, Clemente CD. Anatomy of the Human Body. Philadelphia: Lea & Febiger; 1985.)*

COLUMN A   COLUMN B

84. _____   (A) femoral artery

85. _____   (B) femoral vein

Questions 86–89: Match the structures in Fig. 14–41 with the terms in Column B.

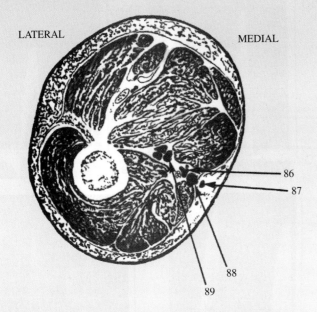

FIGURE 14–41. Cross section proximal thigh. *(Reprinted with permission from Gray H, Clemente CD. Anatomy of the Human Body. Philadelphia: Lea & Febiger; 1985.)*

COLUMN A	COLUMN B
86. _____	(A) profunda (deep) femoral vein and artery
87. _____	(B) femoral artery
88. _____	(C) great saphenous vein
89. _____	(D) femoral vein

Questions 90–93: Match the structures in Fig. 14–42 with the terms in Column B.

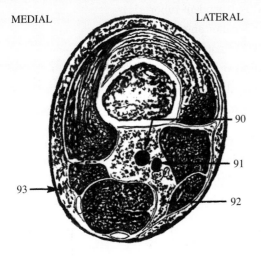

FIGURE 14–42. Cross section of the popliteal space. *(Reprinted with permission from Gray H, Clemente CD. Anatomy of the Human Body. Philadelphia: Lea & Febiger; 1985.)*

COLUMN A	COLUMN B
90. _____	(A) short (lesser) saphenous vein
91. _____	(B) popliteal vein

92. _____	(C) great saphenous vein
93. _____	(D) popliteal artery

Questions 94–100: Match the structures in Fig. 14–43 with the terms in Column B.

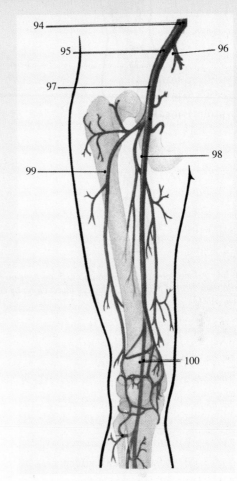

FIGURE 14–43. Arteries of the thigh. *(Reprinted with permission from Abbott Laboratories, North Chicago, IL. Medical Illustrations by Scott Thorn Barrows, AMI.)*

COLUMN A	COLUMN B
94. _____	(A) internal iliac artery
95. _____	(B) popliteal artery
96. _____	(C) superficial femoral artery
97. _____	(D) profunda (deep) femoral
98. _____	(E) common femoral artery
99. _____	(F) distal aorta artery
100. _____	(G) external iliac artery

Questions 101–106: Match the structures in Fig. 14–44 with the terms in Column B.

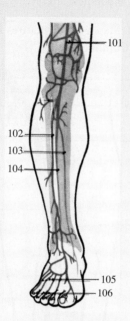

FIGURE 14–44. Arteries of the leg. *(Reprinted with permission from Abbott Laboratories, North Chicago, IL. Medical Illustrations by Scott Thorn Barrows, AMI.)*

COLUMN A	COLUMN B
101. _____	(A) peroneal artery
102. _____	(B) popliteal artery
	(C) plantar metatarsal arteries
103. _____	(D) digital arteries
104. _____	(E) anterior tibial artery
105. _____	(F) posterior tibial artery
106. _____	

Questions 107–110: Match the velocity waveforms in Fig. 14–45 with the terms in Column B.

COLUMN A	COLUMN B
107. _____	(A) 20–40% diameter reduction stenosis
108. _____	(B) 0% diameter reduction stenosis
	(C) 50–99% diameter reduction stenosis
109. _____	(D) 1–19% diameter reduction stenosis
110. _____	

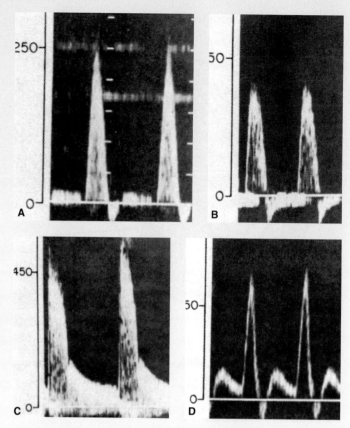

FIGURE 14–45. Velocity waveforms. *(Reprinted from Bergan JJ, Yao JST: Arterial Surgery: New Diagnostic and Operative Techniques. Philadelphia: Grune & Stratton, 1988: 441.)*

111. Signs and symptoms of arterial disease of the lower extremity include

   (A) intermittent claudication
   (B) dependent rubor
   (C) pallor on elevation
   (D) impotence in males
   (E) trophic skin changes
   (F) all of the above
   (G) A, B, D, and E

112. There are many known risk factors that play a part in the development of atherosclerosis of the extremities. These include

   (A) family history
   (B) cigarette smoking
   (C) hypertension
   (D) malignancies
   (E) diabetes mellitus
   (F) all of the above
   (G) A, B, C, and E

113. The acceleration time in Fig. 14–46 is

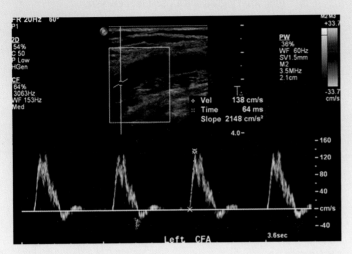

FIGURE 14–46. Doppler signal.

(A) within normal limits

(B) suggestive of a distal stenosis

(C) suggestive of a distal occlusion

(D) consistent with a severe proximal stenosis

114. With a hemodynamically significant, short-segment stenosis, one would expect

(A) an increased peak-systolic velocity and an increased end-diastolic velocity

(B) a decreased peak-systolic velocity and a decreased end-diastolic velocity

(C) an increased peak-systolic velocity and a decreased end-diastolic velocity

(D) a decreased peak systolic velocity and an increased end-diastolic velocity

115. Information obtained from the pulsed-wave Doppler spectral display includes all the following except

(A) the source of origin of the Doppler signal

(B) pulsatility features of the waveform

(C) velocity or frequency shift of the blood flow

(D) direction of flow

116. Spectral broadening results in the loss of the clear spectral window below the peak-systolic velocity spectral waveform in systole. Which of the following statements is *true*?

(A) a small sample volume placed centrally in the artery should decrease the size of the spectral window.

(B) the spectral window filling occurs as flow disturbances produce vortices (swirling eddies) with varying flow direction.

(C) vortices (rotating flow) will show only forward flow and produce a narrow band of velocities demonstrating a clear spectral window.

(D) loss of the spectral window occur only with stenotic lesions of 75% or greater.

117. Appreciable changes in pressure and flow do not occur until the diameter of an artery is reduced by 50% or greater. This degree of narrowing is called

(A) hemodynamically significant

(B) Reynolds number

(C) Bernoulli's principle

(D) Poiseuille's law

118. The principal control mechanisms affecting blood volume changes are

(A) viscosity and blood vessel diameter

(B) cardiac output and peripheral resistance

(C) blood pressure gradients and inertial losses

(D) energy losses and flow-reducing lesions

119. One advantage of using continuous wave Doppler is

(A) the ability to differentiate overlying blood vessels

(B) minimal spectral broadening

(C) high velocities can be displayed without aliasing

(D) control of the depth selection of the sample site

120. Factors affecting the Doppler shift frequency include

(A) Doppler angle

(B) transducer

(C) velocity of the red blood cells

(D) B and C

(E) A, B, and C

121. As an arterial stenosis becomes hemodynamically significant, which statement is *true* about the hemodynamics of the stenosis?

(A) flow volume increases, peak-systolic velocity decreases

(B) flow volume decreases, peak-systolic velocity decreases

(C) flow volume decreases, peak-systolic velocity increases

(D) flow volume increases, peak-systolic velocity increases

122. The highest peak systolic velocity is found

(A) at the narrowest portion of the stenotic lesion

(B) just proximal to the stenotic lesion

(C) just distal to the stenotic lesion

(D) both proximal and distal to the stenotic lesion

123. The flow pattern throughout the stenotic lesion will be

    (A) laminar

    (B) mild scattering

    (C) disturbed

    (D) turbulence only on the outer edges

124. All other factors being constant, the artery with the smallest radius will have

    (A) lower resistance to flow

    (B) higher resistance to flow

    (C) no change in the resistance

    (D) variable resistance

125. Which of the following is *not* used to determine the severity of arterial stenoses?

    (A) peak systolic velocity

    (B) end diastolic velocity

    (C) systolic velocity ratio

    (D) volume flow

126. With a 50–99% diameter reduction in a peripheral artery, the waveform would

    (A) be triphasic with no appreciable spectral broadening

    (B) normal reverse components of waveform with mild spectral broadening

    (C) loss of reverse component with a distal damped monophasic waveform

    (D) proximal waveform will have diminished velocities and a monophasic waveform

127. In Fig. 14–47, color-flow Doppler of the iliac artery shows

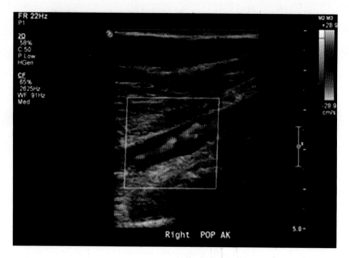

FIGURE 14–47. Color-flow Doppler of the iliac artery.

    (A) normal iliac arterial graft

    (B) iliac artery graft with stenosis

    (C) iliac artery graft with occlusion

    (D) iliac artery graft with pseudoaneurysm

128. Fig. 14–48 is an image of a distal bypass graft. Identify A, B, and C.

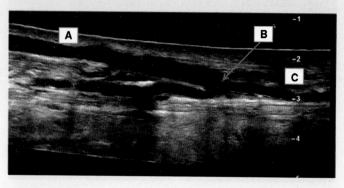

FIGURE 14–48.

    (A) _____

    (B) _____

    (C) _____

129. In Fig. 14–49, segmental pressures and Doppler waveforms of the lower extremities show

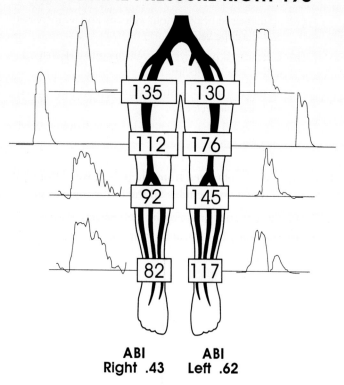

FIGURE 14–49. Arterial segmental pressure study.

    (A) severe occlusive disease of the right lower extremity

    (B) claudication disease of the left lower extremity

    (C) bilateral severe occlusive disease

    (D) bilateral mild claudication disease

    (E) both A and B

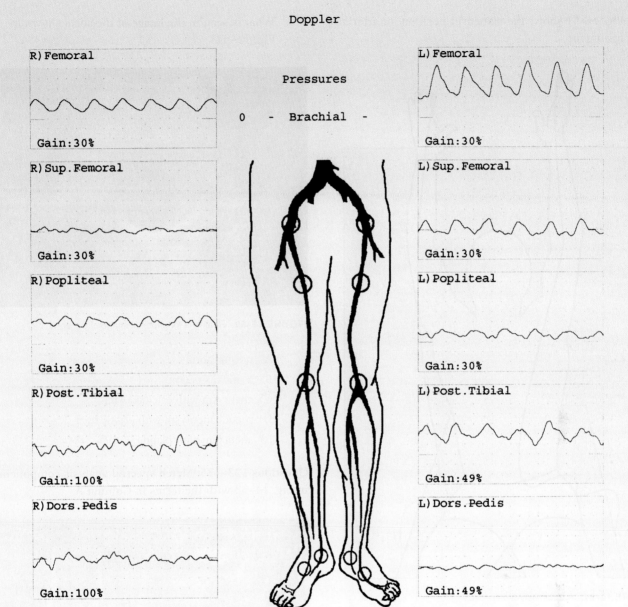

FIGURE 14–50. Arterial segmental pressure study.

130. **In Fig. 14–50, segmental pressures and Doppler waveforms of the lower extremities show**

(A) normal segmental and pressure study

(B) bilateral claudication disease

(C) bilateral iliac artery occlusion

(D) occlusive disease on the right and claudication disease on the left

131. Fig. 14–51 shows the maneuver position for arterial testing for

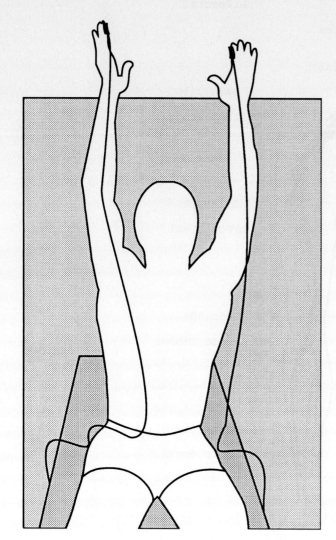

FIGURE 14-51. Arterial testing maneuver.

(A) thoracic outlet compression

(B) Raynaud's disease

(C) Raynaud's phenomenon

(D) subclavian steal syndrome

132. What is seen in the image of the aorta shown in Fig. 14–52?

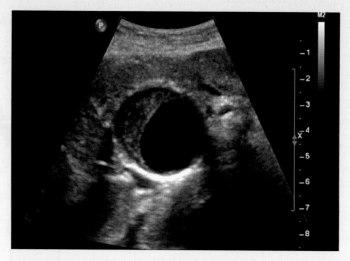

FIGURE 14-52. Real time longitudinal image of the aorta.

(A) normal aorta

(B) aortic dissection

(C) aneurysm with calcified wall

(D) pseudoaneurysm with classic tract

(E) aneurysm with plaque

Questions 133–135: Match spectral analysis components in Fig. 14–53 with the terms in Column A.

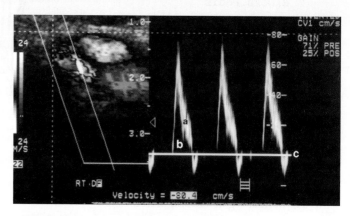

FIGURE 14-53. Spectral analysis waveform.

COLUMN A	COLUMN B
133. _____	(A) bandwidth
134. _____	(B) spectral window
135. _____	(C) zero baseline

Questions 136–145. Match the upper extremity arteries in Fig. 14–54 with the letters in Column B.

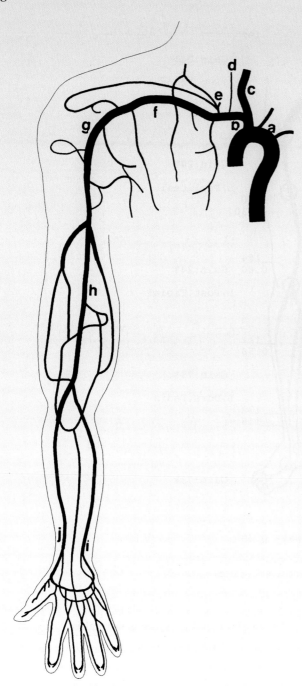

FIGURE 14–54. Upper extremity arterial anatomy.

COLUMN A   **COLUMN B**

136. ulnar artery _____   (A)

137. axillary artery _____   (B)

138. brachial artery _____   (C)

139. radial artery _____   (D)

140. subclavian artery _____   (E)

141. vertebral artery _____   (F)

142. aortic arch _____   (G)

143. thyrocervical artery _____   (H)

144. common carotid artery _____ (I)

145. brachiocephalic artery _____ (J)

146. Fig. 14–55 is a diagram of what type of surgical graft?

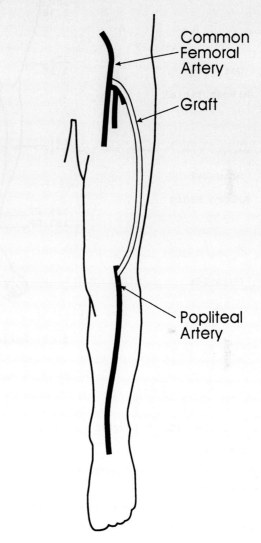

FIGURE 14–55. Surgical graft diagram.

(A) aortofemoral
(B) femoral–popliteal
(C) aorta
(D) femoral–femoral

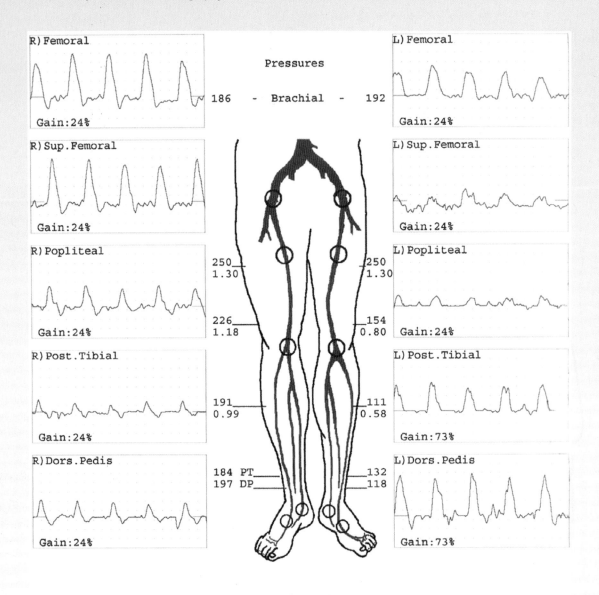

FIGURE 14–56. Arterial segmental pressure study.

147. In Fig. 14–56, the ankle brachial index seen is

(A) normal study

(B) claudication of the right and severe occlusive disease on the left

(C) normal on the right and claudication on the left

(D) bilateral severe occlusive disease

148. Blood flow information from a specific location is obtained by the

(A) velocity range

(B) Doppler angle

(C) field of view

(D) sample volume

149. The digital blood pressure is normally

(A) within 20–30 mm Hg of the brachial pressure

(B) the same as the brachial pressure

(C) within 10–20 mm Hg of the brachial pressure

(D) within 30–40 mm Hg of the brachial pressure

150. Normally, the flow velocity in an artery accelerates

(A) slowly

(B) very rapidly

(C) moderately

(D) variably

151. The image Fig 14–57 represents

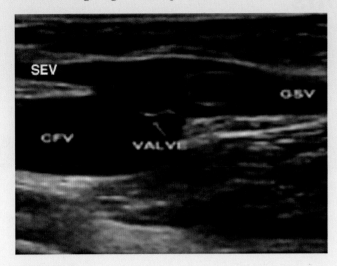

FIGURE 14–57.

- (A) reflux in the femoral vein
- (B) thrombus in the common femoral vein
- (C) thrombus in the proximal great saphenous vein
- (D) normal great saphenous vein

152. The image Fig 14–58 represents

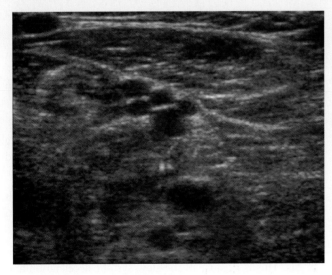

FIGURE 14–58.

- (A) a large Baker's cyst
- (B) a ruptured gastrocnemius muscle
- (C) multiple veins in the calf (posterior tibial and peroneal veins)
- (D) soleal vein thrombosis

153. Identify the image above Fig 14–59

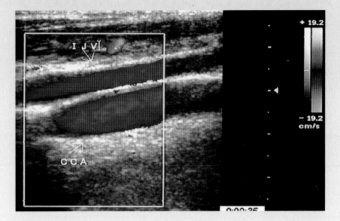

FIGURE 14–59.

- (A) normal flow dynamics of the neck vessels
- (B) partially occluded external jugular vein
- (C) partially occluded internal jugular vein
- (D) retrograde internal jugular vein flow

154. Identify the findings in this image Fig 14–60

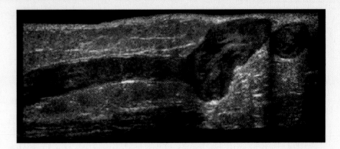

FIGURE 14–60.

- (A) normal appearance of the short saphenous vein in the foot
- (B) occluded, varicose superficial vein
- (C) partially occluded deep vein in the leg
- (D) an occluded popliteal vein behind the knee

Answers and Explanations

At the end of each explained answer, there is a number combination in parentheses. The first number identifies the reference source; the second number or set of numbers indicates the page on which the relevant information can be found.

1. **(C)** The Doppler shift is the difference between the received and transmitted frequencies or the difference between the reflected and transmitted frequencies and is defined in the Doppler equation. *(2:43)*

2. **(A)** The Doppler effect is a change in frequency relative to motion. The frequency received is higher or lower than the transmitted frequency depending on whether the motion is toward or away from the transducer. *(2:44)*

3. **(B)** Continuous-wave Doppler has two inherent crystals in one transducer. One to receive and one to send continuously. *(1:154)*

4. **(D)** Higher. When we think of the Doppler principles we think of motion. For example, as a train moves closer to us the sound is louder, and as it is moves farther away, the sound is lower. The sound frequency increases as it approaches the receiver and decreases as it gets farther from the receiver. *(1:149)*

5. **(A)** It increases. If the Doppler frequency is higher, the Doppler shift frequency will be higher and, conversely, if the Doppler frequency is lowered, the Doppler shift frequency will be lower. This is defined by the Doppler equation, which states the Doppler frequency is proportional to both the reflector frequency and the ultrasound transmitted frequency. *(Study Guide; 1:54)*

6. **(C)** When the flow is toward the transducer at zero degrees the Doppler frequency shift is the greatest and reduced accordingly at other incident angles. A perpendicular or 90° angle of insonation results in no detected Doppler shift. Because zero degree is not feasible in most clinical applications; we avoid the 90° angle and maintain a 30–60° for clinical applications. *(2:46)*

7. **(C)** Plethysmography. Strain gauge plethysmography is one of the older noninvasive vascular techniques for measuring the outflow of venous blood to determine deep vein thrombosis. It has a specificity approximately 60–70% and a positive predictive value of only approximately 50%. Most laboratories now use color flow Doppler. Photoplethysmography is still in use in some laboratories for screening patients for reflux. It demonstrates the filling time of the veins and differentiates between superficial and deep venous incompetency. *(3:779, 780)*

8. **(D)** The spectral analysis displays the frequency distribution on a time scale. To process the Doppler signal and calculate all the frequency components the Fast Fourier Transform method is used. The spectral analysis determines the presence, direction, and characteristics of blood flow. The spectral analysis does provide the quantification and measurements of the blood flow. This cannot be achieved with color-flow imaging alone. *(Study Guide)*

9. **(A)** peak systole; **(B)** early diastolic; **(C)** in diastole. *(Study Guide)*

10. **(B)** Spectral broadening means broadening or increase in the bandwidth with filling of the spectral window. This can range from mild to severe and is caused by disturbed flow. Disturbed flow produces increased frequencies and the formation of small eddies that increase the center stream and produce random motion of the blood cells. Spectral broadening is commonly seen with stenosis. *(1:167; 2:70)*

11. **(D)** The Nyquist limit is controlled by the pulse repetition rate. Aliasing is seen with high velocities that exceed the Nyquist limit or one-half; the pulse repetition rate. It is seen on the spectral analysis waveform display as a wraparound with the higher velocities appearing as a negative reading below the baseline. *(2:49)*

12. **(E)** Triphasic waveform that is consistent with a high-resistance peripheral artery. It demonstrates a rapid systolic rise, prominent flow reversal, and forward flow in diastole. *(2:66)*

13. **(A)** Spectral broadening caused by stenosis of the vessel. There is an increase in the frequencies/velocities causing spreading of the bandwidth. Characteristics associated with disturbed flow and stenotic lesions. *(2:70)*

14. **(B)** Aliasing (exceeding the Nyquist limit) is seen with mild spectral broadening and turbulence of the waveform secondary to a high-grade stenosis. *(Study Guide)*

15. **(D)** Damped monophasic waveform distal to a stenosis. This is because of the slow systolic acceleration and rounding of the systolic peak. The peak systolic velocity will be decreased and the diastolic velocity increased. *(2:48:51)*

16. **(D)** Monophasic waveform *(2:70)*

17. **(A)** Doppler equation where:
    FS = Doppler frequency shift (difference between original transmitted frequency and received frequency)
    V = Velocity of the interface
    Fo = Original transmitted frequency
    Cos = Doppler angle (angle of incidence between the beam and the interface)
    c = velocity of sound in the medium *(2:43, 44)*

18. **(D)** Percutaneous transluminal angioplasty (PTA) is the nonoperative dilatation of arterial stenoses using inflatable balloon-tip catheters. This procedure has been used to dilate or recanalized arteries or grafts in every anatomic region. It has less risks, shorter recovery time, and is less expensive than surgical revascularization. (2:370, 371)

19. **(B)** Embolization is the introduction of a substance or device via a catheter into a vessel to occlude the vessel and eliminate blood flow. (4:605)

20. **(C)** Hemodynamics is the study of the movement of blood and of the forces concerned. This term is commonly used in vascular ultrasound. (4:835)

21. **(A)** Laminar flow is the normal flow pattern usually seen where blood flow is highest in the center and lowest near the walls creating a parabolic flow profile. Turbulent flow is where fast moving blood moves in diagonal directions secondary to sharp turns, tortuosity, or rough surfaces. Eddy currents are whorls or currents seen in rapid moving blood. Boundary layers are the blood adjacent to the arterial wall with slower flow. (Study Guide)

22. **(D)** Photoplethysmography (PPG) uses a light sensor that shines light into superficial skin layers, and a photoelectric detector measures the reflected light. PPG is a simple noninvasive test for assessing chronic venous insufficiency in postphlebitic patients. (3:779, 780)

23. **(B)** Vortice. The poststenotic zone is immediately past an arterial stenosis. The flow becomes disorganized with frank swirling movements, which are called vortices. (Study Guide)

24. **(C)** The Reynolds number (RE) predicts the stability of a fluid and defines the point where flow changes from laminar to turbulent. If the RE exceeds 2,000, laminar flow tends to be disturbed. This is a basic principle in fluid dynamics. (Study Guide)

25. **(E)** 2,000 (2:6)

26. **(A)** Poststenotic turbulence is commonly seen immediately distal to an arterial stenosis. In fact, this is usually one of the diagnostic criteria for identification of stenotic lesions. It is described as the flow stream distal to the stenotic lumen spreads out, the laminar flow pattern is lost, and flow becomes disorganized. (1:23)

27. **(A)** Inversely. The volume flow is proportional to the fourth power of the radius so small changes in the radius can make large changes in the flow. The length of the vessel and the viscosity of blood do not change much in the cardiovascular system, so the changes in blood flow occur primarily as a result of changes in the radius of the vessel and the difference in the pressure energy level. (1:130, 131)

28. **(D)** Blood pressure is the pressure exerted on the wall of a blood vessel by the contained blood and the difference in the blood pressure within the vascular system provides the immediate driving force that keeps the blood moving. Pulse pressure is the difference between the systolic pressure and the diastolic pressure. The mean pressure is the average blood pressure throughout the cardiac cycle and blood flow is the volume of blood flowing through a vessel, organ, or circulatory system for a given period of time. (Study Guide)

29. **(D)** 120/70 mm Hg. The systolic pressure is the peak blood pressure within a large artery approximately 120 mm Hg. The diastolic pressure is the lowest pressure during the cardiac cycle, approximately 70 mm Hg. (Study Guide)

30. **(C)** The pulse is the pressure wave created by the expansion and contraction of the arteries during the cardiac cycle. The pulse pressure is the difference between the systolic pressure and diastolic pressure. (Study Guide)

31. **(A)** Pulse rate or number of pulsations per minute varies and is normally 50 to 100 pulses per minute. (Study Guide)

32. **(F)** Bradycardia. The most significant risk factor is the unavoidable family history. Cigarette smoking, diabetes, aging, and hypertension all lead to the development of atherosclerosis. Bradycardia is slowness of the heart rate and pulse rate. (4:175)

33. **(C)** Pressure is not one of the symptoms of lower extremity arterial disease. Claudication is the most common symptom in lower extremity arterial disease. Other symptoms include coldness, cyanosis or color changes, or the absence of pulses. As the ischemia progresses to severe, symptoms will include rest pain, nonhealing ulcers, microemboli, or gangrene of the foot. (2:256-257)

34. **(C)** The classic six Ps for acute arterial ischemia are; pain, pallor, paresthesias, poikilothermia, paralysis, and pulselessness. If a patient presents with these symptoms, the extremity is examined to assess the severity of the ischemia and to determine the urgency of further tests and treatment. (3:703)

35. **(D)** The ankle brachial index or ankle brachial pressure is used for peripheral arterial examinations and segmental pressure examinations. Normally, the systolic ankle pressure should be equal to or greater than the systolic pressure. The ratio should be 1.0 or greater. (2:279)

36. **(C)** Patients with an ankle brachial index of 0.6–0.9, which falls in the claudication range require exercise testing. These patients with mild arterial disease usually have compensatory collateral flow. Collateral flow provides sufficient flow under resting conditions, but when the extremity is stressed or exercised, there will be claudication pain. Exercise testing normally increases the total limb blood flow; however, with significant arterial disease, ankle pressure will drop after exercise. The time it takes to return to the pre-exercise level is an indication of the severity of disease. (2:279)

37. **(A)** The pressure is recorded at the site where the cuff is inflated and deflated, even though the Doppler probe is maintained in place at the posterior tibial artery. *(2:279)*

38. **(B)** The cuff at each site is inflated until the systolic pressure, sound, or Doppler waveform disappears. The cuff is slowly released until the sound or Doppler waveform returns. The return of the Doppler sound is then recorded. *(Study Guide)*

39. **(C)** The brachial artery systolic pressure is the standard for segmental arterial studies. The bilateral brachial pressures normally should be within 10 mm Hg of each other. The highest value of the two brachial systolic pressures is used. If the bilateral brachial pressures differ by more than 10 mm Hg, then an upper extremity arterial lesion is suspected. *(Study Guide)*

40. **(B)** As stated in the answer to question 39, the brachial systolic pressures should be within 10 mm Hg of each other. If there is a greater difference, an upper arterial lesion is suspected on the side with the lowest value. *(Study Guide)*

41. **(B)** Patients who have intermittent claudication have a pressure index in the range of 0.6–0.9 and are required to have exercise testing to evaluate the severity of the disease. *(2:256-257)*

42. **(C)** An ankle index of 0.5 or less indicates severe arterial occlusive disease and exercise testing is not required. *(Study Guide)*

43. **(D)** Toe pressure. Diabetic patients who have calcified vessels may have systolic pressures at the ankle arteries that exceed 300 mm Hg. This exceeds the limit of the automated units to record the systolic pressure. Toe pressures are required using photoplethysmography and toe cuffs. *(Study Guide)*

44. **(C)** The normal toe pressure is 60% of the brachial pressures. *(2:276)*

45. **(A)** Leg exercise increases blood flow. In the presence of significant arterial disease, the ankle pressure drops after exercise for two reasons: first, increased flow across the stenosis results in turbulence and a pressure drop, and second, blood flow is diverted into the higher resistance collaterals of the leg muscles. *(Study Guide)*

46. **(D)** The internal capsule is located in the brain. The composition of the arteries includes: the tunica intima (inner layer), the tunica media (middle layer), and the tunica adventitia (outer layer). *(Study Guide)*

47. **(C)** Vasoconstriction is the decrease in the caliber of the vessels, especially constriction of arterioles, which leads to decreased blood flow to a part. *(Study Guide)*

48. **(A)** The brachiocephalic or innominate arises on the right from the aortic arch and gives rise to the right common carotid artery and the right subclavian artery. On the left, there is no brachiocephalic artery, the left carotid artery arises from the aortic arch. *(2:416)*

49. **(C)** The axillary artery is a direct continuation of the subclavian artery. The subclavian descends lateral to the lateral margin of the scalenus anterior to the outer border of the first rib and then becomes the axillary artery. *(2:263)*

50. **(C)** Radial and ulnar arteries. The brachial artery is a continuation of the axillary artery. It terminates about a centimeter distal to the elbow joint by dividing into the radial and ulnar arteries. *(2:263)*

51. **(A)** The common femoral artery is a continuation of the external iliac artery. It begins at the inguinal ligament midway between the anterior superior iliac spine and the symphysis pubis. It descends the thigh and becomes the popliteal artery as it passes through the adductor canal. *(2:267)*

52. **(C)** The posterior tibial artery lies posterior to the medial aspect of the tibia and ankle joint. This artery is the one most often used for segmental pressure examination. If the vessel has a low Doppler signal or there is no Doppler signal, alternative vessels are the anterior tibial and dorsalis pedis. *(2:268)*

53. **(C)** Ischemia is defined as a deficiency of blood to a body part because of the functional constriction or obstruction of a blood vessel. Hallett presents several clinical categories of chronic limb ischemia that are common in dealing with lower extremity arterial disease. *(4:958)*

54. **(A)** An embolism is defined as a sudden blocking of an artery by clot or foreign material traveling through the blood stream. There are many origins of embolism, which include; air, coronary, infective, pulmonary, and tumors. *(4:606)*

55. **(B)** Claudication. This is a classical term used to describe peripheral arterial disease and the most common manifestation of peripheral artery occlusive disease. It actually means to "limp." It is described as pain during exercise that ceases when the activity is stopped. *(2:256, 257)*

56. **(B)** Atherosclerosis is the cause of most arterial diseases today. It is defined by the World Health Organization as a combination of changes in the intima and media of the artery. These changes include focal accumulation of lipids, hemorrhage, fibrous tissue, and calcium deposits. *(3:707, 708)*

57. **(C)** The blood flow and pressure are not significantly diminished until at least 75% of the cross-sectional area of the vessel is obliterated. This figure for cross-sectional area can be equated to a 50% reduction in lumen diameter. The formula for the area of a circle (area = 3.14 × radius^2) explains the relationship between the cross section and the vessel diameter. *(Study Guide)*

58. **(E)** All of the above. Although the radius is the greatest influence on a critical stenosis other factors also influence the critical stenosis to a lesser extent. They include: length of stenosis, blood viscosity, and peripheral resistance. *(2:10, 11)*

59. **(C)** The distal superficial femoral artery in the adductor canal is a common location of stenosis or occlusion in the lower extremity. This is one of two common anatomic sites. The other is the distal abdominal aorta and iliac arteries. (*Study Guide*)

60. **(B)** Anterior tibial artery. (*Study Guide*)

61. **(A)** Subclavian steal syndrome. Occurs more often in the left subclavian artery and is a common atherosclerotic lesion. It is usually discovered because the left brachial blood pressure is significantly lower than the right; however, other clinical symptoms may be present such as claudication, dizziness, syncope, visual blurring, or ataxia. Subclavian steal syndrome is characterized by reversal of blood flow within the vertebral artery resulting from a hemodynamically significant stenosis or occlusion in the proximal subclavian or innominate artery. The steal is induced because of the decreased pressure in the vessel distal to the stenotic lesion, which leads to retrograde flow in the ipsilateral vertebral artery. This retrograde vertebral flow on the side of the lesion is taken from the contralateral vertebral artery, which is stealing it from the basilar artery. (*2:214, 215*)

62. **(D)** Reversal of blood flow in the affected vertebral artery is a classic sign of subclavian steal syndrome. It goes through several stages as the stenosis or occlusion progresses. Beginning with the deceleration of the antegrade flow during systole, followed by an alternating flow with reversal of flow in systole and reduced antegrade flow during diastole and culminating with a reversal of flow during the entire pulse. (*2:214, 215*)

63. **(C)** A difference in bilateral blood pressure in the upper extremity of 10–20 mm Hg and a decreased peripheral pulse in the affected upper extremity is a hallmark sign of subclavian steal. (*2:214, 215*)

64. **(B)** Thoracic outlet syndrome is defined as compression of the brachial plexus nerve trunks characterized by pain, paresthesia of fingers, vasomotor symptoms, and weakness of the small muscles of the hand. The subclavian artery leaves the chest by the thoracic outlet. It passes over the first rib, behind the clavicle, and between the anterior and middle scalene muscles. Because of the confines of the thoracic outlet the subclavian artery, the subclavian vein, and the brachial plexus are subject to compression. Noninvasive testing for this entity requires special maneuvers, which include: exaggerated military position, hyperabduction, and Adson maneuver. The rationale is to determine any obliteration of the blood flow, which relates to specific positions. (*3:704, 790*)

65. **(C)** Multimaneuvers are used for the evaluation of thoracic outlet syndrome. These positions are used to demonstrate an obliteration of blood flow relating to specific positions. During the maneuvers, the waveforms are recorded by Doppler or photoplethysmography to identify any change in blood flow. (*3:298–302*)

66. **(A)** Raynaud's disease is an innocuous vasospastic disorder; whereas, Raynaud's phenomenon is an underlying systemic or vascular abnormality with vascular occlusion. (*3:1642*)

67. **(B)** Raynaud's phenomenon is associated with occlusive disease, whereas Raynaud's disease is associated with vasospasm. (*3:1642*)

68. **(C)** Pseudoaneurysms (false aneurysms) do not have a true arterial wall and are usually the result of vascular injury caused by trauma or previous surgical reconstruction. The pseudoaneurysm lies outside the arterial wall; whereas, the true aneurysm is contiguous with the arterial wall. (*3:666*)

69. **(B)** Mycotic aneurysms are secondary to an infectious process that involves the arterial wall. (*3:723–730*)

70. **(C)** Arterial dissection usually develops secondary to a tear in the intimal layer, which allows blood to enter the wall of the vessel and the creation of two lumens. Characteristically, a moving flap is seen in the lumen of the vessel with real-time imaging. (*3:723–730*)

71. **(C)** Ankle brachial index quantitates the blood flow. The segmental pressures combined with the ankle brachial index provide an assessment of arterial disease in the entire extremity. It determines the level of disease and estimates the severity of the disease. This exam is often used for arterial screening of the lower extremities. Duplex and color-flow Doppler provide anatomical detail and hemodynamics but cannot quantitate the flow. (*3:704*)

72. **(D)** A decrease in peak systolic flow velocity to <45 cm/sec would indicate impending graft failure. The normal graft has a hyperemic waveform (forward flow throughout the pulse cycle) and a systolic flow velocity of >45 cm/sec. (*Study Guide*)

73. **(C)** Arteriovenous fistula is an abnormal communication between an artery and a vein. It may be the result of a congenital defect, created by surgical means as seen in the dialysis access graft (Brescia–Cimino), or caused by trauma as seen secondary to percutaneous biopsy procedures in the renal or liver transplant created trauma. (*3:879, 880*)

74. **(B)** The resistive index calculates and quantifies resistance to blood flow. A high-resistance waveform pattern has a high systolic peak and a low diastolic flow. The resistance can be calculated using the resistive index, systolic frequency (S), minus diastolic frequency (D), divided by the systolic frequency. (*2:616*)

75. **(A)** Tachycardia refers to a rapid heartbeat and usually means a heart rate above 100 bpm. (*4:1850*)

76. **(D)** Angiography is an invasive procedure using computerized fluoroscopy for direct visualization of the arterial system after injection of a contrast medium. (*4:83*)

77. **(B)** The ankle brachial index (ABI) is the measurement of the systolic blood pressure at the ankle divided by the brachial systolic pressure. It is used to determine the presence and severity of arterial disease. *(2:279)*

78. **(C)** The patient history should always be obtained before the vascular examination. It provides valuable information as to the patient's symptoms and related problems. It also ensures that a complete evaluation of the patient is performed. In some cases, the clinical history may be incorrect or the wrong examination is ordered. Talking to the patient and acquiring history and clinical information, ensures information is correct and the correct exam is being performed. If they not, then take the necessary time to talk to the clinician to make sure information is correct. *(Study Guide)*

79. **(C)** Segmental arterial pressures can be obtained using three or four cuffs. It is preferred to use four cuffs to differentiate between the common femoral artery and superficial femoral artery lesions. This is not possible with the three-cuff method. *(Study Guide)*

80. **(D)** Microbubbles of air are used for most sonographic contrast agents. The success of the more sophisticated contrast agents has been dependent on stabilization of these micro air bubbles because they are usually short lived in the peripheral circulation, and to transport them within the body by means of a carrier agent. *(2:41)*

81. **(B)** The cardiovascular system has two major pathways, the systemic circulation, and pulmonary circulation. The path of the blood from the left ventricle through the body is the systemic circulation and its passage from the right ventricle via the lungs to the left atrium is the pulmonary circulation. *(Study Guide)*

82. **(D)** Tunica media is the fibromuscular middle layer that extends from the internal to external elastic lamina and is circumferential. It is the thickest layer of the artery and aids in maintaining continuous circulation and appropriate blood pressure by controlling the diameter of the vessel lumen. *(Study Guide)*

83. **(D)** The vertebral artery is the first branch of the subclavian artery. It arises from the superoposterior aspect of the subclavian artery. *(2:211-222)*

84. **(A)** Femoral artery. *(Study Guide)*

85. **(B)** Femoral vein. *(Study Guide)*

86. **(D)** Femoral vein. *(Study Guide)*

87. **(B)** Femoral artery. *(Study Guide)*

88. **(C)** Great saphenous vein. *(Study Guide)*

89. **(A)** Profunda (deep) femoral vein and artery. *(Study Guide)*

90. **(D)** Popliteal artery. *(Study Guide)*

91. **(B)** Popliteal vein. *(Study Guide)*

92. **(A)** Short(small) saphenous vein. *(Study Guide)*

93. **(C)** Great saphenous vein. *(Study Guide)*

94. **(F)** Distal aorta artery. *(Study Guide)*

95. **(G)** External iliac artery. *(Study Guide)*

96. **(A)** Internal iliac artery. *(Study Guide)*

97. **(E)** Common femoral artery. *(Study Guide)*

98. **(C)** Superficial femoral artery. *(Study Guide)*

99. **(D)** Profunda (deep) femoral artery. *(Study Guide)*

100. **(B)** Popliteal artery. *(Study Guide)*

101. **(B)** Popliteal artery. *(Study Guide)*

102. **(E)** Anterior tibial artery. *(Study Guide)*

103. **(F)** Posterior tibial artery. *(Study Guide)*

104. **(A)** Peroneal artery. *(Study Guide)*

105. **(C)** Plantar metatarsal arteries. *(Study Guide)*

106. **(D)** Digital arteries. *(Study Guide)*

107. **(A)** 20–49% diameter reduction stenosis. *(Study Guide)*

108. **(D)** 1–19% diameter reduction stenosis. *(Study Guide)*

109. **(C)** 50–99% diameter reduction stenosis. *(Study Guide)*

110. **(B)** 0% diameter reduction stenosis. *(Study Guide)*

111. **(F)** All of the above. Intermittent claudication is usually the first symptom of arterial disease. As the disease progresses to the point of rest pain, the trophic skin changes, dependent rubor, and pallor on elevation occur. If the level of disease is aorto-iliac, it often renders the male impotent because the penile circulation branches from the internal iliac. *(3:1546–1548)*

112. **(F)** All of the above. Atherosclerosis is a disease process that is influenced by several risk factors: family history, cigarette smoking, hypertension, hyperlipidemia, diabetes mellitus, malignancies, and aging. *(Study Guide)*

113. **(A)** Within normal limits *(Study Guide)*

114. **(A)** A hemodynamically significant lesion is a 50% diameter reduction or greater. As the stenotic segment exceeds 50%, the peak systolic velocities also increase. The ratio of systolic to diastolic velocities begins to fall. *(Study Guide)*

115. **(A)** The source of origin of the Doppler signal is derived from the sample volume location on the 2D image and not from the spectral display. Amplitude of the Doppler signal, pulsatility features of the waveform, velocity or frequency shift of the blood flow, and direction of flow are all obtained from the spectral display. *(Study Guide)*

116. **(B)** A clear spectral window indicates laminar flow with little flow disturbances. A small sample volume placed in the central portion of the normal flow stream will produce a crisp, clear window. Flow disturbances, such as vortices and swirling eddies, will decrease the size of the spectral window and should demonstrate flow reversal as well. Spectral broadening can occur with moderate stenotic lesions as well as severe lesions. (2:70)

117. **(A)** Critical stenosis. The critical stenosis occurs with a diameter reduction of 50% or greater (area reduction of 75%) or greater. This is also called a hemodynamically significant lesion. (2:10, 11)

118. **(B)** The two principal mechanisms that control blood volume are the cardiac output and the peripheral resistance. Cardiac output (milliliter per second) is the rate of blood flow per minute. Two factors that affect cardiac output are heart rate and stroke volume. Peripheral resistance is controlled by the arterioles and arterial capillaries. These tiny vessels control the volume of blood flow. (2:289)

119. **(C)** The major advantage of continuous wave Doppler is that it can display high velocities without the phenomena of aliasing occurring. Unfortunately, it has no range resolution, and its sample size cannot be controlled. (1:150–154)

120. **(E)** Doppler shift frequencies are affected by Doppler angle, transducer frequency, and the velocity of the red blood cells. As the Doppler angle decreases between the Doppler beam and the flow stream, there will be an increase in the frequency shift. If the transducer frequency decreases, the frequency shift will decrease. The velocity of the red blood cells will affect the Doppler shift. As the red blood cells move faster, the frequency shift will increase. (1:137)

121. **(C)** As an arterial stenosis exceeds 60%, the peak systolic velocity will increase and the volume of the flow will decrease. (2:72–74)

122. **(A)** The single most valuable Doppler finding is increased velocity in the stenotic zone for determining the severity of arterial stenosis. (Study Guide)

123. **(C)** Disturbed flow is seen throughout the stenotic lesion and just distal to the stenosis in the poststenotic zone. The maximal flow disturbance usually occurs within 1 cm beyond the stenosis. (2:72–74)

124. **(B)** As the radius of an artery decreases, the resistance to flow will increase. (2:72–74)

125. **(D)** Volume flow is not used in determining the severity of arterial stenosis. There are three stenotic zone velocity measurements commonly used to determine the severity of arterial stenoses: peak systolic velocity, end diastolic velocity, and the systolic velocity ratio (comparison of peak systole in stenoses to peak systole in the proximal normal segment. (2:72–74)

126. **(C)** In a 50–99% diameter reduction of the artery, there will be a loss of reverse flow with forward flow throughout the cardiac cycle and distal to the stenosis the waveform will be damped and monophasic. (2:72–74)

127. **(C)** Iliac artery graft with occlusion. The iliac graft is seen in a longitudinal plane with the characteristic corrugated appearance. Color Doppler identifies adjacent blood flow; however, there is absence of flow in the graft compatible with graft occlusion. (Study Guide)

128. **(A)** vein bypass graft **(B)** distal anastomosis **(C)** outflow artery. (Study Guide)

129. **(C)** Bilateral severe occlusive arterial disease. Bilateral iliac artery stenosis with monophasic waveforms throughout the lower extremity and abnormal segmental pressures. The ankle brachial index is 0.4 on the right and 0.6 on the left indicating severe occlusive arterial disease. Normally, the waveforms would be triphasic, and there would be a pressure gradient of >30 mm Hg between each cuff. The upper thigh pressure should be at least 40 mm HG above the brachial pressure. Usually the cutoff for severe occlusive arterial disease is 0.5 or less; however, the waveforms indicate severe disease and exercise revealed a slow recovery time which would confirm the diagnosis. (1:268, 297)

130. **(C)** Bilateral iliac artery disease. Abnormal Doppler waveforms bilaterally with zero flow or severely damped monophasic flow. The ankle brachial index could not be obtained because of absence of flow in the lower extremities. (Study Guide)

131. **(A)** Thoracic outlet compression. It is the Adson maneuver using attached photo cells for photoplethysmographic recording of the waveform. (Study Guide)

132. **(E)** Fig. 14–52 shows an abdominal aortic aneurysm with internal plaque. (2:542)

133. **(c)** Zero baseline (Study Guide)

134. **(b)** Spectral window (Study Guide)

135. **(a)** Bandwidth (Study Guide)

136. **(I)** (Study Guide)

137. **(G)** (Study Guide)

138. **(H)** (Study Guide)

139. **(J)** (Study Guide)

140. **(F)** (Study Guide)

141. **(D)** (Study Guide)

142. **(A)** (Study Guide)

143. **(E)** (Study Guide)

144. **(C)** *(Study Guide)*

145. **(B)** *(Study Guide)*

146. **(B)** Femoral-popliteal (fem-pop) arterial graft. *(Study Guide)*

147. **(C)** The ankle brachial index (ABI) on the right is 1.03, which is normal. ABI on the left is 0.69, which is in the claudication range. *(Study Guide)*

148. **(D)** Sample volume. The frequency spectrum shows the blood flow information from a specific location using the sample volume. The spectral analysis is the display of the frequency distribution within the signal, but the sample volume denotes the specific location. The Doppler angle governs the intensity of the reflected wave and the field of view governs the viewing area of the vessels. *(1:154)*

149. **(A)** Digital blood pressure is normally within 20–30 mm Hg of the brachial pressure. This usually corresponds to a ratio of finger systolic pressure to brachial systolic pressure of greater than 80%. *(Study Guide)*

150. **(B)** Very rapidly. Flow velocity in a normal artery accelerates very rapidly in systole. It produces an almost vertical deflection of the Doppler waveform at the beginning of systole. *(2:72–74)*

151. **(C)** Thrombus in the proximal great saphenous vein

152. **(C)** Multiple veins in the calf (posterior tibial and peroneal veins)

153. **(D)** Retrograde internal jugular vein flow

154. **(B)** Occluded, varicose superficial vein

References

1. Frederick WK. *Sonography Principles and Instruments.* 8th ed. Philadelphia, PA: Elsevier Saunders; 2011.

2. Zwiebel WJ, Pellerito JS. *Introduction to Vascular Ultrasonography.* 5th ed. Philadelphia, PA: Elsevier Saunders; 2005.

3. Brunicardi CF. *Schwartz's Principles of Surgery.* 9th ed. New York: McGraw-Hill; 2010.

4. *Dorland's Illustrated Medical Dictionary.* 31st ed. Philadelphia, PA: Elsevier Health Sciences; 2010.

15

Neurosonology

*Charles S. Odwin and Chandrowti Devi Persaud**

Study Guide

INTRODUCTION

Neurosonology had its beginning in the late 1960s and early 1970s. One of the first applications was the A-mode, or amplitude mode, to determine midline shifts. If, in fact, the midline was shifted, this was an indication of a tumor or pathology. As newer technology and gray-scale imaging emerged, new applications also emerged. The A-mode midline shift examination was quickly replaced with computerized axial tomography. The realization that the open fontanelles in neonates offered a sonographic window to permit ultrasound scanning of the neonatal brain opened new technological advances. Gray-scale imaging became a mainstay in the neonatal department primarily to detect intracranial hemorrhage and monitor enlargement of the ventricles. Ultrasound was also being utilized in neurosurgery to localize lesions and pathology during the surgical procedure. The introduction of color-flow Doppler added diagnostic capabilities for identifying vascular variances and anomalies in the neonate.[1] It was also a time when transcranial Doppler was introduced using the transtemporal window for examination of the adult patients. The advantages of neurosonology include more easily available, portability, cost-effectiveness, noninvasiveness, and high sensitivity. Neurosonology has been an ongoing expanding specialty for more than 40 years. It now requires the sonographer to have a well-rounded knowledge encompassing anatomy, vascular hemodynamics, positioning, and instrumentation. Transcranial Doppler and vascular studies are included in the cerebrovascular section. This chapter deals primarily with neonatal neurology.

INSTRUMENTATION AND TECHNIQUE

Real-time gray-scale imaging using a 7.5 to 12 MHz frequency is most commonly used in the evaluation of the neonatal brain.

Higher frequencies such as 12 MHz may be used for superficial structures. Duplex and color-flow Doppler sonography are used to evaluate congenital vascular anomalies, cerebral perfusion, and vascular anatomy.[1]

The anterior fontanelle is used as an acoustic window in the first year of life. It starts to close at 9 months and is completely closed in 13 months.[2] Standard scanning planes and views for evaluations of the brain are coronal, sagittal, and axial.

Coronal. These scans are obtained through the frontal fontanelle (Figs. 15–1 A–F). Six standard coronal sonograms taken at the level of:

- frontal horns (anterior to the foramen of Monro)
- foramen of Monro
- posterior aspect of the third ventricle through the thalami
- quadrigeminal cistern
- trigones of the lateral ventricles
- parietal and occipital cortex

Sagittal. These scans are obtained through the frontal fontanelle (Figs. 15–2 A–C). The three standard scans include:

- *Midsagittal plane,* which includes the following anatomical landmarks: cavum septi pellucidi, cavum vergae, corpus callosum, pericallosal artery, cingulate sulcus and gyrus, third ventricle, massa intermedia in the third ventricle, quadrigeminal cistern, and fourth ventricle (Fig. 15–2B).[2]
- *Parasagittal* right planes, which include the following anatomical landmarks: lateral ventricle, choroid plexus, thalamus, and parietal and occipital lobes (Fig. 15–2A).
- *Parasagittal* slightly more lateral than the above on the left, which includes the following anatomical landmarks: the body, occipital and temporal horns of the

*Karen K. Rawls and Carol A. Krebs wrote the previous-edition version.

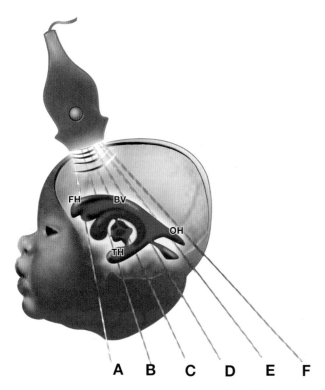

FIGURE 15-1. Schematic of the coronal planes. (**A** to **F**) are scanning planes from anterior to posterior. FH is frontal horn; BV is body of ventricle; TH is temporal horn; OH is occipital horn.

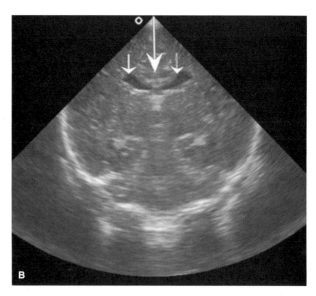

FIGURE 15-1B. Normal coronal sonogram. Corpus callosum (large arrow); anterior horns lateral ventricles (two small arrows).

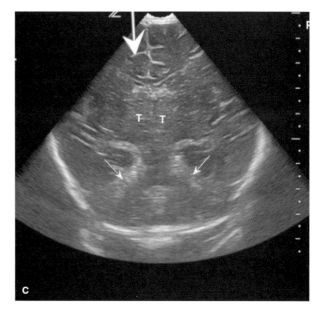

FIGURE 15-1C. Normal coronal sonogram. Cingulate sulcus (large arrow); thalamus (T); tentorium (small arrows).

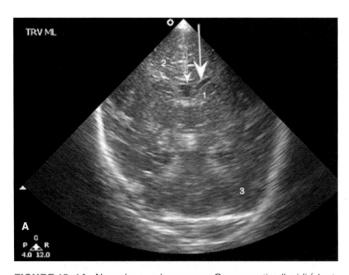

FIGURE 15-1A. Normal coronal sonogram. Cavum septi pellucidi (short arrow); lateral ventricle (long arrow); caudate nucleus (1); frontal lobe (2); temporal lobe (3).

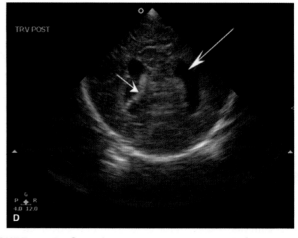

FIGURE 15-1D. Coronal sonogram represents plane D. Short arrow choroid plexus. Long arrow trigone of the lateral ventricle.

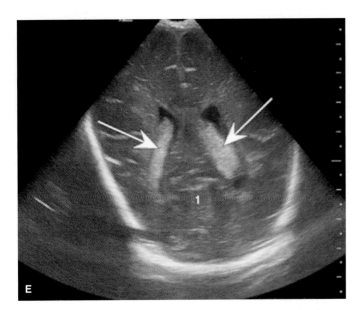

FIGURE 15–1E. Coronal sonogram represents plane E. Arrowhead = to choroid plexus, cb = cerebellum.

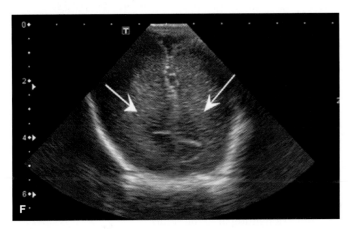

FIGURE 15–1F. Coronal sonogram represents plane F. Area between arrowheads = white matter of the occipital lobe and sulci.

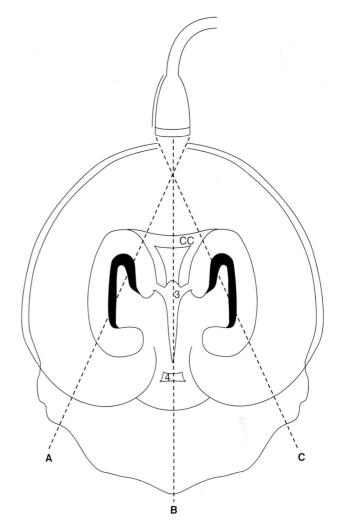

FIGURE 15–2. Schematic of the sagittal planes.

lateral ventricles, and the glomus (largest) part of the choroid plexus. The frontal, parietal, temporal, and occipital lobes are seen surrounding the lateral ventricle (Fig. 15–2C).

Axial. These scans are obtained through the squamosal portion of either temporal bone. To obtain the desired images and anatomical landmarks, the transducer is angled superiorly. The ventricles are seen just above the choroid plexus. The lateral ventricular measurements are obtained in this position or the squamosal fontanelle.

MNEMONICS

Mnemonics are just one of many useful ways to formulate words that will help you remember. How fast you learn, and how much you retain after you learn, may be a big factor in

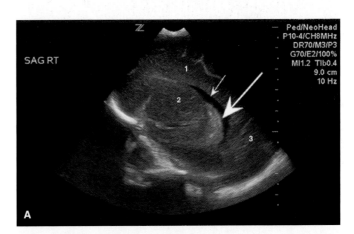

FIGURE 15–2A. Normal parasagittal sonogram. Lateral ventricle (small arrow); choroid plexus (large arrow); parietal lobe (1); thalamus (2); occipital lobe (3).

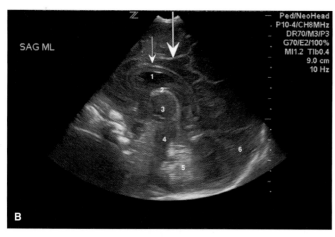

FIGURE 15–2B. Normal sagittal midline sonogram. Corpus callosum (small arrow); cingulate sulcus (large arrow); cavum septi pellucidi (1); choroid plexus (2); third ventricle (3); fourth ventricle (4); cerebellar vermis (5); occipital lobe (6).

taking examinations. The following are study groups. Formulate your own mnemonic device to help you remember them.

The mnemonic "SCALP" serves as a memory key for the five layers of the scalp listed below:

S   skin

C   connective tissue

A   aponeurosis epicranialis

L   loose connective tissue

P   pericranium

The mnemonic "PAD" serves as a memory key for the three layers of membranes called meninges, which cover the brain and spinal cord from inner to outer. The three layers are as follows:

P   pia

A   arachnoid

D   dura

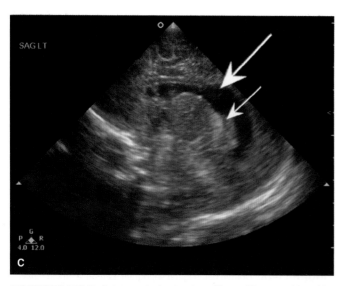

FIGURE 15–2C. Left parasagittal sonogram. Short white arrow choroid plexus; Long white arrow lateral ventricle.

A mnemonic for the 12 cranial nerves is "O,O,O Tell Ted And Frances About Going Vacationing After Halloween."

O   olfactory

O   optic

O   oculomotor

T   trochlear

T   trigeminal

A   abducens

F   facial

A   acoustic

G   glossopharyngeal

V   vagus

A   accessory

H   hypoglossal

The mnemonic "MAPS" serves as a memory key for these fontanelles:

M   mastoidal

A   anterior

P   posterior

S   sphenoidal

The time of closure for the fontanelles varies. The posterior is the first to close at 2–3 months, with the anterior closing at 13 months.[2]

The mnemonic "SAC" serves as a memory key for the three scanning planes used in neonatal cranial sonography.

S   sagittal scan taken along the axis of the sagittal suture (longitudinal in the skull)

A   axial scan taken from a lateral approach through the temporal bone.

C   coronal scan taken along the axis of the coronal suture (transverse in the skull)

TERMINOLOGY

Fontanelles are membrane- covered gaps created when more than two cranial bones are juxtaposed, also called soft spots.[2] There are six fontanelles: one frontal, one posterior, two mastoidal, and two sphenoidal.

The following definitions of the various anatomic structures associated with sonographic neurologic examinations will enhance your understanding of the anatomic diagrams in the subsequent text.

Arachnoid—The middle layer of meninges covering the brain and spinal cord.

Atrium (Trigone) of the Lateral Ventricles—This is where the anterior, occipital, and temporal horns join.

Brainstem—Part of the brain connected to the forebrain and the spinal cord. It consists of the midbrain, pons, and medulla oblongata.[1]

Caudate Nucleus—Consists of a head, body, and tail. It lies next to the lateral wall of the lateral ventricles.

Cavum Septi Pellucidi—A thin triangular cavity filled with cerebrospinal fluid that lies between the anterior horns of the lateral ventricles. If located anterior, it is termed a cavum vergae. The cavum septi pellucidi has also been referred to as a fifth ventricle and the cavum vergae as a sixth ventricle.

Central Nervous System—The central nervous system consists of the cerebellum, cerebrum, spinal cord, pons (brainstem), and medulla.

Cerebellum—Portion of the brain that lies posterior to the pons and medulla oblongata below the tentorium.

Cerebral Hemispheres—These are paired brain matter separated from the midline by the falx cerebri.

Cerebrum—The largest part of the brain, which consists of two hemispheres.[1]

Choroid Plexus—Mass of special cells located in all components of the ventricles except for the cerebral aqueduct. They regulate the intraventricular pressure by secreting or absorbing cerebrospinal fluid.[1]

Cistern—Enclosed space serving as a reservoir for cerebrospinal fluid.

Corpus Callosum—Large group of nerve fibers visible superior to the third ventricle that connects the left and right sides of the brain.[1]

Ependyma—The membrane lining the cerebral ventricles.[1]

Epidural—Lies outside the dura mater.

Falx Cerebri (interhemispheric fissure)—A fibrous structure separating the two cerebral hemispheres.

Germinal Matrix—Periventricular tissue including the caudate nucleus. Before 32 weeks gestation, it is fragile and bleeds easily.[1]

Gyri—Convolutions on the surface of the brain caused by infolding of the cortex.[1]

Massa Intermedia—Also called the interthalamic adhesion, this is the place of fusion between the third ventricle and the medial surface of the thalami.

Meninges—The brain coverings.[1]

Mesencephalon—Midbrain.

Parenchyma—Cortex tissue of the brain.[1]

Pia Mater—The innermost of the three membranes covering the brain and spinal cord.

Pineal Recess—Posterior recess on the third ventricle. There are two posterior recesses: the pineal and the suprapineal recesses.

Prosencephalon—Forebrain.

Rhombencephalon—Hindbrain.

Subdural—Between the dura mater and the arachnoid.

Subependyma—Area immediately beneath the ependyma. In the caudate nucleus, it is the site of hemorrhage from the germinal matrix.

Subarachnoid—Between the arachnoid and the pia mater.

Sulcus—A groove or depression on the surface of the brain, separating the gyri.[1]

Suprapineal recess—One of the two posterior recesses on the third ventricle.

Sylvian Fissure—Lateral cerebri fissure.

Tela Choroidea—Point where the choroid attached to the floor of the lateral ventricles and located behind the foramen of Monro. Most common site of hemorrhage.

Tentorium—V shaped echogenic structure which separates the cerebrum and the cerebellum and is an extension of the falx cerebri.[1]

Thalamus—Two ovoid brain structures situated on either side of the third ventricle superior to the brainstem.[1]

Ventricle—A cavity within the brain containing cerebrospinal fluid.[1]

Vermis Cerebellum—Median part of the cerebellum that lies between the two hemispheres.

ANATOMY

It is essential to know the basic anatomy of the brain. The main parts of the brain are the cerebrum, cerebellum, and the brainstem.

Cerebrum

The cerebrum is divided into two cerebral hemispheres by the longitudinal fissure and connected by the corpus callosum. It is made up of six lobes. The lobes are named according to the skull bones they lie under.

Lobes of the brain and the main functions are:

- One frontal lobe—functions include personality, language, and judgment
- Two parietal lobes—functions include senses and muscle control
- Two temporal lobes—function is auditory
- One occipital lobe—function is vision

The cerebrum consists of an outer thin gray matter called cerebral cortex and inner white matter. On the surface, there are numerous ridges or convolutions gyri and sulci (grooves). Gyri appear hypoechoic and are marked off by sulci. Sulci appear echogenic. Prominent sulci are pericallosal sulcus, cingulate sulcus and the calcarine sulcus. Deep sulci are called fissures. Fissures appear echogenic and are the longitudinal, transverse, fissure of Rolando (central sulcus), and the Sylvian fissure (lateral sulcus).

Cerebellum

The cerebellum is divided by the vermis into two hemispheres and is separated from the occipital lobe by the transverse fissure superiorly. It has an inner white matter and thin gray outer cortex. On the sonogram, it appears echogenic. Functions include muscle coordination and equilibrium.

Brainstem

Superiorly the brainstem includes: diencephalon, midbrain, pons and the medulla oblongata inferiorly. It lies between the base of the cerebrum and the spinal cord. The diencephalon includes the thalamus and the hypothalamus. The midbrain (mesencephalon) includes the cerebral aqueduct, cerebral peduncle, and the corpora quadrigemina. The brainstem functions mainly for automatic survival, controls the heart beat and breathing, and acts as a relay station for sensory impulses and reflexes.

Basal Ganglia

The basal ganglia is the gray matter that lies deep within the cerebral hemispheres. It includes the caudate nucleus, putamen, and globus pallidus. The caudate nucleus is a common site for intracranial hemorrhage.

There are six ventricles. The first and second are called the right and left lateral ventricles. The lateral ventricles are the largest cerebrospinal filled cavities. Each lateral ventricle is arbitrarily divided into the frontal horn, body, occipital horn, and temporal horn. The third and fourth are below the first and second. Between the frontal horns of the lateral ventricle is the cavum septum pellucidum (CSP) the fifth ventricle; posterior to the CSP is the cavum vergae the sixth ventricle. The third

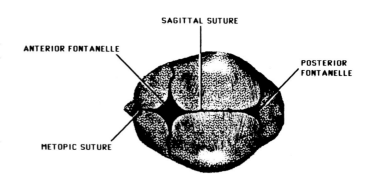

FIGURE 15–4. A diagram of a superior view of the infantile skull.

ventricle is bridged by the massa intermedia. There are several foramens, which include:

Foramen of Monro—Also termed intraventricular foramen, it divides the frontal horn anteriorly from the body of the ventricle posteriorly and connects the third ventricle with the lateral ventricle.

Aqueduct of Sylvius—Also called the cerebral aqueduct, it connects the third and fourth ventricles.

Foramen of Luschka—The opening in the roof of the fourth ventricle for circulation of the cerebrospinal fluid.

Foramen of Magendie—The opening in the roof of the fourth ventricle for circulation of the cerebrospinal fluid.

The following pages contain illustrations of anatomical structures. Study each illustration carefully, then close your examination book and try to form a photographic image of the illustration in your mind. Then draw and label the illustration on a separate sheet of paper without referring to the illustration. Although this process may sound difficult at first, it is a simple method of developing a photographic memory. As sonographers, we see hundreds of sonographic images each day and have probably used photographic memory without even realizing it. Go ahead and try this with the following illustrations (Figs. 15–3 to 15–30).

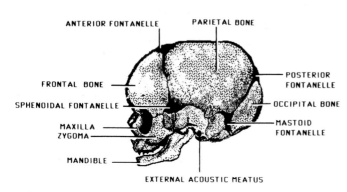

FIGURE 15–3. Diagram of a lateral view of the infantile skull.

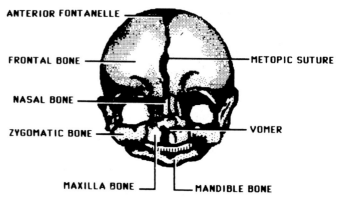

FIGURE 15–5. An anterior view of an infantile skull.

Ventricular System

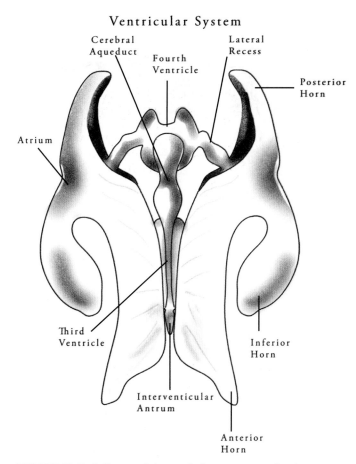

FIGURE 15-6. A diagram of the ventricular system, superior view.

Ventricular System

FIGURE 15-7. A diagram of the ventricular system, lateral view.

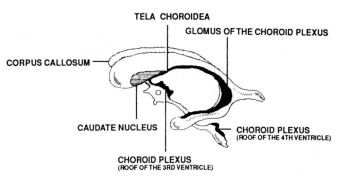

FIGURE 15-8. A diagram of the ventricular system and choroid plexus, lateral view.

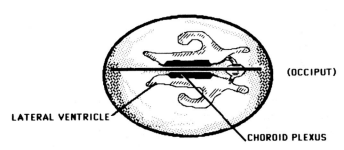

FIGURE 15-9. A diagram of an axial view at the level of the lateral ventricle.

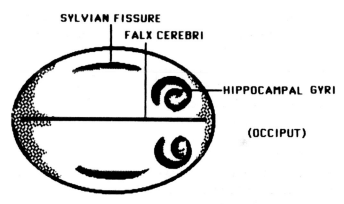

FIGURE 15-10. A diagram of an axial view at the level of the Sylvian fissure.

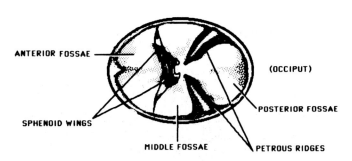

FIGURE 15-11. A diagram of an axial view at the base of the skull.

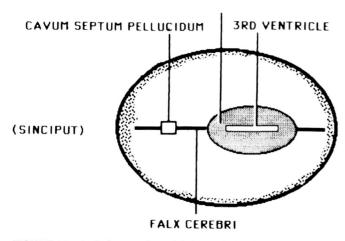

FIGURE 15-12. A diagram of an axial view at the level of the thalami.

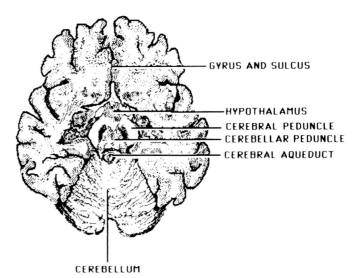

FIGURE 15-15. A diagram of a coronal section of the brain.

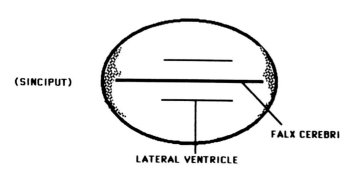

FIGURE 15-13. A diagram of an axial view at the level of the lateral ventricle.

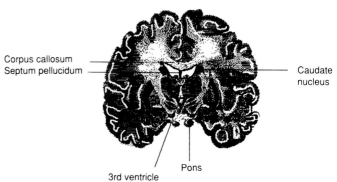

FIGURE 15-16. A diagram of a coronal section of the brain.

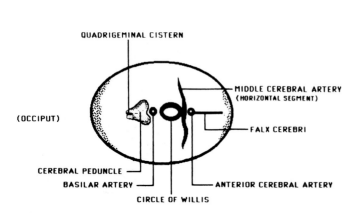

FIGURE 15-14. A diagram of an axial view at the level of the base of the skull.

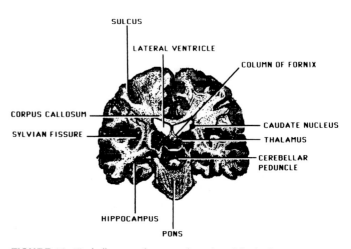

FIGURE 15-17. A diagram of a coronal section of the brain.

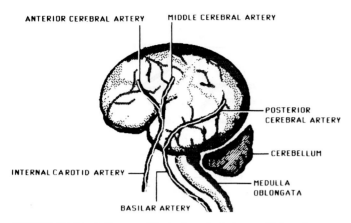

FIGURE 15-18. A diagram of the brain and arteries, sagittal section.

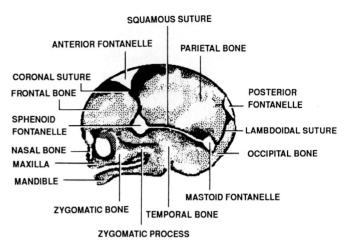

FIGURE 15-21. A diagram of a lateral view of the infantile skull.

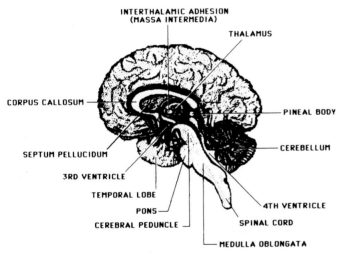

FIGURE 15-19. A diagram of the brain, sagittal section.

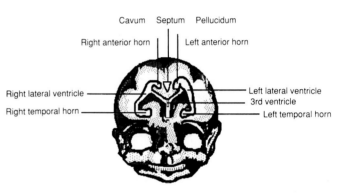

FIGURE 15-22. A diagram of an anterior view of the infantile skull with the ventricular system.

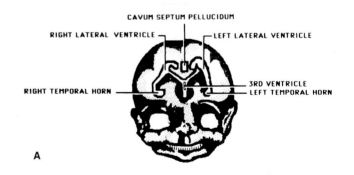

A

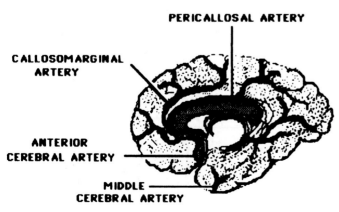

FIGURE 15-20. A diagram of the lateral aspect of the internal carotid artery divisions.

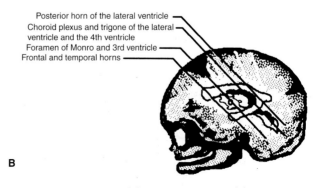

B

FIGURE 15-23. A diagram of (A) an anterior view and (B) a lateral view of the infantile skull with the ventricular system.

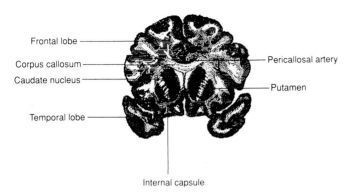

FIGURE 15–24. A diagram of a coronal section of the brain.

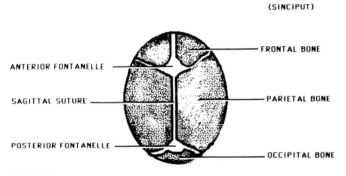

FIGURE 15–25. A superior view of an infantile skull.

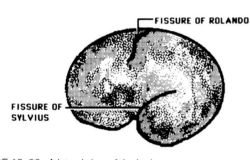

FIGURE 15–26. A lateral view of the brain.

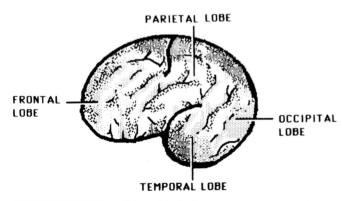

FIGURE 15–27. A lateral view of the brain.

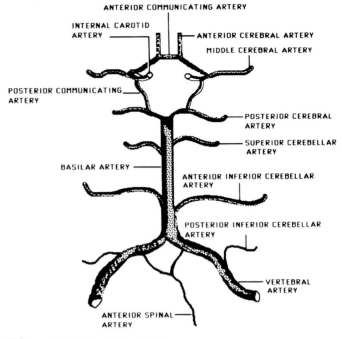

FIGURE 15–28. The circle of Willis.

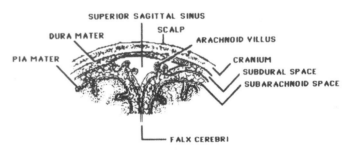

FIGURE 15–29. A diagram of a coronal section of the meninges and cortex.

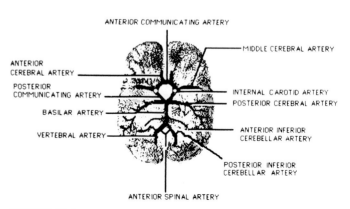

FIGURE 15–30. A diagram of the arteries at the base of the brain.

DISEASE AND PATHOLOGY

Intracranial Hemorrhage

The most common intracranial pathology in neonates and infants is intracranial hemorrhage.

The most common risk factors are prematurity, gestational age of less than 32 weeks, and low birth weight (<1,500 g). Other risk factors include gender (male 2:1), multiple gestations, trauma during delivery, prolonged labor, hyperosmolarity, hypocoagulation, pneumothorax, patent ductus arteriosus, and increased or decreased blood flow. The underlying pathophysiology is hypoxia.[3] Clinical symptoms may include respiratory distress syndrome, hematocrit drop, prematurity (<32 weeks or 1,850 g), or problems during delivery. Most bleeds occur within 72 hours after birth. Later complications of hemorrhage include hydrocephalus and porencephalic cyst.[1]

There are several types of hemorrhages, which are named according to the location.

a. *SEH: Subependymal* hemorrhage occurs in the caudate nucleus and can be seen inferior to the floor of the lateral ventricles[1] (Fig. 15–31).

b. *IVH: Intraventricular* hemorrhage occurs within the ventricles and can completely fill the ventricles forming a cast[1] (Fig. 15–32).

c. *IPA: Intraparenchymal* hemorrhage occurs within the brain substance, usually near the caudate nucleus and lateral to the ventricles. Dilatation of the lateral ventricles is often associated with parenchymal hemorrhage[1] (Fig. 15–33).

d. *CPH: Choroid* and cerebella hemorrhage occur within the echogenic choroid and cerebellum. They may be difficult to distinguish; however, outline irregularity and increased echogenicity will suggest a hemorrhage.[1]

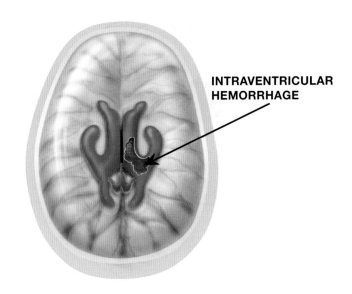

FIGURE 15–32. Intraventricular hemorrhage grade 2.

e. *GMH: Germinal matrix hemorrhage* is the site of many subependymal hemorrhages and is often associated with prematurity.

f. *SAH: Subarachnoid hemorrhage* is located between the arachnoid and pia mater and may be difficult to see on ultrasound unless there is a large amount of blood present.

The sonographic appearance of intracranial hemorrhage changes with time. Early hemorrhages are echogenic and change to decreased echogenicity in a few weeks. The end result is often porencephalic cysts.[1]

g. *SDH: Subdural hemorrhage* is located between the dura mater and the arachnoid. Trauma can cause a tearing of the dural folds or rupture of the medullary veins, which causes blood collection around the periphery of the brain. The cerebral

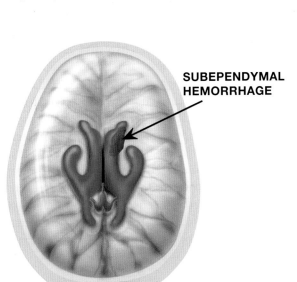

FIGURE 15–31. Subependymal hemorrhage grade 1.

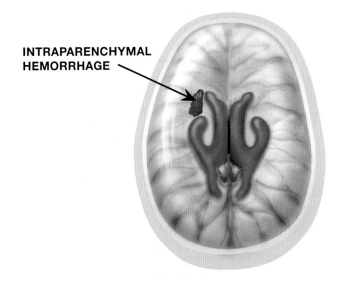

FIGURE 15–33. Intraparenchymal hemorrhage grade 3.

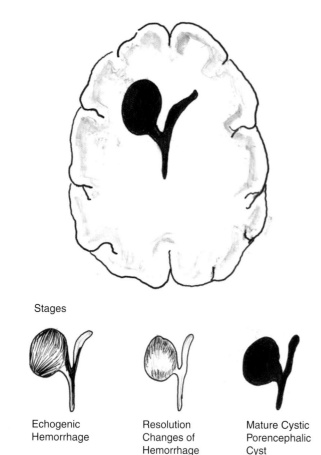

Stages

Echogenic Hemorrhage

Resolution Changes of Hemorrhage

Mature Cystic Porencephalic Cyst

FIGURE 15–34. Intraparenchymal hemorrhage grade 4.

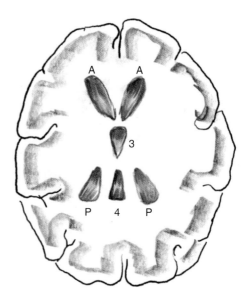

(obstruction with enlargement of the ventricles)
A = Anterior horn
P = Posterior horn
3 = Third ventricle
4 = Fourth ventricle

FIGURE 15–35. Porencephalic cyst.

surface will appear flattened with an echogenic space between the cranium and the cerebrum. On a coronal view, fluid can be seen within the inter-hemispheric fissure, with blood collecting around the brain. The gyri are compressed and become more prominent and closer together.[1]

Grading of Intracranial Hemorrhage[2]

Grade 1. This is a germinal matrix or subependymal hemorrhage. It is seen inferolaterally to the floor of the frontal horn or body of the lateral ventricle and medially to the head of the caudate nucleus (Fig. 15–31).

Grade 2. This is an intraventricular hemorrhage presented with no dilatation and may coexist with germinal matrix hemorrhage (Fig. 15–32).

Grade 3. This is an intraventricular hemorrhage with dilatation of the ventricle and may coexist with germinal matrix hemorrhage (Fig. 15–33).

Grade 4. This is an intraparenchymal hemorrhage, which may coexist with germinal matrix and intraventricular hemorrhage with or without dilatation (Fig. 15–34).

Porencephalic Cyst. This is a cyst arising from the ventricle that develops secondary to parenchymal hemorrhage[1] (Figs. 15–34 and 15–35).

Hydrocephalus. Ventricular dilatation is most often secondary to obstruction of the cerebrospinal flow pathways. This is typically associated with enlargement of the head, brain atrophy, and mental deterioration. It is first seen sonographically in the occipital horn, followed by the body and the anterior horn. It can be a minimal, moderate, or marked degree. The third and fourth ventricles are normally barely seen on the scan, so dilatation is easy to visualize.[1] Ultrasound monitors ventricular enlargement and if a shunt placement is required, it can assist in localization. In addition, ultrasound can provide follow-up examinations for the shunt procedure to ensure patency[1] (Fig. 15–35).

Periventricular Leukomalacia. Periventricular leukomalacia (PVL) occurs in neonates who have had asphyxia.[1] It is a region of coagulation necrosis and rarified neutrophile areas that contain swollen axons or macrophages followed by a reaction of microglia cells and astrocytosis. Hemorrhage may accompany the infarction, and the areas of necrosis may liquefy and cavitate.[4] Sonographically, this condition will present with lesions distinctly separate from the caudate nucleus and usually adjacent to the atrium of the lateral ventricles. There will be increased echoes at the external angle of the lateral ventricles, with extensions radiating anterior to the frontal horns. It may be asymmetrical or bilateral. The echo intensity decreases in 2–4 weeks, and cysts or cavities are seen later in the previously echogenic areas[5] (Fig. 15–36).

Intracranial Infections

Encephalitis and Brain Edema. Encephalitis is inflammation of the brain. It is characterized sonographically with an overall

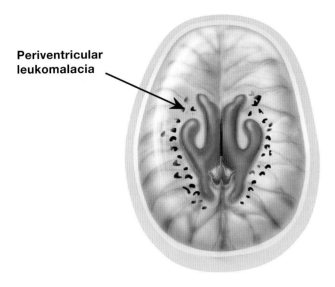

FIGURE 15–36. Periventricular leukomalacia.

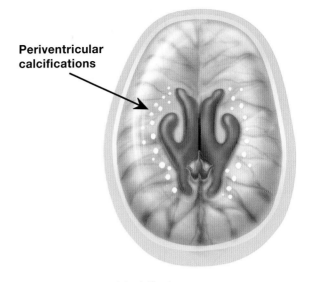

FIGURE 15–37. Intracranial calcifications.

increased echogenicity. Brain edema also shows increased echogenicity but has an additional finding; the ventricles become slitlike as a result of the brain swelling.[1]

Ventriculitis. Infection of the ventricles is usually associated with encephalitis. It causes dilatation of the ventricles, and they may contain septa and debris. The brain becomes more echogenic, and often there are small cystic areas. The lining of the ventricles appears echogenic on ultrasound, and there may be holes in the borders of the ventricles.[1]

Brain Abscess. Abscesses vary in number and size. They may be lobulated and usually appear as cystic-type lesions with nonhomogeneous echogenic material within. There are usually other signs of ventriculitis and encephalitis.[1]

Intracranial Calcifications. Calcifications in the brain may be seen as a result of infections that occurred during pregnancy. For example, cytomegalovirus inclusion disease or toxoplasmosis. Sonographically, echogenic areas may be seen in the brain with associated shadowing[1] (Fig. 15–37).

Cranial Malformations

Arachnoid Cyst. This is an uncommon benign cystic lesion that is lined in arachnoid tissue.[1] The exact etiology of this condition is unknown; however, it can be congenital or caused by previous trauma, infection, or infarction. Common locations of arachnoid cysts include middle cranial fossa anterior to the temporal lobe, the cerebral convexities, the posterior fossa, the suprasellar region, and the quadrigeminal plate cistern. Arachnoid cysts located in the midline may be associated with hydrocephalus. The arachnoid cyst is usually seen on ultrasound as an anechoic mass with well-defined smooth margins. The ventricles may also be dilated[6] (Fig. 15–38).

Agenesis of the Corpus Callosum. The corpus callosum is the tract connecting the right and left cerebral hemispheres. This entity is defined as the absence of the corpus callosum. The corpus callosum may be hypoplastic, partially absent, or totally absent. Agenesis of the corpus callosum can be congenital or acquired. Acquired agenesis, for example, can occur as the result of intrauterine insult with anoxia or infarction in the distribution of the anterior cerebral artery. In the congenital type, the posterior portion of the corpus callosum is generally affected, whereas the anterior portion is affected in the acquired type.[6] Patients may be asymptomatic or have seizures, delayed development, hydrocephalus, or cerebral disconnection syndrome.

Real-time ultrasound shows a wide separation of the ventricular frontal horns with an asymmetrical appearance of the lateral ventricles. The third ventricle is high in position, which produces a "rabbit ear" appearance. The normal prominent corpus callosum is not seen on the midline sagittal scan.[6] CT, MRI, and ultrasound may be used to demonstrate this condition[6] (Fig. 15–39).

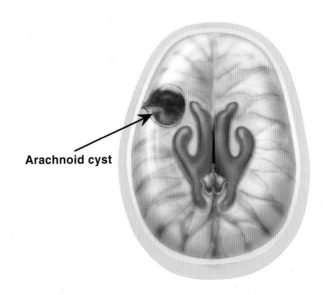

FIGURE 15–38. Arachnoid cyst.

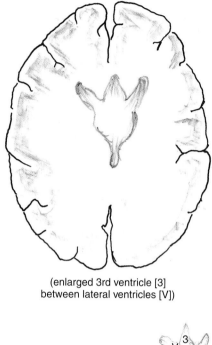

(enlarged 3rd ventricle [3] between lateral ventricles [V])

FIGURE 15–39. Agenesis of the corpus callosum.

Holoprosencephaly. This entity is defined as a congenital malformation with partial or complete failure of the primitive prosencephalon to form the cerebral hemispheres (telencephalon), and a thalamus and hypothalamus (diencephalon). This leads to a midline cleavage defect with failure to form the cerebral hemispheres and the thalamus. There is a common large ventricle with a horseshoe shape. There are three types of holoprosencephaly:

Alobar (severe form)—a single horseshoe-shaped ventricle with a thin cortical mantle. The thalami are fused, and the third ventricle is absent.[1] This type has severe abnormalities and is not compatible with life (Fig. 15–40).

Semilobar (moderate form)—Anterior horns of the ventricles are present. There is a single occipital horn with partial development of occipital and temporal horns. This form is usually associated with mental retardation.[1]

Lobar (mildest form)[1,6]—A less severe variant than the alobar with considerable cortex present.[1]

Risk factors include: maternal diabetes mellitus, toxoplasmosis, trisomies 13, 15, and 18, intrauterine rubella, and Meckel's syndrome. It can be associated with severe facial abnormalities, such as cleft palate, cleft lip, hypotelorism, trigonocephaly, cyclopia, ethmocephaly, and cebocephaly.

Real-time ultrasound demonstrates a large central ventricle draping over a bilobed fused thalamus in a horseshoe-shaped appearance. The third ventricle is usually visible in some form with semilobar and lobar types and is small or absent in the alobar type. The falx cerebri and interhemispheric fissure are present to a variable degree in the semilobar and lobar forms, and are usually absent in the alobar forms. The corpus callosum is absent in the alobar form. There is usually some residual brain tissue, depending on the type, with no differentiation of the frontal, temporal, and occipital horns.[6] CT, MRI, and ultrasound demonstrate holoprosencephaly; however, MRI is superior in showing the structural changes caused by holoprosencephaly.

Arnold–Chiari Malformation. This entity is characterized by inferior displacement of the cerebellum and the fourth ventricle into the upper cervical canal and is usually associated with cerebellar dysplasia.[6] There are four types:

Chiari I Malformation—Low-lying cerebellar tonsils below the foramen magnum. Cisterna magna is small or absent. There can be mild elongation and low position of the fourth ventricle. Complications include hydrocephalus and hydromyelia.

Chiari II Malformation—Inferior displacement of the medulla, fourth ventricle, inferior cerebellar tonsils, and vermis, and the presence of a myelocele or meningomyelocele (Fig. 15–41).

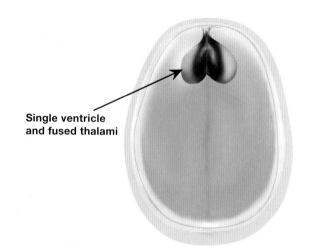

Single ventricle and fused thalami

FIGURE 15–40. Alobar holoprosencephaly.

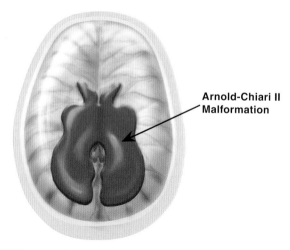

Arnold-Chiari II Malformation

FIGURE 15–41. Arnold–Chiari II malformation.

Chiari III Malformation—Low occiput–high cervical cephalo-cele with a bony defect in the infraocciput, posterior rim of the foramen magnum, and posterior arch of the first cervical vertebra. Herniation of the cerebellum, brainstem, fourth ventricle, and upper cervical cord into the defect may occur.

Chiari IV Malformation—Severe cerebellar dysplasia associated with hypoplastic cerebellum, small brainstem, large posterior fossa, and CSF space not causing pressure effects.[6]

Patients may be asymptomatic or have headache, enlargement of the head from hydrocephalus, ataxia, incoordination, signs and symptoms of increased intracranial pressure, and a cervico-occipital soft tissue mass from encephalocele.[6]

Real-time ultrasound shows the cerebellum low in the posterior fossa. The third ventricle may be obscured by the massa intermedia, and the fourth ventricle may be small or absent. The posterior fossa may be small with the cisterna magna not visualized. Hydrocephalus may be present with the lateral ventricles dilated more than the frontal horns. A myelocele or meningomyelocele may be seen at the cervico-occipital junction.[6]

CT, MRI and ultrasound are used to demonstrate the anomaly. CT and MRI can more effectively demonstrate the bony defects in the occiput, foramen magnum, and C1 and C2 in addition to showing the myelocele or meningomyelocele, fourth ventricle, and brainstem.[6]

Dandy–Walker Malformation or Syndrome. This process is characterized by a cyst in the infratentorial region with absence of the inferior cerebellar vermis and atresia of the foramina of Luschka and Magendie.[7] It is associated with hydrocephalus and presents on ultrasound with a large posterior fossa cyst that communicates with the fourth ventricle and enlargement of the posterior fossa. This condition has been associated with a higher incidence of other anomalies, such as agenesis of the corpus callosum, aqueductal stenosis, porencephalic cyst, encephalocele, holoprosencephaly, and lissencephaly.[7] There will be a small cerebellum and a large posterior fossa[6] (Fig. 15–42).

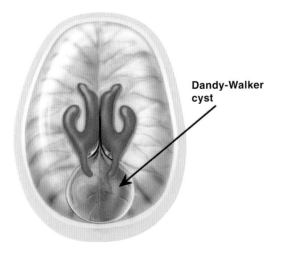

FIGURE 15–42. Dandy–Walker cyst.

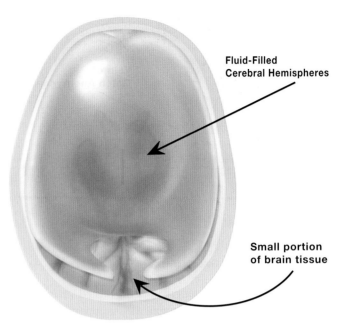

FIGURE 15–43. Hydranencephaly.

Hydranencephaly. This is a severe congenital malformation with a complete or almost complete absence of telencephalic structures. The cerebellum, basal portion of the temporal lobes, occipital lobes, and diencephalon are generally preserved. This anomaly is a result of severe intrauterine destructive process, although the exact etiology is uncertain. Neonates may be asymptomatic or have a large head with marked retardation. Transillumination of the skull is increased because of the thinness of the calvarium and increased intracranial fluid. Cerebral activity may be absent on an electroencephalogram.

Sonographically, this anomaly is seen as large bilateral cystic masses in the supratentorial region. Cerebral tissue may be present in the occipital and basal portions of the temporal lobes. The falx cerebri is usually attenuated and deviated[6] (Fig. 15–43).

Congenital Porencephaly. This anomaly is defined as the presence of cystic cavities within the brain matter. These cystic cavities may communicate with the ventricular system, the subarachnoid space, or both.[4]

Microcephaly. This condition is characterized by a decreased head size and reduction of brain mass. It features a typical disproportion in size between the skull and the face. The forehead slopes with a small brain, and the cerebral hemispheres are affected.[5]

Cranioschisis. This condition is a splitting of the brain caused by failure of the neural tube to close. The level where the neural tube closes determines which anomalies will be present. Various anomalies include anencephaly, encephalocele, and myelomeningocele.

Vein of Galen Aneurysm and Arteriovenous Malformation. The vein of Galen can become dilated or aneurysmal due to an increased flow from a deep cerebral arteriovenous malformation. The enlarged vein of Galen is seen posterior to the third

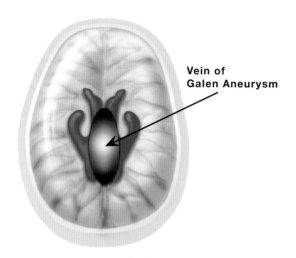

FIGURE 15–44. Vein of Galen aneurysm.

ventricle and draining posteriorly into the dilated straight sinus and torcular herophili.[7] Sonographically, it appears as a cystic midline space with lateral ventricular dilatation.[2] This condition can be differentiated from other cystic anomalies with color-flow Doppler. Schematic of vein of Galen aneurysm (Fig. 15–44).

Tumors

Choroid Plexus Papilloma. That is a benign tumor that causes the choroid plexus to appear enlarged and echogenic. Hydrocephalus may develop because of obstruction of ventricular foramina.[1]

Corpus Callosum Lymphoma. The lymphoma presents as an echogenic mass within the corpus callosum. It has separated anterior horns that are pointed due to the maldevelopment of the corpus callosum.[1]

Teratoma. This benign tumor has typical areas of calcifications and cystic formation. Obstructive hydrocephalus is a common presentation.[1]

References

1. Sanders RC. *Clinical Sonography: A Practical Guide.* 4th ed. Philadelphia, PA: Lippincott Williams & Wilkins; 2006.

2. Kiesler J, Ricer R. The Abnormal Fontanelle. *Am Fam Physician.* 2003; 67:2547-2552.

3. McGahan JP, Goldberg BB. *Diagnostic Ultrasound: A Logical Approach. Philadelphia.* New York : Lippincott-Raven; 1998; 1140-1141.

4. Fleischer AC, Manning FA, Jeanty P, et al. *Sonography in Obstetrics & Gynecology Principles and Practice.* New York: McGraw-Hill; 2001.

5. Babcock DS. *Cranial Sonography of Infants. Syllabus: Categorical Course in Ultrasound.* 70th Scientific Assembly and Annual Meeting of The Radiological Society of North America, November 1984; 123-127.

6. Krebs CA, Giyanani VL, Eisenberg RL. *Ultrasound Atlas of Disease Processes.* Norwalk, CT: Appleton & Lange; 1993.

7. Aletebi FA, Fung KFK: Neurodevelopmental outcome after antenatal diagnosis of posterior fossa abnormalities. *Ultrasound Med.* 1999; 18:683-689.

Questions

GENERAL INSTRUCTIONS: For each question, select the best answer. Select only one answer for each question unless otherwise instructed.

Questions 1–16: Match the structures in Fig. 15–45 with the terms in Column B.

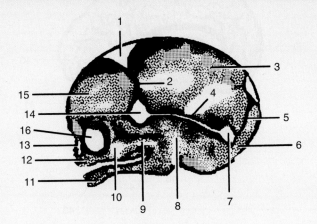

FIGURE 15–45. Lateral view of an infantile skull.

Questions 17–22: Match the structures in Fig. 15–46 with the terms in Column B.

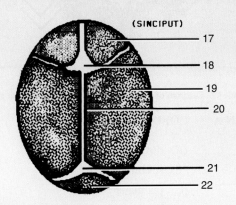

FIGURE 15–46. Superior view of an infantile skull.

COLUMN A	COLUMN B
1. _____	(A) mastoidal fontanelle
2. _____	(B) sphenoid fontanelle
	(C) parietal bone
3. _____	(D) maxilla
4. _____	(E) orbit
5. _____	(F) occipital bone
6. _____	(G) coronal suture
7. _____	(H) frontal bone
8. _____	(I) zygomatic bone
9. _____	(J) nasal bone
10. _____	(K) temporal bone
11. _____	(L) mandible
12. _____	(M) anterior fontanelle
13. _____	(N) squamous suture
14. _____	(O) lambdoidal suture
15. _____	(P) zygomatic process
16. _____	

COLUMN A	COLUMN B
17. _____	(A) occipital bone
18. _____	(B) frontal bone
	(C) sagittal suture
19. _____	(D) anterior
20. _____	(E) parietal bone
21. _____	(F) posterior fontanelle
22. _____	

Questions 23–31: Match the structures in Fig. 15–47 with the terms in Column B.

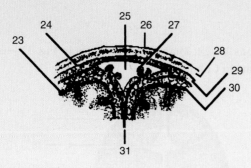

FIGURE 15–47. Diagram of a coronal section of the meninges and cortex.

COLUMN A   COLUMN B

23. _____

24. _____

25. _____

26. _____

27. _____

28. _____

29. _____

30. _____

31. _____

(A) dura mater
(B) subdural space
(C) pia mater
(D) superior sagittal sinus
(E) arachnoid villus
(F) falx cerebri
(G) subarachnoid space
(H) scalp
(I) cranium

Questions 32–37: Match the structures in Fig. 15–48 with the terms in Column B.

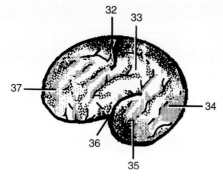

FIGURE 15–48. A lateral view of the brain.

COLUMN A   COLUMN B

32. _____

33. _____

34. _____

35. _____

(A) frontal lobe
(B) Sylvian fissure
(C) fissure of Rolando
(D) occipital lobe

36. _____   (E) parietal lobe

37. _____   (F) temporal lobe

Questions 38–50: Match the structures in Fig. 15–49 with the terms in Column B.

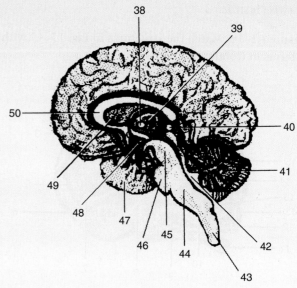

FIGURE 15–49. Diagram of a sagittal section of the brain.

COLUMN A   COLUMN B

38. _____

39. _____

40. _____

41. _____

42. _____

43. _____

44. _____

45. _____

46. _____

47. _____

48. _____

49. _____

50. _____

(A) corpus callosum
(B) thalamus
(C) cerebellum
(D) pineal body
(E) pons
(F) spinal cord
(G) cerebral peduncle
(H) septum pellucidum
(I) medulla oblongata
(J) interthalamic adhesion
(K) fourth ventricle
(L) third ventricle
(M) temporal lobe

Questions 51–59: Match the structures in Fig. 15–50 with the terms in Column B.

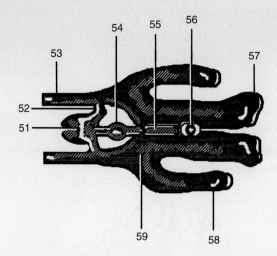

FIGURE 15–50. Diagram of the ventricular system in the superior view.

COLUMN A	COLUMN B
51. _____	(A) third ventricle
52. _____	(B) anterior horn
	(C) inferior horn
53. _____	(D) foramen of Monro
54. _____	(E) lateral recess
	(F) cerebral aqueduct
55. _____	(G) fourth ventricle
56. _____	(H) atrium
	(I) posterior horn
57. _____	
58. _____	
59. _____	

Questions 60–74: Match the structures in Fig. 15–51 with the terms in Column B.

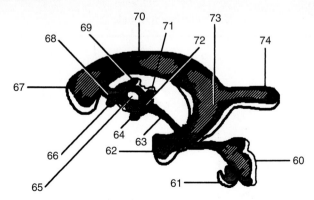

FIGURE 15–51. Diagram of the ventricular system in the lateral view.

COLUMN A	COLUMN B
60. _____	(A) pineal recess
61. _____	(B) body of lateral ventricle

COLUMN A	COLUMN B
62. _____	(C) foramen of Monro
63. _____	(D) posterior horn
	(E) infundibular recess
64. _____	(F) third ventricle
65. _____	(G) preoptic recess
	(H) anterior horn
66. _____	(I) inferior horn
67. _____	(J) collateral trigone
	(K) suprapineal recess
68. _____	(L) foramen of Magendie
69. _____	(M) cerebral aqueduct
	(N) foramina of Luschka
70. _____	(O) interthalamic adhesion
71. _____	
72. _____	
73. _____	
74. _____	

Questions 75–80: Match the structures in Fig. 15–52 with the terms in Column B.

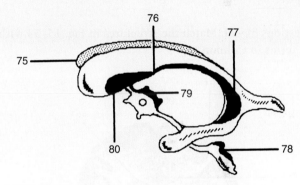

FIGURE 15–52. Diagram of the ventricular system in a neonate.

COLUMN A	COLUMN B
75. _____	(A) caudate nucleus
76. _____	(B) choroid plexus of the third ventricle
	(C) tela choroidea
77. _____	(D) corpus callosum
78. _____	(E) choroid plexus of the fourth ventricle
	(F) glomus of the choroid plexus
79. _____	
80. _____	

Questions 81–84: Identify the structures demonstrated in each scan plane where the lines project in Fig. 15–53, then place in Column A the letter corresponding to the appropriate item in Column B.

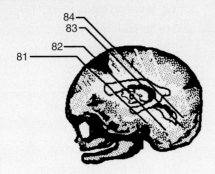

FIGURE 15-53. Diagram of a lateral view of the infantile skull with the ventricular system.

COLUMN A   COLUMN B

81. _____   (A) foramina of Monro and third ventricle

82. _____   (B) posterior horn of the lateral ventricle
              (C) frontal and temporal horns

83. _____   (D) choroid plexus and trigone of the lateral
                  ventricle and the fourth ventricle

84. _____

Questions 85–94: Match the structures in Fig. 15–54 with the terms in Column B.

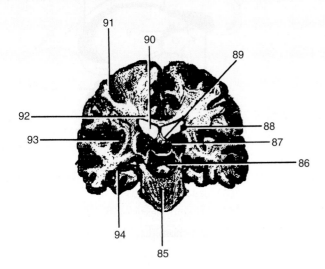

FIGURE 15-54. Diagram of a coronal section of the brain.

COLUMN A   COLUMN B

85. _____   (A) lateral ventricle

86. _____   (B) cerebellar peduncle
              (C) pons

87. _____   (D) corpus callosum

88. _____   (E) caudate nucleus

89. _____   (F) hippocampus

90. _____   (G) Sylvian fissure
              (H) sulcus

91. _____   (I) column of fornix

92. _____   (J) thalamus

93. _____

94. _____

Questions 95–100: Match the structures in Fig. 15–55 with the terms in Column B.

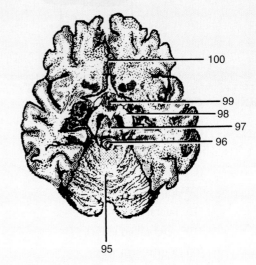

FIGURE 15-55. Diagram of a coronal section of the brain.

COLUMN A   COLUMN B

95. _____   (A) cerebral aqueduct

96. _____   (B) cerebellum peduncle
              (C) cerebellum

97. _____   (D) hypothalamus

98. _____   (E) gyrus and sulcus
              (F) cerebral peduncle

99. _____

100. _____

Questions 101–112: Match the structures in Fig. 15–56 with the terms in Column B.

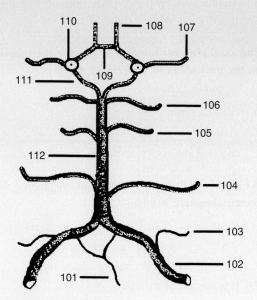

FIGURE 15-56. Circle of Willis.

COLUMN A   **COLUMN B**

101. _____   (A) basilar artery
                (B) posterior cerebral artery
102. _____   (C) middle cerebral artery
103. _____   (D) internal carotid artery
                (E) anterior cerebral artery
104. _____   (F) anterior inferior cerebellar artery
105. _____   (G) vertebral artery
                (H) anterior communicating artery
106. _____   (I) posterior communicating artery
107. _____   (J) anterior spinal artery
                (K) posterior inferior cerebellar artery
108. _____   (L) superior cerebellar artery
109. _____

110. _____

111. _____

112. _____

Questions 113–120: Match the structures in Fig. 15–57 with the terms in Column B.

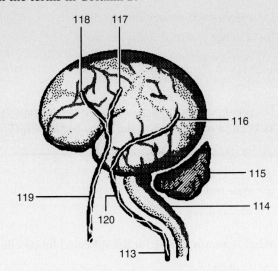

FIGURE 15-57. Diagram of the brain in the sagittal view.

COLUMN A   **COLUMN B**

113. _____   (A) internal carotid artery
                (B) posterior cerebral artery
114. _____   (C) vertebral artery
115. _____   (D) basilar artery
                (E) anterior cerebral artery
116. _____   (F) middle cerebral artery
117. _____   (G) cerebellum
                (H) medulla oblongata
118. _____

119. _____

120. _____

Questions 121–124: Match the structures in Fig. 15–58 with the terms in Column B.

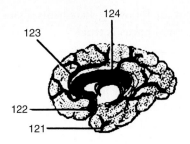

FIGURE 15-58. Diagram of the lateral aspect of the internal carotid artery and its branches.

COLUMN A   **COLUMN B**

121. _____   (A) pericallosal artery
                (B) middle cerebral artery
122. _____   (C) callosomarginal artery
123. _____   (D) anterior cerebral artery

124. _____

125. Which acoustic windows are used most often in neonatal cranial sonography?

    (A) anterior and posterior fontanelle
    (B) anterior and sphenoidal fontanelle
    (C) anterior and mastoidal fontanelle
    (D) posterior and sphenoidal fontanelle

126. On sonography, cytomegalovirus in the neonate is associated with which of the following findings?

    (A) periventricular calcifications
    (B) small cystic lesions
    (C) encephalocele
    (D) anencephaly

127. What is another name for the sphenoid fontanelle?

    (A) lambda
    (B) the anterolateral fontanelle
    (C) the posterolateral fontanelle
    (D) bregma

128. The anterior fontanelle becomes progressively smaller and, in most cases, closes completely by what age?

    (A) 6 months
    (B) 2–3 months
    (C) 12 months
    (D) 18 months

129. What is another name for the mastoidal fontanelle?

    (A) anterior fontanelle
    (B) posterior fontanelle
    (C) lambda
    (D) posterolateral fontanelle

130. Which of the following statements about temporal and occipital horns is true?

    (A) they both diverge laterally as they project from the body of the lateral ventricles.
    (B) they both diverge medially as they project from the body of the lateral ventricles.
    (C) the occipital horn is lateral, and the temporal horns are medial to the body of the lateral ventricles.
    (D) the right temporal horn and the occipital horn are medial, and the left temporal horn is lateral.

131. The lateral ventricular ratio can be obtained by measuring the distance from the

    (A) anterior wall to the posterior wall of the lateral ventricle
    (B) midline to medial wall of the lateral ventricle and from the inner wall of the table of the skull

    (C) medial wall to the lateral wall of the lateral ventricle
    (D) midline to the lateral wall of the lateral ventricle and dividing this by the distance from the midline echo to the inner table of the skull

132. The axial scan is obtained by placing the transducer on the parietal bone just above the

    (A) styloid process
    (B) coronal suture
    (C) glabella
    (D) external auditory meatus

133. Which of the following statements regarding the germinal matrix is false?

    (A) It cannot be visualized as a distinct structure.
    (B) It lies just above the caudate nucleus.
    (C) It disappears between 32 weeks to term.
    (D) It is not a fetal structure.

134. What is the normal location for the germinal matrix after 24 weeks of gestation?

    (A) above the caudate nucleus in the subependymal layer of the lateral ventricle
    (B) within the choroid plexus
    (C) inferior to the caudate nucleus
    (D) within the choroid plexus in the trigone

135. The cisterna magna appears sonographically as

    (A) echogenic space superior to the cerebellum
    (B) echogenic space inferior to the cerebellum
    (C) echo-free space superior to the cerebellum
    (D) echo-free space inferior to the cerebellum

136. Vascular pulsations are sometimes seen in the Sylvian fissure, which most likely represent the

    (A) anterior cerebral arteries
    (B) posterior cerebral arteries
    (C) basilar artery
    (D) middle cerebral arteries

137. Which of the following statements about the fissure and sulci is true?

    (A) fissure and sulci both appear echogenic.
    (B) fissure is echo-free and sulci echogenic.
    (C) sulci is echo-free and the fissure is echogenic.
    (D) fissure and sulci are both echo-free.

138. **Where is the cavum septum pellucidum located?**

    (A) lateral to the corpus callosum

    (B) posterior to the third ventricle

    (C) medial to the thalami

    (D) between the frontal horns of the lateral ventricles

139. **The third ventricle is located between the**

    (A) cavum septum pellucidum

    (B) frontal horns of the lateral ventricles

    (C) thalami

    (D) corpus callosum

140. **Increased echogenicity in the brain parenchyma is seen with**

    (A) subependymal hemorrhage

    (B) intraventricular hemorrhage

    (C) intraparenchymal hemorrhage

    (D) choroid plexus hemorrhage

141. **If dense echogenic material is seen in the ventricle, it is called**

    (A) intraventricular hemorrhage

    (B) intraparenchymal hemorrhage

    (C) subarachnoid hemorrhage

    (D) subependymal hemorrhage

142. **After an intraparenchymal hemorrhage, the clot retracts and may result in a cystic area communicating with the ventricle. What is this termed?**

    (A) holoprosencephaly

    (B) hydranencephaly

    (C) hydrocephalus

    (D) porencephaly

143. **Which of the following is *not* a possible contributing factor to intracranial hemorrhage?**

    (A) maternal ingestion of aspirin during the final weeks of pregnancy

    (B) extrauterine stress

    (C) intrapartum hypoxia

    (D) pleural effusion

144. **A neonate is defined as**

    (A) a child during the first 28 days after birth

    (B) a child from 29 days after birth to 1 year

    (C) a fetus of 20 weeks of gestation to a child 28 days after birth

    (D) conception to birth

145. **What is the most common site for periventricular leukomalacia?**

    (A) white matter surrounding the ventricles

    (B) gray matter surrounding the ventricles

    (C) gray matter around the caudate nucleus

    (D) white matter around the cerebellum

146. **Disruption of organogenesis in brain development causes specific related brain defects. Such defects do *not* include**

    (A) diverticulation

    (B) neural tube closure

    (C) neuronal proliferation

    (D) tuberous sclerosis

147. **Which of the following terms is used to describe any hemorrhage within the cranial vault?**

    (A) subependymal hemorrhage

    (B) germinal matrix hemorrhage

    (C) intraventricular hemorrhage

    (D) intracranial hemorrhage

Questions 148–151: Match the terms in Column B with the types of hemorrhage in Column A.

COLUMN A	COLUMN B
148. cerebrospinal fluid— blood level in the ventricles	(A) intraparenchymal hemorrhage (IPH)
149. echogenic foci in the region of the caudate nucleus	(B) subependymal hemorrhage (SEH)
150. echogenic area in the brain parenchyma	(C) intraventricular hemorrhage (IVH)
151. enlarged irregular and highly echogenic choroid plexus	(D) choroid plexus hemorrhage (CPH)

152. **Which type of intracranial hemorrhage is most common in premature infants?**

    (A) subdural hemorrhage

    (B) intraventricular hemorrhage

    (C) intraparenchymal hemorrhage

    (D) subependymal germinal matrix hemorrhage

153. **True coronal scans are performed at what angle with the orbitomeatal line?**

    (A) 60°
    (B) 90°
    (C) 150°
    (D) They do not have an angle with the orbitomeatal line.

154. **Which of the following does *not* designate the term "acoustic window" in cranial sonography?**

    (A) a procedure to bypass bone interface
    (B) an opening through which ultrasound can travel with little or no obstruction
    (C) an area in which ultrasound is obstructed
    (D) an area in which ultrasound is not obstructed

155. **Which of the following diseases is *not* a common cause of congenital infections of the nervous system?**

    (A) rubella
    (B) toxoplasmosis
    (C) gonorrhea
    (D) syphilis
    (E) cytomegalovirus

156. **Which of the following are *not* sonographic findings of congenital infection of the nervous system?**

    (A) microcephaly with enlargement of the ventricles
    (B) a prominent interhemispheric fissure and brain atrophy
    (C) macrocephaly with enlargement of the ventricles
    (D) calcification in the periventricular regions

157. **According to the computed tomography grading system for intracranial hemorrhage, which of the following is a Grade 1 hemorrhage?**

    (A) subependymal hemorrhage with intraventricular hemorrhage and ventricular dilatation
    (B) subependymal hemorrhage with intraventricular hemorrhage and no ventricular dilatation
    (C) subependymal hemorrhage with intraventricular hemorrhage and intraparenchymal hemorrhage
    (D) isolated subependymal hemorrhage

158. **The foramen between the third and fourth ventricles is the**

    (A) cerebral aqueduct
    (B) foramen of Monro
    (C) foramen of Magendie
    (D) foramen of Luschka

159. **Which of the following is *not* true regarding hydranencephaly?**

    (A) usually only the brainstem and portion of the occipital lobe remain.
    (B) the falx is usually intact.
    (C) the falx is usually not intact because the head is largely filled with fluid.
    (D) there is a severe loss of cerebral tissue.

160. **A Dandy–Walker cyst is usually associated with**

    (A) toxoplasmosis
    (B) dysgenesis of the vermis of the cerebellum
    (C) syphilis
    (D) cytomegalovirus

161. **The current treatment for hydrocephalus with increased intraventricular pressure is**

    (A) Javid's internal shunt
    (B) ventriculoperitoneal (V-P) shunt
    (C) radiation treatment
    (D) ventriculoectomy

162. **Which of the following is *not* a sign of hydrocephalus?**

    (A) skull bones halo sign on x-ray
    (B) anterior fontanelle sinks
    (C) bulging of the frontal bone of the skull
    (D) rapid head growth
    (E) decreasing size of ventricles

163. **The most common cause of congenital hydrocephalus is**

    (A) aqueductal stenosis
    (B) subarachnoid hemorrhage
    (C) interventricular hemorrhage
    (D) intracranial infection

164. **Subperiosteal hematomas are also called**

    (A) cephalohematomas
    (B) subependymal hemorrhages
    (C) intraventricular hemorrhages
    (D) choroid plexus hemorrhages

165. **The cavum pellucidum begins to close at which week of gestation?**

    (A) 40 weeks
    (B) 36 weeks
    (C) 12 weeks
    (D) 24 weeks

166. **Which of the following best defines the Dandy–Walker syndrome?**

(A) a cyst in the posterior fossa that does not communicate with the fourth ventricle

(B) a congenital cystic dilatation of the third ventricle

(C) congenital dilatation of the ventricular system

(D) a posterior fossa cyst that is continuous with the fourth ventricle

167. **Which of the following is a differential diagnosis for hydranencephaly?**

(A) severe hydrocephalus

(B) Dandy–Walker cyst

(C) arachnoid cyst

(D) intracranial teratoma

168. **On cranial sonography, the middle cerebral artery is found in the**

(A) region of the Sylvian fissure and above the corpus callosum

(B) region of the Sylvian fissure and in the circle of Willis

(C) genu of the corpus callosum and Sylvian fissure

(D) genu of the corpus callosum and hippocampal sulcus

169. **What is the most severe form of hemorrhage?**

(A) germinal matrix hemorrhage

(B) intraventricular hemorrhage

(C) subependymal hemorrhage

(D) intraparenchymal hemorrhage

170. **What is another name for the forebrain?**

(A) prosencephalon

(B) mesencephalon

(C) rhombencephalon

(D) myelencephalon

171. **Which of the following vessels does *not* form the circle of Willis?**

(A) posterior cerebral arteries

(B) anterior cerebral arteries

(C) internal carotid arteries

(D) posterior and anterior communicating arteries

(E) external carotid arteries

172. **Which of the following is true regarding noncommunicating hydrocephalus?**

(A) it is also called nonobstructive hydrocephalus.

(B) the cerebrospinal fluid pathways within the brain are blocked.

(C) cerebrospinal fluid is blocked within the ventricular system.

(D) none of the above

173. **A Chiari II malformation is defined as**

(A) a congenital abnormality of the brain with elongation of the pons and fourth ventricle and downward displacement of the medulla into the cervical canal

(B) congenital cystic dilatation of the fourth ventricle caused by atresia of the foramen of Magendie

(C) congenital formation of a holospheric cerebrum caused by a disorder of the diverticulation of the fetal brain

(D) none of the above

174. **The main arteries supplying the brain are**

(A) one vertebral and one carotid artery

(B) one basilar artery and two carotid arteries

(C) two external carotid and two vertebral arteries

(D) two internal carotid and two vertebral arteries

175. **The vertebral artery at the level of the pons is called the**

(A) middle cerebral artery

(B) basilar artery

(C) internal carotid artery

(D) posterior cerebral artery

176. **The greatest proportion of the cerebrospinal fluid is produced by**

(A) choroid plexus

(B) caudate nucleus

(C) lateral ventricles

(D) movement of extracellular fluid from blood through the brain and ventricles

177. **The sonographic findings of ventriculitis do *not* include**

(A) echogenic ventricular walls

(B) septated ventricles

(C) normal-sized ventricles with no debris within

(D) debris within the ventricles

178. How many cranial bones are there?

    (A) 12

    (B) 10

    (C) 8

    (D) 5

179. Blood between the arachnoid membrane and the pia mater is called

    (A) subarachnoid hematoma

    (B) subdural hematoma

    (C) epidural membrane

    (D) intraparenchymal hematoma

180. The amount of cerebrospinal fluid production in children is

    (A) 140 mL/week

    (B) 140 mL/day

    (C) 532–576 mL/day

    (D) 552–576 mL/week

181. The accumulation of blood between the dura mater and the inner table of the skull is called

    (A) subarachnoid hemorrhage

    (B) subdural hematoma

    (C) epidural hematoma

    (D) intraparenchymal hemorrhage

182. Another name for the temporal horn is the

    (A) anterior horn

    (B) posterior horn

    (C) inferior horn

    (D) lateral horn

183. The largest of all the horns is the

    (A) temporal horn

    (B) occipital horn

    (C) frontal horn

    (D) lateral horn

184. Which of the following are *not* midline structures?

    (A) third ventricle and fourth ventricle

    (B) cerebral hemispheres

    (C) cavum septum pellucidum

    (D) falx cerebri

185. The vein of Galen aneurysm is most likely to be located

    (A) anterior to the third ventricle

    (B) posterior to the foramen of Monro and superior to the third ventricle

    (C) posterior to the foramen of Monro and inferior to the third ventricle

    (D) posterior to the fourth ventricle

186. Which of the following is *not* a bacterial cause of intracranial infection?

    (A) Haemophilus influenzae

    (B) herpes simplex

    (C) Diplococcus pneumoniae

    (D) bacterial meningitis

187. The central fissure is also called

    (A) Sylvian fissure

    (B) fissure of Rolando

    (C) lateral fissure

    (D) longitudinal fissure

188. Which of the following is the etiology of a porencephalic cyst?

    (A) intracranial infection

    (B) infarction

    (C) intracranial hemorrhage

    (D) trauma

189. Numerous sulci can normally be identified on the premature brain, particularly in the sagittal scan. Identify the condition that would *least* be likely to obscure the normal sulcal pattern.

    (A) meningoencephalitis

    (B) subdural hematoma

    (C) intracranial infection

    (D) infarction

190. The germinal matrix is largest at which week of gestation?

    (A) 40 weeks (term)

    (B) 24–32 weeks

    (C) 32–40 weeks

    (D) 12–15 weeks

191. Which of the following is *not* an intracranial tumor?

    (A) dermoid tumor

    (B) choroid plexus papilloma

    (C) medulloblastoma

    (D) cyclopia

192. Which of the following *best* describes periventricular leukomalacia?

    (A) ischemic lesions of the neonatal brain characterized by necrosis of periventricular white matter

    (B) a disorder of premature newborns characterized by the increase in vascularity in the periventricular white matter

    (C) a disorder of premature newborns characterized by highly echogenic solid lesions in the parenchyma

    (D) an infection disorder with a decrease in definition of the parenchymal structures

193. Which of the following is *not* a common infection acquired in utero?

    (A) herpes simplex

    (B) leukomalacia

    (C) toxoplasmosis

    (D) cytomegalovirus

194. Which of the following results in the greatest number of neonatal deaths?

    (A) hypoxia

    (B) erythroblastosis

    (C) trauma at birth

    (D) premature placental separation

195. Which of the following is *not* a characteristic of lissencephaly?

    (A) decrease in the size of the Sylvian fissure as the neonatal brain matures

    (B) large ventricles

    (C) less sonographic characteristics because of the inability to differentiate white from gray matter

    (D) large Sylvian fissures

196. If an infant has a ventriculoperitoneal (V-P) shunt and the fontanelles are bulging, the usual position to assist in drainage is the

    (A) Trendelenburg position

    (B) lithotomy position

    (C) semi-Fowler's position

    (D) Sims' position

197. The cerebellum is separated from the occipital lobe of the cerebrum by the

    (A) interhemispheric fissure

    (B) tentorium

    (C) cerebellar vermis

    (D) parieto-occipital sulcus

198. The central nervous system consists of the brain and spinal cord. The spinal cord is referred to as the distal continuation of the central nervous system. The terminal portion of the spinal cord is the

    (A) filum terminale

    (B) conus medullaris

    (C) cauda equina

    (D) pia mater

199. What region of the lateral ventricular system is the first to dilate in hydrocephalus?

    (A) the third ventricle

    (B) occipital horns

    (C) frontal horns

    (D) temporal horns

200. The correct placement for a ventriculoperitoneal (V-P) shunt catheter is

    (A) frontal horns anterior to the foramen of Monro

    (B) frontal horns posterior to the foramen of Monro

    (C) trigone of the lateral ventricle

    (D) the roof of the third ventricle

201. Which of the following is least associated with complete agenesis of the corpus callosum?

    (A) absence of the septum pellucidum

    (B) enlarged septum pellucidum

    (C) wide separation of the lateral ventricle

    (D) displacement of the third ventricle

202. Which of the following is *not* seen in septo-optic dysplasia?

    (A) septum pellucidum

    (B) frontal horns

    (C) thalamus

    (D) occipital horns

203. When scanning neonates, excessive pressure should *not* be applied to the anterior fontanelle because it may

(A) cause increased heart rates

(B) cause slowing of the heart

(C) cause increased body temperatures

(D) cause irregularity of the heart rate

Questions 204 through 214: Match the definitions in Column B with the terms they define in Column A.

COLUMN A

204. periventricular leukomalacia _____

205. tentorium cerebelli _____

206. sulci _____

207. choroid plexus _____

208. cisterna magna _____

209. pia mater _____

210. corpus callosum _____

211. cavum septum pellucidum _____

212. insula _____

213. gyri _____

214. aqueduct stenosis _____

COLUMN B

(A) enclosed space located caudal to the cerebellum, between the cerebellum and the occipital bone, serving as a reservoir for cerebrospinal fluid

(B) folds on the surface of the brain

(C) special cells located in the ventricles that secrete cerebrospinal fluid

(D) softening of the white matter surrounding the ventricles

(E) congenital obstruction of the third and fourth ventricles resulting in ventricular dilation

(F) group of nerve fibers above the third ventricle that connects the left and right sides of the brain

(G) transverse division of dura mater forming a partition between the occipital lobe of the cerebral hemispheres and the cerebellum

(H) a triangular area of cerebral cortex, lying deeply in the lateral cerebral fissure

(I) grooves on the surface of the brain separating the gyri

(J) cavity filled with cerebrospinal fluid that lies between the anterior horns of the lateral ventricle

(K) the inner membrane covering the brain and spinal cord

Each of the following terms has an alternative name. Match the terms in Column A with the alternative term Questions 215 through 222 in Column B.

COLUMN A

215. interventricular foramen _____

216. atrium _____

217. subependymal hemorrhage _____

218. epiphysis cerebri _____

219. posterior horn _____

220. frontal horn _____

221. inferior horn _____

222. interthalamic adhesion _____

COLUMN B

(A) massa intermedia

(B) temporal horn

(C) anterior horn

(D) occipital horn

(E) pineal gland

(F) germinal matrix hemorrhage

(G) trigone

(H) foramen of Monro

223. When evaluating the intracerebral vessels of an infant's brain, the optimal frequency range for a continuous-wave Doppler transducer is

(A) 1–3 MHz

(B) 4–5 MHz

(C) 1–10 MHz

(D) 5–10 MHz

224. When using a transcranial approach with the transducer placed 0.5–1.0 cm anterior to the ear and superior to the zygomatic process, the vessel that can be evaluated most accurately in the neonate's brain is the

(A) middle cerebral artery

(B) anterior cerebral artery

(C) posterior cerebral artery

(D) posterior communicating artery

225. In a normal tracing of a cerebral vessel in a neonate's brain, the maximum systolic velocity is equivalent to the

(A) peak height

(B) area under the curve

(C) slope

(D) minimum height

226. **A Doppler tracing of an anterior cerebral artery in an infant with asphyxia can reveal**

    (A) low pulsatility and high diastolic forward flow

    (B) low pulsatility and low diastolic forward flow

    (C) high pulsatility and high diastolic forward flow

    (D) high pulsatility and low diastolic forward flow

227. **A Doppler tracing of an anterior cerebral artery in an infant with an intraventricular hemorrhage can reveal**

    (A) low pulsatility and low diastolic forward flow

    (B) low pulsatility and high diastolic forward flow

    (C) high pulsatility and high diastolic forward flow

    (D) high pulsatility and low diastolic forward flow

228. **The term craniosynostosis denotes**

    (A) premature fusion of the cranial sutures

    (B) premature separation of the cranial sutures

    (C) a bluish discoloration of the cranium

    (D) a bluish discoloration of the scalp

229. **Hypothermia denotes**

    (A) high memory

    (B) low memory

    (C) high temperature

    (D) low temperature

230. **When the parietal bones are relatively thin, lateral ventricular measurements can be obtained up to**

    (A) 5 years

    (B) 6 months

    (C) 2–3 years

    (D) 6–12 months

231. **In cranial sonography, a real-time linear array transducer is limited. Which of the following statements is *not* true of the linear array limitations?**

    (A) limited field of view

    (B) inability to visualize the inner lateral table of both sides of the calvarium simultaneously

    (C) able to examine only the central portion of the brain

    (D) producing only a 90° pie-shaped image

    (E) low signal-to-noise ratio and artifact

232. **Which of the following sonography planes are *most* comparable with cranial computed tomography?**

    (A) axial

    (B) coronal

    (C) sagittal

    (D) occipital

233. **The choroid plexus is attached to the floor of the lateral ventricle. Its point of attachment is called**

    (A) tela choroidea

    (B) interhemispheric fissure

    (C) pineal body

    (D) caudate nucleus

234. **A structure often confused with the third ventricle in the fetus and neonate is the**

    (A) cavum septi pellucidi

    (B) choroid plexus

    (C) thalamus

    (D) cavum vergae

235. **Between 32 and 40 weeks, the incidence of germinal matrix hemorrhage drops. Approximately what percentage of germinal matrix hemorrhage occurs at 28 weeks of gestation?**

    (A) 25%

    (B) 35%

    (C) 40%

    (D) 67%

236. **The term *isodense* denotes the following**

    (A) same density

    (B) same as sonolucent

    (C) same as echogenic

    (D) same as anechoic

237. **Which of the following is associated with an intracranial hemorrhage?**

    (A) hyaline membrane disease

    (B) sudden change in blood flow to the region of the germinal matrix

    (C) increase in venous and arterial pressure

    (D) expanded volume of plasma

    (E) both B and C

    (F) all of the above

238. **An infant is defined as a child**

    (A) from 29 days after birth to 1 year

    (B) during the first 28 days after birth

    (C) from 1–2 years after birth

    (D) from 2–6 years after birth

239. Which of the following is *not* an imaginary line from the outer canthus to the external auditory meatus?

    (A) orbitomeatal line
    (B) canthomeatal line
    (C) radiographic baseline
    (D) Reid's baseline

240. Posterior fossa scans are performed at what angle with the orbitomeatal line?

    (A) 150° from the orbitomeatal line and perpendicular to the clivus
    (B) 150° from the canthomeatal line and parallel to the clivus
    (C) 90° perpendicular to the orbitomeatal line and parallel to the clivus
    (D) 120° perpendicular to the canthomeatal line and parallel to the clivus

241. If one sees echogenic material within the occipital horn, it would most likely be correct to assume that there is

    (A) a choroid plexus in the occipital horn
    (B) a choroid plexus in the lateral horn
    (C) an intracranial hemorrhage because no choroid extends into this area
    (D) an intracranial hemorrhage because the tail of the choroid extends into the occipital horn

242. Which of the following does *not* describe hydranencephaly?

    (A) the head is largely filled with fluid.
    (B) the falx is usually intact.
    (C) the loss of cerebral tissue is severe.
    (D) the brainstem and a portion of the occipital lobe remain.
    (E) there is a presence of a single midline ventricle.

243. The pericallosal artery is normally seen

    (A) above the corpus callosum
    (B) below the corpus callosum
    (C) in the Sylvian fissure
    (D) between the hippocampal sulcus

244. Approximately how long after ventricular dilatation does the head circumference start to increase?

    (A) 5–7 days
    (B) 3–4 days
    (C) 8 weeks
    (D) 2 weeks

245. If hemorrhage is detected in a newborn on the first examination, studies should be performed

    (A) every 3 days until 2 weeks of age
    (B) every 3 days until 2 months of age
    (C) every 5 days until 3 weeks of age
    (D) every 7 days until 3 weeks of age

246. At which week of gestation is the choroid plexus prominent and may completely fill the lateral ventricle?

    (A) last trimester
    (B) first trimester
    (C) mid trimester
    (D) after birth

247. Hydranencephaly is defined as a

    (A) holospheric cerebrum
    (B) posterior fossa cyst
    (C) congenital cystic dilatation of the fourth ventricle
    (D) head largely filled with fluid and a severe loss of cerebral tissue

248. Which of the following does *not* describe holoprosencephaly?

    (A) formation of a holospheric cerebrum
    (B) disorder of diverticulation of the fetal brain
    (C) cerebral hemispheres and lateral ventricles that develop as one vesicle
    (D) large single midline ventricular cavity
    (E) premature fusion of the cranial sutures either complete or partial

249. Which of the following statements about spinal and cranial nerves is true?

    (A) there are 12 pairs of cranial nerves and 12 pairs of spinal nerves.
    (B) there are 12 pairs of cranial nerves and 31 pairs of spinal nerves.
    (C) there are 15 pairs of cranial nerves and 15 pairs of spinal nerves.
    (D) there are 20 pairs of cranial nerves and 20 pairs of spinal nerves.

250. The spinal cord ends at about what vertebral level?

    (A) L2
    (B) L5
    (C) S2
    (D) S5

251. Which foramen connects the third ventricle to the fourth ventricle?

    (A) foramen of Monro
    (B) foramen of Luschka
    (C) foramen of Magendie
    (D) cerebral aqueduct

252. The two anterior recesses on the third ventricle are the

    (A) supraoptic and pineal recess
    (B) pineal and infundibular recess
    (C) infundibular and suprapineal recess
    (D) supraoptic and infundibular

253. Microcephaly is *not* associated with which of the following?

    (A) diverticulosis
    (B) craniosynostosis
    (C) Meckel–Gruber's syndrome
    (D) chromosomal abnormalities
    (E) exposure to environmental teratogens

254. The two posterior recesses on the third ventricle are

    (A) preoptic and pineal recesses
    (B) pineal and infundibular recesses
    (C) infundibular and suprapineal recesses
    (D) pineal and suprapineal recesses

255. Another name for massa intermedia is

    (A) interthalamic adhesion
    (B) pineal recess
    (C) preoptic recess
    (D) infundibular recess

256. Which structure is *not* a partition of the dura mater?

    (A) falx cerebelli
    (B) falx cerebri
    (C) tentorium
    (D) cerebellum

257. Bleeding within the cerebral parenchyma is called

    (A) subdural hematoma
    (B) intraparenchymal hemorrhage
    (C) cerebellar hemorrhage
    (D) subarachnoid hematoma

258. Another name for the foramen of Monro is the

    (A) interventricular foramen
    (B) cerebral aqueduct
    (C) foramen of Luschka
    (D) foramen of Magendie

259. Which of the following is *not* part of the brainstem?

    (A) spinal cord
    (B) diencephalon
    (C) midbrain
    (D) pons

260. Midline facial anomalies are often associated with holoprosencephaly. These malformations do *not* include which of the following?

    (A) cebocephaly
    (B) cleft palate
    (C) hypoplasia of the ethmoid bone
    (D) cyclopia
    (E) meningomyelocele

261. The meninges covers the brain and spinal cord. Which of the following is *not* one of its layers?

    (A) dura mater
    (B) white matter
    (C) arachnoid membrane
    (D) pia mater

262. Which of the following is *not* an etiology of an arachnoid cyst?

    (A) abnormal mechanism of leptomeningeal formation
    (B) entrapment of subarachnoid space by adhesions
    (C) entrapment of cisternal space by adhesions
    (D) failure of development of the cerebral mantle

263. Which of the following does *not* occur as a result of a vein of Galen aneurysm?

    (A) cardiac failure
    (B) hydrocephalus
    (C) enlarged aorta
    (D) quadrigeminal cyst

264. Which of the following does *not* apply to an arachnoid cyst?

 (A) arachnoid cysts lie between the pia mater and the subarachnoid space.

 (B) arachnoid cysts do not communicate with the ventricles or the arachnoid space.

 (C) arachnoid cysts contain cerebrospinal fluid.

 (D) arachnoid cysts are usually found in the Sylvian fissure, middle fossa, and interhemispheric fissure.

 (E) arachnoid cysts are usually congenital and acquired.

265. Which of the following statements is true about the arachnoid granulations?

 (A) arachnoid granulations lie in the cingulate sulcus.

 (B) arachnoid granulations lie in the pericallosal artery where cerebrospinal fluid is reabsorbed by the blood.

 (C) arachnoid granulations lie in the sagittal sinus and reabsorb cerebrospinal fluid as it circulates.

 (D) arachnoid granulations lie in the ventricular system and reabsorb cerebrospinal fluid as it circulates.

266. Which of the following is *not* a characteristic of schizencephaly?

 (A) absent corpus callosum

 (B) absent septum pellucidum

 (C) unusually shaped ventricle

 (D) dilated septum pellucidum

267. Eight out of 12 neonates with meningitis usually develop which of the following conditions?

 (A) ventriculitis

 (B) intracranial hemorrhage

 (C) abscess

 (D) encephalomalacia

268. Early scans of a preterm infant brain that has periventricular leukomalacia would reveal which of the following findings?

 (A) increased echogenicity at the external angle of the lateral ventricles

 (B) normal echogenicity surrounding the lateral ventricles

 (C) cysts varying from a few small ones to multiple variably sized ones

 (D) markedly decreased vascular pulsations

269. Which of the following arteries is the main nutrient vessel of the subependymal germinal matrix tissue?

 (A) pericallosal artery

 (B) callosal marginal artery

 (C) posterior cerebral artery

 (D) Heubner's artery

270. The most common infections acquired in utero are toxoplasmosis, rubella, cytomegalovirus, and herpes simplex, which is referred to as which of the following terms?

 (A) TORCH

 (B) histogenesis

 (C) cytogenesis

 (D) organogenesis

271. Periventricular leukomalacia (PVL) is a result of infarction in the arterial boundary zones also known as which of the following?

 (A) cervical circulation

 (B) watershed circulation regions

 (C) ventriculofugal artery region

 (D) ventriculopetal parenchymal artery region

272. There are four grades of intracranial hemorrhage. What grade of hemorrhage is demonstrated on the coronal and sagittal sonograms in Figs. 15–59 A and B?

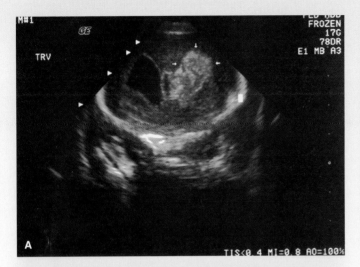

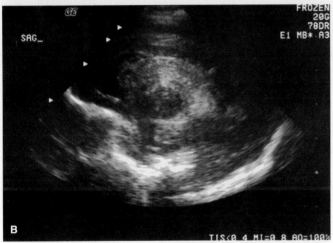

FIGURE 15–59. (A) Coronal sonogram. (B) Sagittal sonogram.

(A) Grade 4
(B) Grade 1
(C) Grade 3
(D) Grade 2

273. Which statement best explains the extent of the intracranial hemorrhage shown in Figs. 15–59 A and B?

(A) an intraparenchymal hemorrhage only is present.
(B) parenchymal and germinal matrix hemorrhages are present.
(C) germinal matrix, and intraventricular hemorrhages are present.
(D) only intraventricular hemorrhage is present.

274. The sonogram shown in Fig. 15–60 was taken from a premature neonate. The sonographic findings demonstrate which of the following findings?

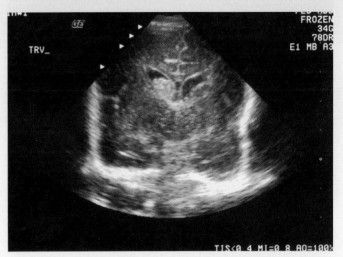

FIGURE 15–60. Coronal sonogram.

(A) lipoma
(B) bilateral germinal matrix hemorrhage
(C) unilateral germinal matrix hemorrhage
(D) none of the above

275. Which of the following is indicated by the abnormal sonographic findings shown in Fig. 15–61?

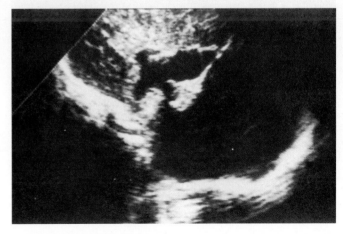

FIGURE 15–61. Midsagittal sonogram.

(A) a Dandy–Walker cyst
(B) dilatation of the fourth ventricle because of obstruction at the foramen of Magendie
(C) atresia of the foramen of Magendie
(D) none of the above

276. What do the arrows in Fig. 15–62 point to?

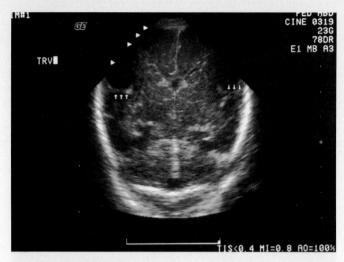

FIGURE 15–62. Coronal sonogram.

(A) choroidal fissure

(B) Sylvian fissure

(C) fissure of Rolando

(D) none of the above

277. What do the arrows in Fig. 15–63 point to?

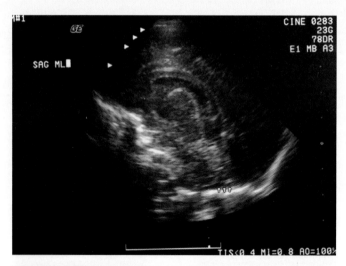

FIGURE 15–63. Sagittal sonogram.

(A) cisterna magna

(B) vein of Galen

(C) vermi of the cerebellum

(D) none of the above

278. The sonograms shown in Figs. 15–64 A and B were taken from a 4-week-old premature neonate. What are the abnormal findings?

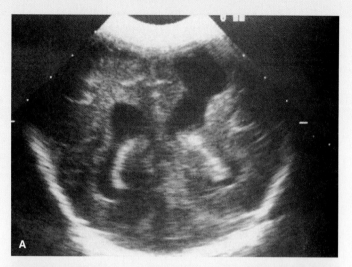

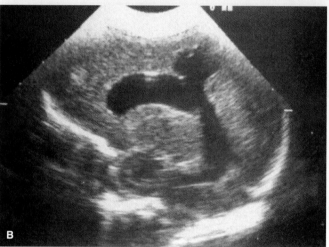

FIGURE 15–64. (**A**) Coronal sonogram. (**B**) Parasagittal sonogram.

(A) arachnoid cyst

(B) enlarged ventricles and an area of porencephaly in the posterior horn of the right lateral ventricle

(C) enlarged ventricles with an area of porencephaly at the region of the body of the left lateral ventricle

(D) isolated porencephalic cyst

279. The abnormal findings in Figs. 15–64 A and B are the result of which of the following?

(A) isolated germinal matrix hemorrhage

(B) resolving intraparenchymal and intraventricular hemorrhages

(C) subarachnoid hemorrhage

(D) none of the above

280. The sonograms shown in Figs. 15–65 A and B were taken from a 1-month-old premature infant. What are the abnormal findings?

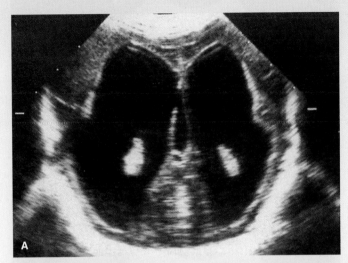

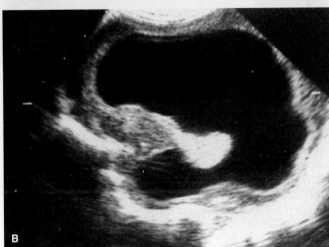

FIGURE 15–65. (A) Coronal sonogram. (B) Parasagittal sonogram.

(A) lobar holoprosencephaly

(B) alobar holoprosencephaly

(C) hydrocephalus

(D) Dandy–Walker cyst

281. What are the bilateral echogenic structures seen in the sonolucent cavities in the coronal view in Figs. 15–65 A and B?

(A) clots

(B) choroid plexus

(C) ethmoid and sphenoid bones

(D) bilateral lipomas

282. The sonogram shown in Fig. 15–66 is a mid-sagittal view of the head of a 1-month-old infant. Which of the following statements best describes the abnormal findings?

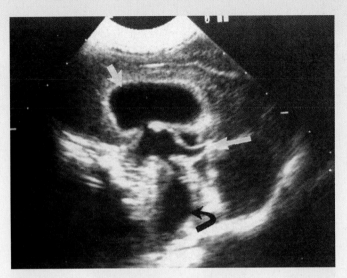

FIGURE 15–66. Midsagittal sonogram.

(A) an enlarged cavum septum pellucidum, enlarged third and fourth ventricles, a dilated foramen of Monro, dilated aqueduct of Sylvius

(B) an enlarged lateral ventricle, an enlarged third ventricle, an enlarged fourth ventricle, a dilated foramen of Monro, and a dilated aqueduct of Sylvius

(C) all abnormalities in (A) plus a posterior fossa cyst

(D) a dilated cavum septum pellucidum only

283. Which of the following structures is the long straight arrow pointing to in Fig. 15–66?

(A) foramen of Monro

(B) supraoptic recess

(C) infundibular recess

(D) pineal recess

284. Identify the enlarged structure the curved black arrow is pointing to in Fig. 15–66.

(A) third ventricle

(B) fourth ventricle

(C) cerebrum

(D) quadrigeminal cistern

285. **Identify the structure the short arrow points to in Fig. 15–66 on the page.**

   (A) one of the lateral ventricles
   (B) cavum septi pellucidi
   (C) cisterna magna
   (D) a cyst in the interhemispheric fissure

286. **What are the two sonolucent areas the arrows point to in Fig. 15–67?**

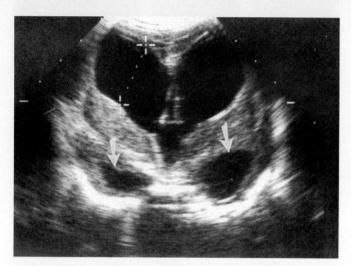

FIGURE 15–67. Coronal sonogram.

   (A) bilateral porencephalic cyst in the temporal lobes
   (B) porencephalic cyst in the frontal lobe
   (C) temporal horns of the lateral ventricles
   (D) frontal horns of the lateral ventricles

287. **What do the sonographic findings in Figs. 15–68 A and B suggest?**

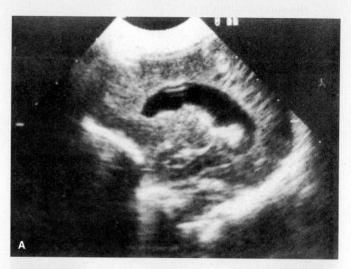

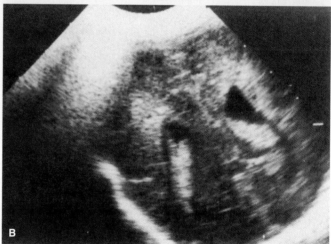

FIGURE 15–68. **(A)** Parasagittal sonogram. **(B)** Coronal sonogram.

   (A) subependymal hemorrhage
   (B) resolving intraventricular hemorrhage and periventricular leukomalacia
   (C) enlarged lateral ventricles
   (D) parenchymal hemorrhage with enlarged ventricles

288. Fig. 15–69 is a mid-sagittal sonogram of the head of a 2-month-old premature infant. The arrow is pointing to a slightly echogenic linear structure in the sonolucent cavity. What is this structure?

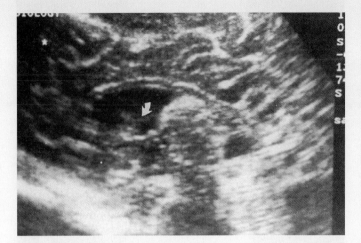

FIGURE 15–69. Midsagittal sonogram.

(A) septal vein
(B) anterior cerebral artery
(C) corpus callosum
(D) pericallosal artery

289. Fig. 15–70 is a sagittal sonogram taken from a 2-week premature neonate born at a gestational age of 31 weeks. What structure is the arrow pointing to?

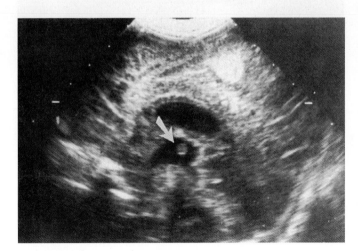

FIGURE 15–70. Sagittal sonogram.

(A) clot in the third ventricle
(B) massa intermedia
(C) interthalamic adhesion
(D) pericallosal artery
(E) both B and C

290. The sonograms in Fig. 15–71 were taken from a 3-week-old neonate born at a gestational age of 31 weeks. Which statement is *not* true of the abnormal findings?

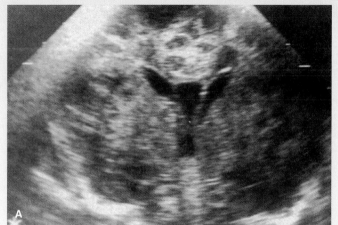

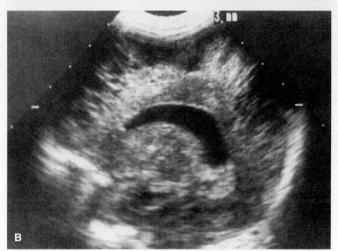

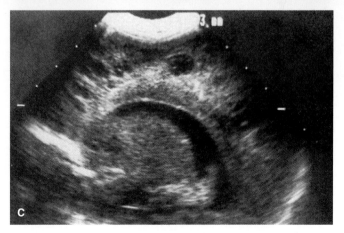

FIGURE 15–71. (A) Coronal sonogram. (B) Parasagittal sonogram. (C) Parasagittal sonogram.

(A) encephalomalacia
(B) diffuse hemorrhagic infarction
(C) periventricular leukomalacia
(D) enlarged ventricles

291. Fig. 15–72 is a magnified coronal sonogram from a full-term neonate with a history of persistent pulmonary hypertension. What is the incidental finding?

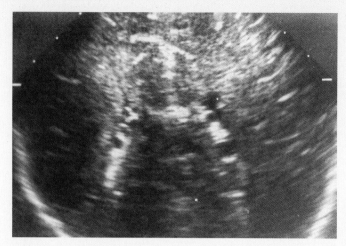

FIGURE 15–72. Coronal sonogram.

(A) arachnoid cysts
(B) multiple irregular-shaped cysts in the glomus part of the choroid plexus
(C) intraventricular hemorrhage
(D) porencephalic cysts

292. What do the bilateral sagittal cranial sonograms in Fig. 15–73 demonstrate?

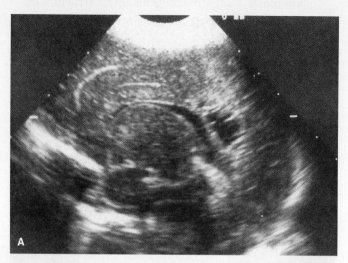

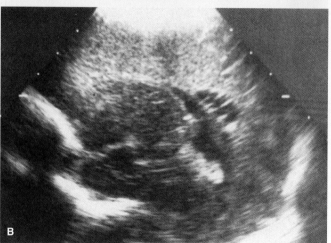

FIGURE 15–73. (**A**) Right parasagittal sonogram. (**B**) Left parasagittal sonogram.

(A) porencephalic cysts that communicate with the ventricles
(B) periventricular leukomalacia
(C) intraventricular hemorrhage
(D) both B and C

293. At what level of the lateral ventricle is the coronal sonogram in Fig. 15–74 taken?

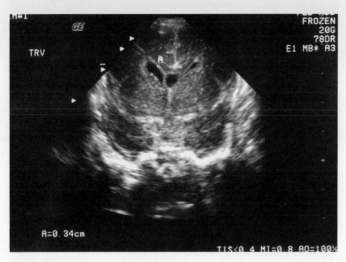

FIGURE 15–74. Coronal sonogram.

(A) occipital horns

(B) body

(C) frontal horns

(D) trigone region

294. Figs. 15–75 A–C were taken from a 2-day-old full-term neonate with abnormal chromosomes, kidneys, and upper and lower extremities. Which of the following are included in the abnormal intracranial findings?

(A) multiple small cysts within the lateral ventricles

(B) septated lateral ventricles

(C) septated cavum septi pellucidi

(D) bilateral porencephalic cysts in the frontal lobe of the cerebrum.

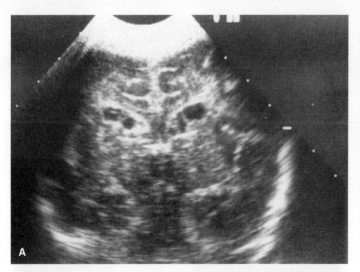

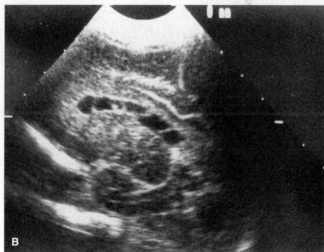

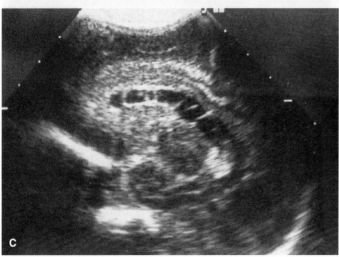

FIGURE 15–75. (A) Coronal sonogram. (B) Right parasagittal sonogram. (C) Left parasagittal sonogram.

295. The echogenic structure the straight arrow points to in Fig. 15–76 is the

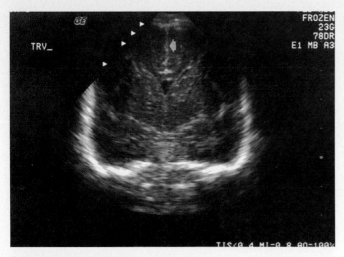

FIGURE 15–76. Coronal sonogram.

(A) interhemispheric fissure

(B) Sylvian fissure

(C) corpus callosum

(D) cingulate sulcus

296. The bilateral sonolucent structures the open arrows point to in Fig. 15–77 represent

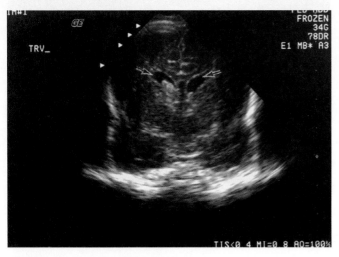

FIGURE 15–77. Coronal sonogram.

(A) trigone region of the lateral ventricles

(B) bodies of the lateral ventricle

(C) frontal horns of the lateral ventricle

(D) porencephalic cysts

297. The straight black arrow in Fig. 15–78 points to

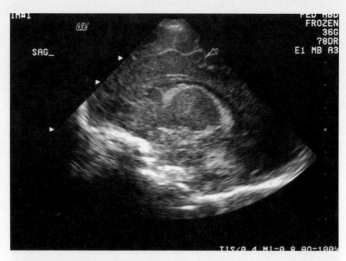

FIGURE 15–78. Sagittal sonogram.

(A) calcarine sulcus

(B) circular sulcus

(C) tentorium

(D) cingulate sulcus

298. The curved arrow in Fig. 15–79 points to

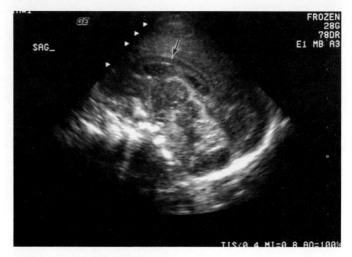

FIGURE 15–79. Midsagittal sonogram.

(A) corpus callosum

(B) interhemispheric fissure

(C) choroid plexus

(D) lateral ventricle

299. The straight arrow in Fig. 15–80 points to an echogenic line called the

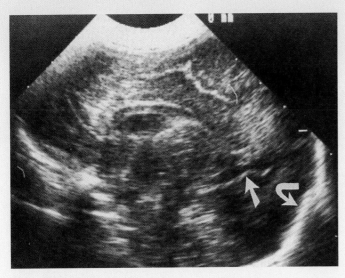

FIGURE 15–80. Sagittal sonogram.

    (A) callosal sulcus

    (B) central sulcus

    (C) parieto-occipital sulcus

    (D) cerebellar vermis

300. The highly echogenic structure that the curved arrow points to in Fig. 15–80 is the

    (A) frontal bone

    (B) temporal bone

    (C) occipital lobe of the cerebrum

    (D) occipital bone

301. A benign mass with areas of calcification and cyst formation in the brain, impinging on the ventricle causing obstructive hydrocephalus is

    (A) Grade 4 intracranial hemorrhage

    (B) Grade 3 intracranial hemorrhage

    (C) cytomegalovirus

    (D) teratoma

302. In adult transcranial Doppler, what is the most common window for scanning?

    (A) transtemporal

    (B) transforaminal

    (C) sphenoidal

    (D) frontal

    (E) both A and B

303. The resistive index for normal arterial Doppler flow in the brain is in which of the following ranges?

    (A) 0.50–0.57

    (B) 0.60–0.67

    (C) 0.70–0.75

    (D) 0.75–0.80

304. What is the most common intracranial artery affected by atherosclerotic disease?

    (A) posterior cerebral artery (PCA)

    (B) internal carotid artery (ICA)

    (C) anterior cerebral artery (ACA)

    (D) middle cerebral artery (MCA)

Answers and Explanations

At the end of each explained answer, there is a number combination in parentheses. The first number identifies the reference source; the second number or set of numbers indicates the page or pages on which the relevant information can be found.

Figure 15–45

1. **(M)** anterior fontanelle
2. **(G)** coronal suture
3. **(C)** parietal bone
4. **(N)** squamous suture
5. **(O)** lambdoidal suture
6. **(F)** occipital bone
7. **(A)** mastoidal fontanelle
8. **(K)** temporal bone
9. **(P)** zygomatic process
10. **(I)** zygomatic bone
11. **(L)** mandible
12. **(D)** maxilla
13. **(J)** nasal bone
14. **(B)** sphenoid fontanelle
15. **(H)** frontal bone
16. **(E)** orbit

Figure 15–46

17. **(B)** frontal bone
18. **(D)** anterior fontanelle
19. **(E)** parietal bone
20. **(C)** sagittal suture
21. **(F)** posterior fontanelle
22. **(A)** occipital bone

Figure 15–47

23. **(C)** pia mater
24. **(A)** dura mater
25. **(D)** superior sagittal sinus
26. **(H)** scalp
27. **(E)** arachnoid villus
28. **(I)** cranium

29. **(B)** subdural space
30. **(G)** subarachnoid space
31. **(F)** falx cerebri

Figure 15–48

32. **(C)** fissure of Rolando
33. **(E)** parietal lobe
34. **(D)** occipital lobe
35. **(F)** temporal lobe
36. **(B)** Sylvian fissure
37. **(A)** frontal lobe

Figure 15–49

38. **(J)** interthalamic adhesion (massa intermedia)
39. **(B)** thalamus
40. **(D)** pineal body
41. **(C)** cerebellum
42. **(K)** fourth ventricle
43. **(F)** spinal cord
44. **(I)** medulla oblongata
45. **(G)** cerebral peduncle
46. **(E)** pons
47. **(M)** temporal lobe
48. **(L)** third ventricle
49. **(H)** septum pellucidum
50. **(A)** corpus callosum

Figure 15–50

51. **(G)** fourth ventricle
52. **(E)** lateral recess
53. **(I)** posterior horn
54. **(F)** cerebral aqueduct
55. **(A)** third ventricle
56. **(D)** foramen of Monro
57. **(B)** anterior horn
58. **(C)** inferior horn
59. **(H)** atrium

Figure 15–51

60. **(L)** foramen of Magendie

61. **(N)** foramina of Luschka

62. **(I)** inferior horn

63. **(M)** cerebral aqueduct

64. **(E)** infundibular recess

65. **(O)** interthalamic adhesion

66. **(G)** preoptic recess

67. **(H)** anterior horn

68. **(C)** foramen of Monro

69. **(K)** suprapineal recess

70. **(B)** body of lateral ventricle

71. **(A)** pineal recess

72. **(F)** third ventricle

73. **(J)** collateral trigone

74. **(D)** posterior horn

Figure 15–52

75. **(D)** corpus callosum

76. **(C)** tela choroidea

77. **(F)** glomus of the choroid plexus

78. **(E)** choroid plexus of the fourth ventricle

79. **(B)** choroid plexus of the third ventricle

80. **(A)** caudate nucleus

Figure 15–53

81. **(C)** frontal and temporal horns

82. **(A)** foramina of Monro and third ventricle

83. **(D)** choroid plexus trigone

84. **(B)** posterior horn of lateral ventricle

Figure 15–54

85. **(C)** pons

86. **(B)** cerebral peduncle

87. **(J)** thalamus

88. **(E)** caudate nucleus

89. **(I)** column of fornix

90. **(A)** lateral ventricle

91. **(H)** sulcus

92. **(D)** corpus callosum

93. **(G)** Sylvian fissure

94. **(F)** hippocampus

Figure 15–55

95. **(C)** cerebellum

96. **(A)** cerebral aqueduct

97. **(B)** cerebellum peduncle

98. **(F)** cerebral peduncle

99. **(D)** hypothalamus

100. **(E)** gyrus and sulcus

Figure 15–56

101. **(J)** anterior spinal artery

102. **(G)** vertebral artery

103. **(K)** posterior inferior cerebellar artery

104. **(F)** anterior inferior cerebellar artery

105. **(L)** superior cerebellar artery

106. **(B)** posterior cerebral artery

107. **(C)** middle cerebral artery

108. **(E)** anterior cerebral artery

109. **(H)** anterior communicating artery

110. **(D)** internal carotid artery

111. **(I)** posterior communicating artery

112. **(A)** basilar artery

Figure 15–57

113. **(C)** vertebral artery

114. **(H)** medulla oblongata

115. **(G)** cerebellum

116. **(B)** posterior cerebral artery

117. **(F)** middle cerebral artery

118. **(E)** anterior cerebral artery

119. **(A)** internal carotid artery

120. **(D)** basilar artery

Figure 15–58

121. **(B)** middle cerebral artery

122. **(D)** anterior cerebral artery

123. **(C)** callosomarginal artery

124. **(A)** pericallosal artery

125. **(A)** Although all of the fontanelles and sutures can be used as an acoustic window to bypass the bone interface, the anterior and posterior fontanelles are used most frequently because of easy access to the paraventricular structures. (1:24, 25)

126. **(A)** periventricular calcifications. Infection of the fetal brain includes toxoplasmosis, other [congenital syphilis and viruses], rubella, cytomegalovirus, and herpes simplex virus. (TORCH). These infections are acquired in utero; however, the diagnoses are usually made in the neonatal-infant period. All TORCH symptoms are characterized by periventricular calcifications. (27:197)

127. **(B)** The anterolateral fontanelle. The sphenoidal fontanelles are positioned anatomically anterior and lateral. (5:345)

128. **(D)** 18 months. The anterior fontanelle is the largest fontanelle and is the last to close. (5:346)

129. **(D)** Posterolateral fontanelle. This is because the mastoidal fontanelles are positioned anatomically posterior and lateral. (5:345)

130. **(A)** They both diverge laterally as they project from the body of the lateral ventricles. The temporal horns (inferior horns) of the lateral ventricles are curved downward and extend laterally from the body of the ventricles. The tip of their inferior end extends around the posterior aspect of the thalamus. The occipital horns (posterior horns) of the lateral ventricles extend laterally from the body of the lateral ventricle and into the occipital lobe. (2:183; 8:29–31)

131. **(D)** The lateral ventricular width/hemispheric width ratio is obtained by measuring the distance from the middle of the falx cerebri (midline echo) to the lateral wall of the lateral ventricle and dividing this by the distance from the falx cerebri (midline echo) to the inner table of the skull. Both measurements are taken from the same image. (2:183; 27:64)

132. **(D)** External auditory meatus. The transducer is placed on the parietal bone above the ear. The tube-like passage in the ear is called the external auditory meatus. (1:29)

133. **(D)** It is a fetal structure. The germinal matrix cannot be depicted as a distinct structure by computed tomography or sonography. The germinal matrix is a structure of the fetus that begins early in gestation and regresses as pregnancy advances. By 32 weeks to term, it may be completely absent. The location of the germinal matrix is above the caudate nucleus in the subependymal region of the lateral ventricle. (2:183; 27:44)

134. **(A)** Above the caudate nucleus in the subependymal layer of the lateral ventricle. The germinal matrix forms the entire subependymal layer of the lateral ventricles in early gestation. After 24 weeks of gestation, the germinal matrix is present only over the head of the caudate nucleus. (2:183; 27:45)

135. **(D)** Echo-free space inferior to the cerebellum. The cisterna magna is anechoic (echo free) and normally can be relatively large. It is located inferior to the cerebellum and should not be confused with a cyst. (2:183; 27:186)

136. **(D)** Middle cerebral arteries. On real-time sonography, a dense echo representing the Sylvian fissure can be seen near the lateral aspect of the brain on most coronal scans. The identification of symmetric pulsation in this fissure is the result of the middle cerebral arteries. (1:95; 27:63)

137. **(A)** The fissure and sulci both appear echogenic. The normal premature brain has numerous echogenic sulci. The echogenicity is caused by normal vascular structures. The fissures and cisterns also are echogenic. (2:187; 27:121)

138. **(D)** The cavum septum pellucidum is located between the frontal horns of the lateral ventricles. (2:187; 27:42)

139. **(C)** The thalami

140. **(C)** An intraparenchymal hemorrhage. Most intraparenchymal hemorrhages appear as increased echogenicity in the brain parenchyma and occur as a result of a subependymal hemorrhage. (2:190; 27:126)

141. **(A)** An intraventricular hemorrhage. These hemorrhages present as high-density echoes in the ventricles. They may present with clots or high-density cerebrospinal fluid blood levels. These findings are more evident with change of head position. (27:123)

142. **(D)** Porencephaly. About 2–3 months after the hemorrhage, necrosis and phagocytosis are completed and an anechoic area termed porencephaly can be depicted (fourth stage). (2:190; 27:128)

143. **(D)** Pleural effusion is not among the many possible causes of intracranial hemorrhage. There are many possible causes of intracranial hemorrhage: maternal ingestion of aspirin, infantile pneumothorax, hypoxia, extrauterine stress, hyaline membrane disease, acidosis, ischemia, hypertension, and hypocarbia. (1:196; 7:100–107)

144. **(A)** a child during the first 28 days after birth (9:2)

145. **(A)** White matter surrounding the ventricles. This is the most common site for periventricular leukomalacia in premature infants. (9:85, 86)

146. **(D)** Tuberous sclerosis. Developmental brain defects in organogenesis are classified in different groups such as neural tube closure, diverticulation, neuronal proliferation and neuronal migration, organization, and myelination. Tuberous sclerosis is a disorder of histogenesis. (27:91–93)

147. **(D)** Intracranial hemorrhage. The term intraventricular hemorrhage was formerly used to refer to all types of cranial hemorrhage and caused some confusion in the terminology. The accepted term now is intracranial hemorrhage, which refers to any hemorrhage within the cranial vault. (8:209; 27:117)

148. **(C)** Intraventricular hemorrhage. This type of hemorrhage is presented as echogenic material within the ventricles. An echogenic clot or elevated levels of blood in the cerebrospinal fluid may be present with a gravitational effect. (27:123)

149. **(B)** Subependymal hemorrhage. This type of hemorrhage originates in the germinal matrix and for this reason is also called a germinal matrix hemorrhage. These hemorrhages present as highly echogenic foci in the region of the caudate nucleus. However, the most common site is the tela choroidea. (27:121)

150. **(A)** Intraparenchymal hemorrhage. This type of hemorrhage is present at first as a homogeneous, highly echogenic focus. However, as hemorrhagic resolution proceeds through its stages, a variety of heterogeneous sonographic appearances can be identified. (27:128)

151. **(D)** Choroid plexus hemorrhage. This type of hemorrhage can be difficult to diagnose because both the normal choroid plexus and a choroid plexus hemorrhage appear echogenic. However, a choroid plexus that is heterogeneous in texture, irregular in contour, and bulbous in the anterior region, with echogenic foci extending from the choroid plexus into the ventricle would strongly suggest hemorrhage. (8:209; 27:126)

152. **(D)** Subependymal germinal matrix hemorrhage is seen primarily in premature infants and is the most common in that age group. (27:121)

153. **(B)** 90°. Coronal scans should be performed at 90° from the orbitomeatal line (canthomeatal line), and the transducer should be angled to sweep from anterior to posterior. (1:49)

154. **(C)** The fontanelles are used as an acoustic window by allowing an opening through which ultrasound can travel with little or no obstruction to bypass bony interfaces. (10:15)

155. **(C)** Gonorrhea. The organisms associated most often with congenital infections of the nervous system are toxoplasmosis, other [congenital syphilis and viruses], rubella, cytomegalovirus, and herpes simplex virus (TORCH). Syphilis is associated but rare. Gonococcal infections are not among the organisms most often associated with congenital infections of the nervous system. (1:186; 27:197)

156. **(C)** The sonographic findings include: periventricular calcifications, ventricular enlargement, and a small head (microcephalus). (1:185; 27:197–199)

157. **(D)** An isolated subependymal hemorrhage. The grades are from Grade I to Grade IV. Grade I is an isolated subependymal germinal matrix hemorrhage. (8:210; 27:131)

158. **(A)** Cerebral aqueduct. The foramen or passage between the third and fourth ventricles also is known as the aqueduct of Sylvius. (8:217)

159. **(C)** Hydranencephaly is a congenital deformity characterized by severe loss of cerebral tissue. The falx, midbrain, basal ganglia, and cerebellum are intact. (8:191)

160. **(B)** Dysgenesis of the vermis of the cerebellum. Dandy-Walker cysts are associated with dysgenesis (defective development) of the cerebellar vermis. (8:191; 27:103)

161. **(B)** A ventriculoperitoneal (V-P) shunt. The purpose of a V-P shunt is to decrease the intraventricular pressure caused by hydrocephalus by shunting the fluid from the ventricle into the peritoneal cavity. (8:242, 246)

162. **(E)** A decrease in the size of the ventricles is not a sign of hydrocephalus. Hydrocephalus is dilatation of the ventricles caused by obstruction of cerebrospinal fluid. X-ray signs include skull bones halo sign and clinical signs include anterior fontanelle sinking, bulging of the frontal bone of the skull and rapid head growth. (9:221–312)

163. **(A)** Aqueductal stenosis. This condition also can be associated with other abnormalities. (8:224)

164. **(A)** Cephalohematomas. These are also called subperiosteal hematomas and refer to hemorrhages beneath the periosteum. (1:194)

165. **(A)** 40 weeks. Between the septum pellucidum is a fluid-filled cavity called the cavum septum pellucidum. The dorsal extension of the cavum septum pellucidum is called the cavum vergae. The fornix is the anatomic landmark dividing this single structure into two cavities. The cavum vergae is the first to start closure at about 24 weeks of gestation. The cavum septum pellucidum begins to close at term (40 weeks). (8:218; 27:42)

166. **(D)** Dandy-Walker syndrome is characterized by continuity of the fourth ventricle with a posterior fossa cyst and hydrocephalus. (8:191)

167. **(A)** Severe hydrocephalus. The differential diagnoses for hydranencephaly are severe hydrocephalus, alobar holoprosencephaly, and massive subdural effusions. (8:191; 27:86)

168. **(B)** Region of the Sylvian fissure and in the circle of Willis. The middle cerebral artery is the continuation of the internal carotid artery. (7:87; 27:63)

169. **(D)** Intraparenchymal hemorrhage. Extension of blood into the brain parenchyma is one of the most severe forms of hemorrhage. (7:101)

170. **(A)** The prosencephalon. During embryologic development, the brain vesicles form the forebrain or prosencephalon, the midbrain or mesencephalon, and the hindbrain or rhombencephalon. (13:370)

171. **(E)** External carotid arteries. The circle of Willis is formed by nine arteries: two posterior cerebral arteries (vertebral arteries), two anterior cerebral arteries, two internal carotid arteries, two posterior communicating arteries, and one anterior communicating artery. (15:12)

172. **(B)** The cerebrospinal fluid pathways within the brain are blocked. Hydrocephalus can be acquired or congenital. It is divided into noncommunicating or obstructive (blockage of cerebrospinal fluid within the brain) and communicating or nonobstructive (blockage of cerebrospinal fluid within the ventricular system). (16:1539)

173. **(A)** A congenital abnormality of the brain with elongation of the pons and fourth ventricle and downward displacement of the medulla into the cervical canal. The elongation of the pons is characterized by displacement of the fourth ventricle. *(27:95)*

174. **(D)** Two internal carotid and two vertebral arteries. These are the two main pairs of arteries that supply the brain with blood. *(15:8)*

175. **(B)** Basilar artery. The pons is the anatomic level at which the vertebral artery changes its name to the basilar artery. *(15:8)*

176. **(D)** Movement of extracellular fluid from blood. Only about 40% of cerebrospinal fluid is elaborated by the choroid plexus. The other 60% is produced by the movement of extracellular fluid from blood through the brain and ventricles. *(27:155)*

177. **(C)** Normal sized ventricles with no debris within them. The sonographic findings of ventriculitis include echogenic ventricular walls, septated ventricles, debris within the ventricles, and ventricular dilatation. *(20:83, 84, 91)*

178. **(C)** Eight. The skull is made up of one frontal bone, two parietal bones, two temporal bones, one occipital, sphenoid, and ethmoid each. *(39:190)*

179. **(A)** Subarachnoid hematoma. Below the arachnoid is the subarachnoid space, which is located between the arachnoid and pia mater. *(18:31)*

180. **(C)** 532–576 mL/day. In an adult, the amount of cerebrospinal fluid produced daily is between 600 and 700 mL. In the child, it is less. *(18:9; 27:156)*

181. **(C)** An epidural hematoma. The accumulation of blood between the dura mater and the inner table of the skull. *(1:194)*

182. **(C)** The inferior horn (cornu) *(18:29)*

183. **(A)** The temporal horn (cornu) *(18:29)*

184. **(B)** Cerebral hemispheres. They are paired brain matter separated from the midline by the falx cerebri. *(20:294)*

185. **(B)** Posterior to the foramen of Monro and superior to the third ventricle *(27:192)*

186. **(B)** Herpes Simples. Intracranial infections can be bacterial or viral

Bacterial	Viral
Diplococcus pneumoniae	toxoplasmosis
Haemophilus influenzae	mumps
Bacterial meningitis	cytomegalovirus
	Herpes simplex *(1:184)*

187. **(B)** The central fissure is also called central sulcus or fissure of Rolando. *(20:295)*

188. **(C)** The etiology of a porencephalic cyst is a subependymal hemorrhage that extends into the brain parenchyma, an infection, an infarction, or trauma. *(1:153; 27:186)*

189. **(B)** Subdural hematoma. The gyri and sulci of the brain are more prominent with a subdural hematoma and are usually obscured in intracranial infections, infarctions, and intracranial hemorrhages. *(27:209)*

190. **(B)** 24–32 weeks. The germinal matrix subsequently regresses in size and is absent at birth. *(1:196)*

191. **(D)** Cyclopia. This is a developmental anomaly, not a tumor. *(1:226)*

192. **(A)** Ischemic lesions of the neonatal brain characterized by necrosis of periventricular white matter. *(21:760)*

193. **(B)** Leukomalacia. The most common infections acquired in utero are toxoplasmosis, other [congenital syphilis and viruses], rubella, cytomegalovirus, and herpes simplex virus (TORCH). *(27:197)*

194. **(A)** Hypoxia and ischemic injuries account for the greatest number of fetal deaths. *(21:752)*

195. **(A)** Decrease in the size of the Sylvian fissure as the neonatal brain matures. Lissencephaly is characterized sonographically by large Sylvian fissures and ventricles. *(27:111)*

196. **(C)** Semi-Fowler's position. This position assists in drainage and prevents pressure on the site. *(28:89)*

197. **(B)** The tentorium. *(39:338)*

198. **(B)** Conus medullaris. The spinal cord is the distal continuation of the central nervous system. It terminates as the conus medullaris at the end of the second lumbar vertebrae. *(44:125)*

199. **(B)** Occipital horns. A change in shape without a change in size occurs first in the frontal horns. However, the occipital horns enlarge first, and the frontal horns enlarge last. *(27:158)*

200. **(A)** Frontal horns anterior to the foramen of Monro. The reason for this position is to avoid obstruction of the shunt tip by the choroid plexus. No choroid plexus extends into the frontal horns or the occipital horns of the lateral ventricle. *(27:166)*

201. **(B)** Enlarged septum pellucidum. In complete agenesis of the corpus callosum, there is no septum pellucidum or corpus callosum. In addition, the third ventricle undergoes upward displacement. *(27:105)*

202. **(A)** Septum pellucidum. In septo-optic dysplasia, schizencephaly, and agenesis of the corpus callosum, the septum pellucidum is absent. *(27:108)*

203. **(B)** Cause slowing of the heart. *(46:5)*

204. **(D)** Periventricular leukomalacia is softening of the white matter surrounding the ventricles. *(58:G8–G54)*

205. **(G)** Tentorium cerebelli is a transverse division of dura mater forming a partition between the occipital lobe of the cerebral hemispheres and the cerebellum. *(58:G8–G54)*

206. **(I)** Sulci are grooves on the surface of the brain separating the gyri. *(58:G8–G54)*

207. **(C)** The choroid plexus comprises special cells located in the ventricles that secrete cerebrospinal fluid. *(58:G8–G54)*

208. **(A)** Cisterna magna is an enclosed space located caudal to the cerebellum, between the cerebellum and the occipital bone, serving as a reservoir for cerebrospinal fluid. *(58:G8–G54)*

209. **(K)** The pia mater is the inner membrane covering the brain and spinal cord. *(58:G8–G54)*

210. **(F)** The corpus callosum is a group of nerve fibers above the third ventricle that connects the left and right sides of the brain. *(58:G8–G54)*

211. **(J)** Cavum septum pellucidum is a cavity filled with cerebrospinal fluid that lies between the anterior horns of the lateral ventricle. *(58:G8–G54)*

212. **(H)** Insula is a triangular area of cerebral cortex, lying deeply in the later cerebral fissure. *(58:G8–G54)*

213. **(B)** Gyri are folds on the surface of the brain. *(58:G8–G54)*

214. **(E)** Aqueduct stenosis is a congenital obstruction of the third and fourth ventricles resulting in ventricular dilation. *(58:G8–G54)*

215. **(H)** Foramen of Monro *(18:30)*

216. **(G)** Trigone *(8:216)*

217. **(F)** Germinal matrix hemorrhage *(1:198)*

218. **(E)** Pineal gland *(58:G42)*

219. **(D)** Occipital horn *(18:30)*

220. **(C)** Anterior horn *(18:30)*

221. **(B)** Temporal horn *(18:30)*

222. **(A)** Massa intermedia *(18:38)*

223. **(D)** 5–10 MHz. The continuous-wave Doppler transducer can either be flat or be a pencil probe with an ultrasonic frequency of 5–10 MHz. *(52:180)*

224. **(A)** Middle cerebral artery. This artery can be evaluated best through the cranial vault because the newborn skull has a single pliable bony layer without the dipole. *(54:499)*

225. **(A)** The peak height *(55:678)*

226. **(A)** The fact that infants with asphyxia have low pulsatility and high diastolic forward flow probably represents a decrease in resistance of the cerebrovascular system in response to the asphyxia. *(57:599)*

227. **(D)** The fact that infants with an intraventricular hemorrhage have high pulsatility indexes and extremely low

diastolic forward flow may represent an increase in resistance in response to the hemorrhage. *(57:599)*

228. **(A)** Premature fusion of the cranial sutures. The prefix cranio relates to the cranium or skull. The suffix synostosis pertains to closure of the sutures. *(27:83)*

229. **(D)** Low temperature. Hypothermia (lowered body temperature) is defined as the reduction of body temperature below 35°C or 95°F. The clinically dramatic consequences of keeping a neonate in a cold environment, such as an air-conditioned ultrasound room could result in shivering and lowered body temperature. *(26:643, 716)*

230. **(C)** 2–3 years. The parietal bones are relatively thin when compared with other cranial bones; therefore, measurements can be obtained up to 2–3 years after birth. *(2:180)*

231. **(D)** Linear array real-time transducer produces a rectangular image. This type of transducer can be used to image the infant's brain. However, in visualizing the neonatal brain, it is limited because of the small size of the fontanelle compared to the size of the transducer. In addition, the rectangular image produced by linear array real-time fails on many occasions to visualize the inner walls of both sides of the calvarium simultaneously. *(2:180–199)*

232. **(A)** Axial. The sagittal and coronal CT views are useful but subject to artifacts; therefore, the axial plane is most compatible with sonography. *(1:24)*

233. **(A)** Tela choroidea. The point at which the choroid attaches to the floor of the lateral ventricles is located behind the foramen of Monro. *(2:187; 27:121)*

234. **(D)** Cavum vergae. The cava septi pellucidi and vergae lie between the frontal horns and bodies of the two lateral ventricles. The fornix divides the cavum septi pellucidi anteriorly and the cavum septum posteriorly. *(2:187; 27:42)*

235. **(D)** 67%. The incidence of germinal matrix hemorrhage varies with age. At 28 weeks, approximately two-thirds of fetuses have such hemorrhages. *(27:135)*

236. **(A)** Same density. The term isodense denotes "same density" as soft tissue. This term is used in computed tomography (CT). A hemorrhage, for example is presented as high density on CT and can become isodense after 5–10 days. *(22; 27:117–119)*

237. **(F)** All of the above. All of the given choices are associated with intracranial hemorrhage. *(7:100–107)*

238. **(A)** From 29 days after birth to 1 year *(9:2)*

239. **(D)** This imaginary line is called the orbitomeatal line, a radiographic baseline, or the canthomeatal line. The Reid's baseline is an imaginary line drawn from the infraorbital rim to the external auditory meatus. *(12:86)*

240. **(A)** 150° from the orbitomeatal line and perpendicular to the clivus. The transducer should be positioned over the

posterior fontanelle and should sweep anterior at 5 mm intervals. *(1:51)*

241. **(C)** An intracranial hemorrhage because no choroid extends into this area. There is no choroid plexus in either the frontal or occipital horn. *(27:44, 166)*

242. **(E)** A single midline ventricle is characteristic of holoprosencephaly not hydranencephaly. The brainstem and a portion of the occipital lobe remain in hydranencephaly. It is a congenital deformity characterized by a fluid-filled head with massive disruption of the cerebral hemispheres. The falx cerebri, cerebellum, and basal ganglia are usually intact. *(8:191; 27:84)*

243. **(A)** Above the corpus callosum. The pericallosal artery is the terminal branch of the anterior cerebral artery. It courses over the superior margin of the corpus callosum. *(8:218)*

244. **(D)** Two weeks. Hydrocephalus occurs first, followed by an increased head circumference approximately 14 days later. *(7:25)*

245. **(A)** every 3 days until 2 weeks of age *(7:117)*

246. **(B)** The choroid plexus nearly fills the entire volume of the lateral ventricles in the first trimester. *(27:74)*

247. **(D)** A head that is largely filled with fluid and a severe loss of cerebral tissue. This congenital deformity of the head is characterized by complete or almost complete absence of the cerebral hemispheres. *(1:152; 8:191)*

248. **(E)** Holoprosencephaly is a developmental abnormality characterized by a single large midline ventricle and diverticulation of the forebrain. A premature fusion of the cranial sutures wither complete or partial is characteristic of craniosynostosis. *(8:191, 192)*

249. **(D)** There are 12 pairs of cranial nerves and 31 pairs of spinal nerves. *(15:4)*

250. **(A)** L2. The spinal cord is shorter than the vertebral column and ends at about the second lumbar vertebra. *(15:4)*

251. **(D)** The cerebral aqueduct. This is also called the aqueduct of Sylvius. *(27:40)*

252. **(D)** The supraoptic recess also called the preoptic recess and the infundibular recess, which lies below the supraoptic recess. *(8:38)*

253. **(A)** Diverticulations are not associated with microcephaly. Microcephaly is associated with Meckel–Gruber syndrome, chromosomal abnormalities, rubella, toxoplasmosis, craniosynostosis, and exposure to environmental teratogens such as radiation. *(27:84, 85)*

254. **(D)** The two posterior recesses on the third ventricle are the pineal recess and suprapineal recesses. *(8:217)*

255. **(A)** Interthalamic adhesion. The place of fusion on the medial surfaces of the thalami on both sides of the third ventricle is called a massa intermedia or an interthalamic adhesion. *(18:38)*

256. **(D)** The cerebellum is not a partition of the dura mater. *(39:338)*

257. **(B)** An intraparenchymal hemorrhage. Any hemorrhage into the brain parenchyma is called intraparenchymal hemorrhage. *(8:209–215)*

258. **(A)** Intraventricular foramen. *(18:29)*

259. **(A)** Spinal cord. The brainstem consists of the diencephalon, the midbrain, the pons, and the medulla oblongata. *(39:357)*

260. **(E)** Meningomyelocele is not associated with holoprosencephaly facial anomalies. The facial anomalies that can be associated with holoprosencephaly are cleft palate(fissure), cleft lip (fissure), cyclopia (single orbital fossa), cebocephaly (characterized by a defective nose and closed eyes), and ethmocephaly (characterized by a defect of the ethmoid bone. *(1:174)*

261. **(B)** The brain is invested by three membranes termed PAD for pia, arachnoid, and dura mater. *(18:1–4)*

262. **(D)** The causes of an arachnoid cyst are arachnoid lesions, entrapment of subarachnoid or cisternal space, and abnormal leptomeningeal formation. *(1:153)*

263. **(D)** A quadrigeminal cyst is not caused by a vein of Galen aneurysm. However, it may be a differential diagnosis because of its location and cystic components. Doppler evaluation should exclude a differential diagnosis. *(27:192)*

264. **(A)** Arachnoid cysts lie between the arachnoid membrane and the dura mater and not between the pia mater and the subarachnoid space. Acquired arachnoid cysts are found in cisterns adjacent to the third ventricle, sella, and posterior fossa. *(27:87, 188, 189)*

265. **(C)** Arachnoid granulations in the sagittal sinus and reabsorb cerebrospinal fluid as it circulates. *(27:155, 156)*

266. **(D)** A dilated septum pellucidum is not a characteristic of schizencephaly. It is characterized by agenesis of the corpus callosum and septum pellucidum in addition to unusually shaped frontal horns of the lateral ventricles. *(27:112)*

267. **(A)** Ventriculitis. These neonates initially develop meningitis, edema, and cerebritis. Eight of 12 neonates with meningitis develop ventriculitis. Late complications include subdural effusion, enlarged ventricles, and ventricular septations. *(27:199)*

268. **(A)** Increased echogenicity at the external angle of the lateral ventricles. Ischemic lesions may occur at the watershed boundary zones of the periventricular white matter and the centrum semiovale as periventricular leukomalacia. *(50:61)*

269. **(D)** Heubner's artery. This is the main nutrient vessel of the subependymal germinal tissue, which is destined to

give rise to much of the glial cell population of the hemisphere. *(49:183)*

270. **(A)** TORCH is the acronym for the most common infections acquired in utero: toxoplasmosis, other [congenital syphilis and viruses], rubella, cytomegalovirus, and herpes simplex virus. *(27:197)*

271. **(B)** In the premature infant, the watershed zones are located in the periventricular white matter adjacent to the external margins of the lateral ventricles. The zones lie approximately 3–10 mm from the ventricular wall. *(27:28)*

272. **(A)** Grade 4 hemorrhage *(27:133)*

273. **(C)** Germinal matrix and intraventricular hemorrhages *(27:133)*

274. **(C)** Unilateral germinal matrix hemorrhage *(27:125)*

275. **(A)** Dandy–Walker cyst *(34:73)*

276. **(B)** Sylvian fissure *(36:821)*

277. **(A)** Cistern magna *(36:821)*

278. **(C)** Enlarged ventricles with an area of porencephaly at the region of the body of the left lateral ventricle *(27:128, 129)*

279. **(B)** Resolving intraparenchymal and intraventricular hemorrhages. The irregularity noted in the choroid plexus region is a sign of intraventricular hemorrhage. *(27:133)*

280. **(C)** Hydrocephalus. The abnormal finding is a severe form of post-hemorrhagic hydrocephalus. *(40:111, 117)*

281. **(B)** Choroid plexus *(20:37)*

282. **(B)** The abnormal findings in Fig. 15–66 revealed an enlarged lateral ventricle, an enlarged third ventricle, an enlarged fourth ventricle, a dilated foramen of Monro, and a dilated aqueduct of Sylvius. *(27:164)*

283. **(D)** Pineal recess. The recess is dilated. The recesses of the third ventricle are as follows: supraoptic, infundibular, pineal, and suprapineal. *(27:40, 41, 44)*

284. **(B)** fourth ventricle *(27:164)*

285. **(A)** One of the lateral ventricles. The ventricle is enlarged. *(41:129)*

286. **(C)** Temporal horns of the lateral ventricles. Both are enlarged. *(41:128)*

287. **(B and C)** A resolving intraventricular hemorrhage and periventricular leukomalacia. The lateral ventricles are enlarged, and small cystic areas are seen in the periventricular regions. *(40:120)*

288. **(A)** Septal vein *(38:623)*

289. **(E)** Massa intermedia. The massa intermedia or interthalamic adhesion, is visualized best in the presence of ventricular dilatation. *(27:41; 40:89)*

290. **(C)** Periventricular leukomalacia. This neonate may have had a generalized cerebral edema that led to multiple areas of infarction termed encephalomalacia or porencephaly. *(27:213)*

291. **(B)** Multiple irregular-shaped cysts in the glomus part of the choroid plexus. A study done with fetuses that had simple choroid plexus cysts revealed a normal karyotype and no significant related abnormalities. Babies were delivered with no neurological abnormalities at the time of the neonatal examination. However, a study involving complex choroid plexus cysts revealed trisomies 18 and 21. *(43:78, 81)*

292. **(D)** (B and C.) The abnormality demonstrated is bilateral periventricular leukomalacia and intraventricular hemorrhage. *(40:12)*

293. **(C)** Frontal horns *(27:17)*

294. **(B)** Septated lateral ventricles. In these sonograms, multiple partitions are seen extending to the lateral walls of the ventricles. This particular case is congenital; however, septated ventricles usually occur in ventriculitis. *(40:83)*

295. **(A)** Interhemispheric fissure. The structure is shown in the coronal view. *(40:34, 36)*

296. **(C)** Frontal horns of the lateral ventricle. The horns are slightly dilated with a unilateral subependymal hemorrhage. *(40:39)*

297. **(D)** Cingulate sulcus *(40:45)*

298. **(A)** Corpus callosum *(40:45)*

299. **(C)** Parieto-occipital sulcus *(40:45)*

300. **(D)** Occipital bone *(41:14)*

301. **(D)** Teratoma *(Study Guide; 27:179)*

302. **(E)** Transtemporal and transforaminal windows *(61:1037)*

303. **(A)** 0.50–0.57. Blood flow in the brain has a low resistive index. *(61:1037)*

304. **(D)** Middle cerebral artery is most commonly affected by atherosclerotic disease. *(61:1040)*

References

1. Babcock DS, Han BK. *Cranial Ultrasonography of Infants.* Baltimore: Williams & Wilkins; 1981.

2. Winsberg F, Cooperberg PL. Real-time ultrasonography: clinics in diagnostic ultrasound. In: Rumack CM, Johnson ML, eds. *Real-Time Ultrasound Evaluation of the Neonatal Brain.* Vol. 10. New York: Churchill Livingstone; 1982.

3. King DL, William McK. *Diagnostic Ultrasound.* St. Louis: CV Mosby; 1974.

4. Ora BA, Eddy L, Hatch G, Solida B, et al. The anterior fontanelle as an acoustic window to the neonatal ventricular system. *J Clin Ultrasound.* 1980; 8:65-67.

5. Williams PL, Warwick R. *Gray's Anatomy.* 36th ed. Philadelphia: WB Saunders; 1980.

6. Bartrum RJ, Crow HC. *Real-time Ultrasound: A Manual for Physicians and Technical Personnel.* Philadelphia: WB Saunders; 1983.

7. Sanders RC, Thomas LS. *Ultrasound Annual.* New York: Raven Press; 1982.

8. Howard WR, William JZ, Babcock DS, et al. *Seminars in Ultrasound.* Vol. 3, No. 3. New York: Grune & Stratton; 1982.

9. Fenichel GM. *Neonatal Neurology.* Vol. 2. New York: Churchill Livingstone; 1980.

10. Haller JO, Shkolnik A, Slovis T. *Clinics in Diagnostic Ultrasound, Vol. 8: Ultrasound Pediatrics.* New York: Churchill Livingstone; 1981.

11. Helen LB, Sandra KM. *The Developing Person: A Life Span Approach.* San Francisco: Harper & Row; 1980.

12. Mallet M. *A Handbook of Anatomy and Physiology for Student X-ray Technicians.* 4th ed. Chicago: American Society of Radiologic Technologists; 1962.

13. Hagen-Ansert S. *Textbook of Diagnostic Ultrasound.* 2nd ed. St. Louis: CV Mosby; 1983.

14. William M. *The American Heritage Dictionary of the English Language.* New York: American Heritage, 1971.

15. Goldberg S. *Clinical Neuroanatomy Made Ridiculously Simple.* Miami: Med Master; 1979.

16. Robbins S, Cortran R. *Pathologic Basis of Disease.* 2 ed. Philadelphia: WB Saunders; 1979.

17. Sutton D. *A Textbook of Radiology and Imaging.* Vol. 2, 3rd ed. New York: Churchill Livingstone; 1980.

18. Carpenter M. *Core Text of Neuroanatomy.* 2nd ed. Baltimore: Williams & Wilkins; 1978.

19. Farmer T. *Pediatric Neurology.* 3rd ed. Philadelphia: Harper & Row; 1983.

20. Hole J Jr. *Human Anatomy and Physiology.* 3rd ed. Dubuque, IA: Wm C Brown; 1984.

21. Gordon BA. *Neonatology, Pathophysiology and Management of the Newborn.* Philadelphia: JB Lippincott; 1975.

22. *Dorland's Illustrated Medical Dictionary.* 26 ed. Philadelphia: WB Saunders; 1981.

23. Schaffer AJ, Avery ME. *Diseases of the Newborn.* 4th ed. Philadelphia: WB Saunders; 1977.

24. Waechter EH, Blake FG. *Nursing Care of Children.* 9th ed. Philadelphia: JB Lippincott; 1976.

25. Hellman LM, Pritchard J, Wynn RM. *Obstetrics.* 14th ed. New York: Appleton-Century-Crofts; 1971.

26. Danforth DN. *Textbook of Obstetrics and Gynecology.* 2nd ed. New York: Harper & Row; 1971.

27. Rumack CM, Johnson MI. *Perinatal and Infant Brain Imaging: Role of Ultrasound and Computed Tomography.* Chicago: Year Book; 1984.

28. Thompson DE. *Pediatric Nursing: An Introductory Text.* 4th ed. Philadelphia: WB Saunders; 1981.

29. Marlow RD. *Textbook of Pediatric Nursing.* 5th ed. Philadelphia: WB Saunders; 1977.

30. Hafen QB, Karren JK. *Prehospital Emergency Care and Crisis Intervention.* 2nd ed. Englewood, CO: Morton; 1983.

31. Fleischer AC, James AE. *Real-time Sonography: Textbook with Accompanying Videotape.* Norwalk, CT: Appleton-Century-Crofts; 1985.

32. Rubin J. Intraoperative ultrasonography of the spine. *Am J Radiol.* 1983; 146:173-176.

33. Grant E, Kerner M, Schellinger D. Evaluation of porencephalic cyst from intraparenchymal hemorrhage in neonates: Sonographic correlation. *Am J Radiol.* 1982;138:467.

34. Grant E, Schellinger D, Richardson J. Real-time ultrasonography of the posterior fossa. *J Ultrasound Med.* 1983; 2:73.

35. Taylor KWJ. Atlas of ultrasonography. In: Mannes E, Sivo J, eds. *The Neonatal Head.* Vol. 1, 2nd ed. New York: Churchill Livingstone; 1984.

36. Shuman W, Rogers J, Mack L. Real-time sonographic sector scanning of the neonatal cranium: technique and normal anatomy. *AJNR Am J Roentgenol.* 1981; 2:349-356.

37. Babcock D, Ball W Jr. Postasphyxial encephalopathy in full-term infants: Ultrasound diagnosis. *Am J Radiol.* 1983;148:417-423.

38. Goldstein R, Filly R, et al. Septal veins: A normal finding on neonatal sonography. *Am J Radiol.* 1986; 161:623-624.

39. Hole JW Jr. *Human Anatomy and Physiology.* 3rd ed. Dubuque, IA: Wm C Brown; 1984.

40. Naidich TP, Quencer RM, eds. *Clinical Neurosonography: Ultrasound of the Central Nervous System.* New York: Springer-Verlag; 1986.

41. Levene M, Williams J, Fawer CL. *Ultrasound of the Infant Brain.* London: Spastics International Medical Publications, and Philadelphia: JB Lippincott; 1985.

42. *Dorland's Illustrated Medical Dictionary.* 26th ed. Philadelphia: WB Saunders; 1985.

43. Hertzberg S, Kay HH, Bowie JD. Fetal choroid plexus lesions. *J Ultrasound Med.* 1989;8.

44. Kapit W, Elson LM. *The Anatomy Coloring Book.* New York: Harper & Row; 1977.

45. Sanders RC. *Clinical Sonography: A Practical Guide.* Boston: Little, Brown; 1984.

46. Martin J. *Ultrasound Technology Series. Cranial Sonography in Infants: Technicare Ultrasound.* New Brunswick, NJ: Johnson & Johnson; 1983.

47. Pilu P, Louis P, Roberto R, et al. The fetal subarachnoid cisterns: an ultrasound study with report of a case of congenital communicating hydrocephalus. *J Ultrasound Med.* 1986; 5.

48. Bowerman RA, Zwischenberger JB, Andrews AF, et al. Cranial sonography of the infant treated with extracorporeal membrane oxygenation. *Am J Radiol.* 1985;145.

49. Wigglesworth JS, Pape KE. An integrated model for haemorrhage and ischaemic lesions in the newborn brain: Early human development. *Early Human Dev.* 1978; 2(2):179-199.

50. Manger MN, Feldman RC, Brown WJ, et al. Intracranial ultrasound diagnosis of neonatal periventricular leukomalacia. *J Ultrasound Med.* 1984; 3:59-63.

51. Christtenen RA, Pinckney LE, Higgins S, et al. Sonographic diagnosis of lipoma of the corpus callosum. *J Ultrasound Med.* 1987; 6:449-451.

52. Perlman JM. Neonatal cerebral blood flow velocity measurement. *Clin Perinatol.* 1985; 12:179-193.

53. Bada HS, Fitch CW. Uses of transcutaneous Doppler ultrasound technique in newborn infants. *Perinatol Neonatol.* 1983; 7:27-35.

54. Raju TNK, Zikos E. Regional cerebral blood velocity in infants: a real time transcranial and fontanellar pulsed Doppler study. *J Ultrasound Med.* 1987; 6:497-507.

55. Gray PH, et al. Continuous wave Doppler ultrasound in evaluation of cerebral blood flow in neonates. *Arch Dis Child.* 1983; 58:677-681.

56. Grant EG, White EM, Schellinger D, et al. Cranial Doppler sonography of the infant. *Radiology.* 1987; 163:177-185.

57. Miles RD, Menice JA, Bashiru M, et al. Relationships of five Doppler measures with flow in vitro model and clinical findings in newborn infants. *J Ultrasound Med.* 1987; 6(10):597-599.

58. Tortora GJ, Anagnostakos NP. *Principles of Anatomy and Physiology.* 6th ed. New York: Harper & Row; 1990.

59. Olds SB, London ML, Ladewig PA. *Maternal-Newborn Nursing: A Family-Centered Approach.* 3th ed. Menlo Park, CA: Addison-Wesley; 1988.

60. Williams PL, Warwick R, Dyson M, et al., eds. *Gray's Anatomy.* 37th ed. New York: Churchill Livingstone; 1989.

61. McGahan JP, Goldberg BB. *Diagnostic Ultrasound: A Logical Approach.* Philadelphia, New York: Lippincott–Raven; 1998: 1140-1141.

Musculoskeletal Ultrasound

Amy E. Wilkinson and Ronald S. Adler

Study Guide

INTRODUCTION

While magnetic resonance imaging (MRI) has been the mainstay of imaging of the soft tissue framework of the musculoskeletal system in the United States,[1] ultrasound provides several distinct advantages. First, ultrasound is a safe modality for those patients who are unable to have an MRI (e.g., those with pacemakers, cochlear implants, or claustrophobia). Second, ultrasound offers the ability to examine ligaments, tendons, and muscle in real-time during provocative maneuvers (e.g., flexion-extension), which can enhance the appearance of a pathological process. Finally, ultrasound is unique in its ability to guide needle placement for interventional procedures.

Ultrasonography is useful in evaluating soft tissue structures, particularly those that are superficial or contain fluid such as joint effusions and ganglion cysts. The normal sonographic appearances of various tissues are described in this chapter, as well as pathological processes and their appearances.

POWER DOPPLER APPLICATIONS TO MUSCULOSKELETAL ULTRASOUND

Power Doppler imaging (PDI) is a technique that displays an amplitude map of the Doppler signal in distinction to conventional color Doppler imaging, which encodes the mean frequency shift in color. PDI has been suggested to be more sensitive in detecting low-flow states.[2] The technique appears exquisitely sensitive to soft tissue hyperemia associated with a number of musculoskeletal lesions. PDI can be used both to detect and to quantify such pathological alterations in vascularity. Moreover, the resolution of hyperemia appears to parallel clinical improvement even with a continued abnormal gray-scale appearance.[3] Thus, the detection of hyperemia may provide additional specificity in the grading of inflammatory

musculoskeletal lesions, as well as a means of following response to therapy.

TENDONS

Normal Sonographic Appearances

While tendons usually have a synovial sheath surrounding them, they can also have a relatively dense connective tissue layer adherence (the paratendon). This is brightly echogenic and sharply demarcates the tendon (Fig. 16–1). The tendon itself consists of dense connective tissue in which collagen fibrils are arranged in bundles surrounded by loose connective tissue.[4] These bundles are further arranged in a parallel linear fashion. The resultant gray-scale ultrasound image reflects this anatomic configuration by displaying marked anisotropy; the tendon is echogenic when scanned perpendicular to its long axis with a linear array transducer. Reduction of the angle by as little as between 2° and 7° produces isoechogenicity relative to muscle, and further reduction produces hypoechogenicity (Fig. 16–2). Due to its fibrillar nature, the tendon is not diffusely echogenic but appears as a series of echogenic parallel linear bands[5] (Fig. 16–3). These features make tendons easy to recognize ultrasonographically.

Pathological Findings

Tendinosis can be diffuse, focal, acute, or chronic. A *diffuse tendinosis* is visualized sonographically as diffuse thickening and hypoechogenicity of the tendon (Fig. 16–4). The appearance of hypoechoic intratendinous clefts may be seen. Measurements of various tendons have been suggested, but it must be remembered that gender, size, and patient training level contribute to tendon thickness, and the final arbiter often relies on comparison to the opposite side. The tendon may lose its normal sharp outline displaying indistinct margins. *Focal tendinosis* will display localized areas of thickening and hypoechogenicity. Symptomatic

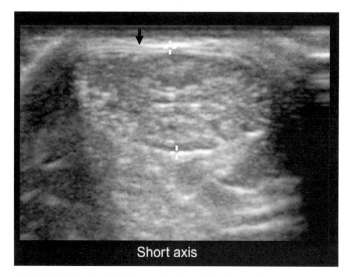

FIGURE 16–1. The Achilles tendon imaged in short axis appears as an echogenic ellipse (between tick marks) surrounded by a thick fibrous layer or paratendon (black arrow).

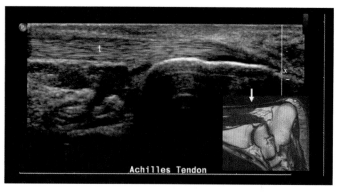

FIGURE 16–3. Fibrillar tendon: On ultrasound, the Achilles tendon (t) is echogenic and fibrillar, as opposed to uniformly low signal as on magnetic resonance imaging (inset image, arrow).

tendinosis has been shown to display areas of increased vascularity on PDI. This is due to infiltrative granulation tissue and has been referred to as an angiofibroblastic response.[6]

A *chronic tendinosis* may slowly calcify. Calcification is recognized sonographically as its signature discrete echogenic area with posterior acoustic shadowing or as merely a nonshadowing amorphous echogenic mass.

An *acute tenosynovitis* is seen as a pathological quantity of fluid or thickening of the tendon sheath.[7] This may be secondary to inflammation, infection, or acute trauma or may be due to an effusion within an adjacent joint. A *chronic tenosynovitis*[8] may be associated with diffuse synovial thickening and secondary inflammation of the tendon, which appears thickened and hypoechoic. Increased peritendinous blood flow is frequently evident on PDI.

Complete rupture is easily recognized in the acute phase both clinically and sonographically. The tendon retracts and the gap between the retracted ends is filled with hematoma.[9] The tendon itself may appear diffusely thickened, heterogeneous, and nodular in contour.

Partial rupture is similar in that there is a discontinuity in the parallel linear echoes of the tendon, with the gap filled by material of variable, but usually decreased echogenicity. Because of the number of intact fibrils, there may only be minimal retraction in a partial tear. This is manifested as a contour deformity or focal thinning (Fig. 16–5). Partial tears may also be manifest as splits paralleling the long axis of a tendon.

ROTATOR CUFF

Though one of the most commonly ordered studies, shoulder sonography is also among the most difficult to master. This is largely because of the challenge it poses to optimally visualize the tendons. The curved surface of the tendons (Fig. 16–6) make them susceptible to anisotropy. This is particularly the case when using the recommended high-frequency linear transducer, when it is necessary to constantly reposition in order to optimally visualize the tendon.

Anatomy is complex in this region particularly postoperatively, when landmarks are skewed. However, recent studies using well-defined techniques and criteria have resulted in very favorable results in detecting rotator cuff pathology.[10]

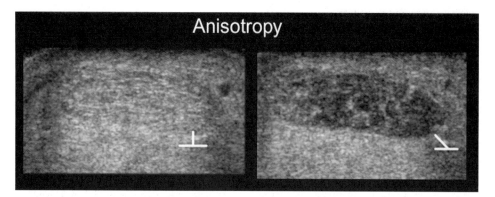

FIGURE 16–2. Anisotropy. When the ultrasound beam insonates the tendon perpendicular to the long axis of the tendon (inset), the tendon appears echogenic. When the beam insonates at an angle, which can be as little as 5–10° (inset), the tendon appears progressively hypoechoic.

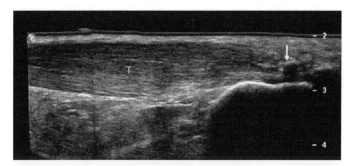

FIGURE 16-4. Diffuse Achilles tendinosis. The tendon (T) is diffusely thickened and heterogeneous. Intrasubstance calcification or ossification (arrow) is present near the tendon insertion.

The indicators of rotator cuff pathology are similar to signs used elsewhere in the musculoskeletal system. The most reliable diagnostic feature of tears relates either to complete absence, focal discontinuity, or contour deformity of the tendon surface[11] (Fig. 16–7). Echogenic areas, which may relate to tears, may also indicate focal calcification, scarring, or at times, normal anatomy, and care must thus be taken. Complex fluid

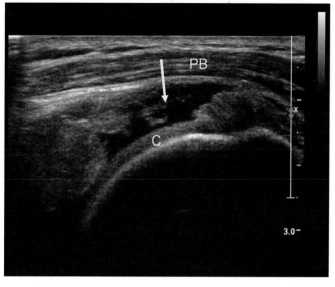

FIGURE 16-7. Rotator cuff tear with discontinuity. Long-axis image of the supraspinatus tendon displays a large full-thickness tear (arrow). The tear appears discretely marginated and filled with hypoechoic fluid and debris. The tear is bounded above by the peribursal fat stripe (PB) and below by articular cartilage (C).

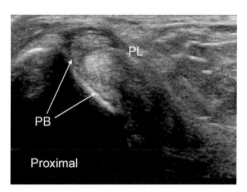
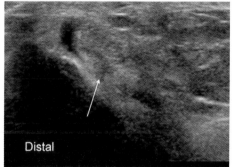

FIGURE 16-5. Longitudinal split of the peroneus brevis tendon in the ankle. The image on the left depicts central thinning of the peroneus brevis tendon (PB) with herniation of the peroneus longus tendon (PL) into the gap. A slightly more distal image (right) shows a central longitudinal split (arrow) within the peroneus brevis, which appears as a hypoechoic fissure within the tendon.

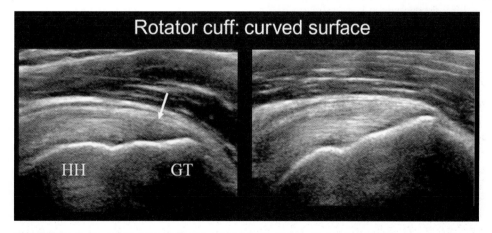

FIGURE 16-6. Normal rotator cuff. The image on the left depicts a long-axis view of the supraspinatus tendon. The deltoid muscle (D), tendon (T), humeral head (HH), and greater tuberosity (GT) are labeled. Because of the convexity of the tendon surface, the distal fibers (arrow) appear less echogenic than the more proximal fibers as a result of anisotropy. Rocking the transducer (image on right) enables one to eliminate the anisotropic effect at the tendon footprint.

filling the gap produced by an articular tear may produce a characteristic cartilage interface sign.[12] Likewise, the loss of the normally convex tendon margin is highly suggestive of a tear. The presence of fluid in the biceps tendon sheath and in the overlying subdeltoid bursa is strong secondary evidence for a tear with a 95% positive predictive value.[13]

MUSCLE

Normal Sonographic Appearances

Normal muscle appears as a homogenous band of parallel echogenic striations (perimysium) with a hypoechoic background corresponding to the muscle fiber bulk (Fig. 16 8). The individual muscle fibers course toward a common aponeurosis and culminate in a tendinous insertion.

Pathological Findings

Muscle can be associated with a number of unique pathologies. *Muscle edema* causes the usual linear striations of the muscle bulk to become rounded and blunt. Echogenicity is transformed from hypoechoic to relatively echogenic (Fig. 16–9). *Pyomyositis* appears as a complex collection within the muscle.[14] The presence of punctate echogenic foci with associated "dirty" shadowing in the nondependent portions of the collection may indicate a gas-forming organism.[15] Likewise, *intramuscular hematoma* may be seen as a complex collection surrounded by granulation tissue. When large, these lesions display an irregular cavity with shaggy borders. The sonographic appearance is dominated by the hematoma and follows typical evolutionary changes with time. *Distraction injuries* differ in that the hematoma is confined usually to a single muscle, and torn fragments of muscle are more likely to be identified within the cavity, producing the "bell-clapper" sign (Fig. 16–10).

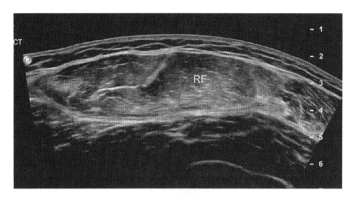

FIGURE 16–9. Muscle edema pattern. Short-axis view of the quadriceps compartment in a professional athlete following a strain injury of the rectus femoris (RF) shows the muscle to display increased echogenicity relative to the adjacent muscles in the thigh.

Ultrasound can be useful to assess healing of these lesions. The cavity gradually decreases in size, and hypoechoic granulation tissue in the margins of the cavity advances to fill in the defect. Eventually, organization can be demonstrated with the reappearance of fibroadipose septa. Sometimes a resolving intramuscular hematoma will undergo peripheral calcification. The presence of calcification along the periphery of an organizing hematoma has been termed *myositis ossificans* (Fig. 16–11).

BURSAE

Normal Sonographic Appearances

Bursae are synovial-lined structures situated about joint capsules, ligaments, and tendinous insertions that help to improve gliding and thus facilitate motion. In fact, they may develop secondarily to sites of abnormal friction and are then referred to as an adventitial bursa. They may communicate with a joint, in which case they are referred to as a synovial cyst (e.g., Baker's cyst).

The synovial-lined sheath surrounding various tendons is another form of specialized bursa. Normal nondistended bursae

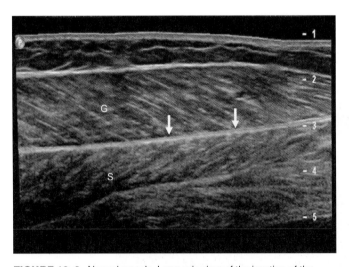

FIGURE 16–8. Normal muscle. Long-axis view of the junction of the gastrocnemius muscle (G) and soleus muscle (S). Each muscle presents a hypoechoic background filled with multiple echogenic linear structures (perimysium). These converge on a central echogenic band (arrows), thereby forming a typical multi-penate architecture.

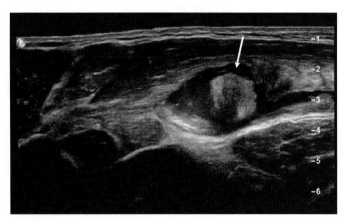

FIGURE 16–10. Muscle hematoma with "bell-clapper" sign. Short-axis image of the hamstring muscles following an acute distraction injury, resulting in a focal tear with hematoma formation. A portion of the tear (arrow) is noted to extend into the hematoma giving rise to a typical bell-clapper appearance. Note the edema pattern in the adjacent muscle.

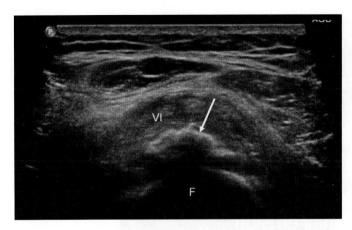

FIGURE 16–11. Myositis ossificans. Following a blow to the thigh, this patient was noted to develop a thigh swelling. Initial radiographs showed the femur to be intact. Follow-up ultrasound showed new curvilinear ossification (arrow) within the injured muscle (vastus intermedius, VI). Note the edema pattern in the adjacent muscle. The femur (F) is labeled.

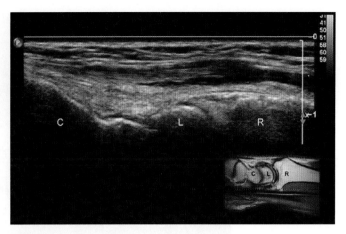

FIGURE 16–13. Normal joint. Long-axis view of a normal dorsal radio-luno-capitate joint (R). The joints appear as the junction of smoothly marginated cortical surfaces of each bone. Articular cartilage generally appears as thin hypoechoic bands overlying the convex surfaces of the lunate (L) and capitate (C) (arrows). Extra-articular fat appears echogenic and overlies the cortical surfaces and can be difficult to distinguish of the adjacent ligamentous stabilizers. A sagittal magnetic resonance image of the wrist showing the same anatomic arrangement is shown in the inset on the right.

may be imperceptible by ultrasound or may be evident as a thin hypoechoic structure, representing a small amount of synovial fluid (Fig. 16–12). The normal bursa should not exceed 2 mm in thickness.

Pathological Findings

Distention of a bursa with fluid or soft tissue is described as bursitis, unless the bursa communicates with the joint. In this way, the distended gastrocnemius/semimembranosus bursa is not thought of as bursitis but is given the title of a Baker's cyst.

In an acute bursitis, the fluid can be anechoic or complex. This may be secondary to inflammation, infection, or acute trauma. Ultrasound is ideal for evaluation of such a mass, demonstrating its cystic nature and enabling a firm diagnosis. It is also an ideal modality for providing guidance for an aspiration and/or injection (as will be discussed later). The presence of hyperemic nodular soft tissue within the collection or in a

peribursal distribution, as assessed by color or PDI, can more readily denote an inflammatory origin.[16]

JOINTS

Normal Sonographic Appearances

A joint is visualized as a synovium-lined space between two cortical surfaces. There should be negligible bulging of the joint capsule and no fluid inside the joint (Fig. 16–13). A thin hypoechoic band of articular cartilage may be evident along the joint margins below the echogenic capsule. Often extra-articular fat is present below the joint capsule.

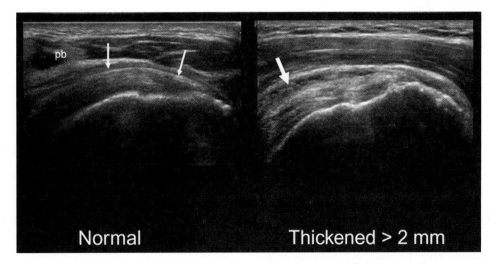

FIGURE 16–12. Normal and thickened bursa. The normal subdeltoid bursa (left, thin arrows) appears as a thin (<2 mm) hypoechoic line deep to the peribursal fat (pb). A thickened bursa (right, thick arrow) can be filled with variable amounts of fluid, soft tissue, and sometimes calcification.

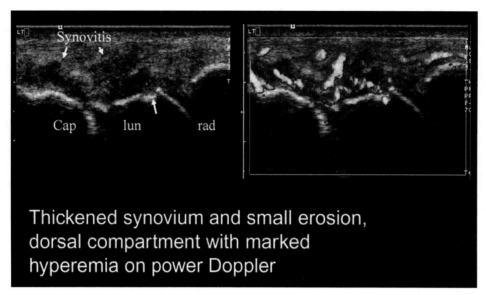

FIGURE 16–14. Inflammatory arthritis. Gray-scale image (left) of a patient with rheumatoid arthritis at the radio-luno-capitate joint (labeled). Abnormal hypoechoic soft tissue along the dorsum of the wrist (synovitis) shows the typical appearance of inflammatory pannus in rheumatoid arthritis. The normal echogenic fat is replaced. A small surface erosion (arrow) in the lunate bone is depicted. The corresponding power Doppler image (right) depicts the extensive hyperemia associated with active inflammation. The vascularity is distributed throughout the abnormal soft tissue.

Pathological Findings

Joint effusions are easily detected sonographically as fluid displacing the joint capsule and fat pad.[17] The presence of low-level echoes, septations, or solid material within the joint fluid may suggest infection, hemarthrosis, or other noninfective inflammatory debris such as fibrin. Fine echoes within the fluid can be seen following intra-articular corticosteroid administration. An anechoic effusion does not necessarily imply a simple synovial collection. In fact, differentiating the various causes of a complex effusion is not usually possible based on the sonographic appearances alone. The major advantages of ultrasound in these circumstances are the demonstration of an effusion, as well as providing guidance for aspiration. With a prosthesis in place, ultrasound may be the only modality to demonstrate the nature and extent of fluid, as both CT and MRI are limited by artifact.[18]

Osteochondral bodies are usually suggested by their sharp margins and they will usually display posterior shadowing. Proliferation and edema of the synovium (Fig. 16–14) are most prominent in the pannus of rheumatoid arthritis but a similar appearance can be seen in other inflammatory arthritides, chronic infections, pigmented villonodular synovitis, synovial osteochondromatosis, and amyloid. Hemophilia can produce a similar picture. The synovium in these cases is hypoechoic and nodular in appearance. Hypervascularity is indicated on PDI.

GANGLION/MISCELLANEOUS CYSTS

Ganglion cysts appear as well-marginated, often multiloculated pseudocysts that may form in relation to joint capsules, tendons, tendon sheaths, ligaments, and muscles. They characteristically contain clear gelatinous material and are often hard to palpation. These are most commonly located along the dorsal surfaces of the wrist (Fig. 16–15) and ankle, although they can occur almost anywhere in the musculoskeletal soft tissues. These are presumably degenerative in nature and may be associated with traumatic origin. While they may be asymptomatic, it is not uncommon for these to produce direct compression of an adjacent neurovascular bundle, tendon, or synovium-lined structure. In these cases, these lesions can produce chronic intermittent pain, weakness, and diminished mobility. While surgery is considered as a definitive treatment, intracystic injection of long-acting corticosteroids is often successful.

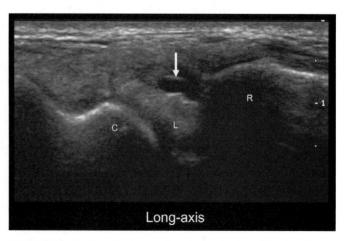

FIGURE 16–15. Dorsal wrist ganglion: Long-axis view of the dorsal scapholunate ligament (L) shows a small unilocular cyst (arrow) superficial to the ligament. The radius (R) and capitate (C) are labeled.

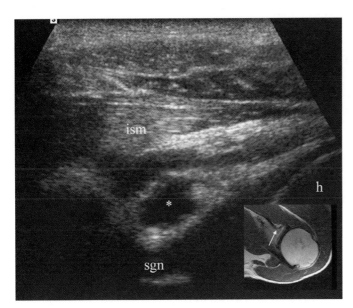

FIGURE 16–16. Spinoglenoid notch (sgn) cyst in the shoulder. The image depicts a hypoechoic cyst (*) in the spinoglenoid notch of the scapula. The humeral head (h) and infraspinatus muscle (ism) are labeled. The inset shows the corresponding anatomic location (arrow) in a representative axial magnetic resonance image of the shoulder.

MENISCAL/PARALABRAL CYSTS

These constitute pseudocysts that form adjacent to a meniscal or labral tear.[19] Similar to synovial cysts, their fluid content presumably relates to a decompressive mechanism in which joint fluid escapes unidirectionally into the collection. These are often multiloculated and can occur either medially or laterally along the femorotibial joint of the knee, spinoglenoid notch in shoulder (Fig. 16–16) and also in variable locations in the hip. The presence of a cyst adjacent to fibrocartilage containing a well-defined hypoechoic defect establishes the diagnosis on ultrasound. While ultrasound can usually identify the nature of the cyst, an MRI is necessary to fully evaluate the extent of internal derangement.

INTERVENTIONAL

Ultrasound is a useful clinical adjunct in the diagnosis as well as treatment of disorders involving the musculoskeletal system. Tendon sheath injections and aspirations, therapeutic injections of interdigital neuromas and plantar fasciitis, joint aspirations, calcific tendonitis aspiration and injections, synovial biopsies as well as aspiration of possible inflammatory collections can all be successfully performed using ultrasound guidance. Either a linear or curved sector transducer can be used depending on local geometry. Using the needle as a specular reflector, passage of the needle tip through the soft tissues into the target of interest can be performed during real-time examination, providing a distinct advantage over such imaging guidance methods as computed tomography (CT).

Injections of tendon sheaths and plantar fascia should be performed under ultrasound guidance, as the needle tip can be placed selectively into either the tendon sheath or perifascial heel fat pad, respectively, thus avoiding direct injection of the tendon itself or plantar fascia, which has been known to cause premature degeneration and rupture.[20]

Ultrasound-guided injection of interdigital neuroma offers an alternative to surgical resection, which often results in stump neuroma formation and consequent return of the patient's clinical symptoms. Neuromas typically appear as hypoechoic nodules in the second and third webspaces, though can sometimes appear in the first and rarely in the fourth (Fig. 16–17).

The ability of ultrasound to identify calcifications in soft tissue allows for direct aspiration and lavage of calcific tendinitis. Mechanical fragmentation of the calcific deposit is performed with aspiration of the fragmented material.

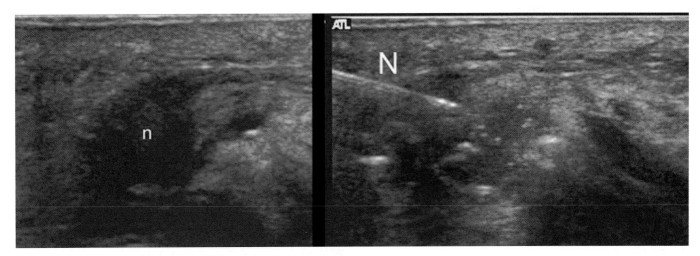

FIGURE 16–17. Neuroma injection. Initial sonogram (left) shows a hypoechoic nodule (n) in the interdigital fat corresponding to a symptomatic neuroma. The image on the right depicts a needle (N) within the neuroma during a guided injection with steroid and anesthetic. Notice that the injected material changes the overall echogenicity of the neuroma and adjacent soft tissue.

CONCLUSION

Because of its noninvasive nature, availability, cost-effectiveness, and exquisite ability to image the soft tissues in both a static and dynamic state, ultrasound has much to offer in imaging of the musculoskeletal system. Normal appearances are, in general, distinct from pathology due to its interruption of the normal soft tissue architecture. Ultrasonography is readily available for the guiding of interventional procedures in the musculoskeletal system. The ability to document exact needle position in real-time facilitates improved accuracy for therapeutic injections, fluid aspiration and soft tissue biopsy.

References

1. Adler RS, Fenzel KC. The complementary roles of MR imaging and ultrasound of tendons. *Radiol Clin North Am.* 2005; 43:771-807.

2. Newman JS, Adler RS, Buder, RO, Rubin JM. Detection of soft tissue hyperemia: value of power Doppler sonography. *AJR Am J Roentgenol.* 1994; 163:385-389.

3. Newman JS, Laing TJ, McCarthy CJ, Adler RS. Power Doppler sonography in synovitis: assessment of therapeutic response: preliminary observations. *Radiology.* 1996; 198:582-584.

4. Fornage BD. *Musculoskeletal Ultrasound.* New York: Churchill Livingstone; 1995.

5. Van Holsbeeck M, Introcaso JH. *Musculoskeletal Ultrasound.* St. Louis: Mosby Year Book; 1991.

6. Riley G. The pathogenesis of tendinopathy. A molecular perspective. *Rheumatology.* 2004; 43:131-142.

7. Jeffrey RB Jr, Laing FC, Schecter WP, Markison RE, et al. Acute suppurative tenosynovitis of the hand: diagnosis with ultrasound. *Radiology.* 1987; 162:741-742.

8. Stephenson CA, Seibert JJ, McAndrew MP, et al. Sonographic diagnosis of tenosynovitis of the posterior tibial tendon. *J Clin Ultrasound.* 1990; 18:114-116.

9. Bouffard JA, Eyler WR, Introcaso JH, Van Holsbeeck M. Sonography of tendons. *Ultrasound Quart.* 1993; 11(4):259-286.

10. Weiner SN, Seitz WH Jr. Sonography of the shoulder in patients with tears to the rotator cuff: accuracy and value for selecting surgical options. *AJR Am J Roentgenol.* 1993; 160:103-107.

11. Middleton WD, Edelstein G, Reinus WR, et al. Sonographic detection of rotator cuff tears. *AJR Am J Roentgenol.* 1985; 144:349-353.

12. Jacobson JA, Lancaster S, Prasad A, van Holsbeeck MT, Craig JG, Kolowich P. Full-thickness and partial-thickness supraspinatus tendon tears: value of US signs in diagnosis. *Radiology.* 2004; 230:234-242.

13. Thain LMF, Adler RS. Sonography of the rotator cuff and biceps tendon: Technique, normal anatomy, and pathology. *J Clin Ultrasound.* 1999; 27,8:446-458.

14. Van Sonnenburg E, Wittich G, Casola G, et al. Sonography of thigh abscess: detection diagnosis and drainage. *AJR Am J Roentgenol.* 1987; 149:769-772.

15. Fornage B, Touche D, Segal P, et al. Ultrasonography in the evaluation of muscular trauma. *J Ultrasound Med.* 1983; 2(12):549-554.

16. Breidahl WH, Newman JS, Taljanovic MS, et al. Power Doppler sonography in the assessment of musculoskeletal fluid collections. *AJR Am J Roentgenol.* 1996; 166:1443-1446.

17. Marchal G, Van Holsbeeck M, Raes M, et al. Transient synovitis of the hip in children: role of ultrasound. *Radiology.* 1987; 162:825-828.

18. Van Holsbeeck M, Eyler W, Sherman L, et al. Detection of infection in loosened hip prosthesis: efficiency of sonography. *AJR Am J Roentgenol.* 1994; 163:381-384.

19. Coral A, Van Holsbeeck M, Adler RS. Imaging of meniscal cyst of the knee in three cases. *Skeletal Radiol.* 1989; 18:451-455.

20. Sofka CM, Collins AJ, Adler RS. Use of ultrasound guidance in interventional musculoskeletal procedures. A review from a single institution. *J Ultrasound Med.* 2001; 20:21-26.

Questions

GENERAL INSTRUCTIONS: For each question, select the best answer. Select only one answer for each question unless otherwise specified.

1. Which of the following modalities has been the mainstay for musculoskeletal imaging in the United States?

    (A) x-ray

    (B) computed tomography (CT)

    (C) magnetic resonance imaging (MRI)

    (D) ultrasound

2. Ultrasonography is most useful in assessing all of the following *except*

    (A) soft tissue

    (B) joints

    (C) dynamic maneuvers

    (D) bone

3. In musculoskeletal ultrasound, what does the term PDI refer to?

    (A) power Doppler imaging

    (B) pre-Doppler imaging

    (C) power dated image

    (D) power duplex indicator

4. PDI has been suggested to be sensitive in detecting low-flow states of soft tissue; therefore, it is useful in monitoring which of the following conditions?

    (A) decreased vascularity with progression of injury

    (B) decreased vascularity with serial exams to demonstrate response to treatment

    (C) increased vascularity demonstrating injury resolution

    (D) the amplitude of blood flow at the injury site

5. Tendons are recognized sonographically by

    (A) the brightly echogenic synovial sheath surrounding the fibers

    (B) the hypoechoic connective tissue surrounding the fibers

    (C) the echogenic bundles of collagen fibrils

    (D) the echogenic anisotropic effect due to the dense connective tissue surround the fibers

6. When does the anisotropic effect occur?

    (A) The probe is placed perpendicular to the tendon of interest.

    (B) The probe is placed parallel to the tendon of interest.

    (C) The probe is placed as little as 2° and 7° away from perpendicular to the tendon of interest.

    (D) The probe is placed <2 or >7 mm away from the tendon of interest.

7. Tendon thickness is often related to gender, size, and training level. For this reason, accurate assessment of tendon size must be made by

    (A) comparison to the contralateral side

    (B) serial measurements to demonstrate the changes associated with healing

    (C) evaluation and comparison to the appropriate chart for each factor

    (D) measuring the tendon with it parallel to the imaging beam

8. Calcification is always characterized sonographically as

    (A) an echogenic focus with a hypoechoic rim

    (B) an echogenic focus with a discrete posterior shadow

    (C) an echogenic focus with a fibrillar pattern

    (D) an echogenic focus with fluid surrounding the muscle fibers

9. Tendinopathy is associated with which of the following ultrasonic findings?

    (A) decreased echogenicity of the tendon

    (B) increased echogenicity of the tendon

    (C) homogeneity of the tendon

    (D) reduction in tendon caliber

10. Complete tendon rupture is sonographically identifiable by which of the following findings?

    (A) tendon thickening and retraction with an adjacent hematoma

    (B) increased echogenicity of the tendon at the tear site

    (C) a discrete gap within the linear echoes of the tendon

    (D) thinning of the tendon and the increased echogenicity of the adjacent inflammatory response

Questions 11–14: The image shown below is a sagittal view of a normal supraspinatus tendon. Match the structures in the image with the terms in Column B.

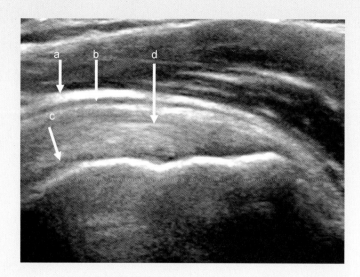

COLUMN A   COLUMN B

11. _____   (A) Subcoracoid-subdeltoid bursa

12. _____   (B) Cartilage

              (C) Supraspinatus tendon

13. _____   (D) Pre-bursal fat stripe

14. _____

15. Which of the following findings indicates strong secondary evidence for a rotator cuff tear?

   (A) increased blood flow in the rotator interval

   (B) presence of fluid in the biceps sheath and overlying subdeltoid bursa

   (C) chronically degenerated cartilage

   (D) presence of tendon calcification

16. Normal muscle has which one of the following sonographic appearances?

   (A) homogenous

   (B) perpendicular echogenic striations

   (C) hyperechoic background

   (D) indistinct individual muscle fibers

17. Pyomyositis is most likely to produce which of the following ultrasonic artifacts?

   (A) ring down

   (B) comet tail

   (C) "dirty" shadow

   (D) acoustic enhancement

18. Ultrasound is useful in the assessment of muscle tissue healing. Which of the following findings best demonstrates organization and healing of the muscle tissue?

   (A) reappearance of fibroadipose septa

   (B) persistent hypoechoic appearance of the intramuscular hematoma

   (C) calcification of the muscle tissue

   (D) internal calcification of the hematoma

19. Myositis ossificans describes which of the following states?

   (A) calcification centrally within an organizing muscle hematoma

   (B) calcification at the torn end of the muscle fibers

   (C) calcification at the healing end of the torn muscle fibers

   (D) calcification along the periphery of an organizing hematoma

20. Normal bursae are best identified sonographically as

   (A) indistinguishable unless pathology is present

   (B) fluid-filled cavities with echogenic walls around the joint capsules only

   (C) immobile echogenic densities adjacent to a joint capsule during manipulation

   (D) synovial fluid-filled structures adjacent to the joint capsule measuring at least 4 mm thick

21. The normal bursa should not exceed which of the following measurements in thickness?

   (A) 2 mm

   (B) 2.5 mm

   (C) 2 cm

   (D) 2.5 cm

22. Synovial fluid seen with acute bursitis is often complex in sonographic appearance. This is most often secondary to which of the following situations?

   (A) inflammation

   (B) early treatment of injury

   (C) delay of diagnosis from the time of injury

   (D) resolution of hemorrhage within the joint capsule

23. In the image below, the structure indicated by the arrow is a distended gastrocnemius/semimembranosus bursa. Which of the following best describes this finding?

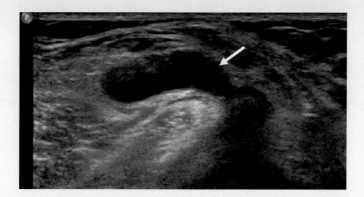

    (A) popliteal bursitis

    (B) non-communicating with the posterior knee joint

    (C) a Baker's cyst

    (D) knee-joint effusion

24. A joint is visualized on ultrasound as:

    (A) a synovium-filled space between two cortical surfaces

    (B) a cartilaginous space between two cortical surfaces

    (C) a synovium filled space between two cartilaginous surfaces

    (D) a cartilaginous space between two cartilaginous surfaces

25. A joint effusion may be indicated on ultrasound by the presence of

    (A) low-level echoes

    (B) septations

    (C) solid material

    (D) displacement of the capsule by fluid

26. Ultrasound for joint effusions would definitely be the preferred imaging modality in patients with which of the following findings?

    (A) adjacent fracture

    (B) joint prosthesis

    (C) rheumatoid arthritis

    (D) adjacent ganglion cyst

27. Ganglion cysts are *not* likely to form in relation to

    (A) joint capsules

    (B) tendon sheaths

    (C) muscles

    (D) joint effusions

28. Which of the following statements is true regarding ganglion cysts?

    (A) They are most commonly located along the volar aspect of the ankle.

    (B) They are most commonly spongy at palpation.

    (C) They are best treated with percutaneous drainage.

    (D) They are often related to prior trauma.

29. Ultrasound can be useful in musculoskeletal disorder treatment as well as diagnosis. What is this due to?

    (A) the ability of ultrasound to be able to capture quicker images of needle placement than CT or MRI

    (B) the ability of ultrasound to be able to discern the gap between the tendon and its sheath avoiding rupture of the sheath

    (C) the ability of ultrasound to better distinguish soft tissue from bony structures than CT or MRI

    (D) the ability of ultrasound to distinguish the needle better than CT or MRI

Questions 30–31: Match the structures indicated in the image below with the terms in Column B.

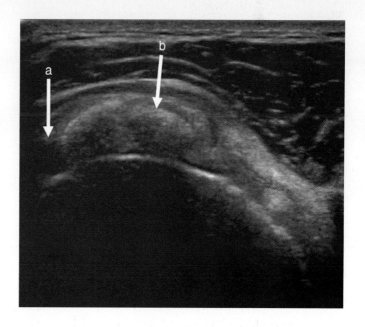

COLUMN A	COLUMN B
30. _____	(A) Calcification
31. _____	(B) Posterior portion of the supraspinatus tendon

Questions 32–34: Match the structures indicated in the image below with the terms in Column B.

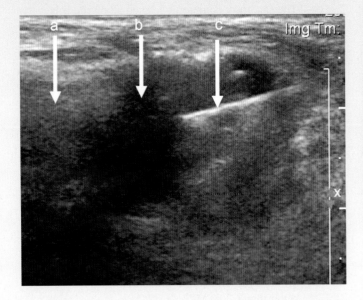

COLUMN A   COLUMN B

32. _____   (A) Neuroma

33. _____   (B) Needle

(C) Interdigital webspace

34. _____

35. Why use the color hue (chroma map) on neuroma studies?

(A) improved visualization

(B) improved specular reflection

(C) reduction in anisotropic effect

(D) reduction of speckle

Questions 36–39: Match the structures indicated in the image below with the terms in Column B.

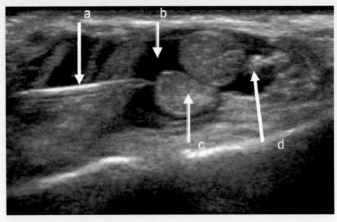

COLUMN A   COLUMN B

36. _____   (A) Peroneal tendons of ankle

(B) Needle

37. _____   (C) Tendon vinculum

38. _____   (D) Distended tendon sheath postinjection

39. _____

40. The needle used in ultrasound-guided therapeutic injections appears:

(A) echogenic with posterior acoustic enhancement

(B) echogenic with posterior reverberation artifact

(C) hypoechoic with posterior acoustic enhancement

(D) hypoechoic with posterior reverberation artifact

41. The following image represents a procedure described in the body of the text. What sort of procedure is it?

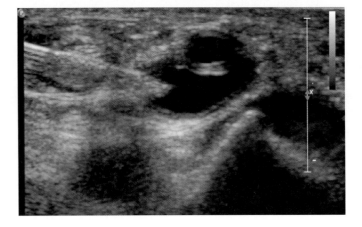

(A) ultrasound-guided biopsy

(B) x-ray-guided injection

(C) diagnostic ultrasound

(D) ultrasound-guided aspiration/injection

Questions 42–44: Match the structures indicated in the image below with the terms in Column B.

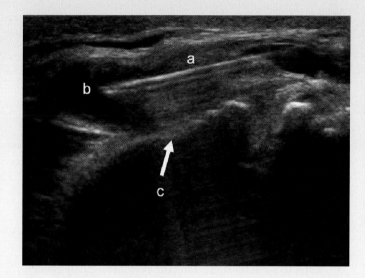

45. The image shown below is an example of which of the following types of sonography?

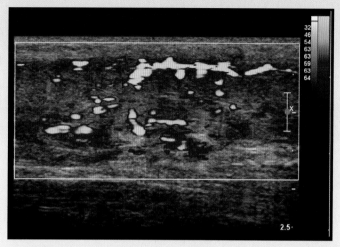

COLUMN A	COLUMN B
42. _____	(A) Cyst
43. _____	(B) Needle
44. _____	(C) Bone

(A) Pulse-wave (PW) Doppler

(B) continuous-wave (CW) Doppler

(C) 2D color Doppler

(D) color power Doppler

Answers and Explanations

1. **(C)** MRI has been the preferred method of evaluating abnormalities of the musculoskeletal system. However, sonography is recognizied as advantageous due to its ability to image in real-time while watching manipulation of the affected anatomy. (*Study Guide*)

2. **(D)** Sonography is unable to delineate information beyond the cortical surface of bony structures due to the acoustic impedance mismatch from the adjacent soft tissue. (*Study Guide; also see Physics Chapter*)

3. **(A)** Power Doppler imaging (PDI) is a technique used to display the detection of blood flow without displaying direction or having dependence on angle of insonation. (*Study Guide*)

4. **(B)** Power Doppler imaging (PDI) has been utilized to assess vascularity associated with low-flow states seen in the musculoskeletal system when assessing degree of injury and its response to treatment. (*Study Guide*)

5. **(C)** Tendons typically demonstrate a surrounding layer of echogenic tissue. However, this is not always representative of a synovial sheath but is sometimes the adherent connective tissue (paratendon). (*Study Guide*)

6. **(C)** The anisotropic effect is an artifact of sonographic imaging when the beam is less than perpendicular to the tissue and a hypoechoic region is identified suggesting an abnormality. (*Study Guide*)

7. **(A)** Multiple factors determine tendon thickness, but the best method for assessing normal versus abnormal thickness for a particular patient is to compare the affected tendon to the unaffected contralateral tendon. (*Study Guide*)

8. **(B)** Calcification within any region of the body is demonstrated sonographically as having an echogenic interface with a discrete shadow posteriorly. (*Study Guide*)

9. **(A)** With diffuse inflammation of the tendon, there is sonographic evidence of diffuse inflammation. (*Study Guide*)

10. **(A)** Complete tendon ruptures often result in the formation of an adjacent hematoma and muscle retraction. (*Study Guide*)

11. **(B)** Cartilage (*Study Guide*)

12. **(C)** Supraspinatus tendon (*Study Guide*)

13. **(D)** Pre-bursal

14. **(A)** Subcorticoid subdeltoid bursa

15. **(B)** Presence of fluid within the biceps sheath has a 95% positive predictive value. (*Study Guide*)

16. **(B)** The sonographic appearance of echogenic striations within hypoechoic bands of is classic for the echogenic perimysium and the hypoechoic muscle fiber bulk. (*Study Guide*)

17. **(C)** The "dirty shadow" appearance is a result of the gas formation within the infected collection of fluid. (*Study Guide*)

18. **(A)** The appearance of an intramuscular hematoma will change over time. With appropriate response to treatment, the resolving injury may often return to a near normal appearance. (*Study Guide*)

19. **(D)** If a hematoma does not resolve entirely, it will often result in a calcification along the periphery. (*Study Guide*)

20. **(D)** Normal bursae are typically too small to identify definitively with sonography. Visualization of this anatomy often suggests pathology immediately. (*Study Guide*)

21. **(A)** The normal bursa is 2 mm thick or less. (*Study Guide*)

22. **(D)** Acute bursitis is most often anechoic in nature due to the recent injury. The appearance of complicated fluid is suggestive of an inflammatory response. This can further be evaluated using PDI to confirm hyperemia. (*Study Guide*)

23. **(D)** If a fluid collection connects with the joint space, it is not considered simply bursitis. Fluid collections along the gastrocnemius muscle communicating with the knee joint is called a Baker's cyst. (*Study Guide*)

24. **(A)** Cartilage should be seen below the echogenic joint margin and a small hypoechoic space between the bony structures of the joint. (*Study Guide*)

25. **(D)** Any sonographic evidence of internal echoes within a joint effusion suggests inflammation or infection of the effusion. Additional imaging modalities may be preferred to further characterize the findings. (*Study Guide*)

26. **(B)** Ultrasound may be utilized effectively on essentially any patient and may be preferred for those patients with prosthesis due to the artifacts seen on CT and MRI. (*Study Guide*)

27. **(D)** Ganglion cysts are often connected the joint capsule but are not a result of a joint effusion. (*Study Guide*)

28. **(D)** Ganglion cysts typically occur on the dorsal aspect of the wrist and ankle and are often presumed to be related to prior trauma. (*Study Guide*)

29. **(D)** Real-time imaging during the insertion of the needle allows for more rapid. Sequential imaging of the advancement of the needle tip during the procedure simultaneously. (*Study Guide*)

30. **(B)** Posterior portion of the supraspinatus tendon (*Study Guide*)

31. **(A)** Calcification (*Study Guide*)

32. **(B)** Needle (*Study Guide*)

33. **(C)** Interdigital webspace (*Study Guide*)

34. **(A)** Neuroma (*Study Guide*)

35. **(A)** Use of a chroma map assists in differentiating adjacent tissues of similar acoustic properties. This allows the subtle differences in the neuroma characteristics to stand out. (*Study Guide*)

36. **(C)** Tendon vinculum (*Study Guide*)

37. **(A)** Peroneal tendons of the ankle (*Study Guide*)

38. **(D)** Distended tendon sheath post injection (*Study Guide*)

39. **(B)** Needle (*Study Guide*)

40. **(B)** When the beam crosses the interface of the metal needle shaft there is strong reflection (echogenic) but the small space between the walls of the lumen often result in the reverberation artifact due to delayed signal return from the far wall of the needle lumen. (*Study Guide*)

41. **(D)** There is a cystic mass present with needle guidance directed toward the mass. Due to the cystic nature of this abnormality, aspiration of its contents would be likely. (*Study Guide*)

42. **(B)** Needle (*Study Guide*)

43. **(A)** Cyst (*Study Guide*)

44. **(C)** Bone (*Study Guide*)

45. **(D)** Color power Doppler provides information obtained by the amplitude of moving blood cells. This method of imaging does not indicate velocity and is not dependent on angle to demonstrate flow making it much more sensitive to low-flow states as seen in the musculoskeletal system. (*Study Guide*)

Index

Note: Page number followed by A, f, Q, and t indicates answer, figure, question, and table respectively.